AF784834

Surgery of the Craniovertebral Junction

Second Edition

Thieme

Surgery of the Craniovertebral Junction

Second Edition

Nicholas C. Bambakidis, MD
Director of Cerebrovascular and Skull Base Surgery
The Neurological Institute
University Hospitals Case Medical Center
Associate Professor of Neurological Surgery
Case Western Reserve University School of Medicine
Cleveland, Ohio

Curtis A. Dickman, MD
Associate Chief, Spine Section
Director, Spinal Research
Division of Neurological Surgery
Barrow Neurological Institute
Phoenix, Arizona

Robert F. Spetzler, MD
Director
J. N. Harber Chair of Neurological Surgery
Barrow Neurological Institute
Phoenix, Arizona
Professor, Department of Surgery
Section of Neurosurgery
University of Arizona College of Medicine
Tucson, Arizona

Volker K. H. Sonntag, MD
Emeritus, Division of Neurological Surgery
Barrow Neurological Institute
Phoenix, Arizona
Professor of Clinical Surgery
University of Arizona College of Medicine
Tucson, Arizona

Thieme
New York • Stuttgart

Thieme Medical Publishers, Inc.
333 Seventh Ave.
New York, NY 10001

Executive Editor: Kay Conerly
Managing Editor: Judith Tomat
Editorial Director: Michael Wachinger
Production Editor: Heidi Grauel, Maryland Composition
International Production Director: Andreas Schabert
Senior Vice President, International Marketing and Sales: Cornelia Schulze
Vice President, Finance and Accounts: Sarah Vanderbilt
President: Brian D. Scanlan
Compositor: Maryland Composition
Printer: Everbest Printing Co.

Library of Congress Cataloging-in-Publication Data

Surgery of the craniovertebral junction.—2nd ed. / [edited by] Nicholas C. Bambakidis ... [et al.].
p. ; cm.
Includes bibliographical references and index.
ISBN 978-1-60406-338-7
I. Bambakidis, Nicholas C.
[DNLM: 1. Atlanto-Axial Joint—surgery. 2. Atlanto-Occipital Joint—surgery. 3. Cervical Vertebrae—surgery. 4. Surgical Procedures, Operative—methods. WE 725]
617.5'8059—dc23

2012006265

Copyright © 2013 by Thieme Medical Publishers, Inc. This book, including all parts thereof, is legally protected by copyright. Any use, exploitation, or commercialization outside the narrow limits set by copyright legislation without the publisher's consent is illegal and liable to prosecution. This applies in particular to photostat reproduction, copying, mimeographing or duplication of any kind, translating, preparation of microfilms, and electronic data processing and storage.

Important note: Medical knowledge is ever-changing. As new research and clinical experience broaden our knowledge, changes in treatment and drug therapy may be required. The authors and editors of the material herein have consulted sources believed to be reliable in their efforts to provide information that is complete and in accord with the standards accepted at the time of publication. However, in view of the possibility of human error by the authors, editors, or publisher of the work herein or changes in medical knowledge, neither the authors, editors, nor publisher, nor any other party who has been involved in the preparation of this work, warrants that the information contained herein is in every respect accurate or complete, and they are not responsible for any errors or omissions or for the results obtained from use of such information. Readers are encouraged to confirm the information contained herein with other sources. For example, readers are advised to check the product information sheet included in the package of each drug they plan to administer to be certain that the information contained in this publication is accurate and that changes have not been made in the recommended dose or in the contraindications for administration. This recommendation is of particular importance in connection with new or infrequently used drugs.

Some of the product names, patents, and registered designs referred to in this book are in fact registered trademarks or proprietary names even though specific reference to this fact is not always made in the text. Therefore, the appearance of a name without designation as proprietary is not to be construed as a representation by the publisher that it is in the public domain.

Printed in China

ISBN 978-1-60406-338-7
eISBN 978-1-60406-339-4

Contents

Preface

It is a pleasure to present the second edition of *Surgery of the Craniovertebral Junction*. Since the publication of the first edition in 1998, the rapid evolution of technological advancements in the field have resulted in innovative modalities of treatment of pathological entities occurring in this complex anatomical region. Such technological adjuncts continue to provide new and safer methods of treating patients with ever-improving rates of safety and efficacy.

The region of the craniovertebral junction continues to challenge surgeons with its great range of pathological entities and anatomical complexities. As with the first edition, this work is the product of a multidisciplinary group of national and international experts in the field of skull base surgery, spinal surgery, and cerebrovascular surgery. New chapters include comprehensive coverage of stereotactic radiosurgery, endovascular surgery, and endoscopic skull base techniques. These advancements are coupled with revised chapters on open surgical methods of treating a vast majority of pathological entities encountered within the craniovertebral junction. These updates are presented so as to continue to offer our patients the best possible outcomes while minimizing the invasiveness in any reasonable way. The inclusion of minimally invasive techniques should not be meant to minimize the importance of open surgical techniques in the management of skull base tumors and cerebrovascular disorders. Indeed, mastery in such open techniques cannot be bought, borrowed, or stolen. It is instead earned through years of rigorous training and experience and has become more important than ever, even as it has become rarer to observe and harder to achieve. It is hoped that such a text can preserve the knowledge gained by so many talented surgeons in the never ending quest to serve the well-being and welfare of our patients.

Our second edition of the book consists of four sections. In Section I, information regarding fundamental anatomy, embryology, neurology, and radiology has been updated and presented to provide a logical basis for the subsequent sections. Section I also includes new material emphasizing the importance of the development of stereotactic radiosurgery in the management of tumors of the craniovertebral junction. Section II provides a comprehensive framework for surgical indications and decision making. New material in this section covers the endovascular treatment of vascular lesions in the craniovertebral junction. In Section III, methods of surgical techniques are summarized, with new chapters on endoscopic skull base techniques. The fixation and fusion techniques in Section IV have been updated as well. Accompanying the second edition is a DVD that includes cadaveric dissections and animations of the various surgical approaches and techniques used in the treatment of lesions of the craniovertebral junction presented in previous chapters. It also includes a selection of narrated cases with short video summaries that are representative of some of the most difficult scenarios that challenge surgeons in this region. We hope that the inclusion of this material may serve as a useful teaching tool in an era of work-hour restrictions and diminishing opportunities to participate in complex, open neurosurgical procedures.

We appreciate the immense support of the contributing authors who volunteered their time in making this volume a success. The contributions of Mark Schornak, MS; Kristen Larson, MS; and Michael Hickman, whose incredible animations and illustrations grace this work, should be particularly acknowledged. Likewise, Marie Clarkson has our special thanks for creating the truly marvelous interactive multimedia presentation on the DVD, by meticulously incorporating videos, animations, still images, text, and virtual reality simulations into a cohesive presentation. This text would have been impossible without the editorial expertise of Kim Duvall, MA, editorial manager at the Neurological Institute at University Hospitals Case Medical Center; and Shelly Kick, PhD, senior editor; Dawn Mutchler, editor; and Jaime L. Canales, production editor at the Neuroscience Publications Office of Barrow Neurological Institute. We thank Kay Conerly, executive editor, and Judith Tomat, managing editor at Thieme Medical Publishers for their continuing faith in the importance of this work.

Nicholas C. Bambakidis, MD
Curtis A. Dickman, MD
Robert F. Spetzler, MD
Volker K. H. Sonntag, MD

Contributors

Felipe C. Albuquerque, MD
Assistant Director, Endovascular Surgery
Professor of Neurosurgery
Division of Neurological Surgery
Barrow Neurological Institute
Phoenix, Arizona

Ossama Al-Mefty, MD, FACS
Director, Skull Base Program
Department of Neurosurgery
Brigham and Women's Hospital
Boston, Massachusetts

Sepideh Amin-Hanjani, MD, FAANS, FACS, FAHA
Professor and Program Director of Neurosurgery
Co-Director of Neurovascular Surgery
University of Illinois at Chicago
Chicago, Illinois

Vijay K. Anand, MD
Clinical Professor of Otolaryngology–Head and Neck Surgery
Weill Cornell Medical College
New York, New York

Paul J. Apostolides, MD
Orthopaedic & Neurosurgery Specialists
Greenwich, Connecticut

Nicholas C. Bambakidis, MD
Director of Cerebrovascular and Skull Base Surgery
The Neurological Institute
University Hospitals Case Medical Center
Associate Professor of Neurological Surgery
Case Western Reserve University School of Medicine
Cleveland, Ohio

Stephen P. Beals, MD
Associate Professor of Plastic Surgery
Mayo Clinic Arizona
Scottsdale, Arizona
Director of Barrow Cleft and Craniofacial Center
Barrow Neurological Institute
Phoenix, Arizona

Kimon Bekelis, MD
Department of Neurosurgery
Dartworth-Hitchcock Medical Center
Hanover, New Hampshire

David M. Benglis, MD
Atlanta Brain and Spine Care
Atlanta, Georgia

Edward C. Benzel, MD
Chairman of Neurosurgery
Neurological Institute
Cleveland Clinic
Cleveland, Ohio

Kristine A. Blackham, MD
Interventional Neuroradiologist
The Neurological Institute
University Hospitals Case Medical Center
Assistant Professor of Radiology and Neurological Surgery
Case Western Reserve University School of Medicine
Cleveland, Ohio

Ruth E. Bristol, MD
Assistant Professor of Pediatric Neurosurgery
Division of Neurological Surgery
Barrow Neurological Institute
Phoenix Children's Hospital
Phoenix, Arizona

Winston T. Capel, MD, FACS
Spinal Surgery/Neurosurgery
Madison, Mississippi

Fady T. Charbel, MD
Professor of Neurosurgery
Head and Chief of Service
University of Illinois Hospital and Health Sciences System
Chicago, Illinois

David Choi, MA, MBChB, FRCS, PhD
Consultant Neurosurgeon
The National Hospital for Neurology and Neurosurgery
London, United Kingdom

Michael D. Coffey, MD
Neuroradiologist
The Neurological Institute
University Hospitals Case Medical Center
Assistant Professor of Radiology
Case Western Reserve University School of Medicine
Cleveland, Ohio

Neil R. Crawford, PhD
Associate Professor of Spinal Biomechanics
Division of Neurological Surgery
Barrow Neurological Institute
Phoenix, Arizona

Hugh Alan Crockard, MB, BCh, DSc, FRCS, FRCP, FDS
Professor of Neurosurgery
University of London
National Hospital of Neurology and Neurosurgery
London, United Kingdom

C. Phillip Daspit, MD
Clinical Professor of Otolaryngology
University of Arizona Health Sciences Center
Tucson, Arizona
Barrow Neurological Institute
Phoenix, Arizona

Bruce L. Dean, MD
Professor of Neuroradiology
Barrow Neurological Institute
Neurology Vice-President
St. Joseph's Hospital and Medical Center
Phoenix, Arizona

Evandro De Oliveira, MD, PhD
Professor and Chief of Neurosurgery
Medical Sciences School
State University of Campinas–UNICAMP
Director, Institute of Neurological Sciences
São Paulo, Brazil

Curtis A. Dickman, MD
Associate Chief, Spine Section
Director, Spinal Research
Division of Neurological Surgery
Barrow Neurological Institute
Phoenix, Arizona

Kadir Erkmen, MD
Assistant Professor of Neurosurgery
Dartmouth Medical School
Surgical Director of Cerebrovascular and Stroke Program
Director of Skull Base Surgery, Medical Director
Neuroscience Unit
Dartmouth-Hitchcock Medical Center
Lebanon, New Hampshire

David J. Fiorella, MD, PhD
Professor of Radiology and Neurosurgery
Stony Brook University Medical Center
Director, Neurointerventional Radiology
Cerebrovascular Center
Stony Brook, New York

Ricardo B. V. Fontes, MD, PhD
Resident in Neurosurgery
Rush University Medical Center
Chicago, Illinois

Mark P. Garrett, MD
Chief Resident
Division of Neurological Surgery
Barrow Neurological Institute
Phoenix, Arizona

Wendy C. Gaza, MS, MD
Assistant Professor of Neurology
Uniformed Services University of the Health Sciences
Lieutenant Commander, United States Navy
Vascular and Interventional Neurologist
Walter Reed National Military Medical Center
Bethesda, Maryland

Venelin M. Gerganov, MD
Associate Neurosurgeon
International Neuroscience Institute
Hannover, Germany

Atul Goel, MD
Professor and Head of Neurosurgery
K.E.M. Hospital and Seth G.S. Medical College
Mumbai, India

Ziya L. Gokaslan, MD, FACS
Donlin M. Long Professor of Neurosurgery
Departments of Oncology and Orthopaedic Surgery
Johns Hopkins University
Neurosurgical Spine Program Vice-Chair
Baltimore, Maryland

Pankaj A. Gore, MD
Neurosurgeon and Co-medical Director
Providence Brain and Spinal Institute
Portland, Oregon

Karl A. Greene, MD, PhD
Chairman of Surgery
Theda Clark Medical Center
Neenah, Wisconsin
Staff Neurosurgeon
NeuroSpine Center of Wisconsin, S.C.
Appleton, Wisconsin

H. Louis Harkey, MD
Professor of Neurosurgery
University of Mississippi Medical Center
Jackson, Mississippi

David J. Hart, MD
Director of Neurosurgery Spine Center
The Neurological Institute
University Hospitals Case Medical Center
Assistant Professor of Neurological Surgery
Case Western Reserve University School of Medicine
Cleveland, Ohio

Roger Härtl, MD
Assistant Professor of Neurological Surgery
Weill Cornell Medical College
Director of Spinal Surgery and Neurotrauma
New York Presbyterian Hospital
New York, New York

Alia Hdeib, MD
Resident in Neurological Surgery
The Neurological Institute
University Hospitals Case Medical Center
Case Western Reserve University School of Medicine
Cleveland, Ohio

John A. Hodak, BS, MD
Former Chairman, Division of Neuroradiology
Barrow Neurological Institute
Phoenix, Arizona

Daniel P. Hsu, MD
Neuroradiologist
The Neurological Institute
University Hospitals Case Medical Center
Assistant Professor of Radiology
Case Western Reserve University School of Medicine
Cleveland, Ohio

Yin C. Hu, MD
Cerebrovascular/Skull Base Fellow
Division of Neurological Surgery
Barrow Neurological Institute
Phoenix, Arizona

Ivo P. Janecka, MD, MBA, PhD
(Former) Professor of Surgery
Harvard University
Foundation for Systems Research and Education
St. Helena Island, South Carolina

Edward F. Joganic, MD
Associate Professor of Plastic Surgery
Mayo Clinic
Consultant, Barrow Cleft and Craniofacial Center
St. Joseph's Hospital and Medical Center
Phoenix, Arizona

Iain H. Kalfas, MD
Center for Spinal Health
Department of Neurosurgery
Cleveland Clinic Foundation
Cleveland, Ohio

Louis J. Kim, MD
Assistant Professor of Neurological Surgery
Associate Chief of Neurological Surgery
University of Washington at Harborview Medical Center
Seattle, Washington

Allan D. Levi, MD, PhD, FACS
Professor of Neurological Surgery
University of Miami Hospital
Miami, Florida

Andrew S. Little, MD
Assistant Professor of Neurosurgery
Division of Neurological Surgery
Barrow Pituitary Center
Barrow Neurological Institute
Phoenix, Arizona

Jonathan H. Lustgarten, MD
Instructor of Clinical Neurological Surgery
Columbia University Medical Center
West Long Branch, New Jersey

Alexander C. Mamourian, MD
Associate Professor of Radiology
Hospital of the University of Pennsylvania
Philadelphia, Pennsylvania

Paul C. McCormick, MD, MPH, FACS
Herbert and Linda Gallen Professor of Neurological Surgery
Director, Spine Center
Columbia University Medical Center
New York, New York

Cameron G. McDougall, MD, FRCSC
Director, Endovascular Neurosurgery
Division of Neurological Surgery
Barrow Neurological Institute
Phoenix, Arizona

Cliff A. Megerian, MD, FACS
Director of the Ear, Nose, and Throat Institute
The Neurological Institute
University Hospitals Case Medical Center
Professor of Otolaryngology—Head and Neck Surgery and Neurological Surgery
Richard and Patricia Pogue Endowed Chair
Case Western Reserve University School of Medicine
Cleveland, Ohio

Arnold H. Menezes, MD
Professor and Vice Chairman of Neurosurgery
University of Iowa Hospitals and Clinics
Iowa City, Iowa

Camilo A. Molina, BA
HHMI Medical Student Fellow
Department of Neurosurgery
Johns Hopkins Hospital
Baltimore, Maryland

Yaron A. Moshel, MD, PhD
Professor of Neurological Surgery
Division of Neuro-Oncology
Thomas Jefferson University
Philadelphia, Pennsylvania

Peter Nakaji, MD, FACS, FAANS
Professor of Neurosurgery
Director, Neurosurgery Residency Program
Director, Minimally Invasive Neurosurgery
Division of Neurological Surgery
Barrow Neurological Institute
Phoenix, Arizona

Ashish Nanda, MD
Assistant Professor of Neurology and Neurosurgery
Co-director Missouri Stroke Program
University of Missouri
Columbia, MO

C. Benjamin Newman, MD
Physician and Surgeon
Department of Neurosurgery
University of California, San Diego
San Diego, California

Joshua W. Osbun, MD
Resident in Neurosurgery
University of Washington
Seattle, Washington

John Piper, MD
Neurological and Spinal Surgery Department
The Iowa Clinic
Des Moines, Iowa

Harold L. Rekate, MD
Professor of Neurosurgery
The Chiari Institute
Director of Hofstra Northshore LIJ College of Medicine
Great Neck, New York

Albert L. Rhoton, Jr., MD
Professor and Chairman of Neurosurgery
University of Florida
Gainesville, Florida

Guilherme R. Ribas, MD
Department of Surgery
University of São Paulo Medical School
Hospital Israelita Albert Einstein
São Paulo, Brazil

John R. Robinson, MD
Director, Back and Spine Institute
Martin Memorial Hospital
Stuart, Florida

Madjid Samii, MD, PhD
Nordstadt Hospital
International Neuroscience Institute
Hannover, Germany

Theodore H. Schwartz, MD
Professor of Neurological Surgery
Weill Cornell Medical College
New York Presbyterian Hospital
New York, New York

Daniel M. Sciubba, MD
Assistant Professor of Neurosurgery
Director of Spine Research
Johns Hopkins University
Baltimore, Maryland

Chandranath Sen, MD
Director of Benign Brain Tumor and Cranial Nerve Disease Program
Department of Neurosurgery
NYU Langone Medical Center
New York, New York

John H. Shin, MD
Attending Neurosurgeon
Harvard Medical School
Massachusetts General Hospital
Boston, Massachusetts

Andrew E. Sloan, MD
Director of Brain Tumor and Neuro-Oncology Center
The Neurological Institute
University Hospitals Case Medical Center
Associate Professor of Neurological Surgery
Peter D. Cristal Chair of Neurosurgical Oncology
Case Western Reserve University School of Medicine
Cleveland, Ohio

Volker K. H. Sonntag, MD
Emeritus, Division of Neurological Surgery
Barrow Neurological Institute
Phoenix, Arizona
Professor of Clinical Surgery
University of Arizona College of Medicine
Tucson, Arizona

Robert F. Spetzler, MD
Director
J. N. Harber Chair of Neurological Surgery
Barrow Neurological Institute
Phoenix, Arizona
Professor, Department of Surgery
Section of Neurosurgery
University of Arizona College of Medicine
Tucson, Arizona

Michael P. Steinmetz, MD
Chairman of Department of Neuroscience
MetroHealth Medical Center
Associate Professor of Neurological Surgery
Case Western Reserve University School of Medicine
Cleveland, Ohio

Marcos Tatagiba, MD, PhD
Chairman and Director of Neurosurgery
Professor of Neurosurgery
University of Tübingen
Tübingen, Germany

Charles Teo, MD
Assistant Professor of Neurosurgery
Prince of Wales Private Hospital
Centre for Minimally Invasive Neurosurgery
Randwick, Australia

Nicholas Theodore, MD, FAANS, FACS
Professor of Neurological Surgery
Chief, Spine Section
Director, Neurotrauma Program
Division of Neurological Surgery
Barrow Neurological Institute
Phoenix, Arizona

B. Gregory Thompson, MD
Professor of Neurological Surgery
University of Michigan
Ann Arbor, Michigan

Bryan J. Traughber, MD
Fellow in Radiology
University Hospitals Case Medical Center
Case Western Reserve University School of Medicine
Cleveland, Ohio

Vincent C. Traynelis, MD
Professor of Neurosurgery
Vice-Chairman and Director of Neurosurgery Spine Service
Rush University Medical Center
Chicago, Illinois

Peter A. Weisskopf, MD, FACS
Head, Neurotology Section
Gamma Knife and CyberKnife Stereotactic Radiosurgery Teams
Co-Director, Acoustic Neuroma Center Skull Base Team
Barrow Neurological Institute
Phoenix, Arizona

Jean-Paul Wolinsky, MD
Associate Professor of Neurosurgery and Oncology
Director of the Johns Hopkins Bayview Spine Program
The Johns Hopkins Hospital
Baltimore, Maryland

Joseph M. Zabramski, MD
Professor of Neurological Surgery
Chief, Section of Cerebrovascular Surgery
Division of Neurological Surgery
Barrow Neurological Institute
Phoenix, Arizona

I Foundations for Surgical Treatment

1 Embryology, Development, and Classification of Disorders of the Craniovertebral Junction

Arnold H. Menezes

The term *craniovertebral junction* (CVJ) refers to the occipital bone that surrounds the foramen magnum, the atlas, and the axis vertebrae. This bony enclosure encompasses the medulla oblongata, the cervicomedullary junction, and the upper cervical spinal cord. Bony abnormalities that affect this complex can result in neural compression along the entire circumference, vascular compromise, and abnormal cerebrospinal fluid (CSF) dynamics.[1,2] The basis for understanding these problems comes from knowledge of the embryology, bony anatomy, and the biomechanics of this region. This chapter discusses the embryology and the normal and abnormal development of the CVJ and the traditional classification of disorders affecting the craniocervical area.[3] Since 1977, the author has investigated 6000 patients with neurological symptoms and signs related to abnormalities of the craniocervical region.[4] A surgical-physiological approach to treatment of the abnormalities is the basis for a practical classification of craniocervical region abnormalities.[5]

Embryology and Development of the Craniovertebral Junction

Congenital anomalies of the CVJ frequently occur with various combinations of neural abnormalities, suggesting an interrelationship, if not a common cause, of its origin and development.[6] A review of the embryology, outlining the developmental sequence and timing of events in this region, follows here.

A definite notochord forms between the ectoderm and the endoderm during the third week of gestation. At the cephalic end of the embryo, the ectoderm immediately overlying the notochord begins to thicken and differentiates into neural ectoderm, which forms the neural plate. This plate begins to buckle along the middle to shape the neural groove, which becomes walled in by the neural folds on each side. While this is occurring, a collection of mesenchymal cells begins to coalesce in three regions. The most medial becomes a solid mass—the paraxial mesoderm—which is just lateral to the notochord and on either side of it. This precursor of bone, skeletal muscle, and skin begins to segment in the cranial and caudal directions.[7–9] The parachordal mesodermal cells migrate to the midline and fuse around the notochord at the level of the jugular foramen.[10]

The bony cranial base is developed by the process of endochondral ossification in which a cartilaginous framework is first developed and subsequently resorbed with further deposition of bone, based on distorting forces such as brain and eye development.[11–13] Suture growth also appears to play a fairly major role. The clivus is elongated by sutural growth of the spheno-occipital synchondrosis and by further sutural growth along the lateral portion of the base. Björk described two sutural growth sites, the petro-occipital and the sphenopetrosal junctions, which result in marked lowering of the occiput and foramen magnum.[11] Thus, the combination of sutural growth and bony accretion is necessary for development in the cranial base.

The majority of the skull and facial bones—including the mandible, maxilla, premaxilla, zygoma, frontal, parietal, vomer, palatine, and nasal bones—develop by intramembranous ossification.[14] This development of intramembranous ossification bypasses the intermediate cartilaginous stage characteristic of the development of the bony cranial base.

During the fourth week of gestation, 42 somites are formed: 4 occipital somites, 8 cervical, 12 thoracic, 5 lumbar, 5 sacral, and 8 to 10 coccygeal pairs. Each somite differentiates into an outer dermatome, an inner myotome, and a medial sclerotome. The sclerotomes are ventromedial in location and destined to form the vertebral bodies. These bilateral ventromedial cells migrate to the midline and surround the notochord. Each sclerotome develops a central cleft called the fissure of von Ebner, which divides a loose collection of cells cranially from a dense cellular area caudally. In the development of the normal spine, cells from the fissure of von Ebner migrate to and encase the notochord to become precursors of the intervertebral disk.[12]

The superior half of one sclerotome (caudal) unites with the lower half of its neighbor (cranial) and thus forms the earliest manifestation of a vertebral body. The first four sclerotomes do not follow this course and eventually fuse to form the occipital bone and the posterior portion of the foramen magnum.[15,16] Vascularization of the occipital bone begins at this time, and differentiation of the ganglia and vascular tissue continues. The hypoglossal and first cervical arteries, although inconspicuous, are present and demarcate the caudal occipital segment.[17]

Simultaneous with this development, there is differentiation of the nervous system process. A tube-like appearance is seen by the end of the third week of gestation, and during the fourth week the neural fold that forms the side wall starts to fuse in the midline to form a tube. This occurs in the region of the future atlanto-occipital junction and corresponds to the fourth somite.[18,19] The fusion of the neural tube proceeds simultaneously in a rostral and caudal dimension with both ends remaining open. During the fifth and sixth weeks, further differentiation of the various parts of the brain and spinal cord occurs.[20] However, the roof of the fourth ventricle thins out in the midline to form the foramen of Magendie and, laterally, the foramen of Luschka. This occurs because an opening forms in the seventh week when a connection between the fourth ventricle and the subarachnoid space is established.

Membrane formation is usually over by 38 to 40 days of gestation. Cartilage formation then begins with chondrification in the basioccipital bone.[13]

The occipital sclerotomes correspond to the segmental nerves that group to form the hypoglossal nerve, with a path through the individual foramina in the bone.[21] The first two occipital sclerotomes ultimately form the basiocciput (**Table 1.1**). The third sclerotome is responsible for the exoccipital center as it forms the jugular tubercles. The key to understanding the CVJ embryology is the proatlas, which is the fourth occipital sclerotome (**Fig. 1.1**).[15,22–24] The hypocentrum of the fourth occipital sclerotome forms the anterior tubercle of the clivus. The centrum of the proatlas forms the apical cap of the dens as well as the apical ligament.[16,17] The neural arch component of the proatlas divides into a rostral ventral component and a caudal dorsal portion. The ventral portion forms the U-shaped anterior margin of the foramen magnum as well as the occipital condyles and the midline third occipital condyle. The cruciate ligament and the alar ligaments are condensations of the lateral portion of the proatlas. The caudal division of the neural arch of the proatlas forms the lateral atlantal masses of C1, as well as the superior portion of the posterior arch of the atlas.

The atlas vertebra is formed by the first spinal sclerotome—a transitional vertebra modified from the remaining spinal vertebra. The centrum is separated to fuse with the axis body forming the odontoid process. At an early stage, a hypochordal bow is found in front of each vertebral segment but subsequently disappears, except for the part that forms the anterior arch of the atlas.[7] The neural arch of the first spinal sclerotome forms the posterior and inferior portions of the atlas arch. The hypochordal bow of the proatlas itself may survive and join with the anterior arch of the atlas to form a variant, such that an abnormal articulation may exist between the clivus, the anterior arch of the atlas, and the apical segment of the odontoid process.[25]

During embryogenesis, the hypocentrum of the second spinal sclerotome disappears. The centrum forms the body of the axis vertebra, and the neural arches develop into the facets and the posterior arch of the axis. Thus, the body of the dens appears from the first sclerotome, whereas the terminal portion of the odontoid process arises from the proatlas.[15] The most inferior portion of the axis body is formed by the second spinal sclerotome. At birth, the odontoid process is separated from the body of the axis vertebra by a cartilaginous band that represents the vestigial disk, referred to as a neural central synchondrosis. It lies below the level of the superior articular facets of the axis and does not represent the anatomical base of the dens.[26] The neural central synchondrosis is present in most children younger than 3 to 4 years old but disappears by age 8. At birth, there should be a recognizable odontoid process that does not fuse to the base of the axis. The tip of the odontoid process is not ossified at birth; hence, it is not seen on the lateral radiograph. It is represented by a separate ossification center, which usually is seen at age 3 and fuses with the remainder of the dens by age 12.[27]

Table 1.1 Embryology and Development of the Craniovertebral Junction

Sclerotomes	Divisions	Subdivisions	Formations
Occipital 1st			Basiocciput
2nd			
3rd			Exoccipital centers (jugular tubercles)
4th "Proatlas"	Hypocentrum		Anterior tubercle clivus
	Centrum		Apical ligament
			Apex of dens
	Neural arch	Ventral rostral	Occipital condyles, third cond.
			U-shape of foramen magnum
			Alar and cruciate ligaments
		Dorsal caudal	Posterior arch of atlas (C1)
			Lateral atlantal masses
Spinal 1st	Hypocentrum persists		Atlas anterior arch
	Centrum		Dens
	Neural arch		Posterior inferior atlas arch
Spinal 2nd	Hypocentrum	Disappears	
	Centrum		Body of axis
	Neural arch		Facets, posterior arch of axis

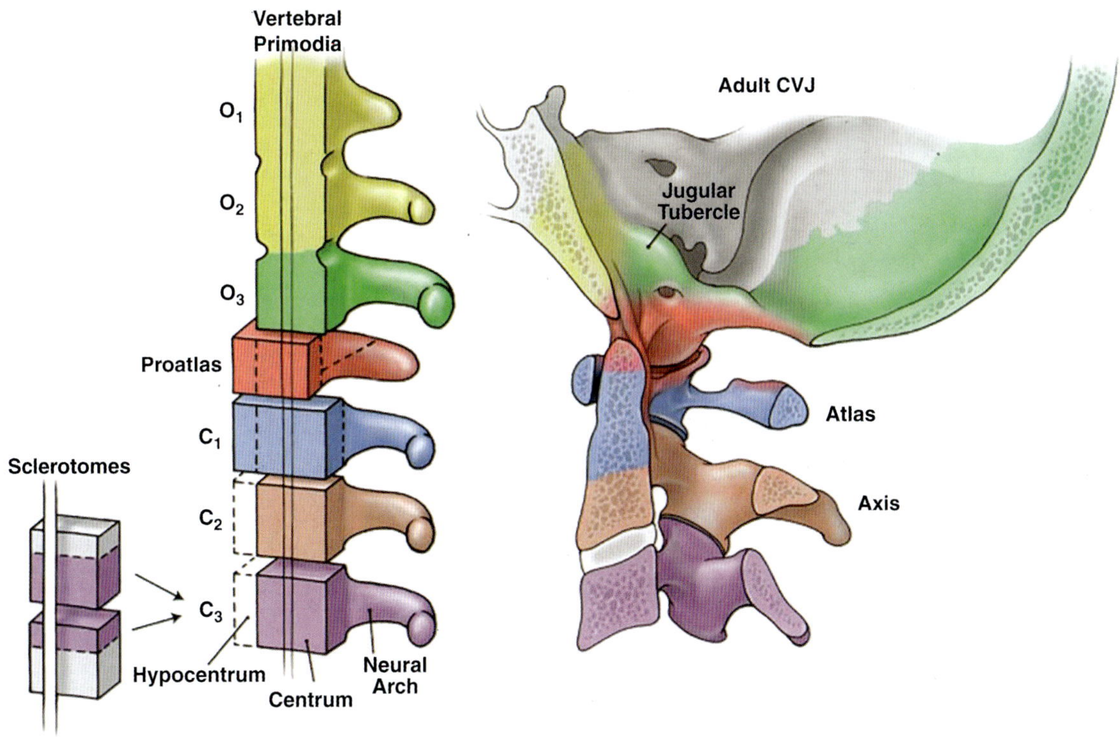

Fig. 1.1 In mammals, the neural arch of the proatlas splits into a rostral and caudal segment; the former is fused into the occipital bone to form the paired occipital condyles. The caudal portion of the proatlas neural arch is incorporated into the atlas and is represented by the paired rostral articulation facets of the atlas and a small portion of the lateral mass. The hypocentrum of the proatlas is reduced into the vestigial condylus tertius or the thin ridge-like anterior prominence of the basicranium. The core of the proatlas centrum is metamorphosized into the apical ligament of the dens. This apical ligament may contain notochordal tissue and can be regarded as a rudimentary intervertebral disk. The paired alar or check ligaments and the transverse ligament of the atlas are derived from the proatlas as unossified tissue. *CVJ*, craniovertebral junction. (Reprinted with permission from Barrow Neurological Institute.)

Expansion in the posterior fossa occurs as a result of a combination of endocranial resorption, sutural growth, and bony accretion.[14] The growth of the basion elongates the basiocciput and lowers the frontal margin of the foramen magnum. There is a comparably matched resorptive drift downward and backward at the opisthion as a result of the cerebellar downward displacement with the rotation of the occipital and temporal lobes of the brain. Thus, the posterior fossa apart from the midline basiocciput relies fairly heavily on endocranial resorption. However, synchondrodial growth is also an important feature in posterior fossa expansion.[11] The sagittal elongation in the spheno-occipital synchondrosis is active into the second decade of life. The fact that the basal angle of the cranial base appears to remain relatively constant throughout life is probably secondary to the mutual interaction between synchondrodial growth at the spheno-occipital synchondrosis and the constant surface remodeling that occurs. Growth in the skull base is interesting in that it coordinates with both brain development and development elsewhere in the body. It has been noted that there are pubertal spurts in the basal growth and that the rostrocaudal orientation parallels the growth in the brain hemispheres. However, despite this gradient of growth in the cranial base, the basicranial inclination of ~130 degrees is maintained throughout postnatal life. This angulation distinctly separates the expanding brain above and the facial complex and nasopharyngeal spaces below. The stability of the craniovertebral articulation with the forward inclination of the top-heavy cranial end of the fetus must then be maintained by the geometry of the articular surfaces of the CVJ, as well as by the ligamentous attachments and, more importantly, by the heavy development of the dorsal and lateral cervical musculature, which provides a clamping action on the craniocervical region.[28,29]

Implications

A wide variety of congenital anomalies of the craniocervical region exists, occurring singularly or as more than one anomaly in the same individual and involving osseous and neural structures.[6,7,30] An insult to both may occur between the fourth and seventh weeks of intrauterine life and may result in a combination of anomalies. A careful look at the embryology and development of the craniocervical region makes it apparent that anomalies in this region would consist of failures of segmentation, failures of fusion of different components of each bone, or hypoplasia and ankylosis.[4,22,31–39]

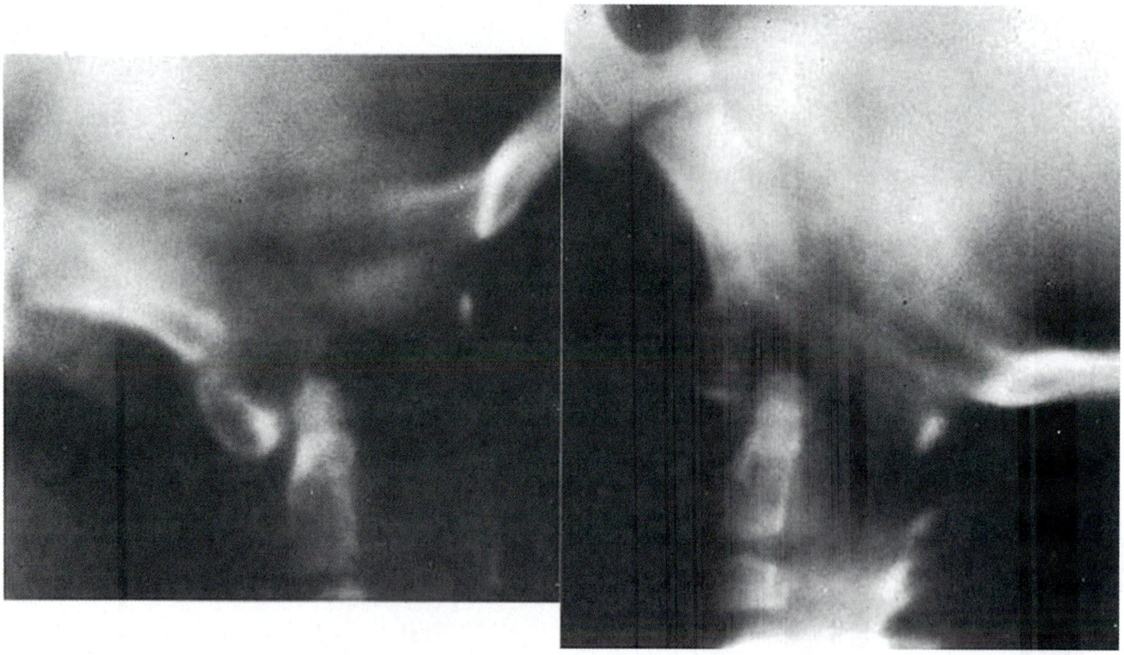

Fig. 1.2 A composite of a midline craniocervical pluridirectional tomogram in the flexed and extended position in an 8-year-old child. Note the atlas assimilation with segmentation failure of C2 and C3 vertebral body. The atlantoaxial dislocation is reducible in extension (*right*).

Understanding the growth of the cranial base and CVJ forms the basis for understanding a variety of anomalous processes: abnormalities of atlas assimilation, occipitalization of the atlas, remnants of the occipital sclerotomes and fusion abnormalities, abnormal fusion between the occiput-C1 and C2, os odontoideum, ossiculum terminale, trauma to the craniovertebral complex in both children and adults, and secondary forms of invagination.[2,39]

It is important to differentiate between an occipital vertebra and atlas assimilation. An occipital vertebra occurs when the third occipital sclerotome fails to be incorporated into the rostral two occipital sclerotomes.[39,40] In this situation, the occipital condyles attach to the vertebra. If the occipital vertebra contains a transverse process, it does not have a foramen for the vertebral artery. In atlas assimilation (sometimes called occipital-atlantal fusion), the transverse process of the atlas bears the bony foramen for the vertebral artery.[41] Segmentation fails between the fourth occipital sclerotome and the first spinal sclerotome (**Fig. 1.2**). Thirty-eight percent of individuals with symptomatic atlas assimilation and segmentation failures of C2 and C3 vertebrae were found to have a Chiari malformation.[4,7] A paramesial invagination, reducible atlantoaxial dislocation, or basilar invagination may exist (**Figs. 1.3** and **1.4**).

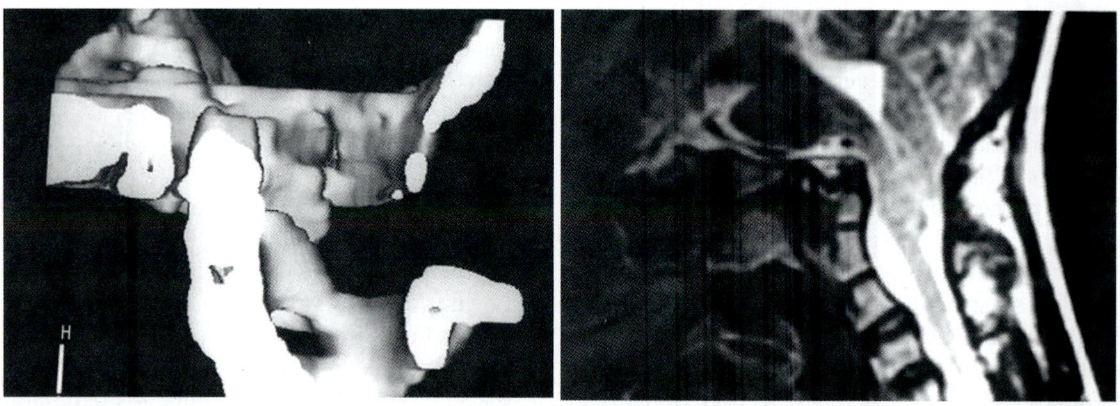

Fig. 1.3 A composite of a midsagittal three-dimensional computed tomography reconstructed image of the craniovertebral junction (*left*) and midsagittal T2-weighted magnetic resonance image through the plane of the craniovertebral junction (*right*), demonstrating atlas assimilation with segmentation failure of C2 and C3. Note the marked acute angle of the clivus-odontoid articulation. The posterior fossa is shallow, and there is hindbrain herniation with ventral indentation of the cervicomedullary junction.

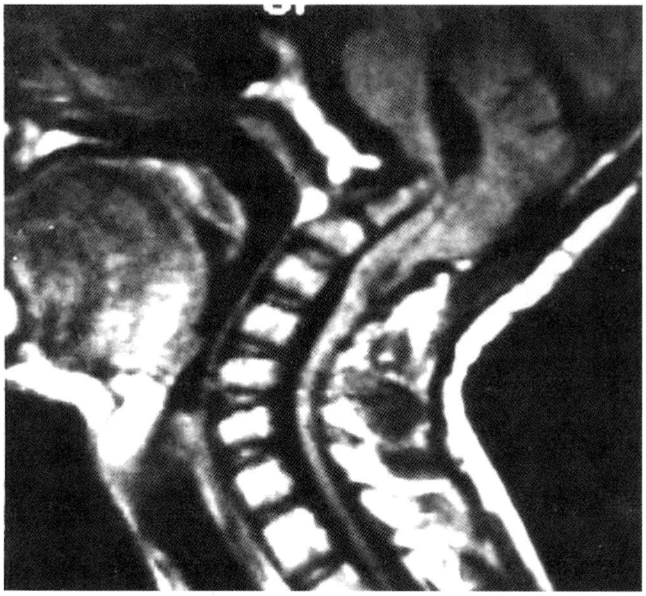

Fig. 1.4 A midsagittal T1-weighted magnetic resonance image of the cervical spine and posterior fossa. Note the extreme basilar invagination of the odontoid process into the medulla. This patient also had a previous posterior fossa decompression for Chiari I malformation.

Os odontoideum was previously considered to be congenital and was described as a failure of fusion between the centrum component of C1 and that of C2.[24] However, the radiographic abnormality always has a hypoplastic dens and the spheno-occipital synchondrosis is a definite visible entity. Thus, os odontoideum cannot be congenital.[26] To be congenital, the defect would have to be below the superior slopes of the C2 facets.[27] Os odontoideum most likely originates as odontoid trauma occurring between ages 1 and 4, with subsequent separation and distraction of the odontoid fragments. The superior segment is distracted upward by the apical and alar ligaments and receives its blood supply from the descending branch of the occipital artery, which courses along the apical ligament.[26,27,42] Thus, there is a hypertrophied, rounded ossicle causing the hypoplastic dens as well as hypertrophy of the anterior arch of the atlas, leading to incompetence of the cruciate ligament and further abnormalities. Aplasia or hypoplasia of the dens is an uncommon feature but has been described (**Fig. 1.5A,B**).

Due to the high fulcrum of neck motion, spinal trauma in children younger than age 8 is mainly at the craniovertebral border,[2] resulting in ligamentous injuries more than fractures. However, odontoid fractures in this age group are usually seen as avulsion injuries with separation of the neural central synchondrosis.

Anomalies and malformations of the caudal occipital sclerotomes are collectively called *manifestations of an occipital vertebra* and result in abnormal bony ridges and overgrowths of the ventral aspect of the foramen magnum.[15,39] At times, segmentation abnormalities of the clivus are recognized and represent a failure of the proatlas to separate from the basiocciput of the clivus. Consequently, bone growth in the anterior aspect of the foramen magnum indents the ventral cervicomedullary junction (**Fig. 1.6**).[7] A third occipital condyle can present in the midline and is called *median occipital condyle* (**Fig. 1.7**).[43–45] Bilateral paramesial compression from hypertrophied occipital condyles represents the ventrorostral neural arch of the proatlas (**Fig. 1.8**).[15,46]

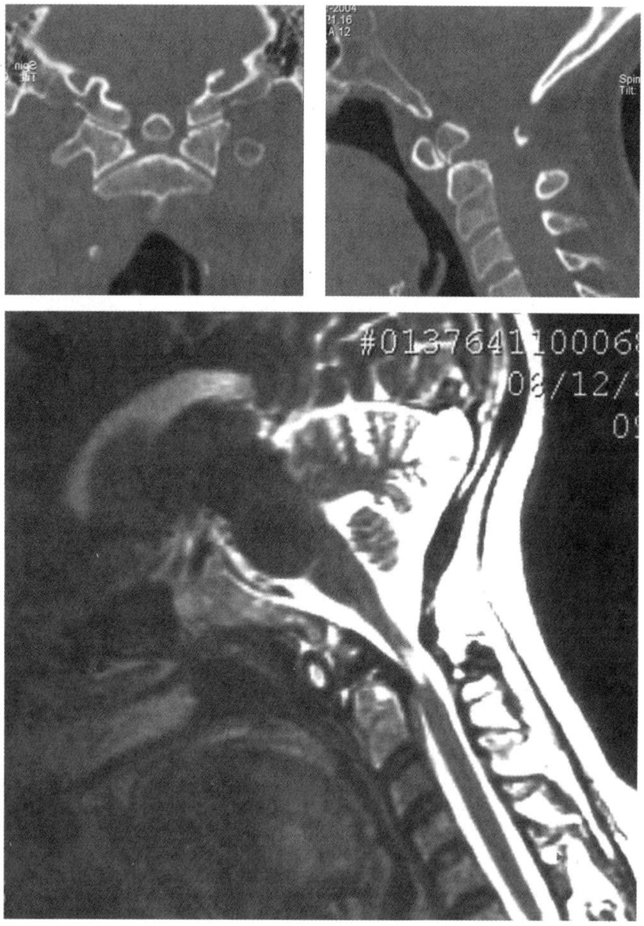

A

B

Fig. 1.5 **(A)** A composite of a two-dimensional computed tomography (CT) scan through the craniovertebral junction. A separate rounded ossicle with smooth borders represents the os odontoideum (*left*). Note that the axis body is not hypoplastic. The neural central synchondrosis is below the level of the defect as seen on the lateral CT scan (*right*). **(B)** There is an unstable dystopic os odontoideum with evidence of previous cord contusion at the cervicomedullary junction with cord atrophy corresponding to the C1-C2 level.

It must be kept in mind that, during development, the occipital sclerotome is functionally a vertebra.[21] In 1981, Marin-Padilla and Marin-Padilla demonstrated that the basichondrocranium of fetuses with hindbrain malformations, such as Chiari syndrome, is shorter than normal and elevated (lordotic) in relation to the axis of the vertebral column.[47] The shortness of the basichondrocranium

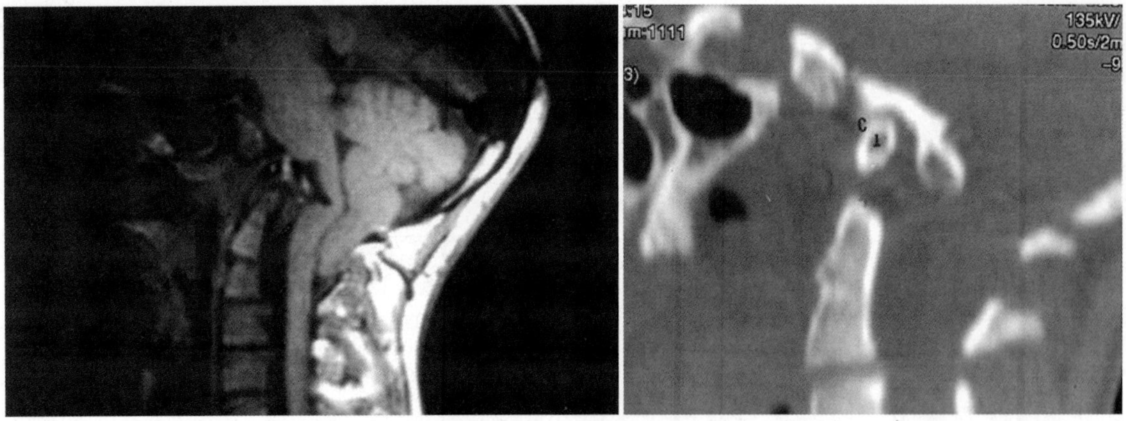

Fig. 1.6 A composite of a midsagittal T1-weighted magnetic resonance image of the craniovertebral junction (*left*) and two-dimensional computed tomography scan through the same plane (*right*). Note the extension of the clivus into the ventral medulla. The posterior fossa volume is small, and there is accompanying significant hindbrain herniation.

A

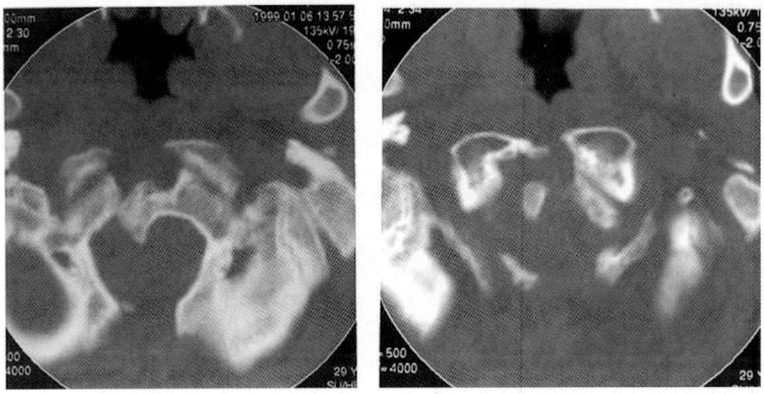

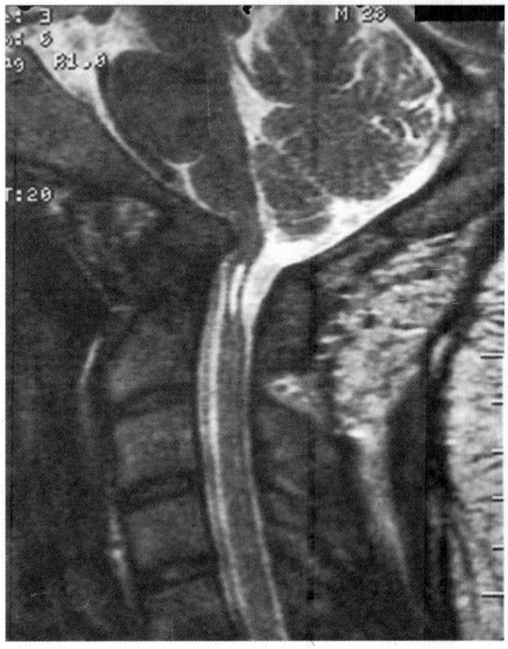

B

Fig. 1.7 **(A)** A composite of an axial computed tomography scan through the plane of the foramen magnum (*left*) and just below it (*right*). Note the hooklike extension from the anterior margin of the foramen magnum representing a median occipital condyle or third condyle. This patient had a previous attempt at anterior decompression prior to evaluation. **(B)** A midsagittal T2-weighted magnetic resonance image of the craniovertebral junction. Note the median occipital condyle with ventral indentation in the cervicomedullary junction.

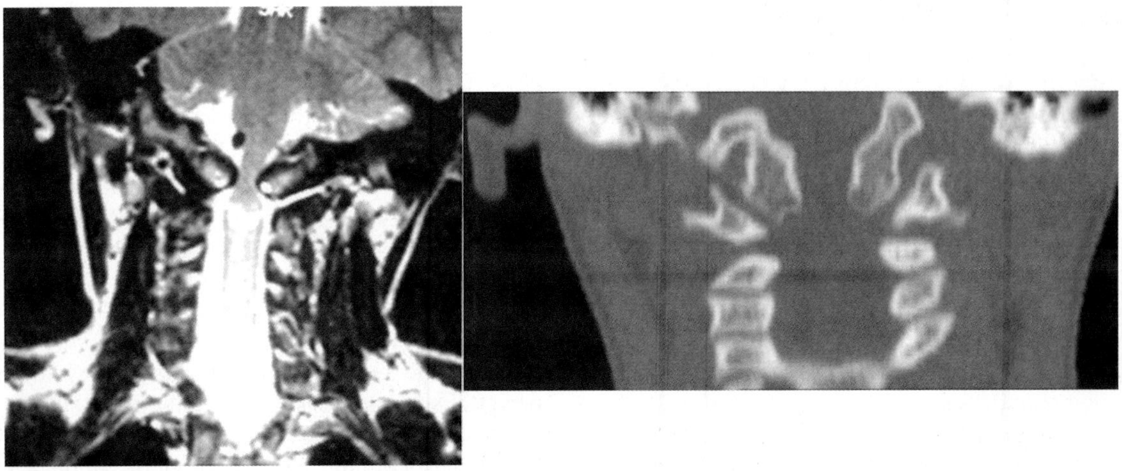

Fig. 1.8 A composite of a T2-weighted magnetic resonance image (*left*) in the coronal plane through the midportion of the spinal canal and two-dimensional computed tomography reconstruction (*right*) through the same plane. Note the hypertrophied occipital condyles causing a pincers-like compression of the cervicomedullary junction.

of these fetuses is attributed to underdevelopment of the occipital bone, especially noticeable in its basal component. The basic defect supposedly results in a short and small posterior fossa, inadequate to contain the developing nerve structures of the region. The authors theorize that the developing cerebellum is displaced downward to an anomalous position just above the foramen magnum, and the developing medulla is compressed and crowded into a small posterior fossa. This lordotic elevation of the basichondrocranium is responsible for the reduction of the pontine flexure and the increased angle of the cervical flexure of the hindbrain in these fetuses. The elongation of the odontoid process could be explained by the depression of the basiocciput, resulting in the basilar impression often seen in clinical Chiari malformations. These changes have been experimentally reproduced in pregnant hamsters by a single dose of vitamin A on the morning of the eighth day of gestation, thus inducing a typical Chiari I and Chiari II malformation as well as various types of axial skeletal-dysraphic disorders known to be associated with the human disease.[48,49]

The ongoing growth of the posterior fossa from birth to later adolescence provides an understanding of the continued need to observe children who have undergone dorsal occipitocervical stabilization or a ventral craniovertebral decompression.[31] The downward growth of the brain, as well as the elongation of the posterior fossa and clivus, may re-create a ventral bony abnormality later in life despite a previous ventral decompression at the CVJ that might have been performed during the first two decades of life. Similarly, patients with known atlas assimilation and basilar invagination tend to become symptomatic toward the end of their first and second decade of life due to developmental changes in the size, structure, and configuration of the foramen magnum.[4,50,51] Basilar impression is due to bone softening states, such as osteogenesis imperfecta, Paget disease, and hyperparathyroidism.[4] The skull base infolds, and the spine ascends (**Fig. 1.9**).

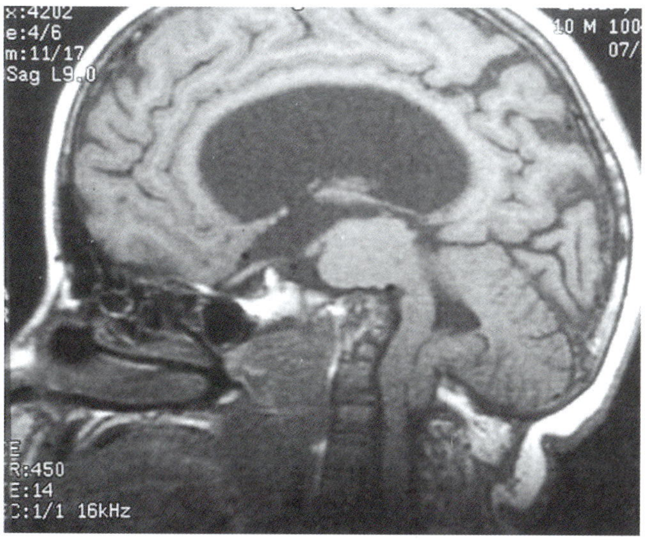

Fig. 1.9 A midsagittal T1-weighted magnetic resonance image of the head and upper cervical spine. This patient had bone softening akin to osteogenesis imperfecta. Note the basilar impression or "secondary basilar invagination." The posterior fossa has buckled upward, and there is marked cerebellar distortion and compression, resulting in significant cerebellar tonsillar ectopia. The invagination at the pontomedullary junction has caused an acute angle of the pontomedullary flexure, resulting in secondary aqueductal stenosis and hydrocephalus.

Classification of Disorders of the Craniovertebral Junction

A wide variety of congenital, developmental, and acquired anomalies exists at the CVJ and may occur as single or multiple anomalies in the same individual. The pathology of these abnormalities is extensive.[4,52–57] Between 1977 and 2009, 6000 symptomatic patients with bony abnormalities of the CVJ were evaluated by the author at the University of Iowa Hospitals and Clinics. A separate database evaluating hindbrain abnormalities (extra-axial and intra-axial neural abnormalities, including vascular malformations and tumors) has been analyzed and forms the basis of the classification of CVJ abnormalities. For the purpose of understanding and discussing these disorders, the entities have been divided into (1) the traditional classification (**Table 1.2**) and (2) the surgical–physiological approach classification.

Surgical–Physiological Approach to the Craniovertebral Junction

A constellation of congenital, developmental, and acquired lesions affects the bony CVJ (**Table 1.2**). In addition, a similar host of intracranial pathologies involves the neural structures, vascular supply and drainage, and CSF pathways. Four factors considered in developing a physiological approach to the surgical treatment of such lesions are (1) reducibility, (2) the direction and manner of encroachment of the lesion in the craniovertebral circumference and its effect on the neural structures, (3) the etiology of the lesion (whether it is bony, soft tissue, extracranial or intracranial, intramedullary or extramedullary), and (4) the growth potential of the area affected. The stability of the region after a surgical approach must be kept in mind as well as the potential for radical resection of benign chemotherapy- and radiotherapy-resistant tumors. Thus, reducible lesions require primary stabilization, whereas irreducible lesions require decompression in the manner in which an encroachment has occurred, whether this is ventral, dorsal, or lateral (**Fig. 1.10**). In any of the circumstances, if instability is present prior to treatment or after the surgical approach, stabilization is paramount.

Table 1.2 Classification of Disorders of the Craniovertebral Junction

A. Congenital

- I. Malformations of occipital bone
  - 1. Manifestations of occipital vertebra
    (e.g., clivus segmentations, remnants around foramen magnum, proatlas remnants)
  - 2. Basilar invagination
  - 3. Condylar hypoplasia
  - 4. Atlas assimilation
- II. Malformations of the atlas
  - 1. Atlas assimilation, atlantoaxial fusion, aplasia of the atlas arches
- III. Malformations of the axis
  - 1. Segmentation failure of C1-C2 or C2-C3; hypoplasia of the dens, ossiculum terminale

B. Developmental and acquired

- I. Traumatic
  - 1. Acute ligamentous and bony injury to CVJ complex
  - 2. Delayed manifestations of CVJ instability; development of os odontoideum
- II. Inflammation leading to instability and granulation masses
  (e.g., rheumatoid arthritis, regional ileitis, psoriasis, scleroderma, pseudogout, ankylosing spondylitis)
- III. Infectious
  (e.g., Grisel syndrome)
- IV. Metabolic
  (e.g., Morquio syndrome, Conradi syndrome, fetal warfarin syndrome, renal rickets)
- V. Genetic transformations
  (e.g., Down syndrome, osteogenesis imperfecta, achondroplasia, Paget disease, neurofibromatosis)
- VI. Neoplastic
  - 1. Benign
    (e.g., aneurysmal bone cyst, osteoblastoma, osteochondroma, chondroma)
  - 2. Malignant
    - a. Primary
      (e.g., chordoma, chondrosarcoma, plasmacytoma)
    - b. Secondary
      (e.g., multiple myeloma, metastatic disease, nasopharyngeal malignancy)

Abbreviation: CVJ, craniovertebral junction.

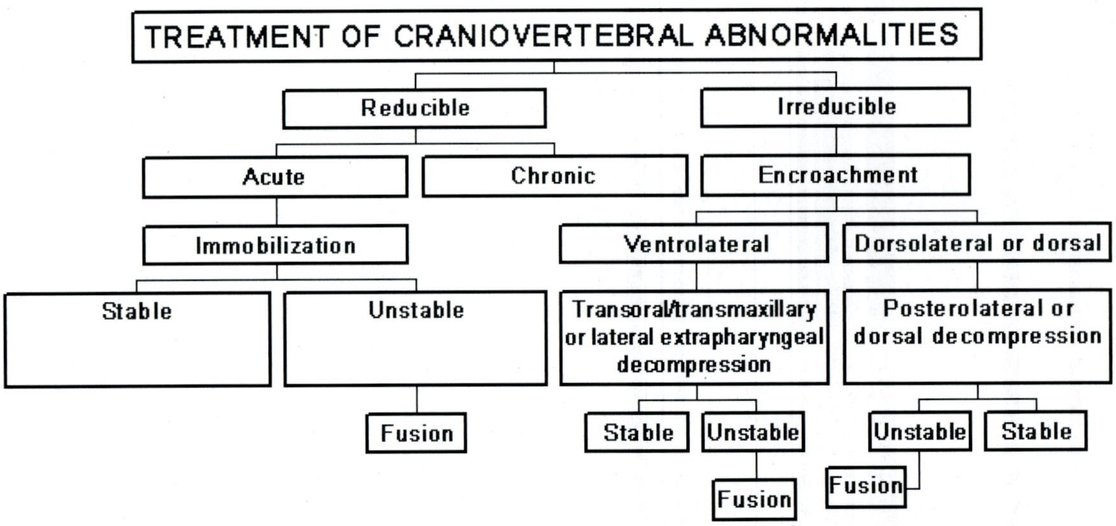

Fig. 1.10 Treatment of craniovertebral abnormalities.

References

1. de Oliveira E, Rhoton AL Jr, Peace D. Microsurgical anatomy of the region of the foramen magnum. Surg Neurol 1985;24(3):293–352
2. Menezes AH. Developmental and acquired abnormalities of the craniovertebral junction. In: VanGilder JC, Menezes AH, Dolan KD, eds. The Craniovertebral Junction and Its Abnormalities. New York, NY: Futura Publishing; 1987:109–158
3. Menezes AH, Graf CJ, Hibri N. Abnormalities of the cranio-vertebral junction with cervico-medullary compression. A rational approach to surgical treatment in children. Childs Brain 1980;7(1):15–30
4. Menezes AH. Craniocervical developmental anatomy and its implications. Childs Nerv Syst 2008;24(10):1109–1122
5. Menezes AH, VanGilder JC, Graf CJ, McDonnell DE. Craniocervical abnormalities. A comprehensive surgical approach. J Neurosurg 1980;53(4):444–455
6. Arey LB. Developmental Anatomy. A Textbook and Laboratory Manual of Embryology. 7th ed. Philadelphia, PA: WB Saunders; 1965:404–407
7. Menezes AH. Normal and abnormal development of the craniocervical junction. In: Crockard A, Hayward R, Hoff JT, eds. Neurosurgery: The Scientific Basis of Clinical Practice. Boston, MA: Blackwell Scientific Publications; 1992:63–83
8. Bardeen CR. Early development of the cervical vertebra and base of the occipital bone in man. Am J Anat 1908;8:181–186
9. Gasser RF. Early formation of the basicranium in man. In: Bosma JF, ed. Symposium on Development of the Basicranium. Bethesda, MD: Department of Health, Education, and Science Publication (NIH); 1976:29–43
10. de Beer GR. The Development of the Vertebrate Skull. Oxford, England: Clarendon Press; 1937:356–373
11. Björk A. Cranial base development. Am J Orthod 1955;41:198–225
12. Melsen B. The cranial base. Acta Odontol Scand 1974;32(Suppl 62):9–111
13. Müller F, O'Rahilly R. The human chondrocranium at the end of the embryonic period, proper, with particular reference to the nervous system. Am J Anat 1980;159(1):33–58
14. Francel PC, Persing JA, Dodson EE. Embryology of craniofacial development. In: Crockard A, Hayward R, Hoff JT, eds. Neurosurgery: The Scientific Basis of Clinical Practice. Boston, MA: Blackwell Scientific Publications; 1992:48–62
15. Menezes AH, Fenoy KA. Remnants of occipital vertebrae: proatlas segmentation abnormalities. Neurosurgery 2009;64(5):945–953, discussion 954
16. Ganguly DN, Roy KKS. A study on the craniovertebral joint in the man. Anat Anz Bd. 1964;114:433–452
17. Gladstone RJ, Wakeley CPG. Variations of the occipito-atlantal joint in relation to the metameric structure of the craniovertebral region. J Anat 1925;59(Pt 2):195–216
18. Hoyte DAN. The role of the cranial base in normal and abnormal skull development. In: Persing JA, Edgerton MT, Jane JA, eds. Scientific Foundation and Surgical Treatment of Craniosynostosis. Baltimore, MD: Williams & Wilkins, 1989
19. Lanier RR Jr. Anomalous cervico-occipital skeleton in man. Anat Rec 1939;73:189–207
20. Macklin CC. The skull of a human fetus of 44 mm. Am J Anat 1914;16:317–426
21. Sensing EC. The development of the occipital and cervical segments and their associated structures in human embryos. Contrib Embryol 1957;36:152–161
22. Garber JN. Abnormalities of the atlas and axis vertebrae: congenital and traumatic. J Bone Joint Surg Am 1964;46:1782–1791
23. Gray SW, Romaine CB, Skandalakis JE. Congenital fusion of the cervical vertebrae. Surg Gynecol Obstet 1964;118:373–385
24. Wollin DG. The os odontoideum: separate odontoid process. J Bone Joint Surg Am 1963;45:1459–1471
25. Macalister A. Notes on the development and variations of the atlas. J Anat Physiol 1893;27(Pt 4):519–542
26. Fielding JW, Hensinger RN, Hawkins RJ. Os odontoideum. J Bone Joint Surg Am 1980;62(3):378–383
27. Menezes AH. Os odontoideum: pathogenesis, dynamics and management. In: Marlin AE, ed. Concepts in Pediatric Neurosurgery. Basel, Germany: Karger; 1988:133–145
28. Chamberlain WE. Basilar impression (Platybasia): a bizarre developmental anomaly of the occipital bone and upper cervical spine with striking and misleading neurologic manifestations. Yale J Biol Med 1939;11(5):487–496
29. Goel VK, Clark CR, Gallaes K, Liu YK. Moment-rotation relationships of the ligamentous occipito-atlanto-axial complex. J Biomech 1988;21(8):673–680
30. Neidengard L, Carter TE, Smith DW. Klippel-Feil malformation complex in fetal alcohol syndrome. Am J Dis Child 1978;132(9):929–930
31. Menezes AH. Evaluation and treatment of congenital and developmental anomalies of the cervical spine. Invited submission from the Joint Section Meeting on Disorders of the Spine and Peripheral Nerves, March 2004. J Neurosurg Spine 2004;1(2):188–197
32. Bystrow A. Assimilation des atlas und manifestation des proatlas. Z Ges Anat 1931;95:210–242
33. Dawson EG, Smith L. Atlanto-axial subluxation in children due to vertebral anomalies. J Bone Joint Surg Am 1979;61(4):582–587
34. Hensinger RN, Lang JE, MacEwen GD. Klippel-Feil syndrome; a constellation of associated anomalies. J Bone Joint Surg Am 1974;56(6):1246–1253
35. Klippel M, Feil A. Un cas d'abence des vertebres cervicales avec cage intoracique remontant jusqu's base du craine. Nouv Icon Salpétrière 1912;25:228
36. McRae DL. The significance of abnormalities of the cervical spine. AJR Am J Roentgenol 1960;84:3–25
37. Nicholson JT, Sherk HH. Anomalies of the occipitocervical articulation. J Bone Joint Surg Am 1968;50(2):295–304
38. Sherk HH, Dawoud S. Congenital os odontoideum with Klippel-Feil anomaly and fatal atlanto-axial instability. Report of a case. Spine 1981;6(1):42–45
39. von Torklus D, Gehle W. The upper cervical spine. Regional anatomy, pathology and traumatology. In: von Torklus D, Gehle W, eds. A Systemic Radiological Atlas and Textbook. New York, NY: Grune & Stratton; 1972:2–77
40. Smith GE. Significance of fusion of the atlas to the occipital bone and manifestations of occipital vertebrae. BMJ 1908;ii:594–600
41. Oetterking B. On the morphological significance of certain craniovertebral variations. Anat Rec 1923;25:339–348
42. Schiff DCM, Parke WW. The arterial supply of the odontoid process. J Bone Joint Surg Am 1973;55(7):1450–1456
43. Rao PV. Median (third) occipital condyle. Clin Anat 2002;15(2):148–151
44. v Lüdinghausen M, Schindler G, Kageyama I, Pomaroli A. The third occipital condyle, a constituent part of a median occipito-atlanto-odontoid joint: a case report. Surg Radiol Anat 2002;24(1):71–76
45. Kotil K, Kalayci M. Ventral cervicomedullary junction compression secondary to condylus occipitalis (median occipital condyle), a rare entity. J Spinal Disord Tech 2005;18(4):382–384
46. Ohaegbulam C, Woodard EJ, Proctor M. Occipitocondylar hyperplasia: an unusual craniovertebral junction anomaly causing myelopathy. Case report. J Neurosurg 2005;103(4, Suppl):379–381
47. Marin-Padilla M, Marin-Padilla TM. Morphogenesis of experimentally induced Arnold-Chiari malformation. J Neurol Sci 1981;50(1):29–55
48. Marin-Padilla M. Notochordal-basichondrocranium relationships: abnormalities in experimental axial skeletal (dysraphic) disorders. J Embryol Exp Morphol 1979;53:15–38

49. Marin-Padilla M, Marin-Padilla T. Developmental abnormalities of the occipital bone in human chondrodystrophies (achondroplasia and tantophoric dwarfism). In: Birth Defects Series. March of Dimes Foundation; 1977;13(3D):7–23
50. Gholve PA, Hosalkar HS, Ricchetti ET, Pollock AN, Dormans JP, Drummond DS. Occipitalization of the atlas in children. Morphologic classification, associations, and clinical relevance. J Bone Joint Surg Am 2007;89(3):571–578
51. Menezes AH. Primary craniovertebral anomalies and the hindbrain herniation syndrome (Chiari I): data base analysis. Pediatr Neurosurg 1995;23(5):260–269
52. Atkinson JL, Kokmen E, Miller GM. Evidence of posterior fossa hypoplasia in the familial variant of adult Chiari I malformation: case report. Neurosurgery 1998;42(2):401–403, discussion 404
53. Crockard HA, Stevens JM. Craniovertebral junction anomalies in inherited disorders: part of the syndrome or caused by the disorder? Eur J Pediatr 1995;154(7):504–512
54. Dietrich S, Kessel M. The vertebral column. In: Thorogood P, ed. Embryos, Genes and Birth Defects. Chichester, England: Wiley, 1997:281–302
55. Kalla AK, Khanna S, Singh IP, Sharma S, Schnobel R, Vogel F. A genetic and anthropological study of atlanto-occipital fusion. Hum Genet 1989;81(2):105–112
56. Lufkin T, Mark M, Hart CP, Dollé P, LeMeur M, Chambon P. Homeotic transformation of the occipital bones of the skull by ectopic expression of a homeobox gene. Nature 1992;359(6398):835–841
57. Nishikawa M, Sakamoto H, Hakuba A, Nakanishi N, Inoue Y. Pathogenesis of Chiari malformation: a morphometric study of the posterior cranial fossa. J Neurosurg 1997;86(1):40–47

2 Anatomical Basis of Surgical Approaches to the Region of the Foramen Magnum

Albert L. Rhoton, Jr. and Evandro De Oliveira

Lesions in the region of the foramen magnum present special problems in operative management because many structures are involved. The structures that must be considered in planning an operative approach to the region include the brainstem and spinal cord, the lower cranial and upper spinal nerves, the vertebral artery and its branches, and the ligaments uniting the atlas, axis, and occipital bone.[1,2]

Osseous Relationships

The osseous structures in the region of the foramen magnum are the occipital bone, the atlas, and the axis. The occipital bone surrounds the foramen magnum (**Fig. 2.1**). The foraminal opening is oval and wider posteriorly than anteriorly. The wider posterior part transmits the medulla, and the narrower anterior part sits above the odontoid process. The occipital bone is divided into a squamosal part located above and behind the foramen magnum, a basal part situated in front of the foramen magnum, and paired condylar parts located lateral to the foramen magnum. The squamous part is an internally concave plate located above and behind the foramen magnum. The internal surface has a prominent ridge, the internal occipital crest, which descends in the midline and serves as the attachment for the falx cerebelli. This crest bifurcates to form paired lower limbs that extend along each side of the posterior margin of the foramen magnum.

The basilar part, which is also referred to as the clivus, is a thick plate of bone that extends forward and upward at an angle of ~45 degrees from the foramen magnum to join the sphenoid bone. The superior surface of the clivus is concave from side to side and is separated on each side from the petrous part of the temporal bone by the petro-occipital fissure. The inferior surface has a small elevation, the pharyngeal tubercle, which gives attachment to the raphe of the pharynx.

The paired condylar parts are situated at the sides of the foramen magnum. The occipital condyles, which articulate with the atlas, are located lateral to the anterior half of the foramen magnum. A tubercle, which gives attachment to the alar ligament of the odontoid process, is situated on the medial side of each condyle. The hypoglossal canal, which transmits the hypoglossal nerve, is situated above and forward of the condyle. The condylar fossa, a depression located on the external surface behind the condyle, is often perforated to form a canal through which an emissary vein passes.

The atlas, the first cervical vertebra, differs from the other cervical vertebrae by being ring shaped and by lacking a vertebral body and a spinous process (**Fig. 2.2**). It consists of two thick lateral masses connected in front by a short anterior arch and behind by a longer curved posterior arch. The position of the usual vertebral body is occupied by the odontoid process (dens). The posterior arch has a groove on the lateral part of its upper outer surface in which the vertebral artery courses. The groove may be partly or fully converted into a foramen by a bridge of bone that arches backward from the superior articular facet to the posterior arch. The upper and lower surfaces of each lateral mass have oval facets that articulate with the occipital condyles and the superior articular facets of the axis. The medial aspect of each lateral mass has a small tubercle for the attachment of the transverse ligament of the atlas. The transverse processes are unusually long and can be felt through the overlying tissues. Each transverse foramen, which transmits a vertebral artery, is situated between the lateral mass and the transverse process.

The axis, the second cervical vertebra, more closely resembles typical vertebrae than the atlas but is distinguished by the odontoid process, which projects upward from the body (**Fig. 2.2**). On the front of the dens is an articular facet, which forms a joint with the back of the anterior arch of the atlas. The dens has a pointed apex that is joined by the apical ligament, a flattened side where the alar ligaments are attached, and a groove at the base of its posterior surface where the transverse ligament of the atlas passes. The dens and body are flanked by a pair of large oval facets that extend laterally from the body onto the adjoining parts of the pedicles and articulate with the inferior facets of the atlas. The superior facets do not form an articular pillar with the inferior facets but are anterior to the latter. The transverse processes are small. Each transverse foramen faces superolaterally, thus permitting the lateral deviation of the vertebral artery as it passes up to the more widely separated foramina in the atlas.

Ligamentous and Articular Relationships

The ligaments and articulations important in planning operative approaches are those joining the atlas, axis, and occipital bone (**Fig. 2.3**). The articulation of the atlas and axis comprises four synovial joints: two median ones on the front and back of the dens and paired lateral ones between the opposing articular facets on the lateral masses of the

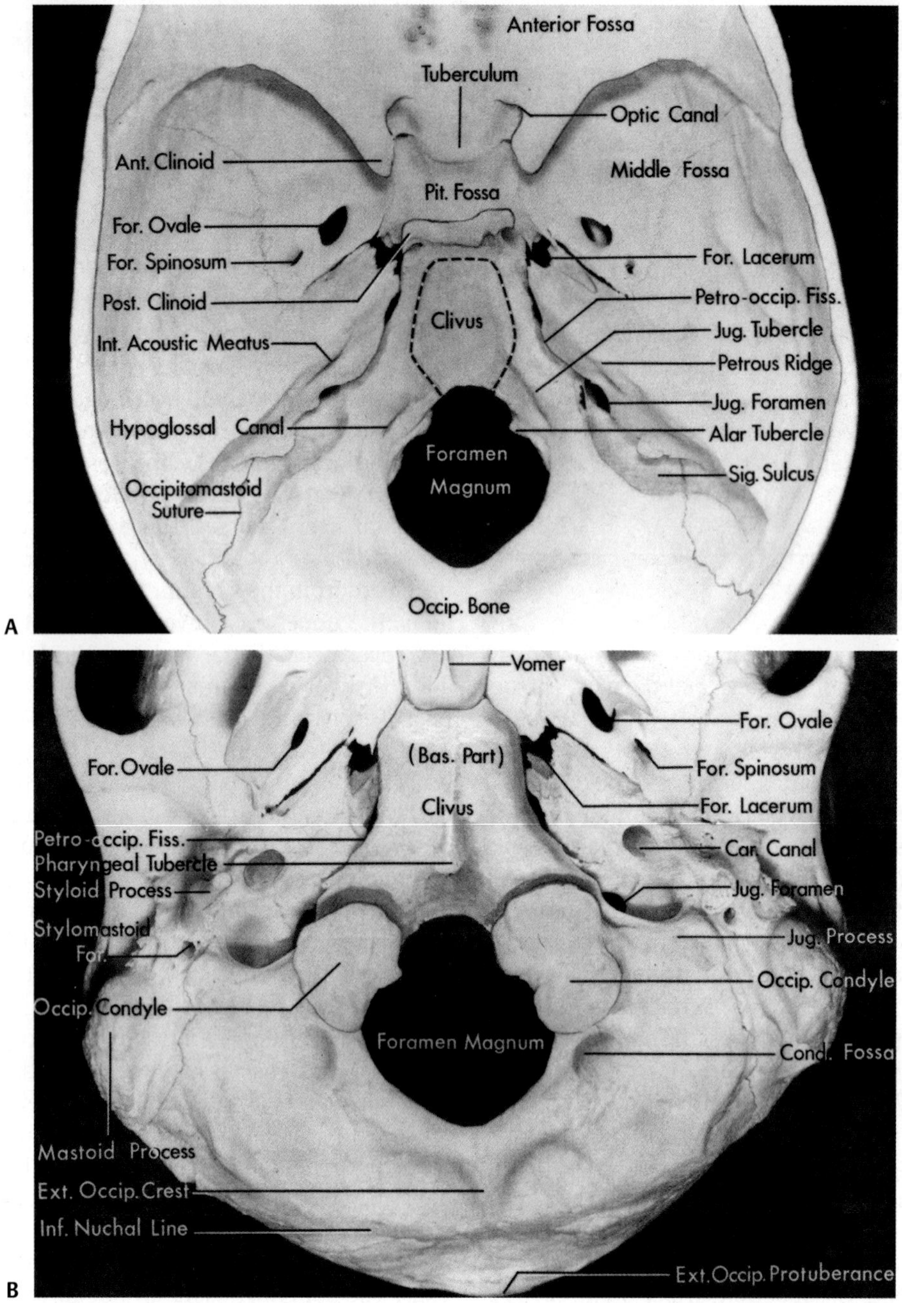

Fig. 2.1 Osseous relationships, base of skull. The occipital bone: **(A)** superior and **(B)** inferior views. The occipital bone (*Occip. Bone*) surrounds the oval-shaped foramen magnum, which is wider posteriorly than anteriorly. The narrower anterior part sits above the odontoid process and is encroached on laterally by **(B)** the occipital condyles (*Occip. Condyle*). The wider posterior part transmits the medulla. **(B)** The basilar part (*Bas. Part*) of the occipital bone is also referred to as the clivus. **(A)** The part of the clivus that can be removed through an anterior operative approach is shown with an interrupted line. *Jug. Foramen*, jugular foramen; *Jug. Tubercle*, jugular tubercle; *Sig. Sulcus*, sulcus of the sigmoid sinus; *Car. Canal*, carotid canal; *For. Lacerum*, foramen lacerum; *For. Ovale*, foramen ovale; *For. Spinosum*, foramen spinosum; *Ant. Clinoid*, anterior clinoid process; *Post. Clinoid*, posterior clinoid process; *Pit. Fossa*, pituitary fossa; *Stylomastoid For.*, stylomastoid foramen; *Int. Acoustic Meatus*, internal acoustic meatus; *Ext. Occip. Protuberance*, external occipital protuberance; *Ext. Occip Crest*, external occipital crest; *Inf. Nuchal Line*, inferior nuchal line; *Petro-occip. Fiss.*, petro-occipital fissure; *Cond. Fossa*, condylar fossa. (From de Oliveira E, Rhoton AL Jr, Peace D. Microsurgical anatomy of the region of the foramen magnum. Surg Neurol 1985;24:293–352. With permission from *Surgical Neurology*.)

atlas and axis. Each joint on the front and back of the dens has its own capsule and synovial cavity. The anterior one is situated between the anterior surface of the dens and the posterior aspect of the anterior arch of the atlas. The posterior one lies between the cartilage-covered anterior surface of the transverse ligament of the atlas and the posterior surface of the dens.

The atlas and axis are united by the cruciform and the anterior and posterior longitudinal ligaments and the articular capsules surrounding the joints between the opposing articular facets on the lateral masses. The cruciform ligament has transverse and vertical parts that form a cross behind the dens. The transverse part, called the transverse ligament, arches across the ring of the atlas behind the dens and is broader behind the dens than where it is attached to a tubercle on the medial side of the lateral masses of the atlas. As it crosses the dens, small longitudinal bands are directed upward and downward. The cranial extension is attached to the upper surface of the clivus between the apical ligament of the dens and the tectorial membrane. The lower band is attached to the posterior surface of the body of the axis.

In front, the atlas and axis are connected by the anterior longitudinal ligament, a wide band fixed to the anterior arch of the atlas and the front body of the axis. The posterior longitudinal ligament is attached above to the transverse part of the cruciform ligament and the clivus. Posterior to the spinal canal, the atlas and axis are joined by a broad, thin membrane that extends from the posterior arch of the atlas to the laminae of the axis (ligamentum flavum).

The atlas and the occipital bone are united by the articular capsules surrounding the atlanto-occipital joints and by the anterior and posterior atlanto-occipital membranes (**Fig. 2.3**). The anterior atlanto-occipital membrane extends from the anterior edge of the foramen magnum to the

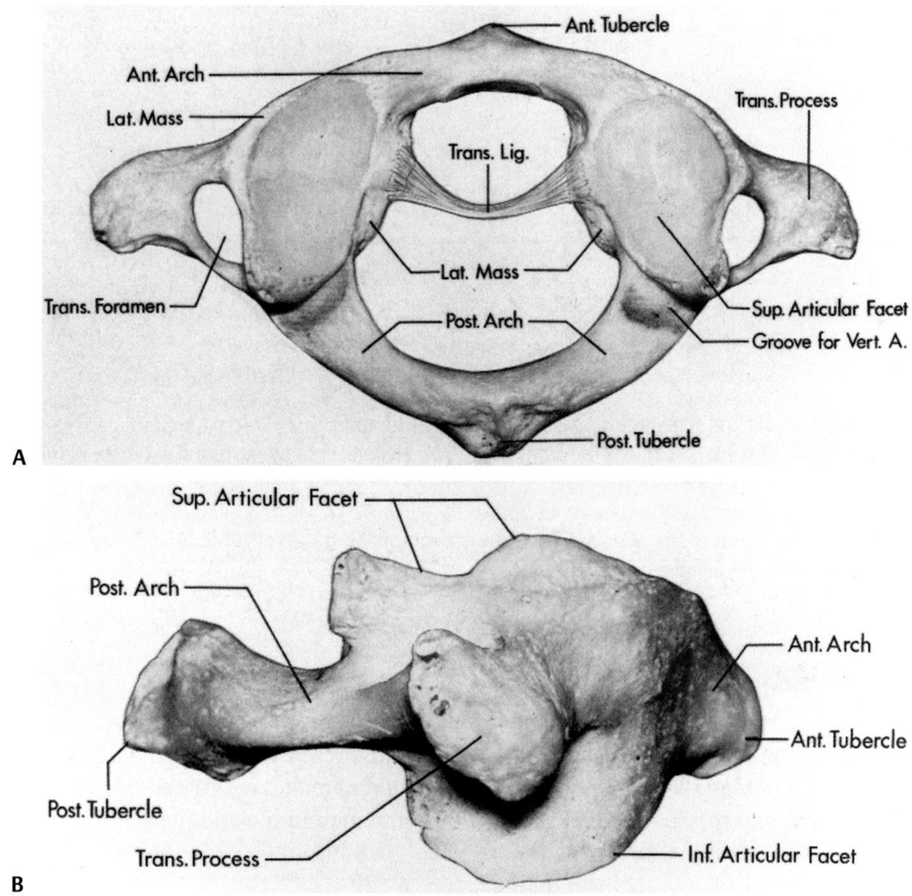

Fig. 2.2 Atlas and axis. The atlas: **(A)** superior and **(B)** lateral views. The atlas consists of two thick lateral masses (*Lat. Mass*), which are connected in front by a short anterior arch (*Ant. Arch*) and posteriorly by a longer posterior arch (*Post. Arch*). The medial aspect of each lateral mass has a small tubercle for the attachment of the transverse ligament (*Trans. Lig.*) of the atlas. The transverse foramina (*Trans. Foramen*) transmit the vertebral arteries. The upper surface of the posterior arch adjacent to the lateral masses has paired grooves in which the vertebral arteries (*Groove for Vert. A.*) course. Other structures include the anterior (*Ant. Tubercle*) and posterior tubercles (*Post. Tubercle*), transverse processes (*Trans. Process*), and the superior (*Sup. Articular Facet*) and inferior articular facets (*Inf. Articular Facets*). *(continued)*

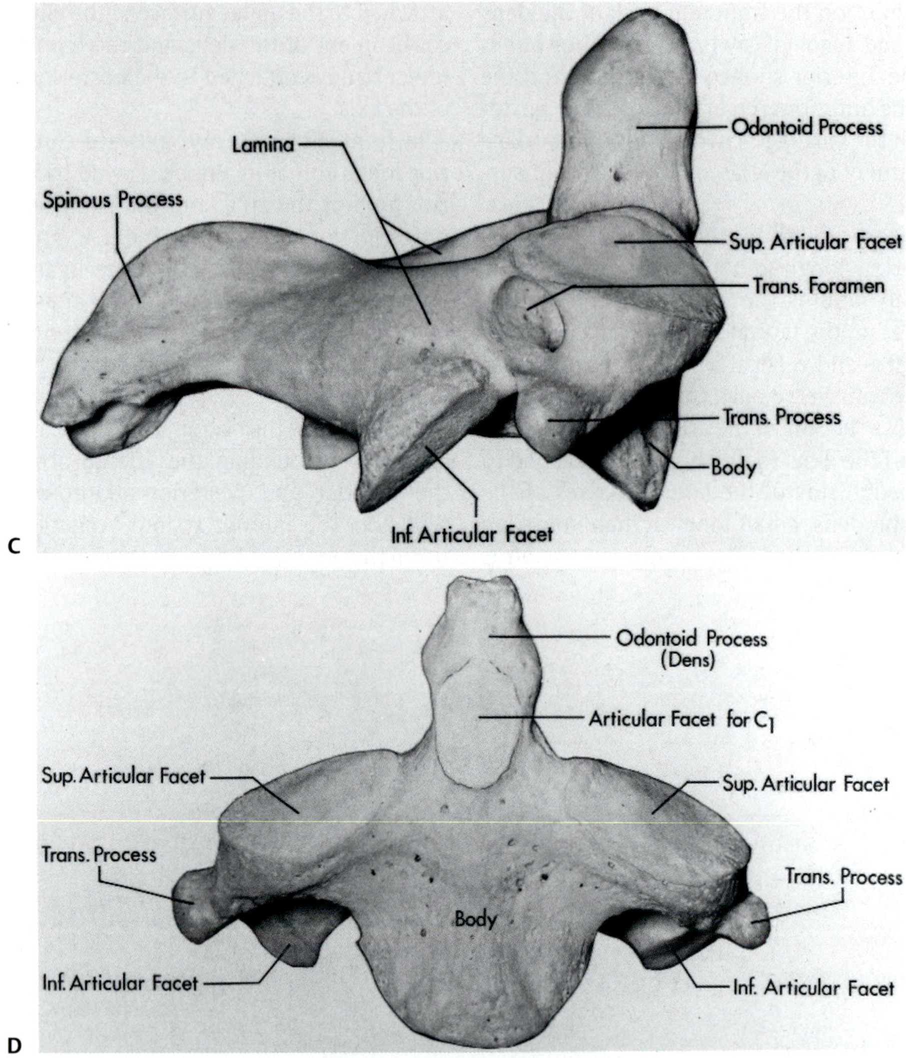

Fig. 2.2 *(continued)* The axis: **(C)** lateral and **(D)** anterior views. The axis is distinguished by the odontoid process (*Dens*). On the front of the dens is an articular facet, which forms a joint with the back of the anterior arch of the atlas. The dens is grooved at the base of its posterior surface where the transverse ligament of the atlas passes. The superior articular facets are anterior to the inferior facets. The transverse foramina are directed superolaterally, thus permitting the lateral deviation of the vertebral arteries as they pass up to the more widely separated foramina in the atlas. (From de Oliveira E, Rhoton AL Jr, Peace D. Microsurgical anatomy of the region of the foramen magnum. Surg Neurol 1985;24:293–352. With permission from *Surgical Neurology*.)

anterior arch of the atlas. The posterior atlanto-occipital membrane extends from the posterior margin of the foramen magnum to the posterior arch of the atlas. The lateral border of this membrane arches behind the vertebral artery and the first cervical nerve root and may be ossified in the area where it arches behind the vertebral artery.

Four fibrous bands—the tectorial membrane, the paired alar ligaments, and the apical ligament—connect the axis and the occipital bone (**Fig. 2.3**). The tectorial membrane is a cephalic extension of the posterior longitudinal ligament that covers the dens and cruciform ligament. It is attached below to the posterior surface of the body of the axis and above to the upper surface of the occipital bone in front of the foramen magnum. The alar ligaments arise on each side of the upper part of the dens and attach to the medial surfaces of the occipital condyles. The apical ligament extends from the tip of the dens to the anterior margin of the foramen magnum and is situated between the anterior atlanto-occipital membrane and the cruciform ligament.

Neural Relationships

The neural structures situated in the region of the foramen magnum are the caudal part of the brainstem, cerebellum, and fourth ventricle; the rostral part of the spinal cord; and the lower cranial and upper cervical nerves (**Figs. 2.4** and **2.5**). The spinal cord blends indistinguishably into the medulla at a

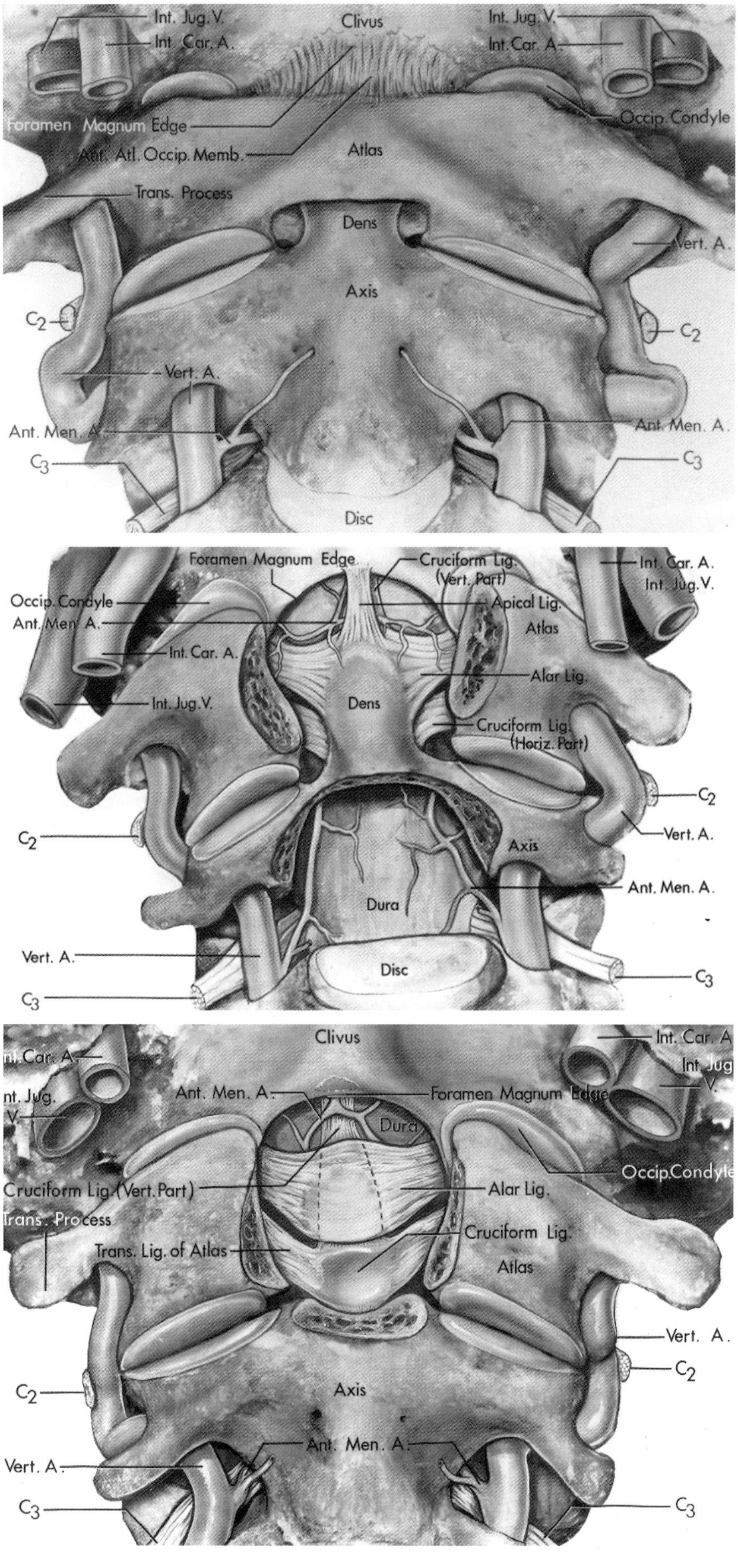

Fig. 2.3 Osseous and ligamentous relationships: **(A–C)** anterior and **(D,E)** posterior views. **(A)** The vertebral arteries (*Vert. A.*) ascend anterior to the cervical nerve roots through the foramina in the transverse processes (*Trans. Process*). The anterior meningeal arteries (*Ant. Men. A.*) send one branch into the axis and another to the dura in the spinal canal. Structures exposed include the anterior atlanto-occipital membrane (*Ant. Atl. Occip. Memb.*), internal jugular veins (*Int. Jug. V.*), internal carotid arteries (*Int. Car. A.*), and occipital condyles (*Occip. Condyle*). **(B)** The anterior arch of the atlas has been removed to expose the apical (*Apical Lig.*), cruciform (*Cruciform Lig.*), and alar ligaments (*Alar Lig.*). The horizontal part (*Horiz. Part*) of the cruciform ligament, which is also called the transverse ligament (*Trans. Lig.*), passes behind the dens, and the vertical part (*Vert. Part*) is seen above the dens. The body of C2 has been removed. The anterior meningeal arteries form an arterial arch above the odontoid process. **(C)** The odontoid process has been removed. The cruciform ligament forms a synovial joint with the odontoid process. The articular cartilage on the cruciform ligament has been preserved. The alar and apical ligaments lie anterior to the cruciform ligament. *(continued)*

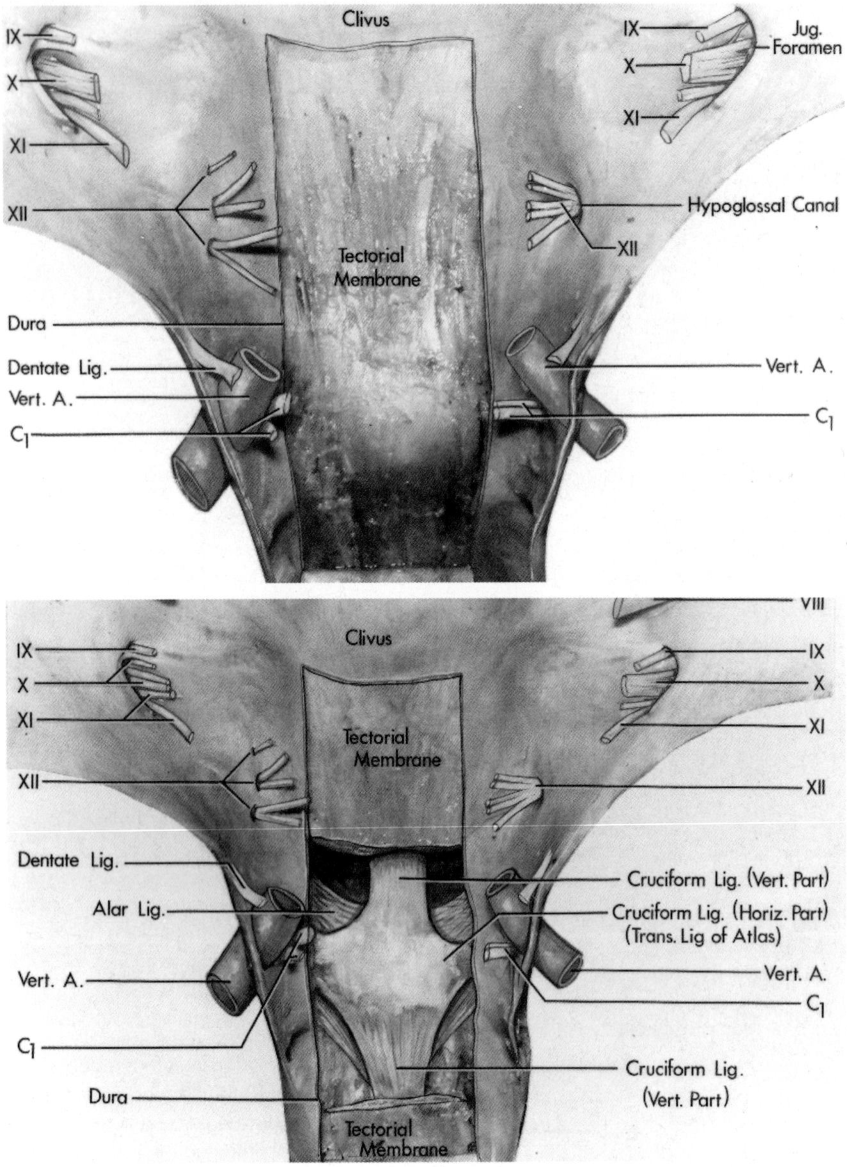

Fig. 2.3 *(continued)* **(D,E)** Posterior views of the anterior margin of the foramen magnum. **(D)** The dura covering the tectorial membrane has been removed. This membrane extends downward from the clivus to insert on the upper cervical vertebrae. Structures in the exposed area include the abducens (*VI*), facial (*VII*), vestibulocochlear (*VIII*), glossopharyngeal (*IX*), vagus (*X*), accessory (*XI*), and hypoglossal nerves (*XII*); internal acoustic meatus (*Int. Acoustic Meatus*); dentate ligament (*Dentate Lig.*); and jugular foramen (*Jug. Foramen*). **(E)** Part of the tectorial membrane has been removed to expose the alar and the vertical and horizontal parts of the cruciform ligament. (From de Oliveira E, Rhoton AL Jr, Peace D. Microsurgical anatomy of the region of the foramen magnum. Surg Neurol 1985;24:293–352. With permission from *Surgical Neurology*.)

level arbitrarily set at the upper limit of the dorsal and ventral rootlets forming the first cervical nerve. It is easier to differentiate this level on the ventral than on the dorsal surface because the ventral rootlets of the first cervical nerve are always present, and the dorsal rootlets are absent in many cases. The fact that the junction of the spinal cord and medulla is situated at the rostral margin of the first cervical root means that the medulla, and not the spinal cord, occupies the foramen magnum. In the upper cervical region the rootlets, which unite to form the spinal part of the accessory nerve, emerge through the lateral funiculus in front of the dorsal roots.

The dentate ligament is a white fibrous sheet that is attached to the spinal cord medially and to the dura laterally (**Fig. 2.4**). Its medial border has a continuous linear attachment to the spinal cord midway between the dorsal and ventral roots. Its lateral border is attached to the dura at intervals by fibrous triangular processes. The most rostral triangular process is attached to the dura at the level of the foramen magnum, and the second one is attached posterior and inferior to the initial intradural segment of the vertebral artery. The lateral border of the dentate ligament between the two most rostral triangular processes is attached to the vertebral and posterior spinal arteries and to the C1 root, making separation of these structures difficult.

The upper spinal cord blends indistinguishably into the lower medulla (**Figs. 2.4** and **2.5**). The anterior surface of the medulla is formed by the medullary pyramids, which face the clivus, the anterior edge of the foramen magnum, and the rostral part of the odontoid process. The anterior median sulcus divides the upper medulla in the anterior midline between the pyramids, disappears on the lower medulla at the level of the decussation of the pyramids (but reappears below the decussation), and is continuous caudally with the anterior median fissure of the spinal cord. The lateral surface of the medulla is formed predominantly by the inferior olives. The posterior surface of the medulla is formed by the inferior

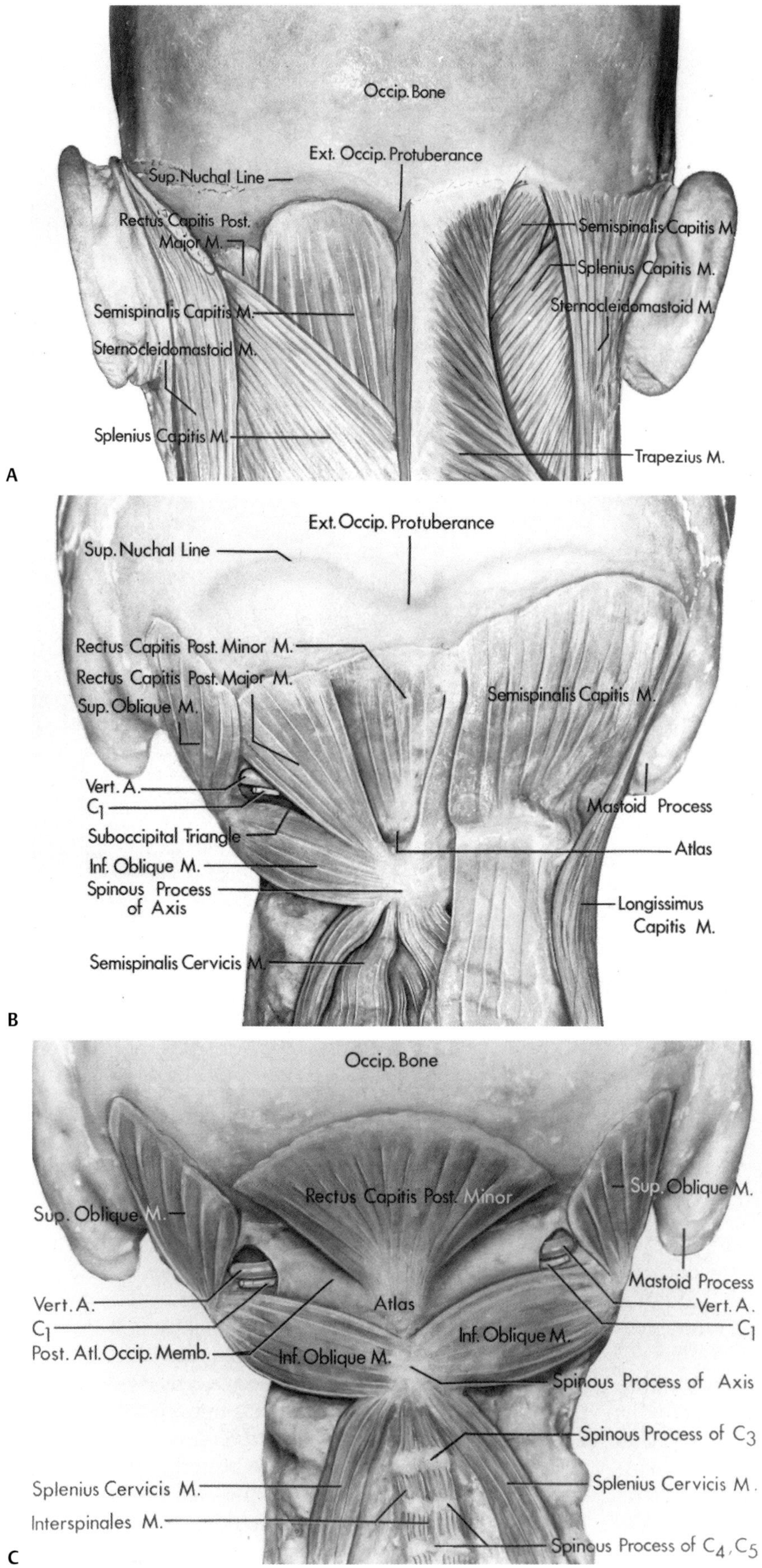

Fig. 2.4 Posterior views. **(A)** The superficial muscles that attach to the occipital bone (*Occip. Bone*) are preserved on the right side and have been removed on the left side. The superficial muscles that are attached to the superior nuchal line (*Sup. Nuchal Line*) and the external occipital protuberance (*Ext. Occip. Protuberance*) are the muscles (*M.*) of the trapezius and sternocleidomastoid. On the left side, the trapezius muscle has been removed, and the upper parts of the splenius capitis and sternocleidomastoid muscles have been reflected laterally to expose the semispinalis capitis and rectus capitis posterior (*Post.*) major muscles. **(B)** The sternocleidomastoid, trapezius, and splenius capitis muscles have been removed on both sides, and the semispinalis and longissimus capitis muscles have been removed on the left side to expose the deep suboccipital muscles. The rectus capitis posterior minor (*Rectus Capitis Post. Minor M.*) arises on the occipital bone above the foramen magnum and inserts on the atlas. The rectus capitis posterior major (*Rectus Capitis Post. Major M.*) extends from the occipital bone to the spinous process of axis. The inferior (*Inf.*) oblique muscle extends from the spinous process of axis to the transverse process of the atlas, and the superior (*Sup.*) oblique muscle extends from the transverse process of the atlas to the occipital bone. The vertebral artery (*Vert. A.*) and the C1 nerve root are seen in the suboccipital triangle, which is situated between the superior (*Sup.*) and inferior (*Inf.*) oblique muscle and the rectus capitis posterior major muscle. **(C)** The semispinalis capitis and rectus capitis posterior major muscles have been removed on both sides. The posterior atlanto-occipital membrane (*Post. Atl. Occip. Memb.*) extends from the arch of the atlas to the posterior margin of the foramen magnum. The vertebral arteries and C1 nerve roots pass anterior to the lateral margin of this membrane. *(continued)*

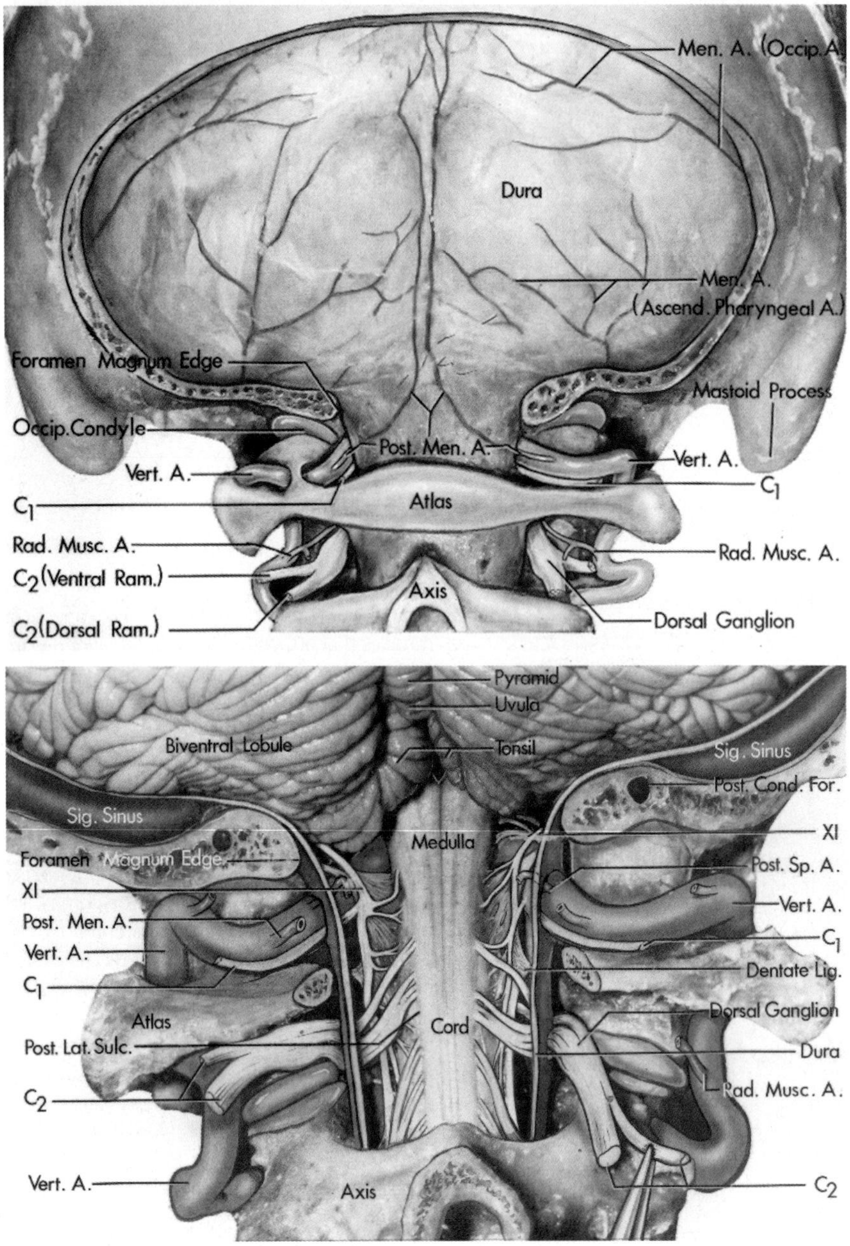

Fig. 2.4 *(continued)* **(D)** The muscles and bone above the foramen magnum have been removed. The posterior meningeal arteries (*Post. Men. A.*) arise below the occipital condyles (*Occip. Condyle*) and ascend on the dura. The occipital (*Occip. A.*) and ascending pharyngeal arteries (*Ascend. Pharyngeal A.*) also give rise to meningeal branches (*Men. A.*). The left vertebral artery passes through a complete ring of bone on the arch of the atlas before entering the dura. Radiculomuscular branches (*Rad. Musc. A.*) arise from the vertebral artery. **(E)** The dura has just been opened. Structures exposed include the posterior spinal artery (*Post. Sp. A.*), accessory nerve (*XI*), sigmoid sinus (*Sig. Sinus*), posterior condylar foramen (*Post. Cond. For.*), dentate ligament (*Dentate Lig.*), and posterolateral sulcus (*Post. Lat. Sulc.*). *(continued)*

cerebellar peduncles, medially by the gracile fasciculus and tubercle, and laterally by the cuneate fasciculus and tubercle. The belly of the pons, which sits on the clivus, is convex from side to side as well as from top to bottom.

The cerebellum rests above the posterior and lateral edges of the foramen magnum. Only the lower part of the hemispheres (formed by the tonsils and the biventral lobules) and the lower part of the vermis (formed by the nodule, uvula, and pyramid) are related to the foramen magnum. The biventral lobule sits above the lateral part of the foramen magnum, and the tonsils rest above the level of the posterior edge.

The cerebellar surface above the posterior part of the foramen magnum has a deep vertical depression, the posterior cerebellar incisura, which contains the falx cerebelli and extends inferiorly toward the foramen magnum. The vermis is folded into and forms the cortical surface within this incisura. The vermian surface within the incisura has a diamond shape. The upper half of the diamond-shaped formation has a pyramidal shape; thus, it is called the pyramid. The lower half of the diamond-shaped formation, the uvula, projects downward between the tonsils, thus mimicking the situation in the oropharynx. Inferiorly, the posterior cerebellar incisura is continuous with the vallecula cerebelli, an opening between the tonsils that extends upward through the foramen of Magendie into the fourth ventricle.

The tonsils, which sit above the posterior edge of the foramen magnum, are commonly involved in herniations through the foramen magnum. Each tonsil is an ovoid structure that is attached along its superolateral border to the

F

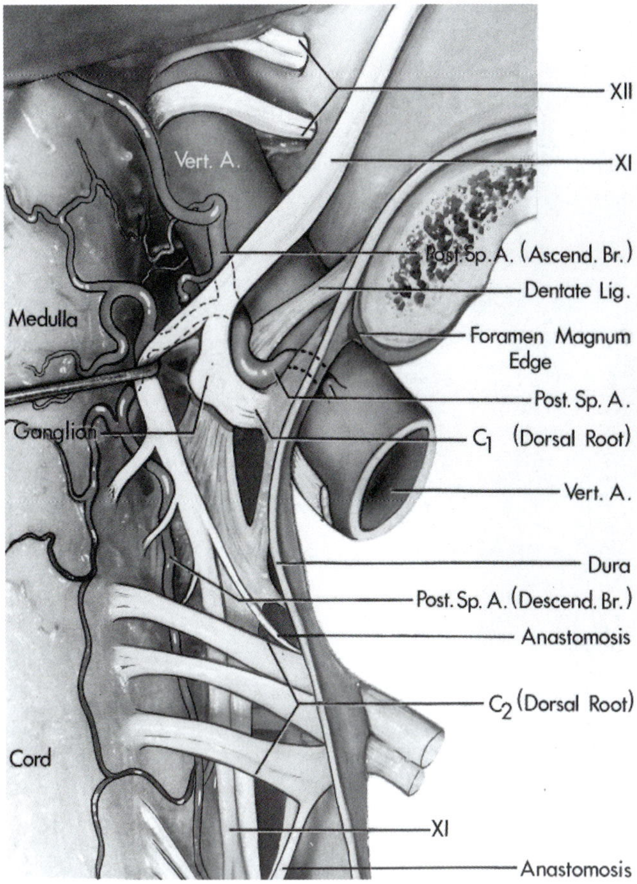

Fig. 2.4 **(F)** *(continued)* Relationships of the dentate ligament and accessory and cervical nerves (enlarged view of another specimen, right side). The spinal portion of the accessory nerve arises from the dorsolateral margin of the spinal cord and ascends between the dorsal roots and the dentate ligament (*Dentate Lig.*). The accessory nerve anastomoses with the C1 and C2 dorsal rootlets. The spinal cord does not contribute a dorsal root to the C1 nerve. The C1 nerve root passes through the dura with the vertebral artery (*Vert. A.*). The most rostral triangular process of the dentate ligament is attached to the dura at the level of the foramen magnum. The posterior spinal artery (*Post. Sp. A.*) splits into ascending (*Ascend. Br.*) and descending branches (*Descend. Br.*). There is a small ganglion in the anastomosis between the accessory nerve and the C1 nerve root. (From de Oliveira E, Rhoton AL Jr, Peace D. Microsurgical anatomy of the region of the foramen magnum. Surg Neurol 1985;24:293–352. With permission from *Surgical Neurology*.)

remainder of the cerebellum. The inferior pole and posterior surface of the tonsils face the cisterna magna and are visible from the suboccipital operative exposure. The lateral surface of each tonsil is covered by the biventral lobule. The medial and anterior surfaces and the superior pole of each tonsil all face, but are separated from, other neural structures by narrow clefts. The anterior surface of each tonsil faces and is separated from the posterior surface of the medulla by the cerebellomedullary fissure. The medial surfaces of the tonsils face each other across the vallecula. The ventral aspect of the superior pole faces the inferior half of the roof of the fourth ventricle.

The cerebellomedullary fissure, which extends superiorly between the cerebellum and the medulla, is situated rostral to the dorsal margin of the foramen magnum. This fissure extends superiorly to the level of the roof of the fourth ventricle and the lateral recesses of the fourth ventricle. The dorsal wall of the fissure is formed by the uvula in the midline and the tonsils and biventral lobules laterally. The ventral wall, formed by the inferior medullary velum and tela choroidea, is exposed by removing the tonsils. The inferior medullary velum is a thin, bilateral, semitranslucent butterfly-shaped sheet of neural tissue that blends into the ventricular surface of the nodule medially and stretches laterally across the superior pole of the tonsil. The tela choroidea, from which the choroid plexus projects, forms the lowest part of the roof of the fourth ventricle.

Cranial Nerves

The lower four cranial nerves are sufficiently close to the foramen magnum that they may be involved in lesions arising there. The rootlets forming the hypoglossal nerve arise from the medulla along a line that is continuous inferiorly with the line along which the ventral spinal roots arise (**Figs. 2.4** and **2.5**). These rootlets exit the medulla along the anterior margin of the olive and pass behind the vertebral artery to reach the hypoglossal canal. The vertebral artery may stretch the hypoglossal rootlets posteriorly over its dorsal surface. The hypoglossal canal may be divided by a bony septum that separates the nerve into two bundles as it exits the skull.

The glossopharyngeal, vagus, and accessory nerves are considered together because they are formed by a series of rootlets that arise in a continuous line along the medulla and spinal cord and exit the skull through the jugular foramen (**Figs. 2.4** and **2.5**). The glossopharyngeal and vagus nerves arise from the medulla along the posterior margin of the olive. The only location where the glossopharyngeal nerve may consistently be distinguished from the vagus nerve is just proximal to a dural septum, which separates these nerves as they penetrate the dura to enter the jugular foramen.[2,3]

The accessory nerve is the only cranial nerve that passes through the foramen magnum (**Figs. 2.4** and **2.5**). It has a cranial part composed of the rootlets that arise from the medulla and join the vagus nerve, and a spinal portion formed by the union of a series of rootlets that arise from the lower medulla and upper spinal cord. In the posterior fossa, the accessory nerve is composed of one main trunk from the spinal cord and three to six small rootlets that emerge from the medulla. The most rostral medullary rootlets are functionally inferior vagal rootlets, as they arise from the vagal nuclei. The lower medullary rootlets join the spinal portion of the nerve. The spinal contribution arises as a series of rootlets situated midway between the ventral and dorsal rootlets. The rootlets contributing to the accessory nerves may arise as low as the C7 root level.[2] These rootlets unite to form a trunk having a diameter of ~1.0 mm, which ascends through the foramen magnum between the dentate ligament and the dorsal roots.

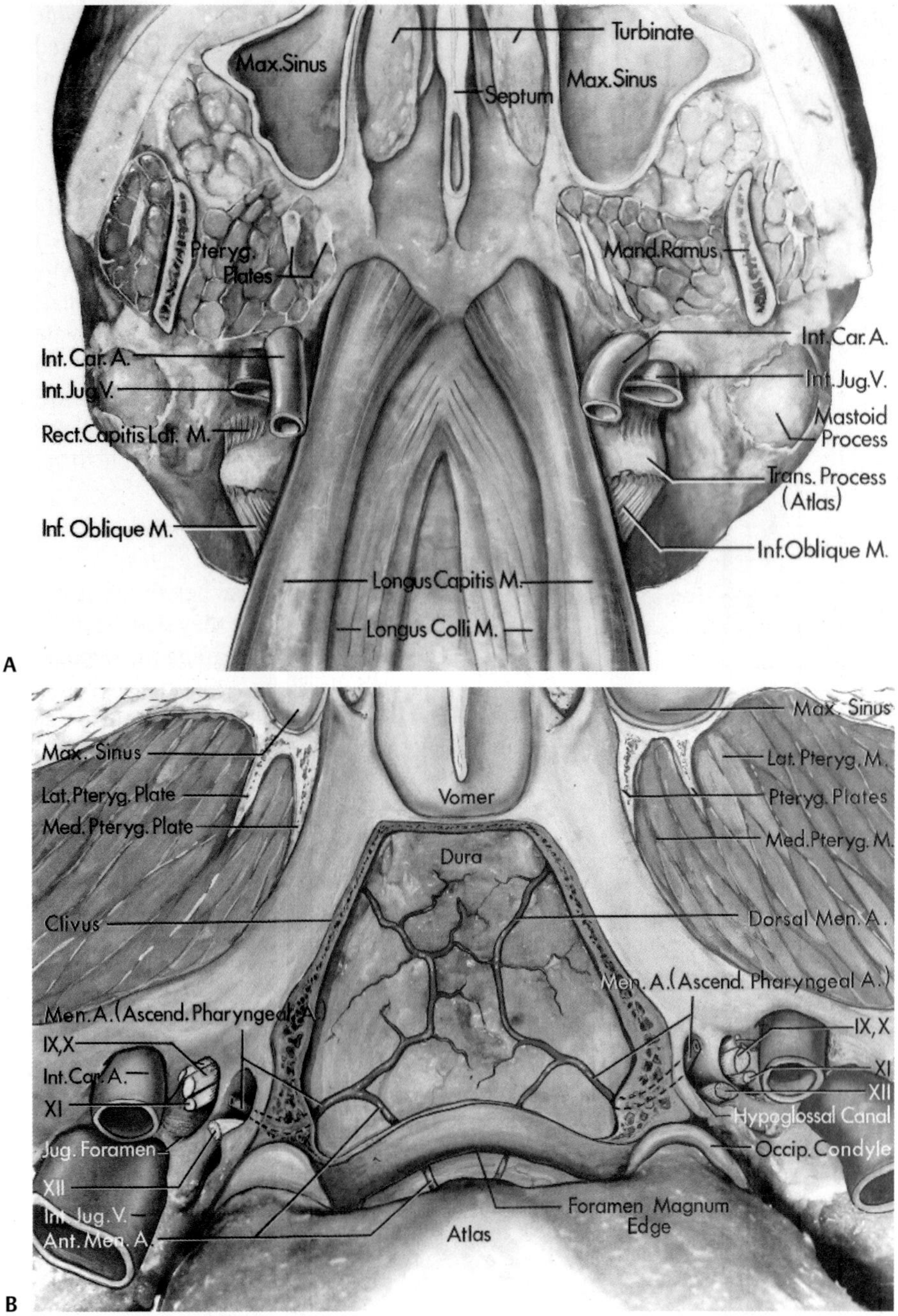

Fig. 2.5 Anterior views. **(A)** The structures anterior to the prevertebral muscles have been removed. Structures exposed include maxillary sinuses (*Max. Sinus*), ramus of the mandible (*Mand. Ramus*), inferior oblique (*Inf. Oblique M.*) and rectus capitis lateralis muscles (*Rect. Capitis Lat. M.*), transverse process (*Trans. Process*), internal carotid artery (*Int. Car. A.*), and internal jugular vein (*Int. Jug. V.*). **(B)** The muscles have been removed. The clivus has been opened above the foramen magnum. The dorsal meningeal branches (*Dorsal Men. A.*) of the meningohypophyseal trunks descend to anastomose with branches of the ascending pharyngeal arteries (*Ascend. Pharyngeal A.*). Structures in the exposure include the medial (*Med. Pteryg. M.*) and lateral pterygoid muscles (*Lat. Pteryg. M.*); medial (*Med. Pteryg. Plate*) and lateral pterygoid plates (*Lat. Pteryg. Plate*); glossopharyngeal (*IX*), vagus (*X*), accessory (*XI*), and hypoglossal nerves (*XII*); and jugular foramen (*Jug. Foramen*). *(continued)*

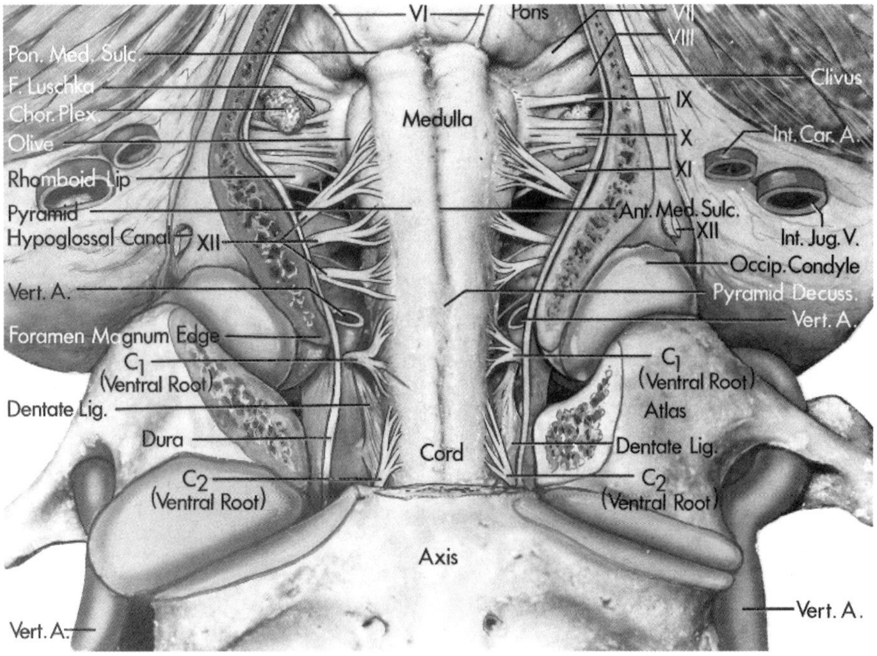

C

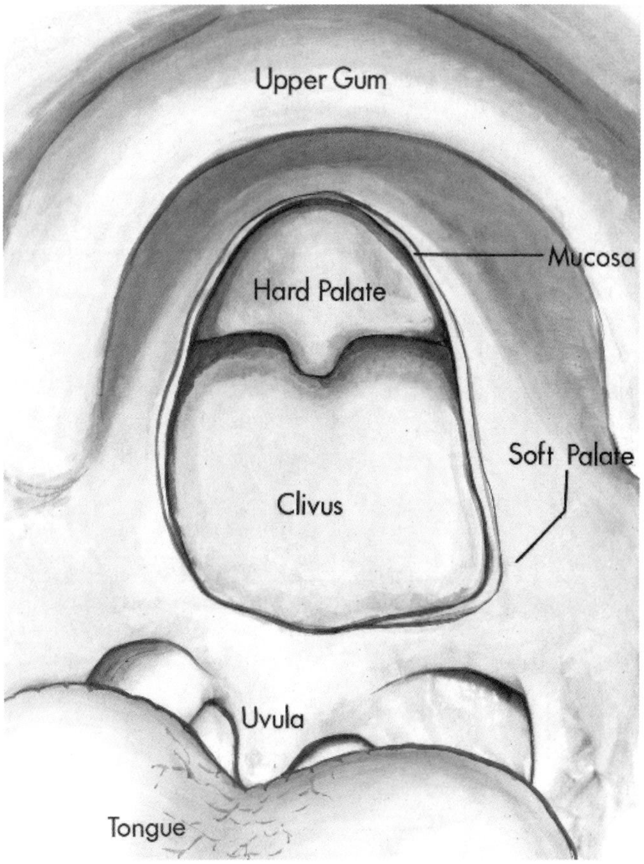

D

Fig. 2.5 *(continued)* **(C)** The clivus, the anterior arch of the atlas, and the dens have been removed. Structures exposed include the abducens (*VI*), facial (*VII*), and vestibulocochlear nerves (*VIII*); anterior median (*Ant. Med. Sulc.*) and pontomedullary sulci (*Pon. Med. Sulc.*); choroid plexus (*Chor. Plex.*); foramen of Luschka (*F. Luschka*); pyramidal decussation (*Pyramid Decuss.*); dentate ligament (*Dentate Lig.*); and occipital condyle (*Occip. Condyle*). **(D–F)** Exposure of the clivus through the pharynx in a cadaver. **(D)** The mucosa on the ventral surface of the hard palate and the adjacent part of the soft palate have been removed to expose the pharyngeal mucosa on the clivus. *(continued)*

Fig. 2.5 *(continued)* **(E)** The lower part of the clivus has been removed to expose the vertebral and basilar arteries (*Bas. A.*) and the origins of the posterior inferior cerebellar (*P.I.C.A.*), anterior inferior cerebellar (*A.I.C.A.*), anterior spinal (*Ant. Sp. A.*), and direct perforating arteries (*Dir. Perf. A.*). **(F)** The vomer has been removed to expose the sphenoid sinus and sellar floor. **(G)** Another specimen. The opening in the clivus exposes tortuous vertebral and basilar arteries. (From de Oliveira E, Rhoton AL Jr, Peace D. Microsurgical anatomy of the region of the foramen magnum. Surg Neurol 1985;24:293–352. With permission from *Surgical Neurology*.)

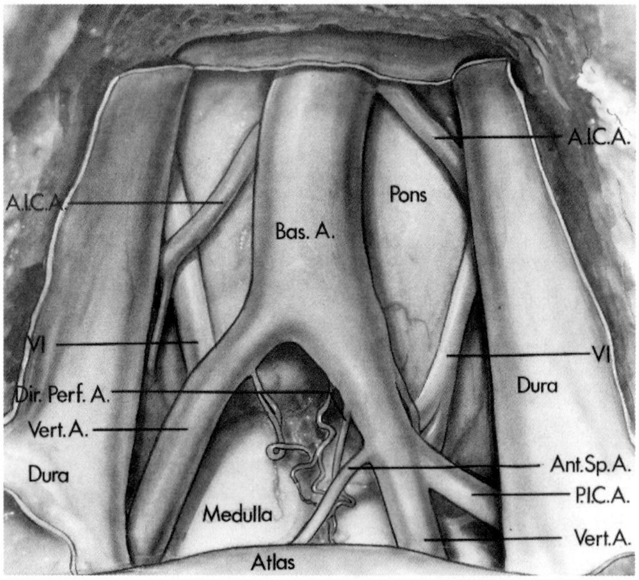

E

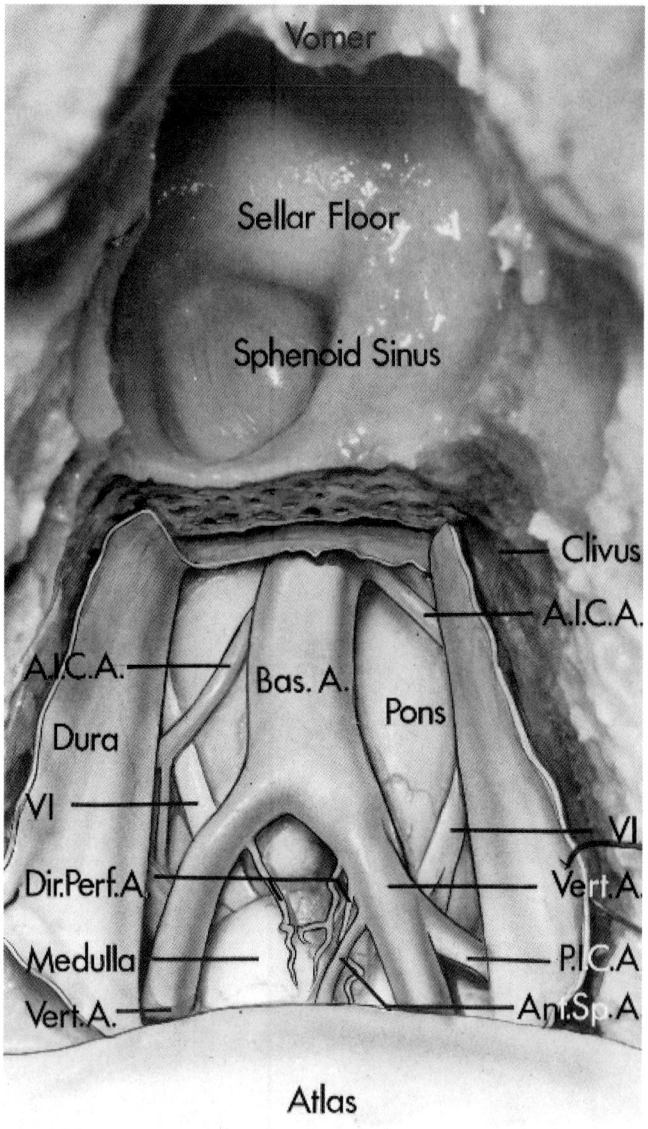

F

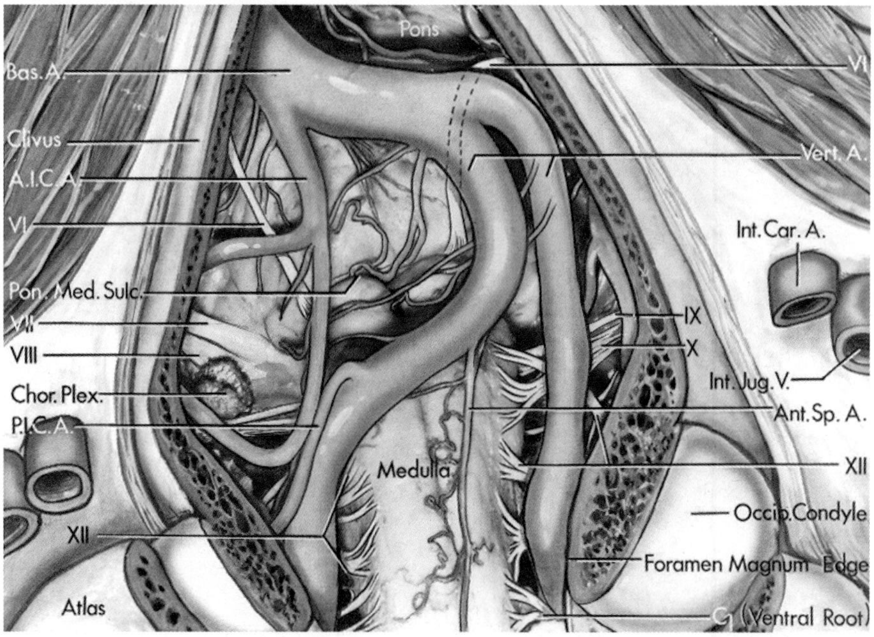

G

All of the 50 accessory nerves examined in our study had connections with the dorsal roots of the upper cervical nerves.[2] The most common and largest anastomosis was with the dorsal root of the first cervical nerve. The C1 dorsal roots frequently arose solely from the accessory nerve without a contribution from the C1 level of the spinal cord. About one third of C1 dorsal roots received rootlets that arose from the spinal cord at the C1 level, but these also had anastomotic fibers from the accessory nerve. The accessory nerves may also have an anastomotic connection with the C2 to C5 dorsal roots.[2,4]

Spinal Nerve Roots

The spinal rootlets in the region of the foramen magnum pass directly lateral to reach their dural foramina (**Figs. 2.3, 2.4,** and **2.5**). The first cervical nerve is located just below the foramen magnum and differs from the other cervical nerves in the consistency and origin of the dorsal rootlets forming the nerve. The C1 ventral root is composed of four to eight rootlets that join and course laterally. Before entering the dural foramen, the C1 ventral root and the corresponding dorsal root, if present, attach to the posterior inferior surface of the initial intradural part of the vertebral artery. They then pass through the funnel-shaped dural foramen around the vertebral artery. The ventral root joins the dorsal root in or external to the dural foramen.

The dorsal root of the first cervical nerve is more complicated than the ventral root because of the variations in its composition and its connections with the accessory nerve. In our study of the 25 spinal cords in which one would expect to find 50 C1 dorsal roots arising from the cord, only 15 were found.[2] The accessory nerve contributed a root to the first cervical nerve in 28 cases of the 35 roots lacking a dorsal root that arose from the spinal cord. In the remaining 7 cases, the C1 dorsal root was absent. Each of the 15 dorsal roots that arose from the spinal cord also had a contribution from the accessory nerve.[2]

■ Arterial Relationships

The major arteries related to the foramen magnum are the vertebral and posterior inferior cerebellar arteries, as well as the meningeal branches of the vertebral and external and internal carotid arteries (**Figs. 2.4, 2.5,** and **2.6**).[2,5–7] The paired vertebral arteries ascend through the transverse processes of the upper six cervical vertebrae, enter the dura behind the occipital condyles, and ascend through the foramen magnum to reach the front of the medulla. The segment most intimately related to the foramen magnum passes medially behind the lateral mass of the atlas and across the groove on the upper surface of the lateral part of the posterior arch of the atlas. This bony groove is frequently transformed into a bony canal that completely surrounds a short segment of the artery (**Fig. 2.4**).

The intradural segment begins at the dural foramen just inferior to the lateral edge of the foramen magnum. The dura in this region forms a funnel-shaped foramen around a 4 to 6 mm length of the artery. The first cervical nerve exits the spinal canal, and the posterior spinal artery enters the spinal canal through this dural foramen with the vertebral artery. These three structures are bound together at the foramen by fibrous dural bands (**Fig. 2.4**). The initial intradural segment of the vertebral artery passes just superior to the dorsal and ventral roots of the first cervical nerve and just anterior to the posterior spinal artery, the dentate ligament, and the spinal portion of the accessory nerve.

The branches arising from the vertebral artery in the region of the foramen magnum are the posterior spinal, anterior spinal, posterior inferior cerebellar, and the anterior and posterior meningeal arteries. The paired posterior spinal arteries usually arise from the vertebral arteries, just outside the dura, but they may also arise inside the dura or from the posteroinferior cerebellar arteries (**Figs. 2.4, 2.5,** and **2.6**). In the subarachnoid space, they course medially behind the rostral-most attachments of the dentate ligament and divide into a branch ascending to the medulla and a branch descending to the spinal cord.

The posteroinferior cerebellar artery usually originates within the dura, but it may infrequently originate from the terminal extradural part of the vertebral artery.[5,8] It may arise at, above, or below the level of the foramen magnum; of the 42 arteries found in 50 cerebella in our study, 35 arose above and 7 arose below the foramen.[2,5] In its course around the anterolateral surface of the medulla, it passes rostral or caudal to or between the rootlets of the hypoglossal nerve, and in its course around the posterolateral medulla it passes above, below, or between the rootlets of the glossopharyngeal, vagus, and accessory nerves. As it passes between the latter nerves, it may be ascending, descending, or passing laterally or medially, or it may be involved in a complex loop that stretches and distorts these nerves. Of the 42 arteries, 16 passed between the rootlets of the accessory nerve, 10 passed between the rootlets of the vagus nerve, 13 passed between the vagus and accessory nerves, 2 passed above the glossopharyngeal nerve between the latter nerve and the vestibulocochlear nerve, and 1 passed between the glossopharyngeal and vagus nerves.[2,5] After reaching the area dorsal to the glossopharyngeal, vagus, and accessory nerves, it passes around the cerebellar tonsil near the roof of the fourth ventricle and bifurcates into a medial and a lateral trunk. The medial trunk supplies the vermis and the adjacent part of the hemisphere, and the lateral trunk supplies the tonsil and the hemispheres.

The anterior spinal artery is formed by the union of the paired anteroventral spinal arteries, which originate from the vertebral arteries (**Fig. 2.5**). One of the anteroventral spinal arteries may continue inferiorly as the anterior spinal artery, and the other may terminate on the medulla. The anterior spinal artery descends through the foramen magnum on the anterior surface of the medulla and the spinal cord in or near the anterior median fissure.

The dura around the foramen magnum is supplied by the meningeal branches of the ascending pharyngeal and occipital

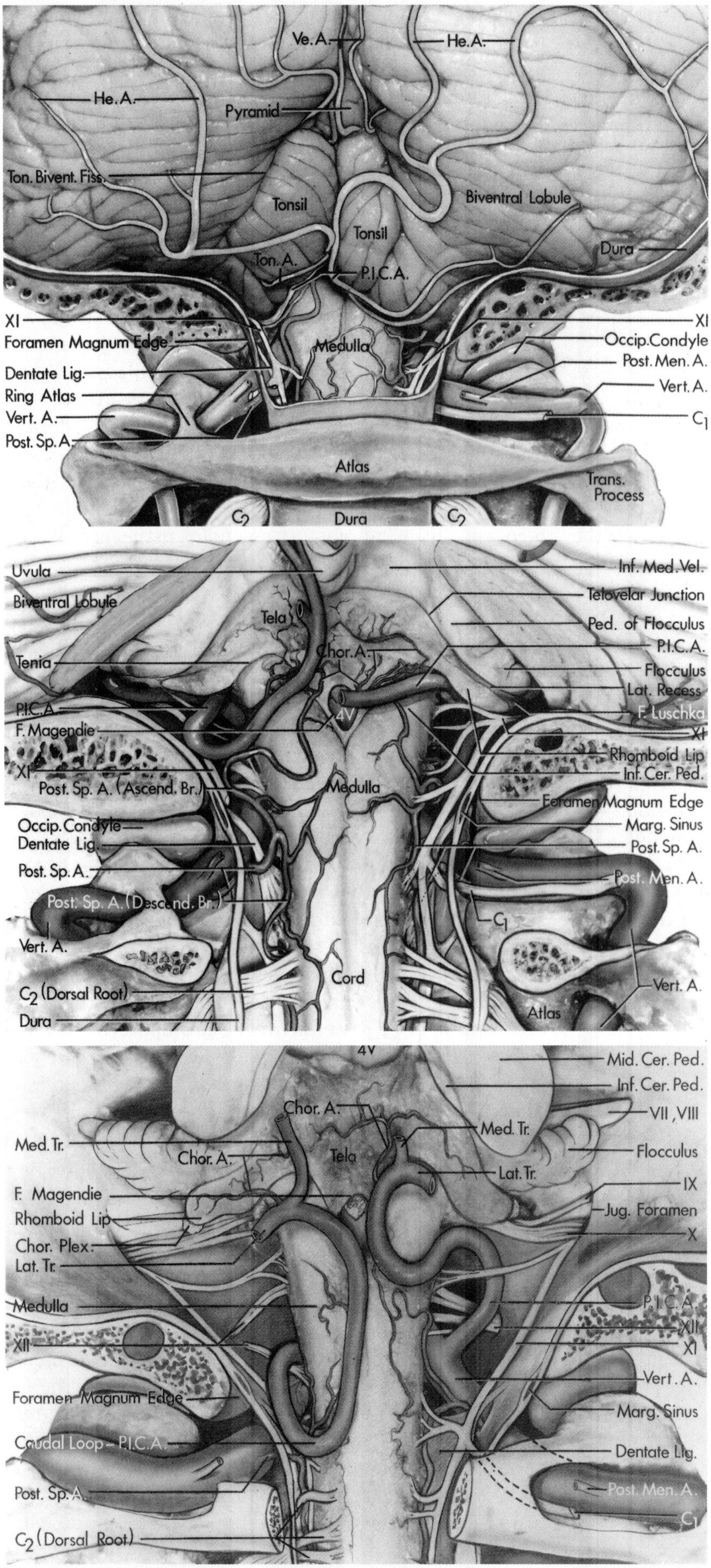

Fig. 2.6 Arterial relationships, posterior views. **(A)** The vertebral arteries (*Vert. A.*) ascend through the foramina in the transverse processes (*Trans. Process*), course below the occipital condyles (*Occip. Condyle*), and give rise to the posterior spinal (*Post. Sp. A.*) and posterior meningeal arteries (*Post. Men. A.*) before entering the dura. The posterior inferior cerebellar arteries (*P.I.C.A.*) course around the tonsils and divide into tonsillar (*Ton. A.*), vermian (*Ve. A.*), and hemispheric arteries (*He. A.*). Structures exposed include the tonsillobiventral fissure (*Ton. Bivent. Fiss.*), dentate ligament (*Dentate Lig.*), and accessory nerve (*XI*). **(B)** The tonsils and adjacent part of the biventral lobule have been removed to show the relationship of the posterior inferior cerebellar arteries to the foramen magnum and roof of the fourth ventricle. The posterior spinal artery splits into ascending (*Ascend. Br.*) and descending branches (*Descend. Br.*). The structures forming the inferior half of the roof of the fourth ventricle (*4V*) are the tela choroidea (*Tela*) and the inferior medullary velum (*Inf. Med. Vel.*). Structures exposed include the peduncles (*Ped.*) of the flocculi, inferior cerebellar peduncles (*Inf. Cer. Ped*), choroidal arteries (*Chor. A.*), marginal sinus (*Marg. Sinus*), lateral recesses (*Lat. Recess*), and the foramina of Luschka (*F. Luschka*) and Magendie (*F. Magendie*). **(C)** The structures forming the inferior half of the roof of the fourth ventricle, except for the most caudal strip of the tela, have been removed in another specimen. The left posterior inferior cerebellar artery passes posteriorly between the rootlets of the hypoglossal and accessory nerves and dips below the level of foramen magnum to form a caudal loop before ascending behind the roof of the fourth ventricle. The right posterior inferior cerebellar artery ascends from its origin without forming a caudal loop. Both posterior inferior cerebellar arteries split into medial (*Med. Tr.*) and lateral trunks (*Lat. Tr.*). Structures exposed include the facial (*VII*), vestibulocochlear (*VIII*), glossopharyngeal (*IX*), vagus (*X*), accessory (*XI*), and hypoglossal nerves (*XII*); middle (*Mid. Cer. Ped.*) and inferior cerebellar peduncles (*Inf. Cer. Ped.*); choroid plexus (*Chor. Plex.*); and jugular foramen (*Jug. Foramen*). (From de Oliveira E, Rhoton AL Jr, Peace D. Microsurgical anatomy of the region of the foramen magnum. Surg Neurol 1985;24:293–352. With permission from *Surgical Neurology*.)

arteries, the anterior and posterior meningeal branches of the vertebral artery, and the dorsal meningeal branch of the meningohypophyseal trunk of the intracavernous segment of the internal carotid artery (**Figs. 2.4, 2.5,** and **2.6**). Infrequently, the posterior inferior cerebellar and posterior spinal arteries and the intradural part of the vertebral artery give rise to meningeal branches. The anterior meningeal branch of the vertebral artery enters the spinal canal through the C2 to C3 intervertebral foramen and ascends between the posterior longitudinal ligament (tectorial membrane) and the dura (**Fig. 2.3A–C**). At the level of the apex of the dens, these paired arteries join to form an arch over the apex of the dens. The posterior meningeal artery arises from the vertebral artery as it courses around the lateral mass of the atlas and ascends in the dura near the falx cerebelli. The ascending pharyngeal branch of the external carotid artery sends branches through the hypoglossal canal and jugular foramen to the dura above the foramen magnum (**Fig. 2.5**). The meningeal branch of the occipital artery is inconstant. It penetrates the cranium through a mastoid emissary foramen.

Venous Relationships

The venous structures in the region of the foramen magnum are divided into three groups: one composed of the extradural veins, another formed by the intradural (neural) veins, and a third constituted by dural venous sinuses (**Fig. 2.7**).[9] The three groups anastomose through bridging and emissary veins.

A

B

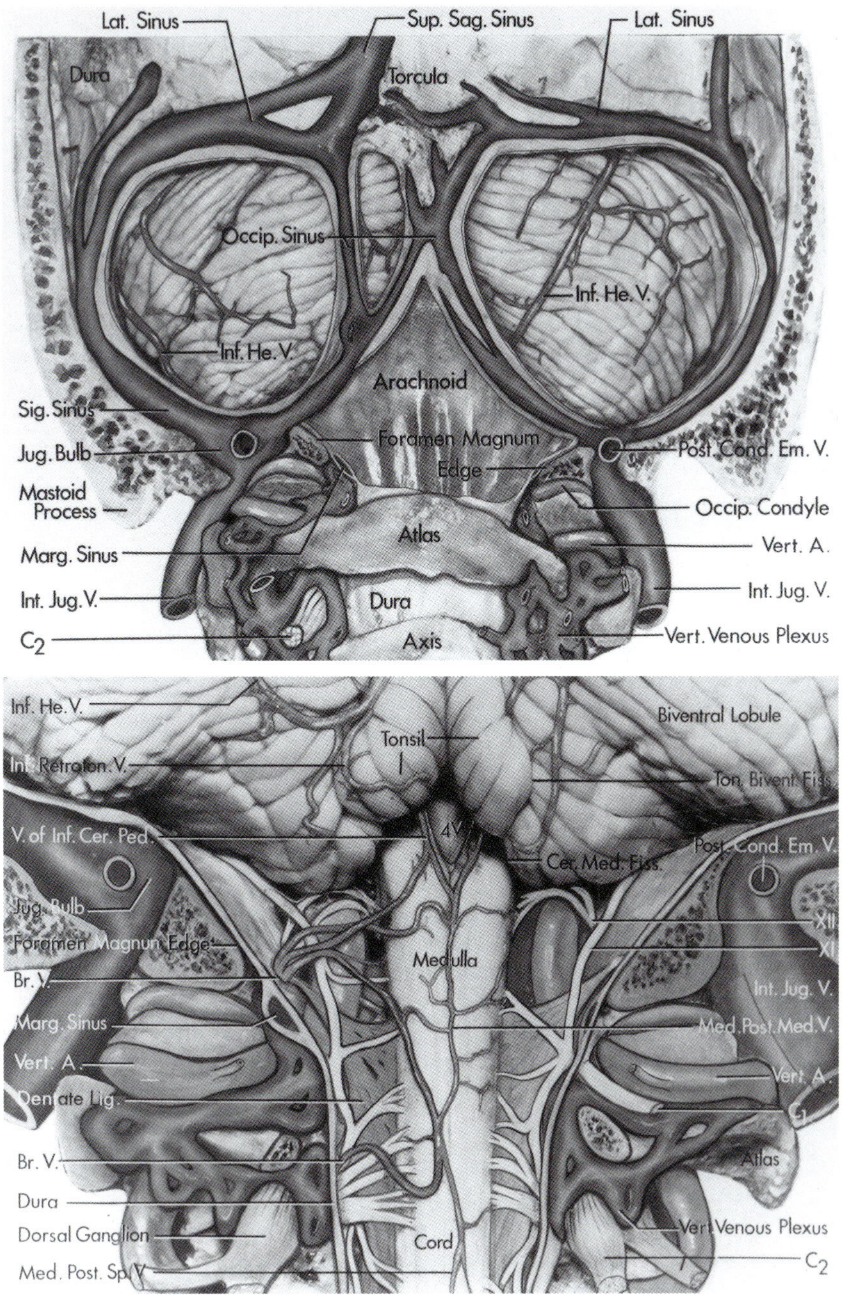

Fig. 2.7 Venous relationships, posterior views. **(A)** The dura over the cerebellum has been removed, except in the area of the venous sinuses. The occipital sinuses (*Occip. Sinus*) join the torcula above and the jugular bulbs (*Jug. Bulb*) below. The vertebral venous plexus (*Vert. Venous Plexus*) anastomoses with the posterior condylar emissary (*Post. Cond. Em. V.*) and internal jugular veins (*Int. Jug. V.*). The marginal sinus (*Marg. Sinus*) courses in the dura at the level of the foramen magnum. Structures exposed include the superior sagittal (*Sup. Sag. Sinus*), lateral (*Lat. Sinus*), and sigmoid sinuses (*Sig. Sinus*); vertebral artery (*Vert. A.*); inferior hemispheric veins (*Inf. He. V.*); and occipital condyles (*Occip. Condyle*). **(B)** The dura below the lateral and sigmoid sinuses has been removed. The median posterior medullary vein (*Med. Post. Med. V.*) splits below the fourth ventricle (*4V*) to form the paired veins of the inferior cerebellar peduncle (*V. of Inf. Cer. Ped.*). Structures exposed include the accessory (*XI*) and hypoglossal nerves (*XII*); dentate ligament (*Dentate Lig.*); cerebellomedullary (*Cer. Med. Fiss.*) and tonsillar biventral fissures (*Ton. Bivent. Fiss.*); and bridging (*Br. V.*), inferior retrotonsillar (*Inf. Retroton. V.*), and median posterior spinal veins (*Med. Post. Sp. V.*). *(continued)*

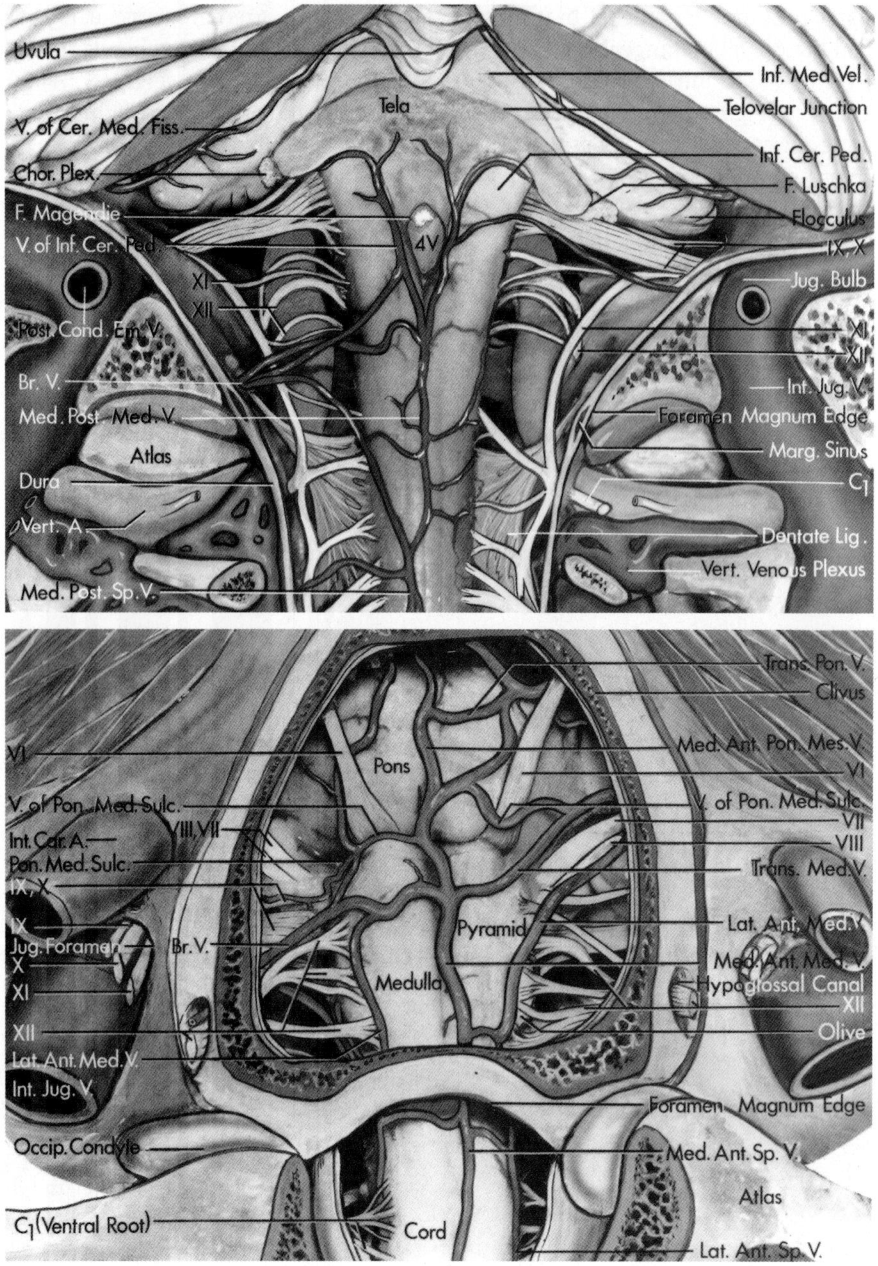

Fig. 2.7 *(continued)* **(C)** The tonsils have been removed to expose the inferior medullary velum (*Inf. Med. Vel.*) and tela choroidea (*Tela*). Structures exposed include the choroid plexus (*Chor. Plex.*), foramina of Luschka (*F. Luschka*) and Magendie (*F. Magendie*), vein of the cerebello-medullary fissure (*V. of Cer. Med. Fiss.*), glossopharyngeal (*IX*) and vagus nerves (*X*), and the inferior cerebellar peduncles (*Inf. Cer. Ped.*). **(D)** The front of the brainstem has been exposed. The veins that cross the front of the brainstem are the median anterior pontomesencephalic (*Med. Ant. Pon. Mes. V.*), median anterior medullary (*Med. Ant. Med. V.*), median anterior spinal (*Med. Ant. Sp. V.*), lateral anterior medullary (*Lat. Ant. Med. V.*), lateral anterior spinal (*Lat. Ant. Sp. V.*), transverse pontine (*Trans. Pons. V.*), and transvers medullary veins (*Trans. Med. V.*), and the vein of pontomedullary sulcus (*V. of Pon. Med. Sulc.*). Other structures in the exposure include the carotid artery (*Int. Car. A.*); abducens (*VI*), facial (*VII*), vestibulocochlear (*VIII*), and hypoglossal (*XII*) nerves; jugular foramen (*Jug. Foramen*); and pontomedullary sulcus (*Pont. Med. Sulc.*). *(continued)*

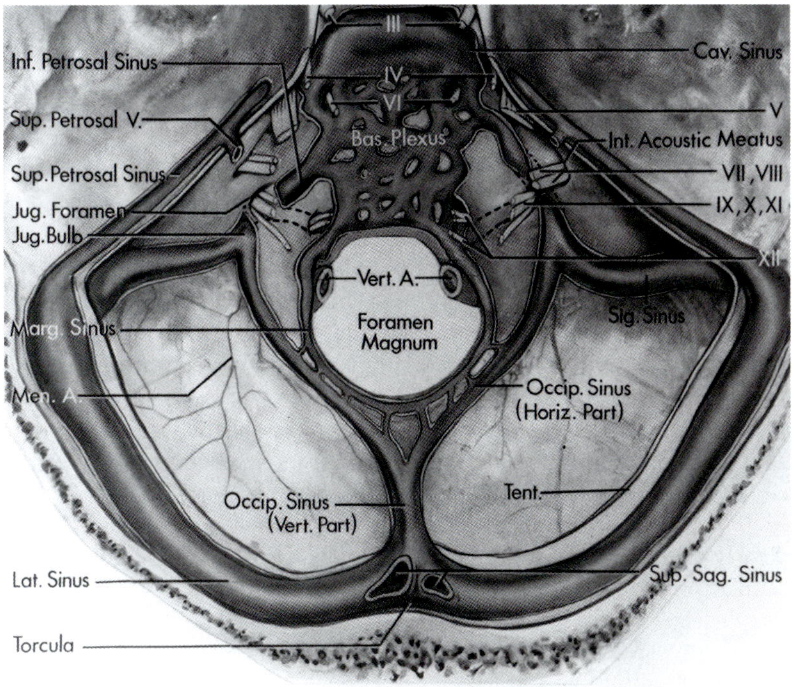

E

Fig. 2.7 *(continued)* **(E)** Superior view. Venous sinuses surrounding the foramen magnum. There are diffuse anastomoses between the venous sinuses around the foramen magnum. Structures exposed include the basilar venous plexus (*Bas Plexus*); superior (*Sup. Petrosal Sinus*), inferior petrosal (*Inf. Petrosal Sinus*), and cavernous sinuses (*Cav. Sinus*); vertical (*Vert. Part*) and horizontal parts (*Horiz. Part*) of the occipital sinus (*Occip. Sinus*); superior petrosal veins (*Sup. Pet.V.*); oculomotor (*III*), trochlear (*IV*), and trigeminal nerves (*V*); internal acoustic meatus (*Int. Acoustic Meatus*); meningeal arteries (*Men. A.*); and tentorium (*Tent.*). Small dural sinuses (*dotted lines*) connect the jugular bulbs with the veins in the hypoglossal canals. (From de Oliveira E, Rhoton AL Jr, Peace D. Microsurgical anatomy of the region of the foramen magnum. Surg Neurol 1985;24:293–352. With permission from *Surgical Neurology*.)

The extradural veins are divided into an extraspinal part, the vertebral venous plexus, which is formed by the veins draining the deep muscles surrounding the cervical vertebrae, and an intraspinal component, the epidural venous plexus, which courses in the epidural space, primarily laterally, with some connections anterior and posterior on the outer surface of the dura. There are anastomotic connections between the epidural and vertebral venous plexus that surrounds the terminal extradural segment of the vertebral artery.

The venous channels in the dura surrounding the foramen magnum are the marginal and occipital sinuses and the basilar venous plexus (**Fig. 2.7**). The marginal sinus is located in the dura, lining the rim of the foramen magnum. The occipital sinus courses in the cerebellar falx. Its lower end divides into paired limbs, each of which courses anteriorly around the foramen magnum to join the sigmoid sinus or the jugular bulb. The basilar venous plexus is located between the layers of the dura on the clivus and extends from the dorsum sellae to the anterior rim of the foramen magnum. It is formed by interconnecting venous channels, which anastomose with the inferior petrosal sinuses laterally, the cavernous sinuses superiorly, and the marginal sinus and epidural venous plexus inferiorly.

The intradural veins in the region of the foramen magnum drain the lower part of the cerebellum and brainstem, the upper part of the spinal cord, and the cerebellomedullary fissure. The veins of the medulla and spinal cord form longitudinal plexiform channels that anastomose at the foramen magnum. The main vein on the posterior surface of the medulla is the median posterior medullary vein. It courses along the posterior median medullary sulcus and divides superiorly, near the obex, into the paired veins of the inferior cerebellar peduncle, each of which courses on the surface of the inferior cerebellar peduncle parallel to and below the lower edge of the fourth ventricle to join veins on the lateral surface of the medulla. The median posterior medullary vein is continuous below with the median posterior spinal vein. Bridging veins connect these veins to the dural sinus in the region of the foramen magnum. The veins draining the tonsils and adjacent part of the cerebellum and brainstem ascend along the vermis to terminate in the sinuses in the region of the torcula. The veins on the anterior and lateral surface of the medulla drain into the veins in the cerebellopontine angle, which form the superior petrosal veins, and empty into the superior petrosal sinus.

Herniations

Herniation of cerebellar tissue into the foramen magnum may cause neural compression and even death. These herniations are commonly referred to as tonsillar herniations; however, the herniation usually involves the tonsils and biventral lobules, both of which are deeply grooved by the edge of the foramen magnum.[2,10] The herniation may compress the medulla and be so severe that the herniated tissue undergoes necrosis. Patients with herniation at the foramen magnum may be asymptomatic or present with pain, signs of neural compression, increased intracranial pressure, and sudden unexpected death. Symptoms caused by dysfunction of the cerebellum, brainstem, and lower cranial and upper spinal nerves include pain in the neck and upper arms, dizziness, ataxia, disturbances of gait, diplopia, dysphagia, tinnitus, decreased hearing, nystagmus, weakness to the degree of quadriparesis, and sensory deficit in the extremities. Coughing or sneezing may aggravate the symptoms and cause syncope. Some patients without prior symptoms who die suddenly are found to have herniations through the foramen magnum at autopsy. The occurrence of sudden death in these patients means that herniation at the foramen magnum is a precarious situation that can be aggravated by minor stresses. The common denominator in these cases of sudden death is herniation of the tonsils and adjacent part of the biventral lobule into the foramen magnum.[10] The herniation may be bilateral and symmetrical, although more commonly symmetry is not strict, and it may be unilateral. The herniated tonsils are tightly pressed against the medulla. Acute or chronic herniations may be seen with space-occupying lesions, such as cerebellar astrocytomas or cystic tumors. Chronic herniation is seen with the Chiari type I malformation.

Tumors

Foramen magnum tumors have frequently eluded early diagnosis because they cause bizarre symptoms simulating cervical spondylosis, multiple sclerosis, or degenerative disease.[11] Tumors arising in the region of the foramen magnum were divided by Cushing and Eisenhardt into a craniospinal group (tumors that arise above and grow downward toward the foramen magnum) and a spinocranial group (tumors that arise below and grow upward toward the foramen magnum).[12] The intradural extramedullary tumors in this region are usually benign, with meningiomas and schwannomas being the most frequent.[12,13] The frequency rate of meningioma to schwannoma is 26:4.[2,12,13] Craniospinal meningiomas tend to originate anteriorly or anterolaterally, and spinocranial meningiomas tend to arise laterally or posterolaterally, close to the initial part of the intradural segment of the vertebral artery. The intramedullary tumors are represented mainly by astrocytomas and ependymomas. Cerebellar tumors, especially those originating in the fourth ventricle (e.g., ependymomas, medulloblastomas, and choroid plexus papillomas), and those arising in the lower part of the cerebellar hemisphere or vermis may extend into or through the foramen magnum into the upper spinal canal. Chordomas and metastases are the most common extradural tumors. The chordomas usually arise at the level of the clivus and may extend caudally into the foramen magnum.

Surgical Approaches

The foramen magnum may be approached anteriorly, posteriorly, or laterally (**Fig. 2.8**). The posterior operative

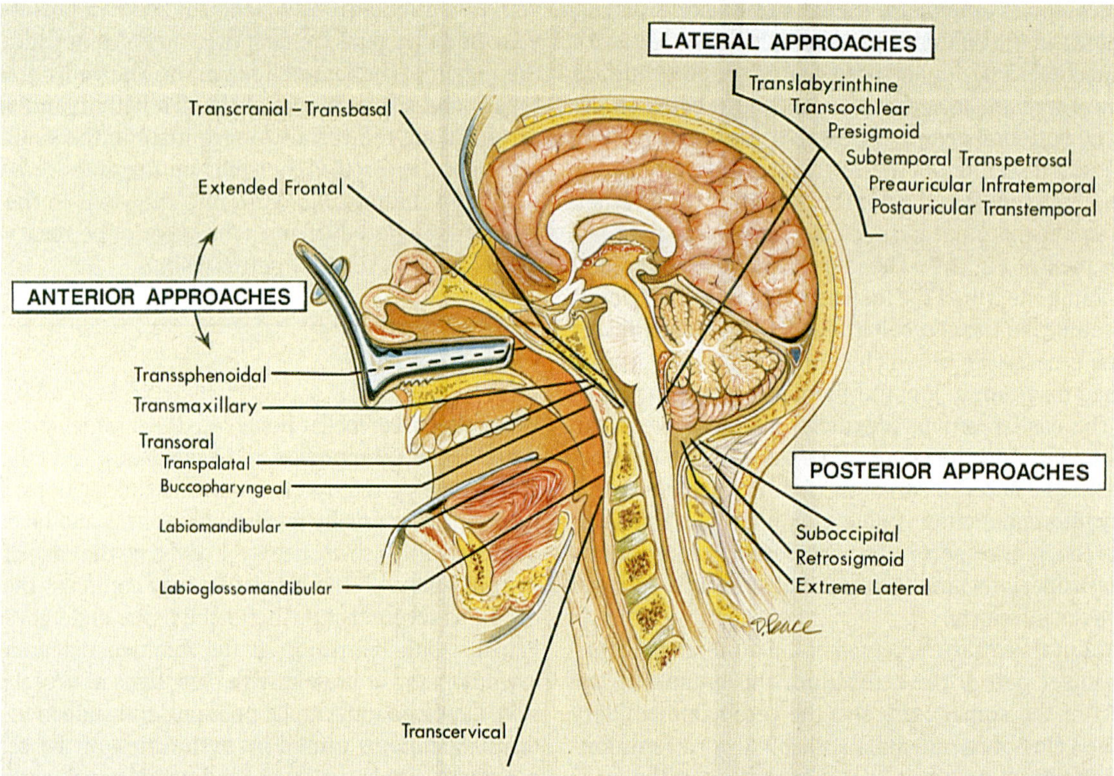

Fig. 2.8 Surgical approaches to the foramen magnum. The posterior operative approach is commonly selected for intradural lesions. An anterior approach is frequently selected for extradural lesions situated anterior to the foramen magnum. A lateral approach may be selected for intradural lesions located lateral to and/or in front of the brainstem, especially if they involve the temporal and sphenoid bones and the clivus. (From de Oliveira E, Rhoton AL Jr, Peace D. Microsurgical anatomy of the region of the foramen magnum. Surg Neurol 1985;24:293–352. With permission from *Surgical Neurology*.)

approach is commonly selected for intradural lesions. An anterior approach is frequently selected for extradural lesions situated anterior to the foramen magnum. A lateral approach may be selected for intradural lesions located lateral to and/or in front of the brainstem, especially if they involve the temporal and sphenoid bones and the clivus.[2]

Anterior Operative Approaches

Anterior approaches are used to reach tumors of the atlas, axis, and clivus; to resect and fixate the odontoid process following ligamentous and osseous injury; to decompress bony malformations of the craniovertebral junction (CVJ), such as basilar invagination; and to approach aneurysms of the vertebral and basilar arteries (**Fig. 2.8**). The greatest advantage of the anterior approach is the direct route to the lesion, and the major disadvantages are the frequency of cerebrospinal fluid (CSF) leaks, pseudomeningocele, and meningitis following the exposure of intradural lesions by this approach.

The transoral route through the mouth and the posterior pharyngeal wall, referred to as the buccopharyngeal approach, is the anterior approach most commonly selected (**Fig. 2.8**). The basic transoral approach may be modified to include a transpalatine approach in which the soft palate or both the soft and hard palates are opened and the labiomandibular or labioglossomandibular approach is used, in which the lip, mandible, and possibly the tongue and floor of the mouth are split to increase the exposure. Other types of anterior approaches are the transcervical approach directed through the submandibular area along the anterior border of the sternocleidomastoid muscle; the transcranial–transbasal and extended frontal approaches, in which the clivus is reached through a bifrontal craniotomy; the transsphenoidal approach, in which the clivus is reached through the sphenoid sinus; and the transmaxillary approaches, in which one maxilla is displaced inferiorly, or both maxillae are displaced inferiorly or split in the midline and each is reflected laterally.

Transoral Approaches

After induction of general endotracheal anesthesia, a tracheostomy is commonly performed, and the mouth is kept opened with a self-retaining retractor (**Fig. 2.9**). To reach the anterior part of the atlas and axis, the posterior pharyngeal wall is incised longitudinally in the midline. The mucosa and prevertebral muscles are elevated as a mucoperiosteal layer, using subperiosteal dissection, and retracted laterally. To expose the clivus, it is often necessary to split the soft palate in the midline. If added cranial exposure is needed, laterally based mucoperiosteal flaps may be elevated from the lower surface of the hard palate, and the posterior part of the hard palate may be removed. The mucosa covering the upper surface of the hard palate should be retracted and not opened. This permits the pharyngeal incision to be extended upward through the vault of the nasopharynx to the posterior border of the vomer. When elevating the mucoperiosteal layer from the clivus, the lateral margins slope dorsally into "gutter-like" depressions in which the tissue becomes thicker and more adherent. Depending on the lesion, the clivus, the anterior arches, the atlas, the dens, and the bodies of C2 and C3 may be removed with a drill and rongeurs. The clival exposure between the occipital condyles is 2 to 2.5 cm wide and 2.5 to 3 cm long. Care must be taken to avoid cranial nerves VI to XII, the internal carotid arteries, the internal jugular veins, and the inferior petrosal sinuses, which are on the margins of the exposure. The most common lesions approached by this route are in an extradural location. Opening the dura will expose both vertebral arteries and the lower end of the basilar artery.

To increase the exposure and reduce the operative depth, the lip and chin may be incised vertically and a step-like mandibular osteotomy accomplished in the midline after removal of a central incisor tooth. Spreading the mandibular edges laterally without splitting the tongue permits the tongue to be depressed downward between the mandibular halves. If the exposure is still inadequate, the tongue and floor of the mouth may be split in the midline. Spreading the mandibular lingual halves exposes the pharyngeal wall down to the level of the arytenoid cartilages.

Transmaxillary Approach

Transmaxillary approaches have been advocated for pathology extending to the upper and middle third of the clivus, which is difficult to reach by the transoral approach (**Fig. 2.10**). Three different types of transmaxillary approaches have been used.[14,15] In one approach, a LeFort I osteotomy is completed, and the maxilla and hard palate are down-fractured into the oral cavity.[15] In the second approach, called the extended maxillectomy, the LeFort osteotomy is combined with a midline incision of the hard and soft palate and the halves of the maxilla are swung laterally.[15] In the third approach, the extended maxillotomy, one half of the maxilla and the hard palate are hinged on the soft palate and folded downward into the floor of the mouth.

In the first approach with a LeFort osteotomy, the upper lip is elevated and a mucosal incision is made along the upper alveolar margin extending around the molars on both sides. The mucosa is stripped off the anterior face of the maxilla below the infraorbital foramen but high enough to avoid the dental roots and extending into the nasal cavity. The saw cuts extend into the maxillary sinuses on both sides, leaving the branches of the internal maxillary artery and the nerves to the maxilla and palate intact. The mucosa on the nasal surface of the maxilla

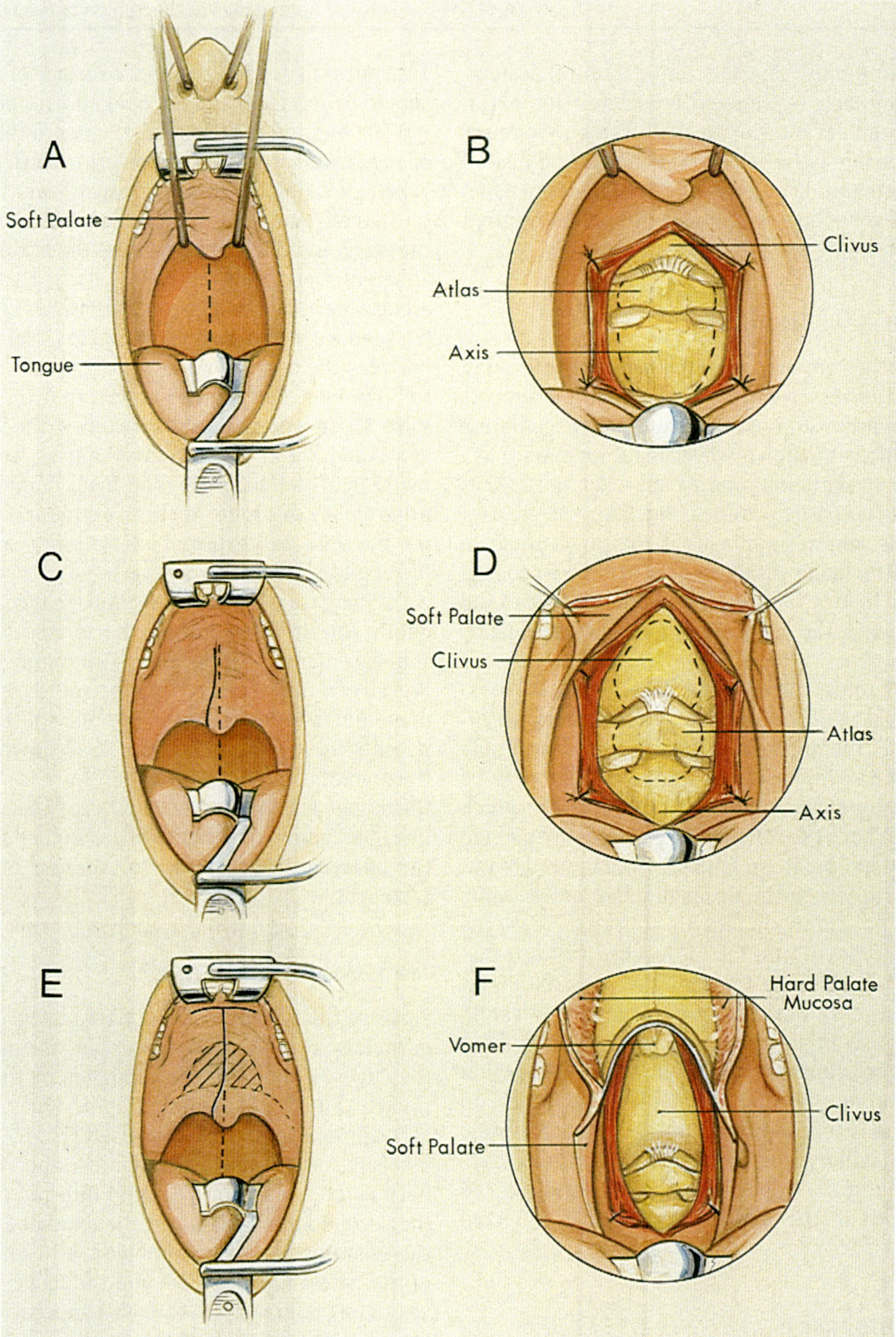

Fig. 2.9 The transoral approach is the anterior approach most commonly selected. Variants of the transoral approach include the transpalatal variant, in which the soft palate or both the soft and hard palates are opened, and the labiomandibular or labioglossomandibular variants, in which the lip, chin, mandible, and possibly the tongue and floor of the mouth are split in the midline to increase the exposure. The transoral approach and its variants permit removal of the clivus, the anterior arch of the atlas, the odontoid process, and the bodies of C2 and C3. **(A)** Transoral approach. The patient is positioned in the Trendelenburg position with the head fixed in a head holder or in traction using cranial tongs so that lateral X-rays or image intensification is available to verify the location. A tracheostomy is commonly performed. Catheters inserted through the nasal passages and brought behind the soft palate and out the mouth or a silk suture brought through the base of the uvula and attached to a nasal catheter may be used to retract the soft palate. The posterior pharyngeal wall is incised longitudinally in the midline (*dotted line*). **(B)** The mucosa and prevertebral muscles are retracted laterally as a single layer, using subperiosteal dissection to reach the atlas, axis, and lower clivus. The anterior arch of the atlas, the odontoid process, and the body of the atlas may be removed (*dotted line*) to expose the dura. **(C)** It may be necessary to split the soft palate in the midline to expose the clivus (palatal incision, *continuous line*; pharyngeal incision, *dotted line*). **(D)** The anterior surface of the clivus has been exposed through the transpalatal approach. The anterior arch of the atlas and the odontoid process may be removed and an opening made in the clivus (*dotted line*). *(continued)*

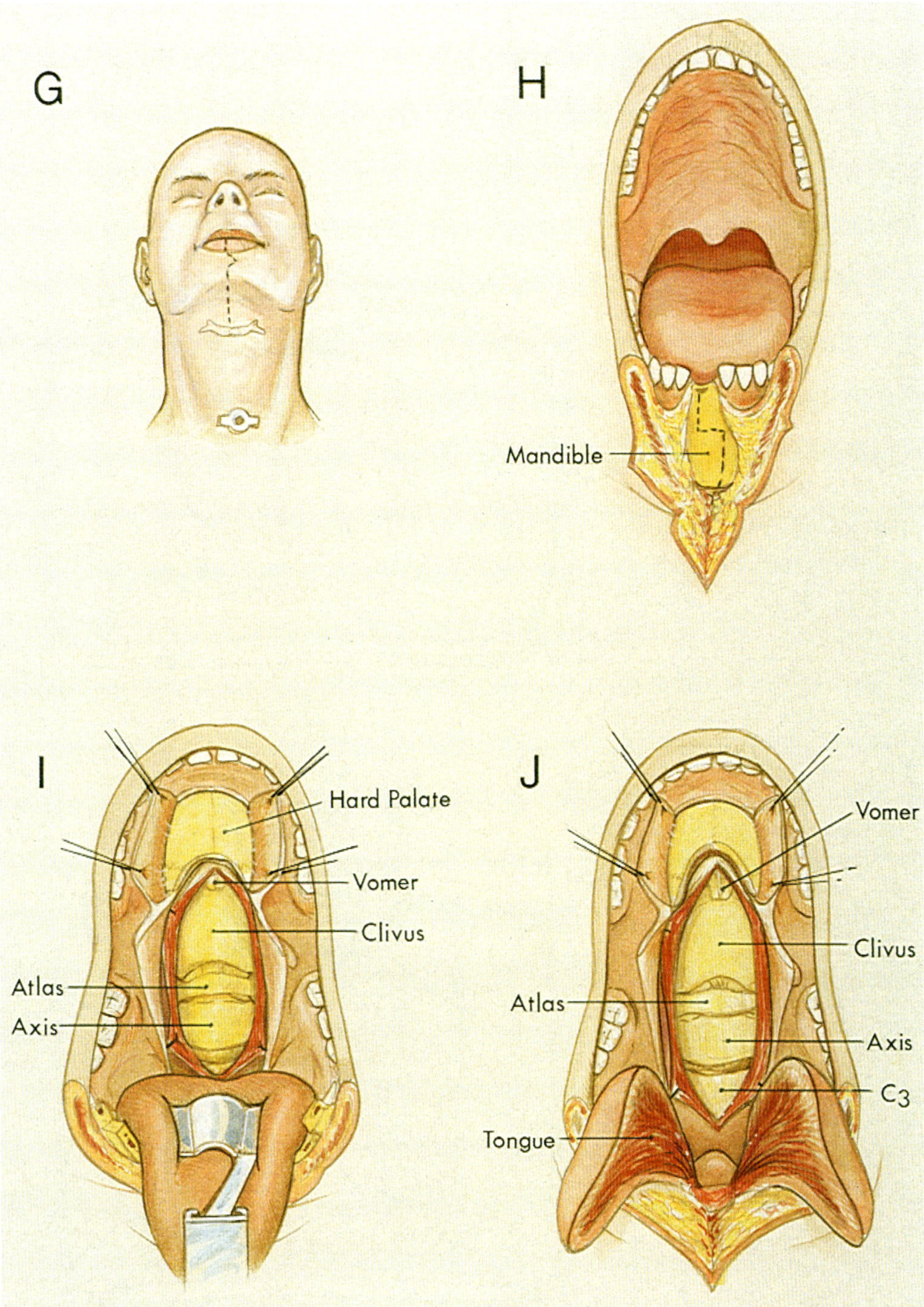

Fig. 2.9 *(continued)* **(E)** If further cranial exposure is needed, laterally based mucoperiosteal flaps may be elevated from the lower surface of the hard palate (*dotted line*), and the soft palate is split in the midline (*continuous line*). The posterior part of the hard palate is removed (*oblique lines*). **(F)** Care is taken to retract rather than open the mucosa lining of the upper surface of the hard palate. The pharyngeal incision is extended upward through the vault of the nasopharynx to the posterior border of the vomer. When elevating the mucoperiosteal layer from the clivus, the lateral margins slope dorsally into gutter-like depressions where the tissue becomes more adherent. The clivus, anterior arch of the atlas, dens, and the bodies of C2 and C3 may be removed. The clival defect is packed with muscle or fat and may be reinforced with a bone graft. The prevertebral muscle and mucosal layers and the palatal openings are closed with absorbable sutures. **(G)** The lower lip and mandible may be split (*dotted line*) to increase the exposure and reduce the operative depth. **(H)** A step-like mandibular osteotomy (*dotted line*) is accomplished in the midline after removal of a central incisor tooth. **(I)** Spreading the mandibular halves laterally without splitting the tongue permits the tongue to be depressed downward between the mandibular halves. **(J)** If the exposure is still inadequate, the tongue and floor of the mouth may be split in the midline. Spreading the mandibular lingual halves exposes the pharynx down to the C3 level. The mucosa and musculature of the tongue and floor of the mouth are reapproximated; the mandibular osteotomy is closed with wire; and the lip, chin, and submandibular region are carefully closed after dealing with the lesion.

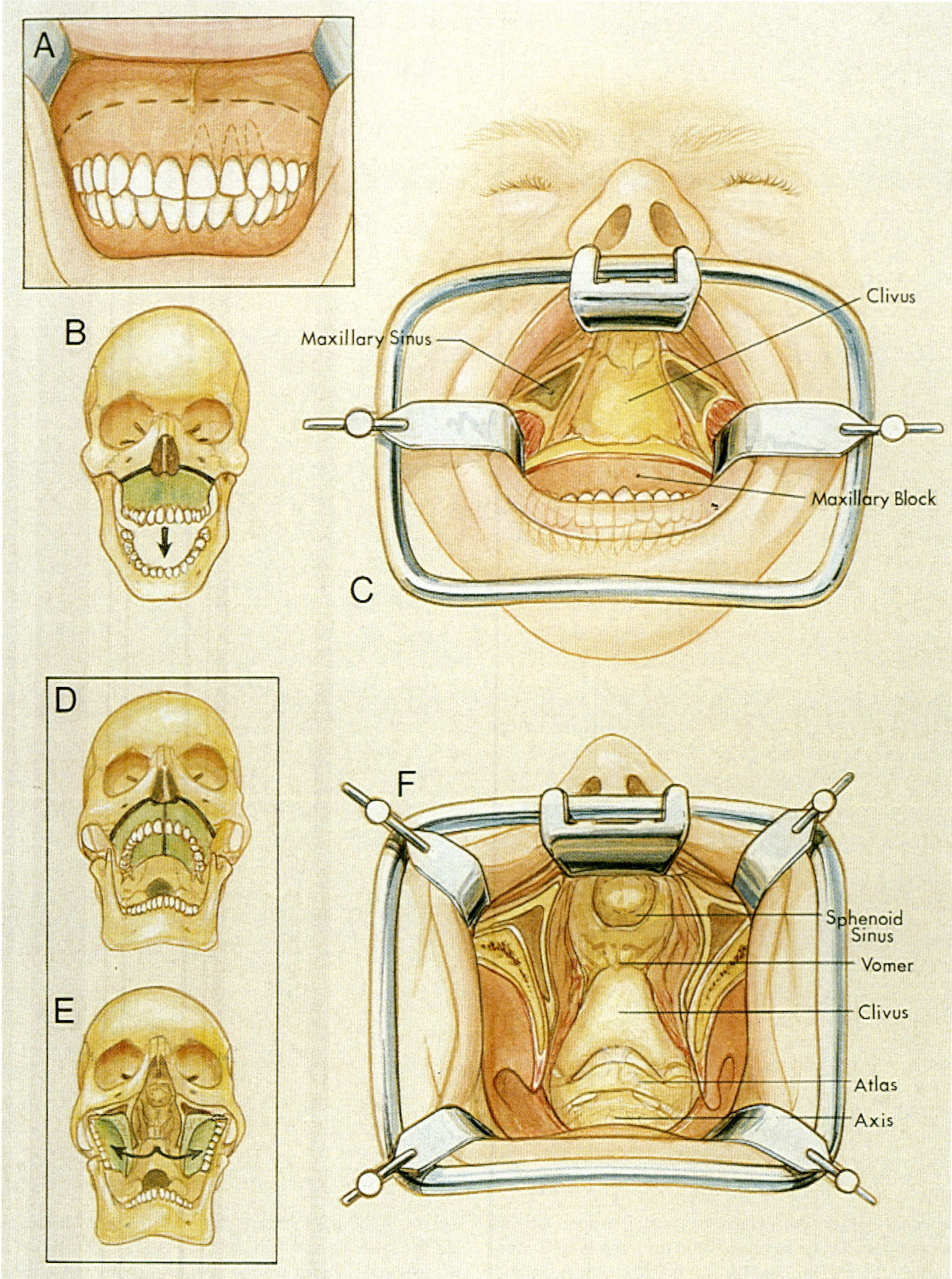

Fig. 2.10 Transmaxillary approaches. Three variants of the transmaxillary approaches are shown. All three can be completed through an intraoral incision with degloving. Another type of incision extending onto the face such as a Weber-Ferguson incision might be considered. **(A)** The upper lip is elevated and the mucosa is incised along the upper alveolar margin around the molars. The mucosa is elevated from the anterior face of the maxilla below the infraorbital foramen, but high enough to avoid the dental roots. The mucosa is elevated from the nasal surface of the maxilla, and the nasal septum is divided above its attachment to the palate. **(B)** The saw cuts (*solid line*) extend into the maxillary sinus on both sides. The free block of maxilla is moved downward (*arrow*) to give wide access to the clivus. **(C)** The intraoral retractor has been placed. Displacing the maxilla downward gives wide access to the clivus. **(D)** Modified technique called the extended maxillectomy includes the LeFort I osteotomy with a midline incision of the hard and soft palate (*solid lines*). **(E)** This allows the halves of the maxilla, which are attached to the muscles and vessels in the infratemporal fossa, to be reflected laterally, providing wider exposure to the clivus and upper cervical spine. **(F)** Retractors have been placed to expose the clivus and upper cervical area. The approach can be extended upward into the sphenoid and ethmoid sinuses and downward to C2 or C3. *(continued)*

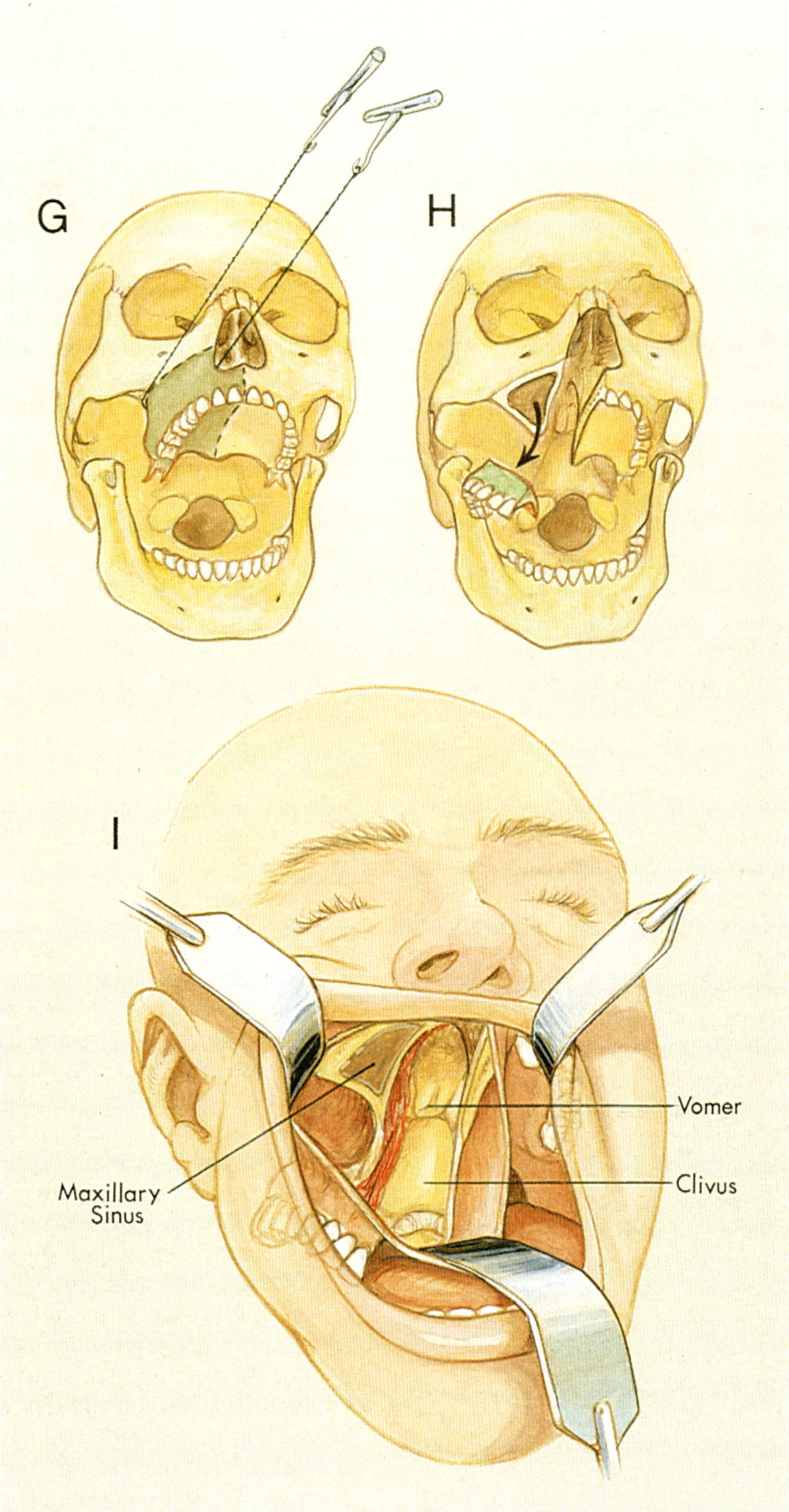

Fig. 2.10 *(continued)* **(G–I)** Unilateral maxillotomy. **(G)** In this approach, one-half of the maxilla is mobilized by a bone cut, which extends back to the infratemporal fossa in the area just below the infraorbital foramen, and the maxilla is divided in the midline. A mucosal incision is made along the lower surface of the hard palate parallel to midline on the side opposite the saw cut through the hard palate, and the anterior face of the maxilla is degloved on one side. The soft palate is left intact. **(H)** The unilateral block of maxilla, which is still attached to the structures in the infratemporal fossa along the pterygoid plates and to the soft palate, which is not interrupted, is folded downward into the floor of the mouth. **(I)** The anterior part of the nasal septum is left undisturbed, but the posterior part is removed along with some of the turbinates and wall of the sinuses to provide a wide exposure of the clivus. This exposure can be enlarged for removal of the walls of the sphenoid and ethmoid sinuses.

is dissected off, and the nasal septum is divided just above its attachment to the palate. The freed bone block includes, in one piece, the part of both maxilla and the maxillary teeth situated below the infraorbital foramen with their intact blood and nerve supply, which enters in the region of the infratemporal fossa and pterygoid plates. The fact that the soft palate is left intact reduces the incidence of speech and swallowing disorders. The intact maxillary block, however, blocks access to the CVJ, although it provides reasonable access to the upper and middle thirds of the clivus. In an effort to increase access to the CVJ, Crockard[15] modified the technique to combine the LeFort osteotomy with a midline incision of the hard and soft palate, thus allowing the maxillary halves, with their attachment, to be reflected laterally. The disadvantage of this procedure is the difficulty in obtaining good dental occlusion and proper functioning of the hard and soft palates.

In a modification recommended by Cocke and colleagues, called the extended maxillotomy, one half of the maxilla is folded into the floor of the mouth on the hinge of the soft tissue, leaving the soft palate intact.[14] This unilateral maxillotomy is attached to a vascular pedicle of tissue, including the internal maxillary artery. The hard palate is divided in the midline, with care being taken to preserve the soft palate.

In each of the three approaches, the posterior part of the nasal septum and turbinates may be removed to expose the posterior pharyngeal wall and to provide access to the clivus and CVJ. These approaches also provide access to the sphenoid and ethmoid sinuses and the sella, and the medial part of the floor of the anterior fossa. The posterior part of the mucosa on both sides of the nasal septum may be prepared to provide flaps that can be folded into the clival defect for closure. In addition, planning will allow for a temporalis muscle graft to be folded into the clival defect for closure. The incidence of swallowing and speech difficulties is significantly greater with those approaches in which the soft palate is divided rather than when it is left intact. In each approach, plates and screws are positioned prior to making the bone cuts to achieve satisfactory dental occlusion following the procedure. The procedure of Robertson and Cocke provides more rapid recovery of oropalatal function because only one half of the maxilla is disturbed, and the soft palate remains intact. That approach to the clivus is slightly oblique but can provide as wide an exposure as is achieved with the approaches involving both halves of the maxilla.

Transcervical Approach

The transcervical approach, as performed by Stevenson and colleagues, is directed through the fascial planes of the neck to the region of the foramen magnum (**Fig. 2.11**).[16] It avoids opening the oropharyngeal mucosa but is selected infrequently because of the depth of the exposure and because it is not a direct midline exposure. A tracheostomy, which allows the jaws to be closed tightly, facilitates the exposure. The T-shaped skin incision includes a submandibular incision from the mastoid tip to the symphysis menti and an inferior extension carried from the midpoint of the submandibular incision across the sternocleidomastoid muscle. The fascial plane between the pharynx and the prevertebral muscles is reached through an exposure directed along the anterior border of the sternocleidomastoid muscle and between the carotid sheath laterally and the esophagus and trachea medially. The prevertebral fascia and muscles are retracted laterally to expose the ventral aspect of the clivus, atlas, and axis. Structures that may be divided from below to above to increase the exposure include the ascending pharyngeal and superior thyroid arteries, external laryngeal nerve, ansa hypoglossi, internal laryngeal nerve, lingual artery, hypoglossal nerve, stylohyoid muscle, anterior belly of the digastric muscle, stylohyoid ligament, glossopharyngeal nerve, and the stylopharyngeus and styloglossus muscles. The anterior arch of the atlas and the odontoid process and a 22-cm width of clivus extending from the foramen magnum to the spheno-occipital synchondrosis may be removed. Deviation laterally may damage the internal jugular vein, internal carotid artery, eustachian tube, and cranial nerves IX to XII.

Transcranial–Transbasal Approach

The transcranial–transbasal approach may be used to approach tumors of the anterior side of the foramen magnum if the tumor also involves and requires resection of part of the ethmoid and sphenoid bones and the clivus (**Fig. 2.12**).[17] The transbasal approach is done through a Souttar scalp incision and a bifrontal free bone flap situated strictly supraorbitally without regard for the frontal sinuses. The subfrontal dura is separated from the orbital roofs; the olfactory nerves are divided at the cribriform plates; and the extradural dissection is carried posteriorly to the lesser wings of sphenoid bone, the tuberculum sellae, and the base of the anterior clinoid processes. The clivus is reached after resecting the posterior part of the floor of the anterior cranial fossa, the upper walls of the ethmoid and sphenoid sinuses, and the floor of the sella. Proceeding downward from the sellar floor, the clivus is removed to open the anterior margin of the foramen magnum. Separation of the pharyngeal mucosa from the front of the spine permits exposure of the anterior arch of the atlas and even the front of the C2 and C3 vertebral bodies. The transbasal approach may be combined with a transnasal–transsphenoidal route to gain access to the sella and to remove all of the clivus below the level of dorsum sellae.

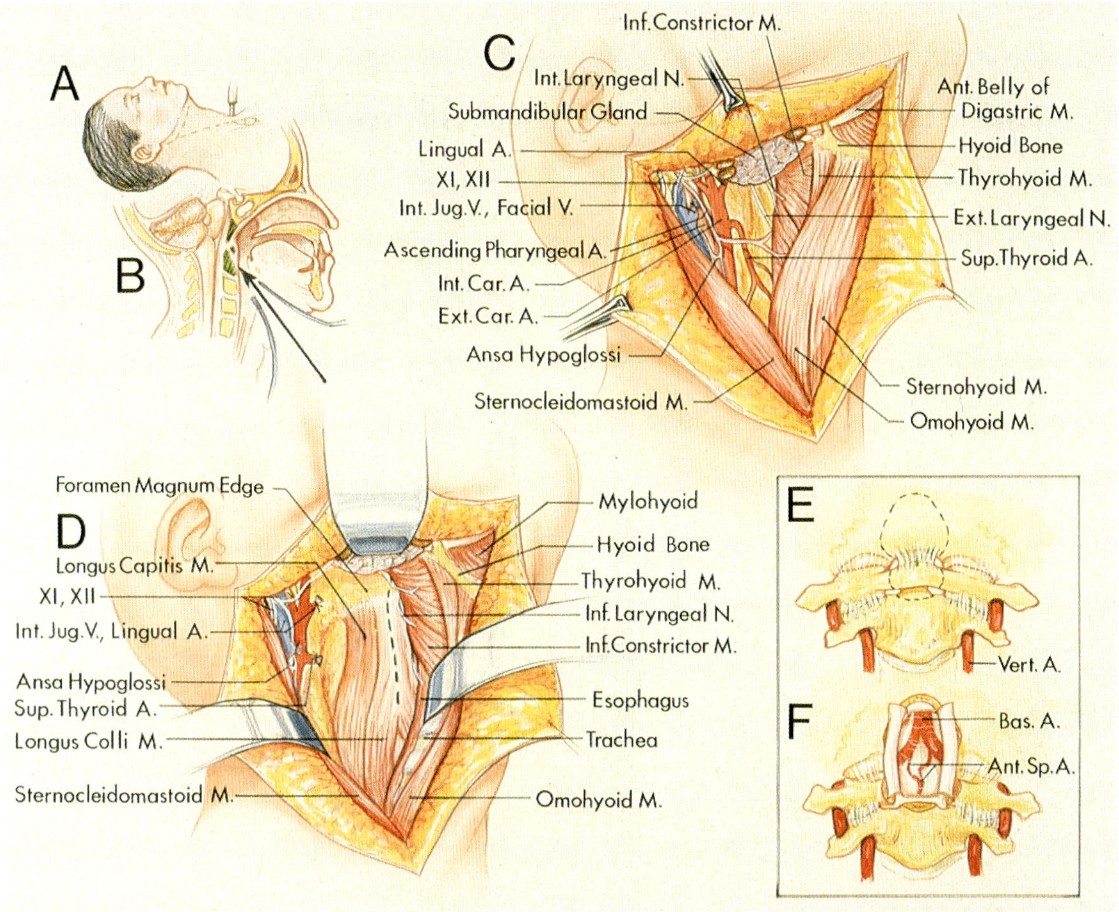

Fig. 2.11 **(A)** Transcervical approach. A tracheostomy allows the jaws to be closed tightly. The T-shaped skin incision (*dotted lines*) includes a submandibular incision extending from the mastoid tip to the symphysis menti and an inferior extension carried downward across the sternocleidomastoid muscle. **(B)** The resectable area (*oblique lines*) includes the clivus, anterior arch of the axis, and the body of the odontoid process of the axis. **(C)** The exposure is directed along the anterior border of the sternocleidomastoid muscle (*M.*) and between the external (*Ext. Car. A.*) and internal carotid arteries (*Int. Car. A.*) and internal jugular vein (*Int. Jug. V.*) laterally, and the esophagus, hypopharynx, and trachea medially. Structures that may be divided to increase the exposure include the ascending pharyngeal and superior thyroid arteries (*Sup. Thyroid A.*), the external laryngeal nerve (*Ext. Laryngeal N.*), ansa hypoglossi, internal laryngeal nerve (*Int. Laryngeal N.*), lingual artery (*Lingual A.*), hypoglossal nerve (*XII*), stylohyoid muscle, anterior (*Ant.*) belly of the digastric muscle, stylohyoid ligament, glossopharyngeal nerve, and the stylopharyngeus and styloglossus muscles. The accessory nerve (*XI*) passes behind the sternocleidomastoid muscle. **(D)** The prevertebral fascia and longus capitis and longus colli muscles are separated in the midline from the clivus to C3 and are retracted laterally using subperiosteal dissection to expose the ventral aspect of the clivus, atlas, and axis. **(E,F)** The anterior arch of the atlas and the odontoid process, and a 2.5-mm width of clivus extending from the foramen magnum to the spheno-occipital synchondrosis may be removed. The basilar (*Bas. A.*), vertebral (*Vert. A.*), and anterior spinal arteries (*Ant. Sp. A.*) are exposed in the dural opening. After dealing with the pathology, the dura is closed, muscle and fat are placed in the clival window, and the prevertebral fascia are sutured in the midline. (From de Oliveira E, Rhoton AL Jr, Peace D. Microsurgical anatomy of the region of the foramen magnum. Surg Neurol 1985;24:293–352. With permission from *Surgical Neurology*.)

Extended Frontal Approach

The extended frontal approach is similar to the transcranial–transbasal approach except that it includes an orbitofrontoethmoidal osteotomy (**Fig. 2.13**).[18] It may also be used to approach tumors of the anterior side of the foramen magnum, especially if the tumor requires resection of part of the ethmoid and sphenoid bones as well as the clivus. The approach utilizes a Souttar scalp incision, bilateral frontal free bone flaps, and an orbitofrontoethmoidal osteotomy in which the supraorbital ridges, upper nasion, part of the roof of the orbits, and the roof of the ethmoid sinuses and the cribriform plate are removed in a single block. The resection of the lesion may involve an extradural or combined intradural–extradural approach. The clivus and foramen magnum are reached after resecting the posterior part of the floor of the anterior cranial fossa, the upper walls of the ethmoid and sphenoid sinuses, and the floor of the sella.

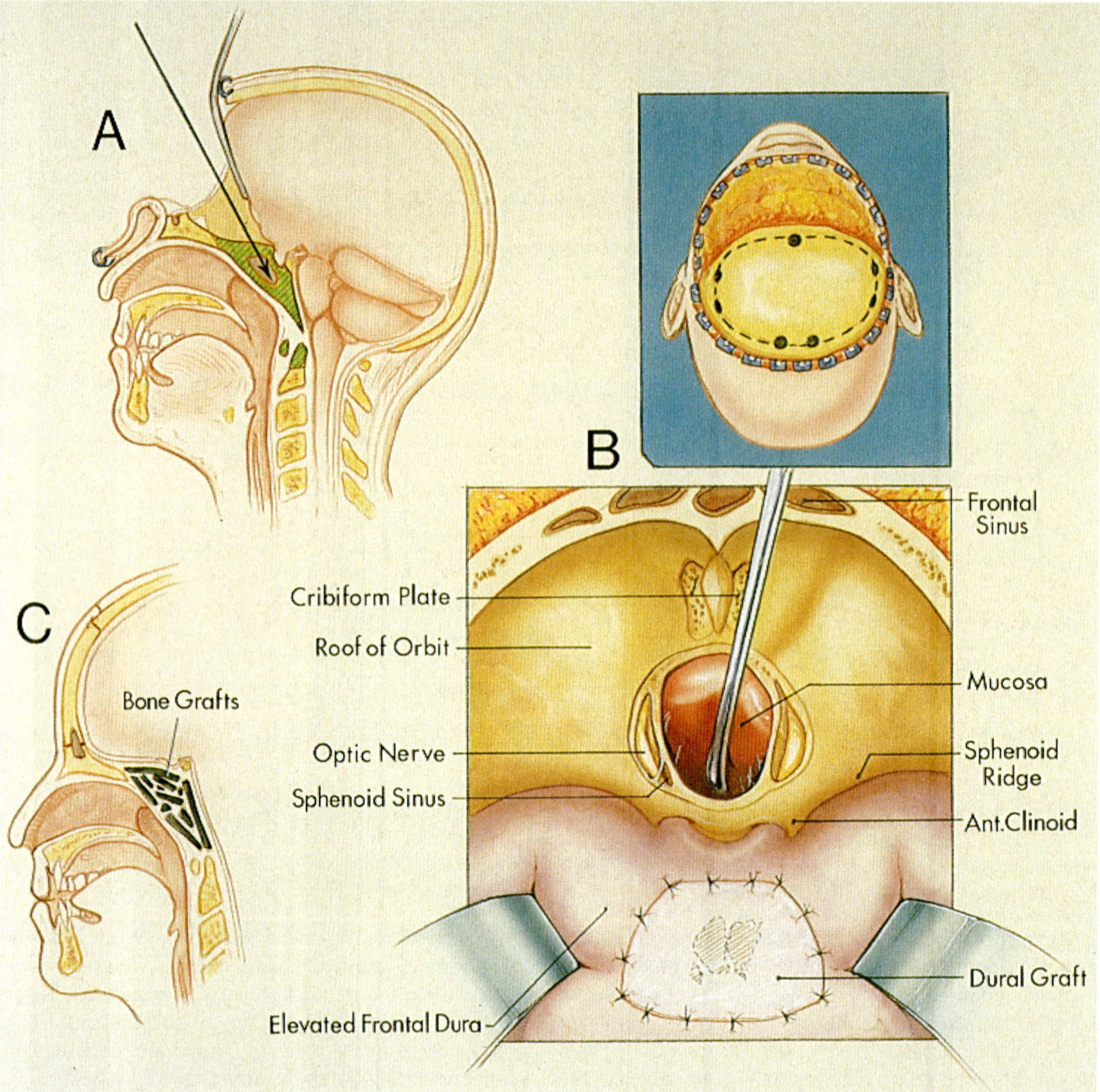

Fig. 2.12 **(A)** The transcranial–transbasal approach may be used to approach tumors of the anterior edge of the foramen magnum if the tumor also involves and requires resection of part of the ethmoid and sphenoid bones (*oblique lines*). **(B)** *Insert*. The Souttar scalp incision is situated behind the hairline, and the bifrontal craniotomy (interrupted lines) is placed strictly supraorbitally without regard for the frontal sinuses (*oblique lines*). **(B)** The subfrontal dura is separated from the orbital roofs; the olfactory nerves are divided at the cribriform plates; and the extradural dissection is carried to the lesser wings of the sphenoid bone, the tuberculum sellae, and the base of the anterior clinoid processes (*Ant. Clinoid*). The clivus is reached after resecting the posterior part of the floor of the anterior cranial fossa, the upper part of the walls of the ethmoid and sphenoid sinuses, and the floor of the sella. Proceeding downward, the clivus is removed to open the anterior margin of the foramen magnum. Separation of the pharyngeal mucosa from the front of the spine exposes the anterior arch of the atlas, and even the front of the C2 and C3 vertebral bodies. The nasal and pharyngeal mucosa should not be opened. Dural defects are closed with a leak-proof dural graft after dealing with the lesion. **(C)** The orbital roof and the remainder of the cranial base are reconstructed using bone grafts. If the clivus has been removed, the graft above the ethmosphenoidal space is fitted into the edge of a vertical graft extending from the anterior margin of the foramen magnum or the anterior arch of the atlas to the floor of the sella. (From de Oliveira E, Rhoton AL Jr, Peace D. Microsurgical anatomy of the region of the foramen magnum. Surg Neurol 1985;24:293–352. With permission from *Surgical Neurology*.)

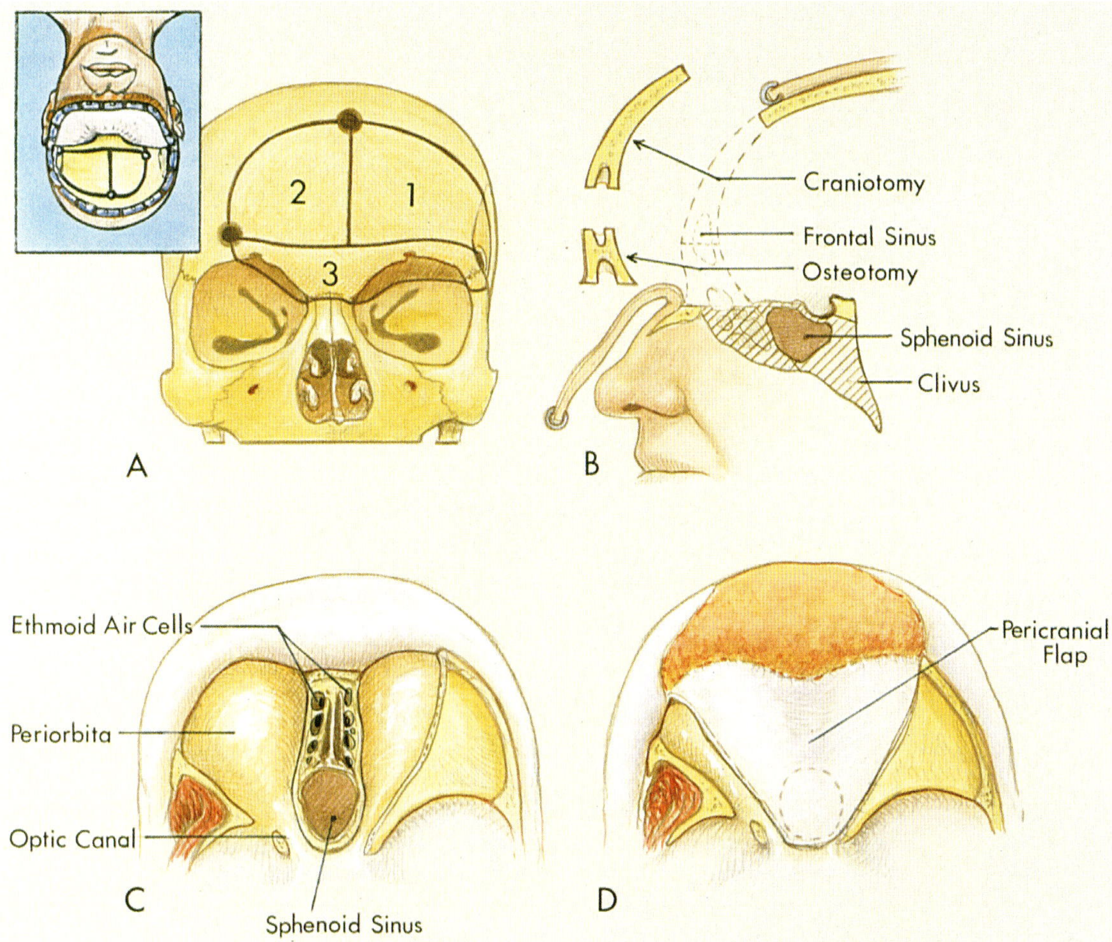

Fig. 2.13 Extended frontal approach. **(A)** The upper left insert shows the scalp flap and the order of the removal of the cranial bones (*1, 2, 3*). The third step, the orbitofrontoethmoidal osteotomy, includes both supraorbital ridges, the anterior part of the roof of the orbits, the frontal sinus, the cribriform plate, and part of the ethmoid air cells in one block. **(B)** Sagittal view. The oblique lines along the skull base show the possible extent of the bone removal. The foramen magnum is reached after removing the posterior part of the floor of the anterior fossa, the ethmoid air cells, walls of the sphenoid sinus, and the clivus. **(C)** The periorbita is exposed along both orbital roofs. The bone removal has been extended into the ethmoid air cells and the sphenoid sinus. The exposure can be extended along the clivus down to the foramen magnum. **(D)** Use of pericranial flap for reconstruction. A fat graft is placed in the ethmoid and sphenoid sinuses prior to reflecting the pericranial flap over them. In addition, a fat graft may also be applied to the inner side of the pericranial flap.

Transsphenoidal Approach

The transsphenoidal approach may be used to expose the upper third of the clivus (**Fig. 2.14**).[19] In approaching the clivus, the floor of the sella is removed and the bony opening is extended downward on the clivus to the inferior margin of the sphenoid sinus. Lesions extending to the upper third of the clivus may be biopsied or partially removed through this approach. The sellar and clival opening is closed with fat or muscle and nasal septal cartilage. The advantage of this approach is the low complication rate, and the disadvantage is the small operative field limited to the superior third of the clivus.

Posterior Approaches

The posterior approaches are preferred for most intradural lesions and especially for those located lateral or posterior to the cervicomedullary junction (**Fig. 2.15A–C**). The patient is most commonly placed in the three-quarter prone (park bench) position. Either a vertical midline or hockey stick suboccipital incision is used. The vertical midline incision is used for lesions situated in the upper spinal canal and posteriorly or posterolaterally in the area at the level of, or above, the foramen magnum. The upper limbs of the Y-shaped muscle incision begin at the level of the superior nuchal line, lateral to the external occipital protuberance, and join several centimeters below the inion, leaving a musculofascial flap along the superior nuchal line for closure. The major extracranial hazard is injury to the vertebral artery as it courses along the lateral part of the posterior arch of the atlas.

The hockey stick incision is selected if the lesion extends anteriorly or anterolaterally to the brainstem

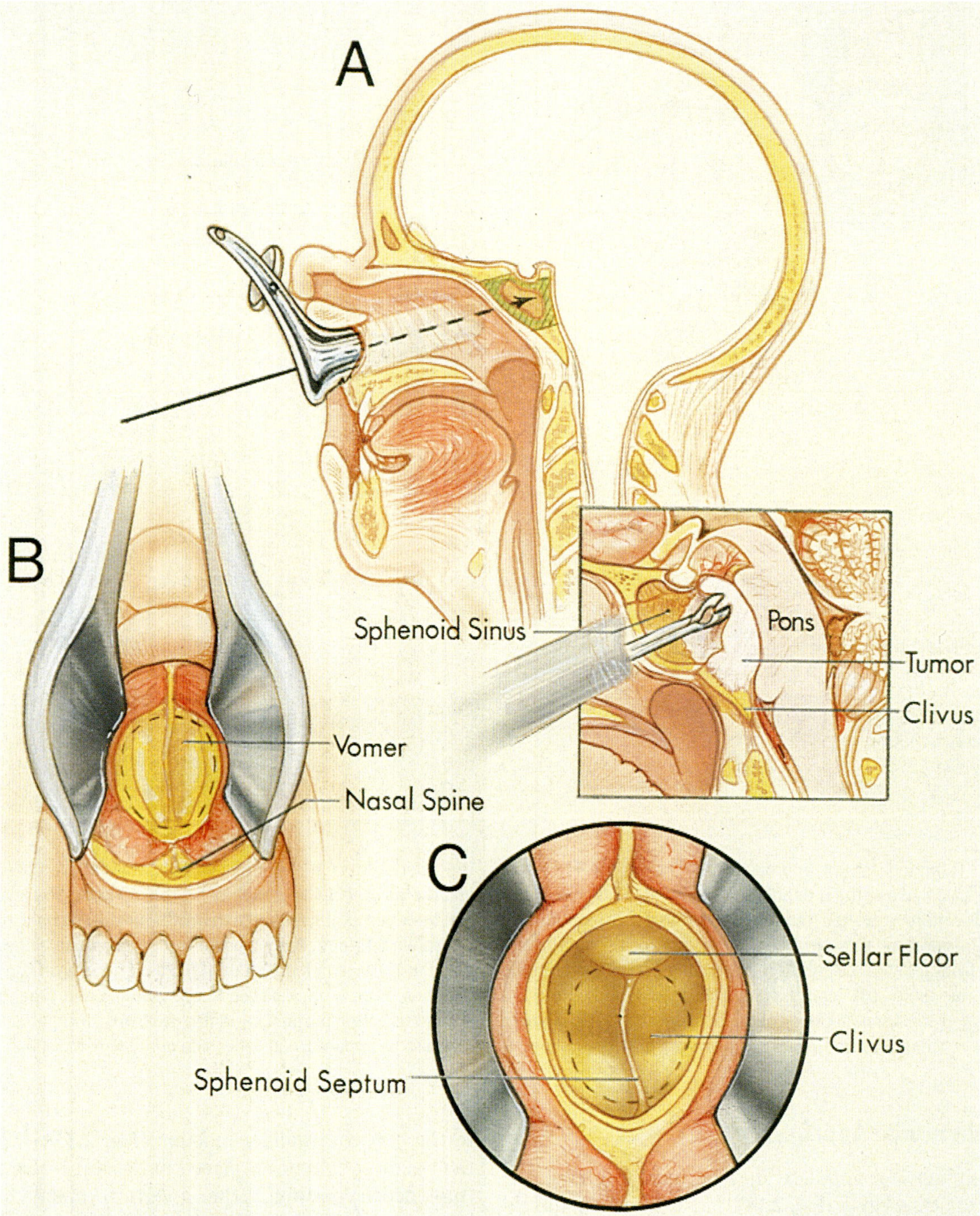

Fig. 2.14 Transsphenoidal approach. **(A)** *Upper left*. This approach directed beneath the upper lip, along the nasal septum, and through the sphenoid sinus may be used to expose the upper third of the clivus. The resectable area (*oblique lines*) includes the floor and anterior wall of the sella, the vomer, and the upper one-third of the clivus. This approach is suitable for biopsying some tumors that extend upward on the clivus from the foramen magnum. *Lower right*. A cup forceps biopsies a clival tumor. **(B)** View through nasal speculum. The anterior nasal spine is preserved and the anterior part of the septal cartilage remains attached to the septal mucosa on one side. The nasal speculum is inserted between the left side of the nasal septum and its mucosa. The nasal septum and the mucosa on the right side of the septum are pushed to the right by the speculum, and the mucosa on the left side of the septum is pushed to the left. The keel on the vomer is exposed. **(C)** Magnified view. The vomer has been removed to open the sphenoid sinus. The sellar floor is above the midline septum. In approaching the clivus, the floor of the sella is removed, and the opening in the bone is extended downward on the clivus (*dotted lines*) to the inferior margin of the sphenoid sinus. (From de Oliveira E, Rhoton AL Jr, Peace D. Microsurgical anatomy of the region of the foramen magnum. Surg Neurol 1985;24:293–352. With permission from *Surgical Neurology*.)

toward the jugular foramen or the cerebellopontine angle. A muscular cuff is left attached along the superior nuchal line to facilitate the closure. This incision permits removal of the full posterior rim of the foramen magnum and the posterior elements of the atlas and axis as well as completion of a unilateral suboccipital craniectomy of sufficient size to expose the anterolateral surface of the brainstem and the nerves in the cerebellopontine angle.

The marginal and occipital sinuses are encountered in opening the dura. Posterior intradural lesions may separate easily from the surface of the brain and spinal cord. Or they may be attached to the nerve roots and spinal cord, or they may extend upward through the cerebellomedullary fissure to be attached to the inferior medullary velum, choroid plexus, or the floor of the fourth ventricle. Resection of one tonsil may facilitate the exposure of tumors in this area. Care is required to avoid injury to the posterior inferior cerebellar artery as it courses around the tonsil.

Laterally situated tumors may be attached to the initial intradural segment of the vertebral artery and to the thick dural cuff around the artery, which also incorporates the posterior meningeal and posterior spinal arteries and the C1 nerve root in fibrous tissue. Dividing the attachments of the upper triangular processes of the dentate ligaments may facilitate the exposure of an anteriorly situated lesion. The most difficult lesions to remove are those situated anterior to the glossopharyngeal, vagus, and accessory nerves and lateral to the medullary segment of the vertebral artery. Exposing these lesions may require the division of a few rootlets of these nerves, but first the nerve rootlets should be gently separated and an attempt made to operate through the interval between the rootlets before dividing any of them. Another route through which it may be easier to reach a lesion anterior to the medulla and pons is the interval between the lower margin of the vestibulocochlear and facial nerves and the upper margin of the glossopharyngeal nerve. The intracapsular contents of the tumor are removed, and the remaining tumor capsule is separated from the surface of the brainstem and nerves, rather than attempting to deliver the whole intact tumor through the limited exposure. Extreme care should be utilized when cutting into tumors, especially meningiomas, which may encase a segment of the vertebral or posterior inferior cerebellar arteries.

A modification of the lateral suboccipital approach, the so-called extreme lateral approach, was devised to provide a better exposure of the structures along the lateral and anterior aspects of the foramen magnum (**Fig. 2.16**).[20] The patient is placed in a modified park bench or three-quarter prone position with the side of the lesion uppermost. A horseshoe incision extends from the lateral aspect of the neck behind the anterior border of the sternocleidomastoid muscle, upward over the base of the mastoid process, curving medially to the inion and downward over the spinous processes of the upper cervical vertebrae. The sternocleidomastoid muscle is detached from the mastoid process and reflected laterally. A narrow cuff of muscle and fascia is left attached along the superior nuchal line to aid in the closure. The splenius capitis, semispinalis, and longissimus capitis muscles are reflected toward the midline. Reflecting the superficial muscles exposes the suboccipital triangle, which is bordered by the superior and inferior oblique and the rectus capitis posterior muscles in which the vertebral artery courses. The superior and inferior oblique muscles are detached from the transverse process of C1 and along the rectus capitis muscles reflected toward the midline.

A retrosigmoid craniectomy, which includes the rim of the foramen magnum, is performed. The posterior arch of C1 is resected up to the transverse foramen, and the posterior half of the two thirds of the occipital condyle and lateral mass of C1 is removed. The dura is opened with the pedicle medially. A small dural incision is directed laterally, below the inferior margin of the sigmoid sinus and immediately above the entrance to the vertebral artery in the dura. This relief incision prevents the dura along the lateral margin of the exposure from hampering the view. The dural incision can be extended completely around the vertebral artery, leaving a cuff of dura encircling the artery. This dural incision, along with removal of the condyle and lateral mass of C1, allows the vertebral artery to be mobilized and gives a more direct approach to the anterior rim of the foramen magnum and the structures ventral to the brainstem and upper cervical cord. Instability is not a concern if the remaining bony elements of the craniospinal junction are left intact. Complete removal of the occipital condyle and lateral mass of C1 may result in instability, necessitating an occipitocervical fusion. Removal of the occipital condyle is done with care to avoid injury to the hypoglossal nerve in the hypoglossal canal, which is located along the anterosuperior margin of the condyle.

Lateral Approaches

The lateral approaches utilize various degrees of resection of the petrous portion of the temporal bone to reach the clival region.[21] The area may be approached laterally directly through the mastoid, labyrinth, and cochlea as in the translabyrinthine and transcochlear approaches; from above through a subtemporal anterior transpetrosal route; or from multiple directions using such combined approaches as the supra- and infratentorial presigmoid approach, to which a translabyrinthine or transcochlear approach may be added. Alternative or extended approaches, most of which include some route through the mastoid and petrous bone, include the anterior and posterior transpetrosal and the subtemporal preauricular infratemporal approaches.

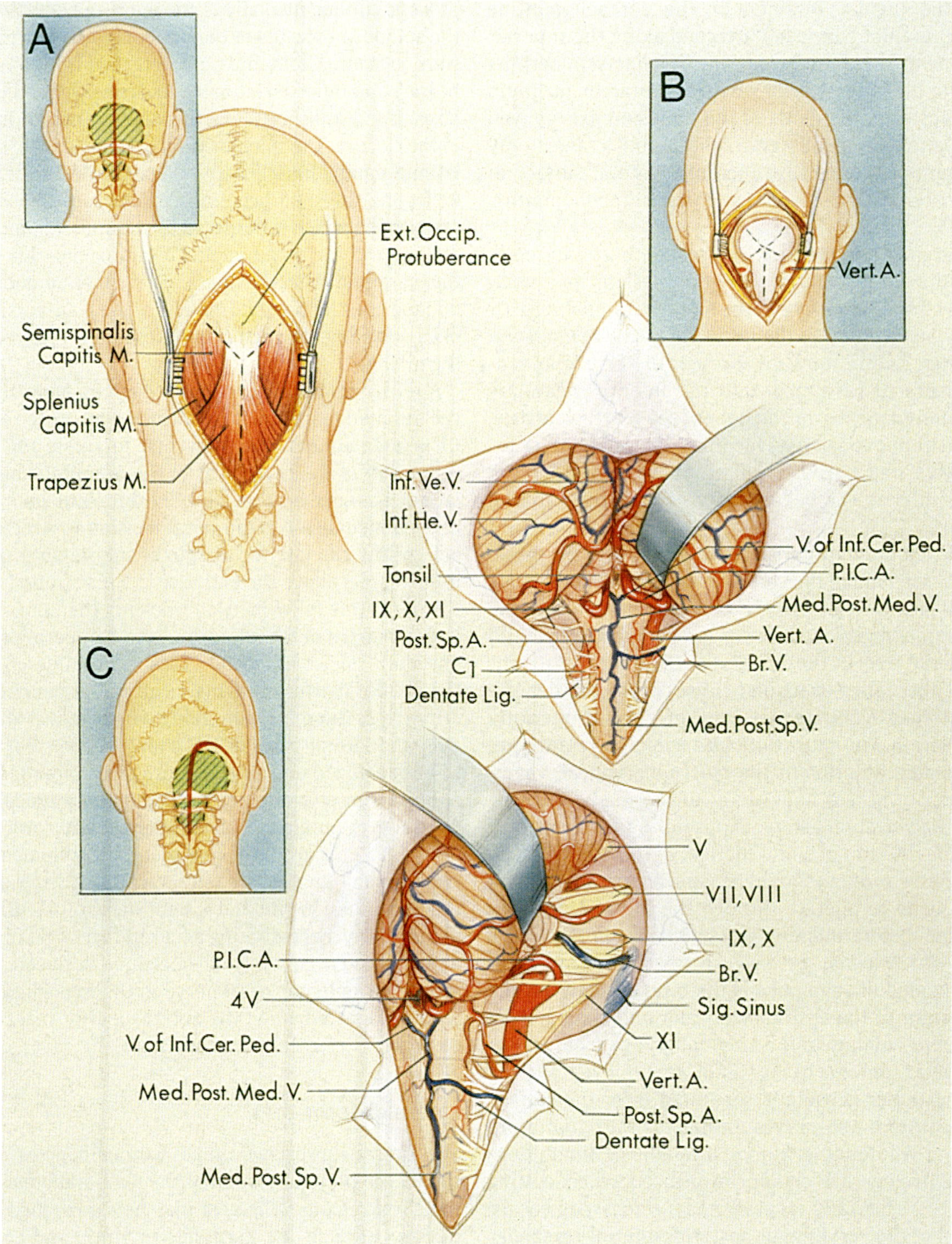
A
B
C
Ext. Occip.
Protuberance
Semispinalis
Capitis M.
Splenius
Capitis M.
Trapezius M.
Vert. A.
Inf. Ve. V.
Inf. He. V.
Tonsil
IX, X, XI
Post. Sp. A.
C1
Dentate Lig.
V. of Inf. Cer. Ped.
P.I.C.A.
Med. Post. Med. V.
Vert. A.
Br. V.
Med. Post. Sp. V.
V
VII, VIII
IX, X
Br. V.
Sig. Sinus
XI
Vert. A.
Post. Sp. A.
Dentate Lig.
P.I.C.A.
4V
V. of Inf. Cer. Ped.
Med. Post. Med. V.
Med. Post. Sp. V.

Translabyrinthine Approach

This approach is directed through a retroauricular incision. The mastoid air cells are removed to skeletonize the sigmoid sinus, middle fossa dura, and mastoid segment of the facial nerve canal to expose the semicircular canals and posterior fossa dura medial to the sigmoid sinus (**Fig. 2.17A–D**).[21] The internal auditory canal is exposed by drilling away the semicircular canals and vestibule, and the bone along the posterior, superior, and inferior margin of the internal auditory canal. The dura in front of the sigmoid sinus and along the internal auditory canal is opened to expose the structures in the cerebellopontine angle.

Transcochlear Approaches

The transcochlear approach is an anteromedial extension of the translabyrinthine approach (**Fig. 2.17**).[21] After exposing the internal auditory canal and facial nerve as described for the translabyrinthine approach, the facial nerve is transposed posteriorly. The cochlea, which is situated anterior and medial to the internal acoustic meatus, and the petrous apex are drilled away to expose and enter the clivus. Extending the dural opening permits visualization of the abducens nerve, the lower margin of the trigeminal nerve, and the nerves entering the jugular foramen.

Combined Supra- and Infratentorial Presigmoid Approach

The presigmoid approach combines a supra- and infratentorial approach with various degrees of petrosectomy, which can vary from a retrolabyrinthine exposure to a translabyrinthine or transcochlear exposure with posterior displacement of the facial nerve (**Fig. 2.18**). The skin incision starts above the zygoma and extends above the ear and downward in the suboccipital region. A temporal and suboccipital craniotomy is performed, and the transverse sinus is exposed. A mastoidectomy with exposure of the middle and posterior fossa dura medial to the sigmoid sinus is completed without entering the labyrinth. The dura is opened in the temporal region, preserving the junction of the vein of Labbé with the transverse sinus. The posterior fossa dural incision, which is located anterior to the sigmoid sinus, is extended medially across the superior petrosal sinus and tentorium and through the tentorial edge. The temporal lobe is elevated and the sigmoid sinus is displaced posteriorly. This exposes the petroclival region from the middle fossa and tentorial incisura to the foramen magnum. The exposure may be improved by various degrees of labyrinthectomy and petrosectomy and transposition of the facial nerve as described for the translabyrinthine and transcochlear approaches.

Subtemporal Anterior Transpetrosal Approach

The subtemporal anterior transpetrosal approach utilizes extradural resection of the petrous apex to reach the side of the

Fig. 2.15 Suboccipital approaches. Either a vertical midline or hockey stick incision is used. The patient is most commonly placed in the semi-sitting position. **(A)** *Upper left*. The vertical midline incision is selected for lesions situated in the upper spinal canal and for those located posteriorly or posterolaterally in the area above the foramen magnum. The incision is of sufficient length to complete a suboccipital craniectomy and a laminectomy of the axis and atlas (*oblique lines*). *Lower right*. The subcutaneous tissues are separated from the underlying fascia near the inion to gain room for a Y-shaped incision in the muscles (*M.*). The upper limbs of the "Y" begin at the level of the superior nuchal line and join several centimeters below the inion. **(B)** *Upper right*. Dural incision (*dotted lines*). *Lower right*. Intradural exposure. The major extracranial hazard is injury to the vertebral artery (*Vert. A.*) as it courses along the lateral part of the posterior arch of the atlas. The vertebral arteries give rise to the posterior inferior cerebellar (*P.I.C.A.*) and posterior spinal arteries (*Post. Sp. A.*). The median posterior spinal (*Med. Post. Sp. V.*) and median posterior medullary veins (*Med. Post. Med. V.*) course in the midline. The vein of the inferior cerebellar peduncle (*V. of Inf. Cer. Ped.*) courses below the fourth ventricle. Inferior hemispheric (*Inf. He. V.*) and inferior vermian veins (*Inf. Ve. V.*) course on the cerebellar surface. Bridging veins (*Br. V.*) pass from the neural surfaces to the adjacent sinuses. The accessory nerve (*XI*) ascends posterior to the dentate ligament (*Dentate Lig.*). The glossopharyngeal (*IX*) and vagus nerves (X) pass toward the jugular foramen. **(C)** *Upper left*. Skin incision (*solid line*) and bone removal (*oblique lines*). *Lower right*. Intradural exposure. The hockey stick incision extends superomedially from the mastoid process along the superior nuchal line to the inion and downward in the midline. This incision is selected if the lesion extends anterolaterally or anteriorly to the brainstem toward the jugular foramen or cerebellopontine angle. This exposure permits the removal of the full posterior rim of the foramen magnum, the posterior elements of the atlas and axis, and, in addition, the ability to complete a unilateral suboccipital craniectomy of sufficient size to expose the anterolateral surface of the brainstem and the nerves in the cerebellopontine angle. Tumors in this area may extend upward through the cerebellomedullary fissure to be attached to the roof or floor of the fourth ventricle (*4V*). Resection of one tonsil may facilitate the exposure. Laterally situated tumors may be attached to the initial intradural segment of the vertebral artery and the thick dural cuff around the artery, which also incorporates the posterior spinal arteries and the C1 nerve root in fibrous tissue. As one moves superiorly along the lateral surface of the medulla, the origin of the posterior inferior cerebellar arteries and the glossopharyngeal, vagus, accessory, facial (*VII*), vestibulocochlear (*VIII*), and trigeminal nerves (*V*) are encountered. The dura is closed with a dural substitute if closure of the patient's dura constricts the cerebellar tonsils or the cervicomedullary junction. The sigmoid sinus (*Sig. Sinus*) is in the lateral margin of the exposure. (From de Oliveira E, Rhoton AL Jr, Peace D. Microsurgical anatomy of the region of the foramen magnum. Surg Neurol 1985;24:293–352. With permission from *Surgical Neurology*.)

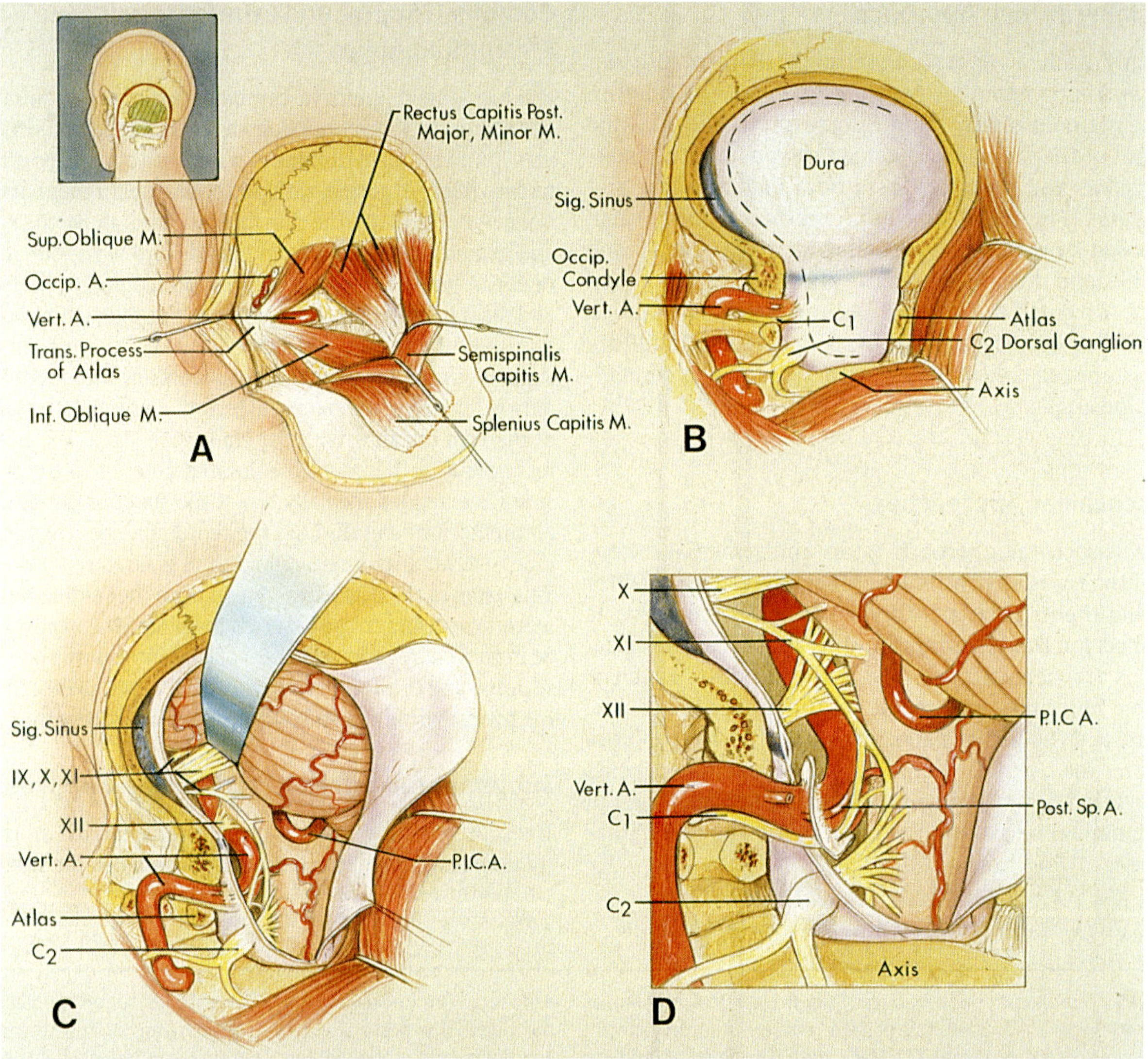

Fig. 2.16 Extreme lateral approach, left side. **(A)** The insert shows the site of the scalp incision. The lateral limb extends below the mastoid tip to reach the transverse process of C1 and C2. A horseshoe scalp flap has been reflected inferiorly to expose the suboccipital muscles (*M.*) and the occipital artery (*Occip. A.*). The more superficial layers of suboccipital muscles have been reflected to expose the superior and inferior oblique and rectus capitis posterior muscles. The vertebral artery (*Vert. A.*) passes medially above the posterior arch of the atlas in the interval between the superior and inferior oblique muscles. **(B)** A suboccipital craniectomy that extends to the foramen magnum and the sigmoid sinus (*Sig. Sinus*) has been completed. The left half of the posterior arch of the atlas has been removed. The C1 nerve root is adherent to the lower margin of the vertebral artery as it passes through the dura. The vertebral artery ascends through the foramina in the transverse processes of the axis and atlas and courses behind the occipital condyle (*Occip. Condyle*) before passing through the dura. **(C)** The dura has been opened and the cerebellum elevated to expose the glossopharyngeal (*IX*), vagus (*X*), accessory (*XI*), and hypoglossal nerves (*XII*), and the posterior inferior cerebellar artery (*P.I.C.A.*). **(D)** The dural incision extends around the vertebral artery so that the artery can be mobilized to increase access to the front of the brainstem. Removal of the occipital condyle will provide access to the skull base up to the level of the hypoglossal foramen but may result in the need for an occipitocervical fusion. The posterior spinal artery (*Post. Sp. A.*) arises from the vertebral artery.

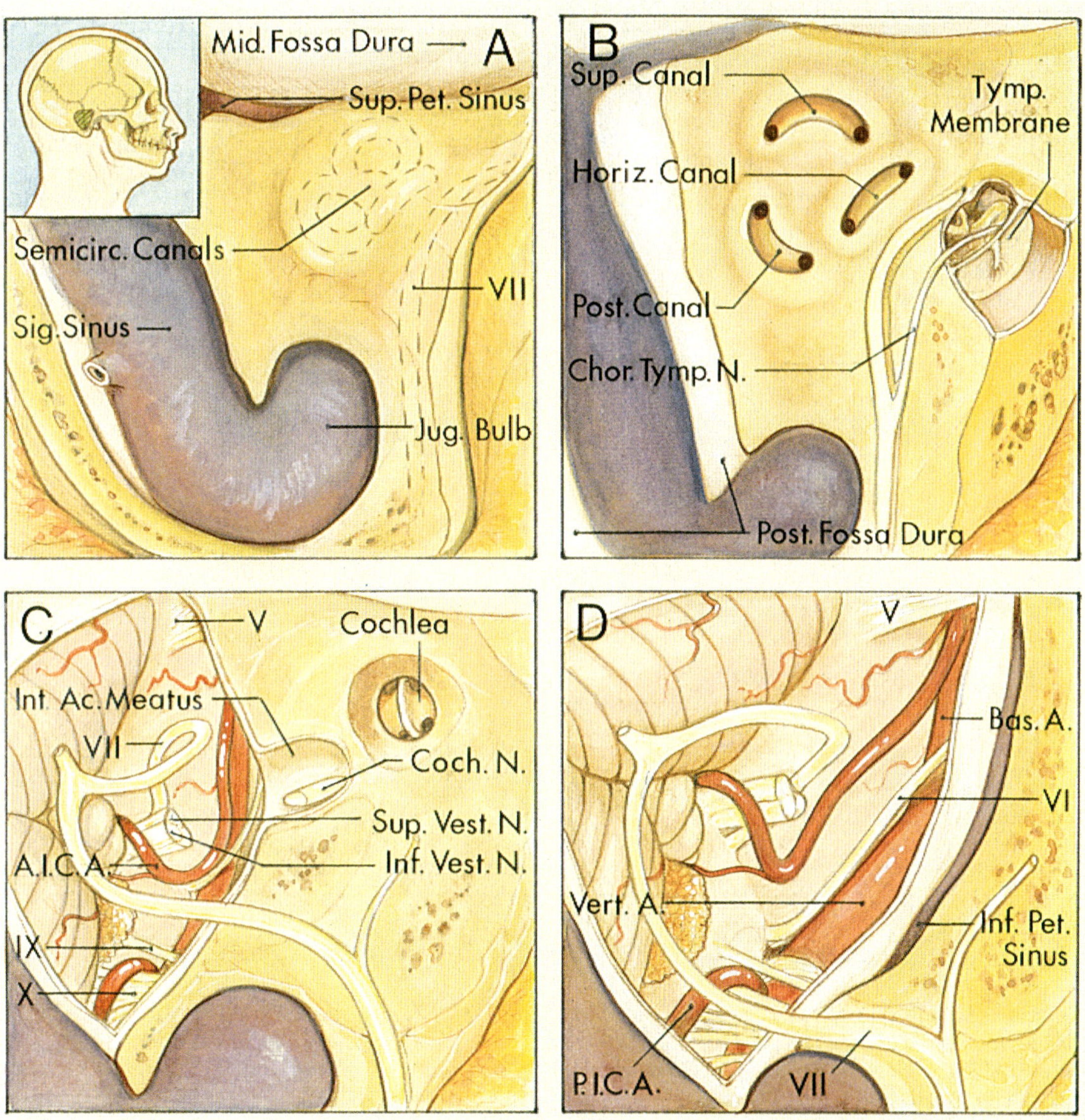

Fig. 2.17 Translabyrinthine and transcochlear exposures, right side. **(A)** The site of the mastoidectomy is shown in the insert (*upper left*). A mastoidectomy has been completed to expose the bone overlying the semicircular canals (*Semicirc. Canals*), facial nerve (*VII*), sigmoid (*Sig. Sinus*) and superior petrosal sinuses (*Sup. Pet. Sinus*), jugular bulb (*Jug. Bulb*), and the dura lining the floor of the middle cranial fossa (*Mid. Fossa Dura*). **(B)** Additional bone has been removed to expose the horizontal (*Horiz. Canal*), posterior (*Post. Canal*), and superior semicircular canals (*Sup. Canal*), and the posterior fossa dura (*Post. Fossa Dura*). The facial nerve passes below the horizontal canal. The chorda tympani (*Chor. Tymp. N.*) crosses the tympanic membrane (*Tymp. Membrane*). **(C)** The semicircular canals have been removed, and the dura lining the internal acoustic meatus (*Int. Ac. Meatus*) and facing the cerebellopontine angle has been opened to expose the trigeminal (*V*), facial, glossopharyngeal (*IX*), and vagus (*X*) nerves. The cochlear (*Coch. N.*), superior (*Sup. Vest. N.*), and inferior vestibular nerves (*Inf. Vest. N.*) have been divided. The facial nerve has been transposed posteriorly. The distal stump of the cochlear nerve enters the cochlea, which has been exposed by additional bone removal. The anterior inferior cerebellar artery (*A.I.C.A.*) courses below the facial and vestibulocochlear nerves. **(D)** The cochlea and part of the petrous apex have been removed to complete the transcochlear exposure of the lateral margin of the clivus and the inferior petrosal sinus (*Inf. Pet. Sinus*). The abducens nerve (*VI*) ascends beside the basilar artery (*Bas. A.*). The posterior inferior cerebellar artery (*P.I.C.A.*) arises from the vertebral artery (*Vert. A.*).

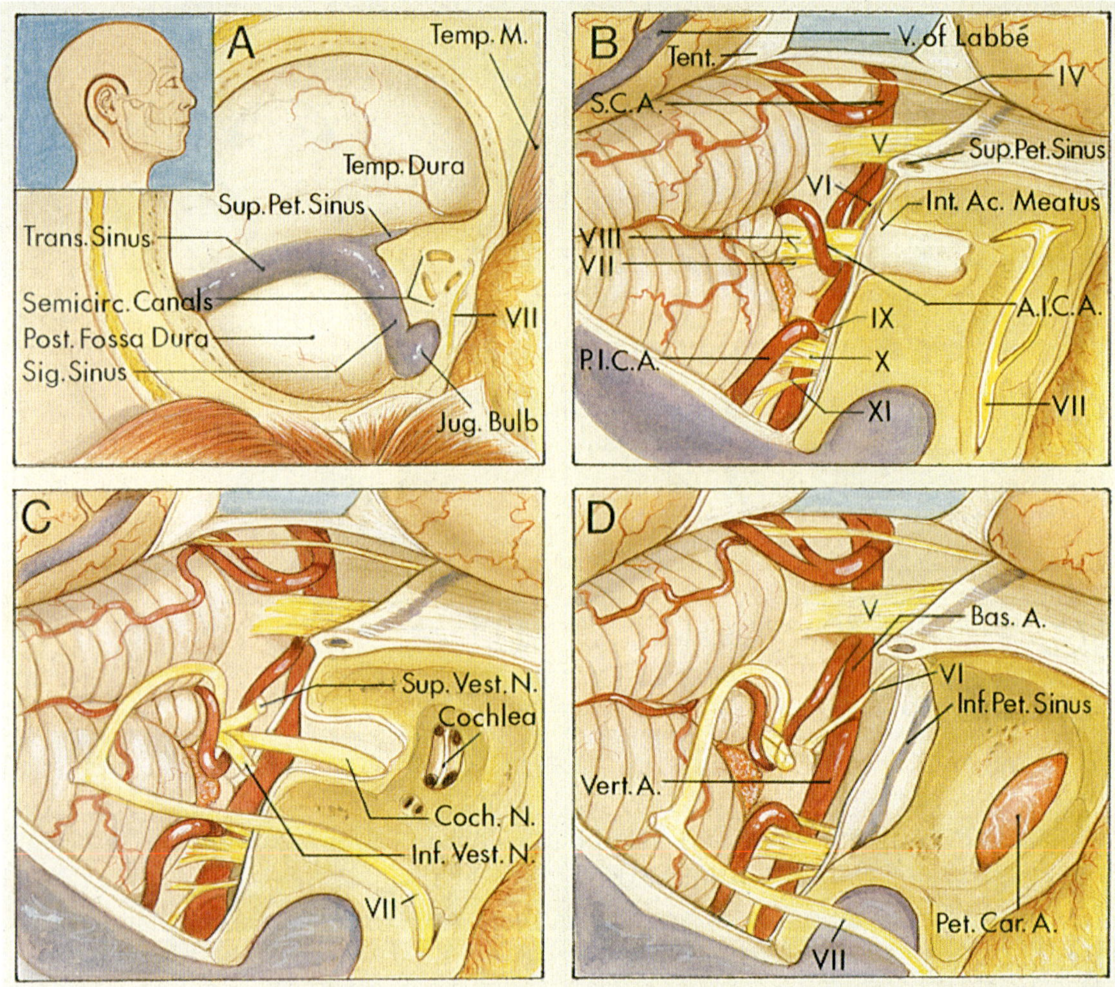

Fig. 2.18 Combined supra- and infratentorial presigmoid approach, right side. **(A)** A temporo-occipital craniotomy has been completed to expose the dura covering the temporal lobe (*Temp. Dura*) and posterior fossa (*Post. Fossa Dura*). The scalp incision is shown in the insert. The temporalis muscle (*Temp. M.*) has been reflected forward. A mastoidectomy has been completed to expose the semicircular canals (*Semicirc. Canals*) and facial nerve (*VII*). Other structures in the exposure include the transverse (*Trans. Sinus*), sigmoid (*Sig. Sinus*), and superior petrosal sinuses (*Sup. Pet. Sinus*), and jugular bulb (*Jug. Bulb*). **(B)** The dura has been opened in front of the sigmoid sinus and over the temporal lobe. The tentorium (*Tent.*) has been divided and elevated. The dural incision extends across the superior petrosal sinus and through the tentorial edge, with care being taken to preserve the trochlear nerve (*IV*) and the junction of the vein of Labbé (*V. of Labbé*) with the transverse sinus. The semicircular canals and vestibule have been removed to expose the dura lining the internal acoustic meatus (*Int. Ac. Meatus*). This exposes the trigeminal (*V*), abducens (*VI*), facial, vestibulocochlear (*VIII*), glossopharyngeal (*IX*), vagus (*X*), and accessory nerves (*XI*), and the superior cerebellar (*S.C.A.*), anterior inferior cerebellar (*A.I.C.A.*), and posterior inferior cerebellar arteries (*P.I.C.A.*). **(C)** The dura lining the internal acoustic meatus has been opened. The facial nerve has been transposed posteriorly, and additional bone has been removed to expose the cochlear nerve (*Coch. N.*) entering the cochlea. The superior (*Sup. Vest. N.*) and inferior vestibular (*Inf. Vest. N.*) nerves have been divided. **(D)** The cochlea has been removed to complete the transcochlear approach and to extend the exposure to the lateral margin of the clivus and the inferior petrosal sinus (*Inf. Pet. Sinus*). This exposure provides access to the vertebral (*Vert. A.*) and basilar arteries (*Bas. A.*) and the front of the brainstem. The petrous segment of the carotid artery (*Pet. Car. A.*) is at the anterior margin of the exposure.

clivus (**Fig. 2.19**). In this approach, directed through a temporal craniotomy, the dura is elevated from the floor of the middle fossa, the middle meningeal artery is transected, and the arcuate eminence and greater petrosal nerve are identified. The petrous segment of the internal carotid artery, which lies beneath the greater petrosal nerve, forms the anterior limit of the exposure, and the trigeminal ganglion forms the medial limit. Drilling is directed behind the carotid artery and through the petrous apex into the clivus. The cochlea, which lies below the floor of the middle fossa near the apex of the angle formed by the greater petrosal nerve anteriorly and the internal auditory canal posteriorly, must be avoided if hearing is to be preserved. The dural incision, which extends across the superior petrosal sinus into the tentorium, exposes the upper clivus from the lower margin of the trigeminal nerve superiorly to the facial nerve inferiorly. The angles of view may be increased if the area is entered through a frontotemporal craniotomy combined with a zygomatic arch resection.

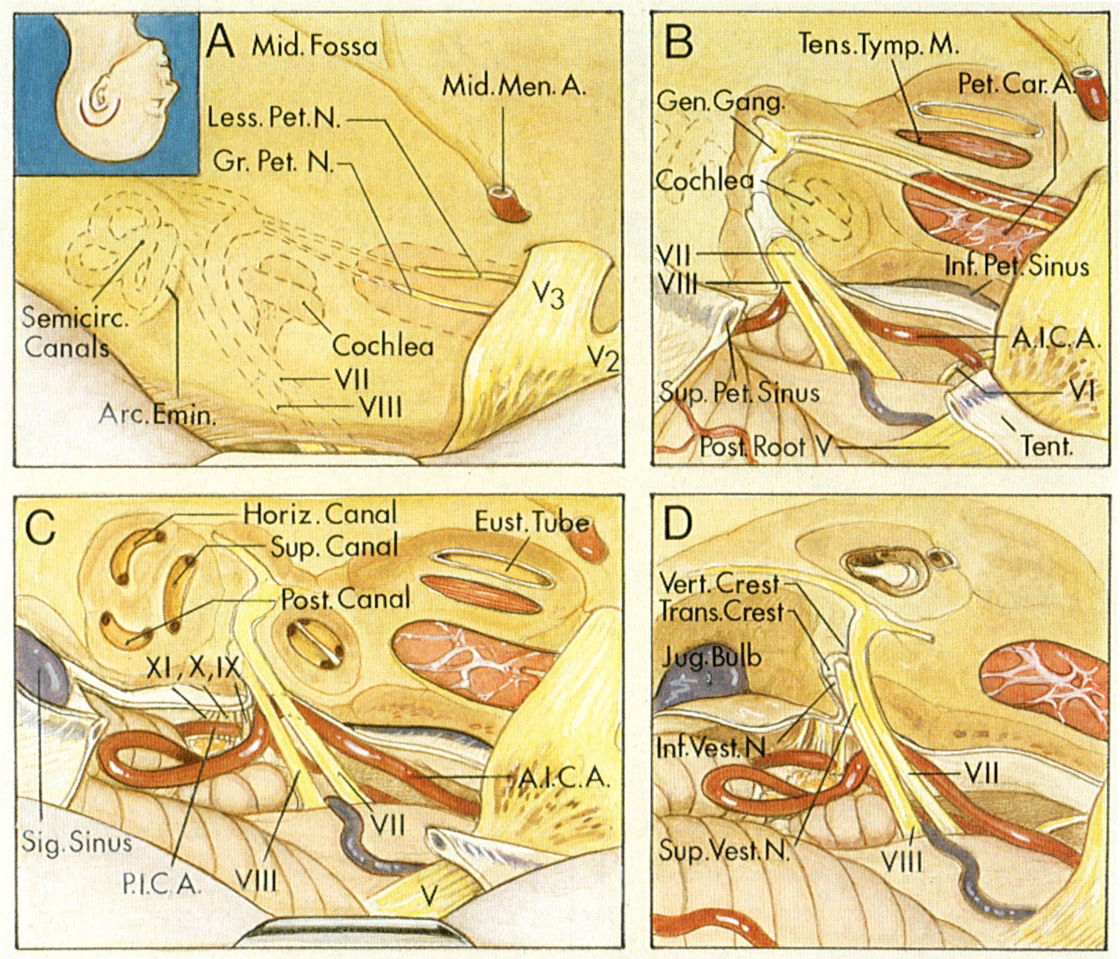

Fig. 2.19 Subtemporal anterior transpetrosal approach, left side. **(A)** The insert shows the site of the scalp incision. The dura has been elevated from the floor of the middle fossa (*Mid. Fossa*) to expose the greater (*Gr. Pet. N.*) and lesser petrosal nerves (*Less. Pet. N.*), middle meningeal artery (*Mid. Men. A.*), and the maxillary (*V2*) and mandibular (*V3*) divisions of the trigeminal nerve. The vestibulocochlear (*VIII*) and facial nerves (*VII*) and the cochlea and semicircular canals (*Semicirc. Canals*) are seen through the floor of the middle fossa. The arcuate eminence (*Arc. Emin.*) overlies the superior semicircular canal. **(B)** Bone of the petrous apex has been removed in the area medial to the internal acoustic meatus and cochlea to expose the geniculate ganglion (*Gen. Gang.*), edge of the clivus, and the inferior petrosal sinus (*Inf. Pet. Sinus*). The petrous segment of the carotid artery (*Pet. Car. A.*) and tensor tympani muscle (*Tens. Tymp. M.*) are situated along the anterior margin of the exposure. The cochlea is located in the angle between the facial and greater petrosal nerves. The dura has been opened to expose the posterior trigeminal root (*Post. Root V*), abducens (*VI*), facial, and vestibulocochlear nerves, and the anterior inferior cerebellar artery (*A.I.C.A.*). The dural incision extends across the superior petrosal sinus (*Sup. Pet. Sinus*) and tentorium (*Tent.*). **(C)** A partial labyrinthectomy and mastoidectomy have been completed from above to expose the superior (*Sup. Canal*), posterior (*Post. Canal*), and horizontal semicircular canals (*Horiz. Canal*), geniculate ganglion, and eustachian tube (*Eust. Tube*). The posterior fossa dura has been opened in front of the sigmoid sinus (*Sig. Sinus*) to expose the glossopharyngeal (*IX*), vagus (*X*), and accessory nerves (*XI*), and the posterior inferior cerebellar artery (*P.I.C.A.*). **(D)** A labyrinthectomy has been completed, thus extending the exposure to the lower part of the clivus and the jugular bulb (*Jug. Bulb*). The transverse crest (*Trans. Crest*) separates the superior and inferior vestibular nerves (*Inf. Vest. N.*), and the vertical crest (*Vert. Crest*) separates the facial and superior vestibular nerves (*Sup. Vest. N.*).

Subtemporal Preauricular Infratemporal Fossa Approach

The subtemporal preauricular infratemporal approach is directed through the part of the anterior surface of the petrous bone located medial to the cochlea (**Fig. 2.20**). The incision extends from the frontal region downward in front of the ear into the neck. The facial nerve and its branches are identified at the stylomastoid foramen and followed to the parotid gland. The zygomatic arch is divided at its anterior and posterior ends, and the temporalis muscle with the overlying segment of the zygomatic arch is reflected downward. The mandibular condyle and capsule of the temporomandibular joint are either dislocated downward or excised. The posterior belly of the digastric muscle is divided, and the styloid process is resected. A frontotemporal craniotomy is then performed, the dura is elevated from the floor of the middle fossa, and the middle meningeal artery is transected. The exposure is carried medially to the foramina ovale and rotundum, the arcuate eminence, and the greater petrosal nerve. Bone is removed along the floor of

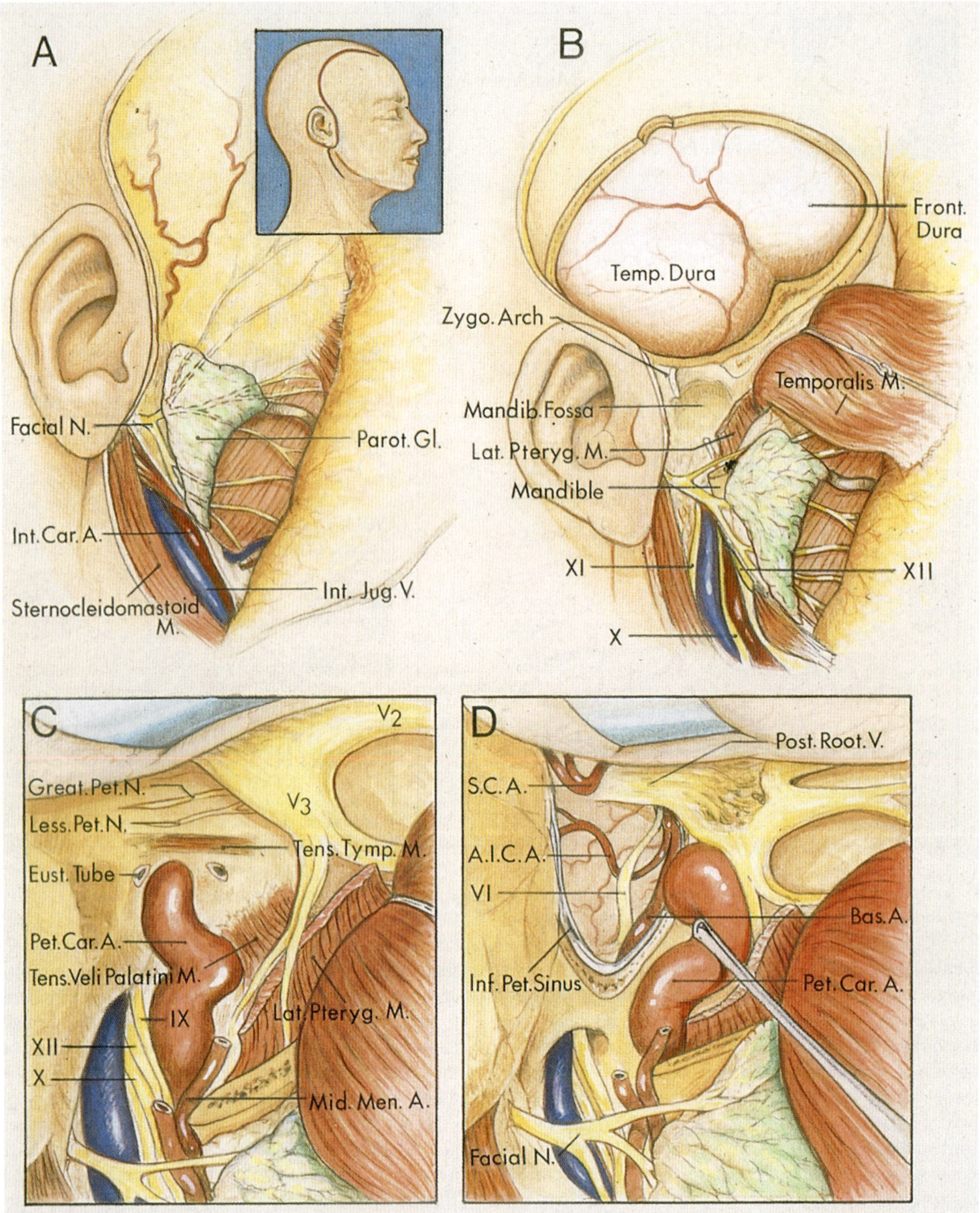

Fig. 2.20 Subtemporal preauricular infratemporal fossa approach, right side. **(A)** The insert shows the site of the skin incision. A preauricular flap, which extends from the temporal region downward in front of the ear along the anterior border of the sternocleidomastoid muscle (*M.*), has been reflected forward. The structures in the exposure include the parotid gland (*Parot. Gl.*), facial nerve (*Facial N.*), internal carotid artery (*Int. Car. A.*), and the internal jugular vein (*Int. Jug. V.*). **(B)** The zygomatic arch (*Zygo. Arch*) has been divided, and the temporalis muscle has been reflected forward. A frontotemporal craniotomy to expose the frontal (*Front. Dura*) and temporal dura (*Temp. Dura*) has been completed. The head and condyle of the mandible have been resected to expose the lateral pterygoid muscle (*Lat. Pteryg. M.*) and glossopharyngeal, vagus (*X*), accessory (*XI*), and hypoglossal nerves (*XII*). The mandibular condyle may be displaced downward rather than being resected in some cases. **(C)** The dura has been elevated from the floor of the middle cranial fossa to expose the greater petrosal nerve (*Great. Pet. N.*) and the maxillary (*V2*) and mandibular divisions (*V3*) of the trigeminal nerve. The tensor tympany muscle (*Tens. Tymp. M.*) and eustachian tube (*Eust. Tube*) are in front of the petrous segment of the internal carotid artery (*Pet. Car. A.*). The tensor veli palatini muscle is attached along the margins of the eustachian tube. The middle meningeal artery (*Mid. Men. A.*) has been divided. **(D)** The petrous segment of the internal carotid artery has been displaced forward, and bone has been removed to expose the lateral part of the clivus in the area behind the inferior petrosal sinus (*Inf. Pet. Sinus*). The dura has been opened behind the carotid artery to expose the posterior trigeminal root (*Post. Root V.*); abducens nerve (*VI*); superior cerebellar (*S.C.A.*), anterior inferior cerebellar (*A.I.C.A.*), and basilar arteries (*Bas. A.*); and the inferior petrosal sinus (*Inf. Pet. Sinus*).

the middle fossa to expose the eustachian tube and tensor tympani muscle, which are resected to expose the petrous carotid artery. The carotid artery is displaced forward, and the petrous apex and clivus are drilled away to provide an exposure limited by Meckel's cave superiorly, the cochlea and internal auditory canal posteriorly, the abducens nerve medially, and the hypoglossal canal inferiorly. The exposure can be extended to include the cavernous sinus and superior orbital fissure.

Postauricular Transtemporal Approach

In this approach, extensive removal of the temporal bone may be combined with an infratemporal fossa approach, transposition of the facial nerve and carotid artery, and resection to the jugular bulb to provide a wide exposure of the petroclival region (**Fig. 2.21**). The incision begins in the temporal region and extends behind the ear onto the neck. The skin flap is

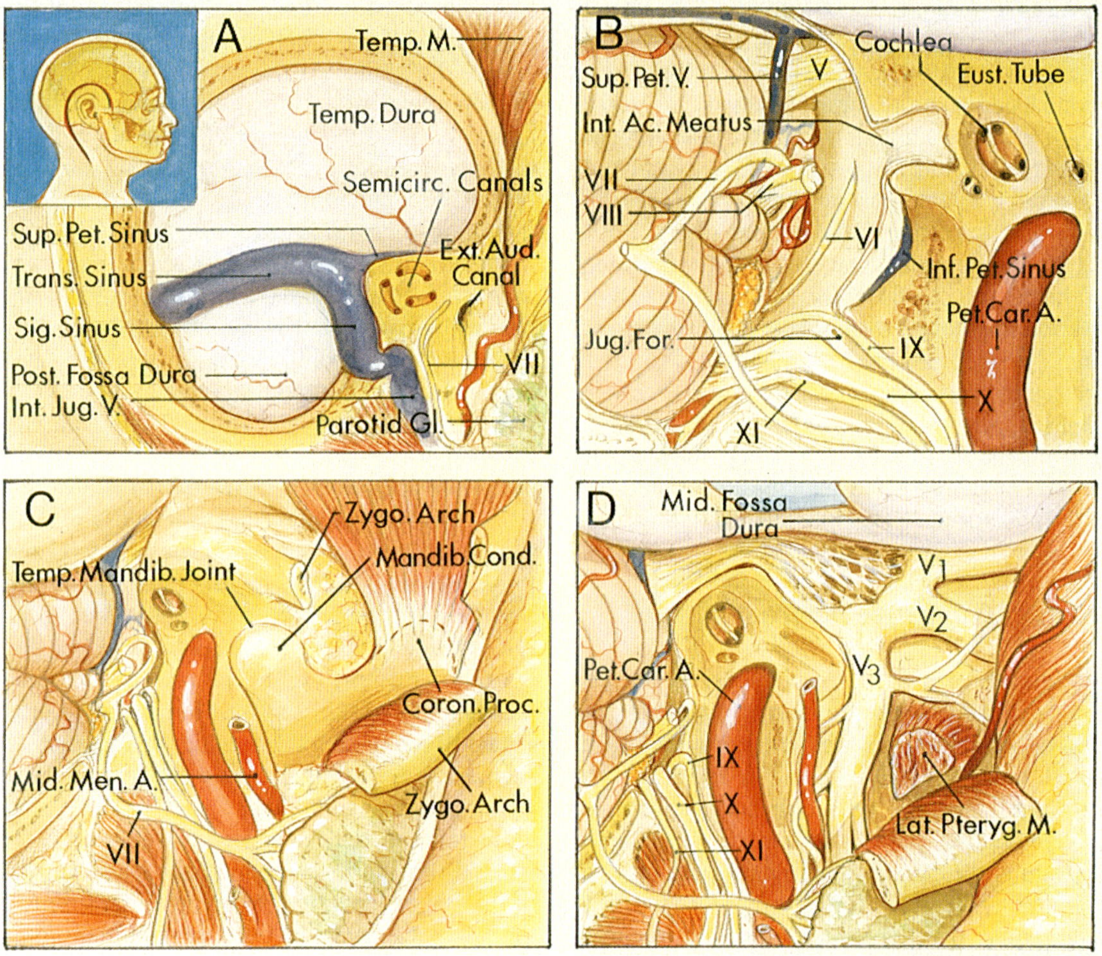

Fig. 2.21 Postauricular transtemporal approach. The scalp incision extends behind the ear (*insert*). **(A)** The external auditory canal (*Ext. Aud. Canal*) is at the center of the exposure. A temporo-occipital craniotomy exposes the transverse sinus (*Trans. Sinus*) and the dura covering the temporal lobe (*Temp. Dura*) and posterior fossa (*Post. Fossa Dura*). A mastoidectomy and partial labyrinthectomy have been completed to expose the semicircular canals (*Semicirc. Canals*). The facial nerve (*VII*) is exposed in the mastoid and into the parotid gland (*Parotid Gl.*). The temporalis muscle (*Temp. M.*) has been reflected forward. Other structures in the exposure include the superior petrosal (*Sup. Pet. Sinus*) and sigmoid sinuses (*Sig. Sinus*) and the internal jugular vein (*Int. Jug. V.*). **(B)** The semicircular canals have been removed, the facial nerve transposed posteriorly, the internal acoustic meatus (*Int. Ac. Meatus*) opened, and the drilling extended into the cochlea. The jugular bulb and the adjacent part of the sigmoid sinus and internal jugular vein have been removed to expose the glossopharyngeal (*IX*), vagus, and accessory nerves (*XI*) at the site at which they pass through the anteromedial part of the jugular foramen (*Jug. For.*). The tympanic end of the eustachian tube (*Eust. Tube*) and the petrous segment of the internal carotid artery (*Pet. Car. A.*) are exposed near the cochlea. The dura has been opened to expose the trigeminal (*V*), abducens (*VI*), and vestibulocochlear nerves (*VIII*), and the nerves passing through the jugular foramen. The inferior (*Inf. Pet. Sinus*) sinus courses along the edge of the clivus. A superior petrosal vein (*Sup. Pet. V.*) empties into the superior petrosal sinus. **(C)** The exposure has been extended forward to include the temporomandibular joint (*Temp. Mandib. Joint*). The zygomatic arch (*Zygo. Arch*) has been divided, and the masseter muscle has been reflected downward to expose the mandibular condyle (*Mandib. Cond.*), middle meningeal artery (*Mid. Mening. A.*), and the attachment of the temporalis muscle to the coronoid process (*Coron. Proc.*) of the mandible. **(D)** The mandibular condyle, coronoid process, floor of the middle fossa, and greater sphenoid wing have been removed. The lateral pterygoid muscle (*Lat. Pteryg. M.*) has been reflected forward. The dura of the middle fossa (*Mid. Fossa Dura*) has been elevated to expose the trigeminal divisions (*V1*, *V2*, and *V3*).

reflected forward and the external auditory canal is divided. The sternocleidomastoid muscle is detached from the mastoid process. The temporalis muscle is reflected anteriorly, and the posterior belly of the digastric muscle is divided and reflected inferiorly. The facial nerve is exposed at the stylomastoid foramen and into the parotid gland. The 9th, 10th, 11th, and 12th nerves are identified in the neck, as are the internal carotid artery and internal jugular vein. Temporal and retromastoid craniotomies and a simple mastoidectomy are performed. The facial nerve is skeletonized from the geniculate ganglion to the stylomastoid foramen and transposed anteriorly or posteriorly as needed to complete the exposure. The sigmoid sinus and jugular vein may be ligated to facilitate dissection of the lower cranial nerves at the jugular foramen. This may be combined with a translabyrinthine or transcochlear approach to expose the clivus. The bony portion of the external auditory canal and the tympanic bone are drilled away to further expose the ascending portion of the petrous carotid artery, and the cochlea may be drilled away to expose the horizontal segment of the petrous carotid artery. The exposure extends from the inferior aspect of the trigeminal ganglion to the foramen magnum. The exposure may be carried medially into the clivus and retropharyngeal space and anteriorly to expose the sphenoid sinus. The approach may be combined with resection of the zygomatic arch and displacement of the temporomandibular joint to give access to all of the areas that can be exposed in the preauricular infratemporal fossa approach.

Selection of Operative Approach

Anterior extradural lesions of the clivus or upper cervical vertebrae are best reached by one of the anterior approaches. The transoral approach is selected for most anterior extradural lesions because it provides a midline exposure and is the most direct route to the pathology. The transmaxillary approaches have been advocated for pathology extending to the upper and middle third of the clivus, which is difficult to reach by the transoral approach. Before selecting an anterior approach, which would require that the dura be opened through the oropharynx, one should consider choosing a posterior or lateral approach, as the incidence of CSF leaks and meningitis is high if the dura is opened through the oropharynx. The transcervical approach has the advantage of reaching the foramen magnum through the deep fascial planes of the neck rather than through the oropharynx; however, the depth of the exposure, the length of the time required to complete the dissection, and the fact that the foramen magnum is not approached from the midline have prevented it from gaining common usage. The transcranial–transbasal and extended frontal approaches offer other anterior routes for reaching the foramen magnum; however, these approaches should not be considered for tumors strictly localized in the region of the foramen magnum, but they might be used for an extensive lesion involving the ethmoid and sphenoid sinuses as well as the clivus and foramen magnum. The transsphenoidal approach provides an easy route for biopsying lesions in the region of the foramen magnum if they extend to the upper third of the clivus, but it does not provide adequate exposure for removing larger lesions in the region.

The posterior approaches are preferred for most intradural lesions. The vertical midline incision and a bilateral suboccipital craniectomy and upper cervical laminectomy are used for lesions situated in the upper spinal canal and posteriorly or posterolaterally in the area above the foramen magnum. The hockey stick incision and a unilateral suboccipital craniectomy and upper cervical laminectomy are selected if the lesion extends anterolaterally or anteriorly to the brainstem toward the jugular foramen or cerebellopontine angle. The extreme lateral modification of the lateral suboccipital approach gives a more direct approach to lesions ventral to the brainstem and along the anterior rim of the foramen magnum, while reducing the need for retraction of neural structures.

The lateral approaches to the region require various degrees of resection of the temporal bone. An advantage of the lateral approaches is that they reach the area through tissue planes outside the oropharynx. They provide another route by which anterior intradural lesions situated medial to the nerves entering the internal acoustic meatus and jugular foramen can be approached without entering the nasopharynx. They also provide an avenue of exposure for lesions that involve the temporal and sphenoid bones in addition to the clivus. One or a combination of the lateral approaches is frequently used to expose intra- or extradural clival lesions that also involve the temporal and sphenoid bones. They also provide access to the anterior aspect of the midbrain, pons, and medulla and to the cerebellopontine angle and nerves in the posterior fossa. They may also provide better access to the temporal bone, jugular foramen, and petrous segment of the internal carotid artery than the other anterior or posterior approaches.

The translabyrinthine approach provides access to the contents of the internal auditory meatus and the adjacent part of the cerebellopontine region, but exposure of the region inferior to the jugular bulb and anterior to the internal acoustic meatus is very poor. The transcochlear approach, when combined with the posterior transposition of the facial nerve, allows visualization of the structures anterior to the internal auditory canal and to the midportion of the clivus. The combined supra- and infratentorial presigmoid approach has the advantage of providing the shortest working distance to clival lesions. It provides access to cranial nerves III through XII and to the major arteries in the posterior circulation. Access to the lower part of the clivus is limited by the height of the jugular bulb, which may be overcome by division of the sigmoid sinus or working posterior to it.

The subtemporal anterior transpetrosal approach provides access to the upper clivus in the area between the trigeminal nerve above and the facial and vestibulocochlear nerves below. The subtemporal preauricular infratemporal approach, when combined with anterior displacement of the internal carotid artery, provides a route for resection of extradural clival lesions situated medial to the cochlea and extending from the level of the trigeminal nerve to the foramen magnum. The postauricular transtemporal approach, when combined with a transcochlear approach, may be used for pathologies involving the lower and middle clivus with extension to the infratemporal fossa and jugular bulb. The sigmoid sinus and jugular vein may be ligated with resection of the jugular bulb to expose lesions that extend into the jugular foramen. When combined with an infratemporal fossa exposure and anterior displacement of the intrapetrous carotid artery, the petrous temporal bone can be completely excised, providing the widest possible exposure to the petroclival region.

References

1. Coin CG, Malkasian D. Foramen magnum. In: Newton TH, Potts DG, eds. Radiology of the Skull and Brain. St. Louis, MO: CV Mosby; 1971:275–286
2. de Oliveira E, Rhoton AL Jr, Peace D. Microsurgical anatomy of the region of the foramen magnum. Surg Neurol 1985;24(3):293–352
3. Rhoton AL Jr, Buza R. Microsurgical anatomy of the jugular foramen. J Neurosurg 1975;42(5):541–550
4. Ouaknine G, Nathan H. Anastomotic connections between the eleventh nerve and the posterior root of the first cervical nerve in humans. J Neurosurg 1973;38(2):189–197
5. Lister JR, Rhoton AL Jr, Matsushima T, Peace DA. Microsurgical anatomy of the posterior inferior cerebellar artery. Neurosurgery 1982;10(2):170–199
6. Newton TH. The anterior and posterior meningeal branches of the vertebral artery. Radiology 1968;91(2):271–279
7. Newton TH, Mani RL. The vertebral artery. In: Newton TH, Potts DG, eds. Radiology of the Skull and Brain. St. Louis, MO: CV Mosby; 1974:1659–1709
8. Matsushima T, Rhoton AL Jr, Lenkey C. Microsurgery of the fourth ventricle: Part 1. Microsurgical anatomy. Neurosurgery 1982;11(5):631–667
9. Matsushima T, Rhoton AL Jr, de Oliveira E, Peace D. Microsurgical anatomy of the veins of the posterior fossa. J Neurosurg 1983;59(1):63–105
10. Friede RL, Roessmann U. Chronic tonsillar herniation: an attempt at classifying chronic hernitations at the foramen magnum. Acta Neuropathol 1976;34(3):219–235 (Berlin)
11. Abbott KH. Foramen magnum and high cervical cord lesions stimulating degenerative disease of the nervous system. Ohio State Med J 1950;46:645–651
12. Cushing H, Eisenhardt L. Meningiomas: Their Classification, Regional Behavior, Life History and Surgical End Results. Springfield, IL: CC Thomas; 1938:169–180
13. Stein BM, Leeds NE, Taveras JM, Pool JL. Meningiomas of the foramen magnum. J Neurosurg 1963;20:740–751
14. Cocke EW Jr, Robertson JH, Robertson JT, Crook JP Jr. The extended maxillotomy and subtotal maxillectomy for excision of skull base tumors. Arch Otolaryngol Head Neck Surg 1990;116(1):92–104
15. Crockard HA. The transmaxillary approach to the clivus. In: Sekhar LN, Janecka IP, eds. Surgery of Cranial Base Tumors. New York, NY: Raven Press; 1993:235–244
16. Stevenson GC, Stoney RJ, Perkins RK, Adams JE. A transcervical transclival approach to the ventral surface of the brain stem for removal of a clivus chordoma. J Neurosurg 1966;24(2):544–551
17. Derome P. The transbasal approach to tumors invading the base of the skull. In: Schmidek HH, Sweet WH, eds. Current Techniques in Operative Neurosurgery. New York, NY: Grune & Stratton; 1977:223–245
18. Sekhar LN, Nanda A, Sen CN, Snyderman CN, Janecka IP. The extended frontal approach to tumors of the anterior, middle, and posterior skull base. J Neurosurg 1992;76(2):198–206
19. Hardy J, Grisoli F, Leclercq TA, Marino R. L'abord trans-sphénoïdal des tumeurs du clivus. Neurochirurgie 1977;23(4):287–297
20. Sen CN, Sekhar LN. An extreme lateral approach to intradural lesions of the cervical spine and foramen magnum. Neurosurgery 1990;27(2):197–204
21. Tedeschi H, Rhoton AL Jr. Lateral approaches to the petroclival region. Surg Neurol 1994;41(3):180–216

3 Biomechanics of the Craniovertebral Junction

Curtis A. Dickman, Nicholas Theodore, and Neil R. Crawford

The craniovertebral junction (CVJ) has unique anatomical characteristics that enable different biomechanical behavior than in other regions of the spine. This biomechanical behavior is characterized by published experimental data collected in both the clinical and laboratory setting. This chapter defines important biomechanical terms; describes the normal biomechanical properties of the CVJ; and summarizes the effects of injury, disease, and fixation on CVJ biomechanics.

Measuring Spinal Motion

Standardized terminology and conventionalized measuring systems are necessary to define spinal kinematics and biomechanics accurately. A three-dimensional Cartesian coordinate system[1] has been accepted as a frame of reference to define spinal motion (**Fig. 3.1**). Spinal movements are characterized by two distinct types of motion: *rotations* (angular motions) and *translations* (linear motions). Each type of motion is described relative to each of the three axes of motion (*x*, *y*, and *z*). Clinically, rotation solely about the *x*-axis is referred to as flexion/extension, *y*-axis rotation is referred to as axial rotation, and *z*-axis rotation is referred to as lateral bending. Clinically, translation without rotation is referred to as subluxation. Both types of movement (translations and rotations) are important for understanding normal and pathological spinal behaviors.

Although usually reported in terms of motion in individual planes, the different spinal motions are linked, or coupled, together. Coupling refers to the simultaneous motions (rotations and/or translations) that occur secondary to the intended main motion (rotation and/or translation).[1–3] For example, axial torque produces primarily axial rotation of C1 on C2, but also produces significant coupled *y*-axis translation, with C1 positioned farther caudally at neutral than when rotated left or right.[3] Similarly, coronal plane torque at the CVJ produces primarily lateral bending at the occipitoatlantal segment (C0-C1) and at the atlantoaxial segment (C1-C2), but it also produces substantial coupled axial rotation.[4] The secondary coupled motions are usually smaller than the primary motion but are sometimes the same order of magnitude.[1,4] Posture, injury, fixation, applied load vector, angle of articulations, and other factors can influence the amount of coupling that occurs.

Biomechanical Flexibility Testing

The majority of information from the laboratory relating to the biomechanics of the CVJ has been derived from an experimental method known as *flexibility testing*. Flexibility testing is performed in vitro, using cadaveric spine segments of two or more vertebrae that have been stripped of muscle tissue, leaving the ligaments and bone structures intact. Although animal models are sometimes used experimentally in other regions of the spine where porcine, equine, or bovine anatomy is similar to human anatomy, the unique anatomy of the CVJ precludes the use of most

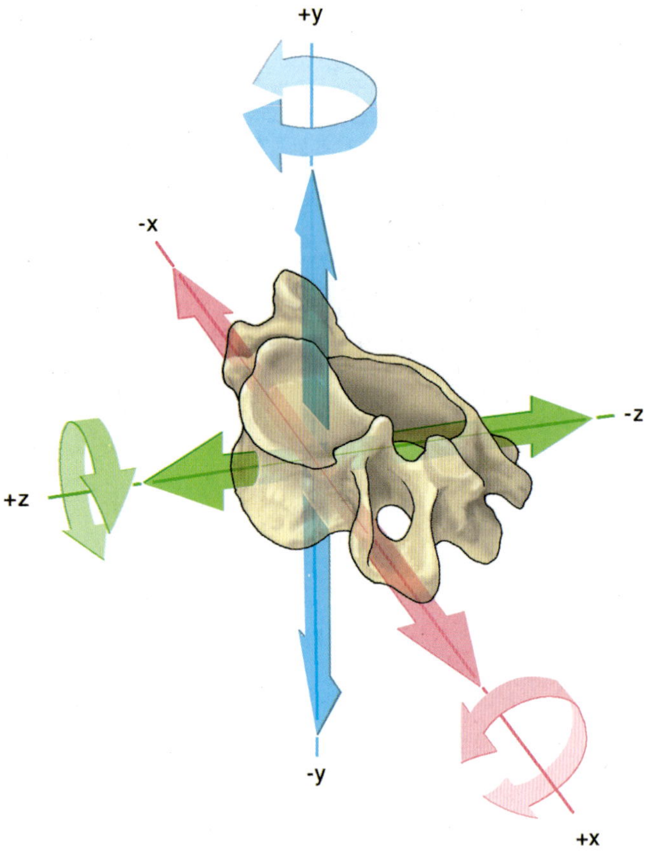

Fig. 3.1 Cartesian coordinate system for analyzing spinal motions. The *x*-axis is oriented laterally, the *z*-axis is oriented anteroposteriorly, and the *y*-axis is oriented cephalocaudally. The *arrows* indicate the vertebra's 6 degrees of freedom (i.e., the vertebra is capable of translating or rotating along each of the three axes). (Reprinted with permission from Barrow Neurological Institute.)

animal models except some primates for studying CVJ biomechanics in vitro.[5]

For a flexibility test, load (torque, linear forces, or combination) is applied to the spinal segments, and the resulting spinal motions are measured.[6] One or several levels of the spine can be examined simultaneously with a flexibility test. Results are usually reported in terms of the motion of a single vertebra with respect to its adjacent inferior vertebra: a *motion segment*, or the sum of motion across the key motion segments. Load-deformation responses can be analyzed for parameters such as stiffness, flexibility, range of motion (ROM), neutral zone (NZ) or lax zone (LZ), elastic or stiff zones (SZ), and axes of rotation.[6,7] All of these biomechanical parameters are distinct and unique for each spinal level, and several parameters are sensitive indices of spinal instability. The information generated from in vitro flexibility testing represents the contributions of the bony articulations and ligamentous attachments between each motion segment without the stabilizing contributions of the muscles. Flexibility testing is only an in vitro technique; technically, it is not possible to perform such testing in living organisms because of ethical and practical limitations.

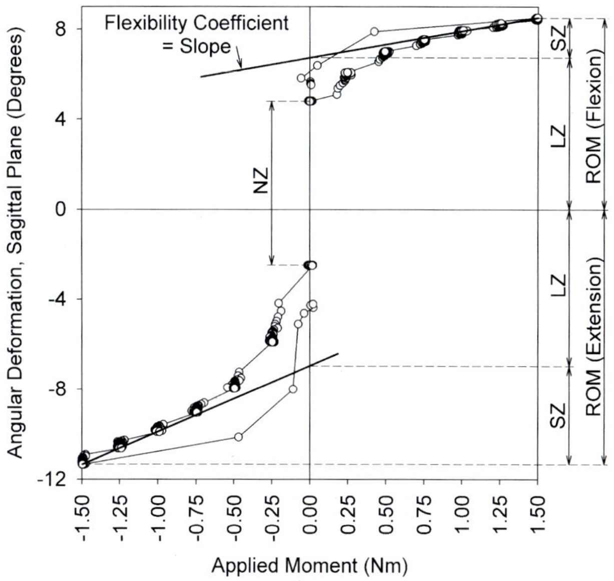

Fig. 3.2 Torque versus angular deformation for C0-C1 in flexion and extension. This load-deformation curve demonstrates how the range of motion (*ROM*), lax zone (*LZ*), stiff zone (*SZ*), neutral zone (*NZ*), and flexibility coefficients are measured. (Reprinted with permission from Barrow Neurological Institute.)

Load-Deformation Responses of the Craniovertebral Junction

Flexibility testing produces load-versus-deformation curves that characterize the unique behavior of the CVJ. These curves show applied load versus angular or linear displacement. Qualitatively, these plots represent a unique biomechanical "fingerprint" of the joint and the specimen being tested. Several parameters may be extracted from these curves for quantitative and qualitative analysis (**Fig. 3.2**).

ROM, LZ, SZ, NZ, flexibility, and stiffness are important parameters that can be measured from the load-deformation curve. ROM is defined as the displacement between the neutral or resting position of the motion segment and the limit of its physiological motion.[7,8] The neutral position is defined as the posture where minimal joint stresses occur and where minimal muscular effort is required to maintain the spatial orientation.[8] This neutral or resting position is best approximated by the halfway point of the bilateral LZ. The LZ is the portion of the ROM where the ligaments are lax and small forces produce large vertebral displacements, represented on the load-deformation curve by the range where load is near zero (**Fig. 3.2**).[7] The NZ is a subset of the LZ, representing where only frictional joint resistance occurs.[7,8] The SZ is the steep portion of the load-deformation curve near the edge of the ROM, where the ligaments become stretched and stiffness increases, causing resistance to any further movement. Flexibility is the amount of deformation in response to a unit load. This parameter is a measurement of the inherent "elasticity" or "stretchability" of the specimen.[6] Flexibility is not constant over the entire ROM of the specimen. Flexibility should be measured from the steeper linear portion (SZ) of the load-deformation curve (**Fig. 3.2**).[5–7] Stiffness is the inverse of flexibility. It is the amount of resistance to a unit increment of displacement in the specimen. Bone-on-bone contact is more stiff/less flexible, whereas a stretching ligament is less stiff/more flexible.

It may seem trivial to extract lax and stiff components from load-deformation curves instead of just evaluating the ROM; however, these separate indices are more sensitive measurements of injury and instability than ROM.[8,9] Pathological conditions may affect the lax and the stiff regions differentially, leaving the total ROM constant. These terms are important for understanding how the spine becomes unstable and how fixation devices behave, even though the terms cannot be measured in vivo.

The normal values for ROM, LZ, and SZ at C0-C1 and C1-C2 are summarized in **Fig. 3.3** and **Table 3.1**. The motion characteristics of the different levels of the CVJ are due to the geometry of the vertebrae and skull base, the shapes of the joints, and the arrangements of the ligaments. Neither the C0-C1 nor C1-C2 joints have an intervertebral disk. The ball-and-socket shaped C0-C1 joints allow slightly more flexion and extension than the other levels of the cervical spine, although they are quite rigid in axial rotation and lateral bending. The biconvex articular surfaces of the C1-C2 joints allow gliding and wide rotation of C1 around the dens. The atlantoaxial motion segment is the most flexible motion segment in the entire spine with respect to axial rotation, allowing a bilateral ROM of 80 degrees or more. More than half of all cervical axial rotation occurs

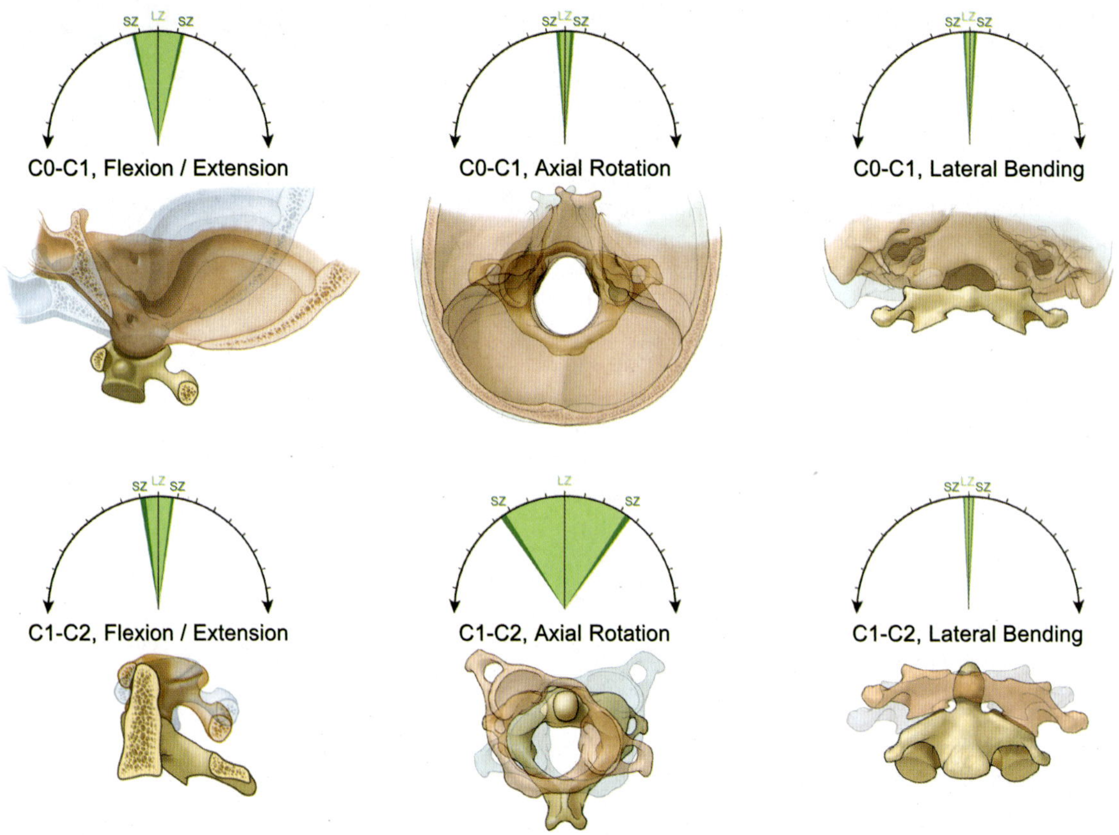

Fig. 3.3 Graphical representation of the normal angular motions at the occipitoatlantal motion segments (C0-C1) and the atlantoaxial motion segments (C1-C2). The lax zone (*LZ, light green*) and stiff zone (*SZ, dark green*) are components of the total range of motion. (Reprinted with permission from Barrow Neurological Institute.)

at the atlantoaxial motion segment, a point surgeons must consider when deciding to fuse the atlantoaxial joints. Both C0-C1 and C1-C2 allow less lateral bending than the subaxial cervical motion segments, which average ~8 degrees unilaterally.[3]

■ Coupled Motion

As mentioned, coupling refers to the secondary motions that occur simultaneously with a primary motion. The coupling patterns can be measured at each motion segment. The coupling patterns can be used to differentiate the normal from the unstable spine. Coupling can be displayed graphically by using individual load-deformation curves that represent the simultaneous motion that occurs in each of the three primary reference planes.

Normally, lateral bending and axial rotation are strongly coupled at the C1-C2 joints.[3,4,10] This pattern is due to the sloping conformation of the C1-C2 articular surfaces, which make these motions interdependent.[3–5] The direction of the coupled motions is often opposite that of the main motion (e.g., left axial rotation is coupled with right lateral bending at C1-C2).

Maintaining different postures affects the direction of the angular coupling patterns at the CVJ.[4,10] For example, when the neck is in a neutral or extended position, coupled right axial rotation occurs during left lateral bending at C1-C2. However, when the neck is in a flexed position, coupled left axial rotation occurs during left lateral bending.

Table 3.1 Angular Motions (degrees) of the Occipitoatlantal and Atlantoaxial Motion Segments

Motion Segment	Flexion			Extension			Axial Rotation			Lateral Bending		
	LZ	SZ	ROM	LZ	SZ	ROM	LZ	SZ	ROM	LZ	SZ	ROM
C0-C1	12.1	1.7	13.8	12.1	1.6	13.7	2.7	1.8	4.5	1.9	1.3	3.2
C1-C2	6.6	3.2	9.9	6.6	1.3	8.0	32.8	3.1	35.9	2.0	0.8	2.7

Abbreviations: LZ, lax zone; SZ, stiff zone; ROM, range of motion. Mean normal in vitro angular motions at C0-C1 and C1-C2 in response to incremental bending moments up to 1.5 Nm (approximate physiological limit) from 50 specimens. Motions are one-sided (unilateral).

Axes of Rotation: Instantaneous Center of Rotation and Helical Axis of Motion

The instantaneous center of rotation,[3] an important parameter that reflects the kinematic behavior of the spine, can be used to differentiate the normal spine from the injured, unstable spine. The instantaneous center of rotation can be measured during flexibility testing. The term center of rotation refers only to rotation in a single plane. It is the point within the plane of motion about which the vertebra rotates. The approximate locations of instantaneous centers of rotations for C0-C1, C1-C2, and C2-C3 are depicted in **Fig. 3.4**.

The three-dimensional analog of the instantaneous center of rotation, called the instantaneous helical axis of motion, measures the axis or line in space (rather than the point on a plane) about which the vertebra rotates at a given instant in time.[3] If the vertebra is also allowed to slide along this axis, the helical axis of motion forms a complete (6 degrees of freedom) description of motion. The motion of a vertebra from one location in space to another can be uniquely described by specifying the orientation of the helical axis of motion, the angle of rotation about it, and the distance of translation along it. The instantaneous center of rotation represents the intersection of the instantaneous helical axis of motion with the plane of interest (**Fig. 3.5**).

A collection of instantaneous centers of rotation or instantaneous helical axes of motion accumulated at intervals during a rotational movement of the spine (the *centrode*) can help assess instability.[11,12] If the joint movement is pure rotation without translation, all instantaneous axes in the centrode will coincide. However, if some sliding (translation) occurs at the joint, the distribution of the points or lines will widen. In addition, if the orientation of the lines of the helical axis of motion is parallel, the rotation is true. If the angles of the lines of the instantaneous helical axis of motion vary widely, the joint is wobbling.[12]

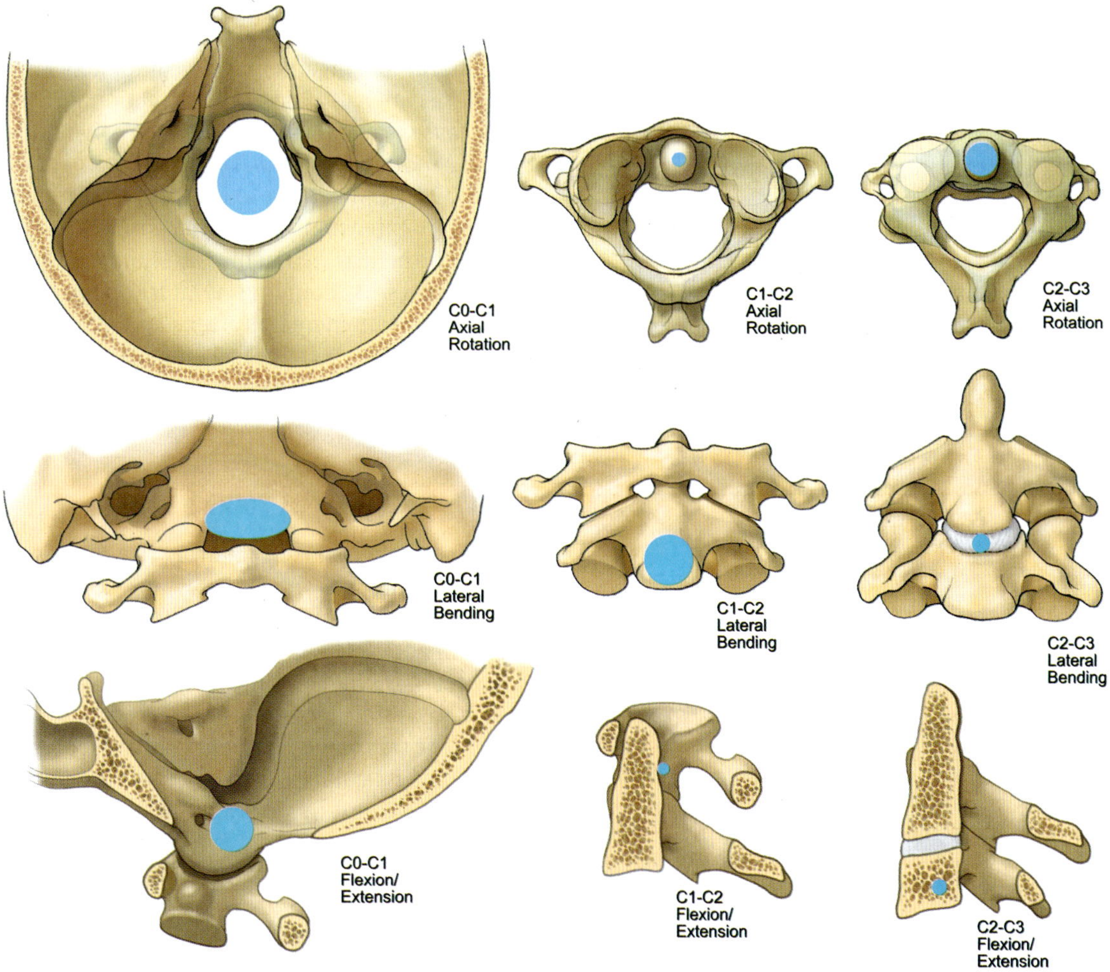

Fig. 3.4 The approximate locations (*blue*) of the instantaneous center of rotation for C0-C1, C1-C2, and C2-C3 during motion in each plane. (Reprinted with permission from Barrow Neurological Institute.)

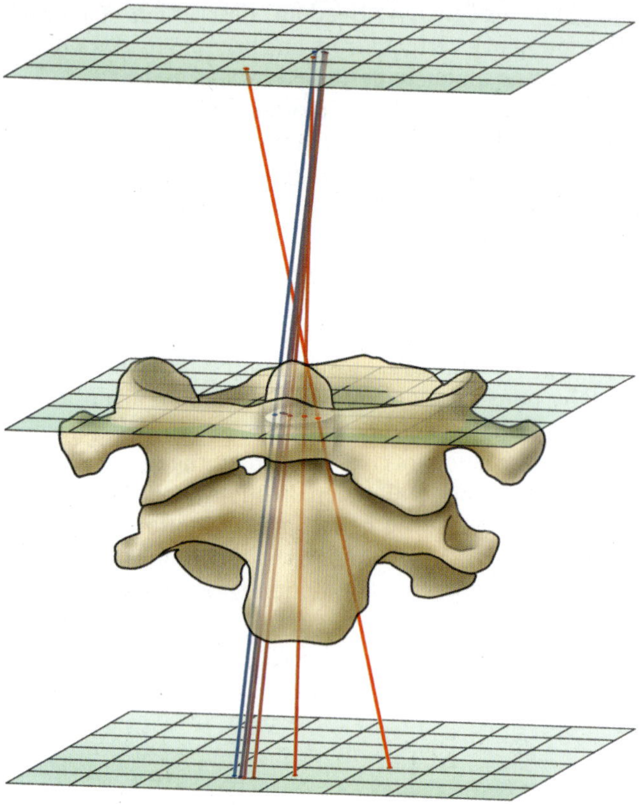

A

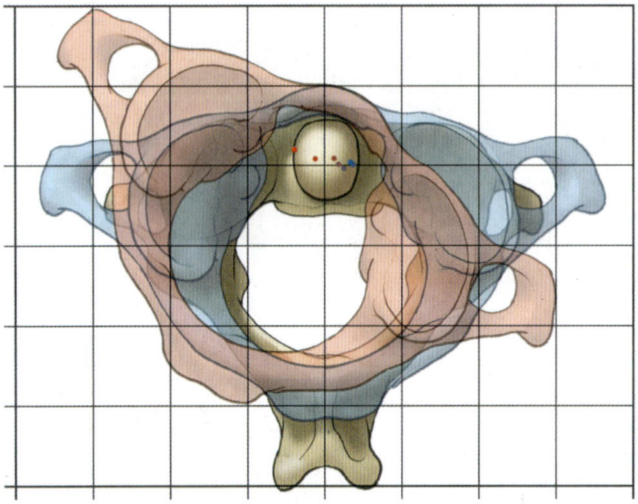

B

Fig. 3.5 The rotational path of axial rotation of C1 on C2 described for a cadaveric specimen undergoing biomechanical testing. **(A)** A centrode (collection) of the instantaneous helical axes of motion is a precise three-dimensional representation of the rotational path. The axes cross the upper, middle, and lower planes at different locations depending on the orientation of each axis. **(B)** A centrode (collection) of the instantaneous centers of rotation is a two-dimensional approximation of the same motion. The instantaneous centers shown here are the intersections of the instantaneous helical axes of motion with the coordinate system plane nearest the plane of motion (the middle plane of Fig. 3.5A). This two-dimensional representation assumes that rotation occurred only in the plane shown. Each line or data point represents a 4-degree interval in the rotation of the specimen from its starting orientation (*blue*) to its final orientation (*red*). (Reprinted with permission from Barrow Neurological Institute.)

Mechanics of Injury

Injuries to the atlantoaxial complex may be described using the concept of major injuring vector, representing a summary of the most important forces and/or moments (torques) applied to the spine and causing the injury in question. A diagram of spinal anatomy with a major injuring vector superimposed provides an easily understood description of the mechanism of injury. Some common injuries to the atlantoaxial complex are illustrated in **Fig. 3.6**.

Alterations in Biomechanical Parameters Induced by Spinal Injuries and Disease

Alar Ligament Failure

Failure of one alar ligament results in modest rotatory atlantoaxial instability. This instability is manifested as an increase in the C1-C2 ROM during axial rotation, predominantly through an increase in the NZ.[13,14] The SZ and flexibility, however, do not change significantly. Alar ligaments are important in limiting axial rotation. In an experimentally induced atlantoaxial hyperrotation, the contralateral alar ligament was completely disrupted in 4 of 14 specimens.[15] Bilateral transection of the alar ligaments causes considerably more extensive alterations of C0-C1-C2 motion than unilateral alar ligament disruption. The NZ and ROM during axial rotation, lateral bending, and flexion-extension are all increased significantly.[13,14] Damage to the alar ligament also significantly affects the coupling patterns. Coupling of lateral bending with flexion and extension increases after sequential transection of the alar ligaments.[14] The alar ligaments primarily function to stabilize the spine during flexion and extension and to limit axial rotation and lateral bending.[3]

Transverse Ligament Failure

The transverse atlantal ligament is the thickest, strongest ligament of the entire spine. It is the predominant stabilizer of the atlas, constraining C1 around the dens. Very high loads with anteriorly directed vectors at C1 are required to disrupt the transverse ligament. The mechanisms of failure of the transverse ligament have been analyzed in vitro.[16] The inelastic transverse ligament fails suddenly, resulting in anterior C1 subluxations up to 12 mm. The accessory ligaments at C1-C2 are relatively weak and stretch with ease after the transverse ligament is rendered incompetent. This characteristic has important clinical consequences. The transverse ligament tears suddenly as an "all-or-nothing" phenomenon because it is stiff and inelastic. It does not tear partially or gradually. When torn, the transverse ligament is incapable of repair. Because the ligament injury renders C1 grossly unstable, C1-C2 fusion must be performed.

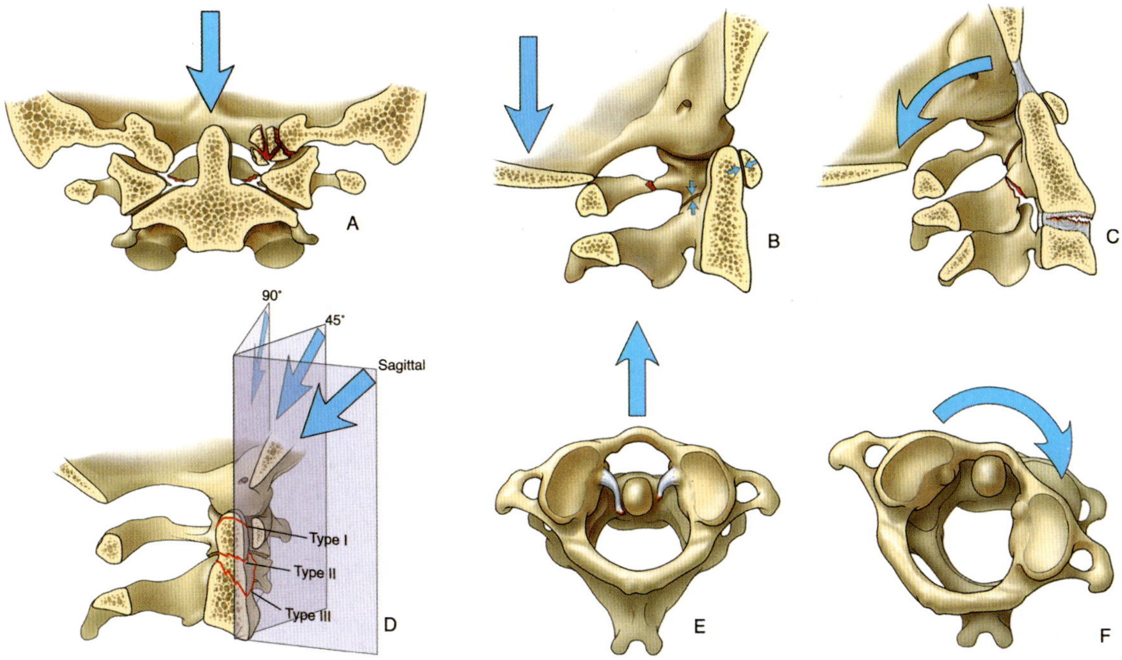

Fig. 3.6 Major injuring vectors (MIVs). **(A)** A neutrally aligned axial compressive MIV is associated with a four-part (Jefferson) fracture of C1 and with occipital condyle fractures.[43] **(B)** A posteriorly positioned axial compressive MIV is associated with fractures of the posterior ring of C1 near the vertebral artery. **(C)** Hangman's fractures of C2 often appear in conjunction with C1 arch fractures. The MIV of the hangman's fracture has a significant bending component. **(D)** MIVs of various angles can produce type I, II, and III odontoid fractures. The MIV for odontoid fractures may occur in any direction. **(E)** Transverse ligament rupture occurs secondary to an anteriorly directed MIV (vector I). **(F)** Rotational subluxations are produced by an MIV, with a significant torque component.[3] (Reprinted with permission from Barrow Neurological Institute.)

Capsular Ligament Failure

Failure of the C1-C2 joint capsular ligaments primarily increases the ROM slightly during axial rotation but has little effect on lateral bending or flexion and extension.[9] Most of the increase in ROM is due to an increase in the SZ. Injury to the capsular ligaments is an important mechanism associated with rotatory C1-C2 subluxations. These ligaments are seemingly the "first line of defense" against hyperrotation; in experimentally induced hyperrotation, 14 of 14 specimens showed disrupted capsular ligaments.[15]

Effects of Transoral Odontoidectomy

Surgical procedures to decompress the ventral brainstem or upper cervical spinal cord can destabilize the CVJ. Our laboratory examined the effects of transoral odontoidectomy on spinal motion in vitro.[17] When the dens and transverse ligament were removed, the rotational ROM at C1-C2 increased due to increases in the LZ. The ROM and LZ increased substantially during flexion, extension, and lateral bending. During axial rotation ROM did not increase. However, C1 axial rotation was associated with significant C1 translation that stretched and pretensioned the ligaments, preventing excessive angular motion. No significant changes occurred in the SZ or flexibility measurements.

Transoral odontoidectomy produced a wide range of unconstrained movement (laxity) of C1. The translational movements of C1 increased significantly, especially in the anteroposterior direction. Postoperatively, the instantaneous center of rotation centrode for C1-C2 angular motion changed from a constrained, focal distribution to an unconstrained, mobile, wide distribution (**Fig. 3.7**). The increased area of the instantaneous center of rotation centrode reflects the change in the articulations from a pivot around the dens to a gliding surface where translational and rotational instability occurs. In a different experiment, we found that an odontoidectomy in which the ring of C1 was transected to gain access to the dens allowed significantly greater lateral spreading of the halves of C1 and basilar invagination than an odontoidectomy in which partial resection of the ring of C1 spared the continuity of the ring.[18] Transoral odontoidectomy significantly alters spinal motion and destabilizes the CVJ. Despite these experimental results, clinically most but not all patients will become unstable after transoral odontoidectomy.[19] Patients with congenital bone malformations and preexisting fusions or assimilations of the joints had only a 50% risk of instability compared with the ~90% rate of instability in patients with rheumatoid arthritis. All patients should be evaluated and monitored for instability after transoral odontoidectomy. If instability develops, internal fixation and fusion should be performed.

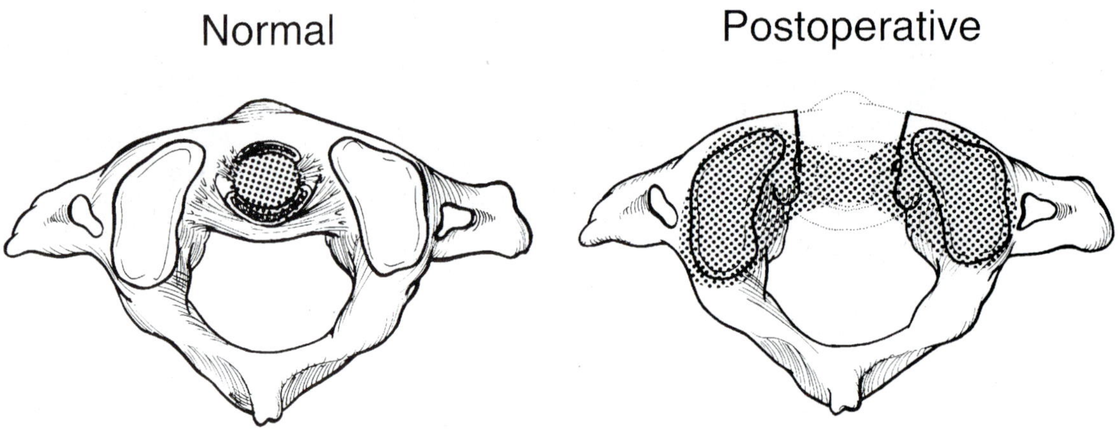

Fig. 3.7 Illustration of the distribution of instantaneous centers of rotation (centrode) during axial rotation before and after transoral odontoidectomy. (Reprinted with permission from Barrow Neurological Institute.)

Biomechanical Effects of Atlas Fractures

Experimental laboratory studies of atlas injuries indicate that burst fractures of the atlas typically result from compressive injuries (**Fig. 3.6A**).[20,21] The instability related to atlantal burst fractures manifests an increase in the NZ and ROM during flexion, extension, and lateral bending. In these studies, in vitro compressive injury caused a 90% increase in the NZ during flexion and extension, a 44% increase in ROM during flexion and extension, and a 20% increase in NZ and ROM during lateral bending. However, no significant changes were seen in axial rotation NZ or ROM. The extent of instability (and the requirement for fixation) after atlas burst fractures primarily depends on the degree of fragmentation of C1.

Rheumatoid Arthritis

Pathological movement patterns occur as a manifestation of instability in rheumatoid arthritis. Basilar invagination and anterior C1-C2 subluxations are classic, common pathological characteristics of rheumatoid spinal involvement. The disease destroys the ligaments, erodes the articular surfaces, softens the bones, and incites inflammatory pannus formation—all of which weaken and distinctly alter the normal motions of the craniovertebral articulations. In an in vivo study of patients with rheumatoid arthritis and anterior atlantoaxial or vertical subluxation, Iai and colleagues[22] found a decrease in the amount of coupling of lateral bending with axial rotation. The full ROM center of rotation for C1-C2 axial rotation in these patients with rheumatoid arthritis differed substantially from that of normal patients because of the destruction of the ligament and bone.[22] Centers of rotation were scattered widely in patients with rheumatoid arthritis. In comparison, the centers of rotation were consistently within the same focal anatomical distribution centered at the dens in normal patients. These findings are similar to our in vitro results of changes in the instantaneous center of rotation centrode after transoral odontoidectomy (**Fig. 3.7**).

Vertical Distraction Injuries

Vertical distraction of the skull relative to the cervical spine can lead to occipitoatlantal dislocation (OAD), atlantoaxial dislocation (AAD), or both.[23] Ligament configuration dictates which injury will occur.[24] In particular, CVJ regions with a smaller cross-sectional area of the caudal vertical band of the cruciate ligament were found to fail as AAD whereas CVJ regions with a smaller rostral cross-sectional area of the vertical cruciate ligament failed as OAD. Other factors related to failure mode were presence or absence of apical ligament (OAD if absent), and left–right symmetry and cross-section of the alar ligaments (more asymmetrical distribution and ovoid cross-section more often failed as OAD).[24]

Biomechanics of Internal Fixation Devices

Several in vitro studies have analyzed the stiffness or flexibility of different fixation techniques for stabilizing the spine after correctable instability (odontoid fracture), C0-C1 instability, C1-C2 instability, or C0-C1-C2.

Odontoid Screws

Odontoid screws are used to treat unstable type II or shallow type III odontoid fractures.[25] Although early techniques using two screws placed through the body of C2 into the dens were described, Sasso and colleagues[25] showed that a single screw provided equivalent mechanical stability to that provided by two screws. Importantly, neither single- nor two-screw fixation techniques restored normal strength to the dens. The failure strength of the fixated specimens was reduced to half of the original strength of the intact specimens. A later study confirmed that fixated specimens can fail again relatively easily by the screws levering out of the C2 body anteriorly during extension.[26] Odontoid screws do not immediately restore full strength to the spine. Permanent stability occurs only after the bone fracture heals satisfactorily. Therefore, surgeons should use a semirigid cervical orthosis to reduce the stress on the spine while the bone heals. The hardware cannot be relied on exclusively to maintain spinal stability immediately after an odontoid screw is placed.

C1-C2 Fixation

Posterior wired bone graft fixation, typically using braided titanium cable, is one method for immobilization of C1-C2. Several wired graft configurations have been described. Biomechanically, techniques where the wired bone graft is wedged between the ring of C1 and lamina of C2 are more effective in limiting motion than onlay techniques where the graft rests dorsal to C1.[27] Immediately after fixation, cable techniques controlled only 20 to 50% of the destabilized motion at C1-C2 in all directions. With cyclic fatigue representing several weeks of normal postoperative wear, C1-C2 cable fixation became significantly looser and more flexible. Posterior wired grafts are insufficient for stabilizing C1-C2 in all directions of loading after injuries such as odontoidectomy, odontoid fracture, or atlantoaxial multiligamentous disruption. The mean ROM during flexion-extension is 2.3 to 2.8 degrees compared with 8.6 degrees or more during axial rotation.[28] Adequate bone graft healing requires adequate control of the destabilized motion. Consequently, some supplemental fixation (i.e., halo brace or screw fixation) is advocated after C1-C2 is fixated with cables.

Atlantoaxial transarticular screws are widely considered the most stable method of fixating C1-C2. These screws are inserted vertically across the atlantoaxial joints to provide an internal anchor that inhibits rotation and translation in all directions. C1-C2 transarticular screws are significantly more rigid than wiring techniques.[29] Of the three planes of loading, transarticular screws are weakest in resisting flexion-extension. The reason for this limitation is that the screws cross the C1-C2 articulations near the center of rotation in the sagittal plane, resulting in flexing and pivoting of the screws at this location. Fortunately, a C1-C2 interspinous wired graft typically accompanies transarticular screw fixation. The wired graft is well posterior to the axis of rotation, effectively serving as a buttress against extension, a tension band against flexion, and a scaffold for new bone growth. Experimentally, addition of the wired graft significantly improved resistance of the construct to flexion-extension.[29] Rigid fixation is particularly important for maximizing the fusion rate at C1-C2 because of the extensive translational and rotational laxity associated with instability of this joint.

Although effective in eliminating motion, transarticular screw fixation is not always feasible due to an aberrant course of the vertebral artery.[30] Other methods that have been devised and tested in vitro for screw fixation of C1-C2 also may be combined with an interspinous wired graft, including posterior cantilevered rod fixation of C1 lateral mass screws to C2 pars screws (Harms/Goel technique)[31] or posterior cantilevered rod fixation of C1 lateral mass screws to C2 intralaminar screws (Wright technique).[32] Biomechanically, these techniques cannot immobilize the joint as effectively as transarticular screws because they fixate the joint farther posterior than transarticular screws. Farther posterior fixation means that both the screw–rod element and graft element of the construct for these other screw types are well posterior to—and on the same side of—the axis of rotation during flexion-extension and axial rotation. In contrast, a greater distance separates elements of the transarticular screw–graft construct, giving it better leverage against all motions. In vitro testing of the different constructs confirms the effectiveness of transarticular screws relative to the other C1-C2 screw techniques in minimizing LZ, SZ, and ROM (**Fig. 3.8**).

C0-C1 Fixation

Because C1-C2 normally allows more than 50% of the axial rotational motion of the neck, multilevel fusion crossing C1-C2

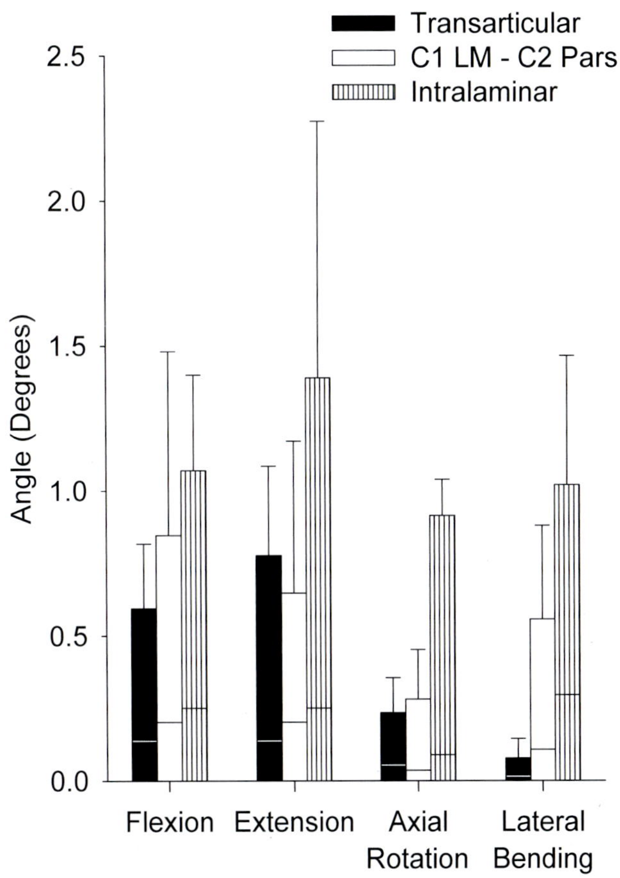

Fig. 3.8 Comparison of C1-C2 motion for three screw constructs, each augmented with a posterior wired graft: (1) transarticular screws, (2) C1 lateral mass screws interconnected via rods to C2 pars interarticularis screws, (3) C1 lateral mass screws interconnected via rods to C2 intralaminar screws. Top-loading polyaxial locking screws were used in Constructs 2 and 3. *Full bars* represent range of motion. On each bar, the portion above the horizontal dividing line represents the stiff zone and the portion below the horizontal dividing line represents the lax zone. *Error bars* show standard deviations. Data compiled from one unpublished experiment and experiments by Härtl et al.[32] and Naderi et al.[29] (Reprinted with permission from Barrow Neurological Institute.)

should be avoided if instability exists only at C0-C1. Gonzalez and colleagues[33] showed the biomechanical feasibility of transarticular screw fixation for immobilizing and fusing C0-C1 without compromising motion at C1-C2 (**Fig. 3.9**). The method was also proven feasible clinically.[34] As with C1-C2 transarticular screw fixation, the proximity of the transarticular screws to the C0-C1 axis of rotation during flexion-extension requires a posterior wired graft between C0 and C1 to ensure good resistance to all modes of loading. An alternative to this technique is the placement of C1 lateral mass screws interconnected via rods to keel screws in the occiput.[35,36] This construct can also be accompanied by a wired graft between the posterior skull base and the posterior arch of C1. During extension and lateral bending, this technique allowed significantly greater ROM and LZ in vitro than C0-C1 transarticular screw fixation, but it may be less technically challenging to perform.

C0-C1-C2 Fixation

Numerous options exist to immobilize the C0-C1 and C1-C2 motion segments simultaneously. Hurlbert and colleagues[37] studied four configurations of occipitoatlantoaxial fixation and found that hardware incorporating transarticular screws at C1-C2 connected via rigid extensions to screws into the skull base restricted motion better than devices utilizing sublaminar wires—both in terms of immediate stability and the amount of loosening at the bony interface that occurs from cyclic fatigue. Newer multiaxial locking cantilevered top-loading systems are now available and provide excellent resistance to loading in all directions. Such devices are effective in limiting motion to less than 15% of normal C0-C2 ROM in any direction of loading.[38] Instead of dorsal fixation, transarticular screws can be inserted at both the occipitoatlantal and atlantoaxial motion segments to provide a more central fixation of the CVJ.[39] As noted, adequate limitation of flexion and extension requires a wired posterior graft at both C0-C1 and C1-C2.

Biomechanical Comparisons of Cervical Orthoses

Orthoses are used as load-sharing devices to reduce the external loads applied to the spine while an injury or a fixated fusion is healing. Orthoses can act as irritative restraints to restrict spinal movement (i.e., soft collar), or they can immobilize the surrounding tissues and facial structures (i.e., molded collars, posture braces). The different types of orthoses have substantially different abilities to control the motions of the cervical spine (**Fig. 3.10**).[40,41] The mechanical effectiveness of the orthosis should be the primary consideration when a device is selected for a particular task. The halo brace is the most effective constraint to cervical motion at all levels, eliminating more than 95% of motion in all directions. At the other extreme, the soft cervical collar provides very little immobilization and acts like a "band-aid" to remind the patient to restrict motion. The various molded rigid braces have intermediate properties for controlling flexion and extension, lateral bending, and axial rotation (**Fig. 3.10**).

The control of spinal motion provided by a halo brace is related to the distance of the spinal segment from the regions of relatively more rigid skull and torso fixation. The halo

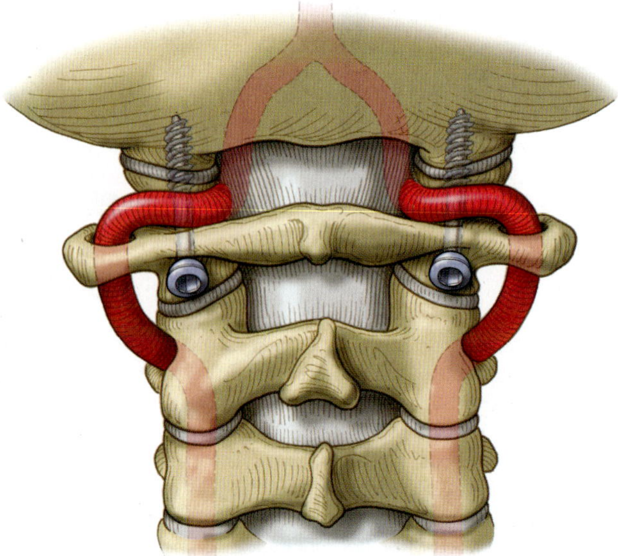
A

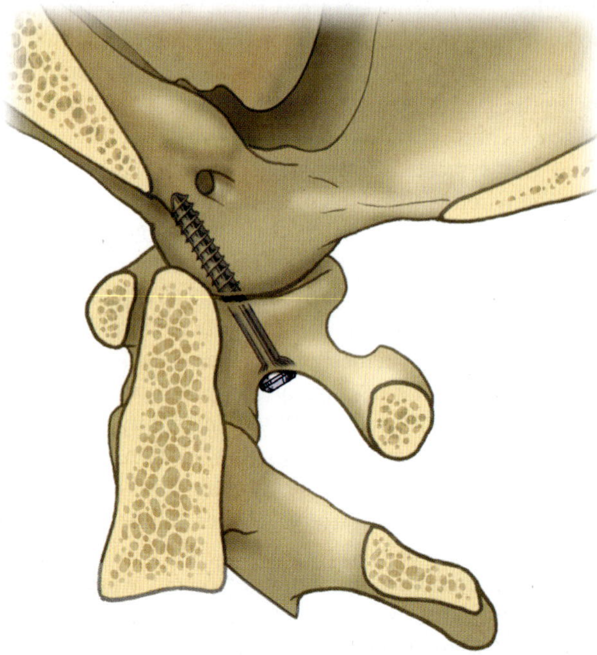
B

Fig. 3.9 Illustrations showing **(A)** anteroposterior and **(B)** lateral views of placement of occipitoatlantal transarticular screws. (Reprinted with permission from Barrow Neurological Institute.)

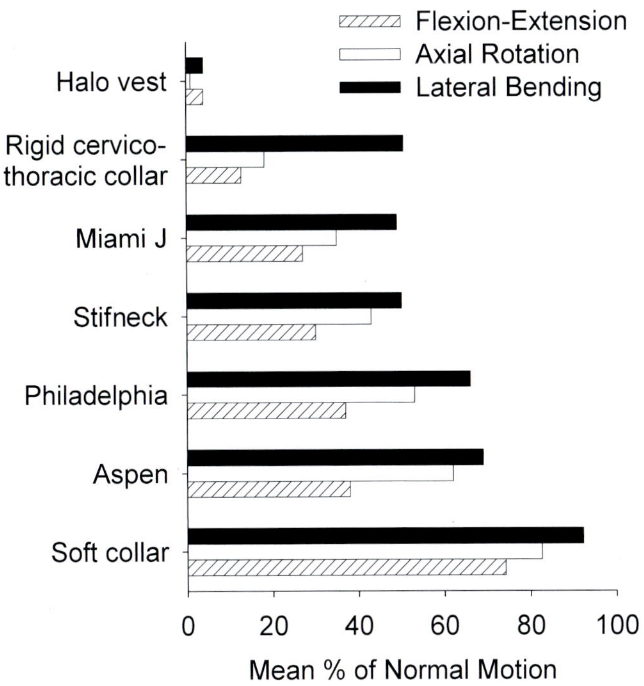

Fig. 3.10 Comparisons in C0-C7 motion allowed by several different types of cervical orthoses (based on data from Johnson et al.[41] and Askins and Eismont[40]). The halo brace was substantially better than any of the other orthoses tested for controlling cervical motion. Soft collars offer very little control of cervical motions. (Reprinted with permission from Barrow Neurological Institute.)

provides worse control of motion at the CVJ (i.e., C0-C1-C2) and cervicothoracic junction and better control of midcervical motion.[42] This pattern reflects snaking movements of the spine, which can occur analogous to the undulations of a snake when it is picked up by its head and tail. The thoracic vest must harness the thorax and fit snugly (like a saddle on a horse) to provide adequate halo fixation.[42]

Conclusion

The biomechanics and kinematics of the CVJ are physiologically interdependent with the configuration and mechanical properties of the bones and ligaments that compose this region. The normal and pathological mechanical responses studied in vitro and in vivo provide an improved understanding of the treatment of clinical spinal instability. Behavior of the occipitoatlantal and atlantoaxial joints is described comprehensively in terms of LZ, SZ, ROM, flexibility, stiffness, instantaneous axes of rotation, and coupling patterns. Injury, diseases, surgical interventions, and orthoses can significantly affect spinal stability. The effects can be measured precisely as alterations in the biomechanical response patterns of CVJ movement. Ultimately, the effectiveness of different fixation devices is measured by their ability to rigidly immobilize the unstable spine, to facilitate bone healing, and to protect neurological function.

References

1. Panjabi MM, White AA III, Brand RA Jr. A note on defining body parts configurations. J Biomech 1974;7(4):385–387
2. Goel VK. Three-dimensional motion behavior of the human spine—a question of terminology. J Biomech Eng 1987;109(4):353–355
3. White AA III, Panjabi M. Clinical Biomechanics of the Spine. 2nd ed. Philadelphia, PA: Lippincott; 1990
4. Panjabi MM, Oda T, Crisco JJ III, Dvorak J, Grob D. Posture affects motion coupling patterns of the upper cervical spine. J Orthop Res 1993;11(4):525–536
5. Dickman CA, Crawford NR, Tominaga T, Brantley AG, Coons S, Sonntag VK. Morphology and kinematics of the baboon upper cervical spine. A model of the atlantoaxial complex. Spine 1994;19(22):2518–2523
6. Panjabi MM. Biomechanical evaluation of spinal fixation devices: I. A conceptual framework. Spine 1988;13(10):1129–1134
7. Crawford NR, Peles JD, Dickman CA. The spinal lax zone and neutral zone: measurement techniques and parameter comparisons. J Spinal Disord 1998;11(5):416–429
8. Panjabi MM. The stabilizing system of the spine. Part II. Neutral zone and instability hypothesis. J Spinal Disord 1992;5(4):390–396, discussion 397
9. Crisco JJ III, Oda T, Panjabi MM, Bueff HU, Dvorák J, Grob D. Transections of the C1-C2 joint capsular ligaments in the cadaveric spine. Spine 1991;16(10, Suppl):S474–S479
10. Crawford NR, Yamaguchi GT, Dickman CA. Methods for determining spinal flexion/extension, lateral bending, and axial rotation from marker coordinate data: analysis and refinement. Hum Mov Sci 1996;15(1):55–78
11. Gertzbein SD, Seligman J, Holtby R, et al. Centrode patterns and segmental instability in degenerative disc disease. Spine 1985;10(3):257–261
12. Winters JM, Peles JD, Osterbauer PJ, Derickson K, Deboer KF, Fuhr AW. Three-dimensional head axis of rotation during tracking movements. A tool for assessing neck neuromechanical function. Spine 1993;18(9):1178–1185
13. Panjabi M, Dvorak J, Crisco JJ III, Oda T, Wang P, Grob D. Effects of alar ligament transection on upper cervical spine rotation. J Orthop Res 1991;9(4):584–593
14. Panjabi M, Dvorak J, Crisco J III, Oda T, Hilibrand A, Grob D. Flexion, extension, and lateral bending of the upper cervical spine in response to alar ligament transections. J Spinal Disord 1991;4(2):157–167
15. Rocha R, Sawa AG, Baek S, et al. Atlantoaxial rotatory subluxation with ligamentous disruption: a biomechanical comparison of current fusion methods. Neurosurgery 2009;64(3, Suppl):137–143, discussion 143–144
16. Fielding JW, Cochran GB, Lawsing JF III, Hohl M. Tears of the transverse ligament of the atlas. A clinical and biomechanical study. J Bone Joint Surg Am 1974;56(8):1683–1691
17. Dickman CA, Crawford NR, Brantley AG, Sonntag VK. Biomechanical effects of transoral odontoidectomy. Neurosurgery 1995;36(6):1146–1152, discussion 1152–1153
18. Naderi S, Crawford NR, Melton MS, Sonntag VK, Dickman CA. Biomechanical analysis of cranial settling after transoral odontoidectomy. Neurosurg Focus 1999;6(6):e7
19. Dickman CA, Locantro J, Fessler RG. The influence of transoral odontoid resection on stability of the craniovertebral junction. J Neurosurg 1992;77(4):525–530
20. Oda T, Panjabi MM, Crisco JJ III, Oxland TR, Katz L, Nolte LP. Experimental study of atlas injuries. II. Relevance to clinical diagnosis and treatment. Spine 1991;16(10, Suppl):S466–S473

21. Panjabi MM, Oda T, Crisco JJ III, Oxland TR, Katz L, Nolte LP. Experimental study of atlas injuries. I. Biomechanical analysis of their mechanisms and fracture patterns. Spine 1991;16(10, Suppl): S460–S465
22. Iai H, Goto S, Yamagata M, et al. Three-dimensional motion of the upper cervical spine in rheumatoid arthritis. Spine 1994;19(3): 272–276
23. Gonzalez LF, Fiorella D, Crawford NR, et al. Vertical atlantoaxial distraction injuries: radiological criteria and clinical implications. J Neurosurg Spine 2004;1(3):273–280
24. Yüksel KZ, Yüksel M, Gonzalez LF, et al. Occipitocervical vertical distraction injuries: anatomical biomechanical, and 3-tesla magnetic resonance imaging investigation. Spine 2008;33(19):2066–2073
25. Sasso R, Doherty BJ, Crawford MJ, Heggeness MH. Biomechanics of odontoid fracture fixation. Comparison of the one- and two-screw technique. Spine 1993;18(14):1950–1953
26. Ames CP, Crawford NR, Chamberlain RH, Deshmukh V, Sadikovic B, Sonntag VK. Biomechanical evaluation of a bioresorbable odontoid screw. J Neurosurg Spine 2005;2(2):182–187
27. Dickman CA, Crawford NR, Paramore CG. Biomechanical characteristics of C1-2 cable fixations. J Neurosurg 1996;85(2):316–322
28. Crawford NR, Hurlbert RJ, Choi WG, Dickman CA. Differential biomechanical effects of injury and wiring at C1-C2. Spine 1999;24(18):1894–1902
29. Naderi S, Crawford NR, Song GS, Sonntag VK, Dickman CA. Biomechanical comparison of C1-C2 posterior fixations. Cable, graft, and screw combinations. Spine 1998;23(18):1946–1955, discussion 1955–1956
30. Paramore CG, Dickman CA, Sonntag VK. The anatomical suitability of the C1-2 complex for transarticular screw fixation. J Neurosurg 1996;85(2):221–224
31. Hott JS, Lynch JJ, Chamberlain RH, Sonntag VK, Crawford NR. Biomechanical comparison of C1-2 posterior fixation techniques. J Neurosurg Spine 2005;2(2):175–181
32. Härtl R, Chamberlain RH, Fifield MS, Chou D, Sonntag VK, Crawford NR. Biomechanical comparison of two new atlantoaxial fixation techniques with C1-2 transarticular screw-graft fixation. J Neurosurg Spine 2006;5(4):336–342
33. Gonzalez LF, Crawford NR, Chamberlain RH, et al. Craniovertebral junction fixation with transarticular screws: biomechanical analysis of a novel technique. J Neurosurg 2003;98(2, Suppl):202–209
34. Feiz-Erfan I, Gonzalez LF, Dickman CA. Atlantooccipital transarticular screw fixation for the treatment of traumatic occipitoatlantal dislocation. Technical note. J Neurosurg Spine 2005;2(3):381–385
35. Bambakidis NC, Feiz-Erfan I, Horn EM, et al. Biomechanical comparison of occipitoatlantal screw fixation techniques. J Neurosurg Spine 2008;8(2):143–152
36. Maughan PH, Horn EM, Theodore N, Feiz-Erfan I, Sonntag VK. Avulsion fracture of the foramen magnum treated with occiput-to-c1 fusion: technical case report. Neurosurgery 2005;57(3):E600, discussion E600
37. Hurlbert RJ, Crawford NR, Choi WG, Dickman CA. A biomechanical evaluation of occipitocervical instrumentation: screw compared with wire fixation. J Neurosurg 1999;90(1, Suppl)84–90
38. Cheng BC, Hafez MA, Cunningham B, Serhan H, Welch WC. Biomechanical evaluation of occipitocervicothoracic fusion: impact of partial or sequential fixation. Spine J 2008;8(5):821–826
39. Gonzalez LF, Klopfenstein JD, Crawford NR, Dickman CA, Sonntag VK. Use of dual transarticular screws to fixate simultaneous occipitoatlantal and atlantoaxial dislocations. J Neurosurg Spine 2005;3(4):318–323
40. Askins V, Eismont FJ. Efficacy of five cervical orthoses in restricting cervical motion. A comparison study. Spine 1997;22(11):1193–1198
41. Johnson RM, Hart DL, Simmons EF, Ramsby GR, Southwick WO. Cervical orthoses. A study comparing their effectiveness in restricting cervical motion in normal subjects. J Bone Joint Surg Am 1977;59(3):332–339
42. Ivancic PC, Beauchman NN, Tweardy L. Effect of halo-vest components on stabilizing the injured cervical spine. Spine 2009; 34(2):167–175
43. Anderson PA, Montesano PX. Morphology and treatment of occipital condyle fractures. Spine 1988;13(7):731–736

4 Radiological Evaluation of the Craniovertebral Junction

Bryan J. Traughber, John A. Hodak, Alexander C. Mamourian, Bruce L. Dean, Michael D. Coffey, and Daniel P. Hsu

The craniovertebral junction (CVJ) is composed of the occipital bone, atlas (C1), axis (C2), and soft tissue structures, including the ligaments of the atlantoaxial and atlanto-occipital articulations. The essence of craniovertebral evaluation lies in determining the adequacy of this osseous conduit that the neuraxis, which consists of the spinal cord and the medulla, traverses. Numerous lines and measurements for craniometric assessment of the capacity of this bony canal have been used for plain radiographic analysis. The most common measurements include Chamberlain's line, McGregor's line, Wackenheim's clivus baseline, McRae's line, the atlanto-occipital joint axis angle, the bimastoid line, and the digastric line (**Fig. 4.1**).[1] In addition to positive contrast myelography with and without computed tomography (CT), measuring these lines has been the traditional way to assess the degree of impingement or distortion of the spinal cord or medulla. Magnetic resonance imaging (MRI) has proven to be an invaluable tool for the evaluation of soft tissue anatomy of the CVJ, including neural structures and ligaments.[2] Additionally, preoperative and intraoperative CT multiplanar reconstructions of a patient's anatomy and pathology markedly facilitate surgical planning so that unanticipated findings can be avoided.[3]

■ Osseous Anatomy

The Occipital Bone, Associated Anomalies, and Injuries

The posterior part of the cranium and most of the skull base are composed of the large, dense occipital bone. The occipital bone is composed of the basiocciput, supraocciput, exocciput, and the occipital squamosa, which are separated by synchondroses. The superior half of the clivus is formed by the basiocciput, and the occipital squamosa encompasses the supraoccipital and interparietal calvarium. The lateral margins of the foramen magnum and the occipital condyles are formed by the exocciput.[4–6] The basion and opisthion are terms applied to the anterior and posterior midpoints of the free edge of the foramen magnum. These landmarks are utilized in several measurements that are discussed and illustrated later. Measurements of the foramen magnum in cadaveric skulls have revealed a mean anteroposterior diameter of 34.5 mm (range 29.2 to 40.5 mm) and a mean width of 29.4 mm (range 26.2 to 37.0 mm).[7]

If the primitive elements of the preatlantal vertebrae persist anterior to the foramen magnum, anomalies of the basiocciput may occur. These anomalies manifest themselves in a variety of bony excrescences along the anterior foramen magnum, including the hypocondylar arch and the paramedian third condyle, which articulates with the dens or the anterior arch of the atlas. Occasionally, anomalous remnants form a pseudoarticulation between the occipital bone and the transverse process of the atlas (**Fig. 4.2**). The occipital condyles may be hypoplastic and allow a high position of the atlas and the axis. If the segmentation between the cranium and the first cervical vertebra fails, the atlas will be partially or completely assimilated. Frequently, there are accompanying basilar invaginations as well as other abnormalities, such as fusion of the axis to the third cervical vertebra, Klippel-Feil syndrome, and occipital vertebra and condylar hypoplasia.[4,8–10]

At the posterior lip of the foramen magnum, the remnant of the posterior arch of the atlas may be present as a triangular wedge of bone (**Fig. 4.3**).[11] Atlantoaxial instability is a common associated finding in 50% of patients.[12] Atlanto-occipital assimilation may be a harbinger of other generalized anomalies, such as dwarfism, funnel chest, pes cavus, syndactylies, jaw anomalies, hypospadias, and an occasional defect of the genitourinary tract.[13] Brainstem and cranial nerve signs may occur from anterior encroachment of the neuraxis at the level of the foramen magnum. If the vertebral artery is constricted, syncope, vertigo, and an unsteady gait may result from ischemia.[13]

Clival fractures are generally found with high-force, blunt head trauma and several subtypes have been described. These fractures can be associated with cranial nerve deficits and vascular injury, and resultant mortality is high secondary to brainstem trauma or vertebrobasilar occlusion. The diagnosis of clival fractures is technically difficult on radiographs alone because of the dense petrous bones; however, high-resolution CT with three-dimensional (3D) reconstructions may be helpful for diagnosis.[14]

The Atlas, Associated Anomalies, and Injuries

The first cervical vertebra, the atlas, is ring-shaped and lacks a vertebral and spinous process. Instead, it has two thick lateral masses on the anterolateral aspect of the ring that are connected to the anterior and posterior arches. The inferior surface of each lateral mass articulates with the superior articular facets of the axis.[15] Isolated anomalies of the atlas do not have an abnormal craniovertebral relationship and are not associated with basilar invagination.[4] Paralleling

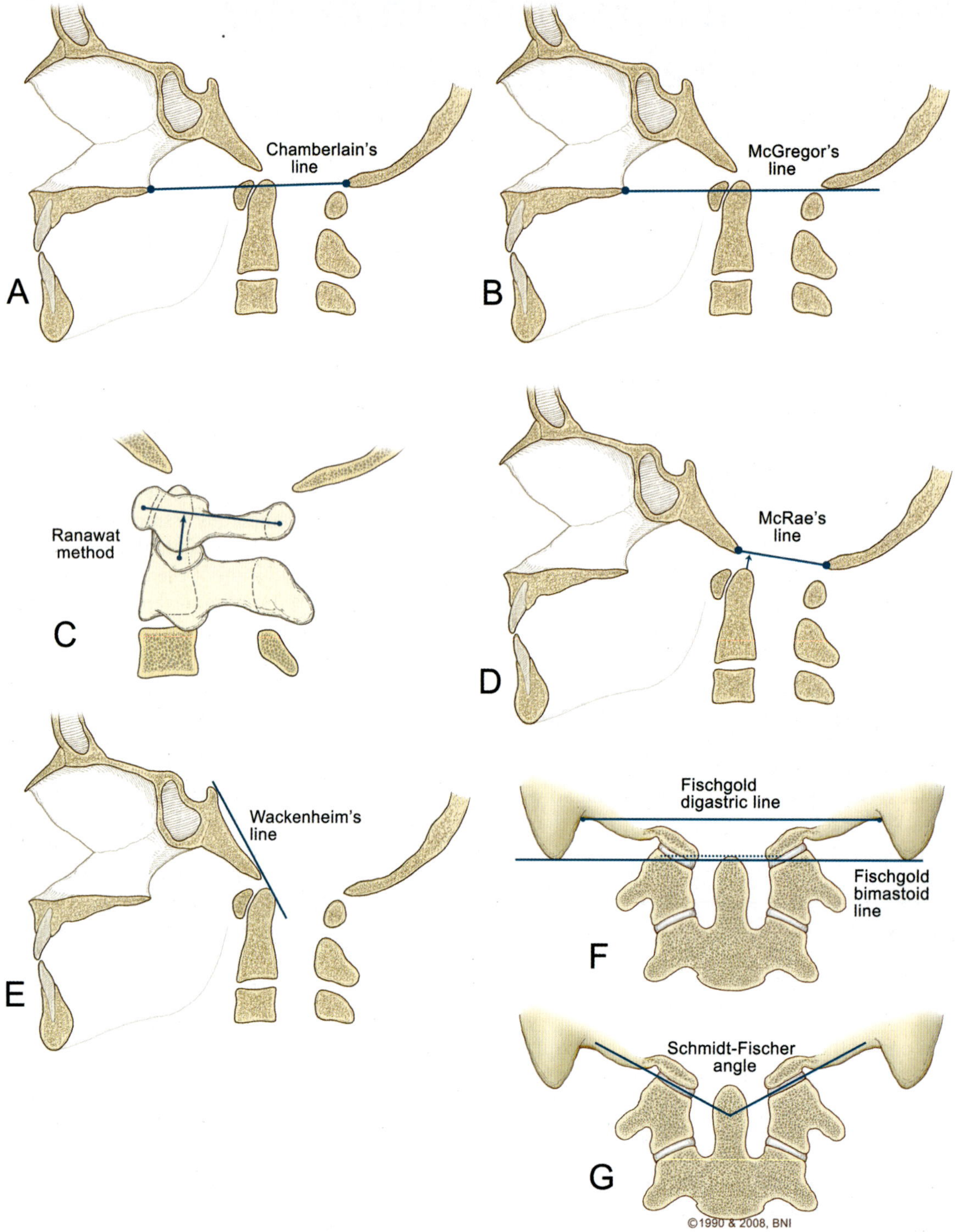

Fig. 4.1 **(A)** Chamberlain's line extends from the hard palate to the posterior margin of the foramen magnum. The odontoid tip is usually below or just tangential to this line. If the odontoid tip is more than 2.5 mm above this line, basilar invagination should be suspected, and it is affirmed if the distance is more than 6.6 mm. **(B)** McGregor's line extends from the hard palate tangent to the undersurface of the occipital bone. The odontoid should lie less than 4.5 mm above this line. **(C)** McRae's line extends from the basion to the posterior border of the foramen magnum. The odontoid should not project above this line. **(D)** Wackenheim's line extends along the posterior margin of the clivus. This line should fall tangential to the tip of the odontoid. **(E)** The bimastoid line joins the mastoid tips. The odontoid lies 3 mm below to 10 mm above this line. **(F)** The digastric line extends between the two digastric grooves, which are medial to the base of the mastoid processes. If the distance between this line and the midoccipital-atlantal joint is less than 10 mm, basilar invagination is present. **(G)** The atlanto-occipital joint angle is formed by intersecting lines drawn parallel to the occipitoatlantal joints. An angle greater than 150 degrees is suspicious for basilar invagination. (Reprinted with permission from Barrow Neurological Institute.)

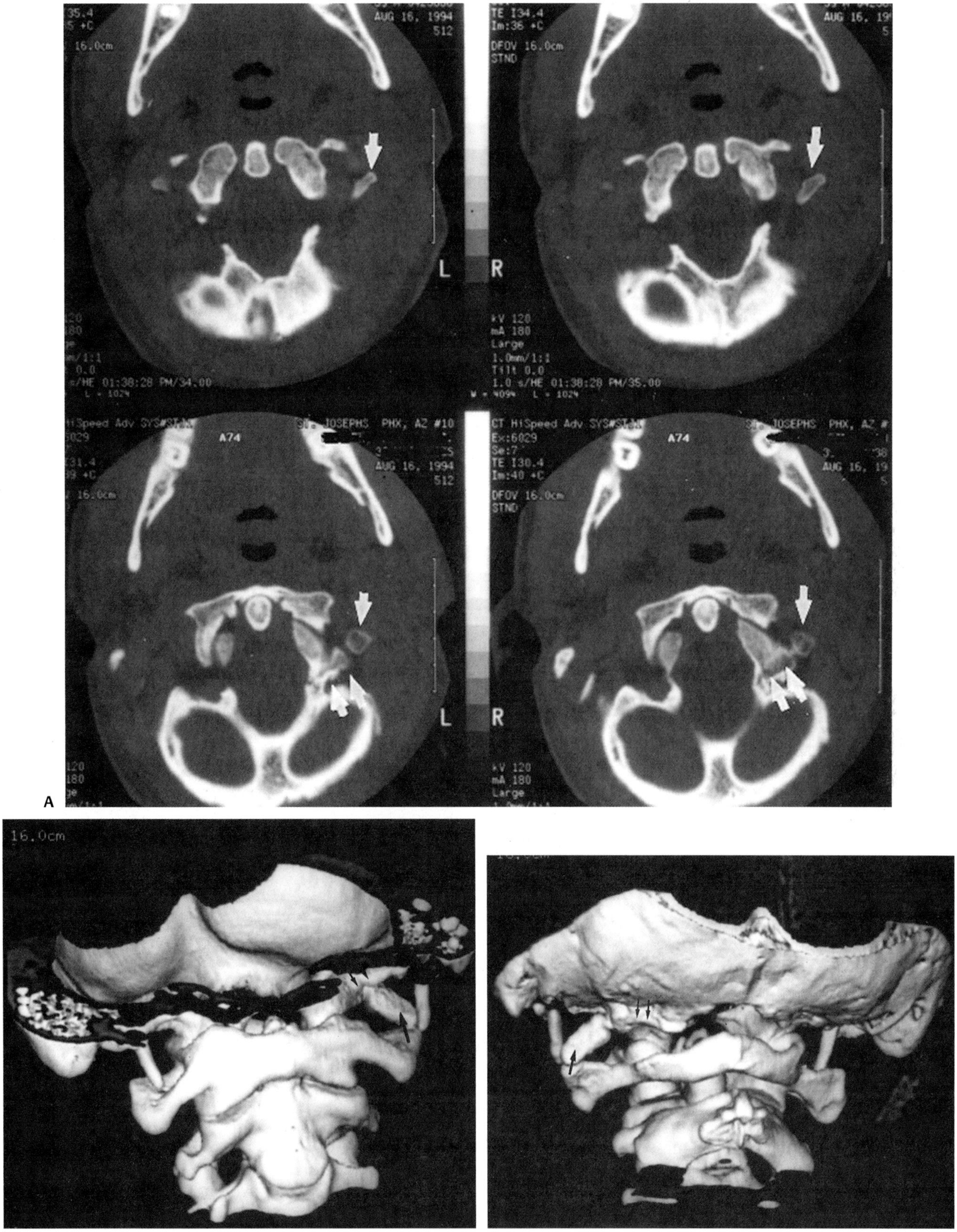

A

B

C

Fig. 4.2 **(A)** Computed tomography (CT) scan performed to rule out a fracture revealed an anomalous remnant of the basiocciput (*arrow*) with a pseudoarticulation between the occipital bone (*double arrows*) and the transverse process of the atlas. **(B)** Anterior and **(C)** posterior views of three-dimensional CT solid modeling of this anomaly demonstrating the spatial relationships of the affected anatomy.

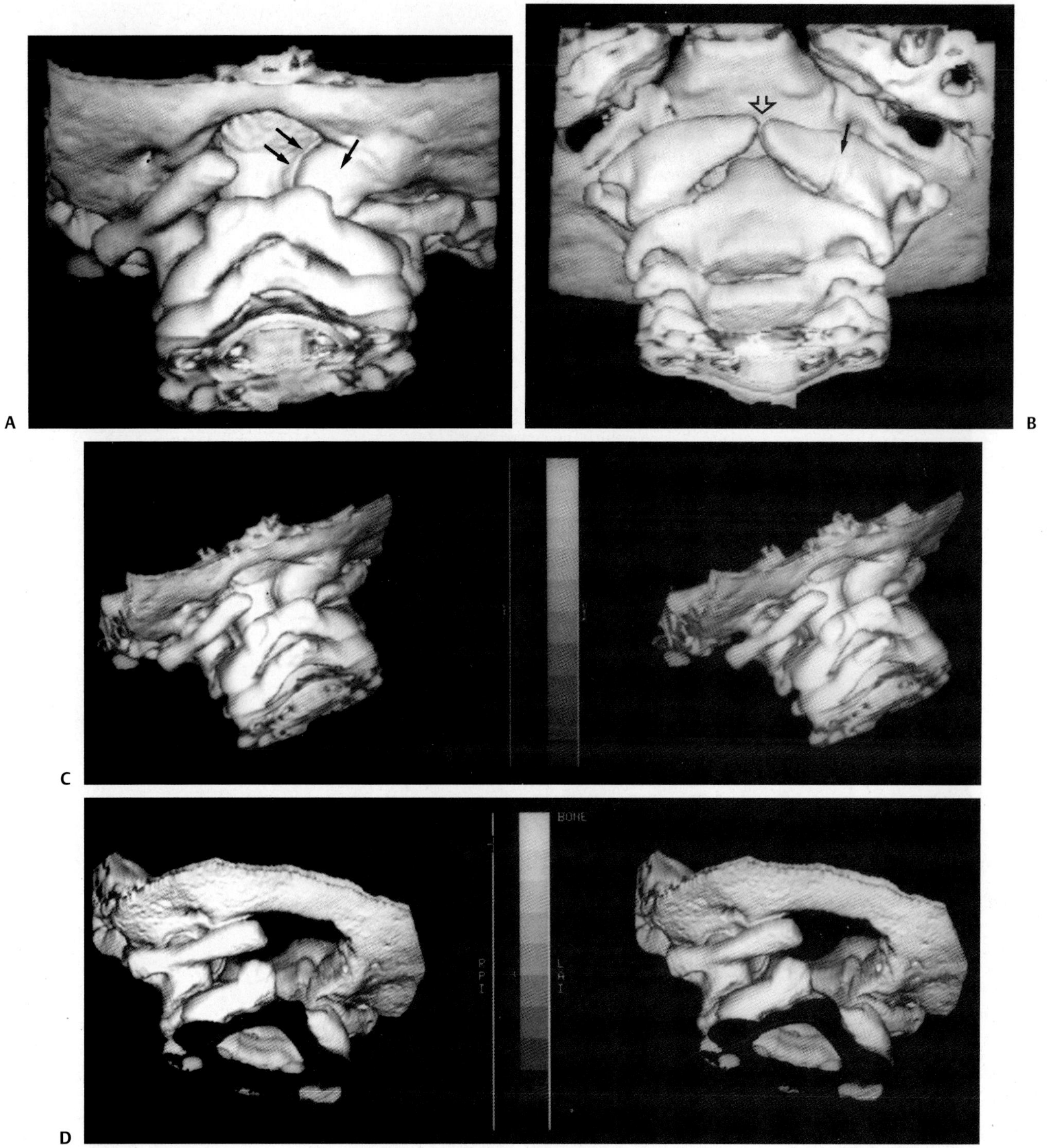

Fig. 4.3 Unilateral atlanto-occipital assimilation in a 3-year-old girl with hemiparesis, initially thought secondary to cerebral palsy. **(A)** Posterior view of three-dimensional (3D) computed tomography (CT) solid modeling, obtained after myelography, demonstrates indentation of the contrast column and cervicomedullary junction (*double arrows*) by the wedge-shaped remnant of the posterior arch of the atlas (*single arrow*). **(B)** Anterior 3D CT view demonstrating associated complete (*open arrow*) and partial (*arrow*) cleft of the anterior arch of the atlas. **(C)** Posterior 3D CT stereo pair for cross-eyed viewing provides additional depth clues of the deforming anomaly. **(D)** Postoperative posterior 3D stereo pair for cross-eyed viewing performed without myelographic contrast medium demonstrates surgical decompression of the posterior foramen magnum and the fusion anomaly.

the atlas ossification centers, these anomalies consist of arch clefts, aplasias, and hypoplasias.[4] The majority of these anomalies are of the posterior arch and include complete aplasia, Keller-type aplasia, aplasia with a unilateral or bilateral remnant, and middle rachischisis, hemiaplasia, or partial hemiaplasia of the posterior arch.[12,16] It is highly important to note that partial hemiaplasias can mimic fractures on plain radiographic examination.[17]

The Jefferson fracture results from axial loading injury with disruption of the anterior and posterior arches of C1 that may be associated with injury to the supporting ligaments. The transverse ligament is crucial in maintaining the integrity of the anatomical position of the odontoid and the anterior arch of C1, which can be avulsed secondary to trauma at the osseous insertion site on C1. The clinical presentation of Jefferson fractures are neck pain, dysphagia, and posterior fossa transient ischemia attack (TIA) or stroke. CT is effective at diagnosis of the osseous avulsion of the transverse ligament, but MRI can be more specific in identifying and assessing the degree of ligamentous injury and possible cord injury.[18]

The Axis, Associated Anomalies, and Injuries

The second cervical vertebra, the axis, forms a pivot for the atlas that allows the head to rotate. The odontoid process projects superiorly from the C2 vertebral body with a facet on its ventral surface that articulates with the dorsal surface on the anterior atlas arch. The axis spinous process is large and is the first bifid vertebra in the cervical spine.[15] Clefts of the axis are rare, as are atlantoaxial fusions, which form a block that usually lacks the anterior arch of the atlas and are associated with a hypoplastic or absent odontoid. Partial fusion may occur between the odontoid and the anterior arch of the atlas or may involve unilateral fusion of the hemiarches of the atlas and axis. These fusions can result in uneven joint surfaces with concomitant impairment of function.[11] An increased incidence of atlantoaxial fusion is present in patients with the Chiari I malformation.[11]

Most anomalies of the axis involve the odontoid process and are not associated with basilar invagination. The tip of the odontoid or os terminale usually appears by the age of 3 and fuses by the age of 12.[4,13] Failure of the os terminale to fuse, also known as Bergman ossicle, originates from failure of fusion of the odontoid process to the proatlas. This important note can be misconstrued as a type I odontoid fracture, although identification of a well-corticated ossicle should make the diagnosis of fracture less likely.[4]

Hypoplasia of the odontoid associated, with an oval ossicle widely separated from C2 and located well above the superior facets of the axis, is termed os odontoideum. The os usually does not preserve the normal shape or size of the odontoid, often being half the normal size and rounded or oval, with a smooth uniform cortex.[13] The anterior arch of the atlas may be hypertrophied, whereas the posterior arch may be hypoplastic in patients with os odontoideum (**Fig. 4.4**).[13,19] These dysplastic states of the odontoid are

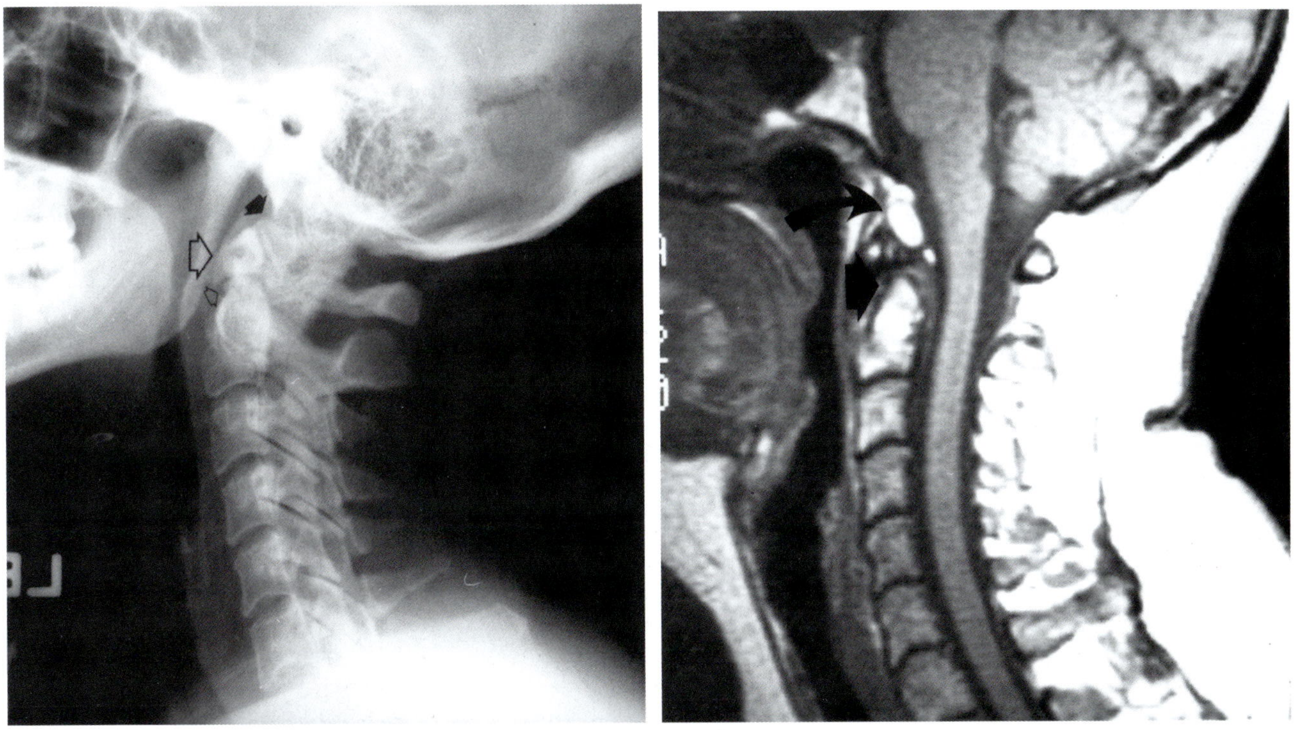

A B

Fig. 4.4 Os odontoideum. **(A)** Lateral plain film radiograph demonstrates well-corticated os (*solid arrow*) well above the blunt sclerotic odontoid (*small open arrow*) displaced anteriorly beneath an enlarged anterior arch of the atlas (*large open arrow*). **(B)** Sagittal T1-weighted magnetic resonance image shows the os (*curved arrow*) well separated from the irregular blunt-shaped base of the odontoid (*arrow*).

uncommon and most often encountered as an isolated phenomenon, but they can be found in several other syndromes involving the bony skeleton, such as Morquio syndrome, mucopolysaccharidoses, spondyloepiphyseal dysplasia congenita, spondylometaphyseal dysplasia, metatrophic dwarfism, and Conradi disease.[20–22] Total aplasia of the odontoid is extremely rare but is often associated with an irregularity of the upper margin of the C2 vertebral body.[23] Compression at the level of the C1 arch can occur in the setting of both hypoplasia and aplasia secondary to the absence of the attachments for the apical and alar ligaments predisposing to atlantoaxial instability.[24]

Basilar Invagination and Platybasia

Primary basilar invagination refers to a developmental anomaly involving an abnormally high vertebral column that prolapses into the cranial base.[25] The condition has numerous causes, including basioccipital hypoplasia, condylar hypoplasia, hypoplasia of the atlas, atlanto-occipital assimilation, odontoid abnormalities, Klippel-Feil syndrome, Chiari malformations (**Fig. 4.5**), syringomyelia, and syringobulbia.[4,13,20] Secondary basilar invagination, which is often termed basilar impression, is a developmental condition associated with softening of the osseous structures at the cranial base. It may be seen in Paget disease, osteomalacia, osteogenesis imperfecta, rickets, renal osteodystrophy, neurofibromatosis, Hurler disease, rheumatoid arthritis, infections of the cranial base, and fractures of the posterior cranial base.[4,13,20] Additionally, platybasia refers to an abnormally flattened cranial base with an increased basal angle. When isolated, platybasia is associated with no signs or symptoms. However, platybasia and basilar invagination or basilar impression often coexist.[4,20]

Occipitoatlantal Joint

To a large degree, occipitoatlantal stability is provided by the contours of this articulation. The orientation of the articular surfaces varies with growth. In children, the surfaces are oriented horizontally and become more vertical with age. This process is thought to account for the greater instability of this joint in children.[26,27] The joint capsules provide additional stability, which increases with age as the capsules become less elastic.

The tectorial membrane and alar ligaments provide ligamentous support to the occipitoatlantal joint. The tectorial membrane represents a cephalad continuation of the posterior longitudinal ligament. It extends from the posterior margin of the body of C2 to the anterior foramen magnum, coursing over the dens and cruciform ligament (**Fig. 4.6**). Functionally, the tectorial membrane limits extension of the occiput-C1-C2 complex and, to a lesser degree, flexion.[28] However, the membrane does not significantly limit axial motion, which is the function of the alar ligaments (**Fig. 4.7**). These ligaments arise from the lateral apex of the dens and insert on the medial inferior aspect of the occipital condyles.

Atlanto-occipital dislocation occurs with disruption of the ligaments between the occiput and upper cervical spine after a hyperextension injury. Injury to the alar ligaments and tectorial membrane can result in anterior dislocation of

A

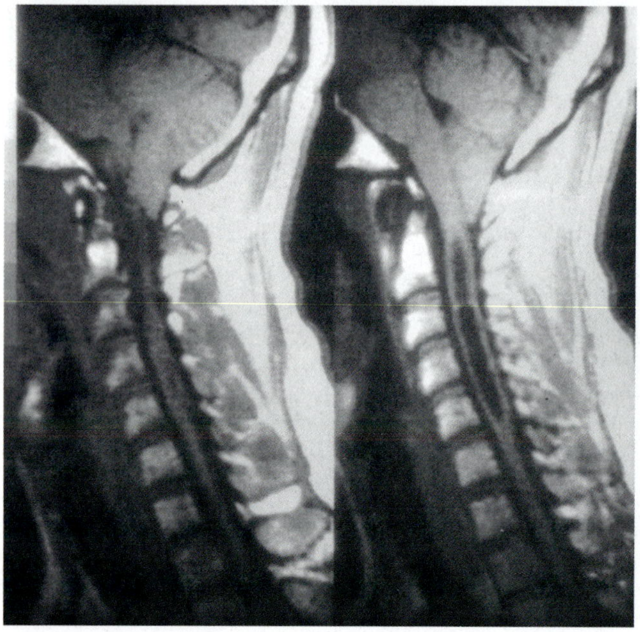

B

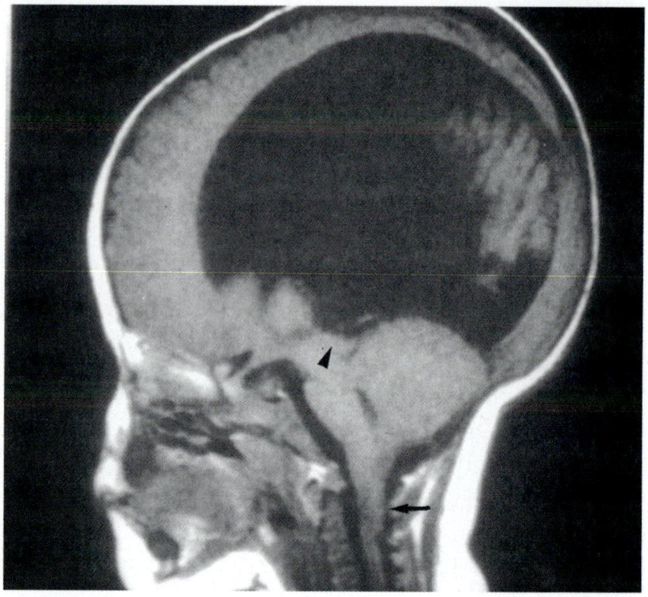

Fig. 4.5 **(A)** Sagittal T1-weighted magnetic resonance image (MRI) of a patient with a Chiari I malformation, demonstrating low-pointed cerebellar tonsils and associated syringohydromyelia. **(B)** Sagittal T1-weighted MRI of a patient with a Chiari II malformation shows marked lateral ventricular enlargement, beaking of the tectum (*arrowhead*), and a vermian peg (*arrow*).

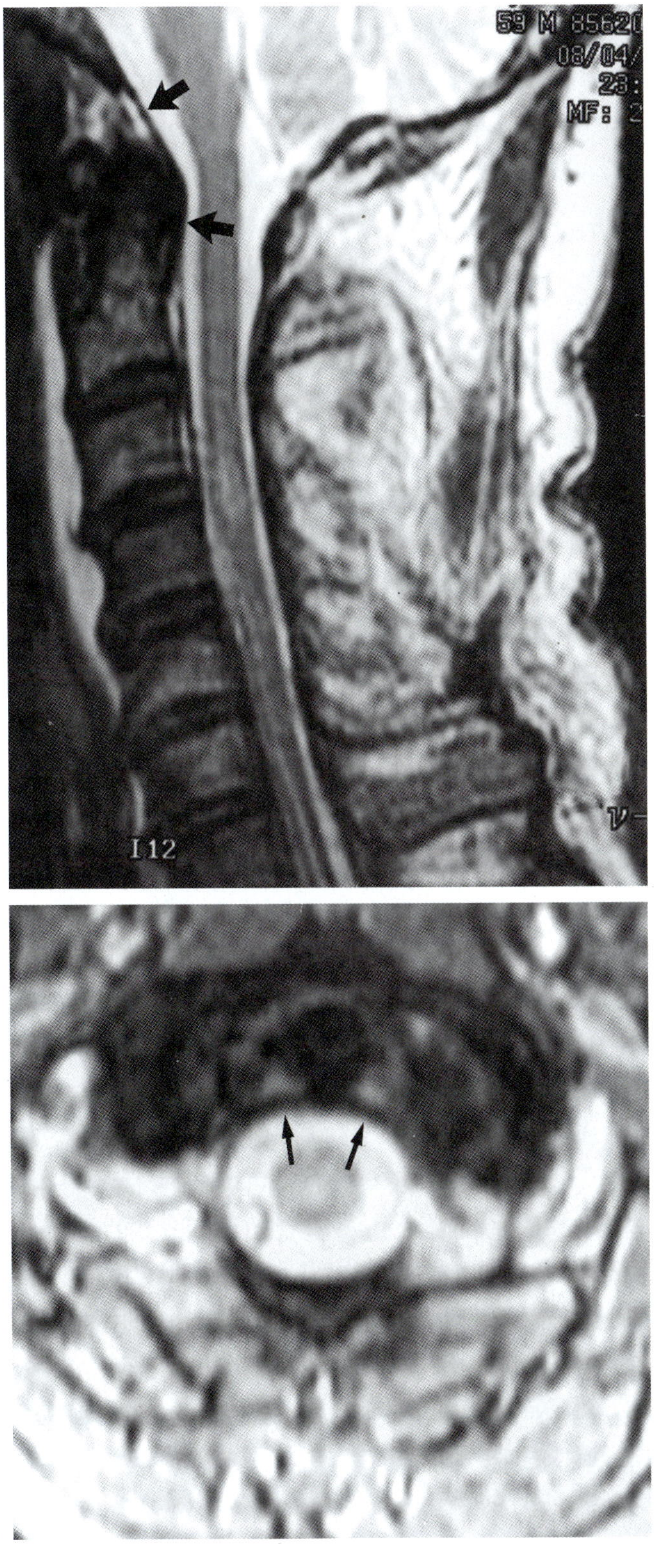

A

B

Fig. 4.6 **(A)** Sagittal T2-weighted magnetic resonance image (MRI) demonstrating the tectorial membrane extending from the body of C2 to the anterior foramen magnum (*arrows*). **(B)** Axial T2-weighted gradient-echo MRI demonstrating the low-intensity signal of the tectorial membrane posterior to the dens. The tectorial membrane is concave posteriorly (*arrows*) compared with the transverse ligament, which is concave anteriorly.

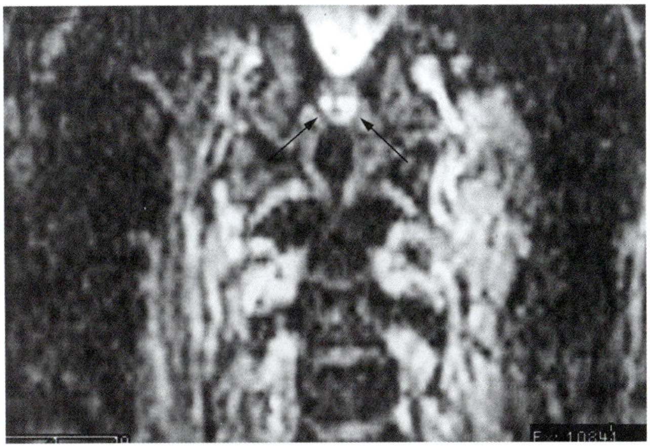

Fig. 4.7 Gradient echo coronal magnetic resonance image demonstrating the alar ligaments (*arrows*) extending from the lateral aspect of the dens to the medial occipital condyles.

the skull base and cervical spine with possible associated odontoid fractures. Dislocation is often accompanied by head injury with high mortality related to brainstem injury. High-resolution CT is effective for accurate diagnosis, and MRI can be utilized to evaluate alar and tectorial ligamentous injury as well as the joint capsule.[29]

Atlantoaxial Joint

Atlantoaxial joint stability requires osseous and ligamentous integrity. Whereas the tectorial membrane and alar ligaments constrain bending and axial movements, anterior subluxation is limited by the transverse ligament. This ligament represents the largest bundle of the cruciform (cross-shaped) ligament that lies just under the tectorial membrane. The cruciform ligament has a craniocaudal element that extends from the base of the dens to the anterior foramen magnum. The larger axially oriented fiber bundle, the transverse ligament, inserts on the medial aspect of the lateral masses of C1 (**Fig. 4.8**). There are often small osseous tubercles at this insertion. The transverse ligament courses posteriorly to the dens, separated from it by a small synovial-lined space. The transverse ligament is ~10 mm thick and has no elastic fibers.[30] Deep to the cruciform ligament are the odontoid ligaments (i.e., the alar and apical ligaments). The apical ligament arises at the tip of the dens and inserts on the anterior margin of the foramen magnum. It confers little ligamentous support for occipital-C1-C2 stability.[28]

The transverse ligament provides the primary stability at the C1-C2 junction. Secondary support is provided by the alar ligaments.[31] In a normal adult with an intact transverse ligament, the space between the posterior margin of the anterior ring of C1 and the anterior cortex of the dens (the atlantodental interval) should be no more than 2 to 3 mm on a lateral cervical radiograph. The alar ligaments do not have sufficient strength to provide stability at the atlantoaxial joint if the transverse ligament ruptures.[28]

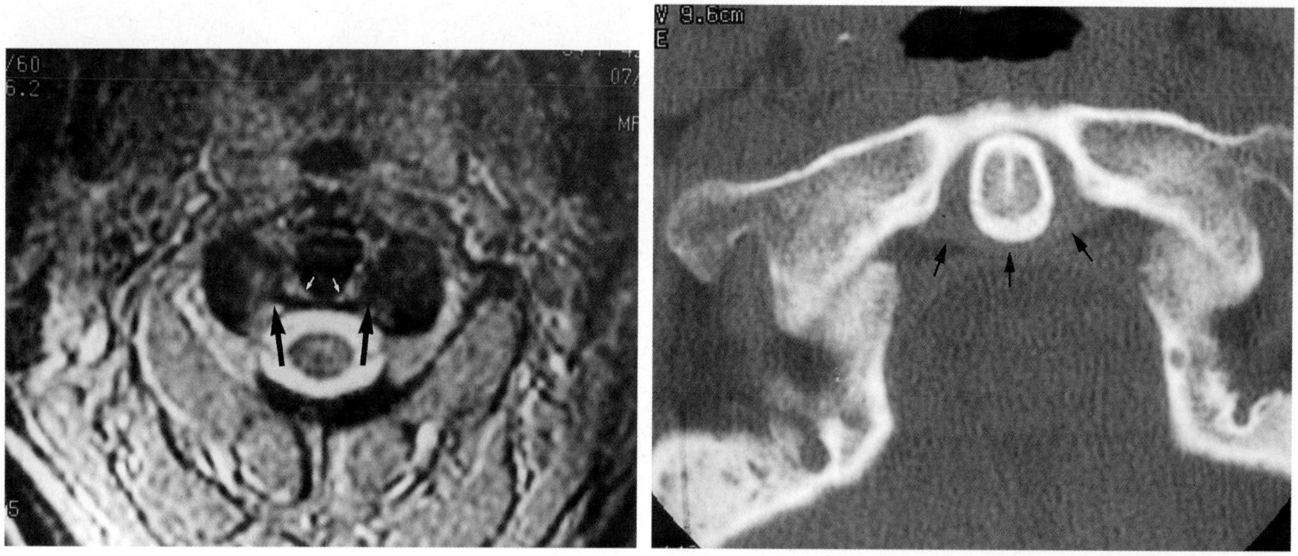

Fig. 4.8 (A) Axial gradient echo magnetic resonance image demonstrating the low-intensity signal of the transverse ligament attached to the medial aspect of the lateral masses of C1 (*black arrows*). The dens is anterior to the transverse ligament separated by the thin high-intensity signal of the synovial space (*white arrows*). **(B)** Thin-section axial computed tomography scan demonstrating the transverse ligament as a relatively high attenuation structure (*arrows*).

Because the transverse ligament is inelastic in the normal individual, it will rupture when sufficiently stressed. In vitro biomechanical studies have shown considerable variation in the strength of the transverse ligament. In one study, the force required for rupture ranged from 12 to 180 kilopounds.[31] When the transverse ligament fails, its midbody may rupture or tear away from its bony insertion on C1—sometimes still attached to a fragment of cortex. The transverse ligament can rupture without associated fracture of the dens. In such cases, there may be anterior subluxation or rotatory dislocation of C1 on C2.[32] Conversely, fractures of the dens or ring of C1 do not indicate in all cases that the transverse ligament is injured. Because the transverse ligament is so important for stability of the atlantoaxial joint and because subluxation may have devastating neurological effects (**Figs. 4.4** and **4.9**), the integrity of the transverse ligament must be assessed.[33]

The integrity of the ligament can be inferred from osseous landmarks. For example, in cases with C1 burst fractures, measurements indicate that the transverse ligament is very likely to be ruptured if the lateral masses of C1 are spread more than 7 mm (**Fig. 4.10**).[30] It is difficult to predict the integrity of the transverse ligament based on the C1-dens space on lateral cervical radiographs. The transverse ligament is presumed to be ruptured in trauma cases when the C1-dens space is 5 mm or more. However, in patients with rheumatoid arthritis, this space may be significantly widened with an intact but lax transverse ligament (**Fig. 4.11**) with varying degrees of atlantoaxial subluxation.[34] In patients with anterior displacement of C1 on C2, the transverse ligament is presumed to be ruptured (**Fig. 4.12**). Conversely,

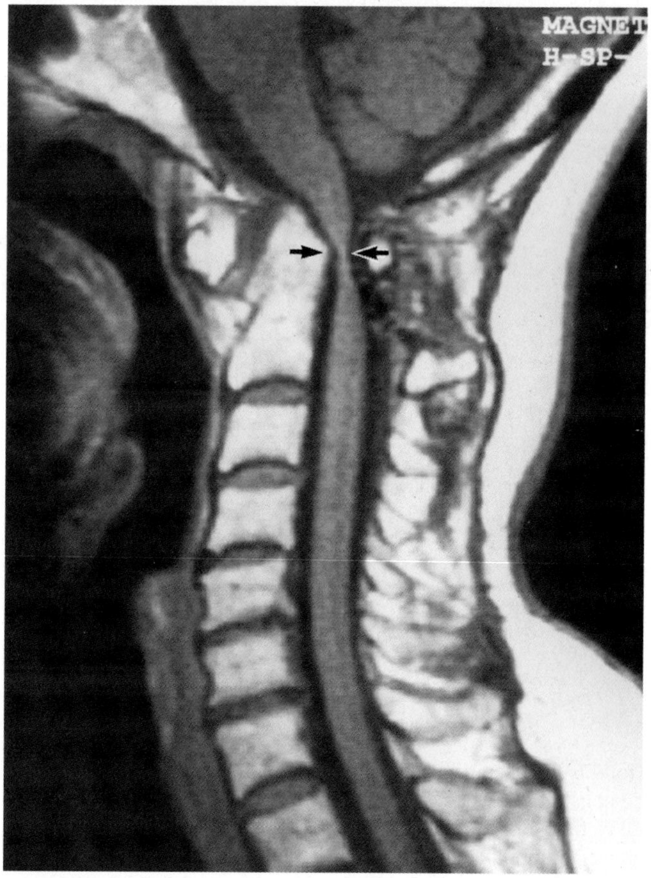

Fig. 4.9 Sagittal T1-weighted magnetic resonance image showing severe compression of the upper cervical spinal cord (*arrows*) in a patient with rheumatoid arthritis and C1-C2 subluxation.

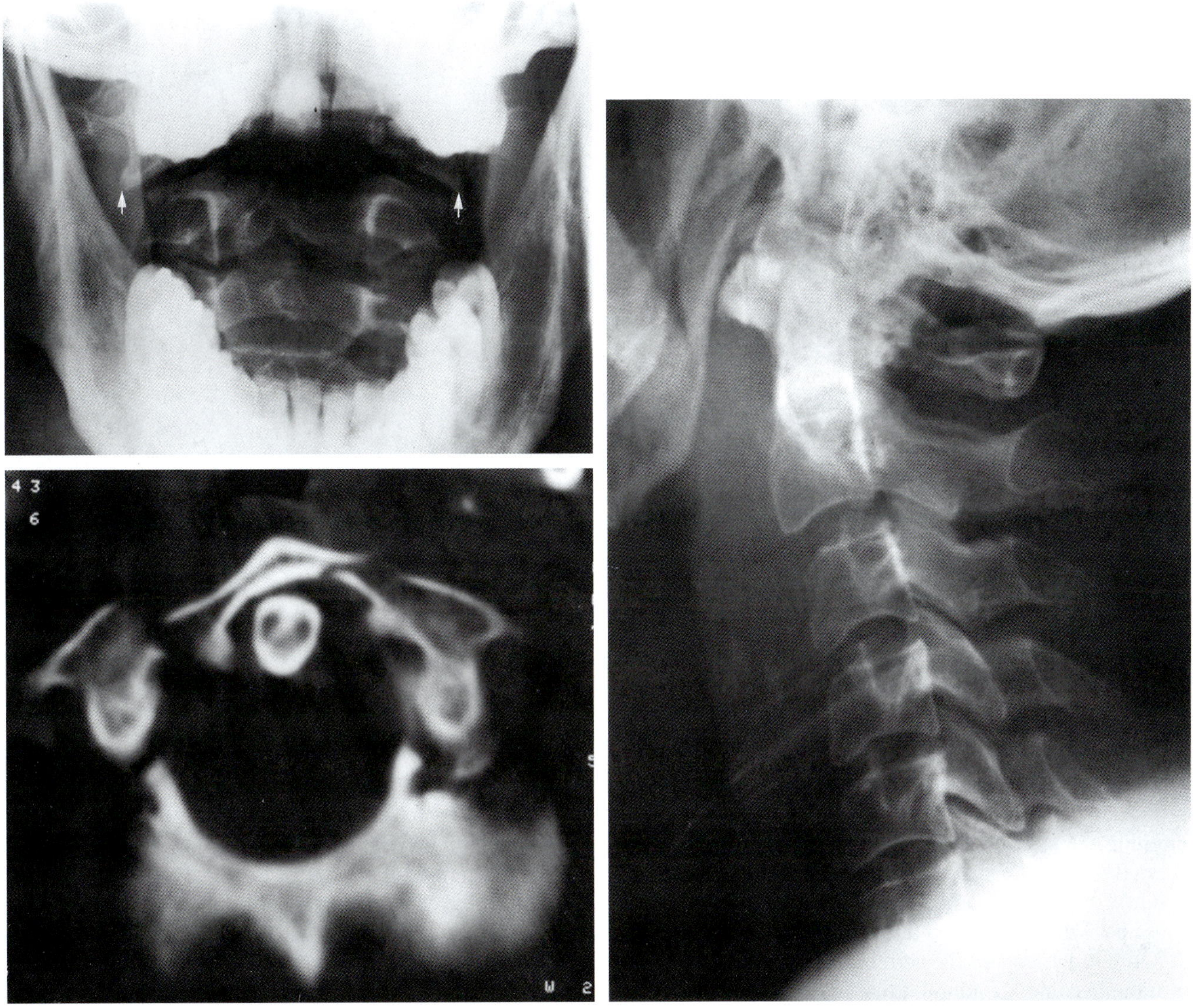

A C B

Fig. 4.10 **(A)** Transoral odontoid plain film radiograph demonstrating lateral splaying of the lateral masses of C1 (*arrows*). The cumulative displacement measures more than 7 mm. **(B)** Lateral plain film radiographs of the upper cervical spine show widening of the predental space, consistent with disruption of the transverse ligament. **(C)** Axial computed tomography scan demonstrating fractures of the anterior ring of C1 in a patient with a Jefferson burst fracture.

when there is combined anterior displacement with contralateral posterior displacement, the transverse ligament is presumed to be intact because the axis of rotation is around the dens.

This inherent assumption in assessing the integrity of the transverse ligament based on osseous relationships suggests a role for more sensitive soft tissue imaging techniques, such as CT and MRI. CT is capable of demonstrating the transverse ligament and, although it is excellent for demonstrating the osseous anatomy of the spine, soft tissue resolution may be limited if fractures and hemorrhage are in the region of the ligament. Using only CT, definitive assessment of the transverse ligament is not possible in all cases. Because MRI is capable of greater soft tissue contrast than CT, MRI can demonstrate the relationship of the spinal cord with surrounding spinal structures. MRI has been shown to be of value in demonstrating the ligamentous structures in patients with traumatic injuries of the CVJ.[2,33,35]

Vascular Anatomy

Normal Vascular Anatomy

The arterial anatomy of the CVJ is primarily composed of the vertebral arteries, its branches, and various anomalies. The embryological formation of the vertebral arteries is complex. They are primarily longitudinal anastomoses between the first seven segmental arteries.[36] Anatomically, the vertebral artery is divided into four segments (**Fig. 4.13**). When discussing the CVJ, we are primarily concerned with the third and fourth segments.

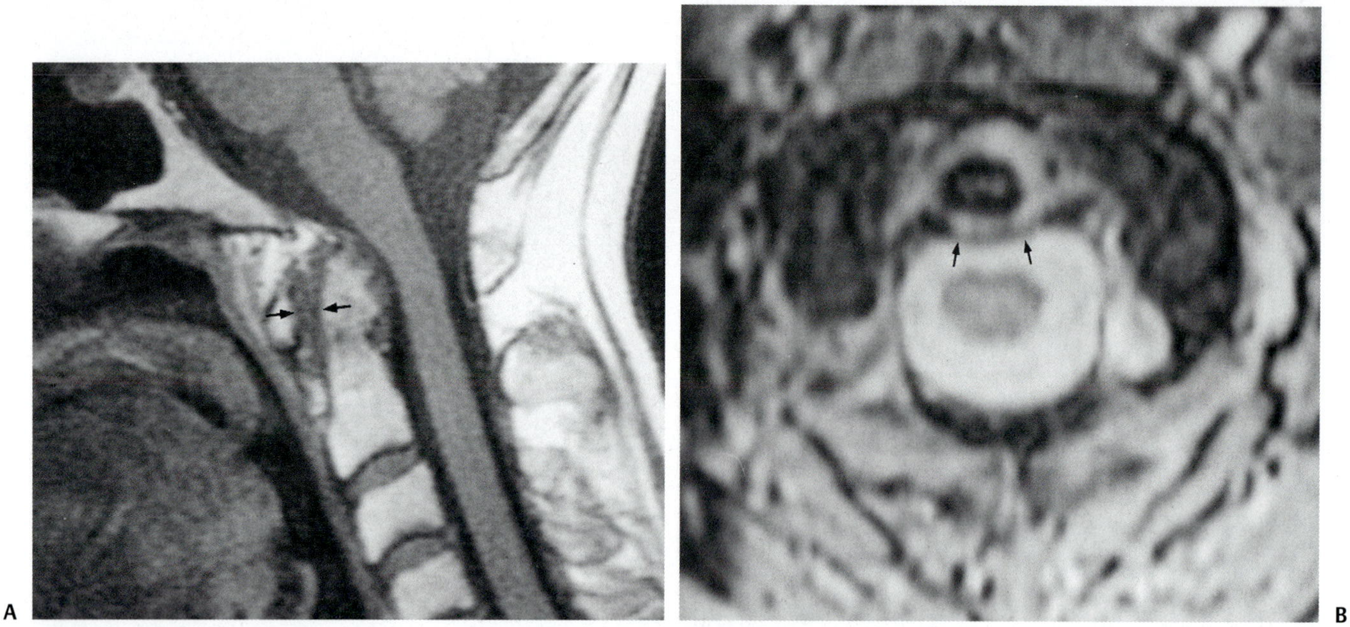

Fig. 4.11 **(A)** In a patient with rheumatoid arthritis, a sagittal T1-weighted magnetic resonance image shows abnormal widening of the space between the anterior arch of C1 and the dens (*arrows*). A band of low-intensity signal in the tissue surrounding the dens reflects pannus formation. **(B)** Axial T2-weighted gradient echo image demonstrating a lax but intact transverse ligament (*arrows*).

The third segments of the vertebral arteries begin as the arteries exit the transverse foramen of C2 (**Fig. 4.14**). The arteries course laterally and superiorly through the transverse foramina of C1 and then posteromedially on the upper surface of the atlas along its posterior ring. The arteries abruptly assume a superoanteromedial course to traverse the atlanto-occipital membrane and dura. This area demarcates the V3 and V4 segments of the vertebral arteries, which, at this location, become intradural. Intradurally, the vertebral arteries join at the clivus, where they form the basilar artery.

The major branches of the V3 and V4 segments include the segmental vessels of C1 (variable) and C2 as well as the anterior and posterior meningeal vessels. More distally, the anterior spinal artery and the posterior inferior cerebellar artery (PICA) arise (**Fig. 4.14**). Posterior spinal branches may arise at all segmental levels, including the PICA branch. There is a plethora of collateral anastomoses between the external carotid and vertebral arteries at this level. The most frequent collaterals are the segmental musculoskeletal branches of the vertebral arteries and the occipital branch of the external carotid artery. Additional anastomoses include the ascending pharyngeal and the posterior auricular branches from the external carotid artery to meningeal branches of the posterior fossa. The thyrocervical and costocervical arteries also may serve as collateral supply to the distal distribution of the vertebral artery.

Anomalies

Vascular anomalies are rare at the CVJ. The hypoglossal and proatlantal arteries represent uncommon persistent fetal anastomoses between the anterior and posterior circulation at this level (**Fig. 4.15**). These embryonic vessels connect the vertebral artery to the anterior circulation. After the trigeminal artery, the hypoglossal artery is the second most common persistent fetal anastomosis.[37] It connects the internal carotid artery with the proximal basilar artery by coursing through the hypoglossal canal. The proatlantal artery most often anastomoses to the external carotid artery and, occasionally, to the internal carotid artery, coursing along the superior border of C1 to anastomose with the ipsilateral vertebral artery. A persistent first intersegmental artery that courses between the atlas and axis in the C2 nerve root space has been reported in the literature unilaterally and bilaterally.[38–40] Additionally, fenestrations are common in the basilar artery but seldom occur in the vertebral artery, although they have been described (**Fig. 4.16**).[38]

Variations of the normal anatomical patterns or positions of vessels are frequently seen and are much more common than anomalies. The course of the V4 segments may be quite variable in elderly hypertensive patients. Typically, the left vertebral artery is the dominant vessel if one is larger than the other. In contrast, 0.2 to 1% of vertebral arteries will end in a PICA terminal branch.[41] One vertebral artery will be small or hypoplastic in up to 40% of patients,[42] with small contributions of blood flow to the distal basilar artery.

Pathology

Dissections at this location are often caused by the mobility of this segment of the vertebral artery (**Fig. 4.17**). Dissections, occlusions, or both may be associated with trauma

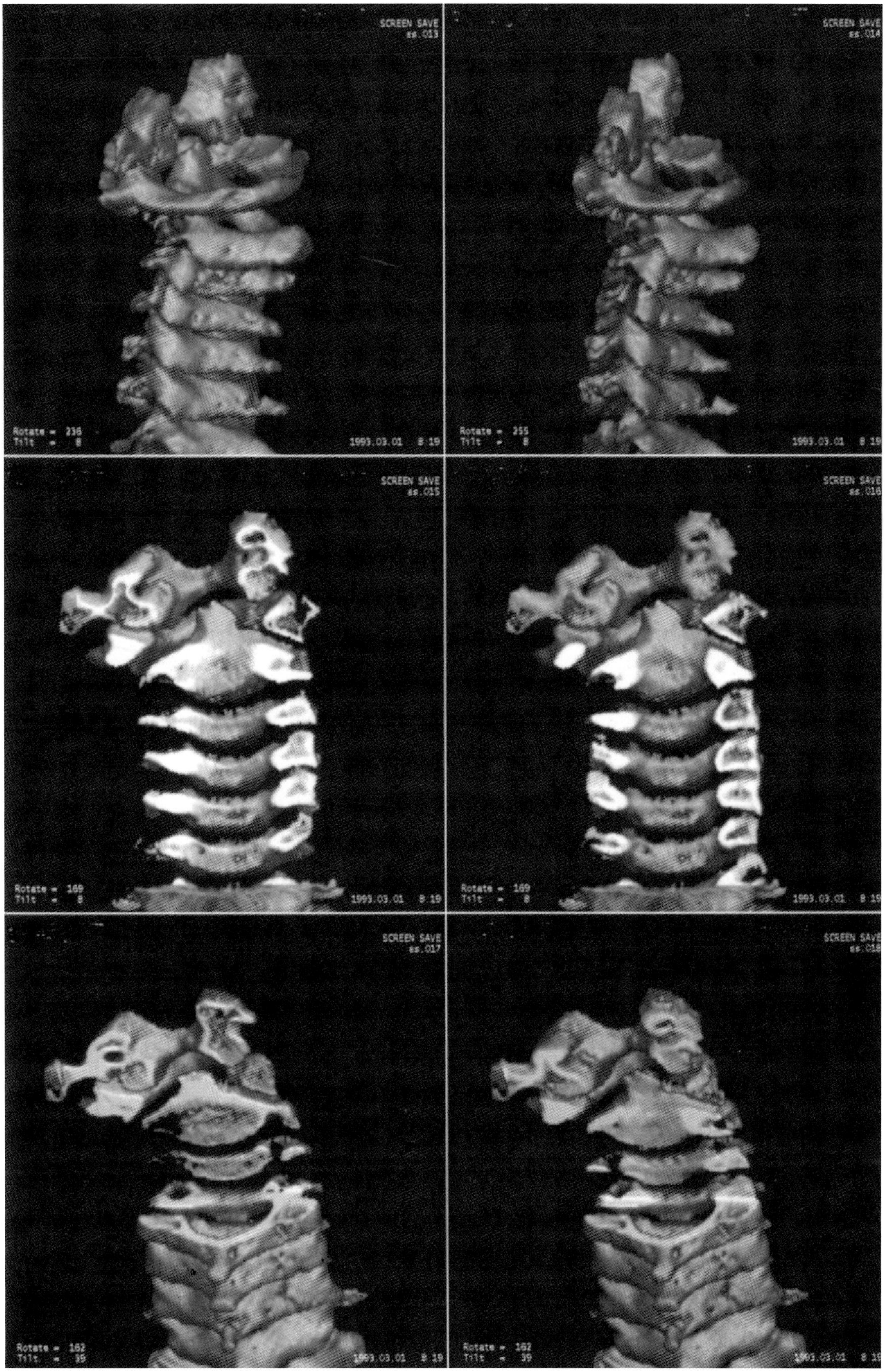

Fig. 4.12 Three-dimensional reconstruction of computed tomography data demonstrating a unilateral anterior subluxation of C1 on C2.

to the cervical spine. Fractures to transverse foramen, in particular, are vulnerable.[43] In addition, rotatory subluxations or rotational injuries can compromise the vertebral arteries at this level.[43,44] In the setting of a vertebral artery occlusion and ischemia of the posterior fossa or spinal cord, a thorough knowledge of vascular collaterals is imperative. Surgical intervention can exacerbate the ischemia if collateral vessels are interrupted.[45] With atlantoaxial or atlanto-occipital dislocations, brainstem injuries can be caused by direct mechanical injury to the medulla or cervical cord, and medullary ischemic injuries can be associated with traumatic dissections of the vertebral artery.[46] Anecdotal cases of recovery of clinical function have been reported in patients with ischemic brainstem injuries.[47]

Occasionally, vertebral artery injuries are seen in patients with rheumatoid arthritis after trauma or in patients with overt subluxations.[48,49] Also, weak to moderate evidence suggests vertebral artery dissections or occlusions with associated stroke can occur with cervical manipulations of the

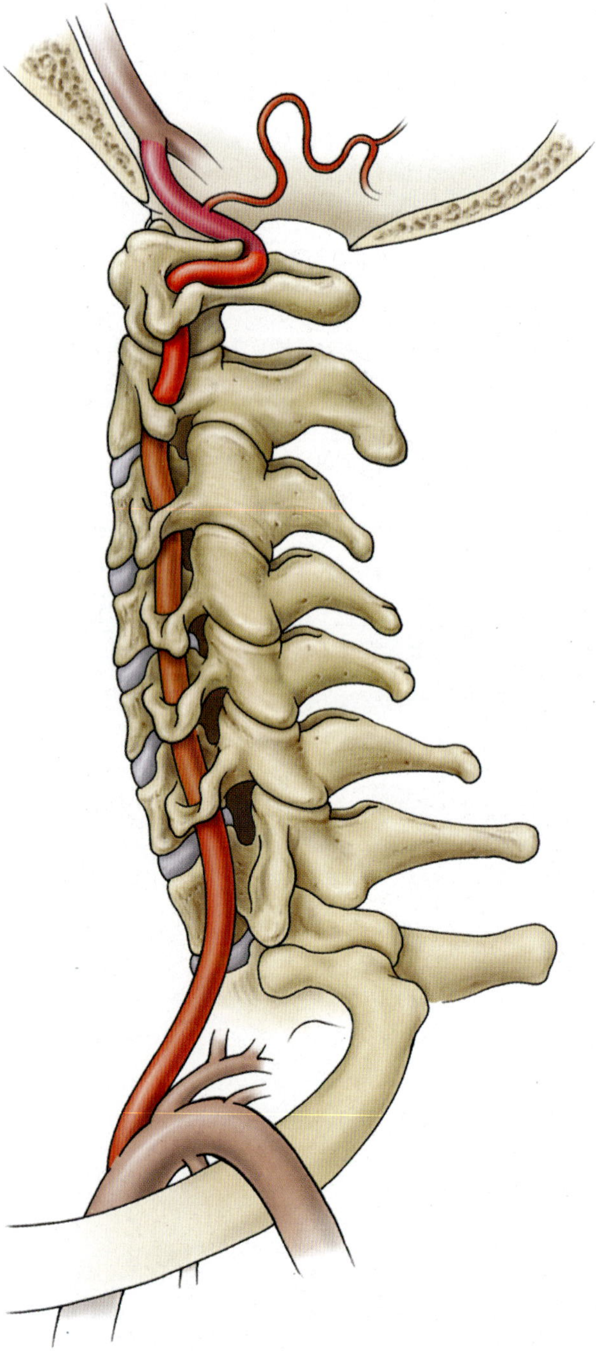

Fig. 4.13 Segments 3 and 4 constitute the components of the vessels at the craniovertebral junction. The primary demarcation between segments 2 and 3 is the transverse foramen of C2; the atlanto-occipital membrane denotes the boundary between segments 3 and 4 where the vertebral arteries become intradural. (Reprinted with permission from Barrow Neurological Institute.)

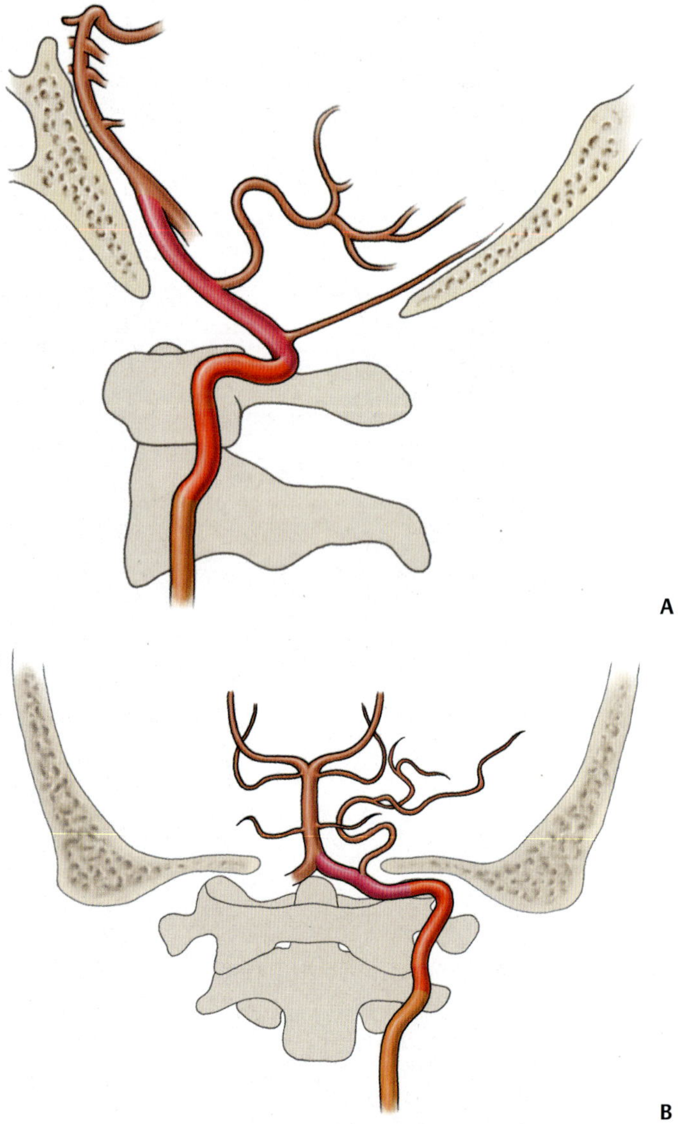

Fig. 4.14 The relationships of segments 3 and 4 of the vertebral artery to the skull base and posterior inferior cerebellar artery are displayed in **(A)** lateral and **(B)** anteroposterior projections. (Reprinted with permission from Barrow Neurological Institute.)

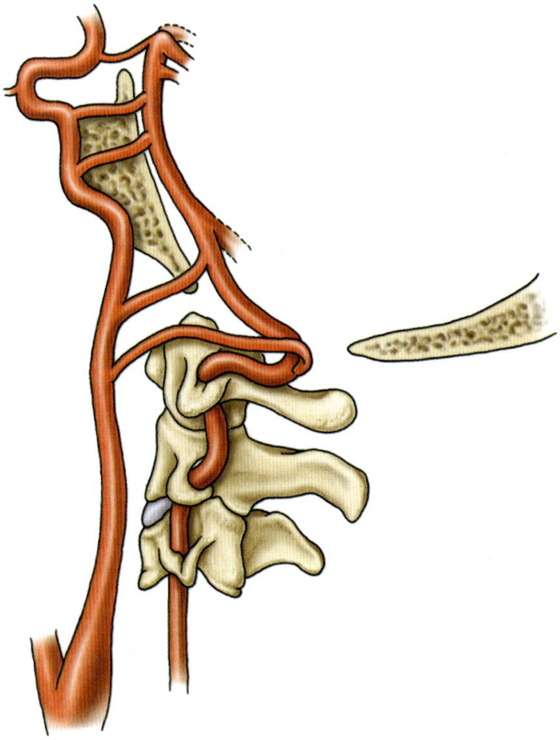

Fig. 4.15 The hypoglossal and proatlantal arteries occur at the skull base and may complicate surgery in this region. The hypoglossal and proatlantal arteries are the second and third most common persistent fetal anastomoses. (Reprinted with permission from Barrow Neurological Institute.)

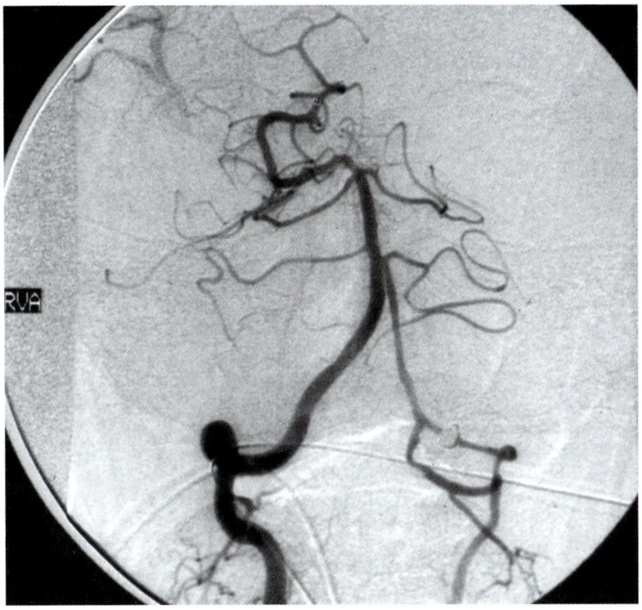

Fig. 4.16 Angiography shows a fenestrated (duplicated) V3 segment of the left vertebral artery.

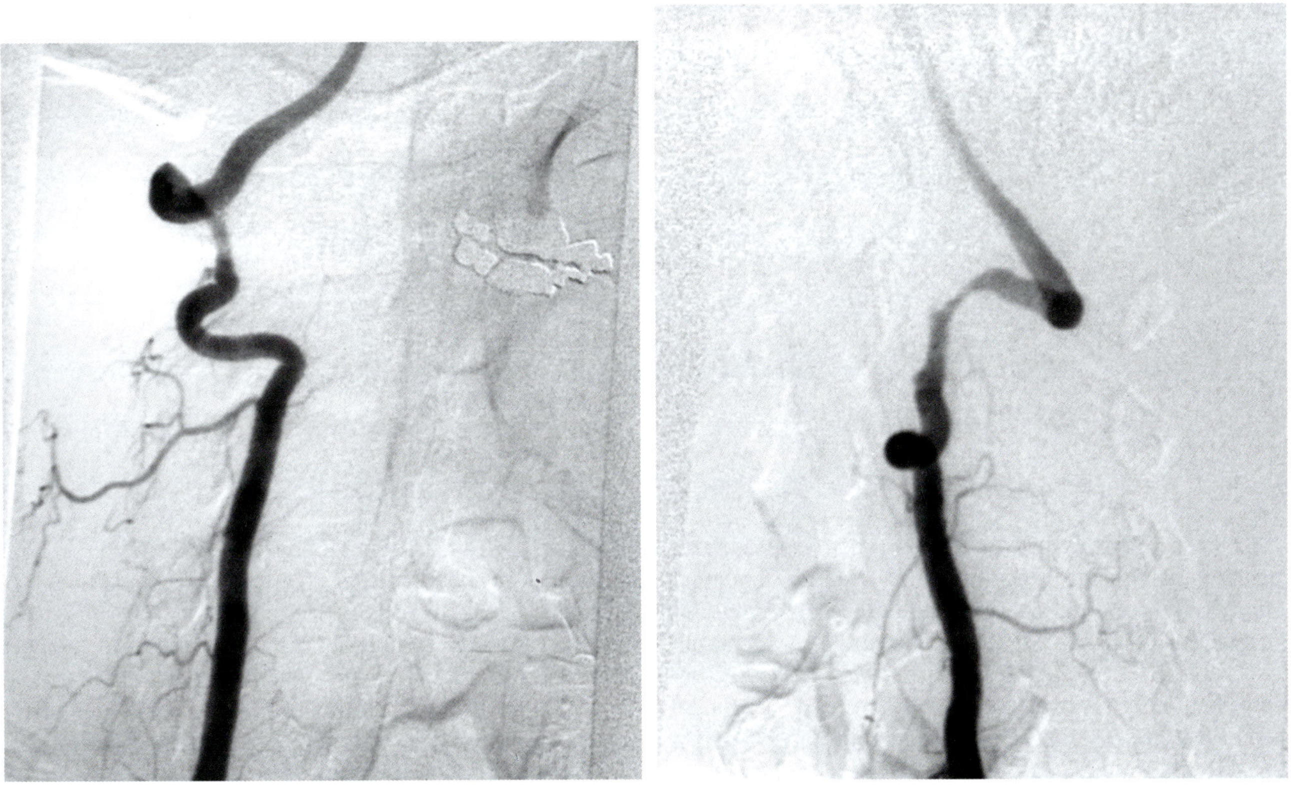

A B

Fig. 4.17 **(A)** Anteroposterior and **(B)** lateral angiographic views display a dissection of the V3 segment of the vertebral artery after chiropractic manipulation.

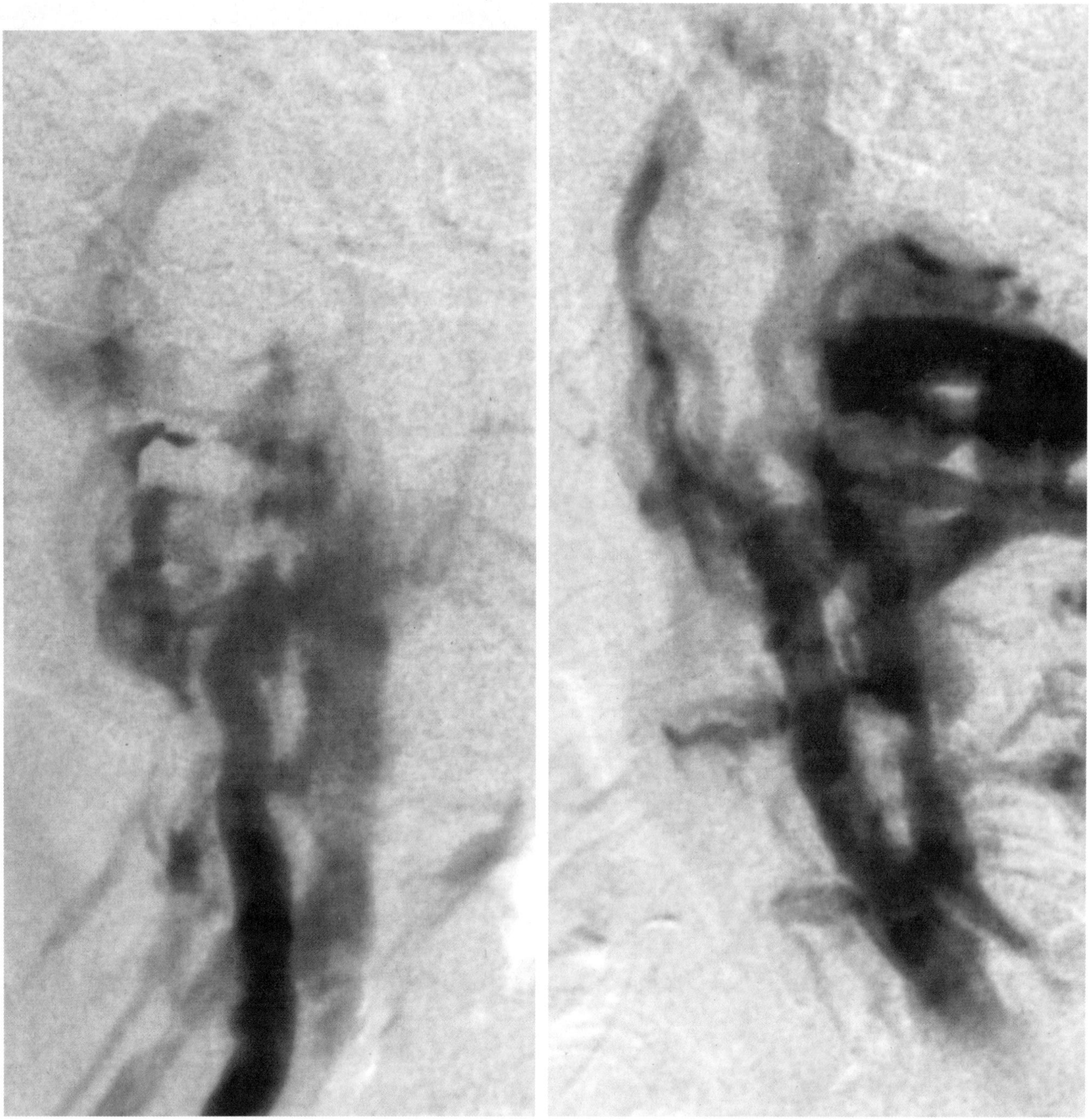

Fig. 4.18 **(A)** Anteroposterior and **(B)** lateral angiographic views depict an arteriovenous fistula after a penetrating trauma near the region of the skull base.

C1-C2 level.[50] Compromise of the vertebral arteries has been documented with head rotation.[51–53] The rotation appears to compress the vertebral artery mechanically, contralateral to the head turn at C1-C2. Some patients with asymmetrically sized vertebral arteries or hypoplastic arteries can become symptomatic from extreme head rotations when the larger vertebral artery is compromised by the rotation.

Penetrating injuries can cause arteriovenous (AV) fistulae because the vertebral arteries are surrounded by a rich venous network and drain directly into the vertebral veins (**Fig. 4.18**).[54] AV fistulae, pseudoaneurysms, and dissections also can be encountered at this level, secondary to fibromuscular dysplasia (FMD).[55,56] Typically, FMD is found in the cervical carotid arteries when the neck vessels are involved. However, the V3 and V4 segments of the vertebral arteries are the second most common area of involvement of the head and neck, found in up to 10% of patients with FMD.[57,58] Occasionally, the occipital and intracranial arteries are involved.[59] Although patients with FMD of the vertebral arteries may present with AV fistulae, they more commonly present with sudden neurological deficits associated with dissections, thromboembolic events, or occlusive ischemia involving the structures of the posterior fossa or spinal cord.[60] There is an increased incidence of intracranial aneurysms.[61] Patients with FMD may present with subarachnoid hemorrhage related to "berry" type aneurysms or dissecting aneurysms.[62,63]

Atherosclerotic disease often involves the origins of the vertebral arteries or the basilar artery, but significant disease is unusual at the CVJ.[64] Aneurysms and AV malformations are also rare at this level, but there is an increased incidence of aneurysms in the vertebrobasilar system in patients with Moyamoya disease.[65,66] Pseudoaneurysms caused by dissections are rare, and "berry" aneurysms near the PICA origin comprise 2 to 3% of intracranial aneurysms.[67] Patients with persistent fetal anastomoses, such as the hypoglossal and proatlantal arteries, may present atypically with posterior fossa ischemic symptoms when the ipsilateral carotid artery is compromised.[68]

Because they are supplied by small segmental branches directly from the vertebral arteries, vascular tumors at the CVJ tend to be more difficult to embolize than those at other spinal levels. Occasionally, these segmental branches have unidentified coexisting posterior spinal artery branches, and larger embolization particles may be needed. The vascular supply from the occipital, ascending pharyngeal, posterior auricular, thyrocervical, and costocervical arteries is usually more amenable to embolization.

Numerous other vascular disorders can compromise the vertebral arteries at the CVJ or vertebrobasilar system. Patients with type I neurofibromatosis and those who have undergone radiation therapy can present with stenosis and vertebrobasilar compromise.[69] Patients with Klippel-Feil deformities may present with vertebral artery occlusions.[70,71] Spondylosis often compromises the vertebral artery in more proximal locations, but rarely at the level of the CVJ.[72,73]

Conclusion

MRI has superior soft tissue discrimination, allowing visualization of the neuraxis without intrathecal contrast medium. The degree of impingement or distortion of the neuraxis can be readily evaluated and analyzed in any imaging plane. New thin-section, high-resolution techniques show promise in the evaluation of the supporting ligaments about the CVJ. It is hoped that these techniques will be important determinants of treatment planning and prognosis. The imaging modalities described here and familiarity with the various anomalies and pathologies that affect the CVJ enable accurate assessment and appropriate treatment planning.

References

1. Dolan KD. Cervicobasilar relationships. Radiol Clin North Am 1977;15(2):155–166
2. Krakenes J, Kaale BR, Rorvik J, Gilhus NE. MRI assessment of normal ligamentous structures in the craniovertebral junction. Neuroradiology 2001;43(12):1089–1097
3. Fox WC, Wawrzyniak S, Chandler WF. Intraoperative acquisition of three-dimensional imaging for frameless stereotactic guidance during transsphenoidal pituitary surgery using the Arcadis Orbic System. J Neurosurg 2008;108(4):746–750
4. Smoker WR, Khanna G. Imaging the craniocervical junction. Childs Nerv Syst 2008;24(10):1123–1145
5. Engelman ED, Schnitzlein HN, Hilbelink DR, et al. Imaging anatomy of the cranio-vertebral junction (occipito-atlanto-axial joint). Clin Anat 1989;2:241–252
6. Schweitzer ME, Hodler J, Cervilla V, Resnick D. Craniovertebral junction: normal anatomy with MR correlation. AJR Am J Roentgenol 1992;158(5):1087–1090
7. de Oliveira E, Rhoton AL Jr, Peace D. Microsurgical anatomy of the region of the foramen magnum. Surg Neurol 1985;24(3):293–352
8. Bewermeyer H, Dreesbach HA, Hünermann B, Heiss WD. MR imaging of familial basilar impression. J Comput Assist Tomogr 1984;8(5):953–956
9. Harwood-Nash D. Anomalies of the craniovertebral junction. In: Hoffman AJ, Epstein F, eds. Disorders of the Developing Nervous System. Boston, MA: Blackwell; 1986
10. Bernini FP, Elefante R, Smaltino F, Tedeschi G. Angiographic study on the vertebral artery in cases of deformities of the occipitocervical joint. Am J Roentgenol Radium Ther Nucl Med 1969;107(3):526–529
11. Naidich TP, McLone DG, Harwood-Nash DC. Malformations of the craniocervical junction. In: Newton TH, Potts DG, eds. Modern Neuroradiology. Computed Tomography of the Spine and Spinal Cord. San Anselmo, CA: Clavadel Press; 1983:355–366
12. von Torklus D, Gehle W. The Upper Cervical Spine, Regional Anatomy, Pathology and Traumatology. A Systematic Radiological Atlas and Textbook. New York, NY: Grune & Stratton; 1972
13. Hensinger RN. Congenital anomalies of the cervical spine. Clin Orthop Relat Res 1991;264(264):16–38
14. Menkü A, Koç RK, Tucer B, Durak AC, Akdemir H. Clivus fractures: clinical presentations and courses. Neurosurg Rev 2004;27(3):194–198
15. Menezes AH, Traynelis VC. Anatomy and biomechanics of normal craniovertebral junction (a) and biomechanics of stabilization (b). Childs Nerv Syst 2008;24(10):1091–1100
16. Gehweiler JA Jr, Daffner RH, Roberts LJ Jr. Malformations of the atlas vertebra simulating the Jefferson fracture. AJR Am J Roentgenol 1983;140(6):1083–1086
17. Dorne HL, Lander PH. CT recognition of anomalies of the posterior arch of the atlas vertebra: differentiation from fracture. AJNR Am J Neuroradiol 1986;7(1):176–177
18. Chen YF, Liu HM. Imaging of craniovertebral junction. Neuroimaging Clin N Am 2009;19(3):483–510
19. Holt RG, Helms CA, Munk PL, Gillespy T III. Hypertrophy of C-1 anterior arch: useful sign to distinguish os odontoideum from acute dens fracture. Radiology 1989;173(1):207–209
20. Sherman J. The craniovertebral junction. In: Rao KCVG, Williams JP, Lee BCP, Sherman JL, eds. MRI and CT of the Spine. Baltimore, MD: Williams & Wilkins; 1994:71–97
21. Shohat M, Lachman R, Rimoin DL. Odontoid hypoplasia with vertebral cervical subluxation and ventriculomegaly in metatropic dysplasia. J Pediatr 1989;114(2):239–243
22. Thomas SL, Childress MH, Quinton B. Hypoplasia of the odontoid with atlanto-axial subluxation in Hurler's syndrome. Pediatr Radiol 1985;15(5):353–354
23. VanGilder JC, Menezes AH, Dolan KD. The Craniovertebral Junction and Its Abnormalities. New York, NY: Futura Publishers; 1987

24. McManners T. Odontoid hypoplasia. Br J Radiol 1983;56(672): 907–910
25. Goel A, Bhatjiwale M, Desai K. Basilar invagination: a study based on 190 surgically treated patients. J Neurosurg 1998;88(6):962–968
26. Pang D, Wilberger JE Jr. Traumatic atlanto-occipital dislocation with survival: case report and review. Neurosurgery 1980;7(5): 503–508
27. Farley FA, Graziano GP, Hensinger RN. Traumatic atlanto-occipital dislocation in a child. Spine 1992;17(12):1539–1541
28. White AA III, Panjabi MM. The problem of clinical instability in the human spine: a systematic approach. In: White AA III, Panjabi MM, eds. Clinical Biomechanics of the Spine. Philadelphia, PA: JB Lippincott; 1978:191–271
29. Traynelis VC, Marano GD, Dunker RO, Kaufman HH. Traumatic atlanto-occipital dislocation. Case report. J Neurosurg 1986;65(6): 863–870
30. Spence KF Jr, Decker S, Sell KW. Bursting atlantal fracture associated with rupture of the transverse ligament. J Bone Joint Surg Am 1970;52(3):543–549
31. Fielding JW, Cochran GB, Lawsing JF III, Hohl M. Tears of the transverse ligament of the atlas. A clinical and biomechanical study. J Bone Joint Surg Am 1974;56(8):1683–1691
32. Wollin DG, Botterell EH. Symmetrical forward luxation of the atlas. Am J Roentgenol Radium Ther Nucl Med 1958;79(4):575–583
33. Dickman CA, Mamourian AC, Sonntag VKH, Drayer BP. Magnetic resonance imaging of the transverse atlantal ligament for the evaluation of atlantoaxial instability. J Neurosurg 1991;75(2):221–227
34. Vetti N, Alsing R, Kråkenes J, et al. MRI of the transverse and alar ligaments in rheumatoid arthritis: feasibility and relations to atlantoaxial subluxation and disease activity. Neuroradiology 2010;52(3):215–223
35. Baumert B, Wörtler K, Steffinger D, Schmidt GP, Reiser MF, Baur-Melnyk A. Assessment of the internal craniocervical ligaments with a new magnetic resonance imaging sequence: three-dimensional turbo spin echo with variable flip-angle distribution (SPACE). Magn Reson Imaging 2009;27(7):954–960
36. Padget DH. Development of cranial arteries in human embryo. Contrib Embryol 1948;32:205–262
37. McCartney SF, Ricci MA, Labreque P, Symes JF. Persistent hypoglossal artery encountered during carotid endarterectomy. Ann Vasc Surg 1989;3(3):257–260
38. Hong JT, Lee SW, Son BC, et al. Analysis of anatomical variations of bone and vascular structures around the posterior atlantal arch using three-dimensional computed tomography angiography. J Neurosurg Spine 2008;8(3):230–236
39. Tokuda K, Miyasaka K, Abe H, et al. Anomalous atlantoaxial portions of vertebral and posterior inferior cerebellar arteries. Neuroradiology 1985;27(5):410–413
40. Sato K, Watanabe T, Yoshimoto T, Kameyama M. Magnetic resonance imaging of C2 segmental type of vertebral artery. Surg Neurol 1994;41(1):45–51
41. Morris L. Non-union of the vertebral arteries: case report. Br J Radiol 1962;35:496–498
42. Burrows PE, Tubman DE. Multiple extracranial arterial lesions following closed craniocervical trauma. J Trauma 1981;21(6):497–498
43. Fassett DR, Dailey AT, Vaccaro AR. Vertebral artery injuries associated with cervical spine injuries: a review of the literature. J Spinal Disord Tech 2008;21(4):252–258
44. Yang PJ, Latack JT, Gabrielsen TO, Knake JE, Gebarski SS, Chandler WF. Rotational vertebral artery occlusion at C1-C2. AJNR Am J Neuroradiol 1985;6(1):96–100
45. Horváth M, Jólesz F, Pásztor E. Development of bilateral collateral circulation after fracture of the axis. Acta Chir Acad Sci Hung 1980;21(1):69–76
46. Rothrock JF, Hesselink JR, Teacher TM. Vertebral artery occlusion and stroke from cervical self-manipulation. Neurology 1991;41(10): 1696–1697
47. Cabezudo JM, Olabe J, Lopez-Anguera A, Bacci F. Recovery from locked-in syndrome after posttraumatic bilateral distal vertebral artery occlusion. Surg Neurol 1986;25(2):185–190
48. Howell SJ, Molyneux AJ. Vertebrobasilar insufficiency in rheumatoid atlanto-axial subluxation: a case report with angiographic demonstration of left vertebral artery occlusion. J Neurol 1988; 235(3):189–190
49. Loeb M, Bookman A, Mikulis D. Rheumatoid arthritis and vertebral artery occlusion: a case report with angiographic and magnetic resonance demonstration. J Rheumatol 1993;20(8):1402–1405
50. Miley ML, Wellik KE, Wingerchuk DM, Demaerschalk BM. Does cervical manipulative therapy cause vertebral artery dissection and stroke? Neurologist 2008;14(1):66–73
51. Hedera P, Bujdáková J, Traubner P. Blood flow velocities in basilar artery during rotation of the head. Acta Neurol Scand 1993;88(3):229–233
52. Natello GW, Carroll CM, Katwal AB. Rotational vertebrobasilar ischemia due to vertebral artery dynamic stenoses complicated by an ostial atherosclerotic stenosis. Vasc Med 2009;14(3):265–269
53. Dabus G, Gerstle RJ, Parsons M, et al. Rotational vertebrobasilar insufficiency due to dynamic compression of the dominant vertebral artery by the thyroid cartilage and occlusion of the contralateral vertebral artery at C1-2 level. J Neuroimaging 2008;18(2):184–187
54. Herrera DA, Vargas SA, Dublin AB. Endovascular treatment of traumatic injuries of the vertebral artery. AJNR Am J Neuroradiol 2008;29(8):1585–1589
55. Bahar S, Chiras J, Carpena JP, Meder JF, Bories J. Spontaneous vertebro-vertebral arterio-venous fistula associated with fibro-muscular dysplasia. Report of two cases. Neuroradiology 1984;26(1):45–49
56. Hieshima GB, Cahan LD, Mehringer CM, Bentson JR. Spontaneous arteriovenous fistulas of cerebral vessels in association with fibromuscular dysplasia. Neurosurgery 1986;18(4):454–458
57. Osborn AG, Anderson RE. Angiographic spectrum of cervical and intracranial fibromuscular dysplasia. Stroke 1977;8(5):617–626
58. Manns RA, Nanda KK, Mackie G. Fibromuscular dysplasia of the cephalic and renal arteries. Clin Radiol 1987;38(4):427–429
59. So EL, Toole JF, Dalal P, Moody DM. Cephalic fibromuscular dysplasia in 32 patients: clinical findings and radiologic features. Arch Neurol 1981;38(10):619–622
60. Reddy SV, Karnes WE, Earnest F IV, Sundt TM Jr. Spontaneous extracranial vertebral arteriovenous fistula with fibromuscular dysplasia. Case report. J Neurosurg 1981;54(3):399–402
61. Mettinger KL, Ericson K. Fibromuscular dysplasia and the brain. I. Observations on angiographic, clinical and genetic characteristics. Stroke 1982;13(1):46–52
62. Vles JS, Hendriks JJ, Lodder J, Janevski B. Multiple vertebro-basilar infarctions from fibromuscular dysplasia related dissecting aneurysm of the vertebral artery in a child. Neuropediatrics 1990;21(2):104–105
63. Perez-Higueras A, Alvarez-Ruiz F, Martinez-Bermejo A, Frutos R, Villar O, Diez-Tejedor E. Cerebellar infarction from fibromuscular dysplasia and dissecting aneurysm of the vertebral artery. Report of a child. Stroke 1988;19(4):521–524
64. Caplan LR. Bilateral distal vertebral artery occlusion. Neurology 1983;33(5):552–558
65. Nagamine Y, Takahashi S, Sonobe M. Multiple intracranial aneurysms associated with moyamoya disease. Case report. J Neurosurg 1981;54(5):673–676
66. Bucciero A, Carangelo B, Vizioli L. Giant basilar artery aneurysm associated with moya-moya disease. Case report and review of the literature. Acta Neurol (Napoli) 1994;16(3):121–128

67. Peluso JP, van Rooij WJ, Sluzewski M, Beute GN, Majoie CB. Posterior inferior cerebellar artery aneurysms: incidence, clinical presentation, and outcome of endovascular treatment. AJNR Am J Neuroradiol 2008;29(1):86–90
68. Kolbinger R, Heindel W, Pawlik G, Erasmi-Körber H. Right proatlantal artery type I, right internal carotid occlusion, and left internal carotid stenosis: case report and review of the literature. J Neurol Sci 1993;117(1-2):232–239
69. Grill J, Dhermain F, Habrand JL. Risks of radiation therapy in patients with neurofibromatosis. Int J Radiat Oncol Biol Phys 2009;75(2):632
70. Hadeishi H, Ishikawa T, Suzuki A, Yasui N. [A case of Klippel-Feil syndrome with crossed renal ectopia with fusion and unilateral vertebral artery occlusion]. No Shinkei Geka 1991;19(2):191–195
71. Hasan I, Wapnick S, Kutscher ML, Couldwell WT. Vertebral arterial dissection associated with Klippel-Feil syndrome in a child. Childs Nerv Syst 2002;18(1-2):67–70
72. Chin JH. Recurrent stroke caused by spondylotic compression of the vertebral artery. Ann Neurol 1993;33(5):558–559
73. Bulsara KR, Velez DA, Villavicencio A. Rotational vertebral artery insufficiency resulting from cervical spondylosis: case report and review of the literature. Surg Neurol 2006;65(6):625–627

5 Neurological Findings of Craniovertebral Junction Disease

David M. Benglis and Allan D. Levi

Neurological manifestations of craniovertebral junction (CVJ) disease may result from various etiologies, therefore making the localization of pathology to this region in the neuraxis challenging.[1,2] The importance of this region as an entrance and exit for vital neural pathways cannot be underestimated. Upper cervical spinal cord damage can manifest in the form of pain, sensory or motor disturbances, proprioceptive derangement, gait imbalance, abnormalities in coordination, and respiratory insufficiency. Although an in-depth history and physical exam are paramount in differentiating the type of insult into a specific category (e.g., traumatic, tumor, vascular, or syrinx), a level and modern diagnosis is also greatly facilitated by imaging, specifically magnetic resonance imaging (MRI) of the CVJ. MRI is the modality of choice for this region due to its multiplanar capability, resolution of soft tissues, and ability to delineate disease process from normal tissue.

The temporal quality of a patient's presentation can also be suggestive of a particular cause. For example, vascular injuries are acute, whereas slow-growing tumors such as meningiomas and schwannomas often have a relentlessly progressive course over many years. General mechanisms in which neurological deficits may occur include traction or direct compression on tissues, interruption in blood flow resulting in ischemia or stroke, and aberrant changes in normal cerebrospinal fluid (CSF) dynamics leading to hydrocephalus and syrinx formation.

Neuropathological Mechanisms of Injury at the Craniovertebral Junction

Trauma

Following spinal cord injury, one of the most important questions concerning the neurological exam is whether the patient has a complete or incomplete spinal cord injury. As treatment and prognosis differ remarkably between these two conditions, the distinction is crucial. Complete motor and sensory disruption below the level of injury (American Spinal Injury Association [ASIA] class A) signifies a catastrophic deficit with future ambulation rates of only 1 to 3%.[3–5] These injuries at the CVJ carry with them a poor prognosis. There are no reported cases of ASIA A patients recovering ambulatory function following atlanto-occipital dislocation.[6]

Due to the larger canal diameter at the CVJ when compared with the subaxial spine, traumatic injuries in this region often cause bony or ligamentous injury while sparing the neural parenchyma.[7] Spinal injuries at the CVJ have a wide range of clinical presentations (**Table 5.1**). Neurological problems range from those with absent voluntary motor control and slight sensory preservation in the lowest sacral dermatomes (ASIA B) to patients with only mild motor or sensory deficits. Bell's cruciate paralysis is a specific type of incomplete spinal cord injury that involves the upper extremities disproportionately compared with the lower. Past explanations for these neurological findings were assumed to be due to a somatotopically organized corticospinal tract. However, evidence from experimental work in primates and observations in humans support alternative explanations and refute this commonly accepted pathophysiological theory.[8] Acute central cord syndrome (ACCS) may also present with disproportionate weakness of the upper extremities. Although difficult to distinguish clinically, the spinal cord pathology surrounding these two syndromes differs and is explained in the following text.[9,10]

Bell's Cruciate Paralysis

Cruciate paralysis was first described clinically by Bell as a syndrome characterized by "paralysis in both arms without weakness in the legs."[11–15] Causative mechanisms are typically due to cervical fractures in the region of the CVJ.[15] The basis for the clinical presentation was thought to be due to midline damage to the rostral portion of the pyramidal decussation that would selectively injure the fibers of the corticospinal tract subserving hand and arm function.[7] In 1901, Wallenberg reported on the complex anatomy present at the CVJ, including the illustration that fibers serving function to the arms decussate more rostrally than those subserving the legs.[16] He described a patient in his report with "hemiplegia cruciata" or ipsilateral arm weakness and contralateral leg weakness. Wallenberg's presumption was that this injury could be explained by rostral unilateral damage to the recently crossed corticospinal fibers of the arm and uncrossed fibers of the legs (**Fig. 5.1**). This observation suggested a somatotopical organization of these fibers

Table 5.1 Types of Fractures of the Craniovertebral Junction

Clival fractures
Atlanto-occipital fractures
Occipital condyle fractures
Atlas fractures
Odontoid fractures (types I, II, IIa, and III)
Hangman's fracture
C2 vertebral body fractures

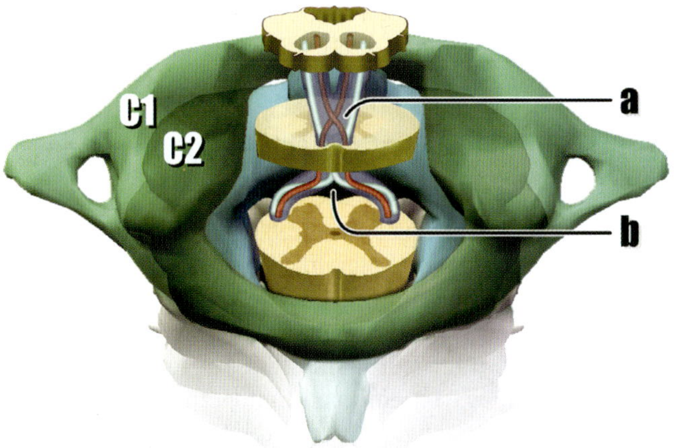

Fig. 5.1 Diagram illustrating Bell's hypothesis (1972), which proposed that (*a*) arm fibers decussate more rostrally in the cervicomedullary junction than (*b*) the fibers supplying motor function to the leg. An injury localized to this level could theoretically produce the clinical symptoms associated with cruciate paralysis whereby there is a disproportionate weakness of the upper versus lower extremities. (Adapted with permission from Marano SR, Calica AB, Sonntag VKH. Bilateral upper extremity paralysis [Bell's cruciate paralysis] from a gunshot wound to the cervicomedullary junction. Neurosurgery 1986;18[5]:642–644.)

at the CVJ.[17] Although this theory has prevailed in neuroanatomical texts, no evidence to date has supported the presence of a somatotopically organized corticospinal tract at the CVJ.[18,19]

Central Cord Syndrome

Schneider and colleagues initially described central cord syndrome as a neurological ailment of the CVJ that caused disproportionate arm versus leg weakness similar in clinical presentation to Bell's cruciate paralysis.[20] The syndrome is reported more frequently among older persons with cervical spondylosis and spinal stenosis and accounts for 9% of the total incidence of spinal cord injuries.[21] The proposed pathophysiological mechanism was thought to be due to selective injury to the medial based arm fibers of a somatotopically organized corticospinal tract within the posterolateral funiculus of the spinal cord.[22]

The Evidence Against Somatotopical Organization of the Corticospinal Tract

Neuroanatomical studies in primates have never supported the theory that there is a somatotopic organization of the corticospinal tract (CST). Pre- and post-decussation fibers are diffusely located within the pyramids and corticospinal tract, respectively, in the posterolateral funiculus as demonstrated by Marchi degeneration studies and modern tracer techniques.[23–26] Similar evidence can be extracted from human reports where lesions of the central nervous system cause retrograde degeneration of the CST in the brainstem and spinal cord.[27,28] Although there appears to be laminar organization spanning the motor cortex, internal capsule, and pons, it is lost at the levels of the medulla and spinal cord. Therefore, the manner in which both Bell's cruciate paralysis and central cord syndrome (CCS) were once thought to have occurred via injury to a somatotopically organized CST must be rethought.

One potential theory to explain the differential findings between upper and lower extremity function in these syndromes, which does not require somatotopic organization of the CST, may be that the CST is more important for the function of the hands and arms than the lower extremities. This difference could explain the observation that an injury at the CVJ could present as a disproportionate weakness of the upper extremities versus the lower. As one ascends the phylogenetic scale, the CST assumes a more important role in movements associated with hand function.[29–32] In higher order mammals with upright postures and complex hand functions, the CST becomes larger in diameter due to an increased number of axons that synapse on motor neurons in the ventral horn of the spinal cord at these associated upper levels.[29–31,33] Sherrington was so impressed with this increase in size of the CST that he remarked, "There is no other system which shows such increase in relative size as traced from lower to higher mammalian types."[34] Following an injection of an anterograde tracer into the primate motor cortex, Pappas and colleagues confirmed that the CST lacks a somatotopical organization at the level of the medullary decussation.[26]

Two alternative mechanisms have been proposed to explain the clinical findings in cruciate paralysis. The first includes selective injury to the ventral CST, which can serve as a significant outflow for the CST that is absent below the cervical enlargment.[28,35] Focal damage to this tract from an anterior spinal fracture could explain the findings in cruciate paralysis. The other mechanism consists of an injury to the collateral fibers of the CST to the brainstem, central gray matter, and dorsal column nuclei. Although the importance of these collateral fiber tracts has yet to be determined, they appear to be segregated from fiber terminations supplying the hind limb.

Selective Primate Corticospinal Tract Lesioning and the Importance of Hand Function

Several studies have focused on the effects following transection of one or both CSTs at the level of the medullary pyramids or cerebral peduncles in the primate.[36–39] In primates, the CST is isolated from other tracts in the brainstem and spinal cord and can therefore be selectively injured. In general, incomplete lesions of the CST do not produce catastrophic motor deficits and recover over time. The predominate deficit following selective lesions of the CST in primates is greater hand and arm weakness when compared with the distal extremities (e.g., elimination of discrete finger movements, diminished general usage, loss of initiative, defective contact placing and grasping, and difficulty in the release of a grasp once initiated).[36,40] Bucy and colleagues described the return of function in these primate studies in a similar manner as that observed with Bell's cruciate paralysis and CCS in observed in humans ("recovery began in the proximal musculature and progressed to the distal musculature as the lower extremities usually recovered before the upper extremities").[41]

Recent data published by Jimenez and colleagues investigated whether there was a reduction in the large α motor neurons at C7, C8, and T1 following traumatic central cord syndrome in postmortem human cervical spinal cord specimens. The spinal cords were divided into acute/subacute (less than 5 weeks, $n = 2$) and chronic (greater than 5 weeks, $n = 3$) depending on the time of death after the initial injury. The chronic group was further subdivided into a high-level cervical group (injury at C2, $n = 1$) and low-level cervical group (injury at C5-C6, $n = 2$). They found a significant reduction in α motor neurons at C7-T1, with respect to the chronic low-level cervical injury group, and attributed this finding to the proximity of the initial injury to these structures.

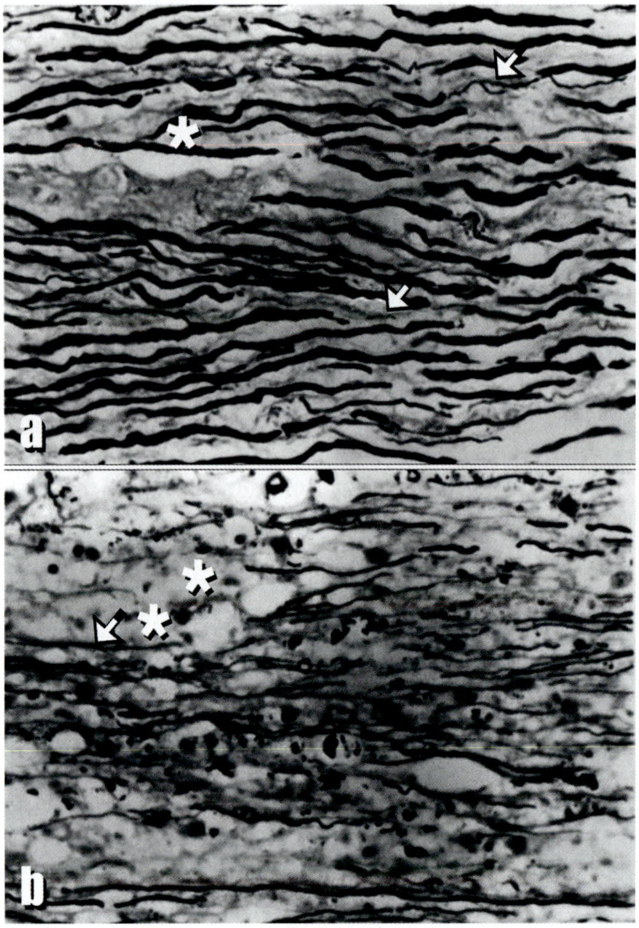

Fig. 5.2 (A) Normal human spinal cord specimen showing large myelinated corticospinal tract (CST) fibers (*asterisk*) and small myelinated CST fibers (*arrows*). **(B)** Wallerian degeneration in the CST in a patient with acute central cord syndrome following trauma with fragmentation of myelin around large (*asterisks*) and small CST fibers (*arrow*). (From Jiminez O, Marcillo A, Levi AD. A histopathological analysis of the human cervical spinal cord in patients with acute traumatic central cord syndrome. Spinal Cord 2000;38:532–537, with permission from Nature Publishing Group.)

Jimenez and colleagues also noted that CCS can occur following a more rostral injury to the CST without affecting these lower α motor axons controlling hand function (**Fig. 5.2**).[42]

Cortical and Spinal Plasticity Following Experimental Selective Lesioning

Nishimura and colleagues explored the mechanism for recovery in hand function following distinct lesions in the CST of macaque monkeys at the C4/5 levels. They theorized that alternate indirect corticomotoneuronal pathways (e.g., subcortical or spinal interneuronal systems) were responsible for this recovery. Positron emission tomography (PET) postinjury revealed that activity increased in a similar pattern to preinjury early in the postinjury period. Yet later, new areas of brain activity were documented. To confirm whether these increased regions of activity observed in PET contributed to hand-directed activity, Nishimura and colleagues selectively inhibited these areas with a gamma-aminobutyric acid type A receptor agonist. Their work suggests that alternate pathways are activated late in the recovery phase with the end result of the restoration of hand function.[43]

Maier and colleagues have examined spinal cord plasticity following transection of the CST at the level of the brainstem in rats.[44] They restricted movement of the unaffected limb, forcing the animals to use the impaired one. This forced rehabilitation of the affected limb was followed by a fuller behavioral recovery on physical tasks in the experimental group. Histologically the group demonstrated lesion-induced growth in the CST from the unlesioned side across the midline via CST collaterals.

Lesioning Alternative Primate Subcortical Spinal Motor Tracts

The inability to completely paralyze monkeys, even with bilateral pyramidal lesions, suggests the existence of alternative descending pathways that are important for voluntary limb function.[37,38] After recovering from bilateral pyramidotomies, Lawrence and Kuypers performed additional anterior or lateral subcortical spinal pathway lesions to further delineate the influence of these alternative tracts on motor function.[37,45] Subcortical pathways were separated into medial (e.g., vestibular nuclei and pontine/medullary reticular formation) and lateral (e.g., pars magnocellularis of the red nucleus) nuclear origins in the brainstem. Terminations of these fiber tracts were on interneurons of the spinal cord. Medial lesions did not worsen distal hand function, whereas lateral lesions exacerbated distal forelimb dysfunction. Remarkably, the monkeys had little difficulty in standing and walking.

Evidence Against Somatotopical Organization of the Corticospinal Tract in Humans

Findings from lesion studies at the CVJ in primates can be extrapolated and applied to clinical and anatomical data available in humans to help explain alternative mechanisms for the neurological findings observed in Bell's cruciate paralysis and CCS. There is a size difference when comparing the CST in humans versus primates. Napier has attributed this increase in size and number of fibers in humans to further refinements of hand dexterity and function.[46] Thus, it is plausible that an injury to this tract may result in greater hand and arm dysfunction in humans when compared with a similar injury in primates.

Furthermore, injuries would also have to be localized to a region of small area located at the medullary decussation or cervical spinal cord to produce differences in the closely packaged hand, arm, and leg fibers. Neuropathological studies of patients following spinal cord injury reveal that focal injuries of the cervical and medullary region are quite uncommon and that wide variations exist between lesion volumes. Thus, in humans, Bell's cruciate paralysis and CCS may be explained by an injury to the entire corticospinal tract. A case report of a 72-year-old patient with cruciate paralysis (0/5 strength in the upper extremities versus 3/5 in the lower) following a fracture of the C2 vertebrae revealed anterograde degeneration of the spinal cord as far down inferiorly as the lumbar cord on pathological examination.[13] This finding suggests that fibers supplying the lower extremities were not spared as previously assumed by Bell.

Composition of the corticospinal tract includes 60% of fibers arising from the primary motor cortex (Brodmann area 4).[47] The diameter of the largest axons ranges from 10 mm to 25 mm. They arise from the pyramidal cells of Betz, which account for only 4% of the total fibers in the corticospinal tract.[48] Large-diameter fibers synapse directly on α motor neurons that tend to supply distal musculature of the upper extremities.[33,48,49] However, most of the fibers in the CST are of small diameter, conduct signals at slow rates, and synapse with interneurons.[49] Because traumatic injuries are more likely to injure large fibers than injure small ones, a diffuse injury could selectively affect them and cause a disparate injury to hand function.[50,51]

Neurological Presentation of Tumors at the Craniovertebral Junction

The presentation of tumors at the CVJ can mimic more common central or peripheral nerve diseases such as cervical spondylosis, carpal tunnel syndrome, multiple sclerosis, or infectious and inflammatory lesions.[52] Rapidity of growth of the tumor and its specific location dictate the presenting symptoms. Tumors may arise from neural structures, their coverings, or surrounding bone. Pain in the distribution of the C2 dermatome is the most frequent initial symptom with exacerbation upon movement. The C2 nerve root can be compressed intradurally or extradurally, and torticollis may be present.[53] Erosive bony tumors produce neck pain not defined to a specific dermatomal region.

Common motor symptoms include weakness and clumsiness of the hands with associated spasticity of the extremities (caused by compression of the CST) (**Fig. 5.3**).[54] In experimental models of upper cervical spinal cord compression,

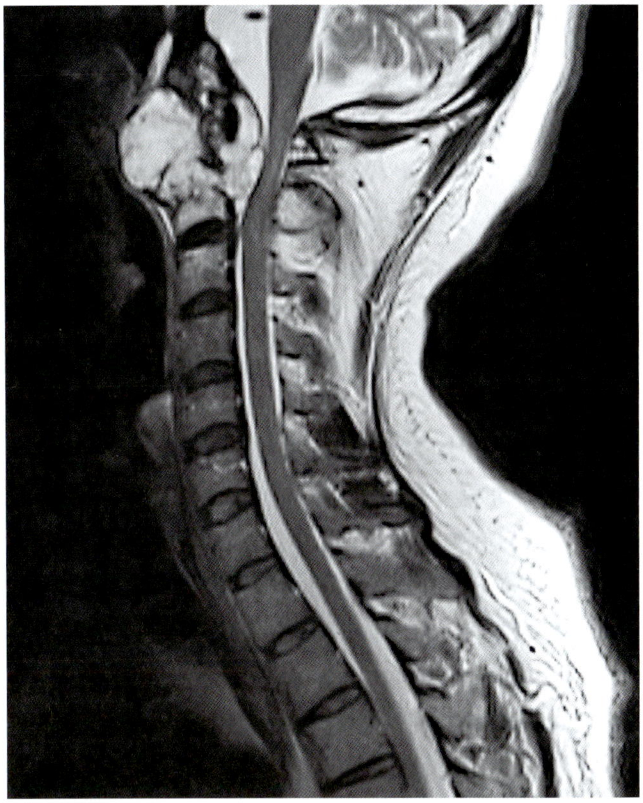

Fig. 5.3 Chordoma involving the craniovertebral junction. This patient presented with long tract symptoms and clumsiness of hands.

a loss of motor neurons in the anterior horns at C7 and T1 is observed.[55] One explanation of this observation of neuronal loss at C7/T1 is that the loss is from an impairment of venous drainage due to high cervical compression; however, MRI evidence refutes this hypothesis.[56] Patients with paramedian, slow-growing tumors (e.g., meningiomas, schwannomas, neurofibromas) may present with a classic syndrome described as a clockwise progression of neurological deficits that first involve the ipsilateral arm, followed by the ipsilateral leg and then the contralateral leg and arm.[57,58] Patients with central intramedullary lesions may present with myelopathy or suspended, dissociated sensory loss. When a syrinx is present, it may be associated with atrophy of upper extremity musculature, Charcot joints, or sensory disturbances.

Cranial Nerve Deficits from Compressive Lesions

Various cranial nerve deficits can manifest from pathology localized to the CVJ. Lesions may affect the nuclei, tracts, or foramen in which the cranial nerves travel. Bilateral cranial nerve involvement may arise from intramedullary tumors associated with a syrinx. The spinal trigeminal nucleus deserves special consideration due to its large size and resultant vulnerability from intramedullary or extramedullary compressive lesions involving the mid pons, medulla, or rostral cervical region. In addition, some cutaneous branches (e.g., proximal to the ear) of the facial, glossopharyngeal, and vagus nerves send pain and temperature fibers to the spinal sensory nucleus. This nucleus and tract mediate pain, temperature, and deep pressure sensation to the facial region, and the fibers are concentrically oriented (e.g., lateral facial sensory fibers enter the nucleus at lower levels). Lesions involving this nucleus may be associated with a classic "onion skin" pattern of deficits with the nose region involved lastly.

The spinal division of the accessory nerve arises from the anterior horn cells of C1 to C5 and travels rostrally through the subarachnoid space between the ventral and dorsal rootlets. It then passes through the foramen magnum where it joins the cranial division, which travels with the vagus before this junction point. This particular nerve is prone to iatrogenic injury during surgery in addition to compression from a mass. Tumors localized to the ventral portion of the foramen magnum may compress the hypoglossal nerve, resulting in subsequent ipsilateral tongue paralysis and atrophy. Similar deficits in tongue function can result from tumors localized in the hypoglossal canal.

The jugular foramen contains the lower cranial nerves and, when encroached upon by lesions, distinct neurological syndromes may arise (**Table 5.2**).[59] Vernet syndrome was classically described as the "syndrome of the jugular foramen." Common tumors affecting this region include glomus jugulare tumors, schwannomas, metastatic lesions, meningiomas, and epidermoids.[59] Involvement of the jugular foramen can cause deficits in taste on the posterior third of tongue (glossopharyngeal nerve), vocal cord and palatal paralysis associated with sensory loss in the pharynx (vagus nerve), and motor deficits of the sternocleidomastoid and trapezius muscles (accessory nerve). Tumors in the carotid canal may affect these nerves that ascend with the carotid artery and may cause Horner syndrome. Intracranial extension of any of these tumors can compress the brainstem and cause long tract symptoms.

Neurological Syndromes Due to Vascular Compromise at the Craniovertebral Junction

Anatomical Description of the Posterior Circulation

A detailed anatomical understanding of the vertebral arteries is paramount for surgeons operating in the CVJ. Stroke syndromes are included in the differential of CVJ pathology, and these vessels are prone to iatrogenic injury during surgery in this region. The vertebral arteries arise as the first branches off the subclavian arteries. They course upward in a superior to medial direction until entering the foramen transversarium at C6, after which they take a relatively vertical path from C6 to C2. After exiting the C1 transverse foramen, they commonly course superolaterally around the atlanto-occipital joint and come to lie in a horizontal groove along the posterior arch of C1, ultimately approaching midline and entering the foramen magnum in a cephalad progression.

Each vertebral artery gives rise to several important intracranial and extracranial branches that supply structures to the upper cervical and caudal brainstem. They cross toward the ventral portion of the spinal cord and medulla, ultimately joining to form the basilar artery. The extracranial portion of the vertebral arteries gives off segmental branches that supply the vertebral bodies, spinal cord, and muscular tissues, whereas the intracranial portion contains both the anterior and posterior spinal arteries and the posterior inferior cerebellar artery (PICA), which is the largest and most variable branch of these parent vessels. The PICA usually arises 1–2 cm below the origin of the basilar artery. The basilar artery bears main branches to the pons, the cerebellum (anterior inferior cerebellar arteries [AICA] and superior cerebellar artery [SCA]), and the mesencephalon, tectum, and posterior temporal and occipital lobes (posterior cerebral arteries [PCA]).

Vascular Occlusive Syndromes of the Posterior Circulation

Occlusive syndromes affecting the vertebrobasilar circulation may arise from an arterial dissection (intracranial or extracranial); atherosclerosis leading to thrombus, embolism, or hemorrhage of large and small vessels (i.e., lacunes); or vasospasm from resultant subarachnoid hemorrhage. Fibromuscular dysplasia, radiation-induced vascular stenosis, and external vascular compression from tumor are less common causes of pathology in this region. Neurological syndromes affecting the vertebrobasilar circulation are discussed in detail in the following section.

Vertebral Artery and Branches

Occlusion of the extracranial portion of the vertebral artery rarely results in neurological deficit.[60] Collateral branches from the external carotid artery and thyrocervical trunk as well as retrograde flow from the distal vertebral artery prevent ischemic complications from extracranial occlusion. On the contrary, intracranial occlusions result in neurological deficits due to infarcts, especially if the parent vessel is dominant.

PICA occlusion can result in Wallenberg syndrome or lateral medullary syndrome.[18] However, this syndrome more

Table 5.2 Cranial Nerve Involvement in Jugular Foramen Syndromes

Syndrome	Glossopharyngeal Nerve	Vagus Nerve	Accessory Nerve	Hypoglossal Nerve	Sympathetic
Vernet	X	X	X		
Collet-Sicard	X	X	X	X	
Villaret	X	X	X	X	X
Jackson		X	X	X	
Schmidt		X	X		

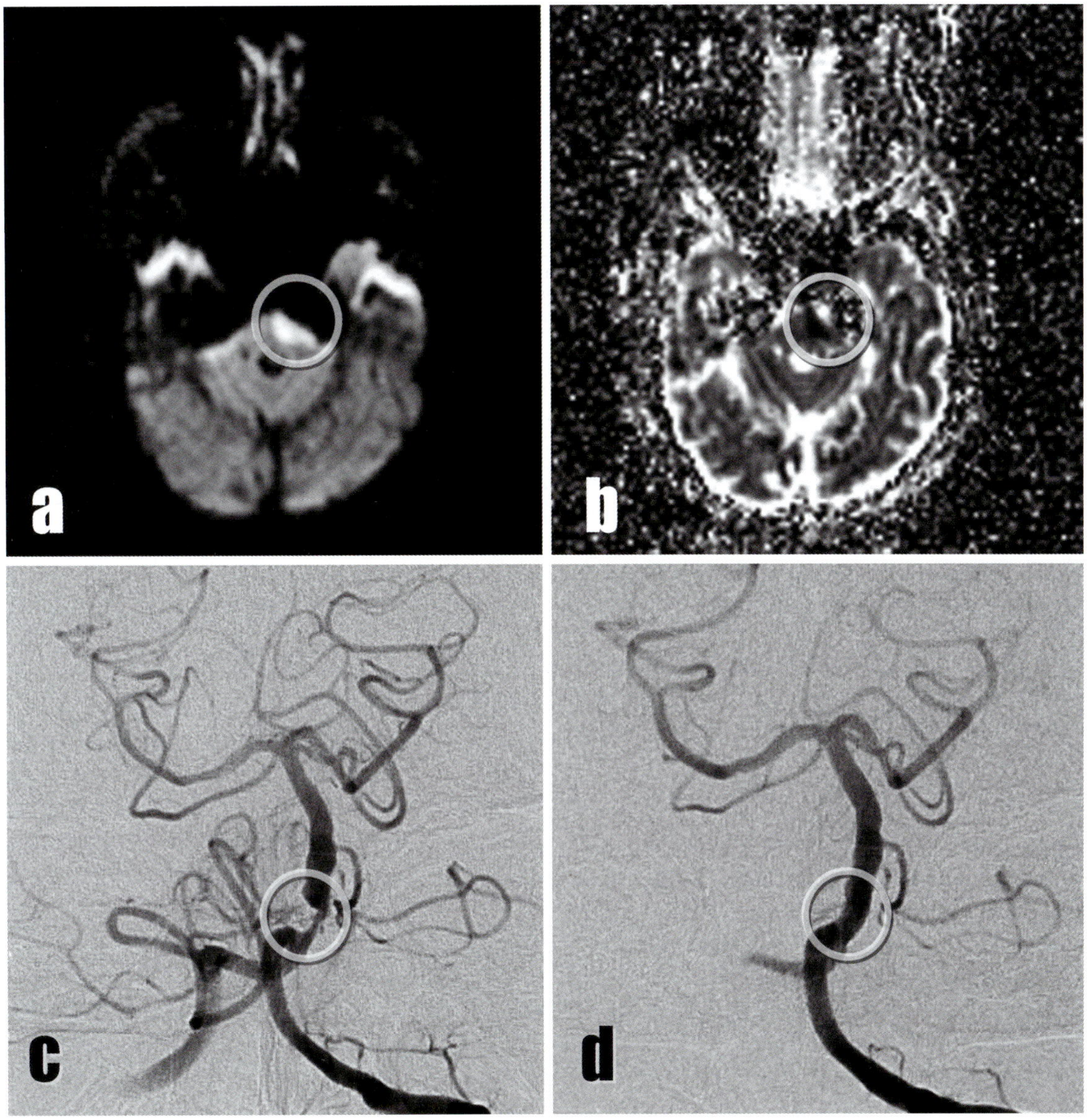

Fig. 5.4 **(A)** Magnetic resonance diffusion-weighted image and **(B)** apparent diffusion coefficient of an infarct in the left pons. Patient presented with sudden onset of skew deviation of the eyes and motor weakness on the opposite side. **(C)** Left vertebral injection revealing severe stenosis at the vertebrobasilar junction (*ring*). **(D)** Left vertebral injection following balloon angioplasty and stent placement showing reestablishment of blood flow. (Courtesy of H. Farhat and A. Sultan, University of Miami.)

commonly results from infarction of the territory supplied by short circumferential arteries originating from the vertebral artery (80 to 85% of the time) (**Fig. 5.4**).[61,62] Patients present with ipsilateral pain and temperature loss to the face and contralateral loss of pain and temperature in the body without pyramidal symptoms. These findings are consistent with damage to the trigeminal tract/nucleus and the prior crossed spinothalamic tract. Consciousness is preserved, and dizziness/vertigo (vestibular nuclei), loss of taste (tractus solitarius), dysphagia (nucleus ambiguous), and Horner syndrome (descending sympathetics in dorsal longitudinal fasciculus) may be found on exam. When the inferior cerebellar peduncle or spinocerebellar tract is involved, gait ataxia and nystagmus may be present.

Infarcts of the inferior cerebellum can result from vertebral artery or PICA occlusion. This syndrome can usually be defined temporally and separated into three distinct phases. The first set of symptoms result from direct damage to the medial (e.g., truncal ataxia, nystagmus, dysarthria) or lateral (e.g., appendicular ataxia, intention tremor) structures of the cerebellum. Second, increased swelling can cause compression of the fourth ventricle with the development of hydrocephalus that causes agitation, nausea, vomiting, and headaches. Third, the swelling progresses to mild brainstem compression, affecting the sixth and seventh cranial nerve nuclei, and causes a lateral gaze palsy and facial weakness, respectively. Severe brainstem compression may ultimately result in coma and death. Surgical decompression is often warranted when early signs of brainstem compression or hydrocephalus are present.[63–65]

Medial medullary syndrome involves the ventromedial structures within the medulla and can result from interruption of blood supply from either the anterior spinal artery or the vertebral artery (**Fig. 5.4**). The medullary pyramids, medial lemniscus, and hypoglossal nerve fibers are affected, leading to neurological symptoms of ipsilateral tongue weakness, contralateral hemiparesis and dysfunction in vibration, and proprioception. Bilateral involvement of the medulla is common.[66]

Basilar Artery and Branches

Basilar artery occlusive syndromes are divided into diseases of the main trunk and diseases of its respective branches. Lacunar infarcts are common in this region and involve vessels measuring less than 200 mcm and produce several distinct clinical syndromes. They include pure motor hemiplegia, dysarthria-clumsy hand syndrome, ataxic hemiparesis, and pure sensory deficits. Infarct sizes are usually small (1–3 mm) compared with cortical-based strokes. Weber syndrome involves interruption of blood flow from a perforating branch of the PCA that supplies the midbrain. The CST and ipsilateral occulomotor nerve fibers are affected. Benedict syndrome is similar to Weber syndrome but additionally involves the red nucleus. Patients are left with a contralateral intention tremor even after the hemiparesis resolves.

Larger basilar branches vulnerable to ischemia are the thalamogeniculate, AICA, SCA, and PCA. Dejerine-Roussy syndrome occurs after occlusion of the medium-sized thalamogeniculate branches and is characterized by contralateral limb and facial numbness, dystonic posturing of the contralateral limb, and contralateral transient hemiparesis. Intense pain may also arise in the paresthetic limb.[67] Although not prone to atherosclerotic disease, the AICA may be injured during tumor resections at the cerebellopontine angle.[68] Cranial nerves located in the mid pons (facial and vestibulocochlear) are usually affected as well as a small area of the anteromedial cerebellum.[62,69] The SCA supplies the lateral tegmentum of the upper pons and midbrain as well as the superior cerebellar vermis. Symptoms of isolated infarction of this vessel include ipsilateral limb and gait ataxia, Horner syndrome, static tremor, contralateral pain and temperature loss on the face and body, and trochlear nerve palsy. However, occlusion of this branch alone is extremely rare, and most insults are associated with concomitant occlusion of the basilar apex.[70]

The severity of symptoms observed with main trunk basilar artery occlusion depends upon both the acuteness of infarct development and the presence of collateral circulation. Thus, a wide range of presentations can be expected, ranging from complete absence of symptoms to transient ischemic attacks; to a complete stroke evolving from nonspecific headache, dizziness, and confusion; to neurological deficits (e.g., cranial nerve palsies, hemiplegia, or quadriplegia); and, ultimately, a locked-in syndrome or coma (**Fig. 5.5**). Common eye findings include internuclear ophthalmoplegia, conjugate horizontal gaze palsy (e.g., toward the lesion), ocular bobbing, pontine pupils, nystagmus, and skew deviation. The locked-in syndrome was originally described by Plum and Posner and is associated with basilar artery thrombosis, which can result in extensive infarction of the ventral pons yet spare the pontine tegmentum that contains the centers for consciousness. Thus, all four limbs as well as the lower cranial nerves are paralyzed and, typically, patients retain the ability only to blink or move their eyes in a vertical plane.[71]

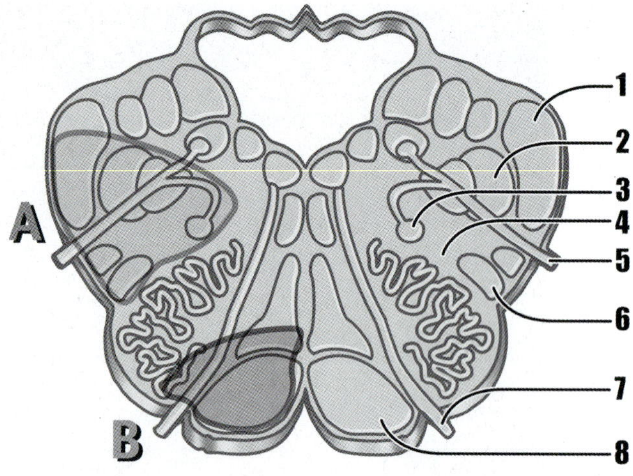

Fig. 5.5 Illustration of a cross-sectional view of the medulla demonstrating the various sensory and motor tracts. *1*, restiform body; *2*, spinal trigeminal tract; *3*, nucleus ambiguous; *4*, descending sympathetic tract; *5*, vagus nerve; *6*, lateral and ventral spinothalamic tracts; *7*, hypoglossal nerve; *8*, corticospinal tract. Lateral medullary syndrome (*zone A*), and medial medullary syndrome (*zone B*). (Adapted from the Barrow Neurological Institute [BNI] with permission from BNI.)

"Top of the basilar" syndrome exists as a clinically distinct entity from the occlusions described previously. The rostral basilar artery gives rise to the SCA, PCA (supplying the midbrain, inferior temporal lobes, and occipital lobes), and perforators that supply the medial diencephalon, including the hypothalamus. Early features of infarction may manifest with behavioral changes and occulomotor findings. Initial delirium or cognitive changes often progress to depressed consciousness and coma. Pupillary abnormalities range from fixed and dilated pupils, to mid-position fixed pupils, or irregularly shaped pupils with poor reactivity. Vertical gaze centers in the mesencephalon are commonly affected.

Chiari Malformations/Syrinxes

Chiari malformations are developmental abnormalities that affect both the bony and neural structures of the CVJ and may alternatively affect the flow of CSF with or without formation of a syrinx.[72,73] The most common types of Chiari malformations are types I and II. Neurological presentations may develop from pathology localized to the cerebellum, brainstem, or upper spinal cord.

Chiari I

Chiari I malformations are presumed to be a disorder of paraxial mesoderm.[74] The cerebellar tonsils are displaced inferiorly through the foramen magnum (**Fig. 5.6**). Patients present

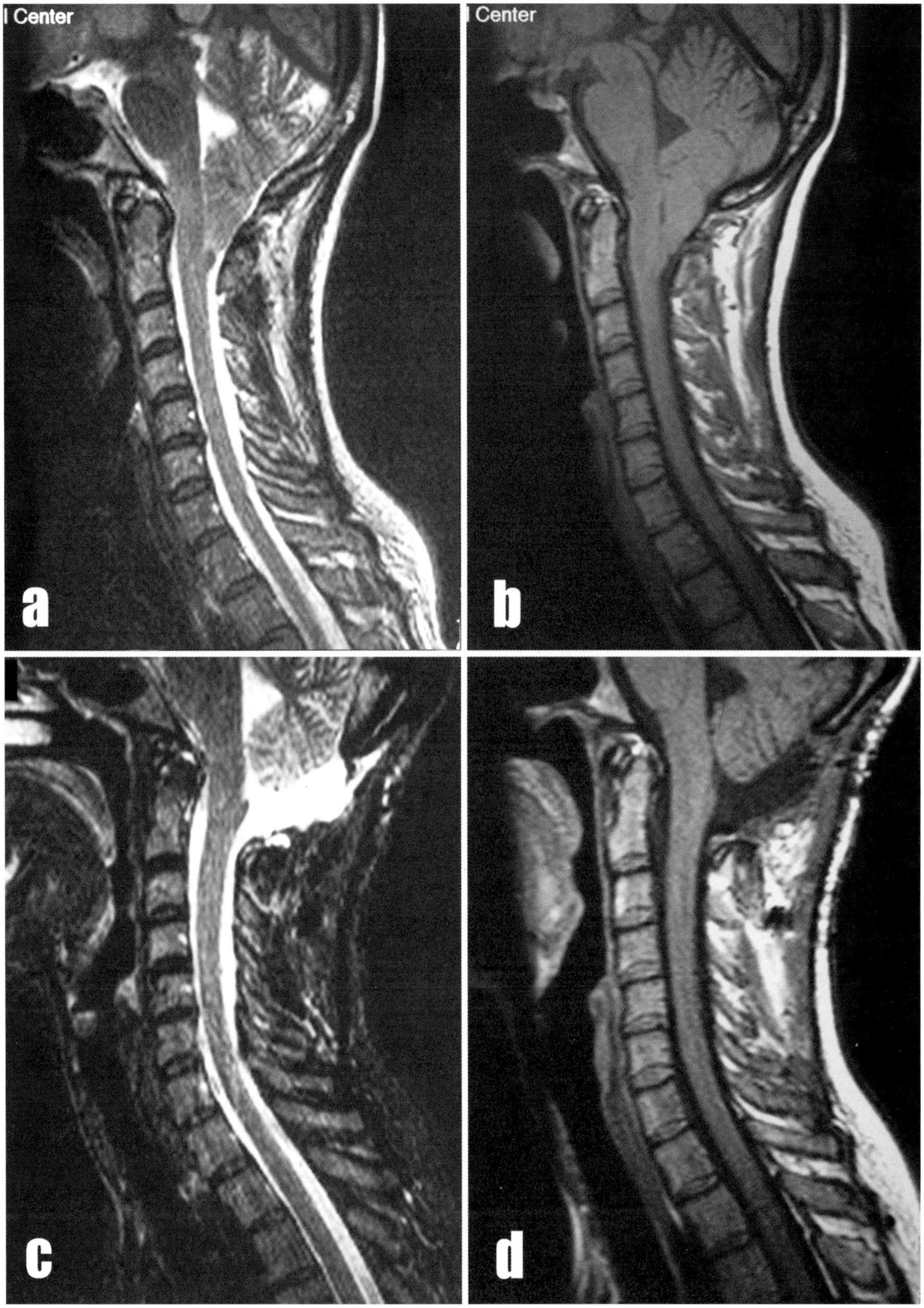

Fig. 5.6 Preoperative **(A)** T1-weighted and **(B)** T2-weighted magnetic resonance images (MRIs) in a patient with Chiari I malformation and significant cerebellar tonsillar herniation through the foramen magnum. The patient presented with typical Chiari-like headaches. Postoperative **(C)** T1-weighted and **(D)** T2-weighted MRIs following a suboccipital decompression.

in adulthood, and the most common symptom is pain referred to either the occipital or neck region. Valsalva maneuvers, coughing, sneezing, or straining tend to worsen the headaches. Motor weakness, spasticity, and numbness may also be present due to compression of the long descending tracts within the spinal cord.[74] Disturbances in gait coordination can also be attributed to cerebellar dysfunction. Pain in the upper or lower extremities as well as diplopia, dysphagia, and tinnitus have also been described.[75] Nystagmus, when present, is downbeat on vertical gaze and rotary in the horizontal plane.

A syrinx complicates the clinical picture, producing additional deficits that include dissociated sensory loss, segmental weakness (upper > lower), hyperactive reflexes (lower > upper), long tract symptoms, and cranial nerve palsies if it dissects into the brainstem. In children, the formation of a syrinx may lead to scoliosis. The direction of the curve is usually to the left and should alert the clinician to consider this particular entity. Syrinx development is correlated with the severity of tonsillar herniation below the foramen magnum. However, in one study, more than half of patients with less than 5 mm of tonsillar herniation had development of a syrinx ($n = 17$ of 32).[74]

Chiari II

The major distinguishing feature in patients harboring Chiari II malformations is caudal displacement of the cerebellar vermis and lower brainstem through the foramen magnum producing a kink-like deformity at the level of the CVJ. Patients commonly present in infancy with Chiari I malformations. Chiari II malformations are likely due to primary neural dysgenesis.[76,77] Infants may also have hydrocephalus with a myelomeningocele, syringomyelia, and lower cranial nerve nuclei degeneration (e.g., presenting with stridor, apnea, weak cry, feeding difficulty, or fixed retrocollis).[78,79] Older children tend to present with spasticity, ataxia, motor weakness, opisthotonos, nystagmus, or oscillopsia.[80]

Conclusion

The CVJ serves as a vital entry and exit point for various neural pathways. Pathology localized to this region may present in a variety of ways. The four most common causes of insults to this region arise from trauma, tumors, ischemia, and abnormal flow of CSF. The history, the neurological exam, and specific imaging modalities help define a particular cause and direct further clinical management. In this chapter, we describe some of the more common neurological presentations of these common categories of CVJ disease.

References

1. Levi AD, Tator CH, Bunge RP. Clinical syndromes associated with disproportionate weakness of the upper versus the lower extremities after cervical spinal cord injury. Neurosurgery 1996;38(1):179–183, discussion 183–185
2. Levi AD. Neurological syndromes of the craniovertebral junction. In: Dickman CA, Spetzler RF, Sontag VKH, eds. Surgery of the Craniovertebral Junction. New York, NY: Thieme; 1998
3. Hansebout RP. A comprehensive review of methods of improving cord recovery after acute spinal cord injury. In: Tator CH, ed. Early Management of Acute Spinal Cord Injury. New York, NY: Raven Press; 1982:181–196
4. Levi L, Wolf A, Rigamonti D, Ragheb J, Mirvis S, Robinson WL. Anterior decompression in cervical spine trauma: does the timing of surgery affect the outcome? Neurosurgery 1991;29(2):216–222
5. Heiden JS, Weiss MH, Rosenberg AW, Apuzzo ML, Kurze T. Management of cervical spinal cord trauma in Southern California. J Neurosurg 1975;43(6):732–736
6. Dickman CA, Papadopoulos SM, Sonntag VK, Spetzler RF, Rekate HL, Drabier J. Traumatic occipitoatlantal dislocations. J Spinal Disord 1993;6(4):300–313
7. Hadley MN, Dickman CA, Browner CM, Sonntag VK. Acute axis fractures: a review of 229 cases. J Neurosurg 1989;71(5 Pt 1):642–647
8. Levi AD, Tator CH, Bunge RP. Clinical syndromes associated with disproportionate weakness of the upper versus the lower extremities after cervical spinal cord injury. Neurosurgery 1996;38(1):179–183, discussion 183–185
9. Schneider RC, Crosby EC, Russo RH, Gosch HH. Chapter 32. Traumatic spinal cord syndromes and their management. Clin Neurosurg 1973;20:424–492
10. Schneider RC, McGillicuddy JE. Concomitant craniocerebral and spinal trauma with special reference to the cervicomedullary region. In: Vinken PJ, Bruyn GW, eds. Injuries of the Brain and Skull. Handbook of Clinical Neurology. Amsterdam, Netherlands: North-Holland Publishing Company; 1975:149–152
11. Marano SR, Calica AB, Sonntag VK. Bilateral upper extremity paralysis (Bell's cruciate paralysis) from a gunshot wound to the cervicomedullary junction. Neurosurgery 1986;18(5):642–644
12. Dumitru D, Lang JE. Cruciate paralysis. Case report. J Neurosurg 1986;65(1):108–110
13. Bell HS. Paralysis of both arms from injury of the upper portion of the pyramidal decussation: "cruciate paralysis." J Neurosurg 1970;33(4):376–380
14. Bell HS. Cruciate paralysis. In: Vinken PJ, Bruyn GW, eds. Injuries of the Brain and Skull. Handbook of Clinical Neurology. Amsterdam, Netherlands: North-Holland Publishing Company; 1975:391–392
15. Dickman CA, Hadley MN, Pappas CT, Sonntag VK, Geisler FH. Cruciate paralysis: a clinical and radiographic analysis of injuries to the cervicomedullary junction. J Neurosurg 1990;73(6):850–858
16. Wallenberg A. Anatomischer Befund in einem als "acute Bulbarrafection (embolie der Art. cerebellar post. inf. sinsistr?)" beschrieben Falle. Arch Psychiatr 1901;34:923–959
17. Landau WM. Cruciate paralysis. Neurosurgery 1986;19(4):676
18. DeJong RN. The Neurologic Examination. Incorporating the Fundamentals of Neuroanatomy and Neurophysiology. 2nd ed. New York, NY: Hoeber-Harper; 1958
19. Crosby EC, Humphrey T, Lauer EW. Correlative Anatomy of the Nervous System. New York, NY: Macmillan; 1962
20. Schneider RC, Cherry G, Pantek H. The syndrome of acute central cervical spinal cord injury; with special reference to the mechanisms involved in hyperextension injuries of cervical spine. J Neurosurg 1954;11(6):546–577
21. McKinley W, Santos K, Meade M, Brooke K. Incidence and outcomes of spinal cord injury clinical syndromes. J Spinal Cord Med 2007;30(3):215–224

22. Foerster O. Symptomatologie der erkrankungen des ruckenmarks und seiner wurzeln. In: Bumke U, Foerster O. Handbuch der Neurologie. Berlin, Germany: J Springer-Verlag; 1935:83
23. Barnard JW, Woolsey CN. A study of localization in the cortico-spinal tracts of monkey and rat. J Comp Neurol 1956;105(1):25–50
24. Coxe WS, Landau WM. Patterns of Marchi degeneration in the monkey pyramidal tract following small discrete cortical lesions. Neurology 1970;20(1):89–100
25. Liu CN, Chambers WW. An experimental study of the cortico-spinal system in the monkey (macaca mulatta). The spinal pathways and preterminal distribution of degenerating fibers following discrete lesions of the pre- and postcentral gyri and bulbar pyramid. J Comp Neurol 1964;123:257–283
26. Pappas CT, Gibson AR, Sonntag VK. Decussation of hind-limb and fore-limb fibers in the monkey corticospinal tract: relevance to cruciate paralysis. J Neurosurg 1991;75(6):935–940
27. Nathan PW, Smith MC, Deacon P. The corticospinal tracts in man. Course and location of fibres at different segmental levels. Brain 1990;113(Pt 2):303–324
28. Nathan PW, Smith MC. Long descending tracts in man. I. Review of present knowledge. Brain 1955;78(2):248–303
29. Heffner R, Masterton B. Variation in form of the pyramidal tract and its relationship to digital dexterity. Brain Behav Evol 1975;12(3): 161–200
30. Kuypers H. Anatomy of the descending pathways. In: Brookhart JM, Mountcastle VB, eds. Handbook of Physiology. The Nervous System. Baltimore, MD: Williams & Wilkins; 1981
31. Phillips CG, Porter R. Corticospinal Neurones: Their Role in Movement. Monographs of the Physiological Society. London, England: Academic Press; 1977
32. Romer AS. The Vertebrate Body. 3rd ed. Philadelphia, PA: WB Saunders; 1962
33. Bortoff GA, Strick PL. Corticospinal terminations in two new-world primates: further evidence that corticomotoneuronal connections provide part of the neural substrate for manual dexterity. J Neurosci 1993;13(12):5105–5118
34. Sherrington CS. The spinal cord. In: Schafer EA, ed. Textbook of Physiology. Vol 2. Edinburgh, Scotland: Young J. Pentland; 1900
35. Nyberg-Hansen R, Rinvik E. Some comments on the pyramidal tract with special reference to its individual variations in man. Acta Neurol Scand 1963;39:1–30
36. Schwartzman RJ. A behavioral analysis of complete unilateral section of the pyramidal tract at the medullary level in Macaca mulatta. Ann Neurol 1978;4(3):234–244
37. Lawrence DG, Kuypers HG. The functional organization of the motor system in the monkey. I. The effects of bilateral pyramidal lesions. Brain 1968;91(1):1–14
38. Tower SS. Pyramidal lesion in the monkey. Brain 1940;63:36–90
39. Bucy PC. Is there a pyramidal tract. Brain 1957;80(3):376–392
40. Hepp-Reymond, Trouche E, Wiesendanger M. Effects of unilateral and bilateral pyramidotomy on a conditioned rapid precision grip in monkeys (Macaca fascicularis). Exp Brain Res 1974;21(5):519–527
41. Bucy PC, Ladpli R, Ehrlich A. Destruction of the pyramidal tract in the monkey. The effects of bilateral section of the cerebral peduncles. J Neurosurg 1966;25(1):1–23
42. Jimenez O, Marcillo A, Levi AD. A histopathological analysis of the human cervical spinal cord in patients with acute traumatic central cord syndrome. Spinal Cord 2000;38(9):532–537
43. Nishimura Y, Onoe H, Morichika Y, Perfiliev S, Tsukada H, Isa T. Time-dependent central compensatory mechanisms of finger dexterity after spinal cord injury. Science 2007;318(5853):1150–1155
44. Maier IC, Baumann K, Thallmair M, Weinmann O, Scholl J, Schwab ME. Constraint-induced movement therapy in the adult rat after unilateral corticospinal tract injury. J Neurosci 2008;28(38):9386–9403
45. Lawrence DG, Kuypers HG. The functional organization of the motor system in the monkey. II. The effects of lesions of the descending brain-stem pathways. Brain 1968;91(1):15–36
46. Napier J. The evolution of the hand. Sci Am 1962;207:56–62
47. Jane JA, Yashon D, DeMyer W, Bucy PC. The contribution of the precentral gyrus to the pyramidal tract of man. J Neurosurg 1967;26(2):244–248
48. Lassek AM, Rasmussen GL. A comparative fiber and numerical analysis of the pyramidal tract. J Comp Neurol 1940;72:417–428
49. Davidoff RA. The pyramidal tract. Neurology 1990;40(2):332–339
50. Quencer RM, Bunge RP, Egnor M, et al. Acute traumatic central cord syndrome: MRI-pathological correlations. Neuroradiology 1992;34(2):85–94
51. Bunge RP, Puckett WR, Becerra JL, Marcillo A, Quencer RM. Observations on the pathology of human spinal cord injury. A review and classification of 22 new cases with details from a case of chronic cord compression with extensive focal demyelination. Adv Neurol 1993;59:75–89
52. Howe JR, Taren JA. Foramen magnum tumors. Pitfalls in diagnosis. JAMA 1973;225(9):1061–1066
53. Symonds CP. Compression of the spinal cord in the neighborhood of the foramen magnum. Brain 1937;6:52–84
54. Crockard HA, Heilman AE, Stevens JM. Progressive myelopathy secondary to odontoid fractures: clinical, radiological, and surgical features. J Neurosurg 1993;78(4):579–586
55. Taylor AR, Byrnes DP. Foramen magnum and high cervical cord compression. Brain 1974;97(3):473–480
56. Levi AD, Tator CH, Bunge RP. Clinical syndromes associated with disproportionate weakness of the upper versus the lower extremities after cervical spinal cord injury. Neurosurgery 1996;38(1): 179–183, discussion 183–185
57. Meyer FB, Ebersold MJ, Reese DF. Benign tumors of the foramen magnum. J Neurosurg 1984;61(1):136–142
58. Stein BM, Leeds NE, Taveras JM, Pool JL. Meningiomas of the foramen magnum. J Neurosurg 1963;20:740–751
59. Svien HJ, Baker HL, Rivers MH. Jugular foramen syndrome and allied syndromes. Neurology 1963;13:797–809
60. Alexander A. The treatment of epilepsy by ligature of the vertebral arteries. Brain 1885;5:170–187
61. Fisher CM, Karnes WE, Kubik CS. Lateral medullary infarction-the pattern of vascular occlusion. J Neuropathol Exp Neurol 1961;20: 323–379
62. Barnett HJM. Stroke: Pathophysiology, Diagnosis, and Management. 2nd ed. New York, NY: Churchill Livingstone; 1992
63. Fisher CM, Picard EH, Polak A, Dalal P, Pojemann RG. Acute hypertensive cerebellar hemorrhage: diagnosis and surgical treatment. J Nerv Ment Dis 1965;140:38–57
64. Duncan GW, Parker SW, Fisher CM. Acute cerebellar infarction in the PICA territory. Arch Neurol 1975;32(6):364–368
65. Sypert GW, ALvord EC Jr. Cerebellar infarction. A clinicopathological study. Arch Neurol 1975;32(6):357–363
66. Ho KL, Meyer KR. The medial medullary syndrome. Arch Neurol 1981;38(6):385–387
67. Dejerine J, Roussy G. Le syndrome thalamique. Rev Neurol (Paris) 1906;14:521
68. Atkinson WJ. The anterior inferior cerebellar artery; its variations, pontine distribution, and significance in the surgery of cerebello-pontine angle tumours. J Neurol Neurosurg Psychiatry 1949;12(2): 137–151
69. Adams R. Occlusion of the anterior inferior cerebellar artery. Arch Neurol Psychiatry 1983;49:765–770
70. Amarenco P, Hauw JJ, Gautier JC. Arterial pathology in cerebellar infarction. Stroke 1990;21(9):1299–1305
71. Plum F, Posner JB. The Diagnosis of Stupor and Coma. 3rd ed. Philadelphia, PA: FA Davis Company; 1980

72. Stovner LJ, Rinck P. Syringomyelia in Chiari malformation: relation to extent of cerebellar tissue herniation. Neurosurgery 1992;31(5): 913–917, discussion 917
73. Dyste GN, Menezes AH, VanGilder JC. Symptomatic Chiari malformations. An analysis of presentation, management, and long-term outcome. J Neurosurg 1989;71(2):159–168
74. Milhorat TH, Chou MW, Trinidad EM, et al. Chiari I malformation redefined: clinical and radiographic findings for 364 symptomatic patients. Neurosurgery 1999;44(5):1005–1017
75. Paul KS, Lye RH, Strang FA, Dutton J. Arnold-Chiari malformation. Review of 71 cases. J Neurosurg 1983;58(2):183–187
76. Gilbert JN, Jones KL, Rorke LB, Chernoff GF, James HE. Central nervous system anomalies associated with meningomyelocele, hydrocephalus, and the Arnold-Chiari malformation: reappraisal of theories regarding the pathogenesis of posterior neural tube closure defects. Neurosurgery 1986;18(5): 559–564
77. Greenberg MS, Arredondo N. Handbook of Neurosurgery. 6th ed. New York, NY: Thieme Medical Publishers; 2006
78. Bell WO, Charney EB, Bruce DA, Sutton LN, Schut L. Symptomatic Arnold-Chiari malformation: review of experience with 22 cases. J Neurosurg 1987;66(6):812–816
79. Oakes W. The Chiari malformations of the child. In: Menezes AH, Sonntag VKH, eds. Principles of Spinal Surgery. New York, NY: McGraw Hill; 1996
80. Hoffman HJ, Hendrick EB, Humphreys RP. Manifestations and management of Arnold-Chiari malformation in patients with myelomeningocele. Childs Brain 1975;1(4):255–259

II Surgical Indications and Decision Making

6 Congenital Malformations of the Craniovertebral Junction

Ricardo B. V. Fontes, Vincent C. Traynelis, and John Piper

The craniovertebral junction (CVJ) is a complex transition zone between the skull base and cervical spine composed of the occiput, axis, and atlas. It is the most mobile region of the spine, and its unique embryological development may lead to anomalies not found elsewhere along the vertebral column. These pathologies are addressed in this chapter along with pertinent aspects of the embryology, clinical presentation, radiological evaluation, and treatment.

■ Occipital Congenital Anomalies

Basilar Invagination and Platybasia

Basilar invagination and platybasia both refer to occipital anomalies described by Chamberlain in 1938.[1] Unfortunately, Chamberlain and several other authors utilized both terms interchangeably, creating confusion over the years. Basilar invagination is a congenital form of occipital hypoplasia manifested by prolapse of the spinal column into the skull base (**Fig. 6.1**). Platybasia is an anthropological term describing an abnormally obtuse ($>$140 degrees) angle between the anterior skull base and the clivus—the normal range of which lies between 120 and 140 degrees (**Fig. 6.2**).[1,2] Platybasia alone causes no neurological symptoms and may be associated with other conditions, such as Klippel-Feil syndrome and occipitalization of the atlas. It should be noted that basilar invagination is distinct from basilar impression—the latter is an acquired condition secondary to osseous disorders.[3]

Occipital hypoplasia may affect the basiocciput, the exoccipital bone, and the squamous occipital bone. Two extreme forms of invagination have been identified. Anterior (or ventral) invagination results when there is shortening of the basiocciput and clivus with concomitant platybasia and a shallow posterior fossa, whereas paramedian invagination is a consequence of hypoplasia of the exoccipital bones with normal clival development and is often accompanied by an element of posterior displacement.[4] Paramedian invagination may be unilateral or bilateral; it may be associated with torticollis (when unilateral), compensatory downward curvature of the squamous occipital bone, and condylar hypoplasia. Usually features of both forms of basilar invagination are combined to produce a mixed clinical picture.[3] Basilar invagination is occasionally associated with Down syndrome and skeletal dysplasia as well as segmentation defects. It should not, however, be confused with other

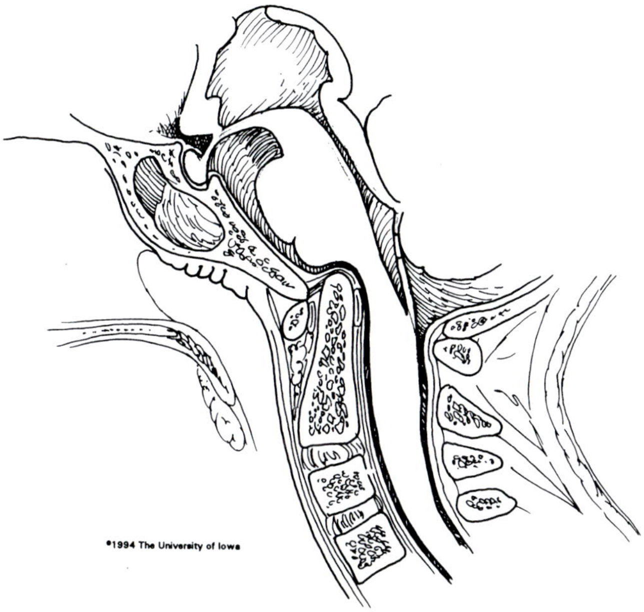

Fig. 6.1 Midsagittal section of the craniovertebral junction reveals characteristic features of basilar invagination. There is congenital prolapse of the cervical spine into the skull base resulting in foramen magnum narrowing and ventral cervicomedullary junction compression.

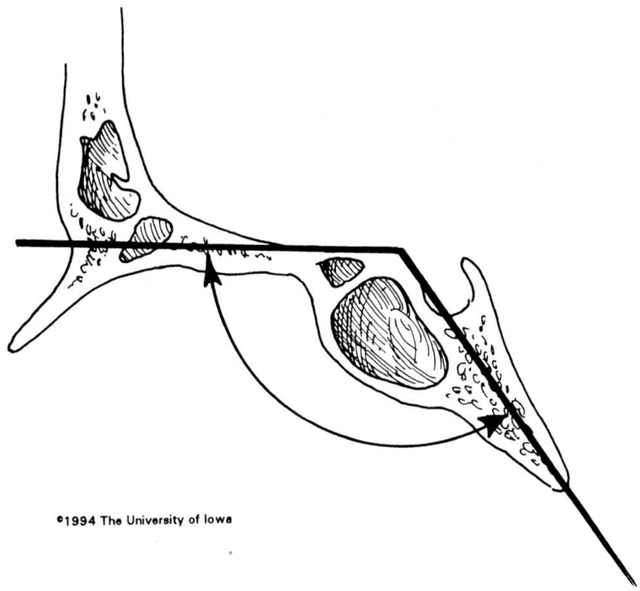

Fig. 6.2 Midsagittal section of the skull base demonstrates the proper technique for measuring the basal angle. A normal angle measures 120 to 140 degrees. Definitions of platybasia differ slightly but, in general, are characterized by basal angles that exceed 140 degrees.

proatlas segmentation anomalies that may include the anterior masses and cause cervicomedullary compression; these are much rarer, have a different embryological basis, and are treated differently.[5]

The radiological findings of basilar invagination were classically described using standard radiographs. Plain films have been supplanted by more sophisticated imaging techniques but the reference perspectives originally developed for them may still be applied to sagittal and coronal reconstructions of high-quality axial computed tomography (CT) scans.[6] On coronal views, invagination is suggested by cephalad displacement of the atlantoaxial articulations—the tip of the dens should extend no more than 10 mm rostral to the bimastoid line.[7] Invagination is more clearly appreciated on sagittal reconstructions: the tip of the odontoid should project no more than 2.5 mm above Chamberlain's line (hard palate to opisthion). Wackenheim's line, which courses down the posterior clivus, represents another classic means of diagnosing invagination. Posterior protrusion of the odontoid, with respect to Wackenheim's clival line, is abnormal.[1,8] The presence of these abnormal skeletal relationships mandates magnetic resonance imaging (MRI) of the CVJ to obtain a clear understanding of their relationship to the neural structures.

Symptoms of basilar invagination ensue when the midsagittal diameter of the foramen magnum is reduced to less than 20 mm (normal range, 35 ± 4 mm).[3] Most patients present with neck pain (80 to 85%), whereas myelopathy is by far the most common finding on clinical examination.[2] A variant of a central cord syndrome related to venous stagnation in the lower cord may occur because these vessels, which normally drain cephalad toward the CVJ, are compressed. Additionally, myriad neuro-ophthalmological signs, such as internuclear ophthalmoplegia and downbeat nystagmus, are possible.[3]

Specific details of the surgical management of the pathologies described herein are discussed elsewhere in this textbook, yet the principles of treatment of basilar invagination lie in the assessment of reducibility and the degree and location of the neural compression at the CVJ. Low weight traction for 48 to 72 hours is an important first step of treatment. Reduction can be achieved in ~20 to 30% of patients with acquired cranial settling. Although no precise data define it, the overall reduction rate is clearly age-dependent, and ~80% of patients age 14 years or younger will be satisfactorily reduced with traction.[3] If reduction is achieved, occipitocervical fusion will prevent recurrent invagination. Irreducible lesions with significant anterior neural compression usually require a decompression through the endonasal or transoral route followed by posterior occipitocervical fusion. Some patients may require additional rostral or caudal extensions for adequate anterior decompression.[9] Certainly, any persistent symptomatic posterior compression with or without reduction should be treated with a decompression of the foramen magnum, posterior fossa, or upper cervical spine, as necessary.

Vertebralization of the Occiput (Occipital Vertebrae)

Other segmentation defects of the occiput occur and are collectively called "manifestations of occipital vertebrae."[3] They derive from the failure of the third occipital sclerotome and proatlas to fuse with the skull base during development. Rarely do they form completely independent spinal segments; most frequently, they are noted as osseous processes around the foramen magnum.[10] Transverse fissures of the basiocciput, third occipital condyle, paracondylic process, epitransverse process, and bipartite atlantal facets are all part of this group. Technically, persistent ossiculum terminale is embryologically related, but this entity is grouped under anomalies of the dens for convenience and historical reasons (**Figs. 6.3, 6.4,** and **6.5**). Vertebralization

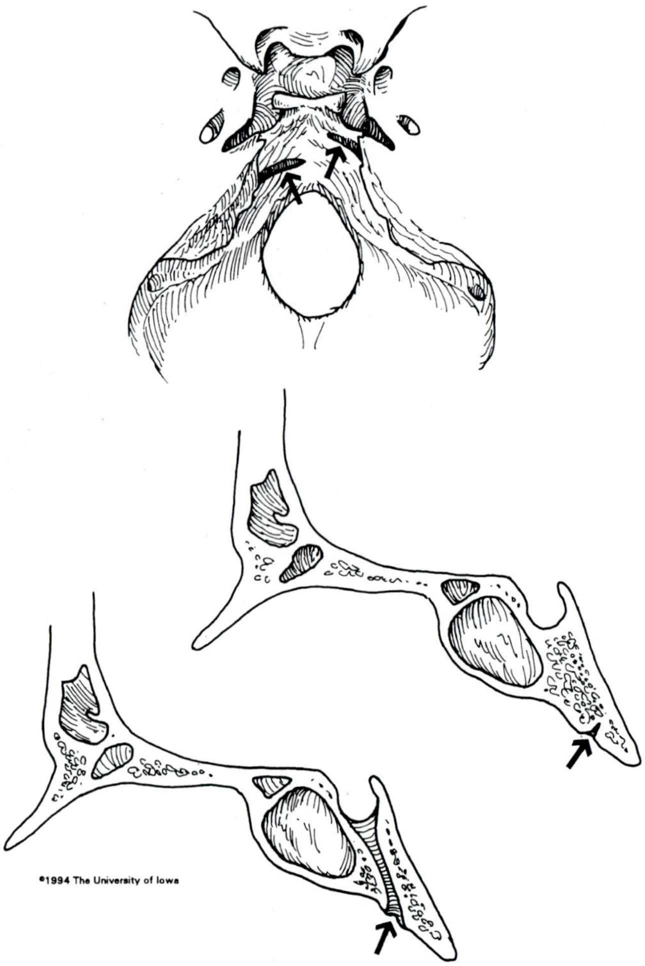

Fig. 6.3 Examples of transverse basioccipital clefts are demonstrated. The uppermost diagram shows the interior aspect of the skull base, revealing the posterior and middle fossae. Small clefts are visible in the region of the clivus (*arrows*). The lower two drawings are of the skull base in the midsagittal plane. Transverse basioccipital clefts may take the form of minimal clefting at the lower portion of the clivus to a cleft of increased severity connecting the base of the clivus and the sella turcica (*arrows*).

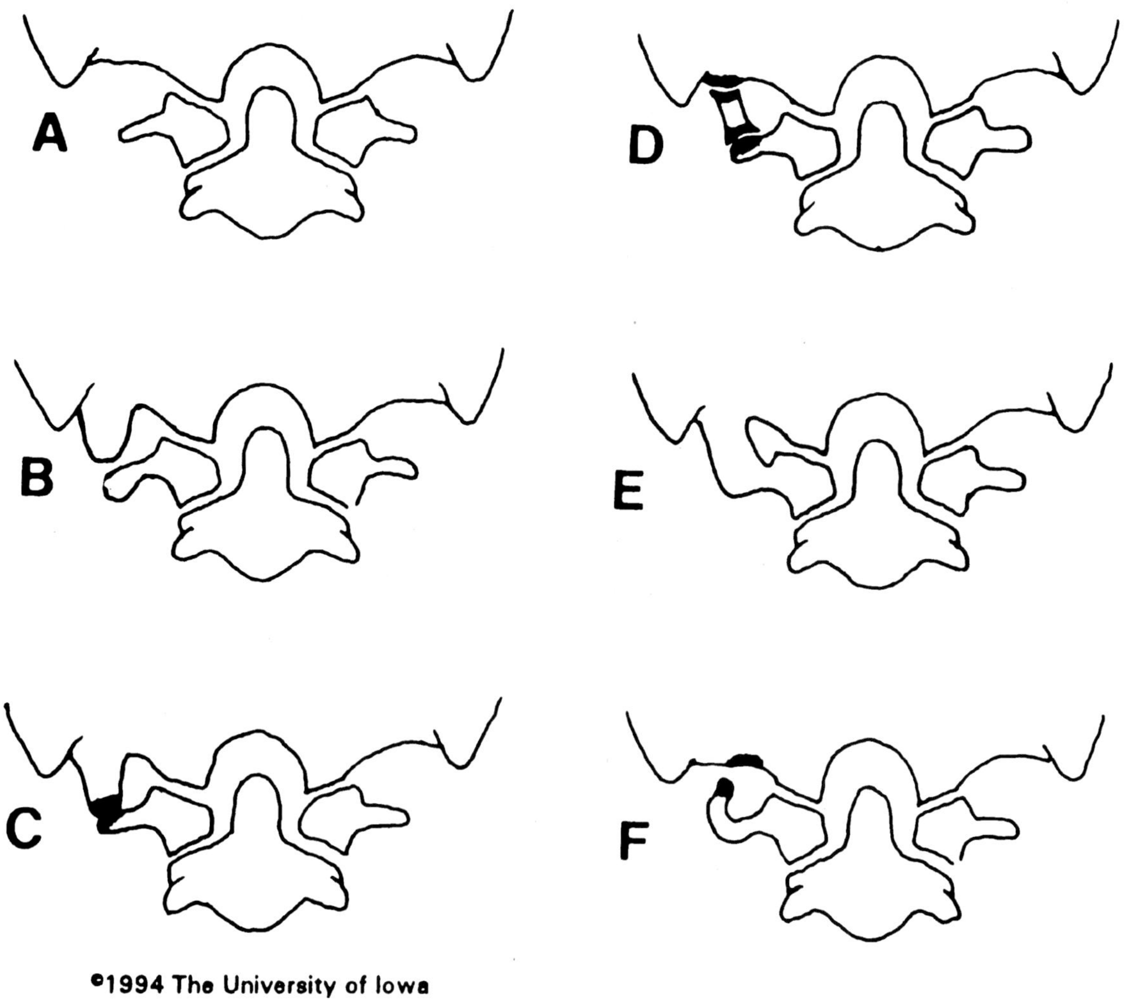

Fig. 6.4 Unusual manifestations of occipital vertebrae include variations of paracondylic masses and processes as well as epitransverse processes. **(A)** A coronal section through the normal craniovertebral junction is shown for reference. **(B)** A paracondylic tubercle is shown extending to the transverse process of the atlas. **(C)** Severe involvement may lead to an articulation between the paracondylic process and a component of the transverse process of the atlas. **(D)** A separate paracondylic mass may articulate with the skull base and the transverse process of the atlas. **(E)** This paracondylic mass was completely incorporated into the skull base and transverse process of C1, causing a complete fusion between these two structures. **(F)** An epitransverse process may extend from the transverse process of C1 to the skull base with which it may articulate.

of the occiput should not be confused with assimilation of the atlas (fusion of C1 sclerotome with the proatlas). The distinguishing feature between these two is the presence in the latter of a foramen through which the vertebral artery and suboccipital nerve traverse.[3,10]

Unilateral or bilateral transverse fissures of the basiocciput (**Fig. 6.3**) are transverse clefts in the region of the clivus resulting from incomplete assimilation of occipital somites. These anomalies may be detected by CT as radiolucent clefts in the clivus, occasionally extending into the hypoglossal canal, in which case the term "bipartite hypoglossal canal" is applied. The third occipital condyle is an osseous protuberance coursing from the basiocciput along the anterior margin of the foramen magnum, typically articulating with the anterior arch of C1 or the dens. If multiple, these ossicles are called basilar processes. This anomalous articulation is commonly associated with basilar invagination, and it often further contributes to neural compression and limitation of movement at the occipital-C1 junction.[11]

A plethora of exotic atlanto-occipital calcifications, pseudoarticulations, and fusions have been described, and new case reports appear regularly.[12,13] Usually these malformations involve the persistence of bony growths protruding lateral to the occipital condyles to the transverse process of C1. Although these osseous masses have been termed "paramastoid," "paraoccipital," or "anomalies of the styloid process," they occur because of the persistence of the transverse processes of the proatlas and, thus, have no embryological relation to the styloid or mastoid processes.[12] They may receive different names according to size, the mildest form of which is a paracondylic tubercle, a small protuberance of the skull base (**Fig. 6.4B**). Paracondylic processes articulate or are fused with the C1 transverse process (**Fig. 6.4C**). When an independent ossicle lies between and articulates with a tubercle and

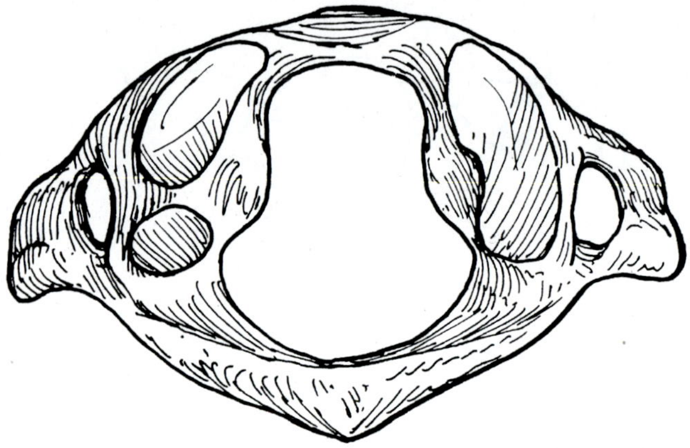

Fig. 6.5 The atlas vertebra as viewed from the top reveals bipartite atlantal facets on the left. The right shows a normal atlantal facet for comparison.

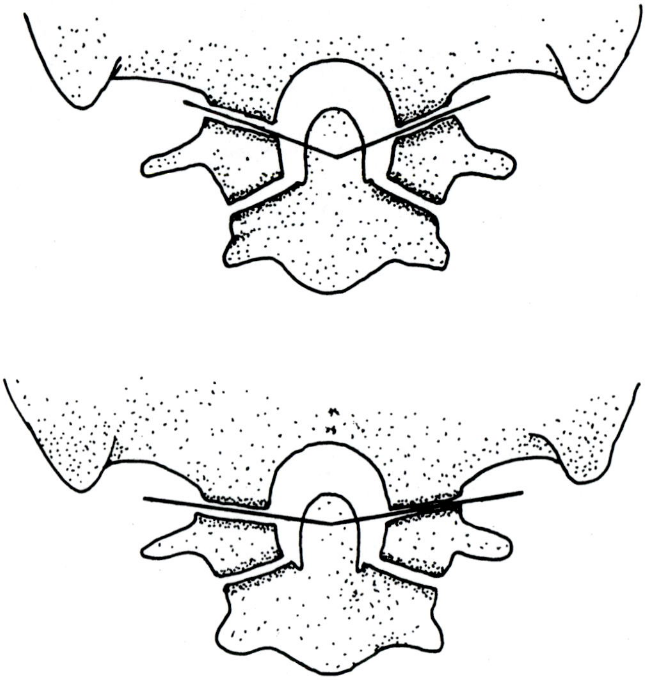

Fig. 6.6 **Top:** A coronal section through the craniovertebral junction demonstrates proper measurement of the Schmidt-Fischer angle at the intersection of two lines passing through the occipitoatlantal articulations. **Bottom:** With hypoplasia of the occipital condyles, the Schmidt-Fischer angle becomes more obtuse.

the transverse process of C1, it is called a paracondylic "mass" (**Fig. 6.4D**). These entities can even lead to complete fusion via a laterally placed osseous trabecula (**Fig. 6.4E**). Epitransverse processes are similar to paracondylic processes except that they are rostral extensions of the C1 transverse processes and articulate with either a paracondylic process or mass (**Fig. 6.4F**). It is evident that the different names describe only nuances of the same problem and can create some confusion. Nonetheless, all of these entities are usually asymptomatic, although such abnormal articulations or fusions may rarely be associated with headache and limitation of motion, necessitating surgical removal.[14]

Bipartite superior atlantal facets are defined by the presence of a small cleft in the superior articulating facets of the atlas. A corresponding division of the occipital condyles may occur in conjunction with these clefts. This anomaly results from the failure of the proatlas to fuse with the lateral part of the C1 sclerotome. The normal process leads to the formation of the C1 lateral mass; when there is incomplete fusion, the vestiges of the superior aspect of the C1 sclerotome give rise to these supernumerary articular facets, with a typically larger anterior surface (**Fig. 6.5**).[15]

Occipital Condylar Hypoplasia

The occipital condyles are derived from the proatlas. Flattened hypoplastic occipital condyles result in superior migration of the atlas and axis relative to the skull base.[15] Hypoplastic occipital condyles may occur unilaterally or bilaterally, and they often accompany paramedian basilar invagination. Both disorders result from hypoplasia of the occipital somites, which form the lateral aspect of the foramen magnum.[3] Although this disorder may occur in isolation, it has been associated with Morquio disease, Conradi syndrome, and spondyloepiphyseal dysplasia. Radiological confirmation of occipital condylar hypoplasia is confirmed by an abnormal increase in the Schmidt-Fischer angle. Measured using an open mouth odontoid view or coronal CT reconstructions, the Schmidt-Fischer angle is defined as the angle at the intersection of two lines passing through the occipitoatlantal joints (normal range, 124–127 degrees) (**Fig. 6.6**).[8]

Congenital Anomalies of the Atlas

Assimilation of the Atlas

Atlas assimilation, also called occipitalization of the atlas, is one of the most common anomalies of the CVJ, affecting 0.14 to 2.76% of individuals. Atlas assimilation is defined by congenital osseous fusion between the skull base and the atlas; relative movement alone is not enough to make this diagnosis. This malformation is caused by persistence of continuity between the hypochordal arch of the atlas and the basal plate of occipital sclerotomes.[3] Assimilation of the atlas was classically thought to primarily involve the anterior arch of C1 and the foramen magnum with the cortex and/or medullary component of the bones being in continuity; however, at times these may be joined only by a thin bony plate.[16] A recent compilation of cases studied with CT scans by Gholve and colleagues revealed that there are a variety of sites that may fuse alone or in a combined fashion.

The condylar fusions are usually asymmetrical, with one side having a cephalad horizontal facet and the opposite side with an inferior oblique facet. Often a remnant of the posterior arch of C1 can be identified along the posterior aspect of the foramen magnum.[12,17] Assimilation of the atlas may also be associated with other conditions, such as Klippel-Feil syndrome, basilar invagination, and Chiari malformations.[16] Rarely, cervicomedullary compression may ensue from congenital canal stenosis or canal compromise, secondary to a thickened posterior dural band.

Atlas assimilation associated with posterior displacement of the dens producing myelopathy is the most common presentation. Neurological symptoms typically arise when the atlantodental interval is ≥4 mm.[2,5,16] Many patients suffer from neck pain. Myriad other symptoms may affect adults and children, including ataxia, tinnitus, nystagmus, dizziness, and bulbar dysfunction. Acute onset often occurs when atlantoaxial instability is associated with the congenital anomaly.[3,16,17]

Atlas assimilation per se requires no treatment; when any of the previously mentioned symptoms develop, surgical treatment aimed at decompression and stabilization is necessary. The treatment of these specific conditions (atlantoaxial instability, basilar invagination, dorsal compression, and Chiari malformation) is addressed in separate sections of this chapter.

Aplasia and Hypoplasia of the Anterior/Posterior Arch of the Atlas

The development of hypoplasia or aplasia of the anterior or posterior arches of the atlas (**Fig. 6.7**) depends on whether the congenital anomaly originates from the proatlas or the first spinal sclerotome. The lateral masses and the superior part of the posterior arch are derived from the proatlas, whereas the anterior arch and the inferior portion of the posterior arch arise from the first spinal sclerotome.[3,11,16] Two ossification centers in the lateral masses of the atlas develop at the 7th week of gestation, and ossification gradually proceeds medially into the anterior and posterior arches. Secondary ossification centers may form in the posterior tubercle and the anterior arch of C1. Ossification of the posterior arch is complete by 3 to 5 years of age, and complete fusion of the anterior arch is achieved by 6 to 10 years.[3]

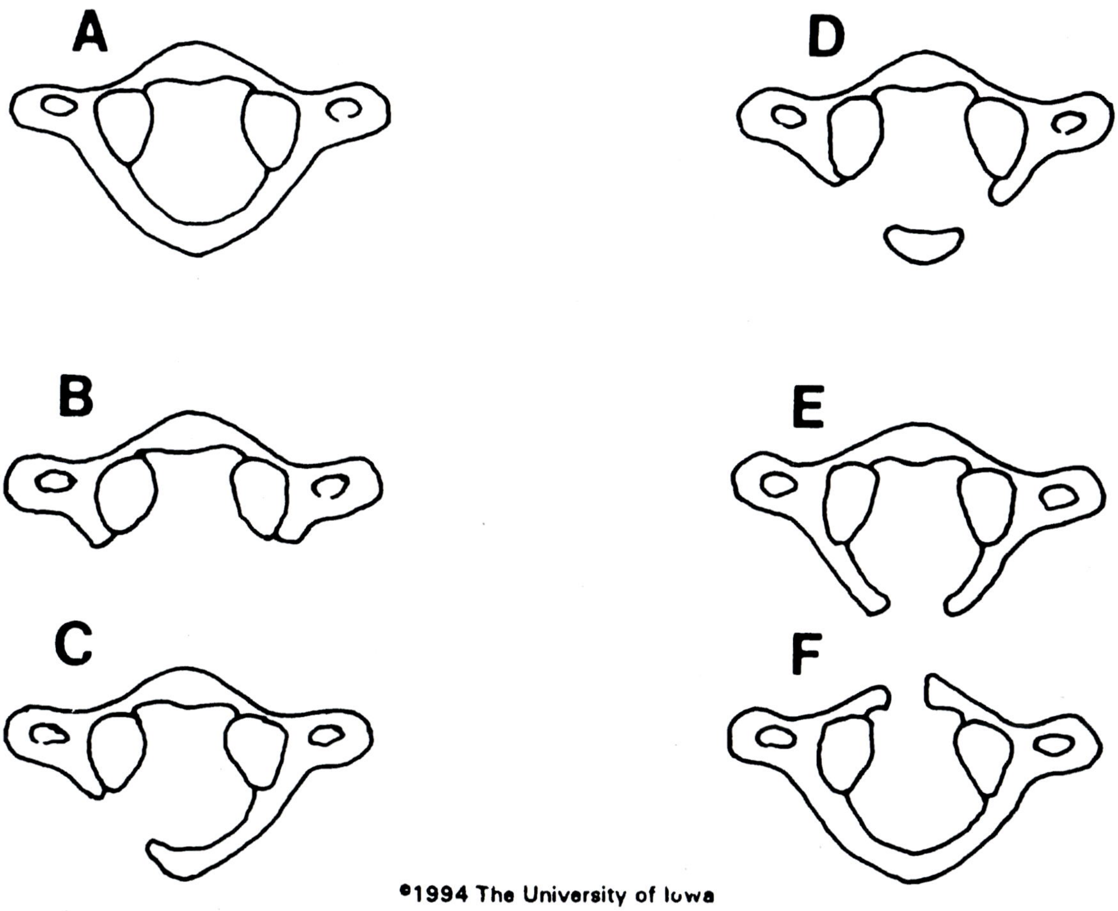

Fig. 6.7 Superior views of the atlas vertebra reveal the range of hypoplastic and aplastic defects of the arches of C1. **(A)** A normal atlas vertebra is shown for comparison. **(B)** Complete aplasia of the posterior arch of the atlas. **(C)** On rare occasions, the hypoplastic defect may be positioned posterolaterally. **(D)** A small ossicle may form posteriorly, being separated from the remaining atlas vertebra by clefts bilaterally. **(E,F)** Hypoplasia of the arches of C1 is often located in the midline, more commonly affecting the posterior arch than the anterior arch.

Several explanations have been proposed to explain the development of a cleft in the arch of the atlas. Currently, the most prominent theory relates to deficient cartilaginous preformation of the atlas, which is supported by the observation that gaps in the atlas are filled with connective tissue and not cartilage. Clefts are much more common than complete aplasia, and they affect the posterior arch (0.5 to 5.0% of anatomical specimens) more frequently than the anterior ring (0.1% of adult specimens).[18] The clefts are usually (97%) on the midline, and these defects are frequently associated with other congenital anomalies such as Klippel-Feil and spina bifida of the axis.[3,19]

Aplasia and hypoplasia of the arches of the atlas have been misinterpreted as fractures with plain radiography. These anomalies may produce lateral offset of the atlantoaxial articular processes as seen in the open-mouth X-ray view or CT coronal reconstructions. The offset for the congenital anomaly is only 1 to 2 mm, whereas that seen with Jefferson fractures is usually at least 3 mm. Hypoplasia of the atlas may be confused with basilar invagination on plain radiographs. In summary, it is difficult to define congenital anomalies of the atlas without obtaining high-quality CT and MRIs.[3,18]

The hypoplastic malformations of the atlas noted here are usually asymptomatic and discovered during cervical spine screening for a variety of reasons, including trauma and spondylosis, and no specific treatment is indicated for such incidentally detected anomalies.[11,18,19] Rarely, severe malformations may be unstable, causing local symptoms, and there are a few reports of spinal compression from a persistent posterior tubercle. Treatment, when indicated, must be tailored to the symptoms: fusion to correct instability and decompression and to treat myelopathy. More extensive procedures may be necessary when congenital atlas malformations are associated with conditions such as anomalies of the dens or basilar invagination.

Aplasia and Hypoplasia of the Atlas

Hypoplasia or aplasia affecting one side of the atlas is a rare congenital anomaly.[20] It has been established that the primary ossification centers for C1 are located in the lateral masses, and perichondral ossification spreads medially along anterior and posterior arches.[3] Absence or hypoplasia of one dominant ossification center in the lateral mass results in hemiaplasia or hemihypoplasia of the atlas. This malformation may occur in isolation or associated with other congenital abnormalities, including Klippel-Feil syndrome, occipitoatlantal fusion, odontoid anomalies, Chiari malformation, plagiocephaly, and other spinal and facial anomalies with a discrete female predominance. The classic description by Dubousset included torticollis as the presenting symptom—headaches, vertigo, and myelopathy may be present, usually at a young age, although symptom onset in mid-adolescence is not uncommon.[20] When minimal hypoplasia is present and there is no evidence of instability, expectant treatment is the norm. Severe torticollis and instability are the most common indications for surgical intervention. Alignment may be restored preoperatively using gentle halo traction. Definitive treatment is achieved via a dorsal occipital-cervical fusion. In the past, there has been concern regarding the creation of such fusions in very young children, which led some surgeons to recommend bracing until 5 to 8 years of age, but it has subsequently been shown that fusion can be safely performed even in very young patients.

Atlantoaxial Fusion and Segmentation Anomalies

Congenital C1-C2 fusions are very rare and appear in the literature as case reports as opposed to series. Fusion of both the anterior and posterior aspects of the atlas and axis is often associated with aplasia or hypoplasia of the anterior arch of the atlas and hypoplasia or aplasia of the dens. Partial fusions can take the form of synostosis between the anterior arch of C1 and the dens, and a case of atlantoaxial arch fusion has been reported. Irregular segmentation of the atlantoaxial complex has also been described. This condition often creates asymmetry in the CVJ articulation with the joint spaces displaced one-half segment cranially or caudally, which may impair the stability of this segment.[11]

■ Congenital Anomalies of the Axis

Anomalies of the Dens

A diverse spectrum of congenital anomalies can affect the dens, ranging from mild forms of hypoplasia to complete aplasia (**Fig. 6.8**).[21] Embryologically, the dens originate from three ossification centers. The majority of the odontoid process is formed from two paramedian ossification centers that are separated centrally by the notochord. These ossification centers are derived from the centrum of the C1 sclerotome and lie close to the base of the dens. The third ossification center, located at the tip of the odontoid process, is called the ossiculum terminale. This ossification center arises from the centrum of the proatlas, which is itself derived from the fourth occipital sclerotome.[22] Failure of the basal ossification centers to fuse in the midline produces a bicornuate dens, in which case a vertical radiolucent line is seen on coronal CT reconstructions. The ossiculum terminale is normally fused to the base of the dens by the age of 12. Failure to fuse leads to "ossiculum terminale persistens," a condition noted by a small radiodense ossicle at the tip of the dens, which should not be confused with os odontoideum (**Fig. 6.8C**). In general, both bicornuate dens and ossiculum terminale persistens do not cause instability and require no treatment.

Congenital anomalies of the base of the dens are of more significance. The dens is joined to the body of C2 by a vestigial disk space called the neurocentral synchondrosis, which is located caudal to the C2 superior facets; thus, the body of C2 receives an important contribution from the two ossification

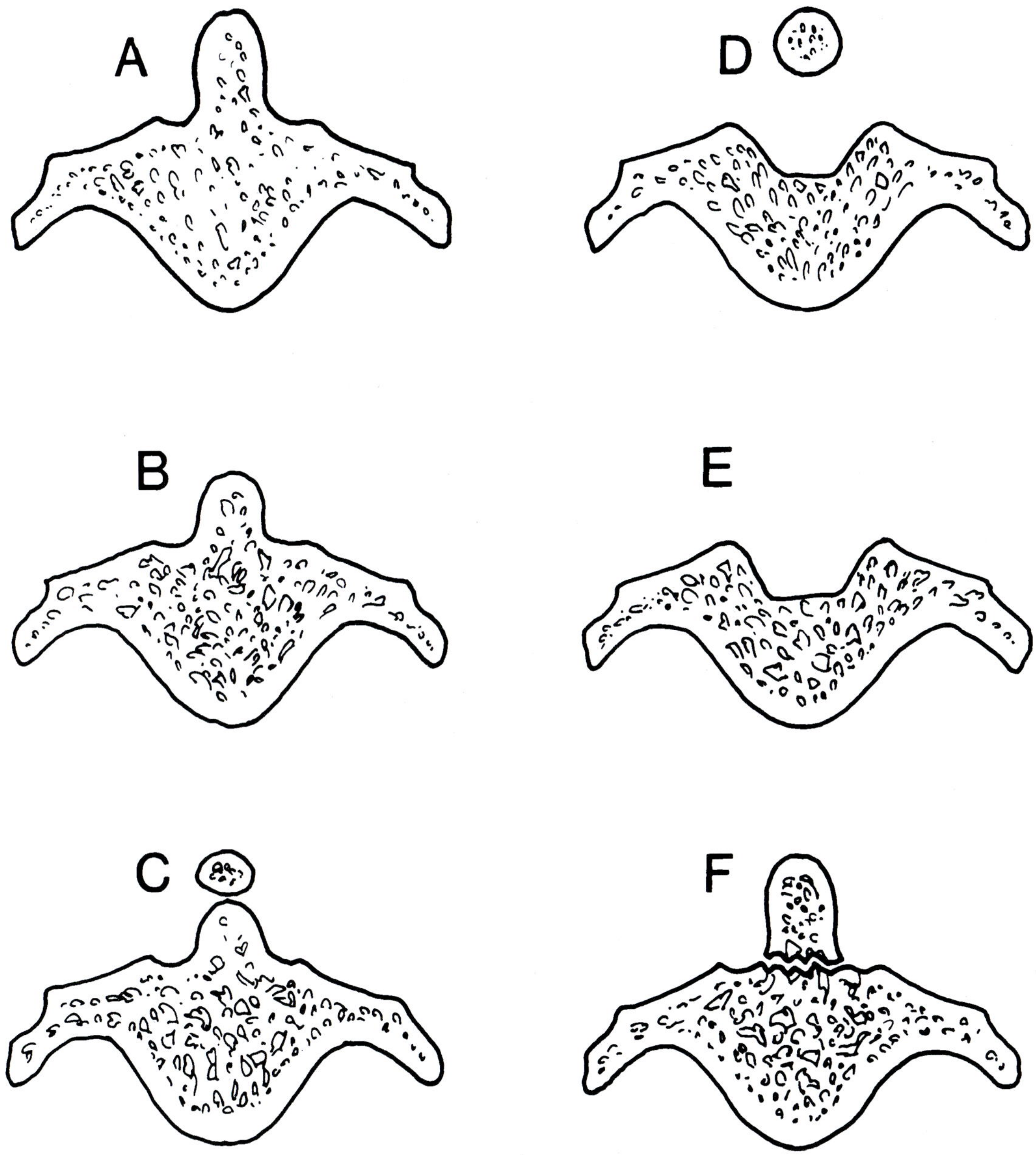

©1994 The University of Iowa

Fig. 6.8 Coronal sections through the C2 vertebra demonstrate the spectrum of congenital anomalies affecting the dens. **(A)** A normal C2 vertebra is shown for comparison. **(B)** With hypoplasia of the dens, the odontoid process is shorter than typical length. **(C)** If the ossiculum terminale fails to fuse with the remaining ossification centers forming the C2 vertebra, an ossiculum terminale persistens results. **(D)** If the ossification centers that form the dens fail to fuse to the remainder of C2, os odontoideum results. Note the smooth characteristic of the ossicle and the indentation in the superior aspect of the body of C2 representing the location of the neurocentral synchondrosis. **(E)** With complete aplasia of the dens, no bony structures can be identified above the level of the neurocentral synchondrosis. **(F)** With traumatic odontoid fracture, the ossicle has an irregular inferior surface corresponding to the remainder of the C2 body that lies above the level of the neurocentral synchondrosis. If the traumatic odontoid fracture is old, sclerotic margins may appear.

centers at the base of the dens. This important caveat helps distinguish congenital anomalies as a result of dens-C2 body fusion failure from traumatic injuries to a normally formed dens. Commonly reported as an anomaly of embryological development of the base of the dens, os odontoideum has been increasingly correlated with trauma and vascular injury in recent years. McRae initially postulated that failure of fusion through the neurocentral synchondrosis would cause os odontoideum.[16] A definite cause has not yet been established, but if this were the case, the cleft between the os odontoideum and the axis would be located below the level of the superior facets. However, most cases present a hypoplastic dens and an ovoid radiodense mass with smooth edges immediately rostral to it. Nonhealing of a simple odontoid fracture is inconsistent with the development of the hypoplastic dens, and the fragment usually has an irregular edge at the base (**Fig. 6.8F**). Over time, the base of the os may become sclerotic but, in general, remains closely approximated to the C2 body. Another explanation for the development of an os odontoideum relates to the tenuous vascular supply of the dens, which consists of anterior and posterior ascending arteries that arise from the vertebral arteries and anastomose in the apical arcade next to the alar ligaments in that same area in which some branches from the carotid arteries also anastomose. This vascular supply could become compromised in the setting of trauma, and an unrecognized fracture may develop a form of avascular necrosis followed by contraction of the alar ligaments, which ultimately leads to a radiographic picture consistent with an os odontoideum. This attractive theory has gained support from several authors.[23] Other congenital and acquired conditions could potentially compromise the vascular supply as well and generate os odontoideum. This abnormality has been reported to occur with viral upper respiratory infections, Morquio disease, and Down syndrome.[24]

Isolated hypoplasia and aplasia of the dens represent a continuum of dysfunction of the ossification centers of the dens (**Fig. 6.8B,E**).[21] Hypoplasia is used to describe a small but normally positioned dens whereas complete aplasia refers to complete absence of the odontoid above the neurocentral synchondrosis. This is extremely rare. In fact, McRae identified no examples of this malformation at the Montreal Neurological Institute prior to 1960.[16] Hypoplasia and aplasia of the dens may also occur in conjunction with systemic conditions, such as Down syndrome, spondyloepiphyseal dysplasia, and some mucopolysaccharidoses.[25]

Symptomatic patients with abnormalities of the odontoid process almost always have instability across the C1-C2 junction. Their symptoms can be mechanical (i.e., neck pain or torticollis) or neurological due to compression of the rostral spinal cord (i.e., quadriparesis or modified Brown-Sequard syndrome). Brainstem or cerebellar compression or ischemia due to vertebral artery compromise has been rarely described.[26] Mild or severe symptoms may be precipitated by relatively minor trauma, and there should be a low threshold to investigate the CVJ in all trauma patients with such complaints.

Diagnostic imaging of these patients should include static neutral views and dynamic images when possible. CT scans and MRIs with sagittal and coronal reconstructions together provide good detail of the osseous and soft tissue components of the CVJ. A complete investigation should include anteroposterior (AP), lateral flexion, neutral, and extension radiographs if the patient is not significantly unstable.[27] Close analysis of the bone window on CT should allow proper visualization of the odontoid cortex and differentiation between acute fractures and an os odontoideum. The instability induced by these dens anomalies is unpredictable and neural compression may occur in flexion or extension, depending on the particular biomechanical characteristics of each patient. Such films are important for preoperative planning.[3] Treatment of patients with symptomatic atlantoaxial instability usually consists of obtaining proper alignment, decompressing the neural elements if needed, and C1-C2 fusion. Persistent neural compression may need to be treated with a dorsal or ventral approach.[9,28] The controversial aspect is how to manage asymptomatic patients found to have os odontoideum through radiological screening. Although some advocate limitation of activity for patients with abnormal motion across the C1-C2 segment, a more pragmatic approach involves analysis of flexion-extension radiographs. It has been recommended that patients with 8 mm or more of atlantoaxial AP translation as detected on flexion-extension lateral radiographs should be treated with fusion. Still, a more aggressive approach is that os odontoideum poses an unacceptable risk of neurological injury in even the mildest form of trauma—these surgeons indicate fusion for each newly diagnosed os odontoideum.[29]

Klippel-Feil Syndrome

Klippel-Feil syndrome (KFS), first described in 1912, is a disorder characterized by congenital fusion of the cervical vertebrae.[30] Approximately half of patients with this condition exhibit the full triad of symptoms characteristic of KFS: short neck, a low posterior hairline, and a restricted neck range of motion. The latter is the most common symptom presenting in isolation but may be evident only if three or more segments are fused.[31] The presence of only one fused segment at an unusually young age is sufficient to make the diagnosis of KFS.[30,32] There may be extraspinal manifestations of KFS, such as a cleft palate, a hearing deficiency, and neurological, cardiac, and genitourinary malformations. KFS is frequently detected in the context of routine imaging for trauma or cervical spondylosis.[33] Its pathogenesis is not totally clarified as some doubt still exists regarding the timing of and the intricacies of fusion in KFS, but the underlying molecular mechanism is related to the diminished expression of the *Pax-1* gene in the skeleton, leading to segmentation defects between the 3rd and 8th weeks of gestation.[32,33]

In addition to congenital fusion of one or more levels, numerous other spinal abnormalities can be present in KFS. Hemivertebrae are identified in 74% of cases, and scoliosis is present in 60% of affected patients. Atlas assimilation and basilar invagination have also been described at the CVJ as has iniencephaly (congenital absence of the posterior elements of the cervical spine with enlargement of the foramen magnum), which is frequently associated with fixed hyperextension across the CVJ. Spina bifida and Chiari malformation have been seen with KFS. Another related finding is Sprengel's deformity, manifested by a high-riding scapula sometimes connected to the cervical spine via an omovertebral bone. Sprengel's deformity is found in ~30% of cases and may be bilateral in the same percentage.[30,32]

The imaging evaluation of patients with KFS generally begins with plain radiographic surveys of the spine (**Fig. 6.9**).

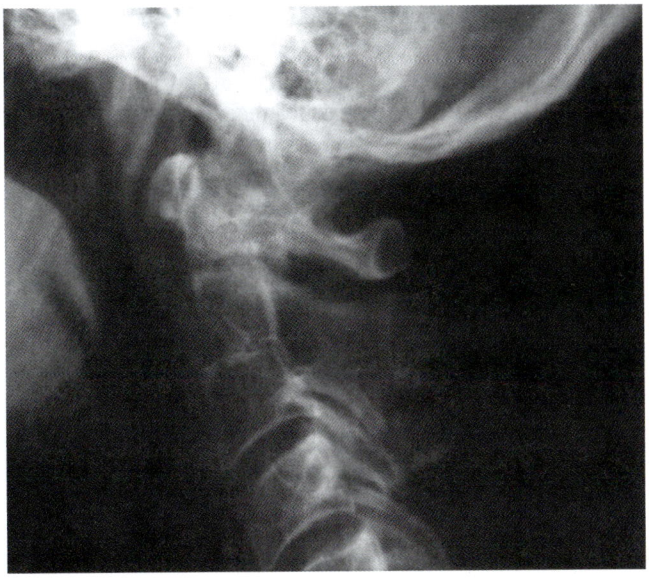

Fig. 6.9 Radiograph of the lateral cervical spine of a 46-year-old man with Klippel-Feil syndrome, demonstrating fusion between the C2 and C3 vertebrae.

These studies frequently demonstrate fusion involving the cervical spine and may reveal other abnormalities such as scoliosis, hemivertebrae, spina bifida, and iniencephaly; however, the high frequency of abnormalities combined with the severity of these lesions often makes plain radiographs difficult to interpret. CT with two- and three-dimensional reconstructions can provide excellent detail in the axial plane; however, the presence of scoliosis, hemivertebrae, and other abnormalities can make interpreting these scans difficult. MRI may be employed to evaluate spinal cord and nerve root impingement, but this technique can be limited by the previously mentioned fixed deformities.[27]

Symptoms and signs associated with spinal involvement from KFS often result from hypermobility at segments adjacent to the fused section of the cervical spine. This hypermobility can produce instability and degenerative changes and increase patient susceptibility to minor trauma. Mechanical symptoms, especially localized pain, are common. Neurological symptoms such as nerve root and spinal cord impingement produce a spectrum of symptoms ranging from simple radiculopathies to quadriparesis. In general, there is less risk of neurological deficit in patients with fusions involving the lower cervical spine and those with fewer involved segments.[33]

Summarizing surgical options is difficult due to the myriad characteristics of KFS. These patients may develop excessive degeneration and instability at levels adjacent to congenital fusions. When needed, surgical treatment usually consists of decompression of the neural elements and arthrodesis across the unstable segments. Atlantoaxial instability may occur when there is a fusion at C2-C3 and assimilation of the atlas, which together predispose the patient to developing hypermobility at C1-C2. Additionally, this combination of abnormalities may lead to facet arthrosis and neural compression. Surgical fusion in KFS extends the already abnormally long moment arm and, thus, may accelerate degeneration at adjacent levels, which may predispose patients to requiring further extension of the fusion. Some authors have tried to obviate the need for additional surgery by performing arthroplasties at levels adjacent to congenital fusions, and the initial reports describing the results of this treatment strategy are promising.[32,33]

Unique Conditions: Down Syndrome and Chiari Malformation

Down syndrome (trisomy 21) is the most common chromosomal abnormality affecting humans, occurring in 1 in 700 live births. Typical characteristics are well-known and include a distinctive facies, mental retardation, and palmar creases whereas other associated abnormalities can include cardiac and bowel malformations, an immunocompromised state, and an increased incidence of leukemia.[34] Of particular interest to spine surgeons is the presence of ligamentous laxity, which is especially common at the CVJ. Almost one third of patients with Down syndrome have some radiological evidence of atlantoaxial instability.[35] Several other CVJ malformations may occur in association with Down syndrome, including C1-C2 rotatory luxations, odontoid malformations, vertebral fusions, hypoplasia of the atlas, and basilar invagination.[34,36] Occipitocervical instability has been increasingly recognized in patients with trisomy 21, and recent studies suggest that there may be radiological indications of occipito-C1 instability in 44 to 61% of affected individuals. It is unclear how many of these patients develop symptoms, and the timeline over which these changes occur is unknown, although atlantoaxial and occipito-C1 instabilities may become symptomatic at a young age.[34]

Although CVJ malformations appear to be equally distributed relative to gender, females are apparently overrepresented in symptomatic cases for unclear reasons. Prior to the adoption of CVJ screening for Down syndrome patients, adult patients occasionally presented with neurological signs and symptoms referable to CVJ instability. With the widespread recognition of these malformations in the Down syndrome population, radiological screening is commonplace, and most patients will present to the spine surgeon with few or no symptoms. Screening for atlantoaxial instability started with the Special Olympics in the mid-1980s, although there has never been an upper cervical injury in a Down syndrome patient during the Special Olympics nor has it been shown that screening prevented any lesions.[36,37] Screening has been extended to all children with Down syndrome at ages 3 and 5. The American Academy of Pediatrics does not recommend additional imaging if initial screening is normal, but in the face of subsequent degeneration, additional imaging may be considered on an individual basis.[37] Radiological screening is commonly performed with simple flexion and extension lateral cervical radiographs. Further investigation with CT and MRI may be warranted if an abnormality is found. Initially negative screening should be repeated as it is known that spondylosis progresses more quickly in Down syndrome patients and instability may become apparent over time. Patients with mild symptoms from CVJ instability or neural compression should undergo fusion and decompression as necessary—the decision to operate on asymptomatic cases is not so straightforward.

Overt C1-C2 instability is generally considered to be indication for fusion even when asymptomatic. High-functioning individuals with mild mental retardation usually have a lower threshold for fusion. If occipito-C1 instability is present, fusions should be extended rostrally to the occiput. Several radiological measurements may be used to detect occipito-C1 instability, two of which are the condyle-C1 distance on coronal CT reconstructions larger than 4 mm or Powers ratio above 1.[36,38] Specific findings in each patient can be broken into separate entities and addressed as in any other patient. Surgical experience with Down syndrome patients was initially poor due to a lack of understanding of CVJ abnormalities in these patients, inadequate fusion techniques, and concerns over infection in immunocompromised patients. Advances over the past two decades have allowed for surgical results comparable to the normal population.[36]

Frequently associated with CVJ abnormalities, Chiari malformation is a complex form of neurodysgenesis first described by Nicolaes Tulp in the 17th century. As many as 25 to 30% of these patients will have basilar invagination,[39] and KPS and atlas assimilation may occur in conjunction with a Chiari malformation.[3] A highly complex abnormality, there is no single theory that adequately explains all aspects of the Chiari malformation.

CVJ congenital anomalies present as a challenging and heterogeneous condition (**Fig. 6.10**). They are common

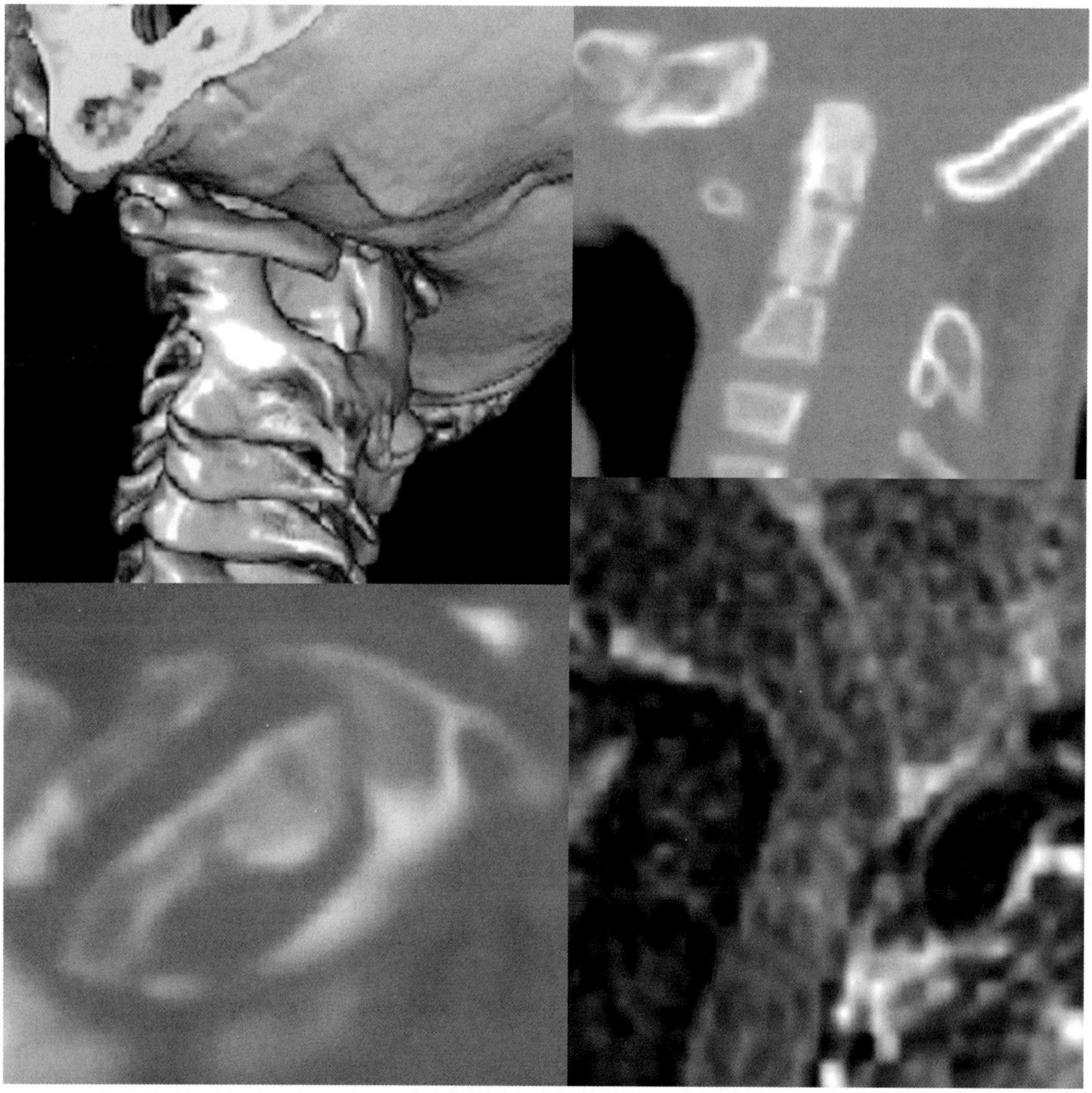

Fig. 6.10 Complex deformity in a 7-year-old boy, including occipital condyle hypoplasia leading to basilar invagination, anterior and posterior spina bifida of the axis, C2-C3 Klippel-Feil, and a Chiari malformation. This patient was successfully treated with traction, realignment, posterior decompression, and dorsal occipital-cervical fusion.

enough that general neurosurgeons will occasionally face these problems in clinical practice, but due to their complexity some patients may require referral for specialized treatment. Advances in diagnostic imaging, surgical technique, and instrumentation, along with a greater understanding of the normal and pathological anatomy, have enabled spine surgeons to offer significantly better treatment options than those available 20 years ago.

References

1. Chamberlain WE. Basilar impression (platybasia). A bizarre developmental anomaly of the occipital bone and upper cervical spine with striking and misleading neurologic manifestations. Yale J Biol Med 1939;11(5):487–496
2. List CF. Neurologic syndromes accompanying developmental anomalies of occipital bone, atlas and axis. Arch Neurol Psychiatry 1941;45:577–616
3. Menezes AH. Craniocervical developmental anatomy and its implications. Childs Nerv Syst 2008;24(10):1109–1122
4. Spillane JD, Pallis C, Jones AM. Developmental abnormalities in the region of the foramen magnum. Brain 1957;80(1):11–48
5. Menezes AH, Fenoy KA. Remnants of occipital vertebrae: proatlas segmentation abnormalities. Neurosurgery 2009;64(5):945–953, discussion 954
6. Pappas CTE, Rekate HL. Role of magnetic resonance imaging and three-dimensional computerized tomography in craniovertebral junction anomalies. Pediatr Neurosci 1988;14(1):18–22
7. Hensinger RN. Osseous anomalies of the craniovertebral junction. Spine 1986;11(4):323–333
8. Wackenheim A. Cervico-Occipital Joint (RX, CT). New York: Springer-Verlag; 1985
9. Perrini P, Benedetto N, Guidi E, Lorenzo ND. Transoral approach and its superior extensions to the craniovertebral junction malformations: surgical strategies and results. Neurosurgery 2009;64(5): ONS331–ONS42
10. Gladstone RJ, Erichsen-Powell W. Manifestation of occipital vertebrae and fusion of the atlas with the occipital bone. J Anat Physiol 1915;49(Pt 2):190–209
11. Naidich TP, McLone DG, Harwood-Nash DC. Malformations of the craniocervical junction. In: Newton TH, Potts DG, eds. Computed Tomography of the Spine and Spinal Cord. San Anselmo, CA: Clavadel Press; 1983:355–366
12. Macalister A. Notes on the development and variations of the atlas. J Anat Physiol 1893;27(Pt 4):519–542
13. McCall T, Coppens J, Couldwell W, Dailey A. Symptomatic occipitocervical paracondylar process. J Neurosurg Spine 2010;12(1):9–12
14. de Graauw N, Carpay HA, Slooff WB. The paracondylar process: an unusual and treatable cause of posttraumatic headache. Spine 2008;33(9):E283–E286
15. Torklus DV, Gehle W. The Upper Cervical Spine. New York, NY: Grune & Stratton; 1972
16. McRae DL. The significance of abnormalities of the cervical spine. AJR Am J Roentgenol 1960;84:3–25
17. Gholve PA, Hosalkar HS, Ricchetti ET, Pollock AN, Dormans JP, Drummond DS. Occipitalization of the atlas in children. Morphologic classification, associations, and clinical relevance. J Bone Joint Surg Am 2007;89(3):571–578
18. Gehweiler JA Jr, Daffner RH, Roberts L Jr. Malformations of the atlas vertebra simulating the Jefferson fracture. AJR Am J Roentgenol 1983;140(6):1083–1086
19. Dorne HL, Lander PH. CT recognition of anomalies of the posterior arch of the atlas vertebra: differentiation from fracture. AJNR Am J Neuroradiol 1986;7(1):176–177
20. Dubousset J. Torticollis in children caused by congenital anomalies of the atlas. J Bone Joint Surg Am 1986;68(2):178–188
21. Kline DG. Atlanto-axial dislocation simulating a head injury; hypoplasia of the odontoid. Case report. J Neurosurg 1966;24(6): 1013–1016
22. Davis D, Gutierrez FA. Congenital anomaly of the odontoid in children. A report of four cases. Childs Brain 1977;3(4):219–229
23. Menezes AH. Pathogenesis, dynamics, and management of os odontoideum. Neurosurg Focus 1999;6(6):e2
24. Crockard HA, Stevens JM. Craniovertebral junction anomalies in inherited disorders: part of the syndrome or caused by the disorder? Eur J Pediatr 1995;154(7):504–512
25. Fielding JW, Hensinger RN, Hawkins RJ. Os odontoideum. J Bone Joint Surg Am 1980;62(3):376–383
26. Fukuda M, Aiba T, Akiyama K, Nishiyama K, Ozawa T. Cerebellar infarction secondary to os odontoideum. J Clin Neurosci 2003; 10(5):625–626
27. Smoker WR, Khanna G. Imaging the craniocervical junction. Childs Nerv Syst 2008;24(10):1123–1145
28. Ahmed R, Traynelis VC, Menezes AH. Fusions at the craniovertebral junction. Childs Nerv Syst 2008;24(10):1209–1224
29. Klimo P Jr, Kan P, Rao G, Apfelbaum R, Brockmeyer D. Os odontoideum: presentation, diagnosis, and treatment in a series of 78 patients. J Neurosurg Spine 2008;9(4):332–342
30. Klippel M, Feil A. Un cas d'absence des vertebres cervicales. Avec cage thoracique remontant jusqu'a la base du crane (cage thoracique cervicale). Nouv Icon Salpetriere 1912;25:223–250
31. Tracy MR, Dormans JP, Kusumi K. Klippel-Feil syndrome: clinical features and current understanding of etiology. Clin Orthop Relat Res 2004;424(424):183–190
32. Samartzis D, Kalluri P, Herman J, Lubicky JP, Shen FH. The extent of fusion within the congenital Klippel-Feil segment. Spine 2008; 33(15):1637–1642
33. Yi S, Kim SH, Shin HC, Kim KN, Yoon DH. Cervical arthroplasty in a patient with Klippel-Feil syndrome. Acta Neurochir (Wien) 2007; 149(8):805–809, discussion 809
34. Menezes AH, Ryken TC. Craniovertebral abnormalities in Down's syndrome. Pediatr Neurosurg 1992;18(1):24–33
35. Martel W, Tishler JM. Observations on the spine in mongoloidism. Am J Roentgenol Radium Ther Nucl Med 1966;97(3): 630–638
36. Hankinson TC, Anderson RCE. Craniovertebral junction abnormalities in Down syndrome. Neurosurgery 2010;66(3, Suppl): 32–38
37. Policy statement: AAP publications reaffirmed and retired. Pediatrics 2007;120(3):683
38. Pang D, Nemzek WR, Zovickian J. Atlanto-occipital dislocation—part 2: the clinical use of (occipital) condyle-C1 interval, comparison with other diagnostic methods, and the manifestation, management, and outcome of atlanto-occipital dislocation in children. Neurosurgery 2007;61(5):995–1015, discussion 1015
39. Tulp N. Amstelredamnensis Observationes Medicae. Amsterdam, The Netherlands: Elsevier; 1641

7 The Rheumatoid Neck: Changing Pathology Requires Altering Surgical Strategies

David Choi and Hugh Alan Crockard

Rheumatoid arthritis (RA) is a relatively new disease in the Western world. The first accurate depiction of its effects on the hands can be seen in a Renoir drawing of the artist at work at the end of the 19th century.[1] At the beginning of the 20th century, A.B. Garrod coined the term "rheumatoid arthritis" and his son, A.E. Garrod, reported that the disease involved the cervical spine.[2] The hands, major limb joints, and cervical spine are involved by the acute or chronic systemic inflammatory disorder characterized by an erosive synovitis, ultimately producing joint destruction, deformity, and painful incapacity. However, the introduction of disease-modifying drugs that dampen the inflammatory process and the decreased use of long-term systemic steroids, once the cornerstone of treatment, have considerably reduced the disease's impact on the joints. The change in medical management of the disease coupled with our better understanding of its long-term effects on the cervical spine by the availability of computed tomography (CT) and magnetic resonance imaging (MRI) have resulted in a major shift in surgical management. Operations once performed late in the course of myelopathy have been replaced with prophylactic operations for cervical instability to prevent myelopathy from developing.[3,4] For example, although vertical translocation of the odontoid peg was common 30 years ago, now it is an extremely rare presentation, with few transoral operations performed for rheumatoid disease (**Fig. 7.1**).

Epidemiology of Rheumatoid Arthritis

RA is two to three times more common in females than in males, with a peak age of onset in the fifth decade, although a juvenile form predominantly affects adolescent females.[5] The disease affects 0.5 to 1% of the population in the West, but the incidence around the world varies considerably; RA is about five times more common in the Pima Indians of Arizona in the United States and almost unheard of in South Africa and Nigeria.[6]

Etiology

The appearance of the disease in Europe after the discovery of the Americas led to the hypothesis of an infectious agent, further supported by a decreasing incidence in Caucasians and an increase in Asian populations.[7,8] Epstein-Barr virus, parvovirus, *Proteus*, *Borrelia*, and mycobacteria among others have been implicated as possible candidate agents[6] that theoretically might cause arthritis by direct effects or the induction of an autoimmune response. The incidence of rheumatoid disease in Asians who now live in the West is twice as high compared with Asians living in their native country, suggesting that environmental factors are significant.[5] Other factors include smoking, blood transfusion, and obesity,[9] which increase the risk of RA, whereas a diet rich in omega-3 fatty acids (like those of Eskimos and Pacific Islanders) decreases the risk.[10] Steroids have a disease-modifying effect. Multiparous women and those taking oral contraceptives are at a lower risk of developing the disease, but there is an increased risk postpartum.[6,11] In 75% of pregnancies, symptoms temporarily improve, possibly due to placental steroid production.[12]

RA has a genetic component, and familial clustering is sometimes evident,[13] although a concordance of only 12 to 15% is seen in monozygotic twin studies.[14] About 40% of the genetic contribution may be accounted for by genes in the human leukocyte antigen alleles (HLA) region as well as other non-HLA genes (e.g., coding for interferons, interleukins, and tumor necrosis factors).[14]

Pathology

Although juvenile RA predominantly causes ankylosis, RA in adults causes joint erosion and instability. In the acute phase, synovial tissue in joints becomes hypertrophic and edematous and forms villous projections that invade joint

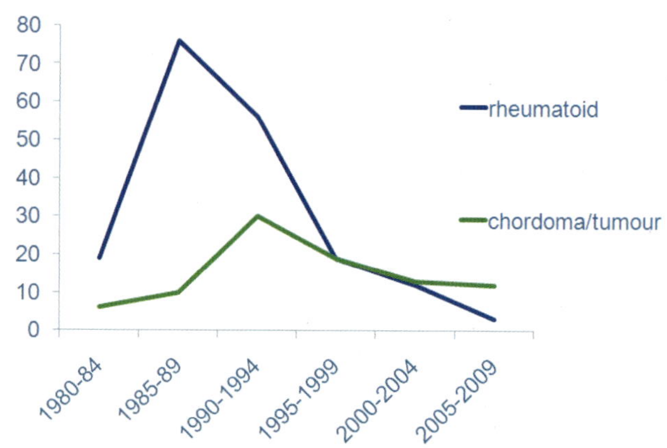

Fig. 7.1 Transoral procedures performed for rheumatoid arthritis patients over the past 30 years at the National Hospital for Neurology and Neurosurgery, United Kingdom, showing a decrease compared with other pathologies, such as chordomas.

cavities, local bone, ligaments, and cartilage. Histological examination of this synovial overgrowth, commonly known as pannus, reveals the accumulation of T cells, B cells, plasma cells, mast cells, macrophages, and natural killer cells that produce proinflammatory cytokines and adhesion molecules. However, O'Brien and colleagues showed that, in patients with cord compression at the craniovertebral junction (CVJ), much of the soft tissue mass consisted of end-stage degenerating ligaments and bone as well as pannus formation.[15] Involvement of cervical bone and joints, particularly at the CVJ, can lead to structural instability and acute cord compression, but as O'Brien has shown, it is more common for the compressive mass to result from undetected or untreated subluxation causing the cord damage over a decade or more.[15] A combination of movement, compression, and stretching of the cord produces edema, axonal swelling, and necrosis principally in the dorsal white matter. It is this repetitive minor trauma associated with the unstable joint—not rheumatoid vasculitis—that leads to clinical myelopathy in most patients.[16] This trauma explains why many patients have asymptomatic atlantoaxial subluxation and why it takes many years of repeated minor trauma to produce symptoms of myelopathy. The therapeutic implication is that medical treatment should be directed at preventing ligamentous damage and joint instability, and surgical fixation should be performed before the onset of myelopathy if possible.

Natural History

RA initially involves the hands and feet, and large joints usually require surgery before the neck does. Wolfe found that one in four patients in the United States had a large joint arthroplasty in the first 6 years of the disease, and Casey and colleagues revealed that cervical disease required surgical treatment in patients who had two to four previous arthroplasties.[17,18] These findings imply that the greater the mobility in a rheumatoid joint, the faster it will degenerate and become unstable. Hence, the cervical spine is affected commonly, particularly the atlantoaxial joint and the CVJ, with the lower spine seldom involved.

The percentage of patients with RA who develop atlantoaxial subluxation varies between series and is largely biased by the source of data collection. Few large, population-based, cohort studies are found in the literature, but from nonsurgical studies over the past decades the percentage of patients with RA with atlantoaxial subluxation varies from 14 to 73%,[19,20] with an average incidence of 35% (21% horizontal and 14% vertical subluxation).[21] More than 30% will have symptomatic atlantoaxial subluxation 5 to 7 years after the onset of the disease. Five percent then become myelopathic a decade later (14 to 17 years after onset).[22–24] Once myelopathy has developed, the outlook is poor with up to 50% mortality within a year. Studies by Sunahara, Hamilton, and Casey and colleagues suggest that life expectancy is ~7 years from the onset of myelopathy and, once bed-bound, death often occurs within 1 year.[17,25,26] Recent studies of atlantoaxial subluxation in nonsurgical European patients, such as the Early Rheumatoid Arthritis Study (ERAS; a multicenter outpatient study), have shown a lower prevalence than before (range 12 to 33%),[27–31] although the incidence of disease presenting to a surgeon remains higher as expected.[32]

The Changing Pattern of Rheumatoid Arthritis

The disease pattern is changing, partly as a result of improved medical treatment and possibly due to altered expression of the disease.[3] Although steroids unquestionably produce relief of symptoms, it is possible that some of the neck problems described in the 1960s, 1970s, and 1980s were caused or exacerbated by steroid treatment itself. In the past few decades, there have been several advances in the development and use of disease-modifying antirheumatic drugs (DMARDs); in the 1980s, cyclosporine became available, then minocycline and leflunomide, and more recently antitumor necrosis factor (anti-TNF) agents (infliximab, etanercept, and adalimumab) and interleukin 1 (IL1) antagonists (anakinra).[33,34] The anti-TNF and anti-IL1 agents have been shown to improve symptoms and signs, decrease radiographic progression, and reduce pain and fatigue.[35–37] Neva and colleagues demonstrated that the use of combination DMARDs has significant advantages over single therapy in reducing the radiological incidence of atlantoaxial subluxation.[38]

We have recently observed a decrease in patients requiring surgery for cervical rheumatoid disease, and similar trends have been reported for large joint replacement in rheumatoid patients in California and in Rochester, Minnesota.[39,40] The observed number of rheumatoid patients presenting for cervical surgery now is much lower than might have been expected based on past decades. Ten years ago, 62,700 patients in the United Kingdom and 220,000 in the United States were predicted to require cervical spinal fixation.[28,41] In 2000, however, Hamilton and colleagues followed up with 3800 rheumatoid patients in western Scotland and detected only 0.7% of patients requiring cervical surgery, a 10-fold decrease in the previously estimated number.[25] Looking at the prevalence of atlantoaxial subluxation and translocation in ERAS, James and colleagues suggested a 5.6% prevalence of subluxation in the first 5 years and translocation in 3.1%,[42] a much lower prevalence of patients at risk in the 21st century.

Evaluation

In the past, the outcome of surgery was reported in terms of operative mortality and major complications. Surgery was performed often in patients with end-stage disease, who did not have an option—quality of life and less serious complications were overlooked. Now that surgery is aimed at

Table 7.1 The Ranawat Classification for Neurological Disability

Grade I	Normal neurological condition
Grade II	Subjective weakness with hyperreflexia and dysesthesia
Grade IIIA	Objective weakness and long-tract signs, but able to walk
Grade IIIB	Objective weakness, unable to walk

prevention of myelopathy, deformity, and treatment of pain, it is essential that internationally accepted objective measures of function and quality of life are used by spine surgeons.

Clinical Assessment

Clinical grading tools have been devised for various spinal conditions, but these are not always suitable for evaluation of rheumatoid myelopathy. The first universally accepted grading, the Ranawat classification (**Table 7.1**), is simple to apply but is a blunt tool that does not distinguish small differences in the severe stages of myelopathy.[43] The move toward using more accurate measures of quality of life rather than physician-reported neurological scales allows comparative health-care studies (e.g., the "short forms" of SF36 and SF12 questionnaires and the EuroQol EQ-5D tool for quality of life and cost effectiveness analysis).[44–46]

Radiological Assessment: Cervical X-rays

Despite a trend in the 1980s and early 1990s to establish radiological criteria for surgery, such methods are now relegated to the archives of history (**Fig. 7.2**) and are not particularly useful for clinical decision making since the advent of CT and MRI (**Fig. 7.3**). Although cervical radiographs were the key to surgical decision making in the past, they are now largely for diagnosis of the at-risk patient rather than directly influencing the management plan. Previously, lively debates around the degree of acceptable subluxation and when to perform fixation[47–53] have been put in perspective by White and Panjabi's demonstration that gross movements occurred

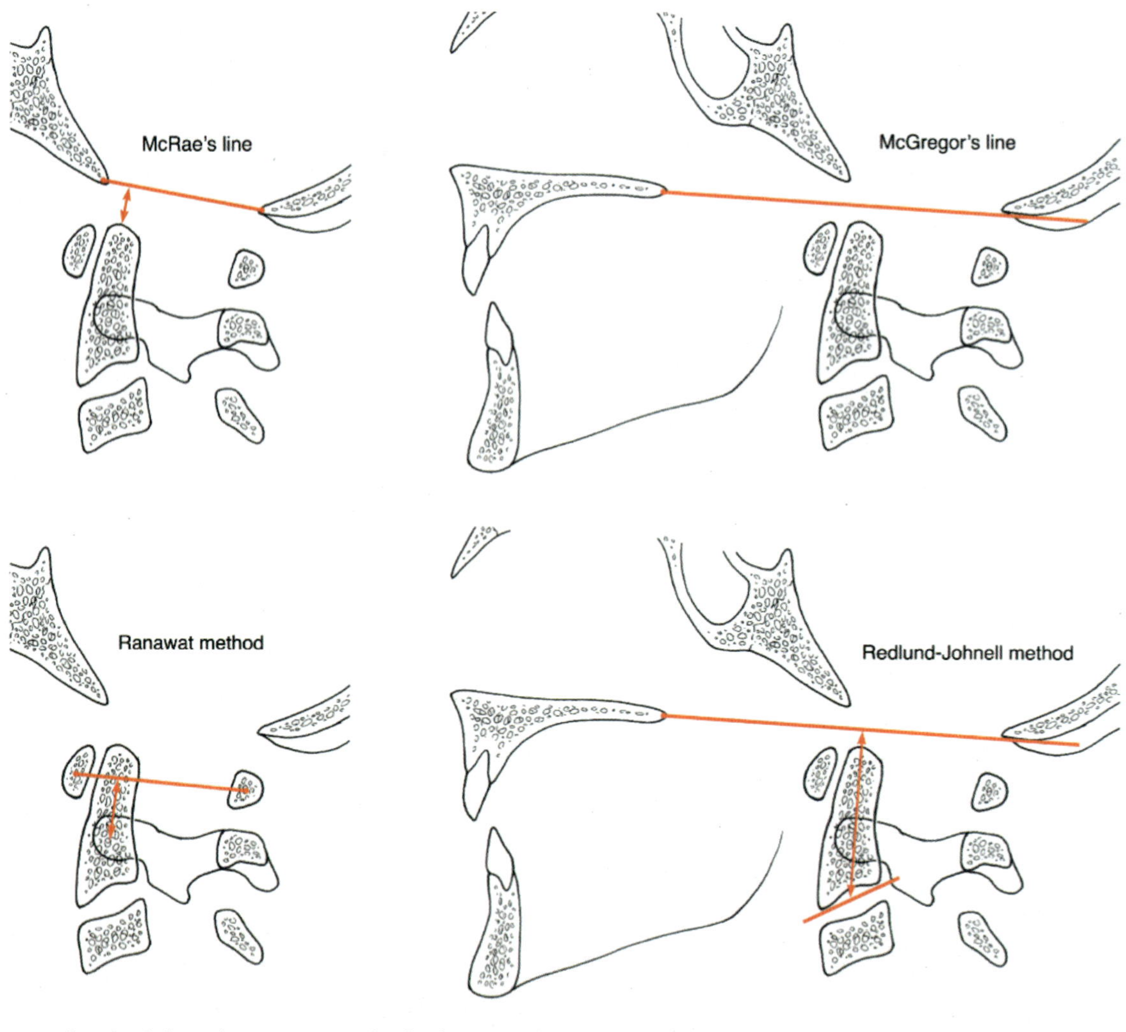

Fig. 7.2 Examples of radiological measurements for the diagnosis of vertical translocation. (Reprinted with permission from Barrow Neurological Institute.)

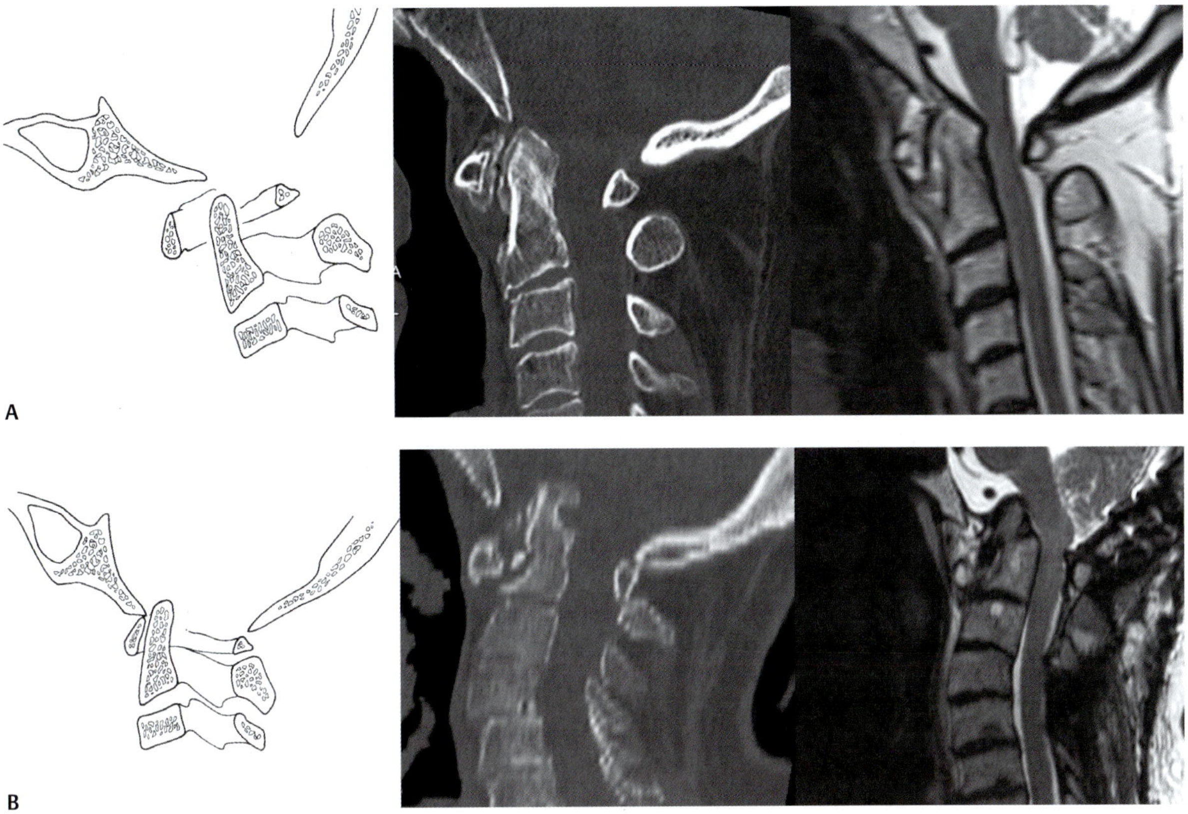

Fig. 7.3 Schematic diagram, magnetic resonance imaging, and computed tomography of **(A)** atlantoaxial subluxation and **(B)** vertical translocation. (**A** [left] and **B** [left] used with permission from Barrow Neurological Institute.)

when the transverse and apical alar ligament complex was damaged.[54] Thus, significant instability should be defined by the point at which these ligaments fail mechanically, and it is incorrect to define a continuous gradation of instability depending on the degree of radiological subluxation. Another fallacy of plain radiographs is that a previously unstable atlantoaxial joint that develops vertical translocation may appear stable. The stability in these cases might be compared with the stability of an impacted fractured neck of the femur. Further evaluation should include MRI and CT scanning to determine the presence of neural compression, soft tissue masses, and malalignment and to estimate bone quality.

Computed Tomography Scans

Although the anterior atlantodental interval on a CT scan is useful in the diagnosis of atlantoaxial subluxation, the posterior atlantodental interval (PADI) is of more practical use and is significant if less than 14 mm. PADIs of less than 10 mm correlate well with MRI findings of significant cord compression but, like plain radiographs, assessment of the PADI does not take into account the effect of local soft tissue or pannus that is not seen, and significant brainstem compression by vertical translocation can be underestimated.[55] CT scans of the CVJ are useful for assessing the degree of joint erosion, bone density, and presence of degenerative cysts and allow an appreciation of the likelihood of good screw purchase.

Magnetic Resonance Imaging

MRI scanning is effective in revealing neural compression by soft tissue masses that is not seen by X-ray or CT and is essential to demonstrate the full extent of brainstem compression caused by vertical translocation. On sagittal scans in flexion, a spinal cord diameter of less than 6 mm was taken as the criterion for diagnosing significant compression in one study.[56] Flexion MRI may diagnose significant cord compression in an additional 26% of patients compared with neutral position MRI.[56] However, MRI findings do not necessarily correlate with clinical findings because myelopathy is usually the result of years of repetitive trauma; therefore, cord compression in itself is not directly associated with clinical signs.[16] Because of this discrepancy, Hamilton and colleagues highlighted the importance of making decisions on the basis of clinical and not radiological findings.[25]

Surgical Decision Making

The current management plan (**Table 7.2**) is entirely different from that in the first edition of this book due to changes in the disease itself that we have mentioned. Of equal importance have been the significant advances in spine stabilization techniques over the past 30 years, affording more exact and safe operations. In this section, we describe the

Table 7.2 Indications for the Surgical Management of Cervical Rheumatoid Disease

C1-C2 fixation should be considered for
Instability and intractable pain
Clinical myelopathy
Occipital neuralgia
Progressive radiological subluxation
Anteroposterior spinal cord diameter <6 mm on flexion magnetic resonance imaging
Posterior atlantodental interval <10 mm on computed tomography
Patients with instability who are unable to wear a hard collar or brace
Fixation of the occiput to cervical spine should be considered for
Vertical translocation
Excessive degeneration or instability of the occipitoatlantal joints
C1 or C2 bone quality that does not allow adequate screw purchase or fixation of a short segment
Disruption of the ring of C1 by fracture or after transoral odontoidectomy
Significant "staircase" deformity or instability in the subaxial spine that requires a longer construct to simultaneously fuse lower levels
Transoral decompression and posterior fixation should be considered for
Irreducible atlantoaxial subluxation or anterior soft tissue mass that causes ventral compression of the neuraxis in the presence of acute neurological deterioration
Marked vertical translocation (>5 mm) that causes brainstem compression

current popular techniques in specialized spine centers around the world.

Fixation and fusion was recommended in the 1960s and 1970s for patients with myelopathy and progressive neurological deficits—sometimes traction was also recommended.[57,58] In the 1970s and 1980s, some surgeons suggested that fixation should not be performed in asymptomatic patients because atlantoaxial instability is common.[2,59] Since then, however, surgical complication rates have decreased. Hamilton and colleagues compared their surgical outcome in the 1970s to the 1990s and found an improvement in mortality from 9 to 0%, a decrease in complication rates, and improvement of symptoms in 89% of patients.[25] It is now accepted that operations for nonambulant myelopathic patients are associated with an unacceptably high complication rate and poor functional improvement and that there is a greater role for prophylactic fixation once a diagnosis of instability has been made rather than waiting until neurological signs manifest.[4,17] Operations are now frequently performed for the treatment of pain in liaison with rheumatologists, radiologists, physicians, and pain clinicians in a much more multidisciplinary fashion than in the past.[3] Also, because operations are now performed more for prophylaxis than for treatment of end-stage disease, fixation should involve good bone fusion with autologous bone graft or bone substitutes with or without bone morphogenic proteins. This recommendation is a change to the previous philosophy of fixation without bone grafting that was commonly practiced in the past.[60] The harvest of bone graft from the iliac crest is associated with significant complications of pain, hip fracture, infection, and hematoma formation,[60] and we are selective in our use of bone graft or artificial substitutes to supplement screw fixation. In older rheumatoid patients, the quality of iliac crest bone graft may be poor; therefore, we prefer to use suboccipital bone dust harvested with a burr; artificial bone substitutes, such as coralline; demineralized bone matrix; or bone morphogenic protein over the lateral masses and screws to aid fusion in these cases.

Postoperatively, external orthoses may be used, although there is no clear data demonstrating their efficacy. We commonly apply a rigid collar after fixation for 6 to 12 weeks to maximize the chances of fusion unless the patient is unable to wear a collar due to pressure sores, poor compliance, or difficulty fitting an adequately shaped collar. One possible disadvantage of using a collar is that neck muscles may atrophy and result in more neck pain or decreased range of movement over time.

Operations for the Rheumatoid Neck

Subaxial Spine

Surgery to the subaxial spine is tailored to the nature of compression as seen on MRI. Radiculopathy can be treated as it would be for other causes of degenerative root compression, but it is more likely that instrumented fusion will be required in rheumatoid patients (**Fig. 7.4A**). Anterior cord compression may be treated by discectomy or corpectomy with insertion of a titanium or carbon fiber cage and adjunctive posterior fixation, whereas posterior compression may be treated by laminectomy and lateral mass fixation alone. Older techniques of rod and wire fixation should be avoided in favor of readily available lateral mass screw systems that are quick and easy to use, affording robust fixation. Patients who have had prolonged steroid treatment will have osteoporotic vertebral bodies.

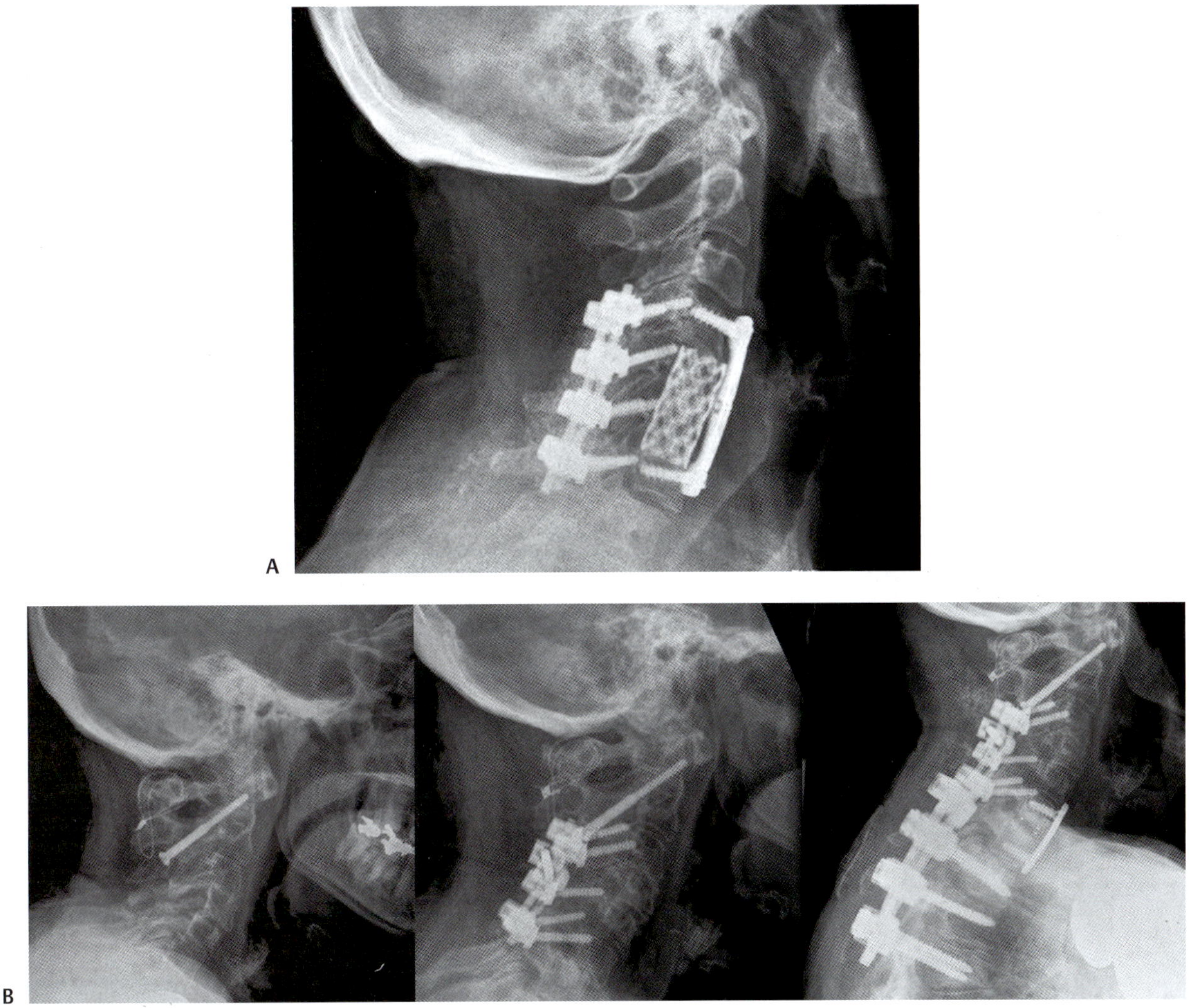

Fig. 7.4 **(A)** Rheumatoid subaxial fixation by anterior and posterior approaches. **(B)** Extension of previous fixations due to adjacent segment disease.

Therefore, anterior fixation alone generally should be avoided due to an increased risk of subsidence and plate failure—additional posterior instrumentation is preferred. Because patients now tend to live longer than they did in previous decades, adjacent segment subluxation is common. If subluxation occurs, then the original fixation is left in place with added fixation above or below as necessary (**Fig. 7.4B**).

C1-C2 Fixation

In patients with horizontal atlantoaxial subluxation, C1-C2 fixation and fusion is recommended to minimize the number of fused segments and spare the occiput in particular. A segment-saving approach minimizes the unacceptable stiffness associated with occipitocervical fixation. It is unusual for rheumatoid disease to affect the occipitoatlantal joints. Malcolm and colleagues showed that head rotation is reduced to 30% and flexion to 40 to 50% of the full range after occipitocervical fixation, which is often sufficient to prevent patients from driving a car (see **Fig. 7.4**).[61]

Historically, silk sutures and malleable wire have been used for fixation and, more recently, the bone graft and wire techniques of Gallie and Brooks as well as Dickman and Sonntag,[62–66] but although effective in limiting flexion and extension, they do not adequately protect against the principal problem of anterior subluxation of C1 on C2 (**Fig. 7.5**). At the end of the 20th century, fixation devices such as the Ti-Frame (DuPuy, Raynham, MA) and Sof'Wire (DuPuy) and posterior Halifax clamps were used, but these too have been replaced by techniques of screw fixation that afford increased rigid fixation in all planes.[21,67–69]

Transarticular screws were first used in 1979, and the Harms technique soon followed.[70,71] These two procedures are the most widely adopted procedures in spine centers around the world. Transarticular C1-C2 screw insertion can be quicker and easier to perform than the Harms technique, with less extensive lateral exposure of the C1-C2 region and associated venous bleeding that may occur. However, the procedure may not be possible in up to 20% of patients due to the presence of a high-riding vertebral artery, which can

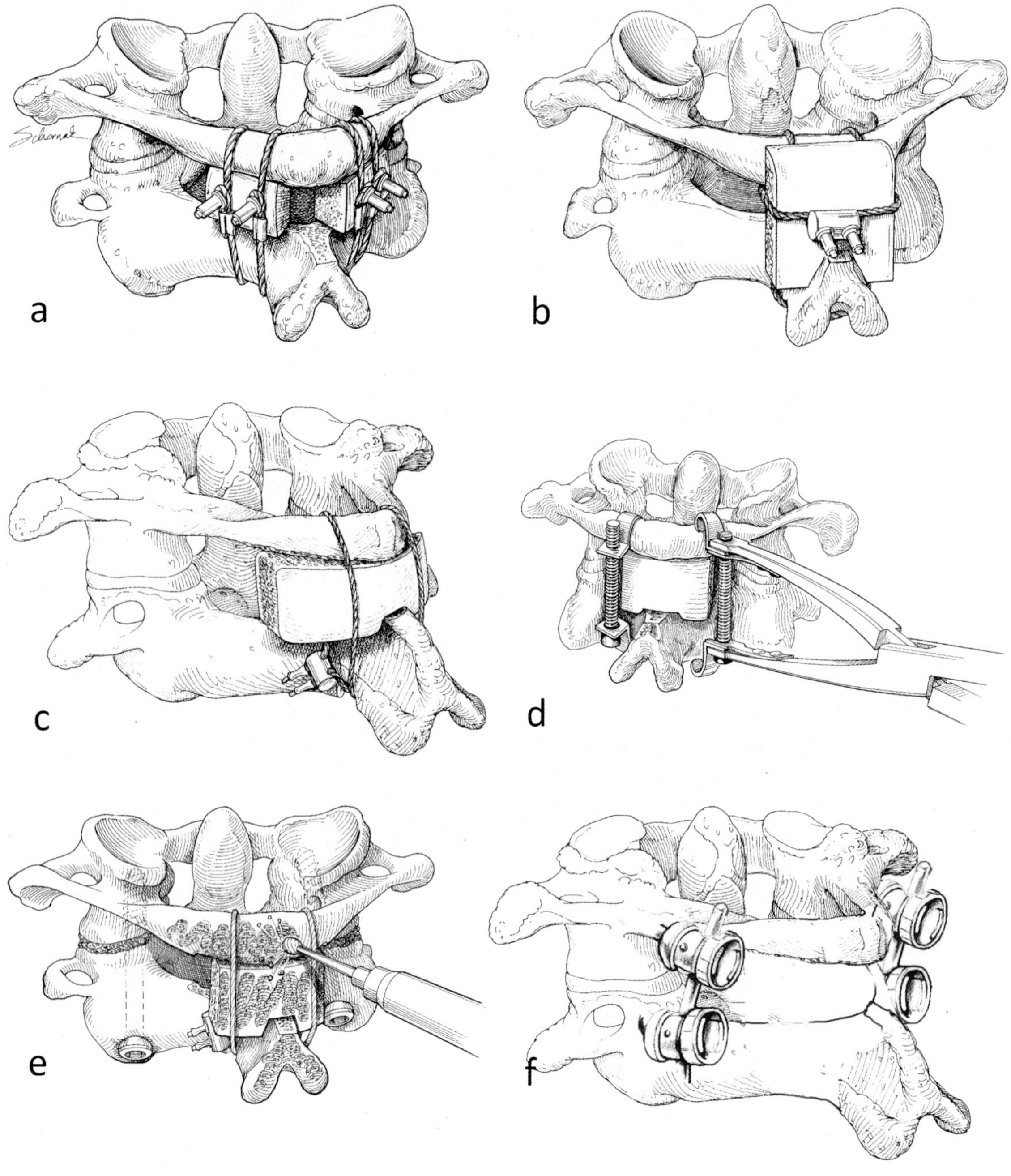

Fig. 7.5 C1-C2 fixation techniques from the past and present: **(A)** Brooks fusion, **(B)** Gallie fusion, **(C)** interspinous fusion, **(D)** Halifax clamps, **(E)** Magerl transarticular screws, and **(F)** Harms technique. (Reprinted with permission from Barrow Neurological Institute.)

lie in the screw trajectory.[71–73] A disadvantage of the transarticular screw technique is that a longer incision often needs to be made, even to the C7 level if there is significant thoracolumbar kyphosis. The procedure also requires a sublaminar wire to be passed under C1 and/or C2 for a simultaneous Gallie or Brooks fusion. The Harms technique of C1 lateral mass and C2 pedicle screw insertion may be performed through an incision smaller than the one used in an equivalent transarticular screw approach and allows intraoperative reduction of C1-C2 deformity. It is also preferable when irreducible subluxation is present or the vertebral artery is abnormally high in the C2 facet.[71–73] However, the Harms technique requires a skilled surgical assistant who understands the anatomy of the vertebral artery, C2 nerve root, and spinal cord. It is necessary for the assistant to protect the vertebral artery using a curved McDonald instrument during drilling while the operating surgeon concentrates on the drilling itself with a two-handed technique. Venous bleeding may partly obscure the surgeon's view but can be controlled by packing with Surgicel fibrillar (Ethicon, Somerville, NJ) or FloSeal (Baxter, Deerfield, IL) and tilting the table to raise the head above the chest.

Transoral Surgery

The only indication for transoral surgery in rheumatoid patients is irreducible vertical translocation with acute myelopathy and rapid onset of neurological symptoms due to anterior compression of the upper cervical cord by odontoid pannus. This surgery is now uncommon for reasons discussed previously but, when performed, posterior occipitocervical fixation is usually required after decompression of the peg and associated ligaments.

Posterior Occipitocervical Fixation

In the past, fusion of the occiput to the upper cervical spine has been achieved by fibular strut graft, malleable wire, or bone cement.[74–76] The use of metal constructs has improved the rigidity of occipitocervical fixation and, during the 1980s and 1990s, techniques involving plates, Luque rods, and loops were developed.[77,78] After fixation with most plates and rods, cranial settling could still occur, leading Ransford to develop a C2 contour to minimize vertical telescoping of the construct, which was attached to the occiput and cervical laminae with wire.[78] However, lateral mass screw systems are now the preferred method for fusing the posterior CVJ using occipital plates.

Reducible vertical translocation, or chronic compression of the upper cervical cord due to odontoid pannus with slowly progressive symptoms and signs, may be treated by occipitocervical fixation alone without anterior odontoidectomy (**Fig. 7.6**). After removal of the dynamic stimulus at C1-C2, the odontoid mass usually regresses with time.

Surgical Results

Surgical outcomes vary considerably among different studies, and the lack of a standardized outcome measure makes it difficult to compare results. Outcomes are also affected by the severity of rheumatoid disease and joint pain, which vary with time, often with an undulating course. Changes in walking or hand function, therefore, cannot always be attributed to the surgery itself.

It is easier to assess and compare mortality rates than symptomatic improvement. In a published series of atlantoaxial and occipitocervical fixations, rates vary from 0 to 18%, and a meta-analysis of 15 studies revealed an overall rate of 6.4%.[21] However, the mortality rate for atlantoaxial fixation in nonmyelopathic patients is now much lower (~1 to 2%), so early surgery can be recommended for asymptomatic patients or C2 nerve root pain. Mortality is related to the degree of preoperative neurological deficit: patients with a Ranawat grading of I or II have a low

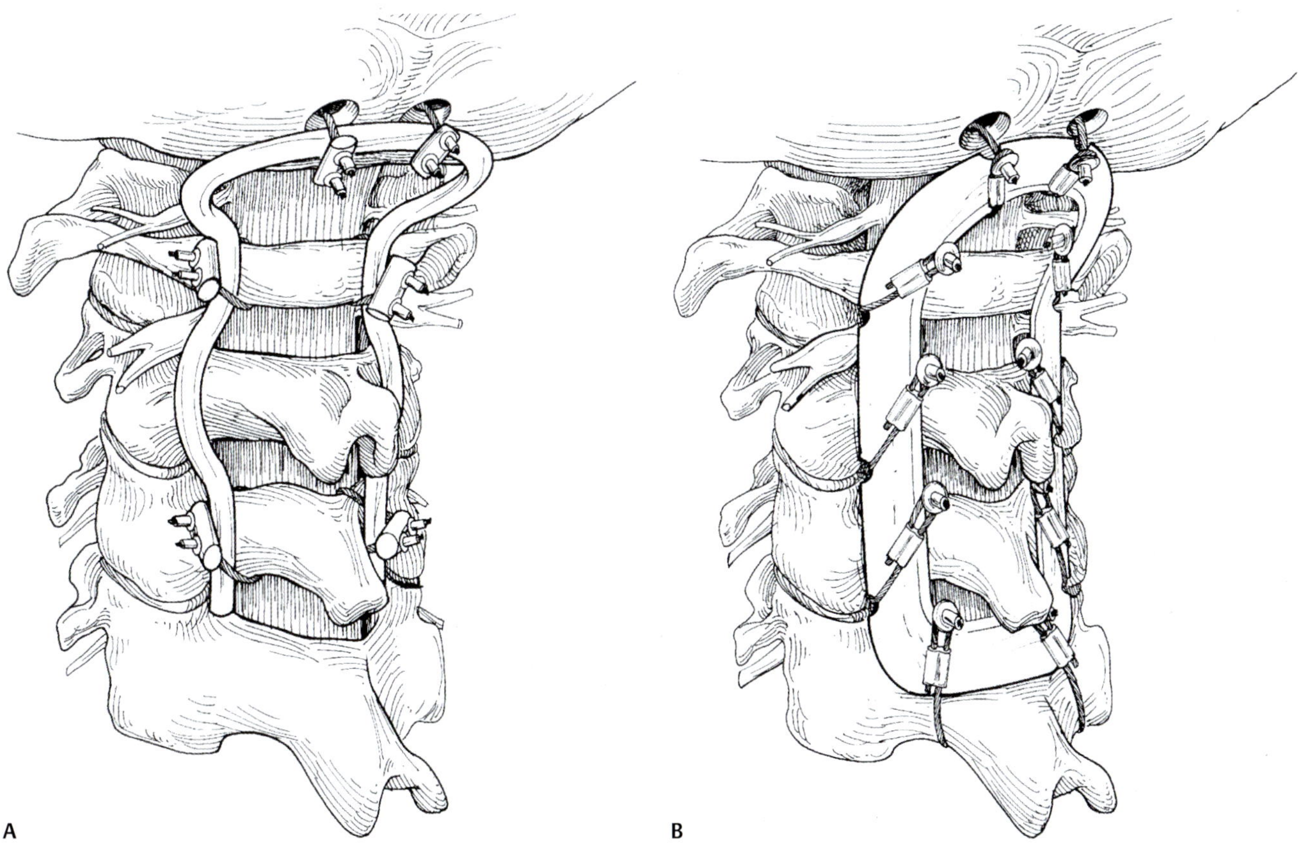

A B

Fig. 7.6 Evolution of occipitocervical fixation: **(A)** Ransford loop, **(B)** Codman Ti-Frame. *(continued)*

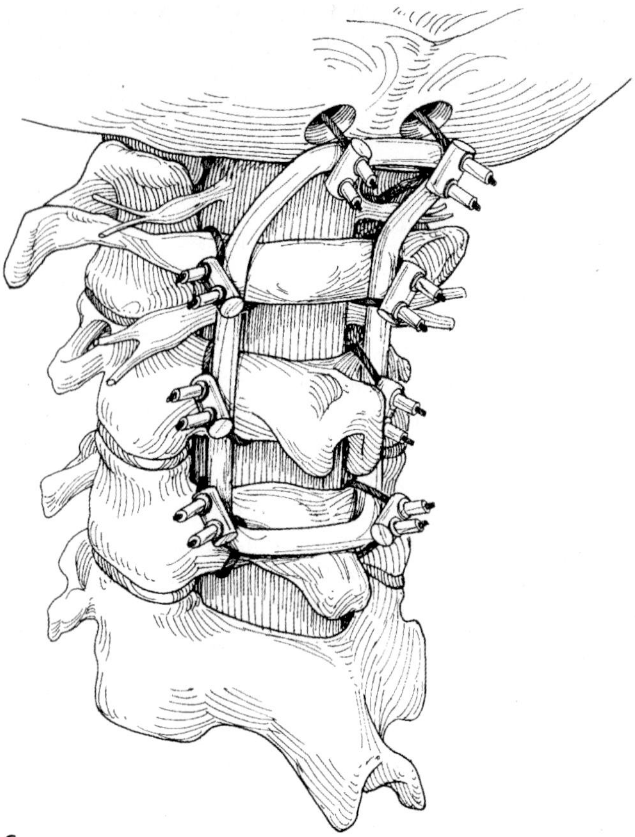

C

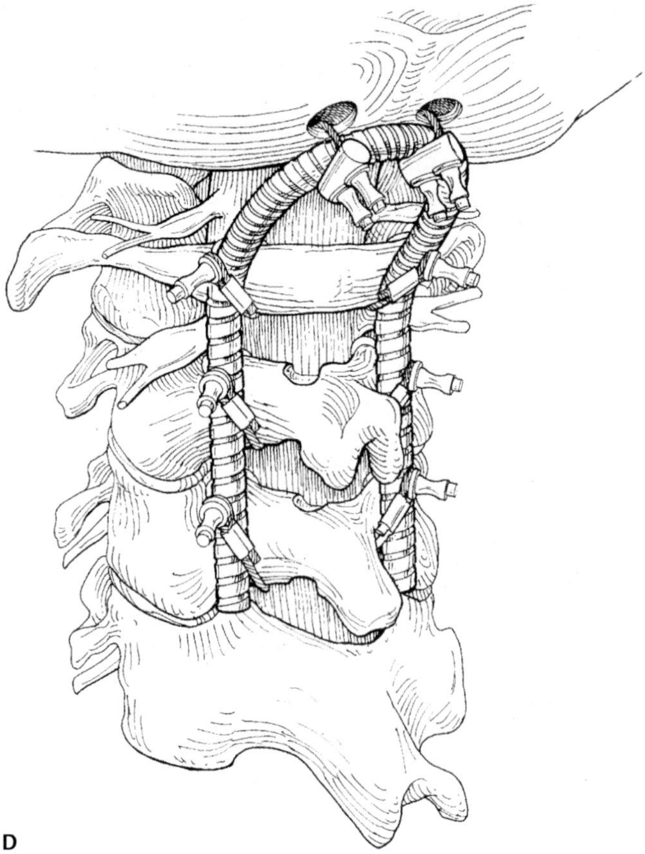

D

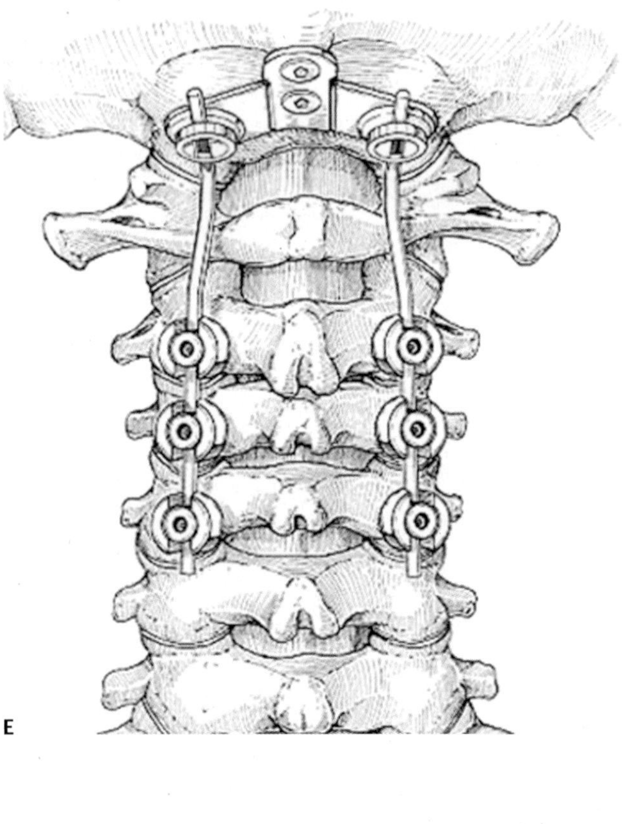

E

Fig. 7.6 *(continued)* **(C)** Hartshill rectangle, **(D)** threaded Steinmann pin, and **(E)** lateral mass–occipital plate fixation. (Reprinted with permission from Barrow Neurological Institute.)

operative mortality (1 to 2%) and 5-year survival of more than 80%,[4] whereas operative mortality in patients with a Ranawat grading of IIIB is 13 to 17%.[4,17,55] With conservative treatment, mortality is as high as 50% within 6 months of the onset of myelopathy and 5-year survival only 11%,[22,60] although one study revealed a similar operative mortality when surgery is performed on patients with Ranawat IIIB myelopathy.[79] Operating at this stage of the disease is often too late.[4]

Symptomatic improvement is difficult to assess. However, in 14 studies, neurological improvement after surgery occurred in an average of 66% of patients with reduction of neck pain in 80%.[21]

Rates of fusion vary from 50 to 92%, with an overall incidence of 83% from a meta-analysis of 13 studies.[21] It is not clear whether the fusion rate has changed significantly with changes in rheumatoid medications and surgical technique. New subaxial subluxation can occur after 5.5% of atlanto-axial fixations and 34 to 36% of occipitocervical fixations within 9 years of surgery,[80,81] although subluxation may also occur in 22% of conservatively treated patients as part of the natural course of the disease.[82] In a small series of patients treated conservatively or by occipitocervical fixation, the surgical group achieved a greater functional improvement.[83]

Conclusion

Rheumatoid disease is changing as a result of advances in medical management, a decline in the long-term use of steroids, and perhaps due to an alteration in the phenotypic expression of the disease itself. As a result, surgical management of the rheumatoid cervical spine has evolved in step with these changes. The disease affects the individual for his or her entire life, and the surgeon should be prepared to re-operate at a later date, extending and adapting constructs as required. Working within a multidisciplinary team of surgeons, physicians, and paramedical professions is mandatory for effective management of cervical rheumatoid disease. A good outcome can be expected when surgery is performed for occipital neuralgia, on patients in Ranawat grades I and II, and by an experienced team. Predictors of a good outcome also include the absence of cord atrophy or compression, satisfactory spinal cord cross-sectional area, young age, and absence of vertical translocation.

References

1. Leden I, Persson E, Persson O. Aspects of the history of rheumatoid arthritis in the light of recent osteo-archaeological finds. Scand J Rheumatol 1988;17(5):341–352
2. Pellicci PM, Ranawat CS, Tsairis P, Bryan WJ. A prospective study of the progression of rheumatoid arthritis of the cervical spine. J Bone Joint Surg Am 1981;63(3):342–350
3. Choi D, Casey AT, Crockard HA. Neck problems in rheumatoid arthritis—changing disease patterns, surgical treatments and patients' expectations. Rheumatology (Oxford) 2006;45(10):1183–1184
4. Casey AT, Crockard HA, Bland JM, et al. Surgery on the rheumatoid cervical spine for the non-ambulant myelopathic patient—too much too late? Lancet 1996;347:1004–1007
5. Calvo F, Alarcon GS. Epidemiology of rheumatoid arthritis. In: Firestein GS, Panayi GS, Wollheim FA, eds. Rheumatoid Arthritis. New Frontiers in Pathogenesis and Treatment. Oxford: Oxford University Press; 2000:15–26
6. Silman AJ, Pearson JE. Epidemiology and genetics of rheumatoid arthritis. Arthritis Res 2002;4(Suppl 3):S265–S272
7. Mijiyawa M. Epidemiology and semiology of rheumatoid arthritis in Third World countries. Rev Rhum Engl Ed 1995;62(2):121–126
8. Gabriel SE, Crowson CS, O'Fallon WM. The epidemiology of rheumatoid arthritis in Rochester, Minnesota, 1955–1985. Arthritis Rheum 1999;42(3):415–420
9. Symmons DP, Bankhead CR, Harrison BJ, et al. Blood transfusion, smoking, and obesity as risk factors for the development of rheumatoid arthritis: results from a primary care-based incident case-control study in Norfolk, England. Arthritis Rheum 1997;40(11):1955–1961
10. Horrobin DF. Low prevalences of coronary heart disease (CHD), psoriasis, asthma and rheumatoid arthritis in Eskimos: are they caused by high dietary intake of eicosapentaenoic acid (EPA), a genetic variation of essential fatty acid (EFA) metabolism or a combination of both? Med Hypotheses 1987;22(4):421–428
11. Doran MF, Crowson CS, O'Fallon WM, et al. The effect of oral contraceptives and estrogen replacement therapy on the risk of rheumatoid arthritis: a population based study. J Rheumatol 2004;31:207–213
12. Nelson JL, Ostensen M. Pregnancy and rheumatoid arthritis. Rheum Dis Clin North Am 1997;23(1):195–212
13. Hameed K, Gibson T, Kadir M, Sultana S, Fatima Z, Syed A. The prevalence of rheumatoid arthritis in affluent and poor urban communities of Pakistan. Br J Rheumatol 1995;34(3):252–256
14. Fife M, Coakley G, Lanchbury J. Current perspectives on the genetics of rheumatoid arthritis. In: Firestein GS, Panayi GS, Wollheim FA, eds. Rheumatoid Arthritis. New Frontiers in Pathogenesis and Treatment. Oxford: Oxford University Press; 2004:3–14
15. O'Brien MF, Casey AT, Crockard A, Pringle J, Stevens JM. Histology of the craniocervical junction in chronic rheumatoid arthritis: a clinicopathologic analysis of 33 operative cases. Spine 2002; 27(20):2245–2254
16. Henderson FC, Geddes JF, Crockard HA. Neuropathology of the brainstem and spinal cord in end stage rheumatoid arthritis: implications for treatment. Ann Rheum Dis 1993;52(9):629–637
17. Casey AT, Crockard HA, Bland JM, et al. Predictors of outcome in the quadriparetic nonambulatory myelopathic patient with rheumatoid arthritis: a prospective study of 55 surgically treated Ranawat class IIIb patients. J Neurosurg 1996;85:574–581
18. Wolfe F, Zwillich SH. The long-term outcomes of rheumatoid arthritis: a 23-year prospective, longitudinal study of total joint replacement and its predictors in 1600 patients with rheumatoid arthritis. Arthritis Rheum 1998;41(6):1072–1082
19. Ornilla E, Ansell BM, Swannell AJ. Cervical spine involvement in patients with chronic arthritis undergoing orthopaedic surgery. Ann Rheum Dis 1972;31(5):364–368
20. Martel W. The occipito-atlanto-axial joints in rheumatoid arthritis and ankylosing spondylitis. Am J Roentgenol Radium Ther Nucl Med 1961;86:223–240

21. Casey AT, Crockard HA. The cervical spine. In: Firestein GS, Panayi GS, Wollheim FA, eds. Rheumatoid Arthritis. New Frontiers in Pathogenesis and Treatment. Oxford: Oxford University Press; 2000:477–487
22. Marks JS, Sharp J. Rheumatoid cervical myelopathy. Q J Med 1981;50(199):307–319
23. Nakano KK. Neurologic complications of rheumatoid arthritis. Orthop Clin North Am 1975;6(3):861–880
24. Winfield J, Cooke D, Brook AS, Corbett M. A prospective study of the radiological changes in the cervical spine in early rheumatoid disease. Ann Rheum Dis 1981;40(2):109–114
25. Hamilton JD, Gordon MM, McInnes IB, Johnston RA, Madhok R, Capell HA. Improved medical and surgical management of cervical spine disease in patients with rheumatoid arthritis over 10 years. Ann Rheum Dis 2000;59(6):434–438
26. Sunahara N, Matsunaga S, Mori T, Ijiri K, Sakou T. Clinical course of conservatively managed rheumatoid arthritis patients with myelopathy. Spine 1997;22(22):2603–2607
27. Carmona L, Gonzalez-Alvaro I, Balsa A, et al. Rheumatoid arthritis in Spain: occurrence of extra-articular manifestations and estimates of disease severity. Ann Rheum Dis 2003;62:897–900
28. Kauppi M, Hakala M. Prevalence of cervical spine subluxations and dislocations in a community-based rheumatoid arthritis population. Scand J Rheumatol 1994;23(3):133–136
29. Naranjo A, Carmona L, Gavrila D, et al. Prevalence and associated factors of anterior atlantoaxial luxation in a nation-wide sample of rheumatoid arthritis patients. Clin Exp Rheumatol 2004;22(4):427–432
30. Neva MH, Isomaki P, Hannonen P, Kauppi M, Krishnan E, Sokka T. Early and extensive erosiveness in peripheral joints predicts atlantoaxial subluxations in patients with rheumatoid arthritis. Arthritis Rheum 2003;48(7):1808–1813
31. Neva MH, Kaarela K, Kauppi M. Prevalence of radiological changes in the cervical spine—a cross sectional study after 20 years from presentation of rheumatoid arthritis. J Rheumatol 2000;27(1):90–93
32. Fujiwara K, Owaki H, Fujimoto M, Yonenobu K, Ochi T. A long-term follow-up study of cervical lesions in rheumatoid arthritis. J Spinal Disord 2000;13(6):519–526
33. Case JP. Old and new drugs used in rheumatoid arthritis: a historical perspective. Part 2: the newer drugs and drug strategies. Am J Ther 2001;8:163–179
34. Fleischmann R, Stern R, Iqbal I. Anakinra: an inhibitor of IL-1 for the treatment of rheumatoid arthritis. Expert Opin Biol Ther 2004;4(8):1333–1344
35. Klinkhoff A. Biological agents for rheumatoid arthritis: targeting both physical function and structural damage. Drugs 2004;64(12):1267–1283
36. Peloso PM, Braun J. Expanding the armamentarium for the spondyloarthropathies. Arthritis Res Ther 2004;6(Suppl 2):S36–S43
37. Yocum D. Effective use of TNF antagonists. Arthritis Res Ther 2004;6(Suppl 2):S24–S30
38. Neva MH, Kauppi MJ, Kautiainen H, et al. Combination drug therapy retards the development of rheumatoid atlantoaxial subluxations. Arthritis Rheum 2000;43(11):2397–2401
39. da Silva E, Doran MF, Crowson CS, et al. Declining use of orthopedic surgery in patients with rheumatoid arthritis? Results of a long-term, population-based assessment. Arthritis Rheum 2003;49:216–220
40. Ward MM. Decreases in rates of hospitalizations for manifestations of severe rheumatoid arthritis, 1983–2001. Arthritis Rheum 2004;50(4):1122–1131
41. Casey AT, Crockard HA. In the rheumatoid patient: surgery to the cervical spine. Br J Rheumatol 1995;34:1079–1086
42. James D, Young A, Kulinskaya E, et al. Orthopaedic intervention in early rheumatoid arthritis. Occurrence and predictive factors in an inception cohort of 1064 patients followed for 5 years. Rheumatology (Oxford) 2004;43(3):369–376
43. Ranawat CS, O'Leary P, Pellicci P, Tsairis P, Marchisello P, Dorr L. Cervical spine fusion in rheumatoid arthritis. J Bone Joint Surg Am 1979;61(7):1003–1010
44. Casey AT, Bland JM, Crockard HA. Development of a functional scoring system for rheumatoid arthritis patients with cervical myelopathy. Ann Rheum Dis 1996;55:901–906
45. King JT Jr, McGinnis KA, Roberts MS. Quality of life assessment with the medical outcomes study short form-36 among patients with cervical spondylotic myelopathy. Neurosurgery 2003;52(1):113–120
46. Ariza-Ariza R, Hernandez-Cruz B, Carmona L, Dolores Ruiz-Montesinos M, Ballina J, Navarro-Sarabia F. Assessing utility values in rheumatoid arthritis: a comparison between time trade-off and the EuroQol. Arthritis Rheum 2006;55(5):751–756
47. Clark CR, Goetz DD, Menezes AH. Arthrodesis of the cervical spine in rheumatoid arthritis. J Bone Joint Surg Am 1989;71:381–392
48. Conaty JP, Mongan ES. Cervical fusion in rheumatoid arthritis. J Bone Joint Surg Am 1981;63:1218–1227
49. Heywood AW, Learmonth ID, Thomas M. Internal fixation for occipito-cervical fusion. J Bone Joint Surg Br 1988;70(5):708–711
50. Kourtopoulos H. von EC: Stabilization of the unstable upper cervical spine in rheumatoid arthritis. Acta Neurochir (Wien) 1988;91(3–4):113–115
51. Papadopoulos SM, Dickman CA, Sonntag VK. Atlantoaxial stabilization in rheumatoid arthritis. J Neurosurg 1991;74(1):1–7
52. Santavirta S, Konttinen YT, Laasonen E, Honkanen V, Antti-Poika I, Kauppi M. Ten-year results of operations for rheumatoid cervical spine disorders. J Bone Joint Surg Br 1991;73(1):116–120
53. Weissman BN, Aliabadi P, Weinfeld MS, Thomas WH, Sosman JL. Prognostic features of atlantoaxial subluxation in rheumatoid arthritis patients. Radiology 1982;144(4):745–751
54. White AA III, Panjabi MM. The basic kinematics of the human spine. A review of past and current knowledge. Spine 1978;3(1):12–20
55. Boden SD, Dodge LD, Bohlman HH, et al. Rheumatoid arthritis of the cervical spine. A long term analysis with predictors of paralysis and recovery. J Bone Joint Surg Am. 1993;75:1282–1297
56. Dvorak J, Grob D, Baumgartner H, Gschwend N, Grauer W, Larsson S. Functional evaluation of the spinal cord by magnetic resonance imaging in patients with rheumatoid arthritis and instability of upper cervical spine. Spine 1989;14(10):1057–1064
57. Newman P, Sweetnam R. Occipito-cervical fusion. An operative technique and its indications. J Bone Joint Surg Br 1969;51(3):423–431
58. Zoma A, Sturrock RD, Fisher WD, Freeman PA, Hamblen DL. Surgical stabilisation of the rheumatoid cervical spine. A review of indications and results. J Bone Joint Surg Br 1987;69(1):8–12
59. Isdale IC, Conlon PW. Atlanto-axial subluxation. A six-year follow-up report. Ann Rheum Dis 1971;30(4):387–389
60. Moskovich R, Crockard HA, Shott S, Ransford AO. Occipitocervical stabilization for myelopathy in patients with rheumatoid arthritis. Implications of not bone-grafting. J Bone Joint Surg Am 2000;82(3):349–365
61. Malcolm GP, Ransford AO, Crockard HA. Treatment of non-rheumatoid occipitocervical instability. Internal fixation with the Hartshill-Ransford loop. J Bone Joint Surg Br 1994;76(3):357–366
62. Mixter SJ, Osgood RB. IV. Traumatic lesions of the atlas and axis. Ann Surg 1910;51(2):193–207
63. Hadra BE. Wiring of the spinous processes in Pott's disease. Trans Am Orthop Assoc. 1891;4:206–207
64. Brooks AL. Atlanto-axial arthrodesis by the wedge compression method. J Bone Joint Surg Am 1978;60(279):284

65. Dickman CA, Sonntag VK, Papadopoulos SM, et al. The interspinous method of posterior atlantoaxial arthrodesis. J Neurosurg 1991;74: 190–198
66. Gallie WE. Fractures and dislocations of the cervical spine. J Bone Joint Surg Am 1939;46:495–496
67. Guyotat J, Perrin G, Pelissou I, Daher T, Bachour E. [Use of Cotrel-Dubousset material in C1 C2 instabilities.] Neurochirurgie 1987; 33(3):236–238
68. Holness RO, Huestis WS, Howes WJ, Langille RA. Posterior stabilization with an interlaminar clamp in cervical injuries: technical note and review of the long term experience with the method. Neurosurgery 1984;14(3):318–322
69. Taggard DA, Kraut MA, Clark CR, Traynelis VC. Case-control study comparing the efficacy of surgical techniques for C1–C2 arthrodesis. J Spinal Disord Tech 2004;17(3):189–194
70. Magerl F, Seemann P. Stable posterior fusion of the atlas and axis by transarticular screw fixation. In: Kehr P, Weidner A, eds. Cervical Spine. New York: Springer-Verlag; 1986:322
71. Harms J, Melcher RP. Posterior C1–C2 fusion with polyaxial screw and rod fixation. Spine 2001;26(22):2467–2471
72. Madawi AA, Casey AT, Solanki GA, Tuite G, Veres R, Crockard HA. Radiological and anatomical evaluation of the atlantoaxial transarticular screw fixation technique. J Neurosurg 1997;86(6):961–968
73. Neo M, Matsushita M, Iwashita Y, Yasuda T, Sakamoto T, Nakamura T. Atlantoaxial transarticular screw fixation for a high-riding vertebral artery. Spine 2003;28(7):666–670
74. Foerster O. Die leitungsbahnen des Schmerzgefu und die chirurgishe Behandlung der Schmerzzustande. Berlin: Urban und Schwarzenberg; 1927
75. Brattstrom H, Granholm L. Atlantoaxial fusion in rheumatoid arthritis. A new method of fixation with wire and bone cement. Acta Orthop Scand 1973;47:619–628
76. Cantore GP, Ciapetta P, Delfini R, et al. Experiences in the use of methacylaten in the stabilization of the cervical spine and the craniocervical junction. Acta Neurochir (Wien) 1982;66:140
77. Grob D, Dvorak J, Panjabi M, Froehlich M, Hayek J. Posterior occipitocervical fusion. A preliminary report of a new technique. Spine 1991;16(3, Suppl):S17–S24
78. Ransford AO, Crockard HA, Pozo JL, Thomas NP, Nelson IW. Craniocervical instability treated by contoured loop fixation. J Bone Joint Surg Br 1986;68(2):173–177
79. van Asselt KM, Lems WF, Bongartz EB, et al. Outcome of cervical spine surgery in patients with rheumatoid arthritis. Ann Rheum Dis 2001;60(5):448–452
80. Kraus DR, Peppelman WC, Agarwal AK, DeLeeuw HW, Donaldson WF III. Incidence of subaxial subluxation in patients with generalized rheumatoid arthritis who have had previous occipital cervical fusions. Spine 1991;16(10, Suppl):S486–S489
81. Matsunaga S, Onishi T, Sakou T. Significance of occipitoaxial angle in subaxial lesion after occipitocervical fusion. Spine 2001;26(2): 161–165
82. Oda T, Fujiwara K, Yonenobu K, Azuma B, Ochi T. Natural course of cervical spine lesions in rheumatoid arthritis. Spine 1995;20(10): 1128–1135
83. Omura K, Hukuda S, Katsuura A, Saruhashi Y, Imanaka T, Imai S. Evaluation of posterior long fusion versus conservative treatment for the progressive rheumatoid cervical spine. Spine 2002;27(12): 1336–1345

8 Traumatic Injuries of the Craniovertebral Junction

Curtis A. Dickman, Karl A. Greene, and Volker K. H. Sonntag

It is useful to classify injuries of the craniovertebral junction (CVJ) as isolated ligamentous injuries, isolated bone fractures, or mixed ligamentous and bony injuries. The extent of the injuries to the bones and ligaments is important for predicting the results of treatment. In this chapter, each category of injury is considered separately. This is an important conceptual framework because ligaments are incapable of repair when disrupted.[1–3] Therefore, ligamentous injuries usually require surgery to restore spinal stability. Bone fractures can usually heal as long as the bones can be reduced and immobilized satisfactorily. However, when the bones are fractured extensively and comminuted widely, or when fractures are accompanied by disrupted ligaments, then nonoperative treatments are likely to fail and surgery is required to restore permanent spinal stability. The mechanisms of injury are reviewed in Chapter 3, Biomechanics of the Craniovertebral Junction. This chapter focuses on the clinical presentation, diagnosis, treatment, and outcome of injuries to the articular and bony structures of the CVJ.

Isolated Ligamentous Injuries

Isolated ligamentous injuries include occipitoatlantal dislocations, transverse ligament disruptions, and rotatory C1-C2 dislocations. Occipitoatlantal dislocations and transverse ligament injuries are highly unstable. These injuries require surgical treatment because the ligaments are avulsed and are incapable of healing. Rotatory C1-C2 dislocations, however, are different, less severe injuries that rarely require surgery.

Occipitoatlantal Dislocations

Occipitoatlantal dislocations are usually caused by high-velocity accidents; they are highly unstable and stretch, compress, and distort the spinal cord.[4–10] They tend to occur in conjunction with severe neurological injuries or cause immediate death (**Table 8.1**). Instability causes mechanical injury by distraction or direct compression of the spinal cord, brainstem, and cranial nerves. Ischemic or vascular injury can occur if the vertebral arteries are stretched. Extensive instability requires immediate rigid spinal fixation to immobilize the ligamentous injury. Occipitoatlantal dislocations should be fixated immediately with a halo brace. Cervical collars (such as a Philadelphia collar) are contraindicated because they reproduce the distractive mechanism of injury and can cause additional severe neurological injury. Cervical traction is likewise contraindicated because it also reproduces the mechanism of injury. Even a halo brace allows significant movement to occur in this form of injury; therefore, urgent operative stabilization is advocated if neurological function can be salvaged. Treatment consists of occipitocervical fixation and fusion.

Occipitoatlantal dislocations can be difficult to diagnose using plain radiographs. Several criteria have been used (**Fig. 8.1**). Most patients with complete spinal cord injuries from occipitoatlantal dislocations have obvious distraction of the occipital condyles from the C1 lateral masses (**Fig. 8.2**). However, if some spinal cord function is preserved, the alignment or gap between the occipital condyles and C1 lateral masses is usually not obvious on plain radiographs because cervical muscle spasm helps to maintain residual alignment. Despite the subtle radiographic clues, patients with incomplete neurological

Table 8.1 Craniovertebral Junction Trauma: Spinal Cord Injury and Mortality Rates*

	Spinal Cord Injury No. (%)	Mortality No. (%)	Total Injuries No.
Occipitoatlantal dislocation	17 (100)	14 (82)	17
Transverse ligament disruption	2 (10)	1 (5)	20
Rotatory atlantoaxial dislocations	0	0	5
Isolated atlas fractures	2 (3)	1 (1.5)	78
Isolated axis fractures	19 (6)	18 (6)	298
Combination atlas-axis fractures	8 (13)	3 (5)	57

*Obtained from 1915 total cervical spine injuries.

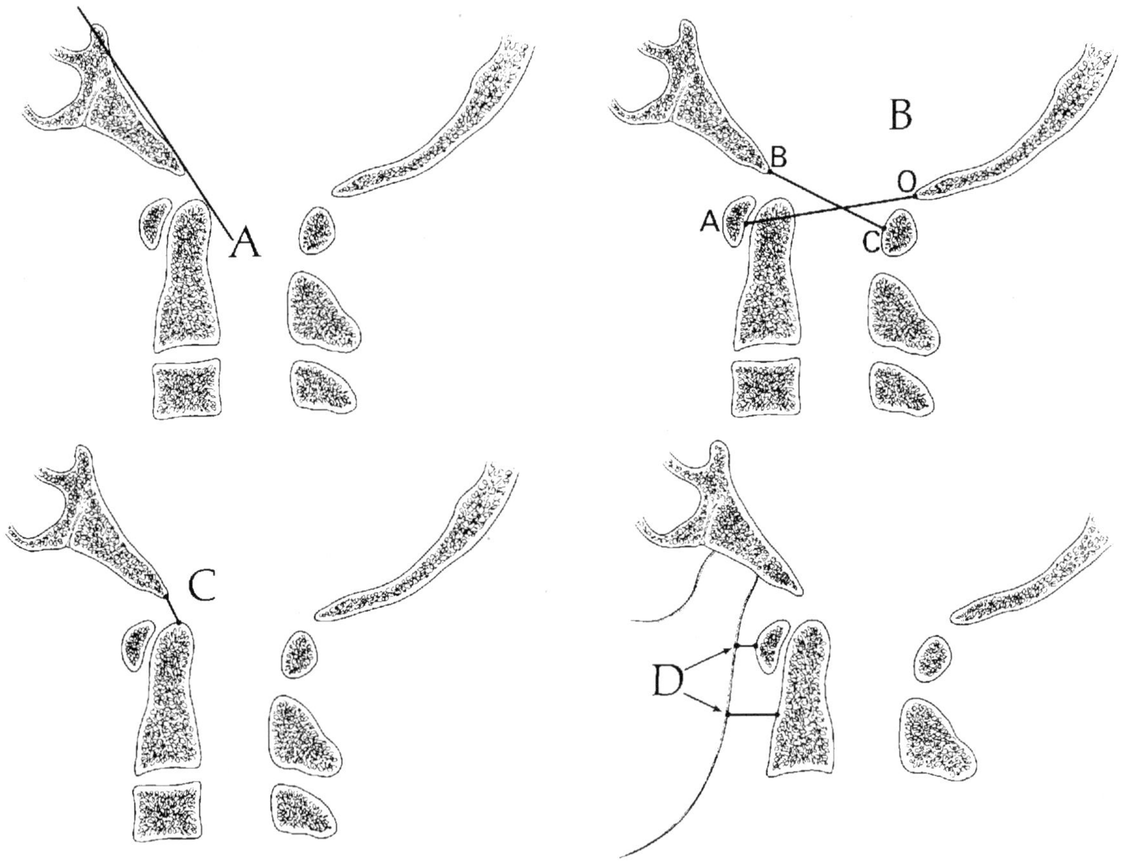

Fig. 8.1 Lateral radiographic criteria for the diagnosis of atlanto-occipital dislocations: **(A)** Wackenheim's line, **(B)** Power's ratio, **(C)** dens-basion distance, and **(D)** Dublin's method. (Reprinted with permission from Barrow Neurological Institute.)

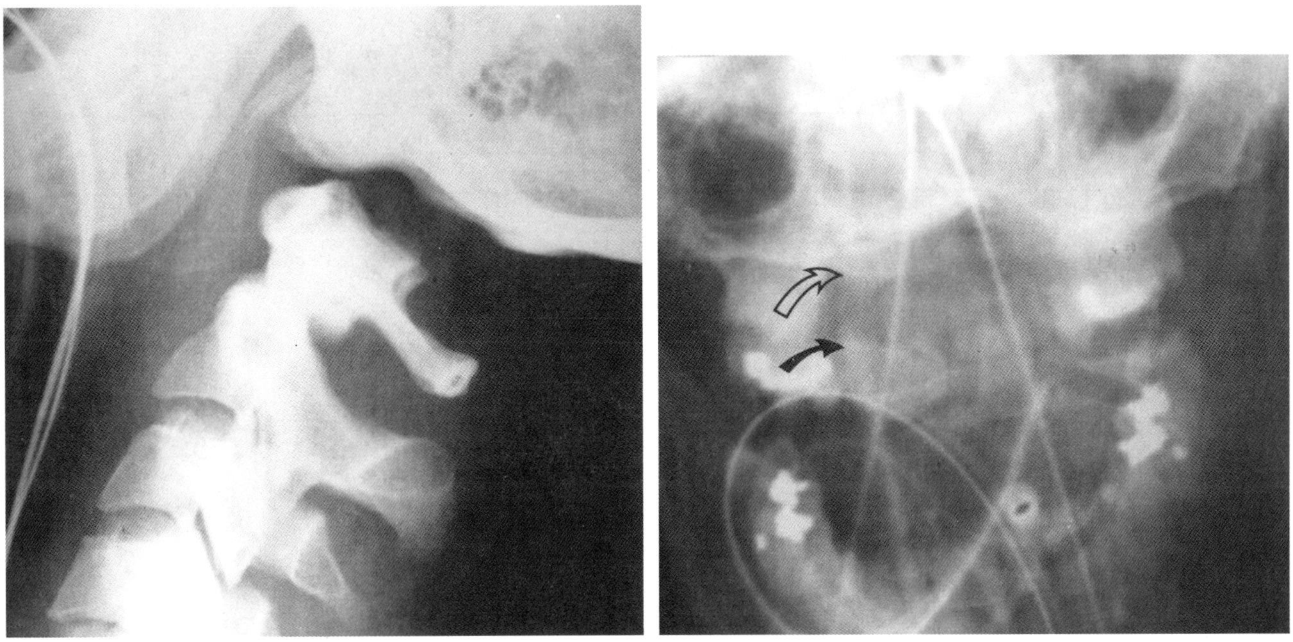

A B

Fig. 8.2 **(A)** Lateral radiographs of an occipitoatlantal dislocation. Severe prevertebral soft tissue swelling is present. The occipital condyles are distracted longitudinally and displaced anteriorly from the C1 lateral masses. **(B)** Open-mouth views demonstrate wide separation of the occipital condyles (*open arrow*) from the upper surface of C1 (*closed arrow*).

injuries are still highly unstable and can deteriorate neurologically. Therefore, it is important to obtain a proper diagnosis and to immobilize the head satisfactorily (i.e., halo brace) until definitive internal stabilization can be performed. Most patients with occipitoatlantal dislocation have a severe head injury that can also obscure the clinical diagnosis.

Plain radiographic diagnostic clues of occipitoatlantal dislocation include severe swelling of the prevertebral soft tissues, widening of the dens-basion distance, and a gap between the occipital condyles and upper surfaces of the C1 lateral masses. Landmarks from the skull base and upper cervical spine can be measured (**Fig. 8.1**), but they are not sensitive or specific enough to detect all occipitoatlantal dislocations (**Table 8.2**).

A variety of plain radiographic measurement techniques may be used to detect dislocations of the CVJ (**Fig. 8.1**). These methods assess the relationships between the skull base and cervical spine on lateral radiographs. Wackenheim's clival line, the dens-basion distance, the Dublin method, the X-line method, and Power's method can be applied.[7,11–19]

Wackenheim's line extends caudally along the posterior surface of the clivus.[19] This line should be tangential to the posterior tip of the dens. If the occiput is displaced anteriorly, the line will intersect the dens. If the occiput is distracted or displaced posteriorly, the line will be separated from the tip of the dens. Traditionally, this technique has been used to assess basilar invagination, but it can provide a general assessment for dislocation.[11,12,19]

Power's ratio assesses the relationship of two lines: the distance between the basion (B) and the posterior arch of the atlas (C) and between the opisthion (O) and the anterior arch of the atlas (A).[17] In normal individuals, BC/OA averages 0.77. A ratio ≥1.0 is a fairly reliable diagnostic indicator of an anterior dislocation. This technique cannot be applied to children or individuals with congenital craniovertebral anomalies, and it can have false-negatives with longitudinal and posterior dislocations. Lee's X-line method is similar to Power's ratio but uses landmarks of C2 (instead of C) in relation to the basion and opisthion as references.[7]

The Wholey dens-basion method measures the interval between the basion and the tip of the dens in a neutral position.[9,12,13,18] In adults, this distance averages 9 mm but varies considerably. Any motion between these landmarks on dynamic radiographs is abnormal.[7] A distance >15 mm in adults or 12 mm in children is abnormal.[7]

Dublin's method measures the distance from the posterior cortex of the ramus of the mandible to the anterior portion of C1 and C2.[14] These measurements must be obtained on 72-cm radiographs with the patient's mouth closed. This is the least reliable method of diagnosis. Normal distances to C1 range from 2 to 5 mm; normal distances to C2 range from 9 to 12 mm. This method is invalid if a mandible fracture is present, and it is unreliable with posterior dislocations.[7]

Plain radiographic measurement techniques are nonspecific and insensitive for diagnosing dislocations for several reasons. True lateral films are needed, and it can be difficult to identify reliably the appropriate landmarks

Table 8.2 Techniques for the Plain Radiographic Diagnosis of Occipitoatlantal Dislocations

		Measurement Technique			
Case	**Types of Dislocation**	**Wackenheim's Line**	**Dens-basion Distance**	**Power's Method**	**Dublin's Method**
1	Longitudinal	+	+	−	0
2	Longitudinal	+	+	+	0
3	Anterior	0	+	+	+
4	Posterior	+	+	−	−
5	Longitudinal	+	+	+	+
6	Anterior and longitudinal	0	+	+	0
7	Posterior	+	−	−	−
8	Anterior and longitudinal	+	+	+	+
9	Rotary	−	−	−	−
10	Longitudinal	+	+	+	+
11	Rotary	−	−	−	−
12	Posterior and longitudinal	+	+	0	0
13	Longitudinal	+	+	+	−
14	Rotary	−	−	−	−
	Total	9	10	7	4

Abbreviations: +, positive for occipitoatlantal dislocation; −, negative for occipitoatlantal dislocation; 0, unable to measure.
Source: Dickman CA, Papadopoulos SM, Sonntag VK, et al. Traumatic occipitoatlantal dislocation. J Spinal Disord 1993;6(4):306. Reprinted with permission from Lippincott-Raven.

(e.g., opisthion, basion). The mastoid processes and mastoid air cells often obscure the visualization of the occipitoatlantal articular surfaces.[7] At best, plain radiographic measurements detect 50 to 75% of dislocations.[7] Wackenheim's clival line and the dens-basion distance are the most sensitive measures for detection of dislocations on plain radiographs. However, only 71% of the cases were detected using the best plain radiographic measurement technique (**Table 8.2**).

Plain radiographic methods of assessing the alignment of the CVJ have additional limitations. Each method is applicable only to specific subtypes of dislocations. None of these methods reliably detect rotational dislocations or minimally displaced subluxations. These techniques are invalid if atlas or axis fractures are present, or if the clivus, atlas, or axis is malformed.[7,10–13,16,19,20]

All suspected occipitoatlantal dislocation injuries should be evaluated rapidly to confirm the diagnosis. Repeat lateral cervical radiographs often display a change in alignment or distraction of the occipital condyles, especially if a cervical collar, which causes distraction (**Fig. 8.3**), has been applied. Thin-section computed tomography (CT) with three-dimensional (3D) reconstruction can be very helpful for demonstrating a dislocated, rotated occipital condyle. Magnetic resonance imaging (MRI) is less useful because it does not clearly depict the osseous anatomy. However, it can confirm the extensive ligament and soft tissue injury in the region and assess the integrity of the spinal cord and brainstem.

Treatment of occipitoatlantal dislocations is based on the extraordinary instability of the ligament avulsions, the risk of delayed neurological injury, and the inability of ligament disruptions to spontaneously heal satisfactorily.

Attempted realignment of dislocations may cause injury and should be instituted cautiously and only under radiographic or fluoroscopic guidance. Axial loading or gentle compression of the head may reduce distractions. Some authors advocate axial traction with low weights to attempt realignment of dislocations.[17,18,21–23] However, these maneuvers are dangerous. Cervical traction or cervical collars reproduce the distractive mechanism of injury, can precipitate additional neurological injury, and are contraindicated. Surgery provides a means to obtain a controlled realignment and to achieve permanent stabilization.

A halo brace alone is inadequate to maintain permanent alignment of the CVJ after an occipitoatlantal dislocation. Acute internal fixation is also needed. However, the halo brace provides a temporary, supplemental means of external stabilization until internal fixation and fusion are attained.

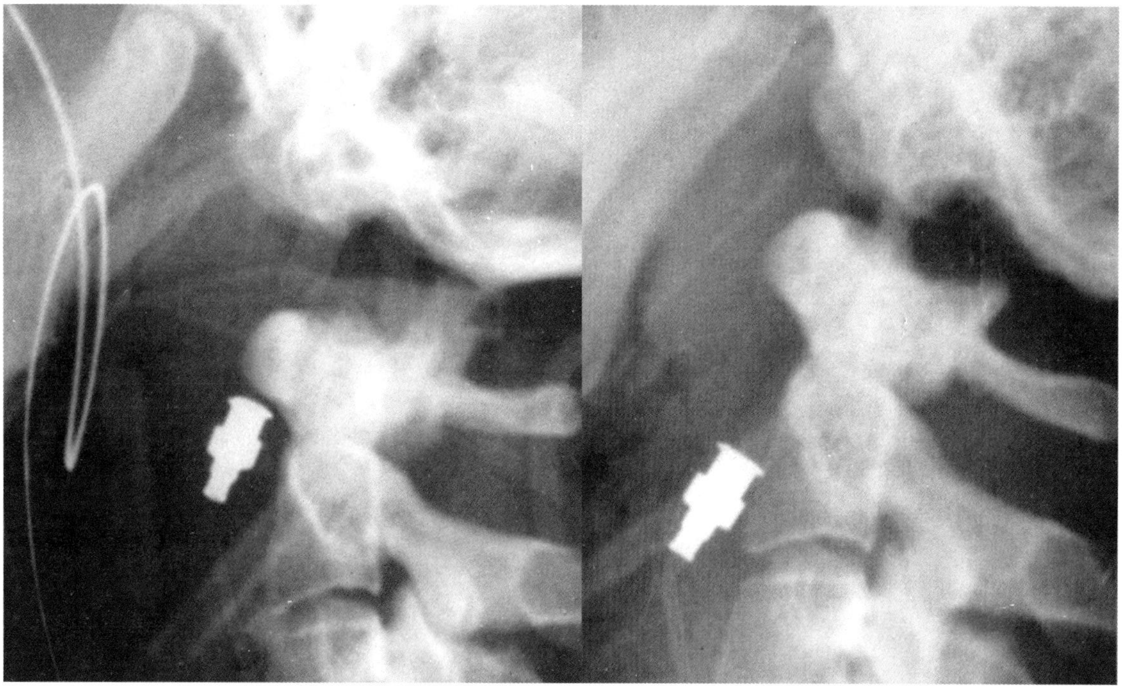

Fig. 8.3 Lateral cervical radiographs of an occipitoatlantal dislocation. The relative position of the occipital condyles and C1 was immediately improved by removing the cervical collar and immobilizing the head in a neutral position on a spine board (*left*). This patient arrived in the emergency department with a Philadelphia collar that was applied at the scene of the accident (*right*). The collar reproduced the distractive mechanism of injury and can cause decompensation of this highly unstable injury.

An aggressive operative treatment strategy is justified if patients have potentially salvageable neurological function. Normal patients or patients with incomplete neurological injuries should be treated urgently because they have a high risk of loss of neurological function due to the extensive instability. Rotational, translational, and distractive injuries are equally unstable. The extreme acute instability and the inadequacy of nonoperative therapy for ligamentous injuries justify the need for early internal fixation. A posterior occipitocervical arthrodesis should be performed for internal fixation to preserve function and to permit the maximal recovery of neurological function.

Transverse Ligament Injuries

Disruption of the transverse atlantal ligament results in anterior C1-C2 subluxation.[24,25] Anterior C1-C2 subluxation, however, can also occur without a disrupted transverse ligament, as with os odontoideum or odontoid fractures. A disrupted transverse ligament is manifested by a widened atlantodental interval (ADI) on lateral cervical radiographs when the neck is flexed. When the head and neck are in a neutral or extended position, the ADI may appear normal. If the ADI exceeds 3 mm in an adult (or 5 mm in children), a transverse ligament disruption should be suspected. MRI with gradient echo sequences can be used to image directly the ligament and to assess its anatomical integrity.[26] Disruption of the ligament appears as high-signal intensity within the ligament, loss of anatomical continuity, and blood at the insertion site of the ligament.

Injuries involving the transverse atlantal ligament can be classified into two distinct categories; each subtype has a separate prognosis and requires different treatments.[25] Type I injuries are disruptions of the substance of the transverse atlantal ligament. Type II injuries are fractures or avulsions that detach the bony tubercle for insertion of the transverse ligament on the C1 lateral mass (**Fig. 8.4**). These two types of injuries can be differentiated using a combination of MRI to assess the soft tissue pathology (i.e., the anatomy of the ligament) in conjunction with thin-section CT to assess the osseous pathology (**Figs. 8.5** and **8.6**). Although plain radiographs are useful to screen for a potential abnormality, plain radiographic indices are unreliable for predicting the status of the transverse atlantal ligament because they do not directly demonstrate its anatomy (**Fig. 8.7**).

Type I injuries are incapable of healing with an orthosis because the ligamentous substance is incapable of repair. These injuries should be treated with early surgery to fixate C1-C2 internally. Type II injuries detach the

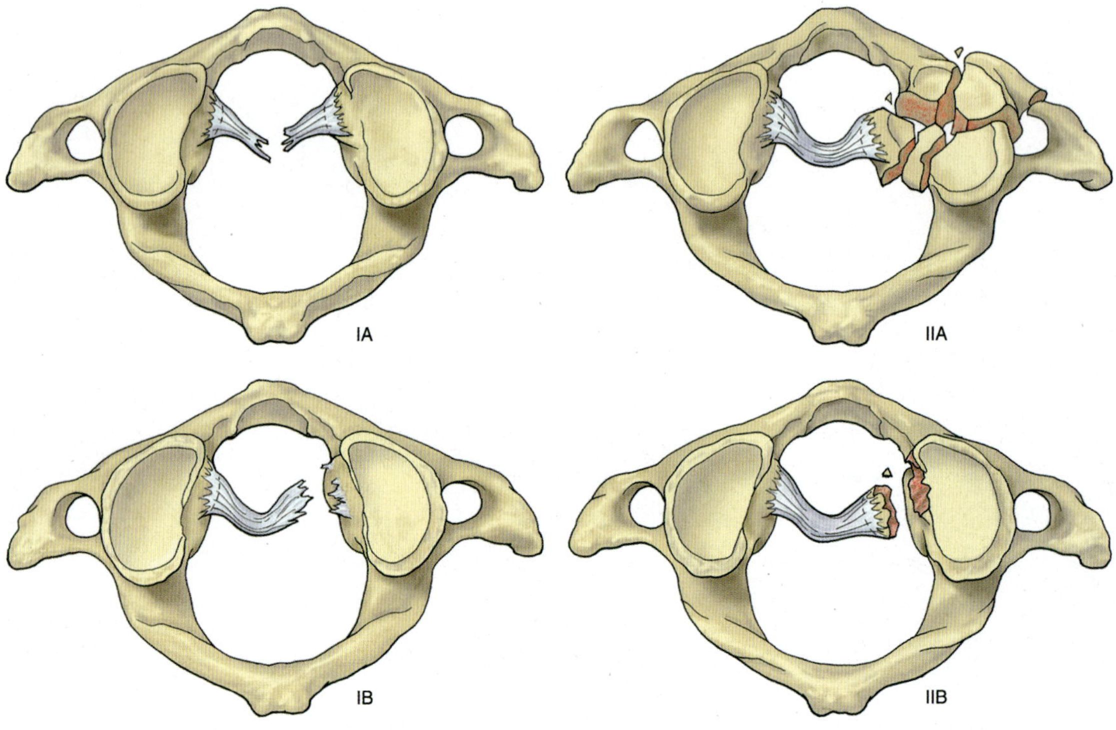

Fig. 8.4 Classification of injuries to the transverse atlantal ligament. Type I injuries disrupt the ligament substance in its midportion (type IA) or at its periosteal insertion (type IB). Type II injuries disconnect the tubercle for insertion of the transverse ligament from the C1 lateral mass involving a comminuted C1 mass (type IIA) or avulse the tubercle from an intact lateral mass (type IIB). (Reprinted with permission from Barrow Neurological Institute.)

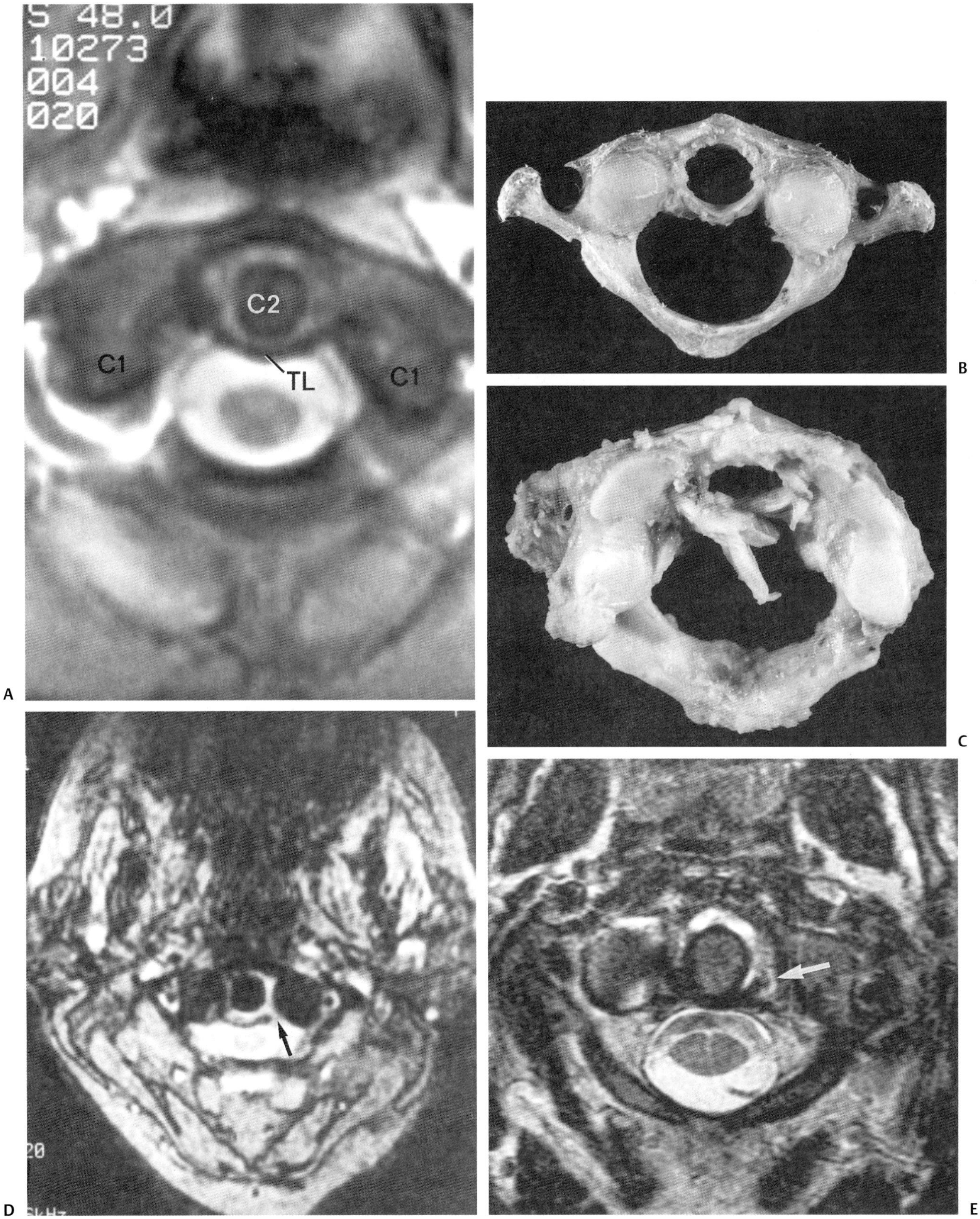

Fig. 8.5 **(A)** The normal transverse atlantal ligament (*TL*) appears on axial gradient echo magnetic resonance imaging (MRI) studies (TR 733 MS, TE 18 MS, flig angle 20 degrees, slice 3 mm) as a homogeneous, continuous, thick, low-signal intensity structure that extends between the medial portions of the lateral masses of C1. The ligament is contrasted by high-signal intensity on both sides—anteriorly by synovium and posteriorly by cerebrospinal fluid. **(B)** Postmortem specimen of C1 demonstrating the structure of the normal transverse atlantal ligament. **(C)** Autopsy specimen demonstrating a midsubstance disruption of the transverse atlantal ligament (type IA injury). **(D,E)** MRI of type IB injuries in which the transverse ligament is torn from its periosteal insertion on the C1 tubercle. The disrupted ligaments demonstrate high-signal intensity within the ligament, loss of anatomical continuity, and blood at the insertion of the ligament (*arrows*).

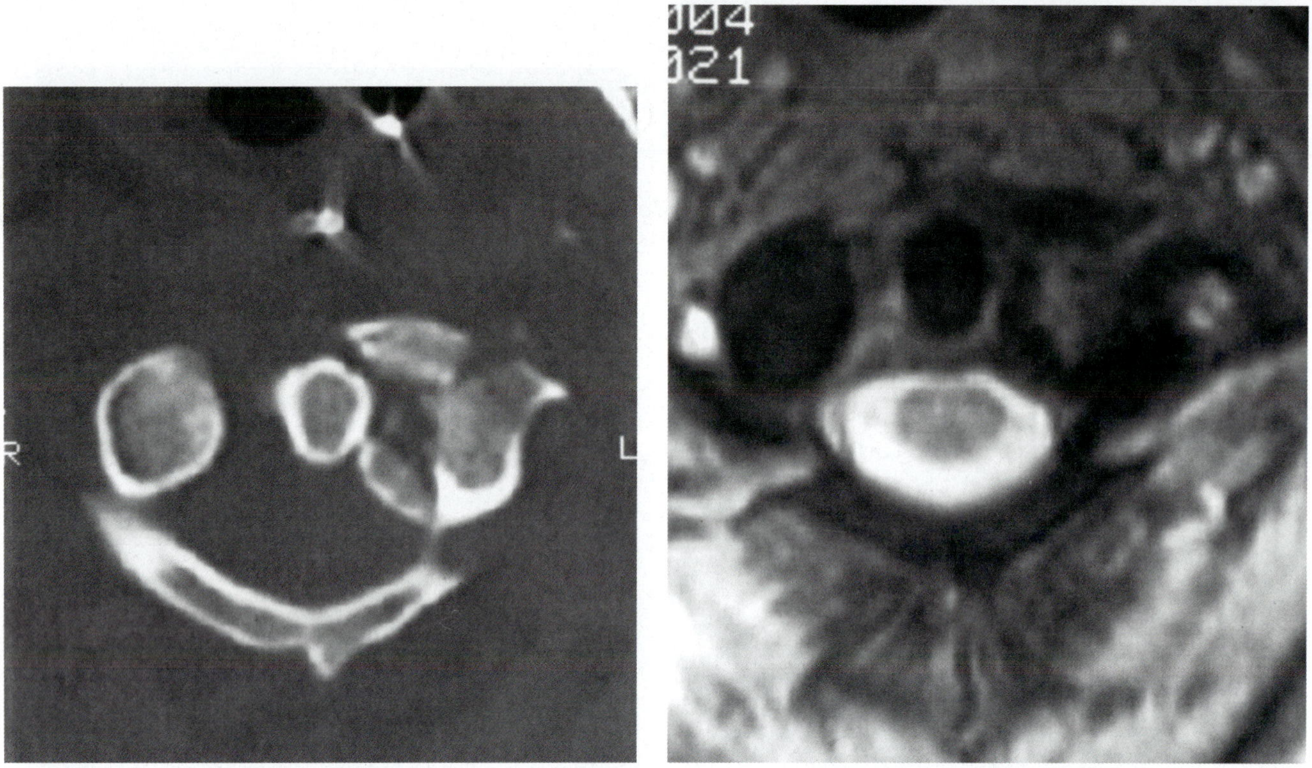

A B

Fig. 8.6 Type II injuries detach the tubercle for the transverse ligament from the C1 lateral mass. **(A)** Computed tomography (CT) scan of a type II injury demonstrates a comminuted fracture of the C1 lateral mass which renders the transverse ligament physiologically incompetent. **(B)** The magnetic resonance image that corresponds to the CT demonstrates that the soft tissue structure of the transverse ligament is preserved.

tubercle and render the transverse ligament physiologically incompetent even though the ligamentous substance is not torn.

Type II injuries have a 74% chance of healing satisfactorily when treated with a rigid cervical orthosis (halo brace) (**Fig. 8.8**). Surgery is reserved for type II injuries that have nonunion with persistent instability after 3 to 4 months of immobilization. Type II injuries have a 26% rate of failure of immobilization; therefore, close monitoring is needed to detect patients who will require delayed operative intervention.

Rotatory C1-C2 Dislocations

Rotatory atlantoaxial dislocations primarily occur in young children and adolescents (**Fig. 8.9**).[3] Children often present with their head fixed in a "cocked robin" position. Open-mouth radiographs demonstrate asymmetry of the lateral masses of C1-C2 on open-mouth views. However, CT is much more helpful for clearly defining the injured anatomy and for ruling out a fracture. Rotation of C1 on C2 of more than 47 degrees in the axial plane is pathognomonic of rotatory C1-C2 dislocation. Two-dimensional and 3D reconstructed CT images are useful for demonstrating the abnormality (**Fig. 8.9**). Treatment consists of reduction with halter traction or Gardner-Wells tongs and subsequent immobilization with a cervical collar for 10 to 12 weeks (**Fig. 8.10**).

MRI studies are recommended to rule out an associated disruption of the transverse atlantal ligament. If the transverse ligament is disrupted, then internal fixation is needed, even if the rotatory dislocation is reducible. If the transverse ligament is normal, external reduction and immobilization represent adequate treatment. The majority of these injuries can be managed nonoperatively with reduction and external immobilization. Surgery is reserved for patients with irreducible or recurrent subluxations, or when the transverse ligament is disrupted (**Fig. 8.10**).

■ Isolated Fractures

Isolated fractures of the atlas, the axis, or combined atlantoaxial fractures are common injuries. Fractures of the first two cervical vertebrae account for one-third of all cervical spine fractures. A substantial proportion of fractures involves both the atlas and axis (i.e., combination atlas-axis fractures) (**Tables 8.1** and **8.3**).

Isolated fractures usually heal nonoperatively as long as the fractures are nondisplaced or minimally displaced

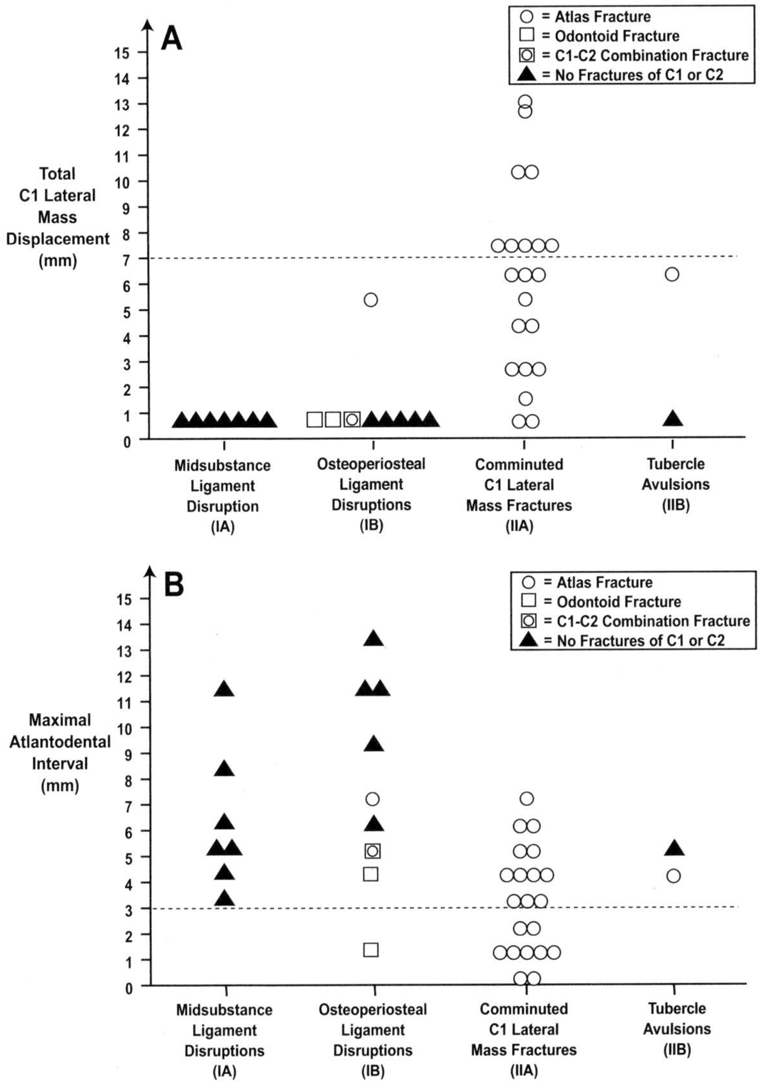

Fig. 8.7 Correlation of plain radiographic findings, with the pathoanatomy of the injury patterns to the bones and ligaments, as visualized using computed tomography and magnetic resonance imaging. **(A)** The type of ligamentous injury in relation to the total amount of displacement of the C1 lateral masses on open-mouth views of C1-C2. If a 7.0-mm criterion is used to presume transverse ligament disruption, more than half of the unstable atlas fractures would have been missed. "Spence's 7.0-mm rule" does not accurately predict the status of the transverse atlantal ligament after an atlas fracture. **(B)** The type of ligament and bone injury in relation to the maximal atlantodental interval on preoperative lateral cervical radiographs. If a 3.0-mm cutoff is used to presume a disrupted transverse atlantal ligament, 10 of the 39 injuries (26%) would not have been detected. Less than 10% of the type I injuries, but almost 40% of the type II injuries, would have been missed. (Reprinted with permission from Barrow Neurological Institute.)

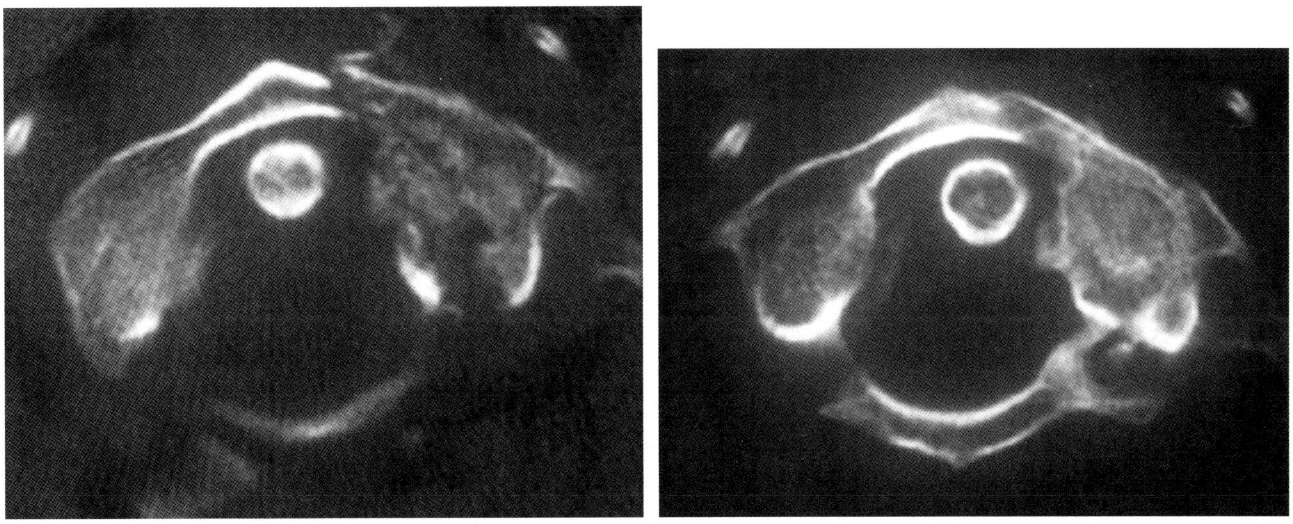

A B

Fig. 8.8 **(A)** This patient sustained a type II injury involving the transverse ligament with extensive crush and comminution of the left C1 lateral mass. **(B)** After 12 weeks of immobilization in a halo brace, the fractures healed with an osseous union and normal motion was restored to C1-C2 without evidence of instability. The tubercle for insertion of the transverse ligament was completely incorporated into the adjacent bone.

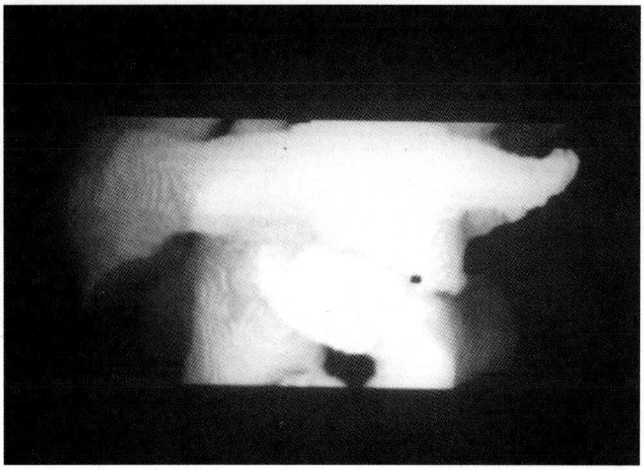

Fig. 8.9 Three-dimensional computed tomography reconstruction of a C1-C2 rotatory dislocation injury.

(**Table 8.3**). The degree of fracture angulation and displacement is a reflection of the extent of the associated spinal ligamentous injury. Minimally or moderately displaced fractures can usually be treated successfully with cervical orthoses (**Table 8.4**). In general, the type of orthosis used for a particular cervical fracture depends on the extent of injury of the bone and ligaments.[27–30] Soft collars or Philadelphia collars are orthoses that restrict cervical motion minimally; these are usually appropriate for nondisplaced fractures. The sternal-occipital-mandibular-immobilization (SOMI) brace and the four-poster brace have intermediate immobilization characteristics and adequately immobilize minimally displaced fractures. A cervicothoracic orthosis, Minerva brace, or halo brace is used for moderately or widely displaced fractures. The relative immobilization characteristics of the different cervical orthoses are discussed in Chapter 3.

Atlas Fractures

A wide variety of atlas fracture patterns exists.[24,25,31–33] Almost any part of the C1 ring can be affected (**Fig. 8.11**). Most C1 fractures heal satisfactorily with an orthosis, except when the anatomical continuity of the transverse ligament is disrupted (**Figs. 8.4, 8.5, 8.6,** and **8.7**) or when an extensively comminuted C1 lateral mass disconnects

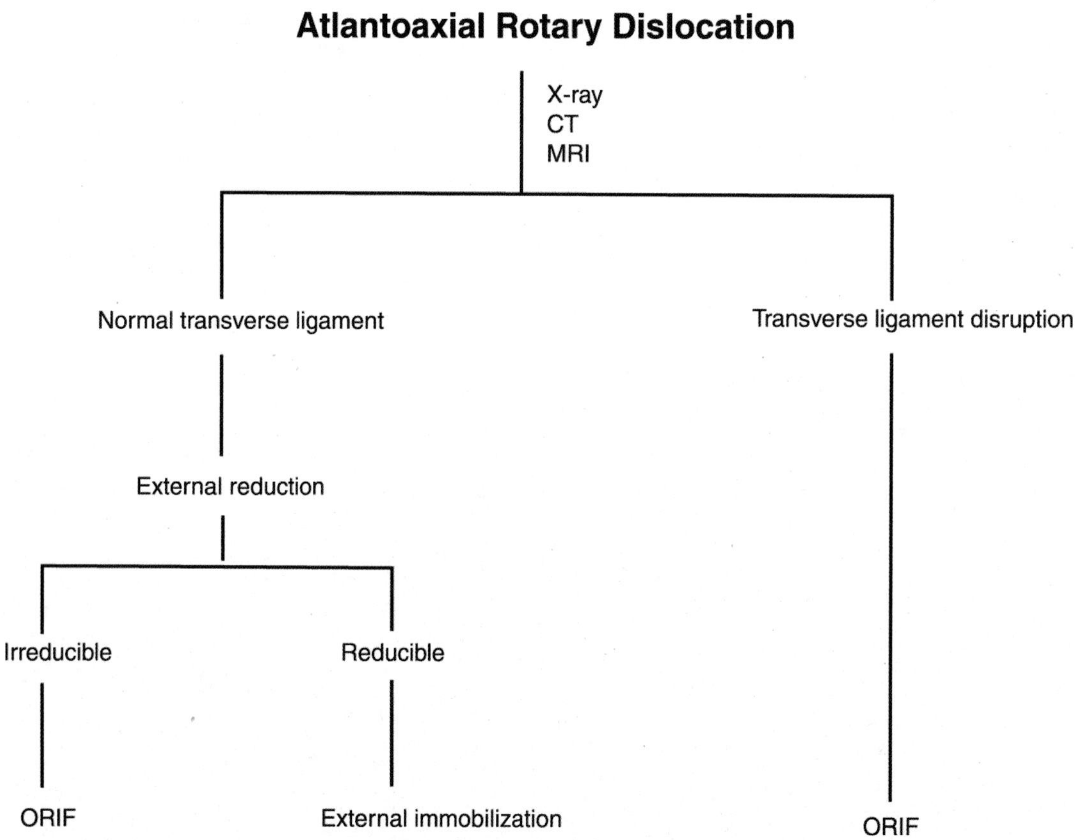

Fig. 8.10 Treatment algorithm for C1-C2 rotatory dislocations. Most patients are treated successfully with reduction and immobilization without surgery. *ORIF*, open reduction and internal fixation. (From Sonntag VKH, Dickman CA. Treatment of cervical spine injuries. In: Rea GL, ed. Spinal Trauma: Current Evaluation and Management. Park Ridge, IL: AANS; 1993:25–74. Reprinted with permission from the American Association of Neurological Surgeons.)

Table 8.3 Treatment and Outcome Among C2 Fractures and C1-C2 Combination Fractures*

	Fracture Type				
	Type I Odontoid	Type II Odontoid	Type III Odontoid	Hangman's	Misc. C2
Isolated C2 fractures, Total (N)	2	134	86	83	75
Initial treatment: (a) external orthosis	2	112	86	80	70
(b) early surgery	0	22	0	0	0
Failures of nonoperative treatment	0	28	2	3	5
Total number requiring surgery	0	50 (36%)	2 (2%)	3 (4%)	5 (7%)
C1-C2 combination fractures, Total (N)	0	23	10	11	13
Initial treatment: (a) external orthosis	0	16	10	11	13
(b) early surgery	0	7	0	0	0
Failures of nonoperative treatment	0	3	0	3	0
Total number requiring surgery	0	10 (43%)	0 (0%)	3 (27%)	0 (0%)

*Data accumulated during an 18-year period at the Barrow Neurological Institute.

the tubercle and renders the transverse ligament physiologically incompetent (**Figs. 8.4, 8.11,** and **8.12**).[24,25] Isolated atlas fractures are best evaluated using a combination of plain radiographs, CT, and MRI. If the transverse atlantal ligament is normal, nonoperative therapy with an orthosis is recommended. However, if the transverse atlantal ligament is disrupted, then C1-C2 fusion is required (**Fig. 8.13**).

Mildly or nondisplaced atlas fractures are treated with a SOMI brace or a Philadelphia collar. A halo brace is used for widely displaced fractures. If the fracture is comminuted and involves the lateral mass of C1 and disconnects the tubercle for insertion of the transverse ligament rendering it incompetent, then a halo brace is recommended. Atlantoaxial stability and functional ligament integrity can be restored as long as the tubercle unites with the C1 lateral mass. This union is best achieved with a halo brace. However, this type of C1 injury has a 26% chance of nonunion when treated with an orthosis.[25] For this injury type, we advocate initial treatment with a halo brace and frequent follow-up. Late surgery may be required if healing is not adequate.

Table 8.4 Orthoses for Cervical Fractures

Fracture Displacement	Orthosis Recommended
Nondisplaced fractures	Soft collar
	Philadelphia-type collar
Minimally displaced fractures	SOMI brace
	Four-poster brace
Moderately or widely displaced fractures	Cervicothoracic brace
	Halo brace

Abbreviations: SOMI, sternal-occipital-mandibular-immobilization.

Axis Fractures

Fractures of the second cervical vertebrae can be characterized as odontoid fractures, hangman's fractures, or miscellaneous C2 fractures (**Table 8.3, Fig. 8.14**).[31,34–38] Odontoid fractures are further subclassified into type I, II, and III injuries. Type I fractures are rare, involve only the tip of the dens, and can be treated adequately with a semirigid orthosis. Type II fractures occur across the neck of the dens and account for two-thirds of all odontoid fractures. Type III fractures extend from the base of the dens into the C2 body and account for one-third of all odontoid fractures. Bone and any associated ligament injuries are best evaluated using thin-section CT and MRI.

Odontoid Fractures

The criteria used for treatment of odontoid fractures are based on the amount of bone displacement and the extent of ligamentous injury (**Figs. 8.15** and **8.16**). Type II odontoid fractures displaced less than 6 mm usually heal adequately when treated with a halo brace. They have an 87 to 93% chance of union when treated with a rigid or semirigid orthosis.[38] Type II odontoid fractures with 6 mm or more of dens displacement or with comminuted fragments of the base of the dens (type IIA fractures) are prone to nonunion and should be treated with internal fixation.[37,38] These widely displaced type II fractures have a 75 to 85% nonunion rate even when treated with a rigid orthosis. We advocate early surgery for widely displaced type II fractures because of their excessively high nonunion rate. Type II fractures can occur in conjunction with a disrupted transverse ligament.[39] When this situation occurs, treatment should consist of immediate surgery for C1-C2 fusion (**Fig. 8.17**). However, an odontoid screw cannot be used if the transverse ligament is incompetent; a posterior fixation must be performed.

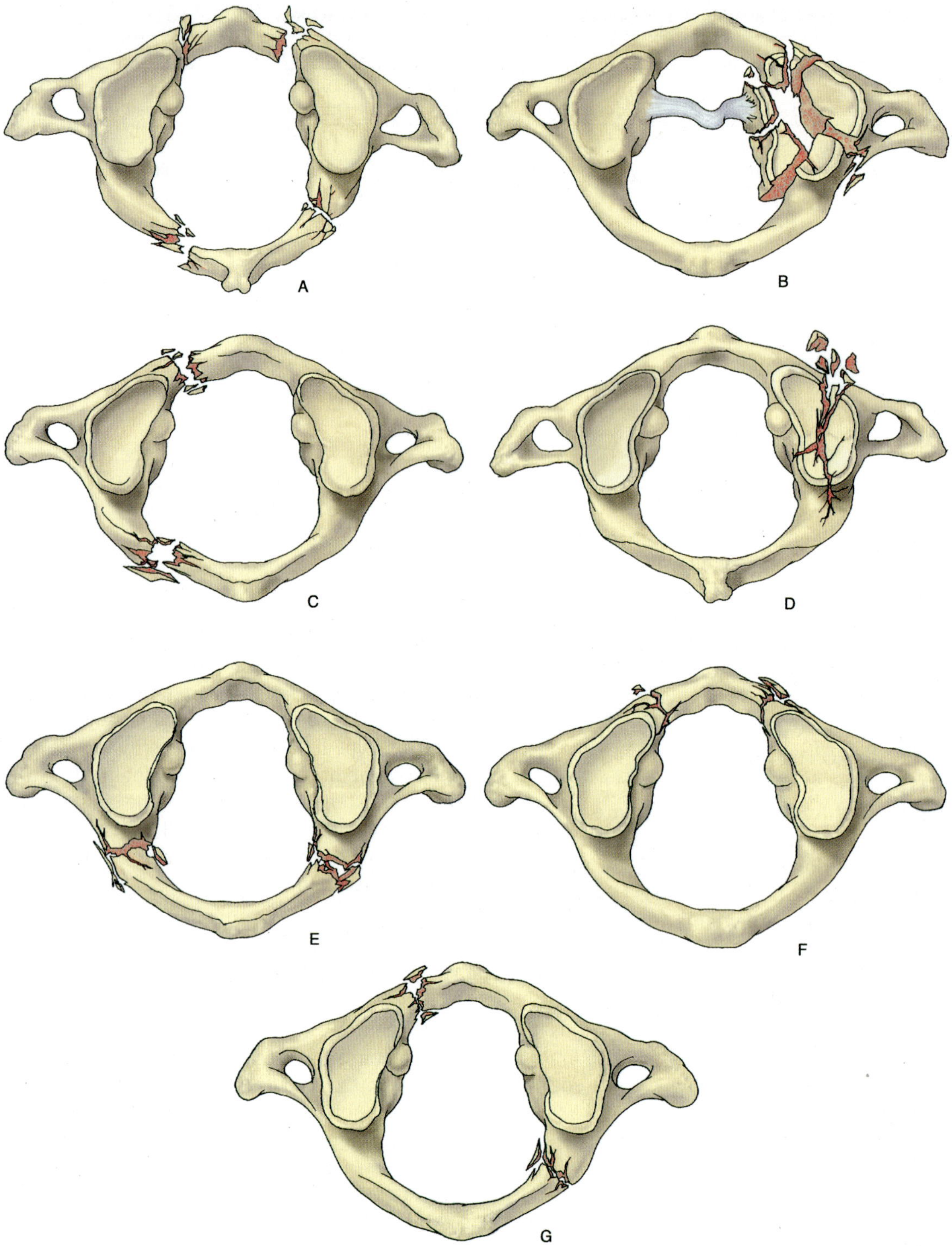

Fig. 8.11 A variety of types of atlas fractures exists. **(A)** The four-part ring or burst fracture is classically referred to as a "Jefferson fracture." **(B)** The comminuted lateral mass fracture is extremely common. It creates C1-C2 instability by rendering the transverse ligament incompetent because it detaches the tubercle for insertion of the transverse ligament. More stable patterns of injury include **(C)** the unilateral ring fracture, **(D)** linear lateral mass fracture, **(E)** posterior ring fracture, **(F)** anterior arch fracture, or **(G)** contralateral ring fracture. The major determinant of stability of these injuries is whether the transverse atlantal ligament is anatomically and physiologically intact. (Reprinted with permission from Barrow Neurological Institute.)

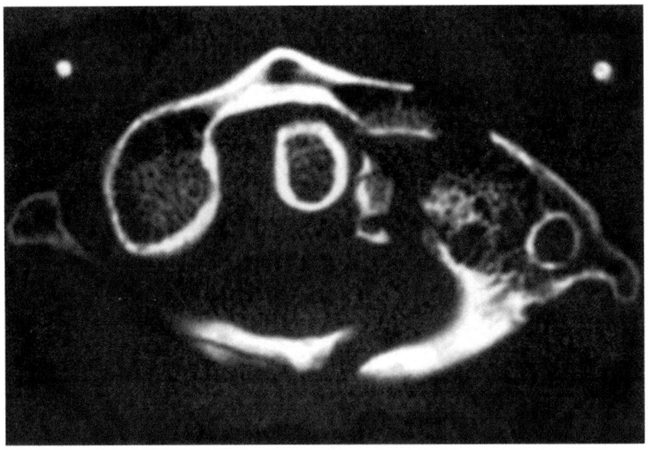

Fig. 8.12 This comminuted C1 lateral mass fracture has detached the tubercle that anchors the transverse ligament, which creates atlantoaxial instability (type II transverse ligament injury). The C1 lateral mass was displaced laterally 9 mm. Despite treatment with a halo brace for 16 weeks, a nonunion developed with persistent C1-C2 instability that required internal fixation.

Type III odontoid fractures usually heal when treated only with an orthosis (**Table 8.3**). If nonunion persists after 12 weeks of halo immobilization, surgery may be necessary. These injuries have only a 2% incidence of nonunion; therefore, early surgery is usually unnecessary for type III fractures.

Hangman's Fractures

Hangman's fractures are vertical or oblique fractures through the pars interarticularis of C2.[35,36,38,40] These injuries disconnect the posterior arch of C2 from the C2 vertebral body. They create a spondylolysis, widen the spinal canal, and are rarely associated with neurological injury. These injuries are most frequently caused by neck hyperextension. When a concurrent C1 fracture occurs, it usually involves the posterior ring of C1 bilaterally due to hyperextension.[34]

The anterior longitudinal ligament and the C2-C3 disk annulus and disk space can be disrupted with hangman's

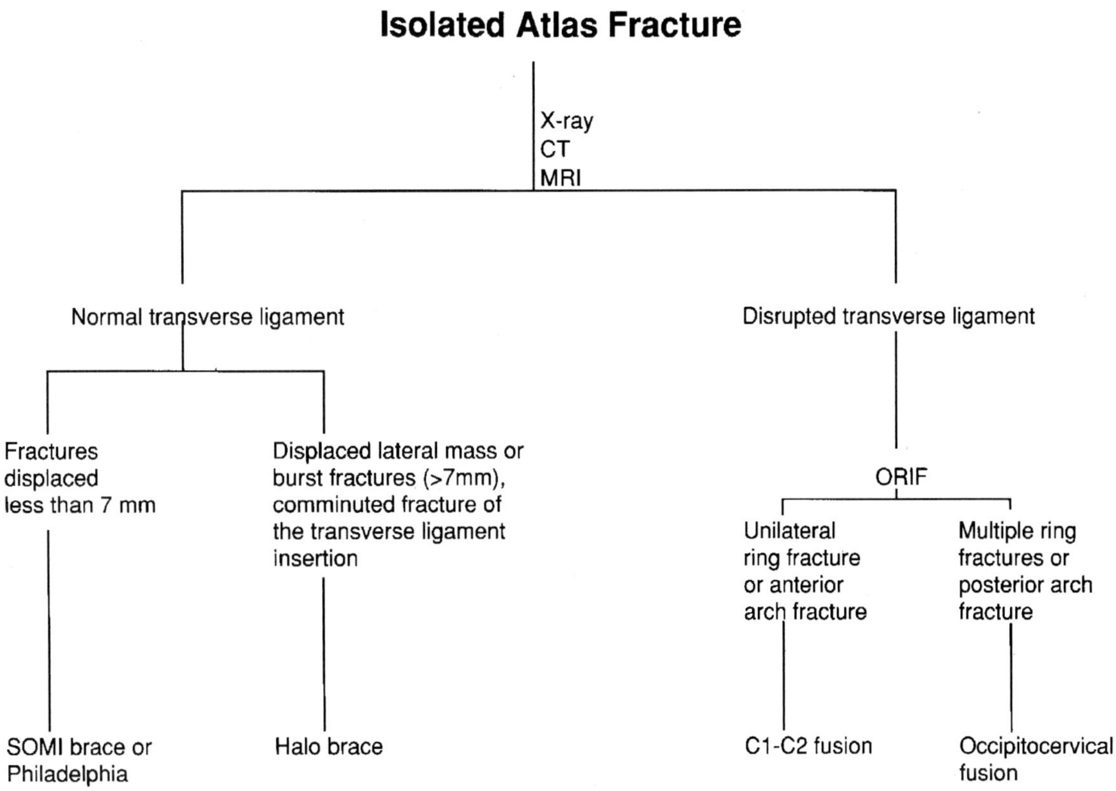

Fig. 8.13 Algorithm for treatment of atlas fractures. The most important factors to consider for treatment are the amount of bone comminution, the width of bone displacement, and whether the transverse ligament is incompetent. If the transverse ligament substance is disrupted (type I transverse ligament injury), surgery is required to restore spinal stability. Widely displaced fractures or comminuted C1 lateral mass fractures (type II transverse ligament injuries) are initially treated with a halo brace, and the majority heal satisfactorily with an orthosis. Surgery is reserved for patients in this category who develop nonunion or persistent instability. Nondisplaced or minimally displaced fractures are treated with nonhalo orthoses. *CT*, computed tomography; *MRI*, magnetic resonance imaging; *ORIF*, open reduction internal fixation; *SOMI*, sternal-occipital-mandibular-immobilization. (From Sonntag VKH, Dickman CA. Treatment of upper cervical spine injuries. In: Rea GL, ed. Spinal Trauma: Current Evaluation and Management. Park Ridge, IL: AANS; 1993:25–74. Reprinted with permission from the American Association of Neurological Surgeons.)

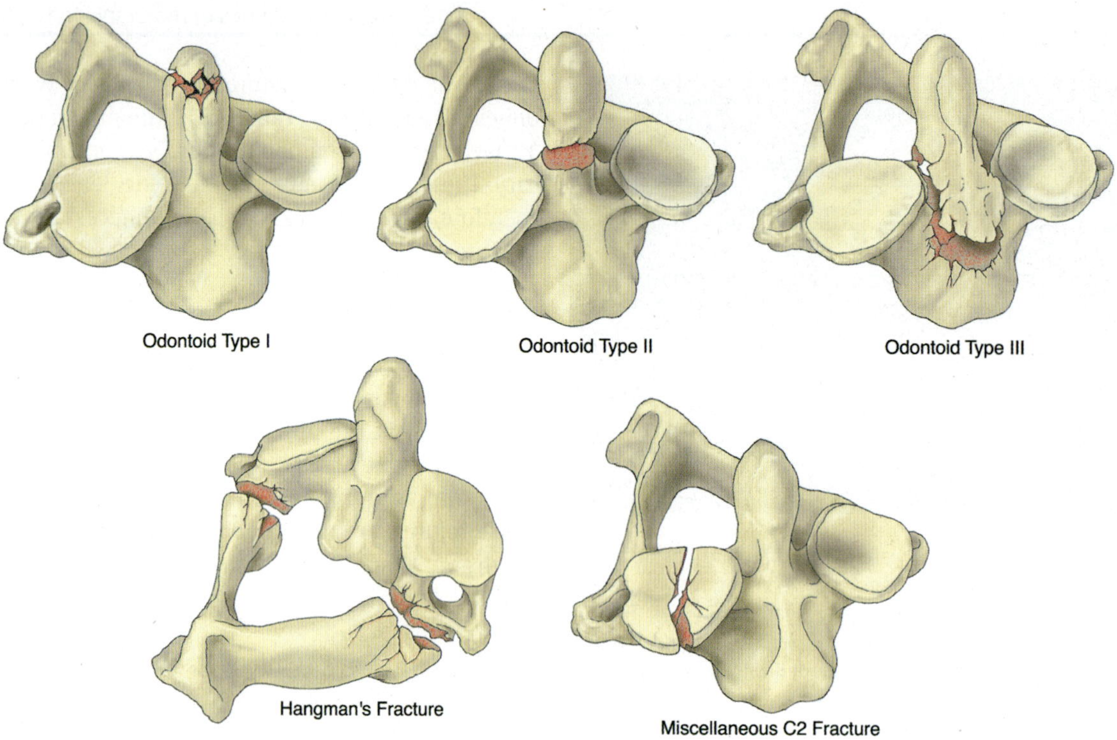

Fig. 8.14 Classification of fractures of the second cervical vertebrae. Type I, II, and III odontoid fractures are, respectively, through the apex of the dens, across the base of the dens, and into the body of C2. Hangman's fractures involve spondylitic fractures bilaterally across the pars interarticularis. Miscellaneous C2 fractures include the laminae, facets, spinous process, or body of C2 (i.e., nonodontoid, nonhangman's fractures). (Reprinted with permission from Barrow Neurological Institute.)

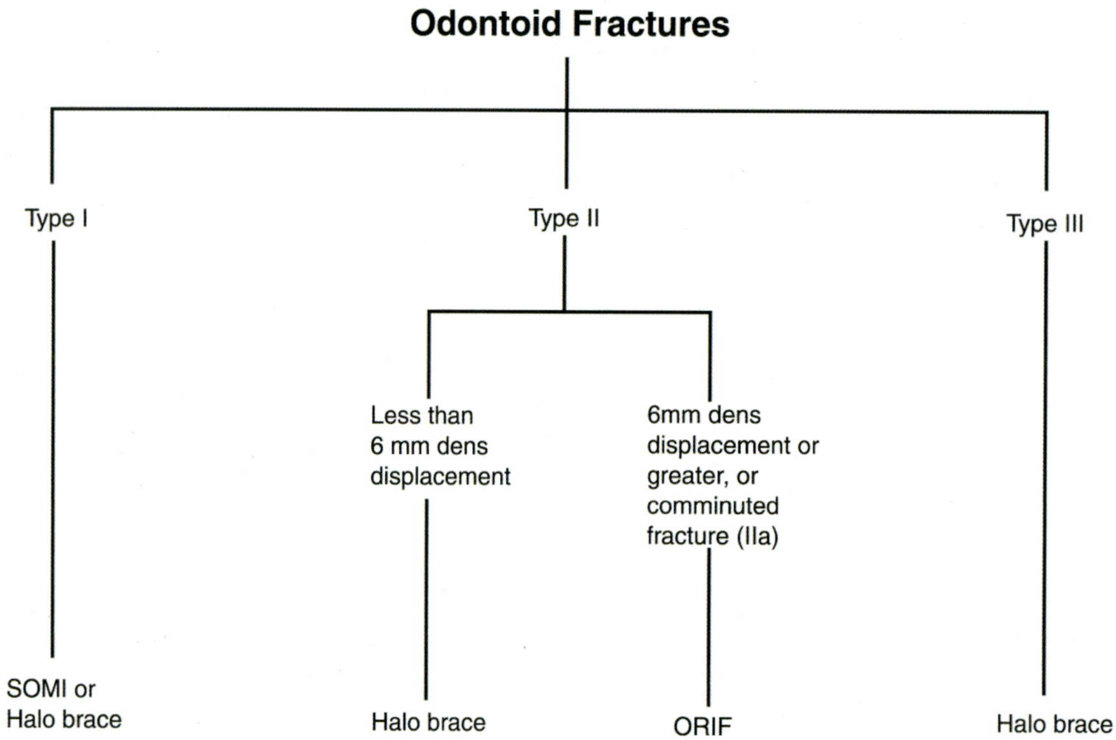

Fig. 8.15 Treatment algorithm for odontoid fractures. Most odontoid fractures heal satisfactorily with an orthosis, except for widely displaced type II odontoid fractures (≥6 mm), which have a 90% chance of nonunion when treated with an orthosis. Rarely, odontoid fractures can be associated with a disrupted transverse ligament; this also requires surgery for internal fixation. *ORIF*, open reduction internal fixation; *SOMI*, sternal-occipital-mandibular-immobilization. (From Sonntag VKH, Dickman CA. Treatment of upper cervical spine injuries. In: Rea GL, ed. Spinal Trauma: Current Evaluation and Management. Park Ridge, IL: AANS; 1993:25–74. Reprinted with permission from the American Association of Neurological Surgeons.)

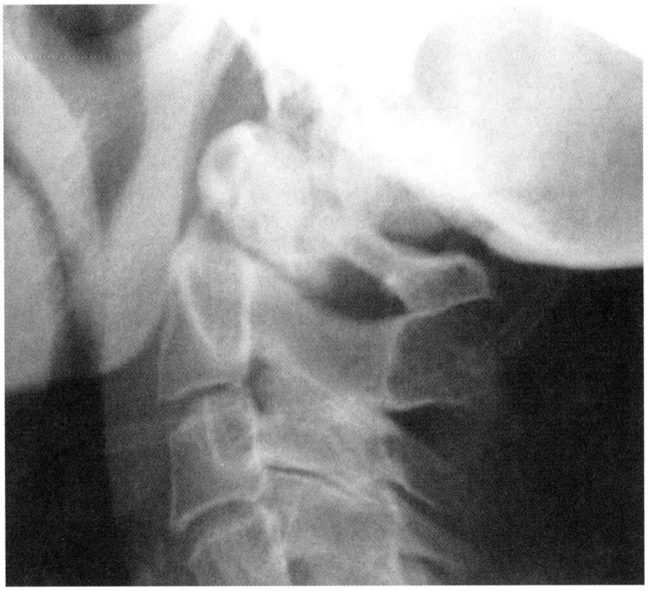

Fig. 8.16 Lateral cervical radiograph of a type II odontoid fracture that is displaced 11 mm posteriorly. This patient was treated with an anterior odontoid screw.

injuries. This disruption can create an unstable subtype of hangman's injury. Injuries associated with more than 4 mm of anterior C2-C3 subluxation or more than 11 degrees of angulation of C2 may not heal with an orthosis.[35,40] The angulation and displacement are manifestations of extensive injuries to the soft tissues of the vertebral column. However, the majority of hangman's fractures heal with just an orthosis (**Table 8.3**). A Philadelphia collar or SOMI brace is recommended for nondisplaced fractures. A halo brace is reserved for displaced hangman's fractures. Surgery is indicated for injuries that cannot be kept aligned satisfactorily in a halo brace, for patients who develop a nonunion, or for hangman's injuries associated with locked C2-C3 facets (**Figs. 8.18** and **8.19**).

Miscellaneous C2 Fractures

Miscellaneous C2 fractures refer to any C2 fracture that does not involve the odontoid process or the pars interarticularis of C2 (i.e., nonodontoid, nonhangman's fracture). These include fractures of the C2 body, C2

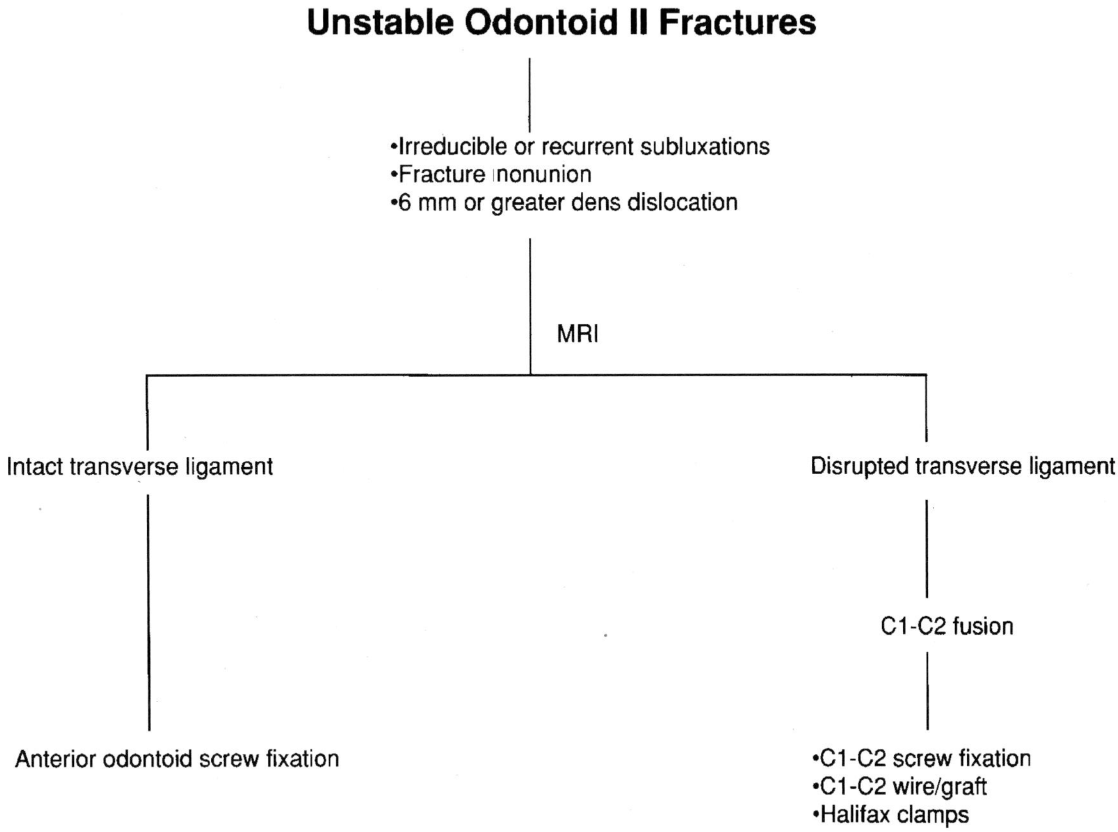

Fig. 8.17 Algorithm for treatment of unstable type II odontoid fractures. Widely displaced fractures (>6 mm) or patients who have failed treatment with an orthosis or who have developed nonunions are candidates for surgery. Odontoid screw fixation can be used only when the transverse atlantal ligament is intact. If the ligament is incompetent, an odontoid screw will not restore atlantoaxial instability even though the fracture is fixated. MRI, magnetic resonance imaging. (From Sonntag VKH, Dickman CA. Treatment of upper cervical spine injuries. In: Rea GL, ed. Spinal Trauma: Current Evaluation and Management. Park Ridge, IL: AANS; 1993:25–74. Reprinted with permission from the American Association of Neurological Surgeons.)

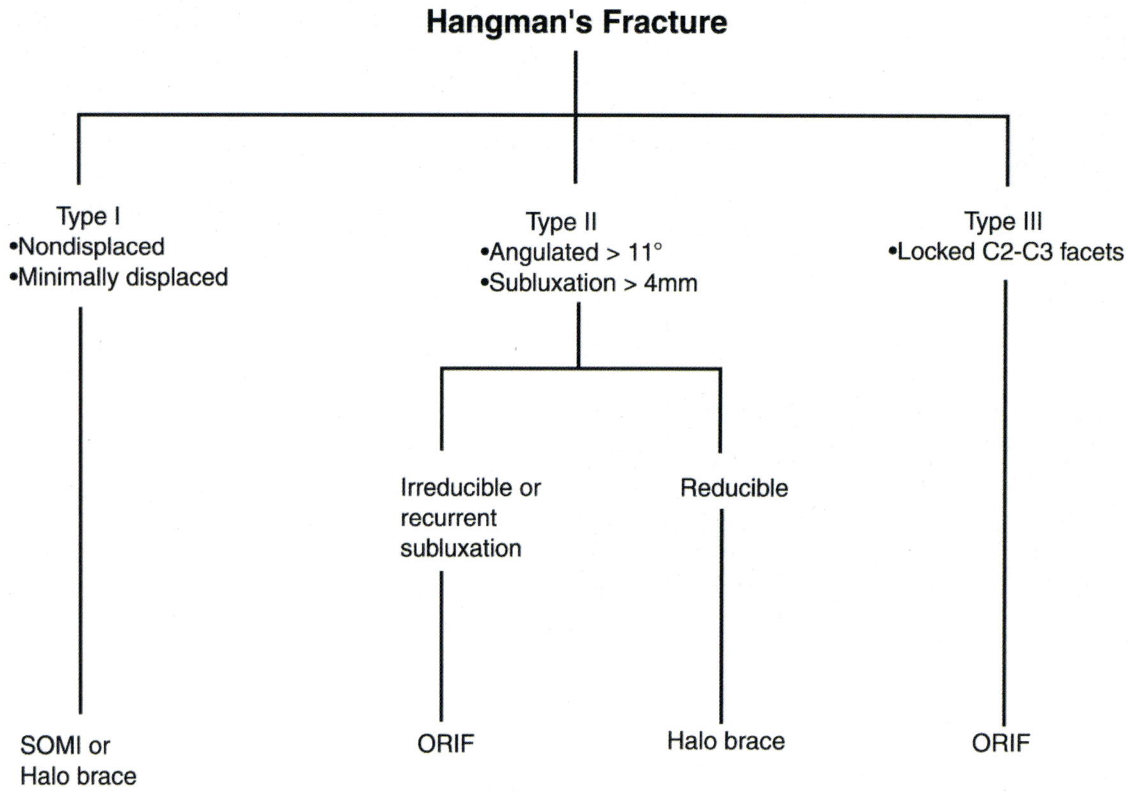

Fig. 8.18 Most hangman's fractures are treated satisfactorily with a sternal-occipital-mandibular-immobilization (SOMI) or halo brace. Surgery is reserved for patients with severe associated ligamentous injury, when orthoses fail to maintain alignment, or when associated with locked C2-C3 facets. *ORIF*, open reduction internal fixation.

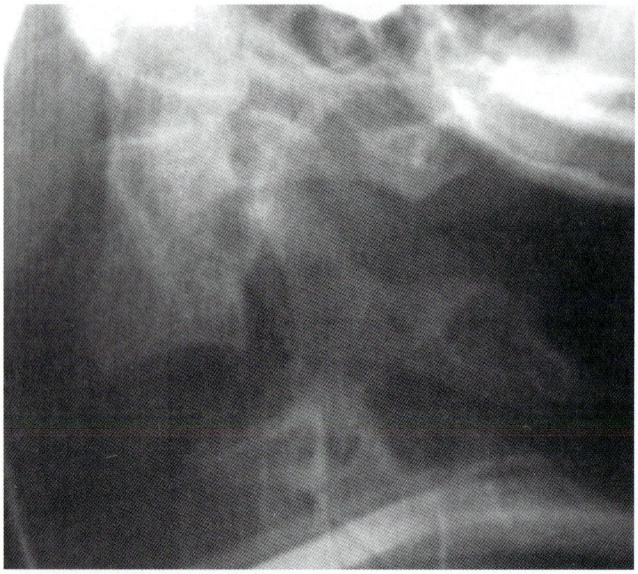

Fig. 8.19 Lateral radiograph of a hangman's fracture associated with bilaterally locked C2-C3 facets. The hangman's fracture creates a spondylolysis, separating the C2 body from the posterior arch. This fracture was reduced surgically because traction would have risked distracting the cervical segments.

laminae, C2 spinous process, or C2 facets. Most of these injuries heal satisfactorily with an orthosis (**Table 8.3**). Nondisplaced, minor fractures are treated with a Philadelphia collar or SOMI brace. Displaced or extensive fractures are treated with a halo brace. Surgery is reserved for cases that fail treatment with an orthosis or develop nonunion.

Combination Atlas–Axis Fractures

Similar to the treatment of isolated C1 or C2 fractures, atlantoaxial fractures are treated according to the extent of bony and ligamentous injuries (**Table 8.3**, **Fig. 8.20**). Combination fractures are relatively common: they account for 44% of all C1 fractures and 16% of all C2 fractures.[34] Combination C1-C2 fractures have a higher rate of neurological injury and a higher rate of nonoperative treatment failure compared with isolated atlas or axis fractures (**Tables 8.1** and **8.3**). These injuries should be evaluated with a combination of plain radiographs, CT, and MRI to determine the extent of bone and ligament injury. When the transverse atlantal ligament is disrupted, early surgery is advocated because the transverse ligament will not heal.

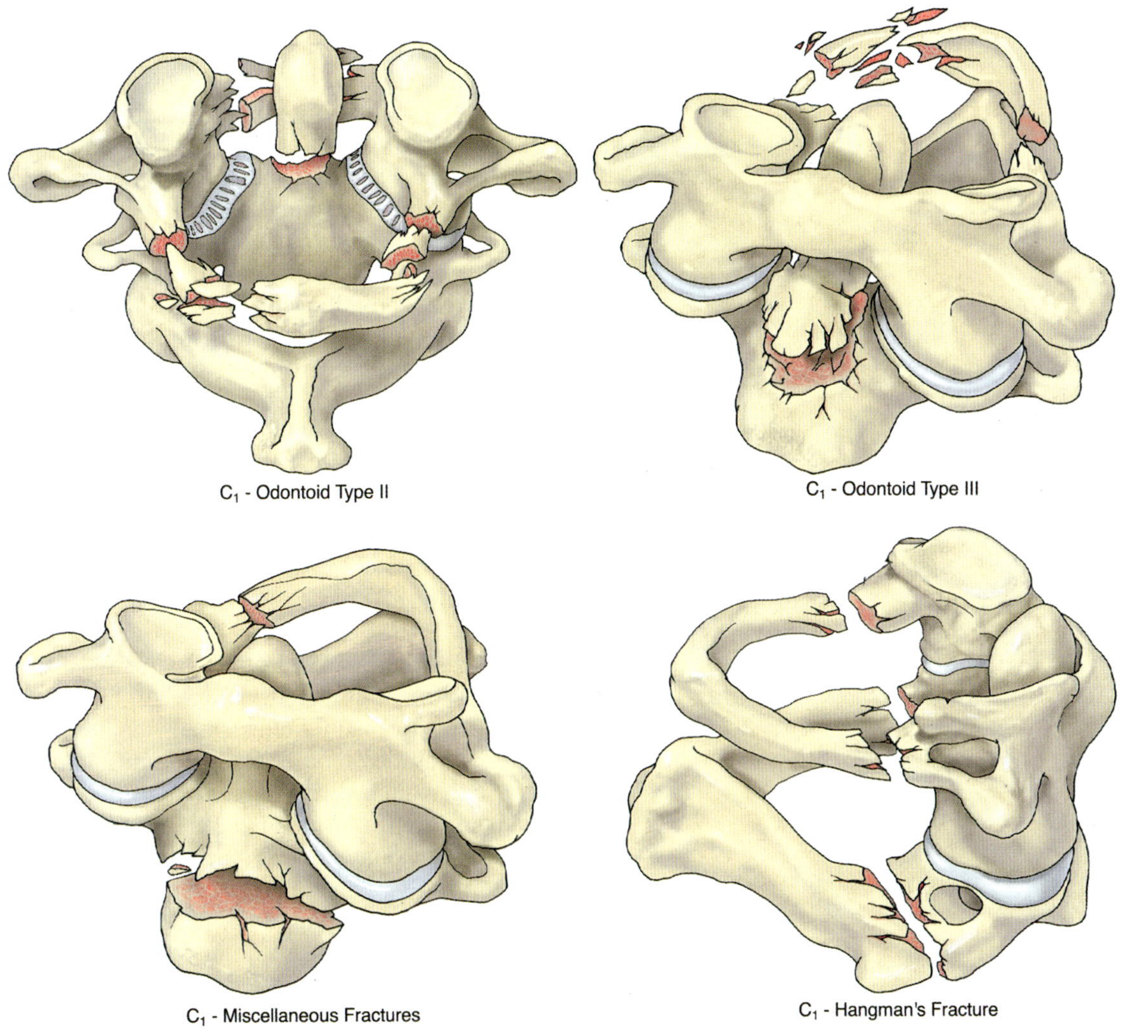

Fig. 8.20 Combination fractures involving both the atlas and axis are treated based on the extent of instability of the C1 fracture (i.e., whether the transverse ligament is incompetent) and the extent of the C2 fracture. Combination atlantoaxial injuries associated with type II odontoid fractures are the most common subtype of injury and also require surgery more often than isolated type II fractures. (From Dickman CA, Hadley MN, Browner C, et al. Neurosurgical management of acute atlas-axis combination fractures. A review of 25 cases. J Neurosurg 1989;70(1):45–49)

The extent of bone injury is the other major determinant of the method of treatment of C1-C2 fractures. Among combination C1-C2 injuries associated with odontoid type II fractures, healing is primarily influenced by the amount of dens displacement (**Fig. 8.21**). If the dens is displaced 6 mm or more, internal fixation is recommended because of the high rate of nonunion associated with widely displaced type II fractures. If the dens is displaced less than 6 mm, a halo brace is adequate. Combination C1-C2 fracture injuries, associated with odontoid type III, hangman's, or miscellaneous C2 fractures, often can be treated successfully with a halo brace. However, combination C1-C2 fractures are more likely to require surgery for internal fixation compared with isolated C1 or C2 fractures (**Table 8.3**).

Injuries Likely to Fail Nonoperative Treatment

Several types of injuries of the CVJ are highly unstable and should be considered for surgical intervention. Such injuries include those that are not immobilized satisfactorily with a halo brace, have recurrent subluxation, reangulation, or malalignment, or result in nonunion after an adequate trial of external immobilization. Extensive crush injuries to the bones or fractures associated with disruption of the major ligamentous stabilizing structures fall into this category of injury. Atlas fractures with a widely comminuted C1 lateral mass,[25] atlas fractures associated with disruption of the transverse

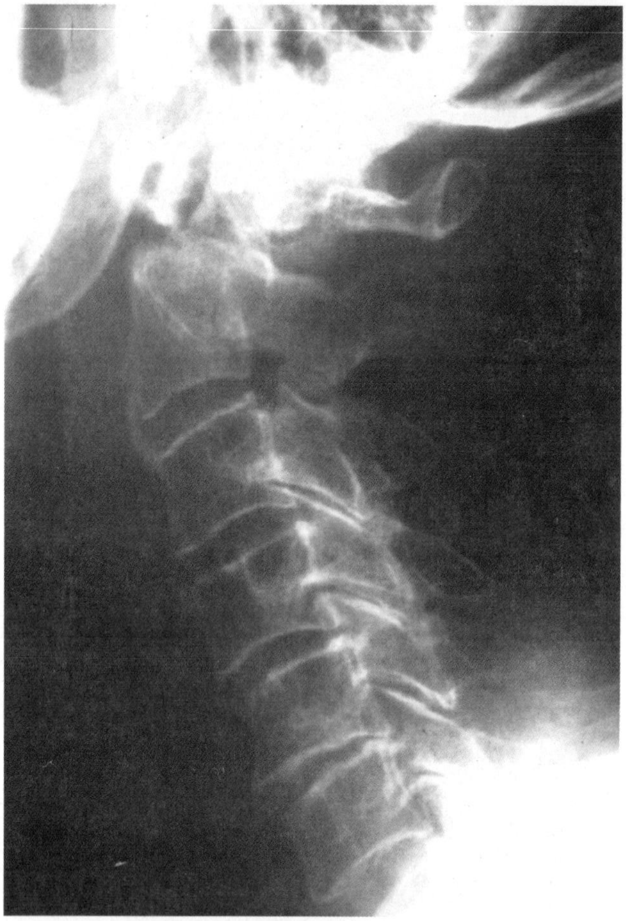

Fig. 8.21 This 10-mm posteriorly displaced type II odontoid fracture was associated with fractures of the lateral mass of C1. The patient was treated with posterior C1-C2 fusion because of the high risk of nonunion associated with his widely displaced odontoid fracture.

atlantal ligament,[24,25] axis fractures associated with transverse atlantal ligament disruption,[39] type II odontoid fractures with 6 mm or greater displacement,[38] extensively comminuted C2 fractures,[38] or hangman's fractures with C2-C3 subluxation more than 4 mm and greater than 11 degrees of C2 body angulation[35,40] exemplify this type of unstable injury. These mixed ligamentous and bony injuries are characterized by wide bone displacement, fracture angulation, subluxation, and extensively comminuted fractures. They are highly unstable and typically have a high rate of nonunion when treated nonoperatively. Alignment of the spine usually cannot be satisfactorily maintained with a halo brace for these injuries. They also tend to develop nonunion or a malaligned union.

Conclusion

Traumatic injuries of the CVJ are treated based on the extent of the injuries to the bone and ligaments that are responsible for maintaining spinal stability. Isolated ligamentous injuries tend to be highly unstable and do not heal with nonoperative management because disrupted ligaments are incapable of repair. Minimally displaced or nondisplaced bony injuries tend to heal satisfactorily with an orthosis. Combined injuries of the bone and ligaments and extensively comminuted, widely displaced fractures tend to require surgery for internal fixation to restore stability to the CVJ. It must be emphasized that although general guidelines can be formulated, treatment options should be individualized.

References

1. Frank C, Amiel D, Woo SL, Akeson W. Normal ligament properties and ligament healing. Clin Orthop Relat Res 1985;196(196):15–25
2. Myklebust JB, Pintar F, Yoganandan N, et al. Tensile strength of spinal ligaments. Spine 1988;13(5):526–531
3. Panjabi MM, Thibodeau LL, Crisco JJ III, White AA III. What constitutes spinal instability? Review Clin Neurosurg 1988;34:313–339
4. Blackwood NJ. III. Atlo-occipital dislocation: a case of fracture of the atlas and axis, and forward dislocation of the occiput on the spinal column, life being maintained for thirty-four hours and forty minutes by artificial respiration, during which a laminectomy was performed upon the third cervical vertebra. Ann Surg 1908;47(5):654–658
5. Bucholz RW, Burkhead WZ. The pathological anatomy of fatal atlanto-occipital dislocations. J Bone Joint Surg Am 1979;61(2):248–250
6. Dickman CA, Papadopoulos SM, Sonntag VKH, Spetzler RF, Rekate HL, Drabier J. Traumatic occipitoatlantal dislocations. J Spinal Disord 1993;6(4):300–313 Review
7. Lee C, Woodring JH, Goldstein SJ, Daniel TL, Young AB, Tibbs PA. Evaluation of traumatic atlantooccipital dislocations. AJNR Am J Neuroradiol 1987;8(1):19–26
8. Pang D, Wilberger JE Jr. Traumatic atlanto-occipital dislocation with survival: case report and review. Neurosurgery 1980;7(5):503–508
9. Papadopoulos SM, Dickman CA, Sonntag VKH, Rekate HL, Spetzler RF. Traumatic atlantooccipital dislocation with survival. Neurosurgery 1991;28(4):574–579
10. Wiesel SW, Rothman RH. Occipitoatlantal hypermobility. Spine 1979;4(3):187–191
11. Chamberlain WE. Basilar impression (platybasia): a bizarre developmental anomaly of the occipital bone and upper cervical spine with striking and misleading neurologic manifestations. Yale J Biol Med 1939;11(5):487–496
12. Dickman CA, Douglas RA, Sonntag VKH. Occipitocervical fusion: posterior stabilization of the craniovertebral junction and upper cervical spine. BNI Q 1990;6(2):2–14
13. Dolan KD. Cervicobasilar relationships. Radiol Clin North Am 1977;15(2):155–166
14. Dublin AB, Marks WM, Weinstock D, Newton TH. Traumatic dislocation of the atlanto-occipital articulation (AOA) with short-term survival. With a radiographic method of measuring the AOA. J Neurosurg 1980;52(4):541–546
15. Kaufman RA, Carroll CD, Buncher CR. Atlantooccipital junction: standards for measurement in normal children. AJNR Am J Neuroradiol 1987;8(6):995–999

16. Lee C, Rogers LF, Woodring JH, Goldstein SJ, Kim KS. Fractures of the craniovertebral junction associated with other fractures of the spine: overlooked entity? AJNR Am J Neuroradiol 1984;5(6):775–781
17. Powers B, Miller MD, Kramer RS, Martinez S, Gehweiler JA Jr. Traumatic anterior atlanto-occipital dislocation. Neurosurgery 1979;4(1):12–17
18. Traynelis VC, Marano GD, Dunker RO, Kaufman HH. Traumatic atlanto-occipital dislocation. Case report. J Neurosurg 1986;65(6):863–870
19. Wackenheim A. Roentgen Diagnosis of the Craniovertebral Region. New York, NY: Springer-Verlag; 1974:660
20. Wiesel S, Kraus D, Rothman RH. Atlanto-occipital hypermobility. Orthop Clin North Am 1978;9(4):969–972
21. Fruin AH, Pirotte TP. Traumatic atlantooccipital dislocation. Case report. J Neurosurg 1977;46(5):663–666
22. Page CP, Story JL, Wissinger JP, Branch CL. Traumatic atlantooccipital dislocation. Case report. J Neurosurg 1973;39(3):394–397
23. Watridge CB, Orrison WW, Arnold H, Woods GA. Lateral atlantooccipital dislocation: case report. Neurosurgery 1985;17(2):345–347
24. Spence KF Jr, Decker S, Sell KW. Bursting atlantal fracture associated with rupture of the transverse ligament. J Bone Joint Surg Am 1970;52(3):543–549
25. Dickman CA, Greene KA, Sonntag VKH. Injuries involving the transverse atlantal ligament: classification and treatment guidelines based upon experience with 39 injuries. Neurosurgery 1996;38(1):44–50
26. Dickman CA, Mamourian A, Sonntag VKH, Drayer BP. Magnetic resonance imaging of the transverse atlantal ligament for the evaluation of atlantoaxial instability. J Neurosurg 1991;75(2):221–227
27. Cooper PR, Maravilla KR, Sklar FH, Moody SF, Clark WK. Halo immobilization of cervical spine fractures. Indications and results. J Neurosurg 1979;50(5):603–610
28. Johnson RM, Hart DL, Simmons EF, Ramsby GR, Southwick WO. Cervical orthoses. A study comparing their effectiveness in restricting cervical motion in normal subjects. J Bone Joint Surg Am 1977;59(3):332–339
29. Koch RA, Nickel VL. The halo vest: an evaluation of motion and forces across the neck. Spine 1978;3(2):103–107
30. Marciano FF, Greene KA, Mattingly LG, et al. Halo brace immobilization of the cervical spine: a review of principles and application techniques. BNI Q 1994;10(1):13–17
31. Hadley MN, Dickman CA, Browner CM, Sonntag VK. Acute traumatic atlas fractures: management and long term outcome. Neurosurgery 1988;23(1):31–35
32. Jefferson G. Fracture of the atlas vertebra. Report of four cases, and a review of those previously recorded. Br J Surg 1920;7:407–422
33. Jónsson H Jr, Bring G, Rauschning W, Sahlstedt B. Hidden cervical spine injuries in traffic accident victims with skull fractures. J Spinal Disord 1991;4(3):251–263
34. Dickman CA, Hadley MN, Browner C, Sonntag VK. Neurosurgical management of acute atlas-axis combination fractures. A review of 25 cases. J Neurosurg 1989;70(1):45–49
35. Effendi B, Roy D, Cornish B, Dussault RG, Laurin CA. Fractures of the ring of the axis. A classification based on the analysis of 131 cases. J Bone Joint Surg Br 1981;63-B(3):319–327
36. Good J. Judicial hanging. Lancet 1913;1:193–194
37. Hadley MN, Browner CM, Liu SS, Sonntag VK. New subtype of acute odontoid fractures (type IIA). Neurosurgery 1988;22(1 Pt 1): 67–71
38. Greene KA, Dickman CA, Marciano FF, Drabier JB, Hadley MN, Sonntag VK. Acute axis fractures. Analysis of management and outcome in 340 consecutive cases. Spine 1997;22(16):1843–1852
39. Greene KA, Dickman CA, Marciano FF, Drabier J, Drayer BP, Sonntag VK. Transverse atlantal ligament disruption associated with odontoid fractures. Spine 1994;19(20):2307–2314
40. Bucholz RW. Unstable hangman's fractures. Clin Orthop Relat Res 1981;154(154):119–124

9 Bone Softening Diseases and Disorders of Bone Metabolism

H. Louis Harkey and Winston T. Capel

Metabolic diseases of the bone are a heterogeneous group of skeletal disorders in which there is an error in formation, remodeling, or absorption of bone. Nearly 400 different conditions fall under the broad heading of constitutional disorders of bone, resulting in complex nosocology and classification.[1] Further complicating matters, modern genomics has blurred the distinction between categories of dysplasia, dysostoses, and metabolic disorders by identifying a limited number of genetic defects associated with this group of bone malformation syndromes. Although the term *metabolic disease* implies a diffuse process, individual bones may be more severely affected than others, and only a few bones with metabolic defects may become symptomatic. It is unusual for a metabolic disease of bone to manifest at the craniovertebral junction (CVJ); when it does occur, the disease typically results in basilar impression and platybasia due to a loss of structural integrity at the skull base. Softening of the bony skull base may produce profound effects on neural structures that it normally supports and protects.

Some bone softening processes of the skull base are primary disorders of metabolism, such as osteogenesis imperfecta, a familial disorder of bone development. Others are secondary and result from a variety of causes, including nutritional abnormalities and hormonal disorders. Although Paget disease is not a metabolic disease, it can involve the skeleton diffusely and occasionally affects the CVJ. All of these diseases have the common feature of skull base deformity arising from the weakened mechanical properties of the skull base.

Certain heritable disorders such as Down syndrome, with inborn errors of metabolism, may not produce bone softening but manifest in the CVJ region. As a result of metabolic errors, osseous development is impaired and, in some cases, results in abnormal craniovertebral architecture. Hereditary connective tissue disorders may be associated with ligamentous laxity in the CVJ region, which can progress to instability. Rather than the basilar impression seen in bone softening metabolic diseases, patients with these inherited disorders present with stenosis at the CVJ from associated kyphotic deformity.

The terms *basilar invagination, basilar impression*, and *platybasia* were used interchangeably by Chamberlain in his original description, leading to some confusion.[2] This chapter follows the convention established by VanGilder, which defines *basilar invagination* as a congenital or primary prolapse of the vertebral column into the skull base.[3] *Basilar impression* refers to a progressive infolding of the skull base or secondary basilar invagination. *Platybasia*, which frequently accompanies both basilar invagination and basilar impression, refers to a flattening of the anterior skull base. In platybasia, the basal angle formed by the plane of the frontal fossa and the plane of the clivus is an abnormally obtuse angle. A characteristic appearance is seen in basilar impression and platybasia associated with bone softening disease affecting the skull base. The bones surrounding the foramen magnum are folded upward and inward around the upper cervical spine, as a ball of putty would deform over the end of a stick. In most cases, the bones are normal in size but distorted in shape. However, in some cases, the molded bones are eroded or even enlarged as a result of the pathological metabolism.

Bone Remodeling

Bone is a specialized form of connective tissue, composed of compact bone and cancellous bone. The histological characteristics are the same for both types, but compact bone lacks the numerous interconnecting cavities of cancellous bone. Cortical bone forms 80% of the volume of the skeleton and is found primarily in long bones. Cancellous bone, constituting 20% of the volume but 70% of the surface area, is found primarily in the vertebrae, the flat bones, and the ends of long bones.[4,5] Bone remodeling occurs only on the surface of bone; therefore, rates of remodeling are greater in cancellous bone because of a higher surface-to-volume ratio. Abnormalities in bone remodeling will differentially affect the weight-bearing bones of the axial skeleton, which have a larger proportion of cancellous bone. Accordingly, the pathological effects of metabolic bone disease are generally manifested in the spine, pelvis, and ends of larger long bones, only rarely affecting the CVJ.

Bone is composed of three types of cells (osteoblasts, osteocytes, and osteoclasts) and a mineralized organic matrix. Osteoblasts cover the surface of bone like an epithelial lining and are responsible for bone apposition. They synthesize the organic components of the bone matrix and deposit the inorganic components. Once the osteoblast is completely surrounded with bone matrix, it becomes an osteocyte. Osteocytes are responsible for maintaining the bone matrix, providing nutrient transportation through the interconnected lacunes and canaliculi in which they lie. Osteoclasts break down bone matrix by secreting enzymes that liberate calcified ground substance and break down the organic matrix. Osteoclasts are found on the surface of bone in excavated depressions called Howship lacunae.

Type I collagen, a fibrous protein, comprises the majority of the organic matrix of bone, accounting for ~90% of bone by weight. The remainder of the organic material, proteoglycans and glycoproteins, forms an amorphous ground substance in bone. Calcium and phosphorus are the two major inorganic components of bone matrix. They exist in the form of hydroxyapatite crystals or amorphous calcium phosphate. Hydroxyapatite crystals lie along the collagen fibrils and are surrounded by amorphous ground substance. This association of hydroxyapatite to the collagen fibers gives bone its characteristic hardness and strength.

Bone formation is a product of bone remodeling, a recapitulating process of osteoclastic stimulation, bone resorption, osteoblastic migration, matrix synthesis, and mineralization. Primary bone, the first bone tissue to appear, contains randomly arranged collagen fibers. This primary bone matures into secondary bone with organized lamellae through a process of bone resorption and subsequent rebuilding. Bone growth is rapid early in life because secondary bone is continually remodeled, with more bone laid down than resorbed. A net increase in bone formation continues until the third decade. Although net bone growth plateaus, remodeling continues throughout life as a perpetual cycle of bone resorption and formation.

In the majority of metabolic diseases of the skeleton, there is a net decrease in bone mass due to an imbalance between bone breakdown and bone remodeling.[6] *Osteoporosis* is a condition in which there is reduced bone mass per unit volume in bone with otherwise normal chemical makeup. Osteoporosis refers to a diverse group of diseases in which the bone is porous or thin but the ratio of mineral to matrix is normal. *Osteomalacia* is a condition in which the organic bone matrix is abnormally mineralized. Rickets and osteomalacia represent the same pathological process; however, *rickets* refers to this process in children whereas *osteomalacia* is generally used to describe defective bone mineralization in adults after the closure of epiphyseal growth plates. The term *osteopenia* is used when the reduction of bone density in osteoporosis or osteomalacia becomes radiographically evident. Osteopenia may be completely asymptomatic but becomes clinically significant when the bone can no longer provide skeletal support and fractures.

Calcium Metabolism and Related Hormones

Calcium and phosphate homeostasis is regulated by bodily need. For instance, growing children are rapidly forming new bone and require additional calcium and phosphate. New calcium is derived through diet and is absorbed through the intestine with the aid of active vitamin D metabolites. Phosphorous is also absorbed through the intestine and is at least partly linked to calcium absorption. Renal filtration is responsible for excretion of plasma calcium. The total amount of calcium excreted by the kidney depends on the rate of reabsorption in the renal tubules. Resorption is increased and excretion decreased by parathyroid hormone (PTH). Phosphate excretion by the kidney is regulated in the opposite way by PTH (i.e., increasing excretion of phosphate). Vitamin D enhances renal tubular resorption of phosphate.

Vitamin D is converted to its active metabolite (1,25-dihydroxycholecalciferol) through a succession of reactions in the skin, liver, and kidney. Physiological levels of vitamin D combined with PTH promote bone resorption by stimulating osteoclastic activity. PTH is secreted by the parathyroid gland in response to decreased plasma calcium levels. In turn, increased PTH increases plasma levels of calcium by releasing it from bone. Calcitonin, secreted by the thyroid gland in response to increases in plasma calcium levels, promotes the movement of calcium and phosphate into bone. Estrogen has an inhibitory effect on bone resorption. As estrogen levels decline following menopause, bone resorption increases.

Calcium and phosphate metabolism as it relates to bone is a twofold process in which one part is involved in the maintenance of plasma calcium equilibrium and the other part is involved in the remodeling of bone. Both parts are intimately related, but the differentiation helps to explain the complex metabolic process and its relationship to metabolic bone disease. Vitamin D and PTH affect plasma levels of calcium and phosphate by altering intestinal absorption and urinary excretion. Calcitonin and PTH alter plasma levels of calcium by affecting the rate of bone resorption. Pathological alterations in calcium homeostasis may result in metabolic bone disease.

Metabolic Disorders

Osteomalacia refers to a diverse group of diseases in which mineralization of newly formed osteoid matrix is deficient. The most common cause of osteomalacia is vitamin D deficiency, but it is also associated with malabsorption syndromes. When osteomalacia occurs in association with chronic renal failure, it is considered to be a form of renal osteodystrophy. The pathogenesis of osteomalacia is complex, but the fundamental problem is one of osteoblast function. A deficiency of phosphate, vitamin D, and/or vitamin D metabolites is responsible for the defective osteoblast function. An abnormality of synthesis, maturation, and mineralization of matrix results in an overall reduced rate of bone formation. The greatest defect, however, is in mineralization, with a net effect of decreased bone mass and markedly diminished mechanical properties.

Skeletal deformities in rickets are more generalized and severe than in adult osteomalacia because the mineralization defect occurs in developing bone. Dwarfism, "pigeon" breast, and bowed legs are general features of rickets that typically do not occur in adult osteomalacia. The spinal manifestations of rickets are not as prominent as those of the long weight-bearing bones because there is less longitudinal growth in vertebrae. The cranial manifestations include craniotabes (thinning and softening of the skull bones) and dolichocephaly (a disproportionately long head).

Basilar impression secondary to osteomalacia has been reported to occur with rickets, nutritional deficiency, renal osteodystrophy, and hyperparathyroidism. Basilar impression occurs more frequently in rickets than in adult onset osteomalacia and is thought to develop during the first 2 years of life, when the rachitic skull base is unable to support the disproportionately large weight of an infant's head.[7,8] In some instances, primary basilar invagination is the result of skull base rickets that has "healed" and, therefore, is secondary rather than congenital. Once the deficiency has been corrected, the bone mineralizes normally and resists further deformation.

Many cases of basilar impression due to osteomalacia are neurologically asymptomatic and are discovered incidentally, particularly if the osteomalacia has "healed." However, if the deficiency persists, basilar impression may be progressive with the gradual onset of neurological symptoms. Neurological deficits stemming from the foramen magnum region are protean, but long tract signs are the predominate finding in basilar impression. Some of these cases may also have a clinical presentation typical of a Chiari I malformation and have ectopic cerebellar tonsils with basilar impression. As a note of caution, nutritional deficiencies can lead to metabolic myopathy in addition to osteomalacia. Therefore, proximal weakness in a patient with osteomalacia may be a manifestation of associated myopathy rather than basilar impression and neural compromise.[9]

Osteogenesis Imperfecta

Osteogenesis imperfecta, or "brittle bone disease," is a familial disorder of type I collagen formation.[10] It is clinically characterized by blue sclera, abnormal dentin in the teeth, and excessive skeletal fragility. Osteogenesis imperfecta denotes a homogenous group of patients with autosomal dominant and recessive inheritance patterns and variable penetrance.[11] Most affected individuals have a mild form of the disease and usually reach adulthood with minimal deformity. However, basilar impression develops in rare cases of osteogenesis imperfecta.[12]

Basilar impression associated with osteogenesis imperfecta may become symptomatic early in life when recognized but in some cases does not present until the third or fourth decade of life. A wide range of neurological symptoms and signs has been attributed to basilar impression and results from direct neural compression, altered flow of cerebrospinal fluid, and/or vascular compromise. Neurological abnormalities include brainstem dysfunction such as central apnea and altered consciousness, lower cranial nerve deficits, myelopathy, and ataxia. Symptoms may be intermittent, and neurological function may decline progressively or in a stepwise fashion. Sudden death has occurred on rare occasion.

The skull shape in patients with osteogenesis imperfecta has been compared with a *tam-o'-shanter*, referring to the floppy beret formerly worn in parts of Scotland. In some cases, however, the overhang is more angular and the interparietal portion of the occipital bone is flattened to produce an appearance reminiscent of the headgear worn by the film character "Darth Vader."[12] The skull base deformity is best demonstrated with two- and three-dimensional reconstructed computed tomography images from which various measurements can be accurately taken (**Fig. 9.1**). The odontoid may be displaced 30 to 40 mm above the McGregor line and 20 mm above the Fischgold digastric line. The caudal clivus is elevated and thinned, in some cases forming a convexity over the tip of the dens. The basal angle of the deformity is obtuse, sometimes exceeding 180 degrees, and the craniovertebral angle is acute, sometimes less than 90 degrees. The petrous ridges are severely elevated, and the basion is infolded, resulting in circumferential deformity of the foramen magnum.

The severe bony invagination in osteogenesis imperfecta dramatically distorts the brainstem as demonstrated on magnetic resonance imaging. The infolding distal clivus contacts the brainstem at the pontomedullary junction, forcing the pons rostrally into the ventral portion of the midbrain (**Fig. 9.2**). The tectum of the midbrain is stretched and rotated into a more horizontal orientation, the middle cerebellar peduncles are draped over the migrating lateral edges of the foramen magnum, and the medulla is elongated. In some cases, a cervicomedullary kink forms dorsally along with herniation of the tonsils beyond the posterior rim of the foramen magnum. Considering the magnitude of distortion of the neural structures that results from the basilar impression, it is remarkable how few neurological deficits are demonstrated by some patients. This observation suggests that the invagination process is very slow, which allows the neural structures to accommodate the deformity as they would a slow-growing tumor.

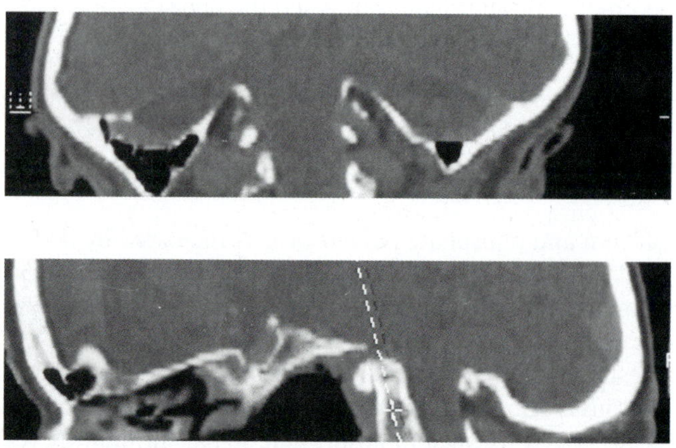

Fig. 9.1 Sagittal and axial computed tomography reformats of a severely distorted skull base due to osteogenesis imperfecta.

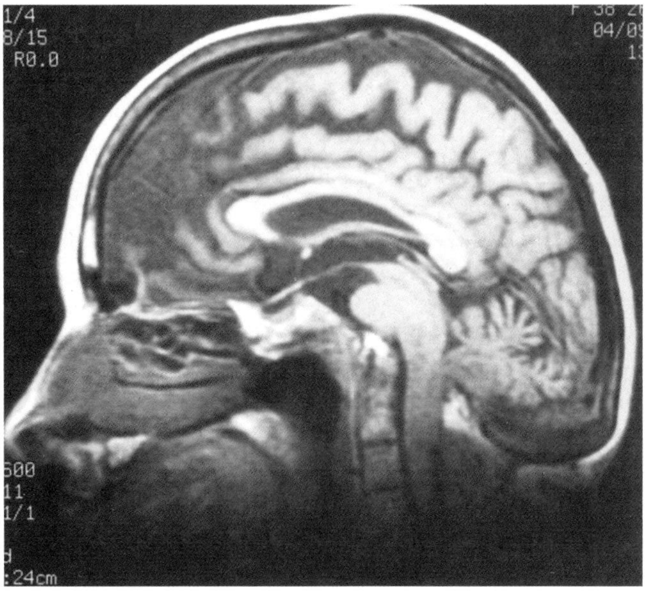

Fig. 9.2 Magnetic resonance imaging of a patient with osteogenesis imperfecta and severe basilar impression distorting the brain stem.

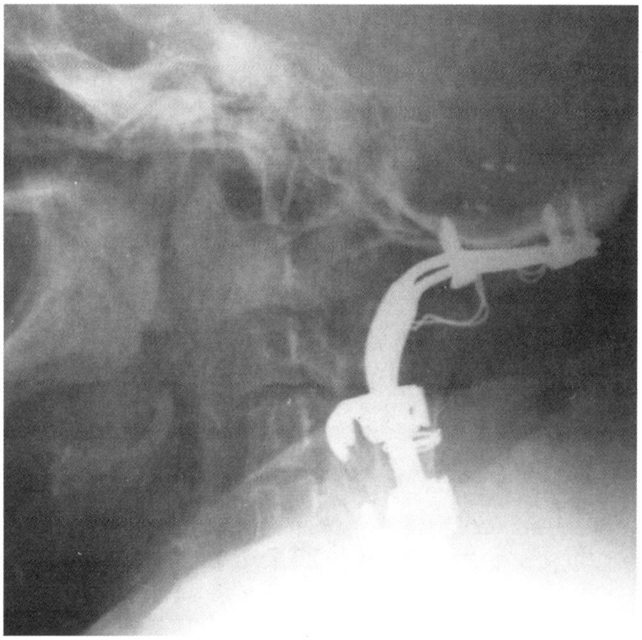

Fig. 9.3 Short-term stabilization is provided by the occipitocervical fixation device following decompression from a copious bone graft that spreads the weight-bearing surface over a larger area of the skull base.

Early reports of the surgical management of basilar impression secondary to osteogenesis imperfecta described decompression by suboccipital craniectomy and upper cervical laminectomy.[13,14] It is now recognized that a more appropriate and effective decompression can be achieved via an anterior approach. Because the offending bony compression is located so far rostrally, a standard transoral approach is inadequate. Only by mobilizing the maxilla can satisfactory exposure be gained anteriorly to remove the infolded clivus and translocated atlas and axis. Even with this approach, the decompression is limited to the anterior bony structures. Further posterior decompression may be necessary but should be performed only after anterior decompression. It should be noted that basilar impression in osteogenesis imperfecta is circumferential and that a 360-degree decompression is not feasible.

Decompression is merely palliative in basilar impression secondary to osteogenesis imperfecta because the basilar impression will invariably progress. To prevent or retard infolding, the weight-bearing surface of the skull base must be redistributed over a larger area. This process can be achieved with internal occipitocervical fixation and copious bone graft, extending as laterally and posteriorly as possible. Bone healing is not impaired in osteogenesis imperfecta, so grafting is typically successful. However, the bone is soft, and fixation devices are prone to failure at any bone/metal interface (**Fig. 9.3**).

Two recent reviews of basilar impression secondary to osteogenesis imperfecta with long-term follow-up have demonstrated that ventral decompression frequently results in symptomatic improvement.[15,16] Both reviews advocate broad-based posterior occipitocervical stabilization to limit the progression of the disease. A greater risk of progression exists in younger patients, probably due to higher rates of bone metabolism. The use of bisphosponates seems to have reduced the incidence of symptomatic basilar invagination in patients with basilar invagination, so one could assume bisphosphonates would improve outcomes following posterior stabilization.

Basilar impression in Hajdu-Cheney syndrome has a similar appearance to basilar impression in osteogenesis imperfecta. Hajdu-Cheney syndrome, also known as acro-osteolysis, is a rare congenital disorder of progressive skeletal dysplasia.[17,18] The hallmark feature of this syndrome is dissolution of terminal phalanges, but skeletal abnormalities are generalized. Affected individuals are short in stature, similar to osteogenesis imperfecta patients, and have progressive cranial deformation as a result of this soft bone disease. Basilar impression in Hajdu-Cheney syndrome is treated as it is in osteogenesis imperfecta.

Paget Disease of Bone

Technically speaking, Paget disease of bone is not a metabolic bone disease but a focal, chronic disease process that may, in some cases, affect multiple bones in the body. However, Paget disease is frequently grouped with other metabolic bone diseases because of similar characteristics, and it is discussed in this chapter because of its association with basilar impression. Paget disease, also known as *osteitis deformans*, is a disease of the elderly and a disease for which the etiology is unknown.[19] Inflammatory, hormonal, autoimmune, neoplastic, and vascular etiologies have been proposed, but the most convincing explanation is that Paget disease may be caused by a slow virus. The pathophysiology is poorly understood but is clearly related to hyperactive osteoclastic activity and abnormal bone reformation, resulting in weakened mechanical properties of the skeleton.[20,21]

Paget disease involves the skull in 65% of cases and primarily affects the calvarium. During the initial phase of osteolysis, large areas of radiolucent bone, termed *osteoporosis circumscripta*, may be present. Subsequent bone reformation appears hyperdense, and the normal cranial outline becomes expanded, obscuring the inner and outer cortical tables. The irregular and patchy appearance of pagetic bone is often referred to as "cotton wool" (**Fig. 9.4**). Cranial thickening is occasionally extensive, leading to compression of neural structures. Pagetic expansion at the skull base may produce cranial nerve and spinal cord deficits by compressing these structures as they exit a foramen. Hearing loss, a relatively common symptom, is usually secondary to compression of the auditory nerve in the internal auditory meatus but may be attributable to pagetic involvement of the ossicles. When the skull base loses its structural integrity due to Paget disease, constant weight-bearing and muscle contraction produce a gradual infolding of the basiocciput (**Fig. 9.4**). Basilar impression occurs in one in three patients with long-standing Paget disease of the skull.[3] The neurological consequences of severe basilar impression are variable and depend on which structures are most severely compromised. Findings may include varying degrees of sleep apnea, nystagmus, and spastic quadriparesis.

Decompressive procedures in Paget disease are technically difficult because the bone is highly vascular and blood loss may be torrential. Decompression should be performed with careful drilling, with frequent stops to wax the bleeding bone edges.[22] The recent bias in surgical treatment of basilar impression due to soft bone diseases is transoral decompression. New developments in anterior approaches to the CVJ permit safe decompression of the lower brainstem and upper cervical cord. Ideally, any surgery should follow a course of suppressive drug therapy (bisphosphonates). Although medical treatment will not reduce expanded bone, it may significantly decrease the highly vascular tissue associated with active Paget disease and the risk of excessive bleeding during surgery. Furthermore, a course of drug therapy before surgery will decrease the risk of postoperative instability due to mechanical failure of bone in the soft phase.

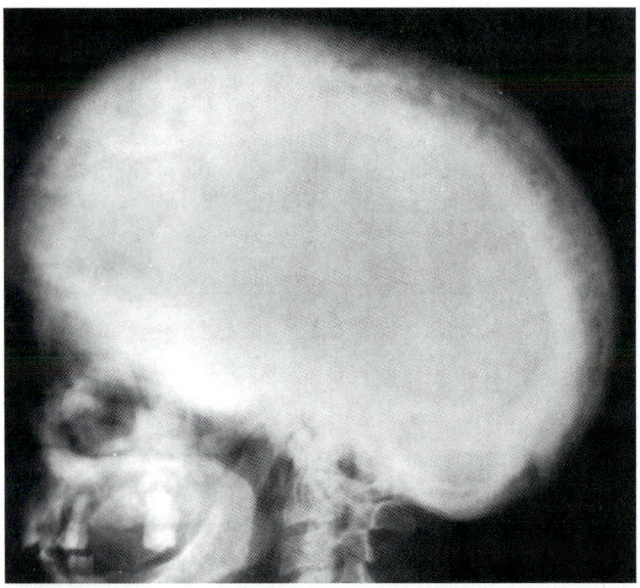

Fig. 9.4 This skull demonstrates the features of Paget disease: thickened calvarium, "cotton wool" appearance, and basilar impression.

Other Metabolic and Genetic Conditions Affecting the Craniovertebral Junction

Down Syndrome

Down syndrome is a genetic form of mental retardation usually caused by trisomy of chromosome 21 and rarely translocation from 13 to 15 groups to chromosome 21. Patients with Down syndrome have an increased incidence of craniovertebral pathology manifested by atlanto-occipital and atlantoaxial instability. The incidence of atlanto-occipital instability is ~10%, and the incidence of atlantoaxial instability is 14 to 24%, which in most cases is asymptomatic.[23–26] Patients may have tandem instabilities of both atlanto-occipital and atlantoaxial joints.[27] Os odontoideum and hypoplastic odontoid process are also associated with Down syndrome and may result in craniovertebral instability. Recognizing the risk of neurological injury due to instability or bony anomaly of the CVJ, the Committee on Sports Medicine of the American Academy of Pediatrics has recommended a screening neurological exam and radiographic studies for children with Down syndrome who wish to participate in contact sports. The committee has also recommended consideration of surgical stabilization when the patient is symptomatic and the atlantodental space exceeds 4.5 mm.[28,29]

Generalized ligamentous laxity is a feature of Down syndrome. Laxity of the craniovertebral ligamentous complex allows for hypermobility of the atlanto-occipital and/or atlantoaxial joints, with resulting craniovertebral instability. Abnormal metabolism of mucopolysaccarides and deficient growth hormone lead to osseous abnormalities,[26] including platybasia and odontoid dysmorphia. In some cases, osseous abnormalities combine with ligamentous laxity to create complex craniovertebral abnormalities. When symptomatic from atlantoaxial subluxation, patients may present with spastic hemiparesis, paraparesis, quadriparesis, torticollis, neurogenic bowel and bladder, or ataxia.[30] Symptoms may develop after an upper respiratory infection, which increases ligamentous laxity due to inflammation.[27]

The surgical management of patients with instability of the atlanto-occipital or atlantoaxial joints depends on the reducibility of the subluxation and on the direction of encroachment in irreducible lesions.[27] For patients with acute instabilities, such as rotary subluxation after upper respiratory infection, the recommended treatment is traction, reduction, and external occipitocervical immobilization for 3 months. Patients with chronic but reducible instability of the atlantoaxial junction require dorsal stabilization. For symptomatic irreducible subluxation, the cervicomedullary junction should be decompressed from the direction of encroachment (i.e., transoral decompression for ventral compression or posterior decompression for dorsal compression). Decompressive procedures should be followed by posterior internal fixation and bone graft fusion, although high rates of bone resorption in such cases have been described.[31]

Achondroplasia

Achondroplasia, the most common form of dwarfism, is associated with stenosis of the CVJ. It is an autosomal dominant condition, but most cases occur as random new mutations. The genetic abnormality results in abnormal endochondral bone formation, but intramembranous and periosteal bone formation remains normal. The net result is foreshortening of long bones that may give rise to the typical dwarf appearance. The skull base develops from cartilage, so it forms abnormally in an achondroplastic dwarf. However, the bones of the convexity are membranous and develop normally. Early synostosis of the vertebral body and posterior arch results in a narrow spinal canal, particularly in the sagittal plane. Neural compression can occur at both the foramen magnum and spinal canal.

Hydrocephalus and cervicomedullary compression from foramen magnum stenosis can result in significant morbidity and mortality, especially in pediatric patients. Clinically, patients with cervicomedullary compression most frequently present with upper and lower extremity paresis, general motor development delay, and respiratory complications.[32,33] Respiratory problems can present a diagnostic dilemma because apnea, tachypnea, cor pulmonale, recurrent pneumonia, and sudden death may result from foramen magnum stenosis or primary pulmonary abnormalities.[33] Similarly, the etiology of weakness may be obscure because hypotonia is a feature of achondroplasia. Sleep studies and somatosensory evoked potentials may help differentiate the cause of such symptoms and dictate the appropriate therapy.[34]

Surgical treatment by suboccipital decompression, when indicated, results in favorable outcomes if performed early after the onset of symptoms.[32,33] Decompression should extend well beyond the level of compression and may require total craniospinal decompression in severe cases.[35] Experience indicates that spinal compression just beyond the laminectomy frequently becomes symptomatic following surgical decompression.

Morquio Disease

Morquio disease is a genetic mucopolysaccharidosis (type IV) resulting in the absence or reduced activity of a lysosomal hydrolase, producing a clinical syndrome that includes severe bony changes leading to dwarfism, ligamentous laxity, and aortic regurgitation. The CVJ develops abnormally in Morquio disease. The odontoid is usually detached from the body of the axis, and the ring of the atlas tends to be narrowed and thickened.[36] Condylar hypoplasia in conjunction with atlantoaxial subluxation allows the posterior arch of the atlas to invaginate the foramen magnum. Chronic instability leads to localized thickening of the anterior extradural soft tissues adjacent to the odontoid. The soft tissue formation in the anterior epidural space is usually reactive ligamentous tissue with or without abnormal deposition of mucopolysaccharide.[37]

Symptomatic patients present with myelopathy with or without history of minor trauma. Patients may lose consciousness after minor trauma due to medullary compression.[36] Aggressive surgical management is advocated because most neurological deficits do not reverse.[38,39] Surgical treatment consists of posterior occipitocervical fusion with or without transoral decompression.

Marfan Syndrome

Marfan syndrome is an autosomal dominate genetic disorder of connective tissue with skeletal, ocular, and cardiovascular abnormalities. Patients have ligamentous laxity and increased kyphoscoliosis and are tall with arachnodactyly. Disorders of the CVJ are rare with isolated case reports of basilar impression and atlantoaxial instability.[40]

References

1. Superti-Furga A, Unger S. Nosology and classification of genetic skeletal disorders: 2006 revision. Am J Med Genet A 2007;143(1):1–18
2. Chamberlain WE. Basilar impression (platybasia): bizarre developmental anomaly of occipital bone and upper cervical spine with striking an misleading neurologic manifestations. Yale J Biol Med 1939;11(5):487–496
3. VanGuilder JC, Menezes AH, Dolan KD. The Craniovertebral Junction and Its Abnormalities. Mount Kisco, NY: Futura Publishing; 1987
4. Lane JM, Beernstein J. Metabolic bone disorders of the spine. In: Herkowitz HN, Garfin SR, Eismont FJ, Bell GR, Balderston RA, eds. Rothman-Simeone The Spine. 4th ed. Philadelphia, PA: WB Saunders; 1999:1259–1280
5. Gartner LP, Hiatt JL. Color Textbook of Histology. 3rd ed. Philadelphia, PA: Saunders Elsevier; 2007:131–156
6. Rodan GA. Introduction to bone biology. Bone 1992;13(Suppl 1):S3–S6
7. Hurwitz LJ, Banerji NK. Basilar impression of the skull in patients with adult coeliac disease and after gastric surgery. J Neurol Neurosurg Psychiatry 1972;35(1):92–96
8. Hurwitz LJ, Shepherd WHT. Basilar impression and disordered metabolism of bone. Brain 1966;89(2):223–234
9. Chakrabarti AK, Johnson SC, Samantray SK, Reddy ER. Osteomalacia, myopathy and basilar impression. J Neurol Sci 1974;23(2):227–235

10. Smith R, Francis MJO, Houghton GR. The Brittle Bone Syndrome. London, England: Butterworths; 1983
11. Sillence DO, Senn A, Danks DM. Genetic heterogeneity in osteogenesis imperfecta. J Med Genet 1979;16(2):101–116
12. Harkey HL, Crockard HA, Stevens JM, Smith R, Ransford AO. The operative management of basilar impression in osteogenesis imperfecta. Neurosurgery 1990;27(5):782–786, discussion 786
13. Fadli ME. Neuropsychiatric complications of osteogenesis imperfecta. "A case with cerebrovascular insufficiency." J Egypt Med Assoc 1968;51(6):528–537
14. Hurwitz LJ, McSWINEY RR. Basilar impression and osteogenesis imperfecta in a family. Brain 1960;83:138–149
15. Sawin PD, Menezes AH. Basilar invagination in osteogenesis imperfecta and related osteochondrodysplasias: medical and surgical management. J Neurosurg 1997;86(6):950–960
16. Ibrahim AG, Crockard HA. Basilar impression and osteogenesis imperfecta: a 21-year retrospective review of outcomes in 20 patients. J Neurosurg Spine 2007;7(6):594–600
17. Williams B. Foramen magnum impaction in a case of acro-osteolysis. Br J Surg 1977;64(1):70–73
18. Van den Houten BR, Ten Kate LP, Gerding JC. The Hajdu-Cheney syndrome. A review of the literature and report of 3 cases. Int J Oral Surg 1985;14(2):113–125
19. Resnick D. Paget's disease. In: Resnick D, ed. Diagnosis of Bone and Joint Disorders. Philadelphia, PA: WB Saunders; 2002:1947–2000
20. Bone HG, Kleerekoper M. Clinical review 39: Paget's disease of bone. J Clin Endocrinol Metab 1992;75(5):1179–1182
21. Kaplan FS. Paget's disease of bone: exploring the questions. Calcif Tissue Int 1992;51(1):1–3
22. Ryan MD, Taylor TKF. Spinal manifestations of Paget's disease. Aust N Z J Surg 1992;62(1):33–38
23. Spitzer R, Rabinowitch JY, Wybar KC. A study of the anomalies of the skull, teeth, and lenses in mongolism. Can Med Assoc J 1961; 84(11):567–572
24. Tishler J, Martel W. Dislocation of the atlas in mongolism: preliminary report. Radiology 1965;84:904–906
25. Pueschel SM, Scola FH. Atlantoaxial instability in individuals with Down syndrome: epidemiologic, radiographic, and clinical studies. Pediatrics 1987;80(4):555–560
26. Michejda M, Menolascino FJ. Skull base abnormalities in down's syndrome. Ment Retard 1975;13(1):24–26
27. Menezes AH, Ryken TC. Craniovertebral abnormalities in Down's syndrome. Pediatr Neurosurg 1992;18(1):24–33
28. Special Olympics. Participation by individuals with Down's syndrome who suffer from atlantoaxial dislocation condition. In: Special Olympics Bulletin. Washington, DC; March 1983
29. American Academy of Pediatrics. Committee on Sports Medicine. Atlantoaxial instability in Down syndrome. Pediatrics 1984;74(1): 152–154
30. Hreidarsson S, Magram G, Singer H. Symptomatic atlantoaxial dislocation in Down syndrome. Pediatrics 1982;69(5):568–571
31. Segal LS, Drummond DS, Zanotti RM, Ecker ML, Mubarak SJ. Complications of posterior arthrodesis of the cervical spine in patients who have Down syndrome. J Bone Joint Surg Am 1991;73(10): 1547–1554
32. Aryanpur J, Hurko O, Francomano C, Wang H, Carson B. Craniocervical decompression for cervicomedullary compression in pediatric patients with achondroplasia. J Neurosurg 1990;73(3):375–382
33. Colamaria V, Mazza C, Beltramello A, et al. Irreversible respiratory failure in an achondroplastic child: the importance of an early cervicomedullary decompression, and a review of the literature. Brain Dev 1991;13(4):270–279
34. Reid CS, Pyeritz RE, Kopits SE, et al. Cervicomedullary compression in young patients with achondroplasia: value of comprehensive neurologic and respiratory evaluation. J Pediatr 1987;110(4): 522–530
35. Uematsu S, Wang H, Kopits SE, Hurko O. Total craniospinal decompression in achondroplastic stenosis. Neurosurgery 1994;35(2): 250–257, discussion 257–258
36. Ashraf J, Crockard HA, Ransford AO, Stevens JM. Transoral decompression and posterior stabilisation in Morquio's disease. Arch Dis Child 1991;66(11):1318–1321
37. Stevens JM, Kendall BE, Crockard HA, Ransford A. The odontoid process in Morquio-Brailsford's disease. The effects of occipitocervical fusion. J Bone Joint Surg Br 1991;73(5):851–858
38. Kopits SE. Orthopedic complications of dwarfism. Clin Orthop Relat Res 1976;114(114):153–179
39. Greenberg AD. Atlanto-axial dislocations. Brain 1968;91(4): 655–684
40. Levander B, Mellström A, Grepe A. Atlantoaxial instability in Marfan's syndrome. Diagnosis and treatment. A case report. Neuroradiology 1981;21(1):43–46

10 Primary Osseous and Metastatic Neoplasms of the Craniovertebral Junction

Daniel M. Sciubba, Camilo A. Molina, Ziya L. Gokaslan, and Jean-Paul Wolinsky

Modern advancements in the understanding of neoplastic spine disease have also significantly improved the diagnosis and treatment of neoplasms at the craniovertebral junction (CVJ). Understanding the CVJ regional anatomy is essential in understanding the presentation, diagnosis, and management of neoplasms in this region. The CVJ encompasses the area of the C2, C1, foramen magnum, and lower clivus. Hence, CVJ tumors are defined as tumors that involve the region extending from the occipital condyles to the atlantoaxial spine.[1] Not surprisingly, tumors in this region are difficult to remove as they are surrounded by the brainstem, vertebral arteries, and lower cranial nerves.[2] Tumors at the CVJ include tumors of osseous origin, tumors that arise from extensions of soft tissue surrounding the region (e.g., hemangiomas), and tumors that arise from nervous system associated tissues (e.g., meningiomas).[3] This chapter discusses the epidemiology, presentation, diagnosis, and management of primary osseous and metastatic bony neoplasms of the CVJ.

Key points for this chapter:

- High-dose steroids are commonly used in the treatment of acute spinal cord injury.
- Significant limitations exist in the both animal and clinical literature supporting the use of steroids in acute spinal cord injury.
- Potential complications exist that are associated with high-dose steroids in patients with acute spinal cord injury.
- Given the risks and benefits, high-dose steroids should be used cautiously, and with careful observation, in patients with acute spinal cord injury.

Incidence and Prevalence

Each year in the United States, an estimated 1.5 million patients are diagnosed with cancer, mainly originating in the breast, prostate, and lung.[4] These tumors have a marked tendency to metastasize. The most frequent sites of distant metastases are the lungs and liver, followed by the bony spine.[5] Cadaveric studies of patients that succumbed to neoplastic illness report that an estimated 30 to 90% of cancer patients are afflicted with bony spine metastasis.[6] Thus, metastatic tumors are the most common bony spine neoplasms, accounting for nearly 90% of such tumors, and primary osseous spine tumors account for the remaining 10% of spinal osseous neoplasms.[7] This relationship applies to bony tumors of the CVJ, where the majority of tumors are of metastatic origin.[1] However, it must be noted that the CVJ is the least affected neoplasm region of the axial skeleton, with only 0.5% of all spine metastases and a comparable proportion of primary tumors localizing there.[8,9]

As stated previously, the most common origins of metastatic spine lesions are breast (35%), prostate (13%), and non-small cell lung carcinomas (10%),[1] all of which most frequently metastasize to the bony spine via hematogenous spread.[10] The mean age of presentation of patients with metastatic lesions of the CVJ is 60 years old.[1]

The prevalence and grade of various types of primary neoplasms of the CVJ correlate to age. In adults, the most common benign primary bone neoplasms in decreasing frequency are aneurysmal bone cysts, giant cell tumors, benign osteoblastomas, eosinophilic granulomas, and solitary plasmacytomas. The most common malignant neoplasms in decreasing frequency are chordomas, myelomas, lymphomas, chondrosarcomas, osteosarcomas, and Ewing sarcomas. In children, the most common primary benign lesions in this region are osteoid osteomas, osteoblastomas, and aneurysmal bone cysts, with the most common malignant tumor being chordomas and Ewing sarcomas.[11] The mean age of diagnosis for benign lesions is 21 and 49 for malignant lesions.[12]

Diagnosis

Presentation

As in the case of any suspected spinal neoplasm, it is essential to perform a detailed physical exam and gather the patient's history to guide the diagnostic process. In the case of CVJ tumors, clinical diagnosis is difficult as it may present similarly to pathologies of degenerative and traumatic origin. Nonetheless, there are several physical signs and reported symptoms that may suggest the presence of a CVJ tumor—the most common symptoms being mechanical and occipital neuralgia. As is the case for lesions in the cervical spine, mechanical pain is present in flexion and extension. However, lesions of the CVJ are distinguished from those in the subaxial spine by eliciting increased pain during rotational motion. It is postulated that the elicited rotational pain is due to stress at the atlantoaxial facet articulations and broad insertion of muscles to C2 and the occiput. Symptoms of occipital neuralgia are thought to originate from compression of the C2 sensory nerve root.[1] Nocturnal pain and persistent, progressive pain are symptoms that may help guide tumor diagnosis. The afflicted segment can be approximated during physical exam via percussion or applied pressure to the symptomatic region. Other reported signs and symptoms include vertigo, dysarthria, dysphagia, and paraspinal muscular pain and spasm, the latter possibly resulting from spinal deformity and collapse.[11]

Signs and symptoms of neurological deficit are less common presentations than mechanical and occipital neuralgia, which may be due to the combination of the generous subarachnoid space at the CVJ (wider canal) and diagnostic advancements such as magnetic resonance imaging (MRI) that allow for the earlier detection of neoplasms during initial noxious presentations. When neurological deficit is present, it is more frequently due to atlantoaxial subluxation than direct tumor compression of the cord and brainstem.[1] Nonetheless, patients may present with neurological deficit. Common signs include hyperreflexia, abnormal plantar responses, bowel and bladder dysfunction, spasticity, paraparesis, and occasionally Brown-Sequard syndrome. The most frequently involved cranial nerve is the spinal accessory nerve and, when compromised, patients present with torticollis and/or weakness of the trapezius and sternocleidomastoid muscles. Cerebellar ataxia may be present if the tumor extends across the foramen magnum.[11]

Laboratory Studies

Blood and serum studies may be useful in the diagnosis of metastatic lesions but have limited utility in the diagnosis of primary tumors. Nonetheless, serum-elevated serum markers such as prostate-specific antigen, carcinoembryonic antigen, and lactate dehydrogenase provide useful information to a diagnosis. In some cases, an elevated erythrocyte sedimentation rate can be found in the setting of a variety of benign and malignant primary tumors; however, this finding is common to any infection. A low hematocrit may suggest a marrow infiltrative process. Lastly, urine and serum electrophoresis should be obtained if a concern for plasmacytoma or multiple myeloma exists.[13]

Imaging

Numerous imaging modalities are helpful in the diagnosis of lesions at the CVJ, including plain radiography, computed tomography (CT), MRI, fluorodeoxyglucose positron emission tomography (FDG-PET), and nuclear scintigraphy. Plain radiography is usually the first imaging modality employed, and it may help in detecting lytic lesions, abnormal masses, pathological fractures, spinal deformities, and subluxation of the upper cervical spine. However, decisions and diagnoses are seldom made on the basis of plain radiography due to its insensitivity in the detection of spinal neoplastic processes.[13]

MRI is the gold standard for diagnosing metastatic and primary spine tumors due to its unmatched sensitivity and ability to exceptionally visualize soft tissue structures and bone–soft tissue interfaces of the CVJ. The latter allows for an anatomically accurate and highly detailed representation of paraspinal, neural, and osseous tumor involvement.[1,13]

CT provides highly detailed representations of the bony anatomy of the spine, providing a sensitive means of assessing lytic bone destruction and spinal alignment. CT is also useful for performing preoperative planning measurements of the bony spine, thereby being an essential tool for planning surgical intervention. CT with myelography can also provide a detailed rendering of the neural elements and thus serves as the imaging of choice for those patients in whom MRI is contraindicated.[1,13]

Bone scans serve as screening tools for tumor identification because they detect osteoblastic activity. However, a positive finding on a bone scan should be confirmed with MRI or CT because positive findings are nonspecific for tumor type. FDG-PET can help in distinguishing benign from malignant processes.[14]

Lastly, it should be mentioned that digital subtraction angiography permits elucidation of lesion vascularization and provides the possibility of embolization. Embolization is indicated for highly vascular tumors, and its use can significantly diminish the amount of intraoperative bleeding in highly vascular tumors, such as aneurysmal bone cysts. This decrease in bleeding allows for more aggressive tumor resection. However, it should be noted that embolization to the cervical spine is difficult because the tumor's blood supply is from the carotid and pharyngeal arteries.[11]

Biopsy

Biopsies can be categorized as excisional biopsies, open incisional biopsies, and needle biopsies and can determine tumor pathology, which is essential for planning appropriate intervention. For example, a biopsy can provide a diagnosis of round cell tumors, such as lymphomas or Ewing sarcoma, where the most primary intervention is chemotherapy. However, the most common percutaneous needle biopsies are difficult to perform for CVJ lesions due to the complex anatomy of this region. Furthermore, these biopsies risk providing a false-negative $<25\%$ of the time. Open incisional and excisional biopsies are alternatives and indicated for establishing the diagnosis, although they are technically challenging in this region. It should be mentioned that transoral biopsies are contraindicated in this region to avoid seeding of the mouth with tumors.[1,15]

Tumor Classification

Tumors of the CVJ can be broadly classified as tumors of metastatic origin or primary origin, with those of metastatic origin being the most prevalent. Primary origin tumors are dichotomized into benign or malignant and further classified according to cellular origin, yielding the two main categories of benign and malignant neoplasm as well as subcategories of osteogenic and cartilaginous tumors. Tumors that fall outside of these subcategories are classified as miscellaneous or tumors of unknown origin. In the following discussion, common adult tumors at the CVJ are categorized according to origin and aggressiveness and presented within their categories in order of decreasing prevalence.

Metastatic Tumors

Although the bony spine is the third most frequent localizing site of distant metastases, metastatic disease to the CVJ accounts for only 0.5% of spine metastases. The mean age at presentation for affected patients is 60 years old, and the majority of tumors derive from carcinomas of the breast, prostate, and lung. Patient history is crucial because any patient with a history of cancer presenting with a constellation of findings suggestive of a neoplasm in the spine should automatically be thought to have a metastatic lesion. Mechanical (flexion, extension, and rotational) pain is most common. Neurological deficit is less common, occurring in only 0 to 22% of cases. MRI is the ideal modality as it provides an excellent visualization of bone and soft tissue interfaces, thereby elucidating tumor extension and involvement of adjacent structures. T2-weighted series are preferential to T1-weighted (without contrast) as they allow for assessing the presence or absence of spinal cord compression. T1-weighted imaging with contrast is an acceptable alternative to T2-weighted imaging. CT imaging can demonstrate lytic bone destruction or sclerotic tumor bone involvement and provides information on spine alignment crucial for preoperative planning.[1] Tumors can be effectively managed through radiation and/or surgery, typically yielding decreased pain and improved function. Survival is variable and dependent on the pathology (i.e., origin) of the metastatic lesion.[6]

Malignant Primary Tumors

Multiple myeloma and plasmacytomas are the most common primary malignant tumors of the bony spine and the second most common to affect the CVJ. Plasmacytomas are considered benign lesions of lymphoid lineage that may differentiate into more aggressive neoplasms collectively known as multiple myeloma. These lesions are characterized by pathognomonic malignant cells in the bone marrow. Patients frequently present with diffuse osteoporosis and osteolytic bone destruction, resulting in local bony pain. Neurological deficits may also be present but are less common. A diagnostic workup of suspected cases consists of laboratory and imaging utilities. The imaging workup should include plain and CT radiographic imaging to reveal the lytic and cystic characteristic appearance of the lesions. A whole body bone scan is also useful in localizing additional lesions in the axial and appendicular skeleton. MRI may be useful in evaluating lesion extension into the spinal canal. A laboratory workup should include a complete blood cell count, electrolyte balance, and serum/urine electrophoresis. Patients afflicted with multiple myeloma are commonly severely anemic and hypercalcemic due to extensive neoplastic infiltration of the bone and marrow. Immune electrophoresis demonstrates monoclonal hypergammaglobulinemia in serum or Bence Jones proteins in urine, both of which are strong indicators of multiple myeloma. It should be noted that to diagnose multiple myeloma (versus a plasmacytoma), characteristic lesions must be in multiple locations. Plasmacytomas themselves have a benign course with a median survival of ~10 years. However, plasmacytomas are capable of transforming into a malignant myeloma, leaving patients with a median survival of 28 months. Optimal treatment of plasmacytomas involves a combination of pharmacotherapy and radiotherapy. The pharmacotherapy includes chemotherapeutic agents such as cyclophosphamide, melphalan, carmustine, and lomustine. It also includes adjuvant bisphosphonates to counteract osteoclastic tumor activity. Low-dose radiation (20 Gy in 10 fractions) is often sufficient to treat cases with absent cord compression. Surgical intervention is indicated in circumstances of bony cord compression not relieved by radiotherapy and in cases of severe spinal instability due to the multiple lesion pattern characteristic of multiple myeloma. Postoperative radiation therapy is also considered beneficial.[11,15–17]

Chordomas are the most common primary malignant tumors that affect the CVJ. They originate from remnants of the primitive notochord. Despite appearing histologically low grade, they are considered malignant due to their high recurrence rate and difficulty to completely resect. Although chordomas can be found throughout the bony spine, they are most commonly found at the two ends of the primitive notochord (35% of them affecting the clivus and CVJ). When occurring at the CVJ, they mostly involve the clivus and extend caudally to C1 and rarely C2. They are more common in males near the fifth to sixth decade than in other populations. When localized to the cervical spine, chordomas primarily present with mechanical neck pain. Occasionally, patients may present with an oropharyngeal mass, airway obstruction, and/or dysphagia due to the extensive soft tissue components of the tumor. On CT, chordomas appear as lytic bone lesions with abnormally large soft tissue components and, in 30% of cases, growth-associated calcification. Chordomas are best visualized on T2-weighted or T1-gadolinium enhanced MRI. On T2-weighted images, chordomas demonstrate a hyperintense signal in comparison to muscular tissue. In diagnostic biopsies, chordomas are known to seed along needle tracts; thus, transoral percutaneous biopsies are generally contraindicated in the suspicion of chordomas. Chordomas are best treated through a wide surgical excision (en bloc resection). In cervical lesions, surgical interventions are multidisciplinary, often requiring the participation of plastic surgeons and otolaryngologists to assist in approach and closure. Transglossal and transmandibular approaches are used because they provide the necessary working room and visualization to achieve complete resection. Lastly, it should be noted that proton beam therapy has recently emerged as an adjunct to surgery for treatment of lesions in difficult locations.[18,19]

Chondrosarcomas are malignant cartilaginous tumors. Although they most frequently affect the thoracic spine (60%), chondrosarcomas also occur in the cervical spine (20%). They typically present during the fifth or sixth decade and affect men twice as often as women. Symptoms develop gradually due to the neoplasm's indolent growth rate. Experienced pain is usually described as focal and dull with a nocturnal exacerbation. A physical exam may yield a palpable mass in the neck as the tumor most frequently involves the posterior elements. Neurological deficit manifests in ~50% of patients at presentation but may be less common in tumors localizing to the CVJ. Chondrosarcoma lesions can be clearly visualized through CT, demonstrating characteristic evidence of lytic and destructive lesions, thickening of the vertebral cortex, bony focal expansion, and exophytic extension into soft tissue. On CT, conventional chondrosarcomas demonstrate a ring-and-arc pattern. Undifferentiated and mesenchymal chondrosarcomas demonstrate bone destruction. Clear cell chondrosarcomas show calcified lytic bone lesions and encompassing sclerosis. MRI may demonstrate soft tissue impingement and invasion by the neoplasm. Prognosis is related to the grade of the lesion. Chondrosarcomas are predominantly resistant to radiotherapy and chemotherapy and are best treated with surgical intervention. En bloc excision is ideal because intralesional (extracapsular) excision has been associated with a high rate of local recurrence. However, high-dose photon radiotherapy and hypofractionated stereotactic radiosurgery are being investigated as alternative therapies, particularly to treat lesions in areas, such as the CVJ, where total tumor removal is difficult. Lastly, angiography and embolization should be considered in the treatment of these highly vascular tumors.[11,20]

Osteosarcomas are among the most frequent malignant conditions that affect bony tissues. However, the majority of osteosarcomas occur in the appendicular skeleton with only 5% occurring in the axial skeleton. Osteosarcomas do not demonstrate a preference for location in the axial skeleton. Tumors most frequently arise during the second and third decade. Studies have found positive associations in patients with a history of Paget disease and hereditary retinoblastoma and in patients previously exposed to ionizing radiation. The majority of patients present with focal pain. When localized to the CVJ, patients less frequently present with neurological symptoms. When radiographically imaged (CT or plain), the lesions show a combination of both lytic and sclerotic growth patterns. The utility of MRI depends on the extent of tumor mineralization. Nonmineralized tumors display high intensity on T2-weighted series and hypointensity in T1-weighted images. In contrast, mineralized tumors are hypointense in both T1- and T2-weighted series. PET may yield the best diagnostic information in the case of osteosarcomas because the imaging utility is particular in detecting the increased bone turnover characteristic of osteosarcomas. Overall, survival prognosis for osteosarcomas is dismal with a median survival time of 2 years. En bloc surgical excision is ideal, and care must be taken to reduce breaching of tumor margins to diminish the incidence of recurrence. Chemotherapy regimens can be coupled to surgical intervention to reduce the incidence of recurrence. Conventional radiotherapy as a primary means of treatment is not recommended because many tumors have been found to be radioresistant. Nonetheless, radiotherapy has been found to be beneficial to treat microscopic postoperative residual tumor.[11,12,15]

Ewing sarcoma is one of the least frequent adult primary osseous malignant neoplasms occurring at the CVJ, although it is one of the most frequently occurring in children and adolescents. The neoplasm is of unknown origin and consists of a small round cell neoplasia. The most commonly presenting symptoms are pain and swelling. Additionally, the condition frequently presents with systemic symptoms, such as fever, and is commonly misdiagnosed as infection. Neurological symptoms may occur but are less common. Conventional radiography yields a mottled, moth-eaten appearance indicative of poorly defined margins and irregular bone destruction. A whole body bone scan is useful to detect additional lesions, which are a common finding in patients afflicted with this neoplasm. Additional diagnostic utilities include a serum lactate dehydrogenase test that suggests the potential presence of this illness. The current treatment of choice is a four-drug chemotherapeutic regimen consisting of dactinomycin, vincristine, cyclophosphamide, and doxorubicin. Recent studies have suggested the addition of etoposide and ifosfamide to the four-drug regimen, reporting increases in survival up to 24%. Conventional radiotherapy (of ~40–65 Gy) can be jointly administered with chemotherapy. The role of surgical intervention in the management of this disease has not yet been established.[11,15,21]

Benign Primary Tumors

Aneurismal bone cysts are derived from vascular structures and account for ~15% of all primary spine tumors. Although they localize mostly to the lumbar spine (45%), they are also found in the cervical spine (30%). In the bony spine, aneurysmal bone cysts most frequently involve the posterior elements. However, lesions are also known to frequently extend onto the vertebral body. They have an unclear pathophysiology and affect most people during their second to third decade. Males are affected slightly more often than females. Surgical intervention can be curative. In addition, embolization should be considered because the tumors are highly vascular and the embolization itself can be curative. Prognosis depends on the rate of recurrence, which can be high (20–30%).[22]

Benign giant cell tumors are locally aggressive, despite their classification as benign. Although occurring primarily in the sacrum, these tumors have been reported in the cervical spine. They are osteolytic and comprised of multinucleated, osteoclastic giant cells, thought to originate from mononuclear cells of macrophage origin. They occur primarily in women in their second and third decades. Pathological fractures may be seen in nearly 30% of patients. En bloc resection is the recommended treatment for these lesions, although it is a difficult task at the CVJ. Intralesional excisions are not recommended because they are associated with a high recurrence rate.[23] However, in sacral lesions, intralesional resection is often performed to minimize neurological sacrifice.

Benign osteoid osteomas and osteoblastomas are benign lesions of osteogenic origin that localize primarily to the lumbar and cervical spine. Osteoid osteomas are four times as frequent as osteoblastomas. The main difference between osteoid osteomas and osteoblastomas is that osteoblastomas are larger and generally more aggressive. However, osteoblastomas are also particular in that they have the potential of malignant transition. Men have a slight predisposition, and onset occurs most frequently during the second decade of life. When localized to the cervical spine, the most common presentation is painful torticollis and reduced range of motion. Primary treatment is complete resection, which frequently has favorable outcomes.[16,24]

Management

Surgical Approach and Technique

Before embarking on a surgical treatment strategy for bony tumors of the spine at the CVJ, it is paramount to understand the pathology of the tumor to be treated. The treatment will be tailored to the goal of the operation. If the treatment is for metastatic disease or recurrent disease, the goal is palliation; if it is for a primary tumor, the goal is to provide a cure or long-term disease-free survival. In this section of this chapter, we describe the surgical strategies for treating metastatic disease separate from those for primary lesions.

The goal of treatment for primary tumors of the spine is to provide a cure or long-term disease-free survival. Most primary tumors of the spine have limited adjunctive treatments in the form of chemotherapy or radiation therapy. If chemotherapy or radiation therapy is to be considered part of the treatment, these modalities need to be incorporated into the surgical plan of treatment. Surgical treatment of primary tumors of the spine usually requires en bloc resection of the tumor to achieve long-term disease-free survival or cure.

In a simplified concept for designing a surgical strategy, the spine can be considered a ring encasing the spinal cord. Primary tumors of the spine will be centered somewhere along this ring. To remove the tumor without violating the margin of the tumor and to preserve the integrity and function of the spinal cord, the ring will need to be cut in two places, releasing the tumor and creating a corridor for the spinal cord so that the tumor can be delivered away from the cord. Resection of the tumor requires two operative stages. The first stage frees the normal spine and spinal cord from the tumor, and the second stage delivers the specimen, which may require one or more surgical approaches. Accomplishing these stages results in complete dislocation of the CVJ, so complex reconstruction techniques are required to stabilize this region.

Critical structures often run through or in close proximity to the tumor and may need to be sacrificed during the first stage of the operation. The location of the vertebral arteries as well as the hypoglossal nerve and cervical roots in relation to the tumor needs to be understood. In addition, the deficit produced by the sacrifice contemplated needs to be evaluated to determine whether it is one the patient will tolerate.

Usually, one vertebral artery is dominant with respect to the other; in our experience, the nondominant artery can be sacrificed without consequence. If the dominant artery is considered for sacrifice, then preoperative evaluation with a balloon test occlusion should be considered to verify that the artery can be sacrificed. If one of the vertebral arteries needs to be ligated, extra care must be taken to avoid manipulation of the remaining artery because vasospasm or vascular injury could be catastrophic.

The hypoglossal nerve exits the hypoglossal canal in the skull base and swings ventrally past the ventral arch of C1 and behind the digastric muscle before entering the tongue. This nerve is usually uninvolved in primary tumors of the spine unless the tumor originates in the skull base and extends caudally into the spine, which can occur with chordomas. The nerve more commonly may be injured during high-cervical approaches, and its anatomy must be fully understood when attacking these tumors. Unilateral injury to the hypoglossal nerve can be tolerated quite well, but bilateral dysfunction will result in tongue immobility, difficulty with swallowing, and aspiration and can result in death.

The first and second cervical roots can be sacrificed bilaterally without significant consequence. Patients may experience numbness in the C2 distribution, but if they are aware of the expected result, they usually have no difficulty with the deficit. Truncation of C3 in isolation is also well tolerated but, if C3 and C4 need to be sacrificed, some diaphragmatic weakness may result, which may be more apparent if bilateral sacrifice is needed. C5, C6, C8, and T1 sacrifice will result in significant functional loss, and the loss has to be weighed against the potential benefit of the tumor resection.

Most primary tumors of the spine at the CVJ arise in the spine ventrally or anterolaterally. Occasionally, these tumors will originate in the posterior aspect of the spine. As the tumor is typically ventral, the first stage of the operation is usually undertaken through a standard posterior approach. The posterior approach allows the surgeon the ability to expose normal areas of the spine and uninvolved areas surrounding the spinal cord so that the normal architecture can be defined prior to coming close to the tumor margin. The soft tissue surrounding the tumor specimen is carefully dissected, leaving a margin of tissue on the tumor. A complete laminectomy is usually performed above and below the levels of tumor involvement—dura, untouched by tumor, is exposed (**Fig. 10.1**).

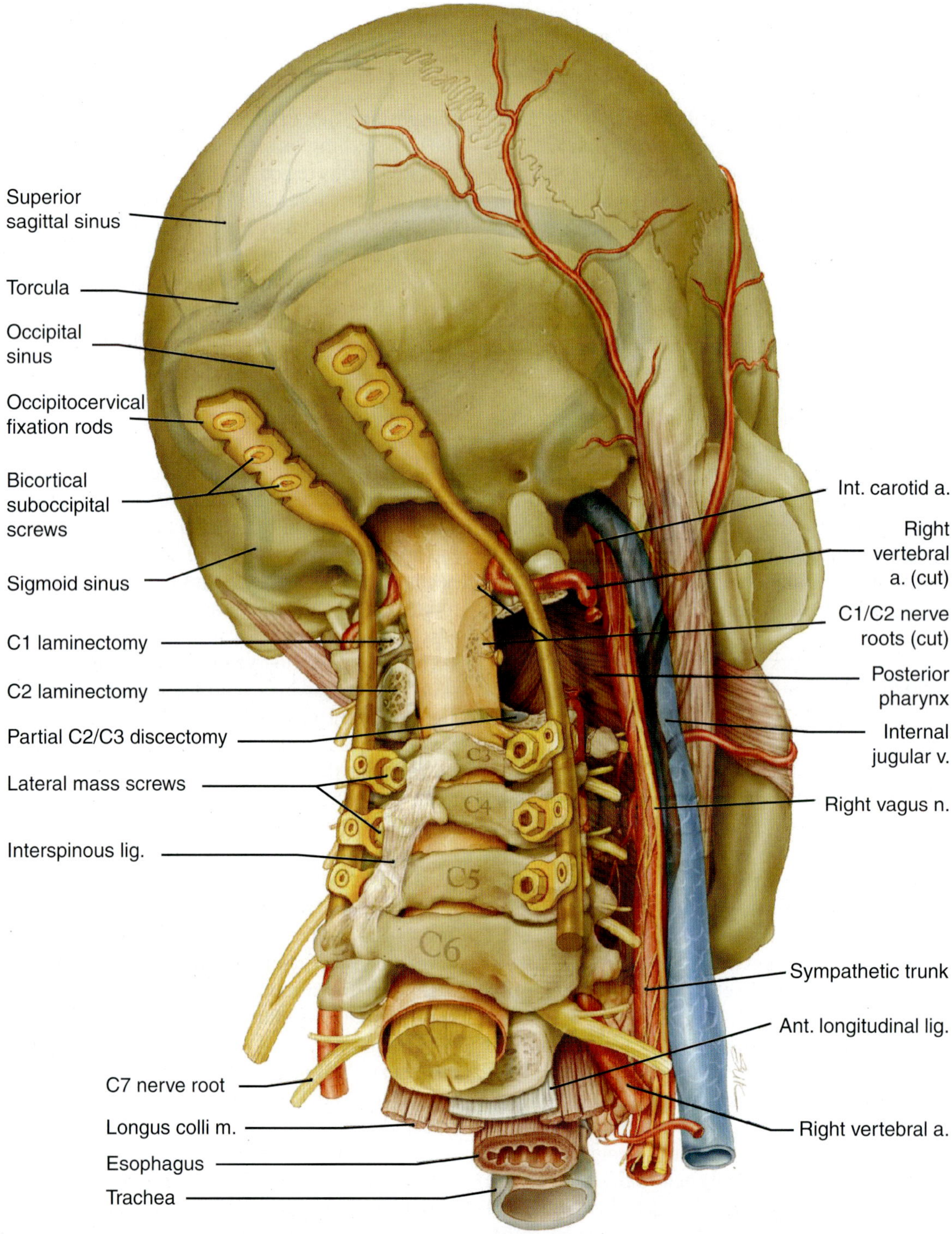

Fig. 10.1 Illustration of posterior cervical approach for en bloc resection of tumors of the craniovertebral junction. (Printed with permission from Ian Suk, Johns Hopkins University.)

The level of interest is identified, and the lamina at the index level is removed, where it is not involved in the tumor. If the entire lamina is uninvolved, it is removed. If part of the lamina or spinous process is involved, only the uninvolved portion is removed, giving access to the spinal canal. The nerve roots to be sacrificed are ligated and cut proximal to the dorsal root ganglion from within the spinal canal.

If the vertebral artery is involved with the tumor or if the vertebral artery will need to be sacrificed, then the artery is skeletonized rostral and caudal to the specimen. After exposing the artery, it is carefully ligated and transected at these points. Care must be taken when exposing the vertebral artery because the vessel is encased in a venous plexus. Injury to the plexus without careful hemostasis can result in life-threatening hemorrhage, without bleeding from the vertebral artery itself (**Fig. 10.2**).

After the neurovascular structures have been controlled, the posteriorly created osteotomies must be completed. On the side of the spine where the vertebral artery has been sacrificed, the remaining portion of the lateral mass and pedicle are removed, both rostral and caudal to the specimen. These transverse osteotomies will eventually be connected to ventral transverse osteotomies through the vertebral body or disk space, ventral to the spinal cord. On the contralateral side, a vertical osteotomy is performed just medial to the transverse foramen, allowing the patent vertebral artery to be preserved in its bony foramen and venous plexus without manipulating the vessel.

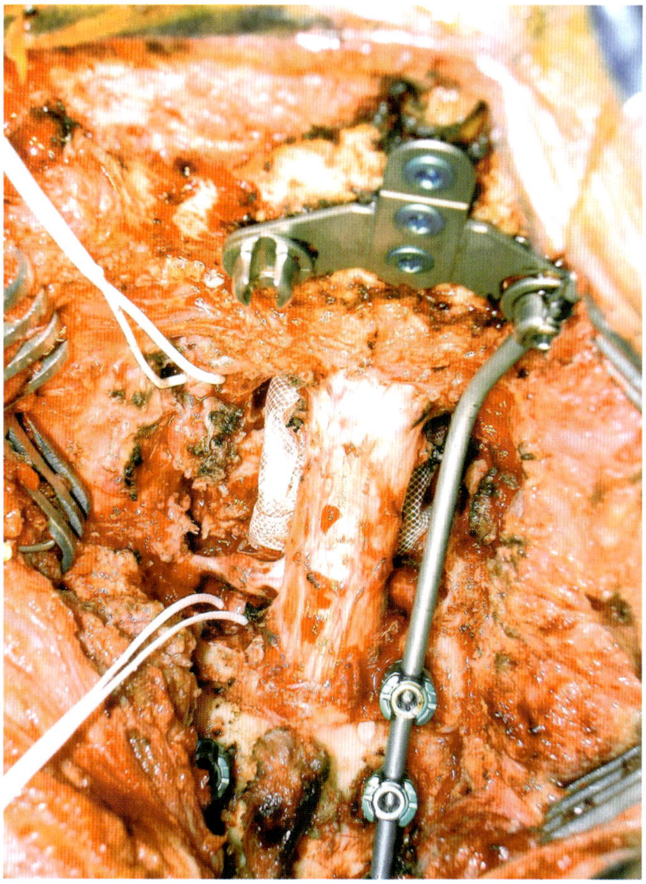

Fig. 10.2 The posterior cervical approach showing isolation of the vertebral artery with vessel loops.

If the rostral aspect of the tumor extends above the C2-C3 disk space, a rostral osteotomy should be attempted from the posterior approach. The region can be accessed by creating a corridor through the C1 lateral mass; the base of the odontoid can then be cut. If the odontoid needs to be delivered as part of the specimen, the transverse ligaments can be cut as they enter the tubercles of C1. The apical ligament can be sectioned at the tip of the odontoid or base of the clivus through an access area created by resecting the lateral mass of C1. Osteotomies rostral to the odontoid for delivery of tumors involving C1 have not yet been described. A rostral osteotomy above the C2-C3 disk space can be performed through a ventral approach but will require some form of a transpharyngeal approach. Given the potential need for postoperative high-dose radiation therapy (proton beam irradiation), this corridor should be avoided because it can present significant problems with pharyngeal dehiscence (**Fig. 10.3**).

Posterior instrumentation is placed to stabilize the spine in anticipation of a complete craniocervical dissociation created by the ventral approach. Some form of occipitocervical or occipitocervicothoracic instrumentation will be needed to provide stability after such a destabilizing procedure. The construct should be designed so that it can withstand significant stress, even if an arthrodesis fails to be achieved. A graft can be placed posteriorly during this stage of the operation or can be later placed after completion of the tumor resection with reopening the posterior wound.

A ventral approach will be needed to complete the transverse osteotomies. If the rostral osteotomy was completed through the posterior approach, then only the caudal osteotomy will need to be completed. If the rostral osteotomy is at C2-C3 or below, then this osteotomy can be completed through a ventral approach without a transpharyngeal approach. Transverse osteotomies are usually performed through the disk space at the margin to the tumor resection. The entire disk needs to be removed, and the posterior longitudinal ligament needs to be completely sectioned as well.

After the transverse osteotomies are completed, the tumor specimen is mobile and the second stage (delivery of the specimen) can be completed (**Fig. 10.4**). The specimen is delivered away from the spinal cord, and care is taken to maintain the integrity of the remaining neurovascular structures.

Once the specimen has been delivered, the anterior reconstruction is performed. If the rostral osteotomy is at or below the C2-C3 disk space, then the anterior

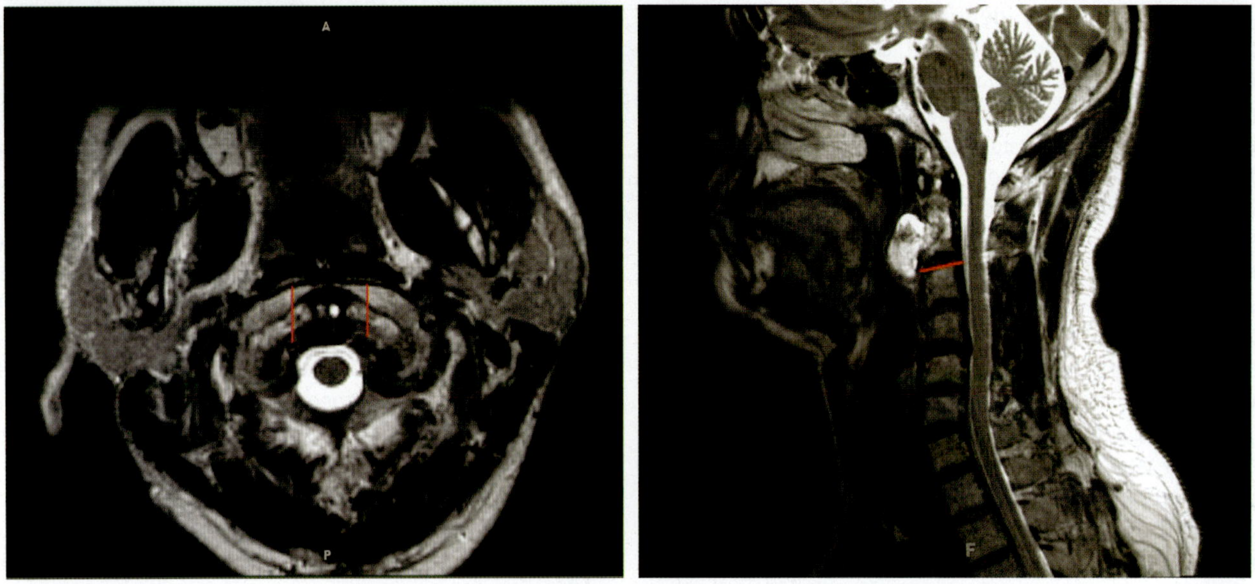

A B

Fig. 10.3 Magnetic resonance images showing planned osteotomies (*red lines*) in the **(A)** axial plane at the transverse ligament and **(B)** sagittal plane at the C2-C3 disk space.

reconstruction is relatively straightforward and can be accomplished with a cage and plate. We tend not to use structural allograft for the anterior reconstruction because we are concerned that there can be resorption of the graft and anterior failure when this technique is used with postoperative radiation therapy. The benefit of cages needs to be balanced against the artifact that will be produced that can make future surveillance MRIs difficult to interpret. If possible, nonmetallic constructs, such as polyetheretherketone (PEEK) or carbon fiber, are used to minimize this problem. When the rostral osteotomy extends beyond the C2-C3 disk space, an anterior reconstruction can be less than satisfying. Custom cages can be placed under the lateral masses of C1 and secured to the anterior arch of C1. In primary tumor surgery, this technique is not ideal because a transpharyngeal approach is needed to place the screws into the anterior arch of C1. To circumvent this problem, we incorporate cages that are placed with a posterior approach. The posterior incision is reopened, and cages are placed from the lateral mass of C1 or condyle down to the remaining lateral mass, caudal to the tumor resection. The cage can be secured by placing lateral mass screws through the cage and attaching it to the posterior instrumentation (**Fig. 10.5**). This construct has proved to be quite robust and redistributes the force created by the head through the cervical spine.

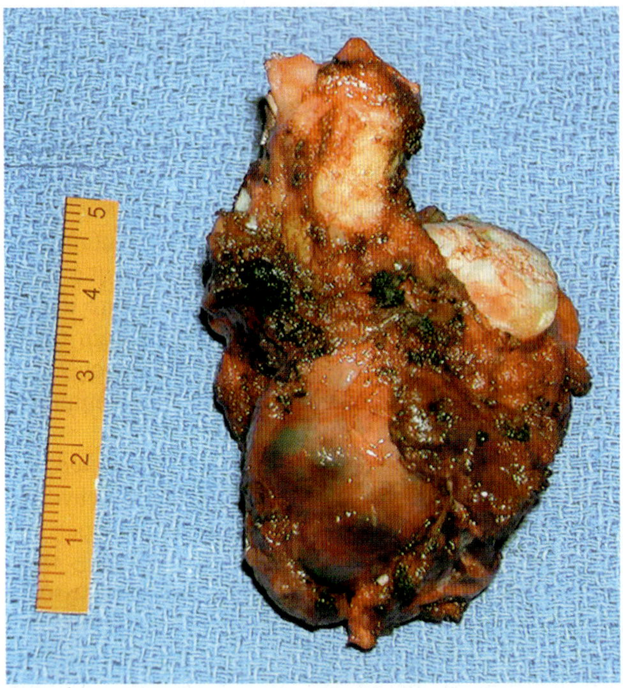

Fig. 10.4 Photograph of the specimen removed en bloc.

The goals of treatment of metastatic disease at the CVJ are distinct from those of primary bony tumors. Metastatic disease treatment pursues palliation of pain and preservation of neurological function. Metastatic tumors at C1 and C2 tend to develop in the ventral aspect of the spine, causing problems by creating spinal instability, which eventually can lead to C1-C2 subluxation and spinal cord compression. The C1-C2 region is quite unique, and unlike other ventral areas of the spine, direct extension of tumor into the dura and spinal cord does not usually occur. The tectorial membrane, transverse ligament, apical ligaments, and cruciate ligaments create a thick and broad barrier that prevents direct extension of the tumor to the dura. This unique anatomy can be an advantage when treating

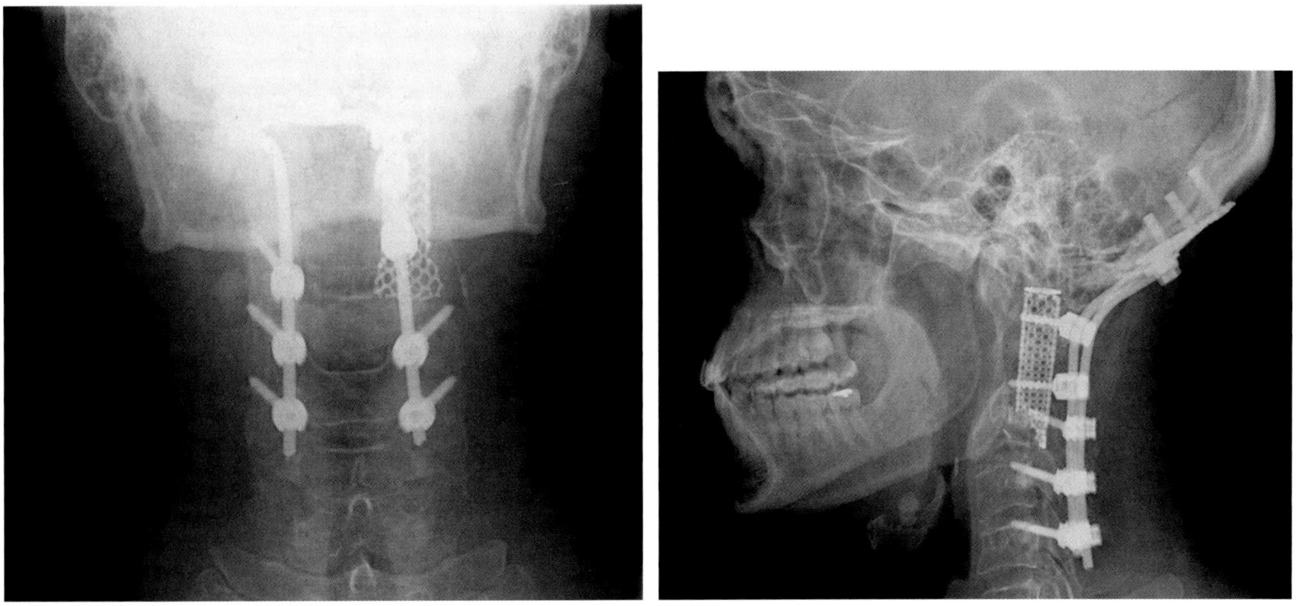

A B

Fig. 10.5 Radiographs following resection showing reconstruction with cage and rod-screw construct in the **(A)** anteroposterior view and **(B)** lateral view.

metastatic tumors of this region. Posterior stabilization, reduction, and postoperative radiation treatment will usually treat these lesions optimally (**Fig. 10.6**). If the ligamentous structures of the CVJ have been previously violated surgically as with a recurrent primary bony tumor, then a ventral resection of the tumor will be required to achieve decompression.

Destruction of the ventral bony structures of the spine can result in instability in the form of C1-C2 subluxation. If it progresses, it can lead to basilar invagination. Correction of this deformity can be performed preoperatively with cranial traction and close monitoring or can be achieved intraoperatively with direct, open reduction of the deformity. Preoperative cranial traction can help to reduce the deformity, but maintaining the alignment while positioning for posterior stabilization can be a challenge. If the alignment is restored and the reduction is retained during positioning, the operation proceeds with a posterior stabilization. Although the instability usually arises from destruction of the C2, we tend to prefer an occipitocervical instrumentation and fusion over a limited construct. These patients will almost always receive postoperative radiation therapy as part of their treatment, and it is the authors' belief that a limited construct places the patient at high risk for failure and neurological decline in the event of a pseudoarthrosis. In addition, extensive instrumentation allows the integrity of the construct to persist, even in the face of progression of the tumor and further destruction of the bony architecture of the CVJ.

If a complete reduction is unable to be achieved or maintained preoperatively, then an intraoperative reduction is an option for treating the subluxation and spinal cord compression. During this procedure, the patient is placed prone on chest rolls and the head is secured to the table by a Mayfield head holder. The patient's neurological status is monitored with somatosensory and motor evoked responses, and a fluoroscopy unit is set up so that the reduction can be viewed as it proceeds. A standard posterior approach is performed. Occipitocervical instrumentation consisting of an occipital plate and lateral mass instrumentation is placed in the usual fashion. Two separate rods are contoured to span the construct. The ends of the rod that will be inserted into the occipital plate are left long. If basilar invagination is present, the rods are loosely attached to the cervical instrumentation and held in place with untightened locking nuts. The rostral ends of the rods are secured tightly to the occipital plate. Gentle distraction is then placed between the cervical instrumentation and the occipital plate bilaterally, reducing the basilar invagination (**Fig. 10.7A**). The cervical instrumentation is tightened to the rod. After reduction of the basilar invagination is completed, the nuts locking the rods to the plate are loosened. C-clamps are placed on the rods, rostral to the occipital plate. Bilateral compression is placed across the plate and the clamps, translating the cervical spine forward in relation to the skull, reducing the subluxation and decompressing the spinal cord (**Fig. 10.7B**). The nuts on the occipital plate are tightened, and the reduction is maintained. The rods are trimmed in situ with a rod cutter, and the arthrodesis is performed. Further decompression can be performed with a laminectomy, if necessary. A laminectomy will also allow evaluation of the spinal cord and ventral compression through intraoperative ultrasound.

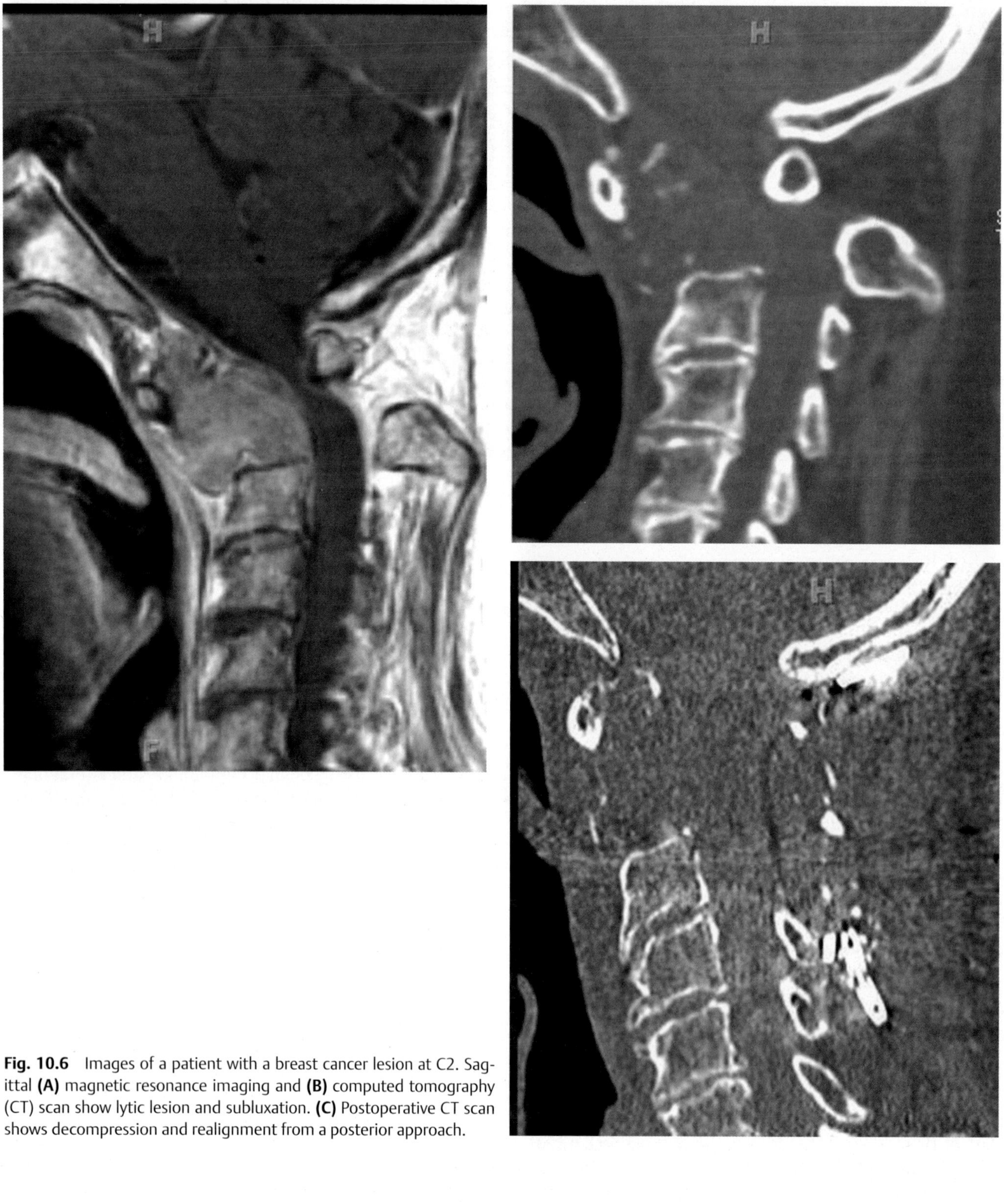

A B C

Fig. 10.6 Images of a patient with a breast cancer lesion at C2. Sagittal **(A)** magnetic resonance imaging and **(B)** computed tomography (CT) scan show lytic lesion and subluxation. **(C)** Postoperative CT scan shows decompression and realignment from a posterior approach.

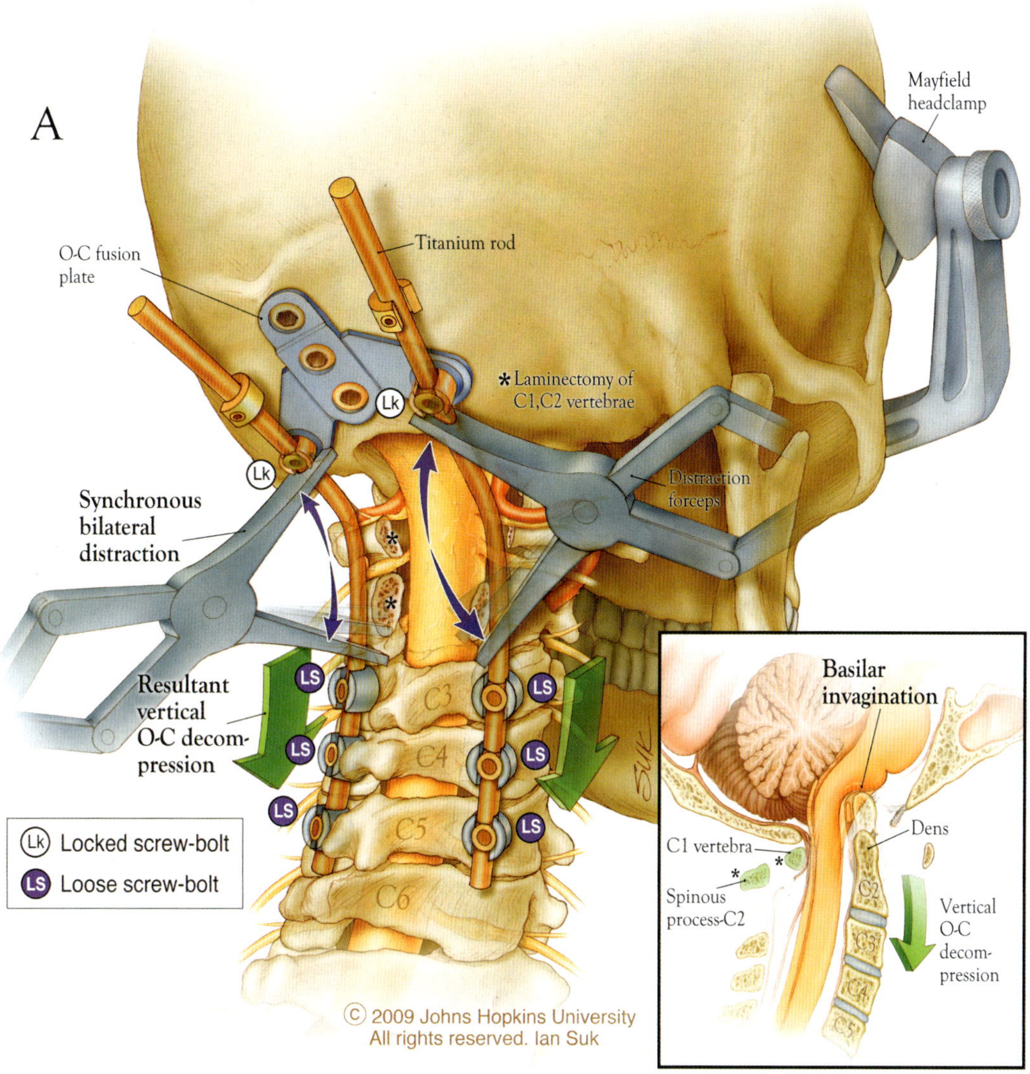

Fig. 10.7 **(A, B)** Illustrations of occipitocervical reduction via manipulation of occipitocervical instrumentation. (From Hsu W, Zaidi HA, Suk I, Gokaslan ZL, Wolinsky JP. A new technique for intraoperative reduction of occipitocervical instability. Neurosurgery 2010;66(2):319–324. Reprinted with permission from Ian Suk, Johns Hopkins University.) *(continued)*

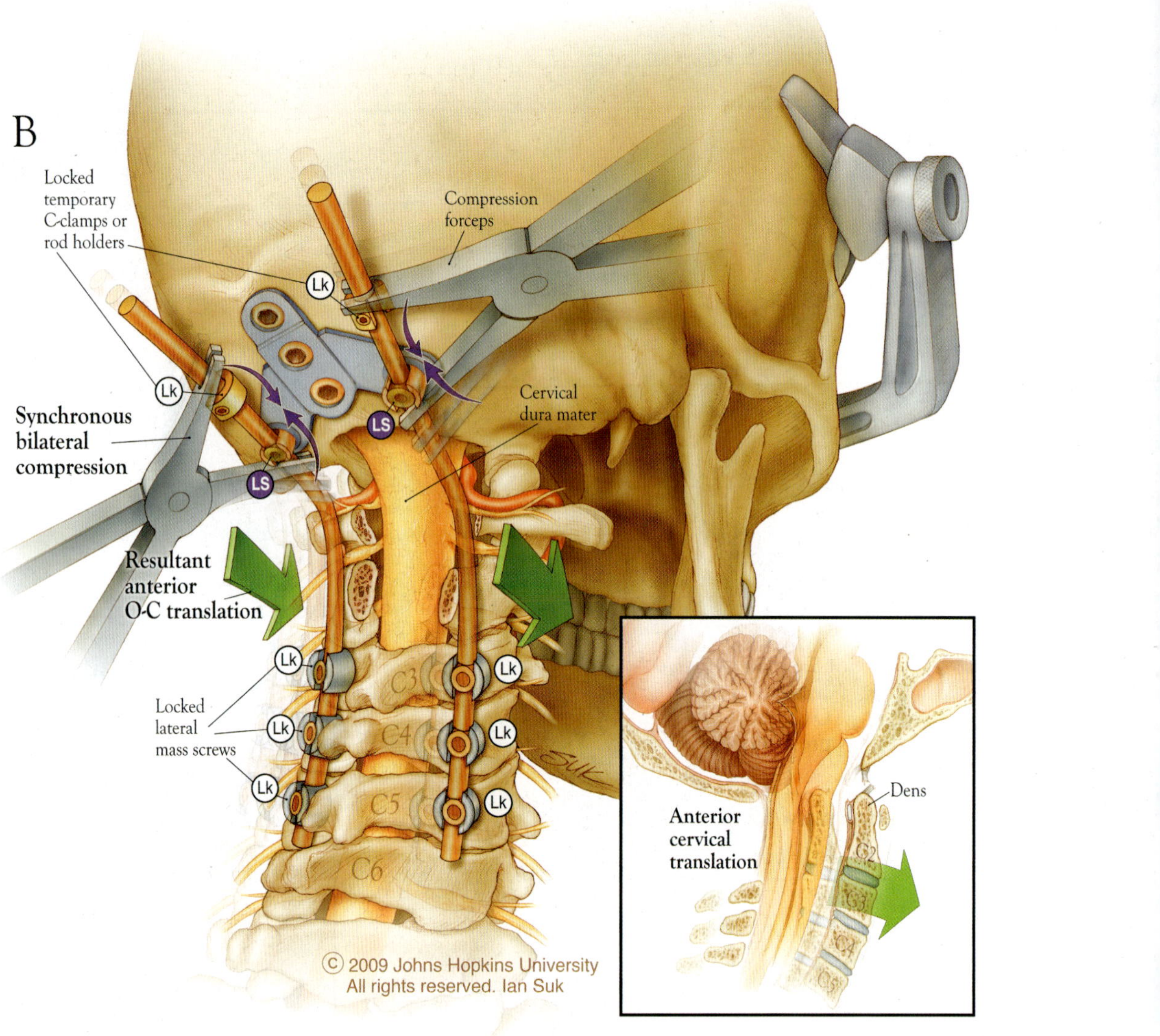

Fig. 10.7 *(continued)*

References

1. Moulding HD, Bilsky MH. Metastases to the craniovertebral junction. Neurosurgery 2010;66(3, Suppl):113–118
2. Sen C, Shrivastava R, Anwar S, Triana A. Lateral transcondylar approach for tumors at the anterior aspect of the craniovertebral junction. Neurosurgery 2010;66(3, Suppl):104–112
3. Menezes AH, Traynelis VC, Fenoy AJ, Gantz BJ, Kralik SF, Donovan KA. Honored guest presentation: surgery at the crossroads: craniocervical neoplasms. Clin Neurosurg 2005;52:218–228
4. American Cancer Society. Cancer Facts and Figures. Atlanta, GA: American Cancer Society; 2005
5. York JE, Wildrick DM, Gokaslan ZL. Metastatic tumors. In: Benzel EC, Stillerman CB, eds. The Thoracic Spine. St. Louis, MO: Quality Medical Publishing; 1999:392–411
6. Sciubba DM, Gokaslan ZL. Diagnosis and management of metastatic spine disease. Surg Oncol 2006;15(3):141–151
7. Sundaresan N, Boriani S, Rothman A, Holtzman R. Tumors of the osseous spine. J Neurooncol 2004;69(1-3):273–290
8. Sherk HH. Lesions of the atlas and axis. Clin Orthop Relat Res 1975;(109):33–41
9. George B, Lot G, Velut S, Gelbert F, Mourier KL. [French language Society of Neurosurgery. 44th Annual Congress. Brussels, 8-12 June 1993. Tumors of the foramen magnum]. Neurochirurgie 1993;39(Suppl 1):1–89
10. Arguello F, Baggs RB, Duerst RE, Johnstone L, McQueen K, Frantz CN. Pathogenesis of vertebral metastasis and epidural spinal cord compression. Cancer 1990;65(1):98–106
11. Dickman CA, Spetzler RF, Sonntag VKH. Surgery of the Craniovertebral Junction. New York, NY: Thieme Medical Publishers, Inc.; 1998:828
12. Chi JH, Bydon A, Hsieh P, Witham T, Wolinsky JP, Gokaslan ZL. Epidemiology and demographics for primary vertebral tumors. Neurosurg Clin N Am 2008;19(1):1–4

13. Donthineni R. Diagnosis and staging of spine tumors. Orthop Clin North Am 2009;40(1):1–7, v
14. Sciubba DM, Gallia GL, McGirt MJ, et al. Thoracic kyphotic deformity reduction with a distractible titanium cage via an entirely posterior approach. Neurosurgery 2007;60(4, Suppl 2):223–230, discussion 230–231
15. Sundaresan N, Rosen G, Boriani S. Primary malignant tumors of the spine. Orthop Clin North Am 2009;40(1):21–36, v
16. Aebi M, Arlet V, Webb JK. AO Spine Manual Clinical Applications. Vol 2. New York, NY: Thieme Medical Publishers; 2007:215–233
17. Bilsky MH, Azeem S. Multiple myeloma: primary bone tumor with systemic manifestations. Neurosurg Clin N Am 2008; 19(1):31–40
18. Sciubba DM, Chi JH, Rhines LD, Gokaslan ZL. Chordoma of the spinal column. Neurosurg Clin N Am 2008;19(1):5–15
19. Singh H, Harrop J, Schiffmacher P, Rosen M, Evans J. Ventral surgical approaches to craniovertebral junction chordomas. Neurosurgery 2010;66(3, Suppl):96–103
20. McLoughlin GS, Sciubba DM, Wolinsky JP. Chondroma/chondrosarcoma of the spine. Neurosurg Clin N Am 2008;19(1):57–63
21. Grier HE, Krailo MD, Tarbell NJ, et al. Addition of ifosfamide and etoposide to standard chemotherapy for Ewing's sarcoma and primitive neuroectodermal tumor of bone. N Engl J Med 2003; 348(8):694–701
22. Burch S, Hu S, Berven S. Aneurysmal bone cysts of the spine. Neurosurg Clin N Am 2008;19(1):41–47
23. Luther N, Bilsky MH, Härtl R. Giant cell tumor of the spine. Neurosurg Clin N Am 2008;19(1):49–55
24. Kan P, Schmidt MH. Osteoid osteoma and osteoblastoma of the spine. Neurosurg Clin N Am 2008;19(1):65–70

11 Primary Extramedullary Tumors of the Craniovertebral Junction

Kadir Erkmen, Kimon Bekelis, and Ossama Al-Mefty

Extramedullary tumors of the craniovertebral junction (CVJ), such as meningiomas, schwannomas, and chordomas, include a wide variety of pathological processes. By definition, tumors that occur at the CVJ involve the foramen magnum, which is a ring-shaped structure that allows passage of neurovascular structures between the brain and the spinal cord. Within the foramen magnum are the brainstem, rostral spinal cord, vertebral arteries and branches, and lower cranial nerves. Tumors can be located anywhere in the ring; thus, surgical approaches to this region need to be tailored to the location of the mass. Posterior tumors of the foramen magnum can be treated safely with standard posterior suboccipital approaches. Once tumors involve the lateral and ventral aspects of the foramen, ventral and lateral approaches are required for safe surgery. Skull base approaches allow access to the tumor without the need for mobilization or retraction of neural structures. The surgeon should be familiar with all approaches to allow optimization of surgery for each patient and each tumor. A commonly used lateral approach is the transcondylar approach, often referred to as the far lateral approach. This approach can be modified based on the location and involvement of the lesion being treated. The extent of condylar removal is dependent on factors such as the patient's anatomy, location of tumor, and preoperative bony involvement. This chapter focuses on the transcondylar skull base approach and its variations.

■ Anatomy

The foramen magnum is made up of the occipital bone, which forms an oval ring (**Fig. 11.1**). The anterior part of the ring is made from the lowest extension of the clivus. The occipital condyles lie in the anterior half of the foramen, allowing access to ventrally located tumor if the condyle is partially removed. The hypoglossal canal traverses the occipital condyle approximately halfway and travels in an anterior to posterior, medial to lateral trajectory as it courses from the intracranial compartment outward. Lateral to the occipital condyle is the jugular foramen, which is posterior to the carotid canal. The stylomastoid foramen and process lie lateral to the jugular foramen. The posterior belly of the digastric muscle attaches at the digastric notch and lies over the facial nerve at its exit point. The condylar vein enters the jugular bulb through the foramen posterior and lateral to the occipital condyle.

■ History

In the past, primary extramedullary tumors of the CVJ have been difficult to diagnose. Their insidious onset and often bizarre symptoms may resemble those of degenerative diseases of the central nervous system (CNS). The clinical course may simulate cervical spondylosis, multiple sclerosis, syringomyelia, or congenital skull base disorders, such as platybasia or Arnold-Chiari malformation. Symptoms may arise only after lesions have grown to a significant size due to the generous subarachnoid spaces of the cervicomedullary junction. The insidious course of these neoplasms can be explained by the anatomical complexity of the area and the decussation of the neural tracts at that level.[1,2]

The first systematic evaluation of tumors of the foramen magnum was done by Elsberg in 1925.[3] Other significant early contributions were made by Abrahamson and Grossman[4] and Elsberg and Strauss.[5] They emphasized the clinical pattern of compression of the cord at the foramen magnum. Further elaboration was provided by Symonds and Meadows.[6] In their 1938 monograph on meningiomas, Cushing and Eisenhardt discussed the compressive nature of spinal cord lesions of the foramen magnum.[7] They divided foramen magnum meningiomas into two subgroups: craniospinal and spinocranial. Craniospinal tumors arise above the foramen magnum ventral to the neuraxis and project downward, displacing the medulla and cervical spinal cord. Spinocranial lesions are found dorsal or dorsolateral to the spinal cord and project upward into the cerebellar cisterns. A posterior fossa syndrome caused by tumors of this region was documented by Castellano and Ruggiero.[8] Their classification was based on the dural site of attachment. Stein and colleagues described 25 cases of mostly spinocranial meningiomas with a stereotypic clinical syndrome.[9]

The first large series of intra- and extra-axial tumors of the CVJ was reported in 1941 by Love and Adson.[10] Later, Love revealed that 30% of lesions were extramedullary tumors amenable to surgical resection.[11] Subsequent reviews limited to benign intradural extramedullary lesions were reported by Dodge and colleagues,[12] Martin and Kleyntjens, and others.[13–15] Yasuoka and colleagues analyzed 57 cases of neurofibromas and meningiomas of the foramen magnum and reported a ratio of 19 neuromas to 37 meningiomas, which was larger than the previously reported ratio.[12,15,16] Meyer reviewed 102 cases of benign extramedullary tumors of the foramen magnum seen between 1924 and 1982.[17] He reported that 40% of these patients had a normal

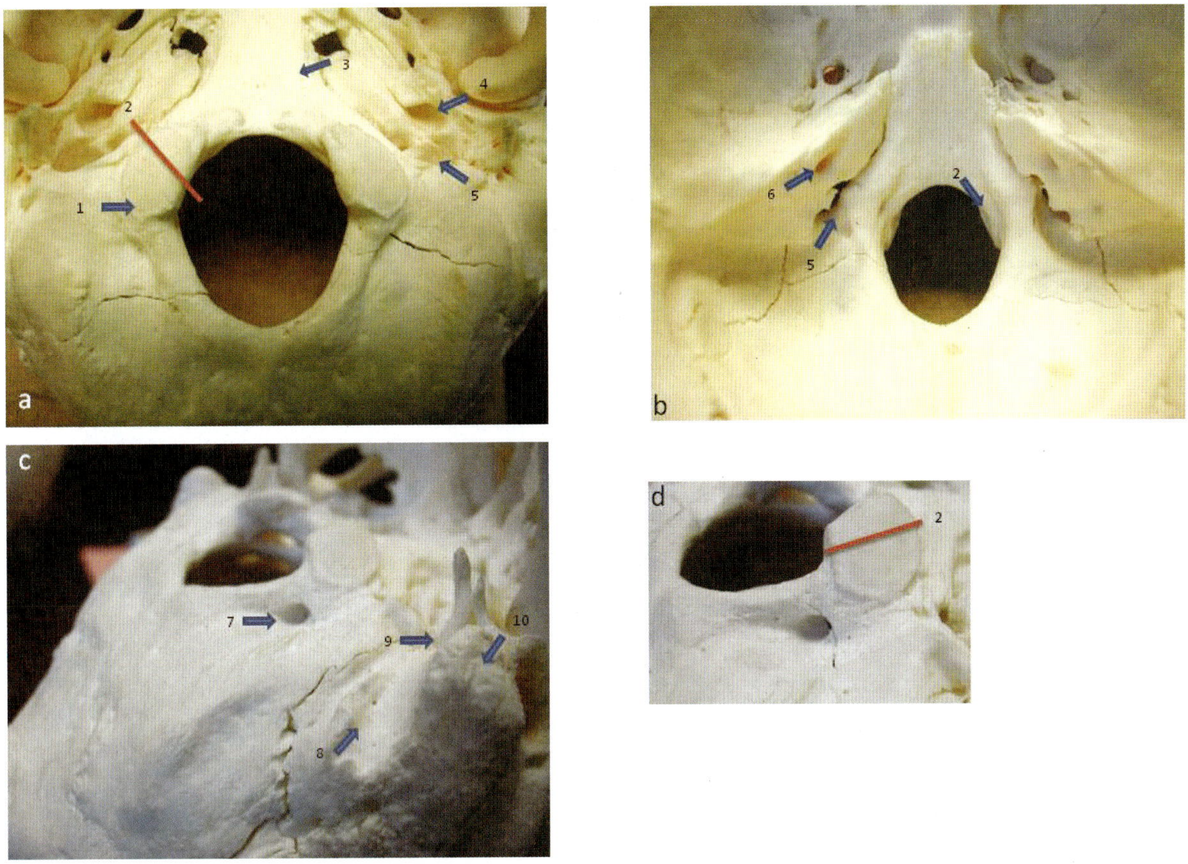

Fig. 11.1 **(A)** Inferior view of the skull demonstrates the oval-shaped ring of the foramen magnum and location of the occipital condyle in the ventral half of the foramen. **(B)** Superior view of the foramen magnum with foramina consists of the internal auditory canal, hypoglossal canal, and jugular foramen. **(C)** Lateral view of the foramen magnum demonstrates the relationship to the mastoid process, stylomastoid foramen, and digastric muscle. **(D)** Higher magnification lateral view demonstrates the course of the hypoglossal canal. *1*, occipital condyle; *2*, course of the hypoglossal canal and nerve; *3*, clivus; *4*, carotid canal; *5*, jugular foramen; *6*, internal auditory canal; *7*, condylar foramen and vein; *8*, digastric notch; *9*, stylomastoid foramen and process; *10*, mastoid process.

neurological examination at first evaluation and that there were no pathognomonic symptoms or physical findings to identify foramen magnum tumors. More recently, Arnautovic and colleagues have supported with their data the efficacy of the transcondylar approach in the resection of foramen magnum meningiomas.[18] Wu and colleagues reported the comparative effectiveness of different surgical techniques in the resection of foramen magnum meningiomas in their group of 114 patients.[19] In the largest series published to date, Menezes has reported his group's experience with CVJ neoplasms in a database of 888 patients seen between 1977 and 2003.[20]

Epidemiology

In an analysis of the University of Iowa Hospitals and Clinics Neurosurgery CVJ registry, 888 patients were evaluated between 1977 and 2003.[20] Of these patients, 382 presented with osseous tumors, 426 had neural tumors, and 179 were treated surgically. A review of several series on the incidence of benign intradural extramedullary tumors of the foramen magnum yielded several cases between 1929 and 2010.[4,17–22] About 75% of these tumors were meningiomas, occurring in a 3:1 ratio to schwannomas. Rare cases of dermoid tumors, teratomas, lipomas, schwannomas, arachnoid cysts, paragangliomas, and intradural extraosseous chordomas have also been encountered. Intramedullary tumors at the cervicomedullary junction include astrocytomas, ependymomas, and cerebellar region tumors such as hemangioblastomas, medulloblastomas, and choroid plexus papillomas. Chordomas, chondromas, chondrosarcomas, and metastases are common extradural intraosseous tumors.

In adults, meningiomas (**Figs. 11.2** and **11.3**) are some of the most common tumors of the foramen magnum.[20] As with other meningiomas of the neuraxis, there is a definite female predominance for meningiomas of the foramen magnum, with ratios from 2:1 to 3.6:1.[8,17,21–23] These lesions usually become symptomatic in the fourth, fifth, and sixth decades of life.[20] The average age of diagnosis reported in a large series is 50.1 years.[20] Lesions are usually located ventrally or ventrolaterally,[20,24] attached to

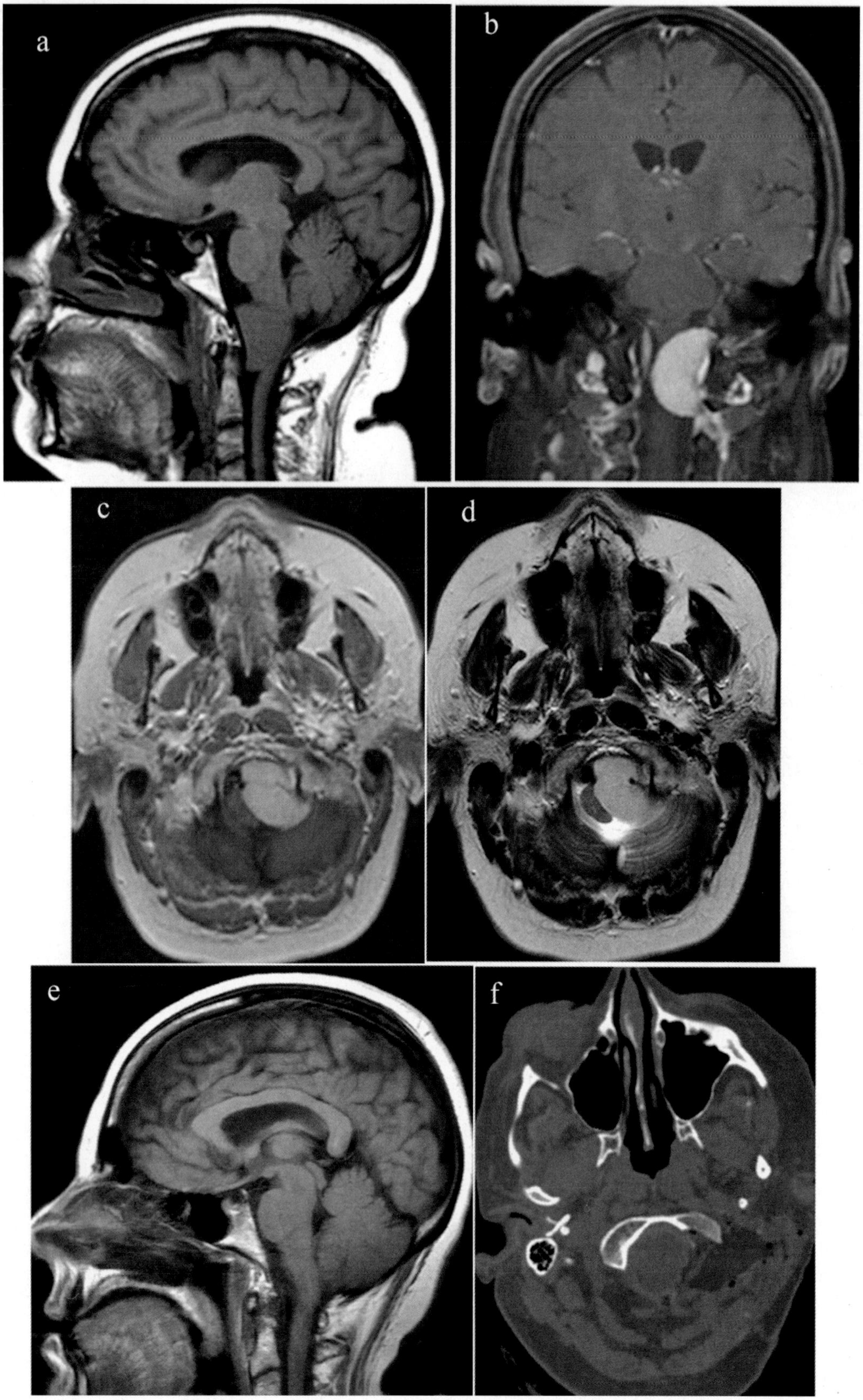

Fig. 11.2 **(A)** Precontrast T1-weighted sagittal magnetic resonance imaging (MRI) demonstrates tumor and brainstem compression associated with a foramen magnum meningioma. **(B)** Postcontrast T1-weighted coronal MRI is shown with homogeneous contrast enhancement. **(C)** Postcontrast T1-weighted axial MRI demonstrates brainstem compression and vascular encasement. **(D)** T2-weighted axial MRI demonstrates the iso- to hyperintense appearance of the meningioma as well as vascular encasement. **(E)** Postoperative sagittal MRI demonstrates complete resection of the tumor through a transcondylar approach. **(F)** Axial computed tomography slice shows the area of condylar removal, allowing ventral access for safe removal of the tumor.

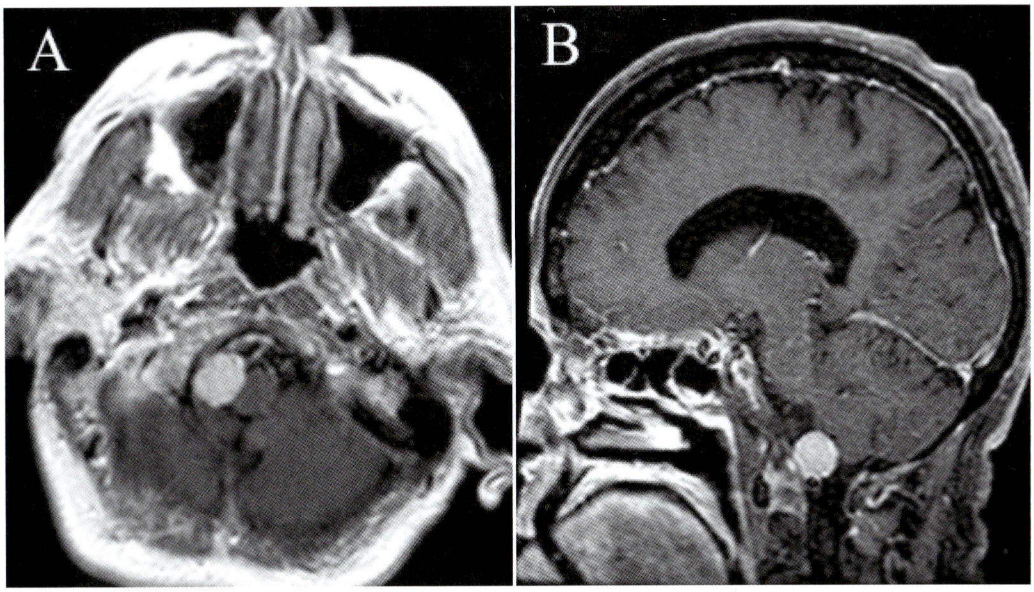

Fig. 11.3 (A,B) In this laterally placed meningioma of the foramen magnum, occipital condyle resection may not be necessary for safe removal due to the location of the tumor in the foramen magnum ring.

the anterior rim of the foramen magnum, and frequently invade the area of the vertebral artery and the exit of the cervical nerve roots.

The occurrence of schwannomas (**Fig. 11.4**) at the region of the foramen magnum is less common than meningiomas in adults.[24] The literature describes the incidence of schwannomas of the CVJ at ~13%. These benign tumors often grow to considerable size before neurological abnormalities manifest. They are seen with roughly equal frequency in men and women. The distribution of patient ages at the time of presentation ranges from adolescence to the seventh decade. In a large series, the average age of presentation was 38 years.[20] Levy and colleagues reported 66 cases of spinal schwannomas, of which 30% were located in the cervical region.[25] Approximately 50% of these tumors are located ventral to the craniospinal axis. Tumors such as chordomas (**Fig. 11.5**), chondrosarcomas, glomus jugulare tumors, and metastases are occasionally observed in this region as well. They are located ventrolateral to the neural structures and are frequently encased in the caudal cranial nerves or vertebral artery.

The epidemiology of the lesions of the CVJ is significantly different in the pediatric population. Menezes has reported chordomas to be the most common tumor of the CVJ in his series of 38 pediatric patients.[1,25–30] Chordomas in children have a slight male predominance with a peak occurrence at 121 months of age.[31] These tumors appear to be very aggressive, with a 68.5% mortality in 25 months, as reported by Borba.[31] By the time chordomas are diagnosed in children, they are usually of a prohibitive size for surgical intervention. However, multidisciplinary treatment of these tumors, including radiation therapy, has resulted in disease-free survival as high as 68% at 5 years.

The second most frequently encountered type of tumor in Menezes' series was meningiomas.[1] In general, meningiomas are rare in children and adolescents, comprising less than 2% of all pediatric intracranial lesions.[27,28] Only a few case series of meningiomas in pediatric patients arising in the region of the foramen magnum exist.[29,30] The operative management of pediatric patients with foramen magnum lesions via the transcondylar approach is similar to that of adults and presents no additional problems. Schwannomas are also encountered in the CVJ, especially in children with familial syndromes. Children with neurofibromatosis type I tend to become symptomatic with multiple bilateral lesions, including plexiform neurofibromas.[1] Most of these lesions occur in a dorsal location, making them easily accessible. Other rare extramedullary lesions of the CVJ encountered in children include fibrous dysplasia of the CVJ, aneurysmal bone cyst, eosinophilic granuloma, primary Ewing sarcoma, and osteoblastoma.[1]

Clinical Presentation

Extramedullary tumors of the foramen magnum may pose a diagnostic dilemma. Their symptoms can be peculiar and fail to fit classic localized findings. They can be intermittent, progressive, and remitting.[1,3–5,7,10,13–19,24,26–52] Diagnosis is often delayed for several years because of these clinical peculiarities. Signs and symptoms can include headaches, occipital radicular pain, cervical pain, phrenic nerve paralysis, lower cranial nerve palsies, hyperreflexia, downbeat nystagmus, atrophy of limb muscles, paralysis of limbs, sensory deficits, cerebellar deficits, sphincter disturbances, Horner syndrome, papilledema, and endocrinopathies.[1,3–5,7,10,13–19,26–52]

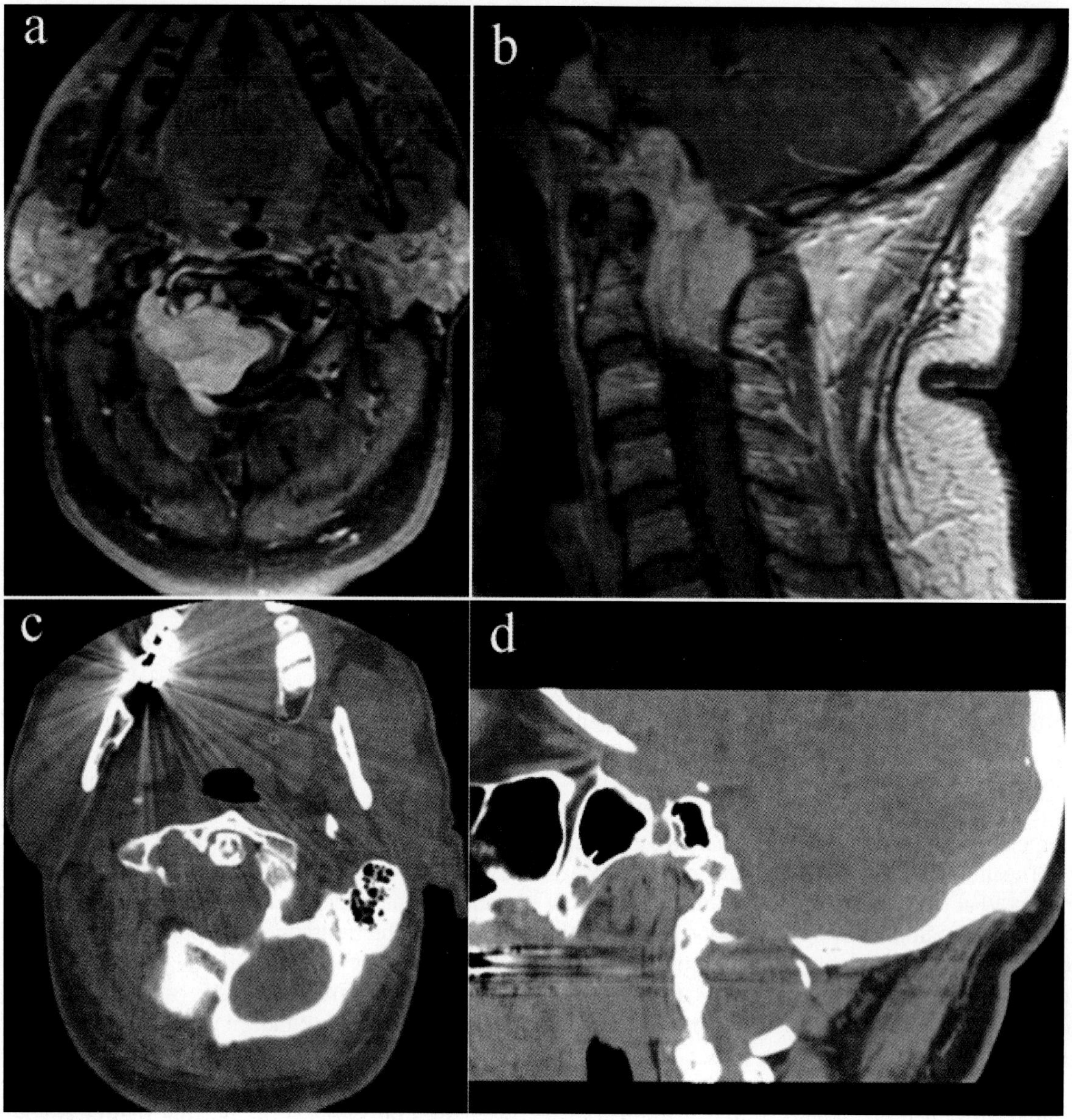

Fig. 11.4 (A,B) Postcontrast T1-weighted magnetic resonance images demonstrate an upper cervical nerve root schwannoma crossing the craniovertebral junction. **(C,D)** Preoperative computed tomography scans demonstrate the bony remodeling as a result of the schwannoma. The scalloping of the bone results in a bony exposure (similar to a transcondylar approach) and in enlargement of the C1 neural foramen.

The most frequent symptom, observed in up to 70% of the patients in a large series, is pain in the C2 nerve root distribution, followed by paresthesias (40% of patients) and cranial nerve palsies (30% of patients), usually manifesting as dysarthria or dysphagia.[21] Children tend to present with involvement of the lower cranial nerves, brainstem dysfunction, and occasionally cerebellar symptoms. They usually maintain their head in a flexed position, resembling torticollis at times.[1]

Supported by classical teaching, partial lesions in this area interrupt decussating pyramidal tract fibers destined for the legs. These fibers cross below those of the arms, resulting in a crural paresis of the lower limbs. Compressive lesions near the foramen magnum may produce weakness of the ipsilateral shoulder and arm followed by weakness of the ipsilateral leg, then the contralateral leg, and finally the contralateral arm (an "around the clock" pattern that may begin in any of the limbs). However, this phenomenon was observed only in 22% of the patients in a large series.[21]

Meningiomas of the foramen magnum are usually symptomatic from involvement of the vertebrobasilar system as well as cranial nerves IX through XII, especially affecting the spinal accessory nerve. Pain and paresthesias are the major symptoms in patients with schwannomas of the foramen magnum. Menezes reports a lower cranial nerve deficit in 38% and myelopathy in 50% of these patients.[21]

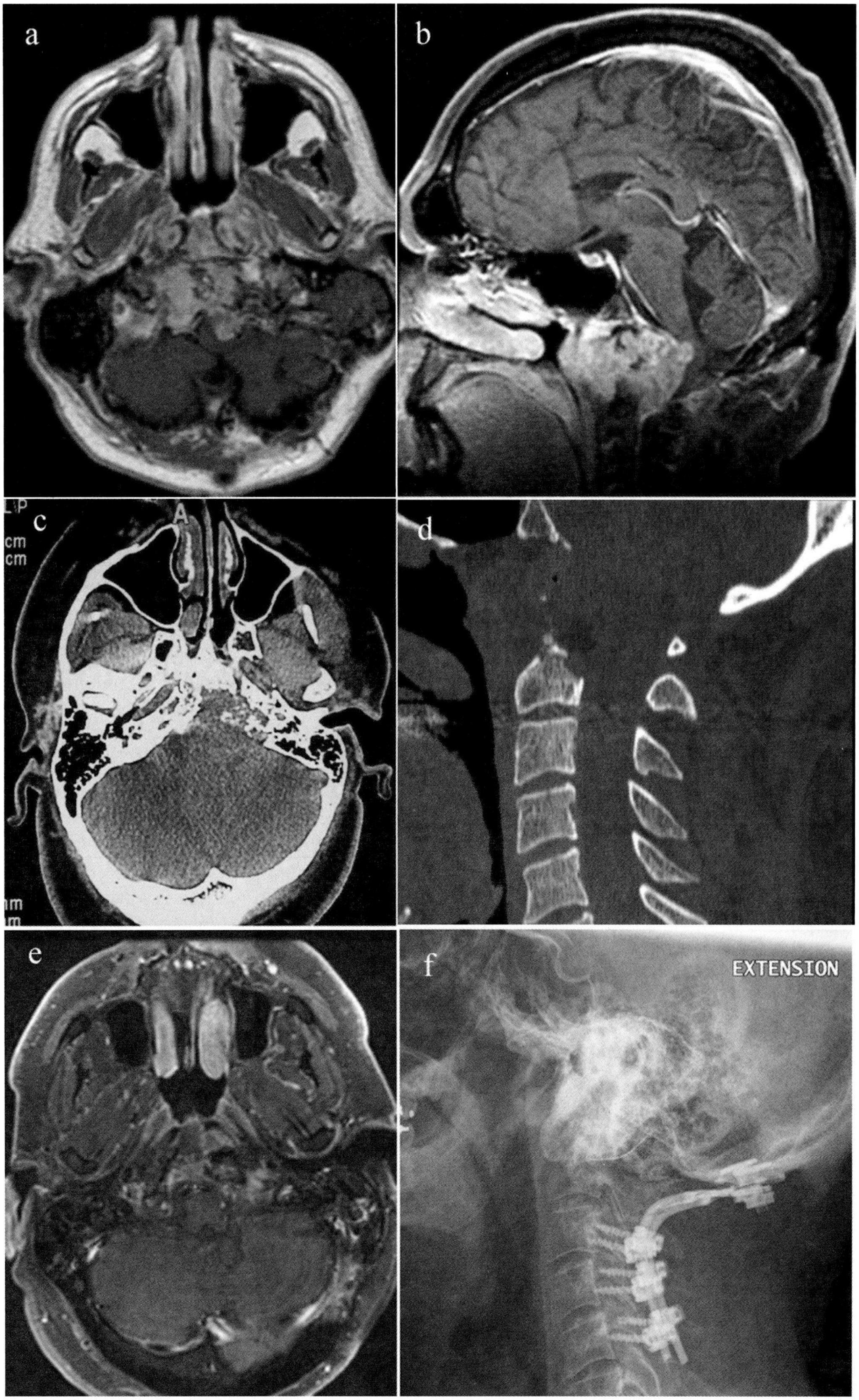

Fig. 11.5 Postcontrast T1-weighted magnetic resonance images (MRI) in **(A)** axial and **(B)** sagittal planes demonstrate the contrast-enhancing mass with brainstem compression in a chordoma. Computed tomography scans in **(C)** axial and **(D)** sagittal reconstructed views demonstrate the bony erosion caused by the tumor. The clivus, anterior arch of C1, and odontoid process have all been enveloped by the tumor. Stipples of calcium represent bone trapped in the tumor mass. **(E)** Postoperative T1-weighted postcontrast MRI demonstrates complete resection of the enhancing mass with elimination of brainstem compression and restoration of brainstem anatomy. **(F)** Lateral radiograph demonstrates the occipitocervical instrumentation used postoperatively to stabilize the spine for fusion.

Operative Techniques

The region of the foramen magnum is the site of many intradural and extradural tumors. Most intradural extramedullary lesions are meningiomas and schwannomas, and most are located anterior to the neuraxis. Malignant lesions such as chordomas, chondrosarcomas, metastases, and glomus jugulare tumors are extradural tumors and frequently found anterior or anterolateral to the cervicomedullary junction. Previously, many surgical approaches have been used to gain access to the skull base for tumor removal. These routes have included transoral, transsphenoidal, transcervical, transbasal, infratemporal, transpetrosal, suboccipital, and retromastoid approaches.[53–61] However, considering the anatomy of the CVJ, there are three main access points:

1. Posterior access with the standard midline posterior approach is the simplest access point and does not destroy important structures, although it is limited to the posterior aspect of the CVJ.
2. Anterior access uses the variants of the transoral approach. At the depth of the mouth, only thin layers of mucosa and muscle are found before reaching the bone. However, anterior access is limited by exposure of the CNS to oral contents and by the difficulty in repairing dura and preventing spinal fluid leakage.
3. Lateral access is directed to the lateral wall of the CVJ and includes the jugular tubercle, occipital condyle, lateral mass of C1, and lateral part of the C2 vertebral body.[60]

The choice of surgical route is based on multiple factors: tumor location and extent of skull base involvement, tumor histology, tumor consistency, the relationship of the tumor to the dura and neurovascular elements, the goal of the operation (i.e., tissue biopsy for diagnosis versus complete resection), the patient's age, craniovertebral stability, and the effect of the lesion on the cord (i.e., syringomyelia). The anterior approaches are recommended for midline extradural tumors. Recently, the addition of flexible or rigid endoscopy with anterior techniques has aided diagnosis and treatment of these lesions. The posterior approaches are recommended for dorsal midline tumors, whereas the lateral (transcondylar) approach permits access to the area of the lower clivus and upper cervical spine and is useful for intradural lesions ventral to the foramen magnum.[53–61] Both extradural and intradural tumors can be extirpated, leaving neurovascular elements intact. This approach offers the advantage of a direct view to the anterior rim of the foramen magnum without requiring brainstem or cerebellar retraction. In fact, depending on whether the route to the CVJ passes posterior (far lateral approach) or anterior (extreme lateral approach) to the sternocleidomastoid muscle, the surgeon acquires access to the inside or outside part, respectively, of the bony canal. In the pediatric population with torticollis and radiographic evidence of rotary subluxation or atlantoaxial dislocation, the need for stabilization and fusion is obvious.[51]

Preoperative Evaluation

The appropriate surgical plan is developed after a complete neurological examination. Preoperative impairment of lower cranial nerve function is important for patient counseling about the possible need for postoperative tracheostomy or gastrostomy. Cardiac and pulmonary function should be assessed preoperatively.

A preoperative workup includes a radiographic examination. Standard X-rays are usually unrevealing, although they may be the first study ordered by primary care physicians in the workup of patients with neck pain. Meningiomas often demonstrate the following findings on plain radiographs: erosion and vascularity, hyperostosis, spicule formation, diffuse thickening, enlargement of meningeal channels, and calcification.[43] Neurofibromas and schwannomas may demonstrate enlarged foramina and scalloping of pedicles.

Computed tomography (CT) with intravenous contrast is routine in the radiographic evaluation of lesions at the cervicomedullary junction. Bone and soft tissue windows provide important planning information. A CT with contrast is diagnostic in 75% of patients with benign intradural extramedullary lesions. Meningiomas, schwannomas, and other tumors may be visualized on an enhanced CT. Bony changes associated with these tumors may allow one to differentiate them. Meningiomas often cause bony hyperostosis or thickening adjacent to the dural site of origin. They often will harbor calcifications within the tumor mass. Schwannomas typically cause bony remodeling, including thinning or scalloping of neural foramina. These tumors follow the course of the nerve of origin and can be dumbbell shaped, growing on both sides of the foramen. Chordomas are evident due to the bony destruction associated with these tumors. Aggressive bony replacement by tumor is common, often with erosion of the clivus, odontoid process, and occipital condyle. These tumors sometimes appear to have calcification, although this is likely calcium remnants within destroyed bony structures.

Magnetic resonance imaging (MRI) is required for all foramen magnum lesions. T1-weighted images demonstrate soft tissue displacement caused by the tumor. Meningiomas may appear isointense, slightly hyperintense, or slightly hypointense relative to normal brain tissue. On T2-weighted images, meningiomas generally show a hyperintense or isointense signal. Administration of the contrast agent gadolinium-diethylenetriamine pentaacetic acid (Gd-DTPA) demonstrates marked enhancement in meningiomas. Differentiation between meningiomas and schwannomas with gadolinium on T1-weighted studies may be possible due to their enhancing characteristics. In addition, schwannomas typically have hyperintense signal on T2-weighted images. The degree of bony erosion or tumor calcification is not well visualized with MRI but can be seen exquisitely with CT as discussed previously. MRI may also allow vascular elements to be evaluated. Arterial encasement, displacement, and occlusion can be seen readily on MRI. Also, the planned route for the surgical resection of the tumor can be aided by the fine detail provided by gadolinium-enhanced axial, coronal, and sagittal views.

Four-vessel cerebral angiography should be considered for patients suspected of having foramen magnum tumors. Angiography reveals the degree of tumor vascularity and its feeding vessels. Preoperative endovascular embolization techniques may be considered, although they are not required for most foramen magnum tumors. The position of major arterial vessels with respect to the tumor is paramount in tumor resection. Foramen magnum tumors often encase or displace the vertebral artery at its insertion into the dura, the posterior inferior cerebellar artery (PICA) at its origin, and the anterior spinal artery at its take-off from the vertebral artery intradurally.

Identification of the venous drainage pattern of the posterior fossa is also beneficial in planning surgical approaches. The side of dominance of the transverse and sigmoid sinuses, the connectivity of the deep and superficial drainage systems, and the height of the jugular bulb are important characteristics of the venous drainage that may alter surgical approaches. This may indicate the side of the surgical route. Patency of the jugular veins, sigmoid, and lateral sinuses and the torcula may be assessed with magnetic resonance (MR) venography without the need for catheter-based angiography in most cases. MR angiography may also be an adequate substitute for angiography, especially in cases where preoperative embolization is not considered. Vertebral and PICA aneurysms can present with foramen magnum syndromes and should be included in the differential diagnosis (**Fig. 11.6**). Identification of these aneurysms as vascular lesions is important preoperatively.

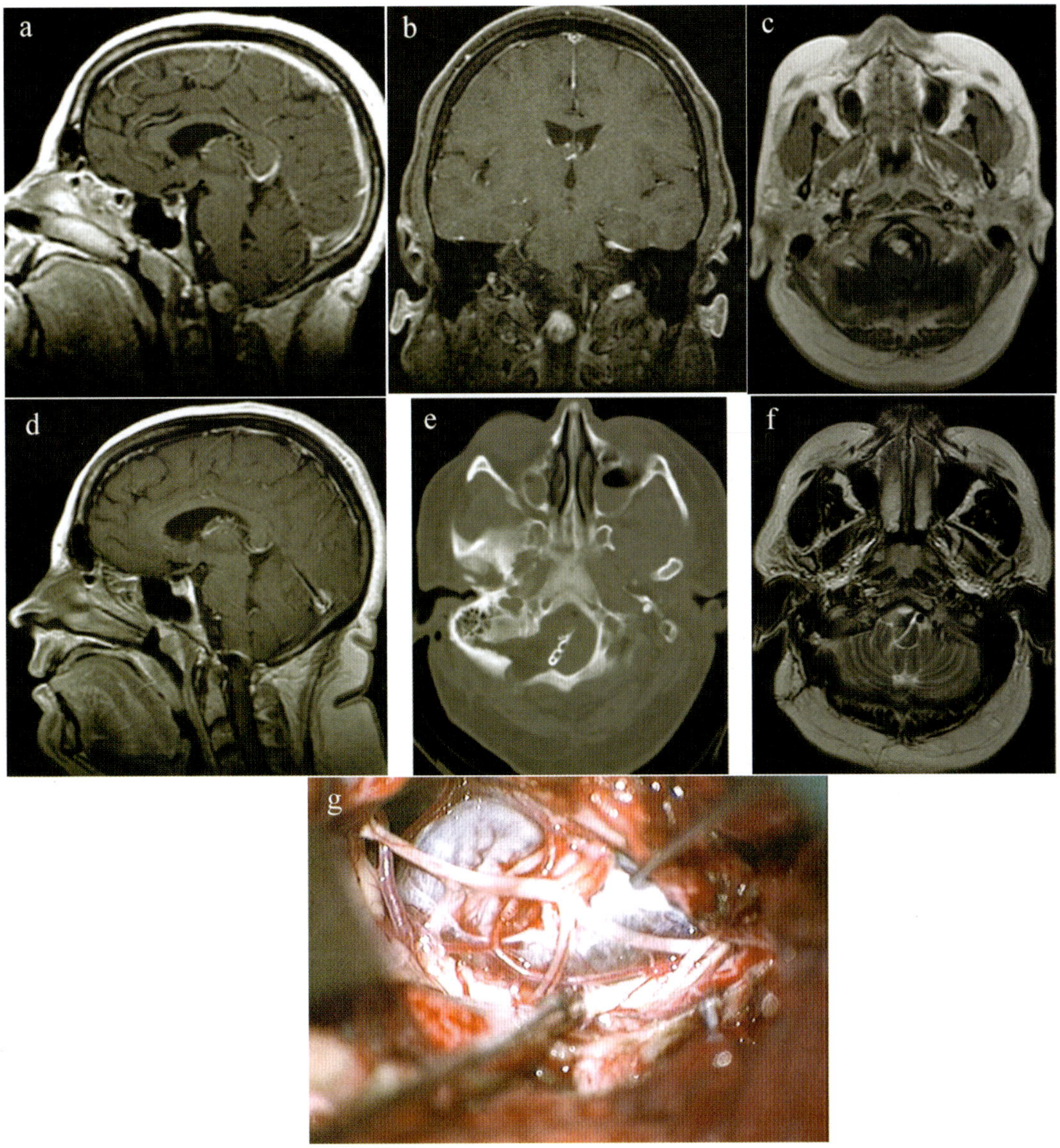

Fig. 11.6 Postcontrast magnetic resonance images in **(A)** sagittal, **(B)** coronal, and **(C)** axial planes demonstrate a vertebral aneurysm mimicking a foramen magnum tumor. **(D–F)** Postoperative images with clip applied to the aneurysm shows decompression of the brainstem. **(E)** A computed tomography image demonstrates the bony resection to allow a lateral approach. **(G)** Intraoperative photograph demonstrates the aneurysm ventral to the brainstem. The lateral transcondylar approach allows visualization ventral to the brainstem without retraction.

Preoperative Considerations

Perioperative considerations of foramen magnum tumors include the administration of corticosteroids immediately preoperatively as well as repeated doses during the surgery and postoperatively. The addition of corticosteroids may minimize brainstem and lower cranial nerve edema during tumor resection. Prophylactic antibiotics are given immediately preoperatively and continued postoperatively. Sequential compression pneumatic boots are used throughout the operation and continued postoperatively until the patient is ambulatory. Electrophysiological monitoring is essential for successful surgery in the foramen magnum. Motor evoked responses, somatosensory evoked responses, brainstem auditory evoked potentials, and lower cranial nerve electromyography signals are monitored during the operation.[62] The larynx can be monitored by intubating the patient using a specialized endotracheal tube that harbors monitoring electrodes. The anesthesiologist places the tube under direct visualization to allow the electrodes to sit at the larynx. Electrodes are also placed in the soft palate, pharynx, and tongue to allow monitoring of lower cranial nerve function. These can be placed safely after the patient is anesthetized, intubated, and positioned properly for surgery. Additional monitors, such as an intra-arterial catheter, central venous or right atrial catheter, and precordial Doppler probe, are used routinely.

Operative Procedure: Transcondylar Approach to Extramedullary Tumors of the Craniovertebral Junction

After the patient is anesthetized, careful positioning is performed. Some surgeons advocate a three-quarter prone or park bench position for this surgery. The position requires the neck to be turned significantly from an anatomical neutral position, which may result in brainstem compression by the tumor and may alter the course of the extradural vertebral artery. In addition, venous return may be compromised with neck turning or with the patient's weight on the chest. We prefer the patient to be placed in a supine position with a large gel roll under the ipsilateral shoulder and hips to allow the patient to be at a 45-degree angle (**Fig. 11.7**). The head, shoulders, and trunk are supported with cushions to maintain a neutral craniospinal axis, allowing the vertebral artery to take a more normal course in the extradural location. The patient's head is fixed with a Mayfield head rest, and the neck is maintained in a neutral position, which effectively makes the head 45 degrees from the floor. In obese patients with a short neck or large shoulders, the ipsilateral shoulder may be pulled down gently and secured to avoid traction on the brachial plexus. The posterolateral aspects of the head, neck, ear, and shoulder are prepared in a sterile manner. The scalp is infiltrated with a 1:100,000 epinephrine solution if there is no contraindication. The location of the tip of the mastoid and the angle of the mandible are marked. The greater auricular nerve is often found bisecting these two points at a perpendicular angle. The incision is planned as a C-shaped arc starting above the pinna of the ear, extending two finger breadths behind the mastoid process and extending two finger breadths behind the ear into a crease in the neck below the tip of the mastoid. The incision is carried through the skin and subcutaneous tissues, and the skin flap is reflected anteriorly and secured with fish-hook retractors.

The approach involves mobilization of the scalp flap anteriorly away from the center of the exposure and allows mobilization of the suboccipital muscles posteriorly. This approach is in contrast to the hockey stick incision and muscle dissection that is described as an alternative in which the scalp and muscles are reflected inferiorly and anteriorly, creating a mass of tissue overlying the center of the exposure. The reported advantage of this approach is the surgeon's familiarity with the midline anatomy, although it creates more distance to the operative site. Two superficial nerves may be identified in the subcutaneous tissues above the surface of the fascia (**Fig. 11.8**). The greater auricular nerve is a large branch located at the midpoint of a line connecting the mastoid eminence and the angle of the jaw. It may be used as a nerve graft for reconstruction if necessary, but the patient will be left with an uncomfortable anesthesia of the auricle if the nerve is cut during the exposure. The lesser occipital nerve is smaller and located medially, exiting under the lateral margin of the sternocleidomastoid muscle. The greater occipital nerve is seldom observed. It is distant from the site of the incision.

The sternocleidomastoid muscle is the most superficial of the three muscle groups of the retromastoid region. It is detached from its insertion on the superior nuchal line and mastoid using subperiosteal dissection and then reflected posteroinferiorly. The splenius capitis muscle, which is partly covered by the sternocleidomastoid muscle, is also freed from its attachment to the mastoid and occipital bones. The intermediate muscular layer consists of the semispinalis capitis and longissimus capitis muscles, which are also freed from the mastoid-occipital margins. As these muscles are released from their insertions on the mastoid and occipital squama, large emissary veins may be encountered. These emissary veins pass through various foramina and establish anastomoses between the cerebral dural sinuses and the deep muscular veins. The bleeding is managed best by careful identification of the origin of the hemorrhage and application of bone wax. Monitoring for air embolism is necessary throughout the operation. The mastoid emissary vein is commonly present as it courses through the mastoid foramen. It interconnects the sigmoid sinus with the posterior auricular or occipital vein. The condylar emissary vein is less constant. This condylar vein passes through the condyloid canal and is an important landmark that indicates the posterior extent of the occipital condyle.

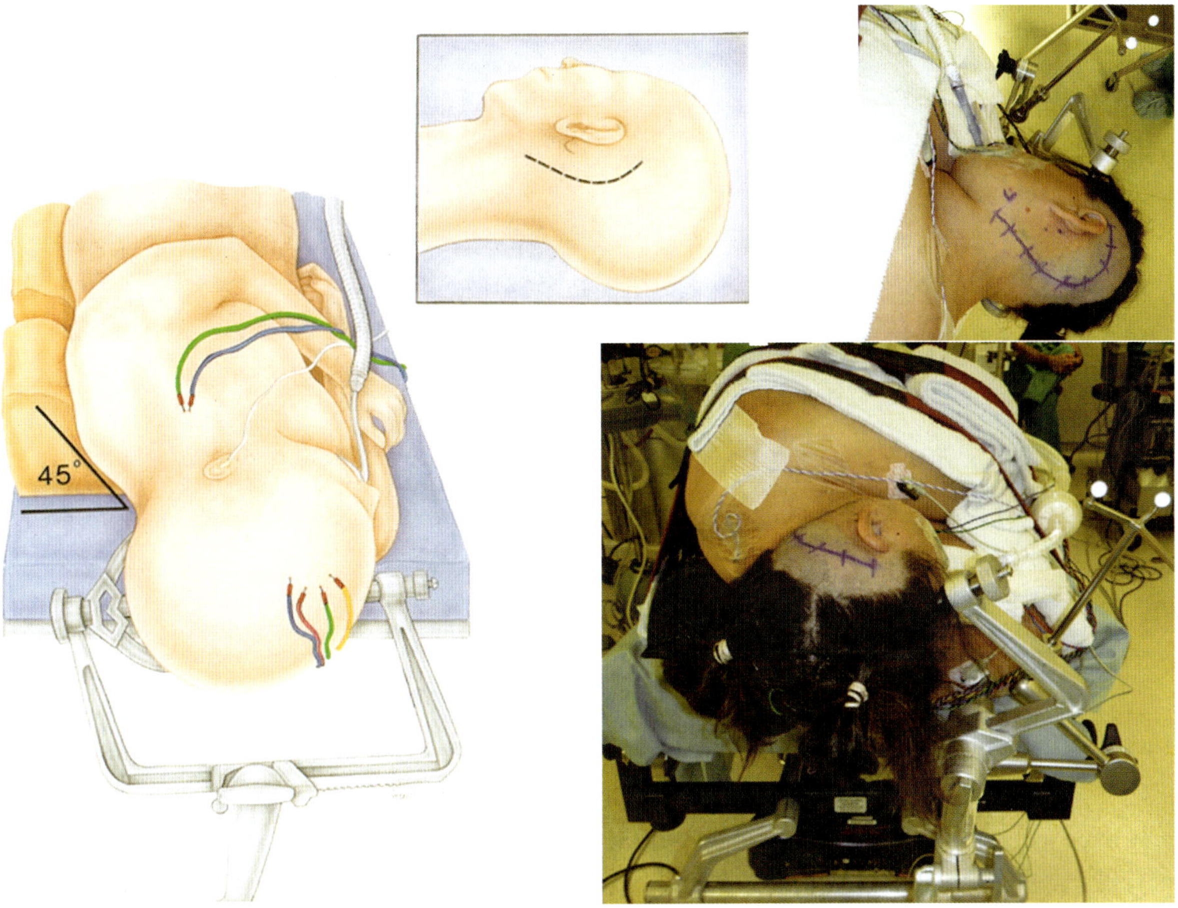

Fig. 11.7 Left and lower right: The patient is placed supine on the bed with a large roll under the shoulder and hips to allow 45-degree elevation of the body. **Upper center and upper right:** The curvilinear incision is shown from above the ear down to a natural crease in the neck. The navigation system tracking device is put out of the surgical corridor. **Left:** Neuromonitoring electrodes are placed for motor evoked potential, somatosensory evoked potential, auditory brainstem response, and electromyography of lower cranial nerves.

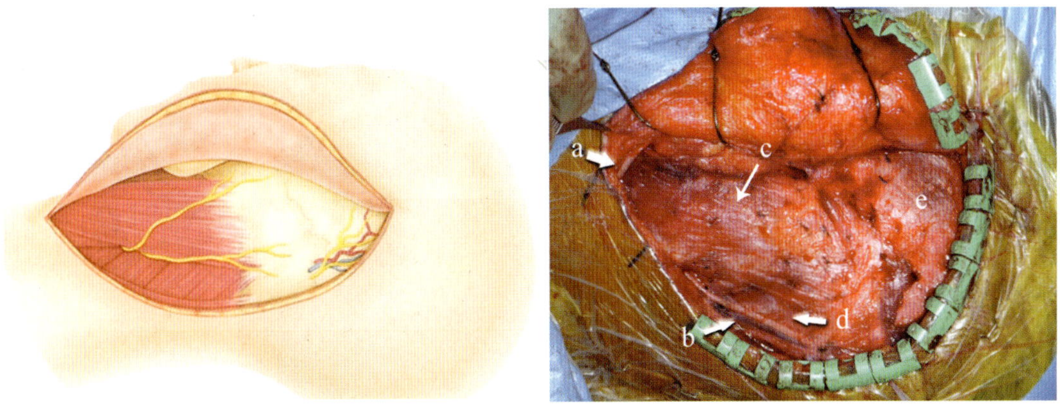

Fig. 11.8 Left: For suboccipital muscles, the skin flap has been rotated anteriorly and away from the surgical corridor. **Right:** Superficial muscles and cutaneous nerves are identified: (*a*) greater auricular nerve, (*b*) occipital nerve, (*c*) sternocleidomastoid muscle, (*d*) splenius capitis and semispinalis capitis muscles seen underlying the sternocleidomastoid muscle, and (*e*) occipitalis muscle.

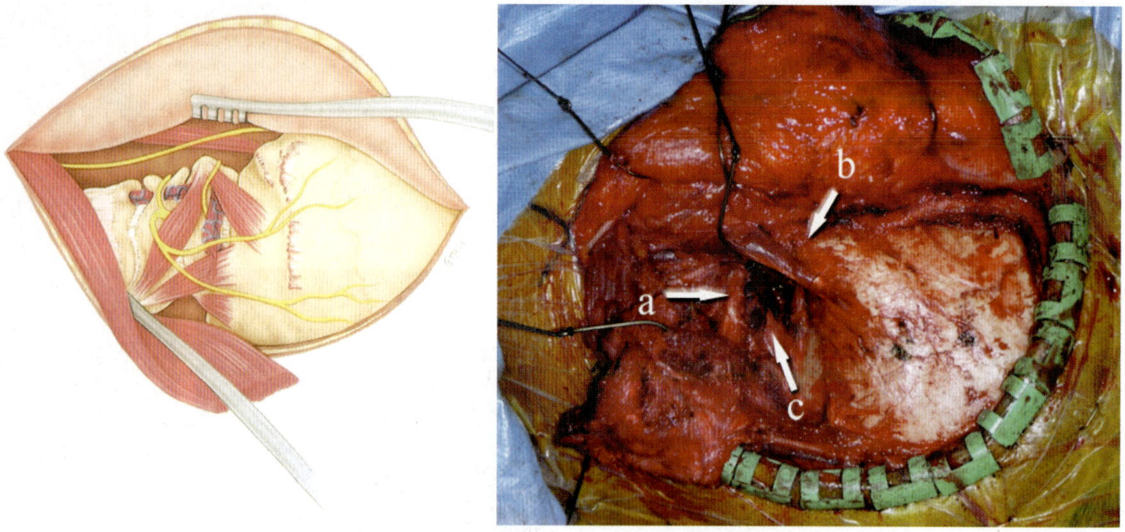

Fig. 11.9 Left: At the suboccipital triangle, the sternocleidomastoid and superficial suboccipital muscles have been swept inferiorly and posteriorly (*left*). **Right:** (*a*) The lateral mass of C1 is identified and (*c*) the vertebral artery is seen within the suboccipital triangle, which is composed of the superior oblique, inferior oblique, and rectus capitis posterior major muscles. (*b*) The posterior belly of the digastric muscle is left in its insertion site on the mastoid digastric groove to protect the facial nerve at the stylomastoid foramen.

The superficial muscular layers are reflected downward and medially, thereby exposing the deep muscular layer, the suboccipital triangle (**Fig. 11.9**). The boundaries of this triangle are formed by three muscles: the rectus capitis posterior major above and medially, the superior oblique capitis above and laterally, and the inferior oblique capitis below and laterally. The vertebral artery and the dorsal ramus of C1 are found in the center of this deep muscular triangle (**Fig. 11.10**).

The lateral mass of C1 and C2 can be easily palpated in the suboccipital triangle ~1 cm below the tip of the mastoid process. The soft tissues overlying the C1 lateral masses are gently dissected free with a periosteal elevator or electrocautery. The vertebral artery can be identified between the lateral masses of C1 and C2 by following the caudal border of the inferior oblique capitis and the ventral ramus of C2 (suboccipital nerve). The foramen transversarium of C1 is drilled open, allowing transposition of the vertebral artery (**Fig. 11.11**). Transposition of the vertebral artery allows drilling of the occipital condyle and C1 lateral mass with safety and allows for an approach lateral to the vertebral artery. To transpose the vertebral artery, it is necessary to expose the artery completely from the foramen transversarium at C1 to its dural entry into the foramen magnum. A venous plexus, which resembles the venous plexuses in the cavernous sinus that encases the carotid artery, encircles the vertebral artery and may be a source of bleeding (**Fig. 11.12**). Hemostasis can

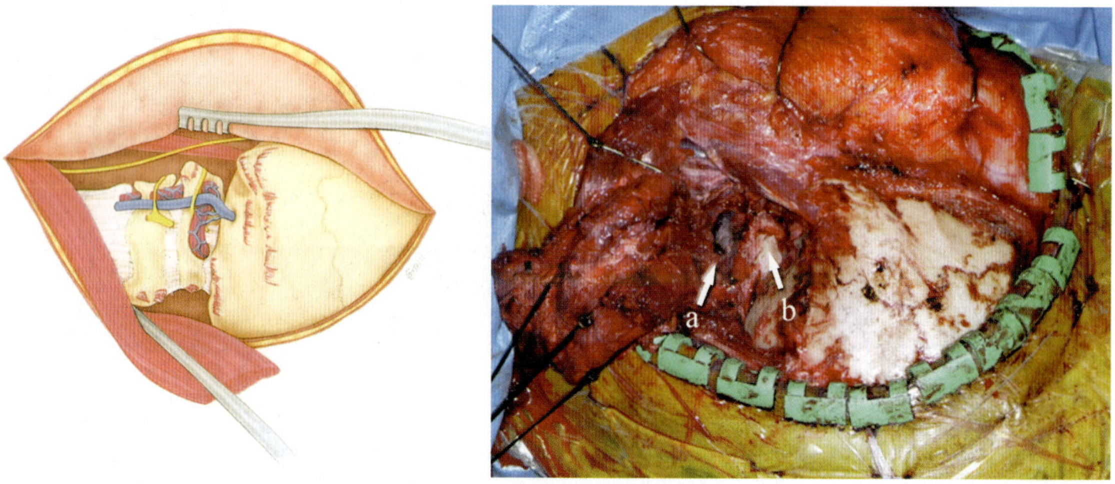

Fig. 11.10 Left: For vertebral artery localization, the muscles of the triangle are reflected or resected to allow access to the lamina and lateral mass of C1 (*left*). The lateral mass of C1 is resected. **Right:** The vertebral artery (*a*) is released from the C1 transverse foramen and (*b*) then transposed posteriorly and inferiorly to allow safe drilling of the occipital condyle.

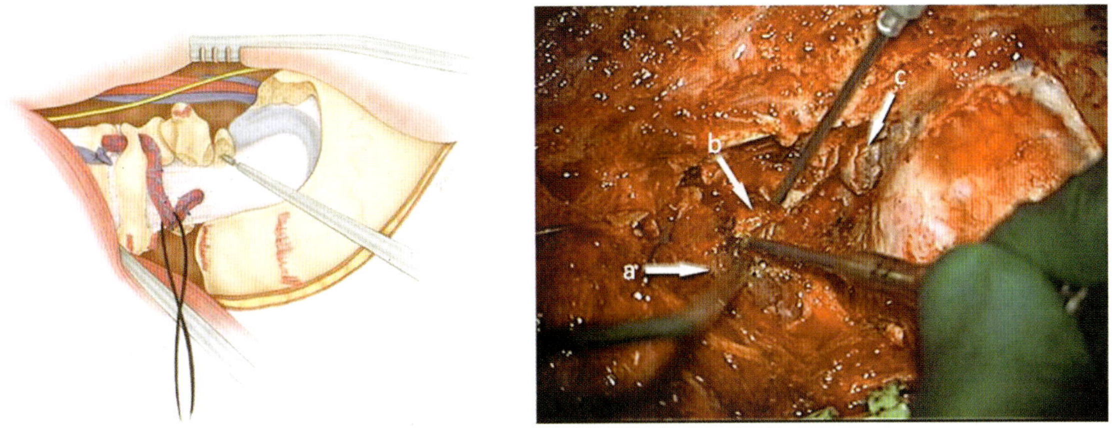

Fig. 11.11 Left: In occipital condyle drilling, the posterior fossa craniotomy has been performed and the transverse-sigmoid sinus junction has been skeletonized. A simple mastoidectomy has been performed to allow access to the jugular bulb. **Right:** (*a*) The vertebral artery is reflected inferiorly and protected with suction during drilling. (*b*) The occipital condyle and C1 lateral mass are drilled to allow for far lateral exposure. (*c*) The jugular bulb is skeletonized and the jugular tubercle is removed to allow dural opening along a straight line across the foramen magnum.

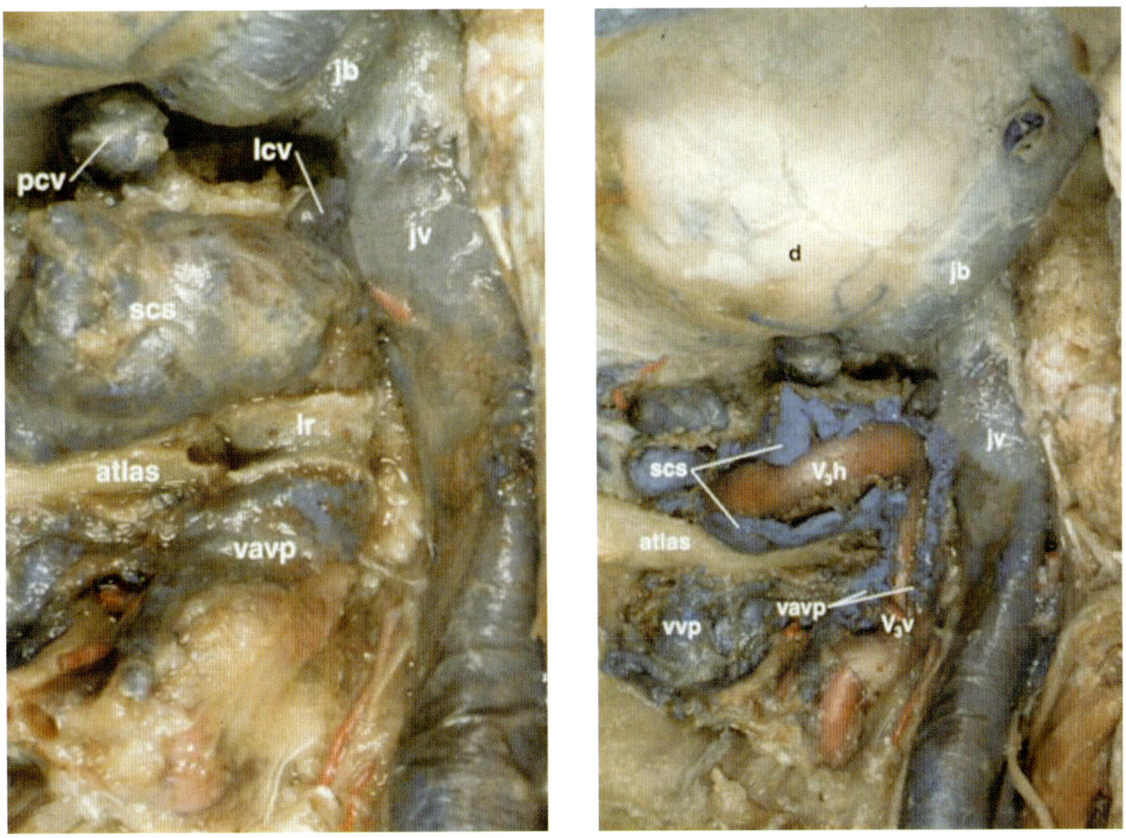

Fig. 11.12 Left: Cadaveric anatomic study of the foramen magnum demonstrates that the vertebral artery is encased in a venous plexus or the suboccipital cavernous sinus (*scs*) as it lies on the ring of C1 until it enters the dura. The jugular vein (*jv*), jugular bulb (*jb*), and posterior condylar vein (*pcv*) are visualized. **Right:** The venous contents of the plexus have been resected to expose the vertebral artery. *lcv*, lateral condylar vein; *lr*, lateral ring of C1; *vavp*, vertebral artery venous plexus around vertical segment; *d*, posterior fossa dura; V_3h, horizontal segment of the vertebral artery; *vvp*, suboccipital epidural venous plexus; V_3v, vertical segment of vertebral artery. (From McLoughlin GS, Sciubba DM, Suk I, et al. Resection of a retropharyngeal craniovertebral junction chordoma through a posterior cervical approach. J Spinal Discord Tech 2010;23(5):359–365.)

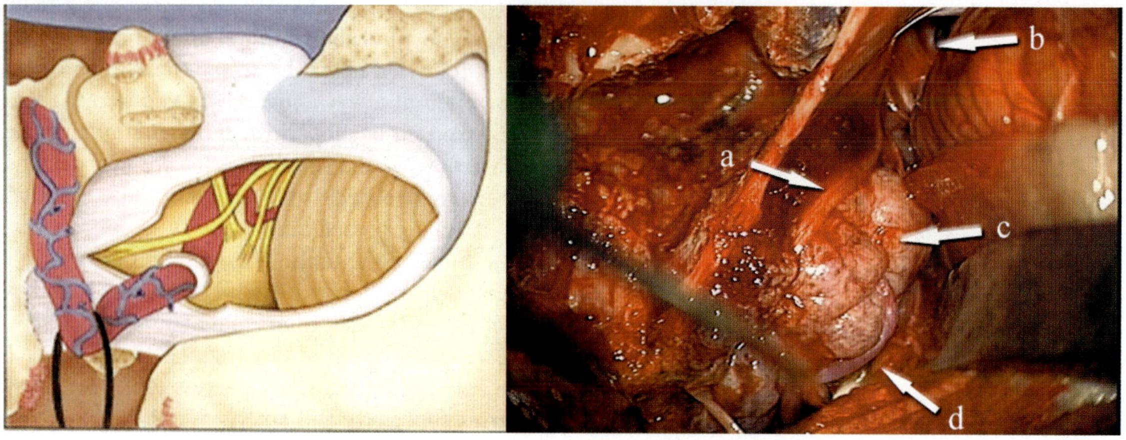

Fig. 11.13 Left: The dura is opened in the posterior fossa and carried across the foramen magnum with a circumferential cut around the vertebral artery at its entry to the subarachnoid space. **Right:** (*a*) The accessory nerve lies over the surface of the tumor, which extends superiorly to (*b*) the jugular foramen where cranial nerves IX, X, and XI exit the cranium. (*c*) The tumor is evident in the foramen magnum. (*d*) The posterior inferior cerebellar artery is encased in the tumor and courses along the ventral aspect of the medulla once it is free of the tumor.

be maintained with small pieces of thrombin-soaked Gelfoam (Baxter, Deerfield, IL) or Surgicel (Ethicon, Somerville, NJ).

The extent of bone removal is individualized based on the dimensions of the foramen magnum tumor. The purpose of any skull base approach is to remove bony obstacles to allow for the most direct approach to the tumor to allow for safe microdissection. For foramen magnum tumors, the goal is bony removal of the condyle and C1 lateral mass to allow a lateral exposure of the ventral foramen magnum to allow tumor resection without brainstem manipulation or retraction. The condyle is drilled away until only a thin shell of cortical bone remains to protect the structures surrounding this restricted space.[63] The transcondylar surgical exposure consists of a mastoidectomy, a suboccipital craniectomy, and removal of the articular surfaces of the occipital condyles and C1. The anterior half of these articular surfaces should be maintained for structural and mechanical stability. The hypoglossal canal transverses the base of the occipital condyle, demarcating its midpoint. It contains the hypoglossal nerve and the meningeal branch of the ascending pharyngeal artery. The tubercle for the alar ligaments is also located at the midpoint of the condyle. Condylar removal anterior to these structures may be performed when necessary but will lead to craniocervical instability and require a fusion. In some chordomas, this bone and occiput-C1 joint are destroyed by the tumor. These patients will all require occipitocervical fusion. Bone removal is carried forward to the vertical segment of the facial nerve and is visualized with the operating microscope. The sigmoid sinus and jugular bulb are gently unroofed and protected. The bony removal provides access to lesions reaching the cerebellopontine angle and internal auditory canal. The retrosigmoid craniectomy extends to the foramen magnum until the bony lip has been completely removed.

Lesions mainly in the posterior fossa that extend rostrally require an extensive mastoid-suboccipital bony removal. However, cervical lesions that extend up to the foramen magnum may not require an extensive suboccipital craniotomy. Bone removal is confined to the posterior half of the articular facets of the occiput and adjacent lamina.

The dura is opened in an oblique incision beginning superolaterally posterior to the sigmoid sinus extending down the midline through the foramen magnum to the level of C2. The dural incision can be made in front and behind the vertebral artery, leaving an elliptical ring of dura that allows mobilization of the vessel during tumor dissection (**Fig. 11.13**). Dural tenting sutures may be used to retract the sigmoid sinus anteriorly. If the jugular bulb is occluded by tumor, it can be removed after the sigmoid sinus is ligated.

This surgical approach brings the surgical view anterior to the cervicomedullary junction. Intracapsular dissection is performed until the tumor capsule is gently removed from the ventral aspect of the medulla and spinal cord (**Fig. 11.14**).

The caudal cranial nerves are identified, skeletonized, dissected from the tumor, and preserved. Electrophysiological monitoring is essential to maintain structural and functional integrity. After the tumor is removed, the dura is closed and the deep muscles are closed in layers. A sterile head dressing is applied.

Postoperative Care

Careful assessment of the lower cranial nerves during the postoperative period is paramount to a successful recovery. Postoperative assessment of cranial nerve function involves evaluation of the voice for hoarseness and swallowing studies, including bedside evaluation and modified barium swallow testing. Patients with tumors that have extensive involvement of the lower cranial nerves may experience dysphagia postoperatively; although usually temporary in

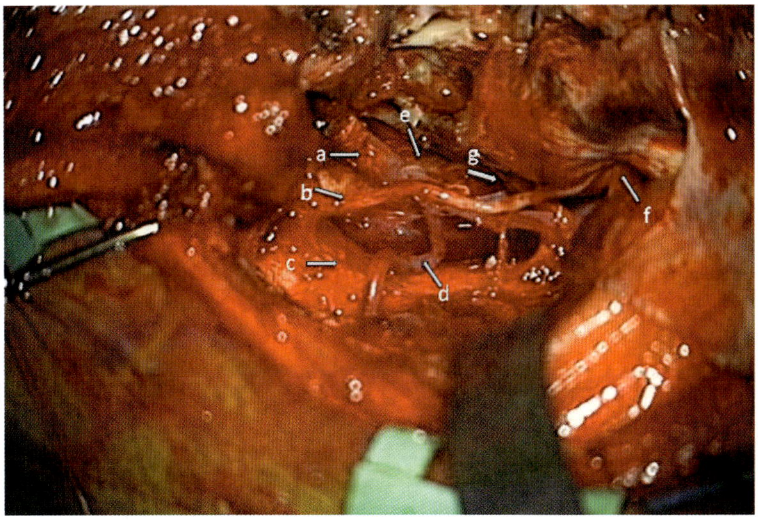

Fig. 11.14 The tumor has been resected, and normal neurovascular structures are visible. (*a*) The vertebral artery at its entry into the dura is visible. The dura is opened around the vertebral artery in a circumferential fashion to show the dural sleeve. (*b*) The accessory nerve courses up from the cervical spine to the jugular foramen. (*c*) The medulla is decompressed by the tumor. (*d*) The posterior inferior cerebellar artery courses along the medulla, having been skeletonized from inside the tumor mass. (*e*) The clivus is the site of origin of the tumor, which has been resected. (*f*) The jugular foramen is free of tumor, and cranial nerves IX, X, and XI exit the foramen. (*g*) The hypoglossal nerve courses into the hypoglossal canal.

nature, it needs to be recognized to avoid aspiration complications. Tracheostomy and feeding gastrostomy tubes may be needed until neural function recovery. Corticosteroids are withdrawn over 7 to 10 days. Sequential compression boots on the lower extremities are used as prophylaxis against pulmonary embolism and continued until the patient is ambulatory. Aggressive pulmonary toilet may include intermittent positive pressure breathing and nebulizer inhalation therapies.

High-resolution CT and MRI are performed with contrast enhancement. These modalities help evaluate the extent of tumor resection and serve as a baseline measurement in case of a recurrence.

Results

Surgery for tumors of the region of the foramen magnum can be associated with several potential complications. Early reports that utilized suboccipital approaches to this region yielded discouraging results, with 34 perioperative deaths in 74 cases.[11] Other reviews also demonstrated high rates of surgical morbidity and mortality. Yasargil and colleagues report an overall mortality rate of 13.2% in their review of foramen magnum meningiomas.[24] Favorable outcomes were described in 69.3%, fair outcomes in 7.9%, and poor outcomes in 9.6%. These disheartening results stimulated research on other routes of surgical access to lesions in this region.

The transcondylar surgical approach has clearly improved operative rates of mortality and morbidity and has enhanced the likelihood of total tumor removal. This success stems from the surgeon's ability to resect the tumor directly without retracting the neural elements of the posterior fossa. The extent of gross total resection and the morbidity and mortality associated with CVJ operations have significantly decreased with these skull base techniques. Pamir and colleagues have reported a 95% rate of gross total resection using the far lateral approach for ventral foramen magnum meningiomas.[56] Menezes has reported a 87% rate of gross total resection for foramen magnum meningiomas with a recurrence rate of 13%.[20] In the same series, gross total resection was achieved for all the patients with CVJ schwannomas with no recurrences. In agreement with these results, Wu and colleagues have demonstrated an 86% gross total resection rate and 1.8% mortality in their series of 114 patients treated mostly with transcondylar approaches.[19]

The most serious complication of surgery to remove tumors of the foramen magnum is injury to the brainstem from manipulating or interfering with its blood supply. This devastating and frequently fatal insult was common before the development of the operative microscope.[8,64] The risk of vascular compromise is increased when the vertebral or basilar artery is embedded in the tumor. The appearance of a neurological deficit may occasionally be delayed in the postoperative period. Vascular spasm is frequently noted as a cause of delayed deficit.

All of the lower cranial nerves are at risk during surgery in this region. Their deficit is a significant cause of morbidity and mortality. Intraoperatively, dissection of these nerves may produce bradycardia and hypotension. Postoperatively, dysphagia, vocal cord paresis, and diminished cough and gag reflex may lead to aspiration and pulmonary complications.

Complications related to disturbances of cerebrospinal fluid (CSF) dynamics include CSF fistulas, hydrocephalus, and pseudomeningocele. Although hydrocephalus may be present before surgery and persist despite total removal of the mass, it also may develop postoperatively. Acute postoperative hydrocephalus usually is obstructive whereas delayed hydrocephalus is communicative and related to poor absorption of CSF or scarring of the basal cisterns.

In our series, we investigated the outcomes of 27 patients with tumors of the foramen magnum who underwent operations via the transcondylar approach during a 7-year period. The vast majority of the lesions were ventral meningiomas (18).[18] The rest of the pathology consisted of rare entities (three chordomas, three chondrosarcomas, one schwannoma, one paraganglioma, and one neuroepithelial cyst). No operative deaths occurred. Transient vocal cord paresis was seen in four patients, with resolution in most cases within 3 to 6 months. Gelfoam injection of the paretic vocal cord was performed in two patients. One patient required a gastrostomy tube for recurrent aspiration due to a poor swallowing reflex. Another patient suffered mild weakness of his hypoglossal nerve, which resolved in 6 weeks. Repeated CSF leakage was seen in two patients. One CSF leak was treated with a lumboperitoneal shunt. The other CSF leak was treated by covering the dura with a trapezius muscle rotational flap. Postoperative wound infection and meningitis were not seen in our series, but vigilance must be constant in the recovery period. One patient developed a clinical picture of aseptic meningitis and was treated successfully without sequelae.

The goal of the surgical approach is to maximize exposure of the tumor affecting the CVJ and involving the brainstem and the spinal cord. At the same time, there is a need to minimize bone removal to maintain stability at the CVJ.

References

1. Piper JG, Menezes AH. Management strategies for tumors of the axis vertebra. J Neurosurg 1996;84(4):543–551
2. Menezes AH. Craniovertebral junction neoplasms in the pediatric population. Childs Nerv Syst 2008;24(10):1173–1186
3. Elsberg CA. Tumors of the spinal cord and the symptoms of irritation and compression of the spinal cord. In: Nerve Roots, Pathology, Symptomology, Diagnosis, and Treatment. New York, NY: Paul B. Hoeber; 1925
4. Abrahamson I, Grossman M. Tumors of the upper cervical cord. Trans Am Neurol Assoc 1921;47:149–168
5. Elsberg CA, Strauss I. Tumors of the spinal cord which project into the posterior cranial fossa: report of a case in which a growth was removed from the ventral and lateral aspects of the medulla oblongata and upper cervical cord. Arch Neurol Psychiatry 1929;21:261–273
6. Symonds CP, Meadows SP. Compression of the spinal cord in the neighbourhood of the foramen magnum. Brain 1937;60:52–84
7. Cushing H, Eisenhardt L. Meningiomas: Their Classification, Regional Behavior, Life History, and Surgical End Results. Springfield, IL: Charles C. Thomas; 1938
8. Castellano F, Ruggiero G. Meningiomas of the posterior fossa. Acta Radiol Suppl 1953;104(suppl):1–177
9. Stein BM, Leeds NE, Taveras JM, Pool JL. Meningiomas of the foramen magnum. J Neurosurg 1963;20:740–751
10. Love JR, Adson AW. Tumors of the foramen magnum. Trans Am Neurol Assoc 1941;67:78–81
11. Love JG, Thelen EP, Dodge HW Jr. Tumors of the foramen magnum. J Int Coll Surg 1954;22(1:1):1–17
12. Dodge HW Jr, Gottlieb CM, Love JG. Benign tumors at the foramen magnum; surgical considerations. J Neurosurg 1956;13(6): 603–617
13. Kreukel W, Friedman G. Diagnose und therapie der kraniospinalen tumoren. Ortschr Neurol Psych. 1967;35:237–262
14. Martin P, Kleyntjens F. Tumeurs sous-durales du trou occipital. Rev Neurol (Paris) 1950;82(5):313–334
15. Tilney F, Elsberg CA. Sensory disturbances in tumors of the cervical spinal cord: arrangements of the fibers in the sensory pathways. Arch Neurol Psychiatry 1926;15:444–454
16. Yasuoka S, Okazaki H, Daube JR, MacCarty CS. Foramen magnum tumors. Analysis of 57 cases of benign extramedullary tumors. J Neurosurg 1978;49(6):828–838
17. Meyer FB, Ebersold MJ, Reese DF. Benign tumors of the foramen magnum. J Neurosurg 1984;61(1):136–142
18. Arnautović KI, Al-Mefty O, Husain M. Ventral foramen magnum meninigiomas. J Neurosurg 2000;92(1, Suppl):71–80
19. Wu Z, Hao S, Zhang J, et al. Foramen magnum meningiomas: experiences in 114 patients at a single institute over 15 years. Surg Neurol 2009;72(4):376–382, discussion 382
20. Menezes AH, Traynelis VC, Fenoy AJ, Gantz BJ, Kralik SF, Donovan KA. Honored guest presentation: surgery at the crossroads: craniocervical neoplasms. Clin Neurosurg 2005;52:218–228
21. Guidetti B, Spallone A. Benign extramedullary tumors of the foramen magnum. In: Symon L, ed. Advances and Technical Standards in Neurosurgery. Vol. 16. Vienna, Austria: Springer-Verlag; 1988: 83–120
22. Guidetti B, Spallone A. Benign extramedullary tumors of the foramen magnum. Surg Neurol 1980;13(1):9–17
23. Smolik EA, Sachs E. Tumors of the foramen magnum of spinal origin. J Neurosurg 1954;11(2):161–172
24. Yasargil MG, Mortara RW, Cureic M. Meningiomas of the basal posterior cranial fossa. In: Krayenbuhl H, ed. Advances and Technical Standards in Neurosurgery. Vol 7. Vienna, Austria: Springer-Verlag; 1980:3–115
25. Levy WJ, Latchaw J, Hahn JF, Sawhny B, Bay J, Dohn DF. Spinal neurofibromas: a report of 66 cases and a comparison with meningiomas. Neurosurgery 1986;18(3):331–334
26. Lot G, George B. Cervical neuromas with extradural components: surgical management in a series of 57 patients. Neurosurgery 1997;41(4):813–820, discussion 820–822
27. Davidson GS, Hope JK. Meningeal tumors of childhood. Cancer 1989;63(6):1205–1210
28. Mendiratta SS, Rosenblum JA, Strobos RJ. Congenital meningiomas. Neurology 1967;7:914–918
29. Bruce DA. Skull base tumors in children. In: Albright AL, Pollack IF, Adelson PD, eds. Principles and Practice of Pediatric Neurosurgery. New York, NY: Thieme; 1999
30. Hanbali F, Tabrizi P, Lang FF, DeMonte F. Tumors of the skull base in children and adolescents. J Neurosurg 2004;100(2, Suppl Pediatrics):169–178
31. Borba LA, Al-Mefty O, Mrak RE, Suen J. Cranial chordomas in children and adolescents. J Neurosurg 1996;84(4):584–591
32. Piehl MR, Reese HH, Steelman HF. The diagnostic problem of tumors at the foramen magnum. Dis Nerv Syst 1950;11:67–76
33. Porras CL. Meningioma in the foramen magnum in a boy aged 8 years. J Neurosurg 1963;20:167–168
34. Saltz SE, Jervis GA. Extramedullary tumors of the upper cervical portion of the spinal cord. Bull Neuro Inst New York. 1937;6:274
35. Bogorodinski IK. Syndrome of the cranio-spinal tumor. State edition USSR (Quoted from Cushing H and Eisenhardt L, Meningiomas) 1936
36. Cadwalader WB. Observations on character on the onset of spinal paralysis with reference to the significance of the apoplectiform type of onset in contrast to the slow progressive development of paralysis. Arch Neurol Psychiatry 1921;6(5):541–549

37. Cohen L, Macrae D. Tumors in the region of the foramen magnum. J Neurosurg 1962;19:462–469
38. Craig WM, Sheldon CH. Tumors of the cervical portion of the spinal cord. Arch Neurol Psychiatry 1940;44:1–16
39. Friedman ED. Compression of the upper cervical cord in the guise of combined system disease. Int Clin 1941;3:102–110
40. Martin JP, Greenfield JG. Tumor in cisterna magna. Proc R Soc Med 1923;16(Neurol Sect):32–35
41. Oppenheim H. Weitere beitrage zur diagnose und differentialdiagnose des tumor medullae spinalis. Mschr Psych Neurol (Berlin) 1913;33:451–493
42. Kimmel DL. Innervation of spinal dura mater and dura mater of the posterior cranial fossa. Neurology 1961;11:800–809
43. Abbott KH. Foramen magnum and high cervical cord lesions simulating degenerative disease of the nervous system. Ohio Med 1950;46(7):645–651
44. Arseni C, Jonesco S. Contribution a l'etude des tumeurs situees au niveau du foramen magnum occipitale. Psychiatr Neurol Neurochir 1960;63:170–183
45. Ferraro A, Barrere SE. Effects of experimental lesions of the posterior columns in Macaca rhesus monkeys. Brain 1934;57:307–332
46. Cushing H. Notes on a series of intracranial tumors and conditions simulating them. Arch Neurol Psychiatry 1923;10:605
47. Beatty RA. Cold dysesthesia: a symptom of extramedullary tumors of the spinal cord. J Neurosurg 1970;33(1):75–78
48. Cloward RB, Kepner RD. Meningiomas of 30 years duration. Arch Neurol Psychiatry 1943;50:327
49. Discussion SB. In: Love JG, Thelen EP, Dodge HW. Tumors of the foramen magnum. J Int Coll Surg 1954;22:14–15
50. Taylor AR, Byrnes DP. Foramen magnum and high cervical cord compression. Brain 1974;97(3):473–480
51. Cogan DG. Down-beat nystagmus. Arch Ophthalmol 1968;80(6):757–768
52. Horrax G. Meningiomas of the brain. Arch Neurol Psychiatry 1939;41:140
53. Menezes AH, Traynelis VC, Gantz BJ. Surgical approaches to the craniovertebral junction. Clin Neurosurg 1994;41:187–203
54. Sen C, Shrivastava R, Anwar S, Triana A. Lateral transcondylar approach for tumors at the anterior aspect of the craniovertebral junction. Neurosurgery 2010;66(3, Suppl):104–112
55. Nanda A, Vincent DA, Vannemreddy PS, Baskaya MK, Chanda A. Far-lateral approach to intradural lesions of the foramen magnum without resection of the occipital condyle. J Neurosurg 2002;96(2):302–309
56. Pamir MN, Kiliç T, Ozduman K, Türe U. Experience of a single institution treating foramen magnum meningiomas. J Clin Neurosci 2004;11(8):863–867
57. Samii M, Gerganov VM. Surgery of extra-axial tumors of the cerebral base. Neurosurgery 2008;62(6, Suppl 3):1153–1166, discussion 1166–1168
58. Shin H, Barrenechea IJ, Lesser J, Sen C, Perin NI. Occipitocervical fusion after resection of craniovertebral junction tumors. J Neurosurg Spine 2006;4(2):137–144
59. Singh H, Harrop J, Schiffmacher P, Rosen M, Evans J. Ventral surgical approaches to craniovertebral junction chordomas. Neurosurgery 2010;66(3, Suppl):96–103
60. Kawashima M, Tanriover N, Rhoton ALJ Jr, Ulm AJ, Matsushima T. Comparison of the far lateral and extreme lateral variants of the atlanto-occipital transarticular approach to anterior extradural lesions of the craniovertebral junction. Neurosurgery 2003;53(3):662–674, discussion 674–675
61. Margalit NS, Lesser JB, Singer M, Sen C. Lateral approach to anterolateral tumors at the foramen magnum: factors determining surgical procedure. Neurosurgery 2005;56(2, Suppl):324–336, discussion 324–336
62. Demonte F, Warf P, Al-Mefty O. Intraoperative monitoring of the lower cranial nerves during surgery of the jugular foramen and lower clivus. In: Loftus CM, Traynelis VC, eds. Intraoperative Monitoring Techniques in Neurosurgery. New York, NY: McGraw-Hill; 1994:205–212
63. Spetzler RF, Grahm TW. The far-lateral approach to the inferior clivus and the upper cervical region: technical note. BNI Q 1990;6(4):35–38
64. Olivecrona H. The surgical treatment of intracranial tumors. In: Olivecrona H, Tonnis W, eds. Handbuch der Neurochirugie. Berlin: Springer-Verlag; 1967:1–301

12 Management of Chiari Malformations

Harold L. Rekate and Ruth E. Bristol

In articles published in 1891 and 1896, Chiari[1,2] described four types of abnormal development of the posterior fossa, which have subsequently been classified as Chiari malformations I, II, III, and IV. Chiari malformation type III is a suboccipital meningoencephalocele, and Chiari malformation type IV is cerebellar agenesis. Both of these problems are exceedingly rare and are not discussed further. The designation of Chiari malformation type II should be reserved for patients with concomitant spina bifida cystica. This complex abnormality of the formation of the posterior fossa structures and contents of the upper cervical spinal canal was probably first described by Cleland.[3] Subsequently, several graduate students reported a case of a Chiari malformation type II and were responsible for the addition of Arnold's name, leading to the name "Arnold-Chiari malformation."[4] For an excellent review of the history of the recognition of this malformation, the reader is referred to Carmel and Markesbery.[5]

Chiari's original articles dealt with hydrocephalus, and it is impossible to distinguish in his writing whether the described hindbrain hernia resulted in the hydrocephalus or resulted from it. However, what has subsequently been described as the Chiari malformation type I describes herniation of the cerebellar tonsils through the foramen magnum. Synonyms for Chiari malformation type I include "the adult Chiari malformation," chronic tonsillar herniation, and hindbrain herniation. There seems to be no logic in continuing to associate the name of Arnold with this malformation. Furthermore, many cases of the Chiari malformation type I are not only acquired but reversible, and the concept of an "acquired" malformation seems oxymoronic; therefore, the term hindbrain hernia would seem to describe this condition best.[6,7]

Is there any reason, then, other than common usage, to retain the term Chiari malformation type I? This term remains useful in that neurosurgeons have a clear idea of what is meant by the term and it leads to an operation that is easily understood by all.

What follows is a description of the surgical management of the Chiari malformation type I with several subtypes as well as of the Chiari malformation type II. There is hardly an issue in neurosurgery that is without its controversial aspects, and it is our intention to highlight areas of significant controversy.

Chiari I Malformation

Anatomy and Pathophysiology

In the Chiari I malformation, the cerebellar tonsils are present within the foramen magnum, usually down to the ring of C1, and occasionally even farther down into the spinal canal to the rings of C2 or C3. Some degree of "hanging" down of the cerebellar tonsils into the cervical spinal canal is considered to be a normal variant. Radiographically, cerebellar tonsillar herniation is clearly abnormal when it is 5 mm below the foramen magnum and, especially, when it has a triangular or "beak-like" appearance (**Fig. 12.1**). Studies using cine magnetic resonance imaging (MRI) lead to a more physiological definition of the Chiari I malformation when alteration of flow of cerebrospinal fluid (CSF) can be found at the foramen magnum. Normally, CSF exits the skull during systole and returns during diastole. This flow can become obstructed, particularly posteriorly, in symptomatic Chiari malformations (**Fig. 12.2**).

Chiari I malformation is found as an isolated phenomenon and is associated with a great variety of other conditions. For the purpose of this discussion, tonsillar herniation secondary to an intracranial mass lesion has been omitted, although in many ways the pathophysiology is the same. Spinal imaging with and without contrast should be considered in a patient presenting with a Chiari malformation

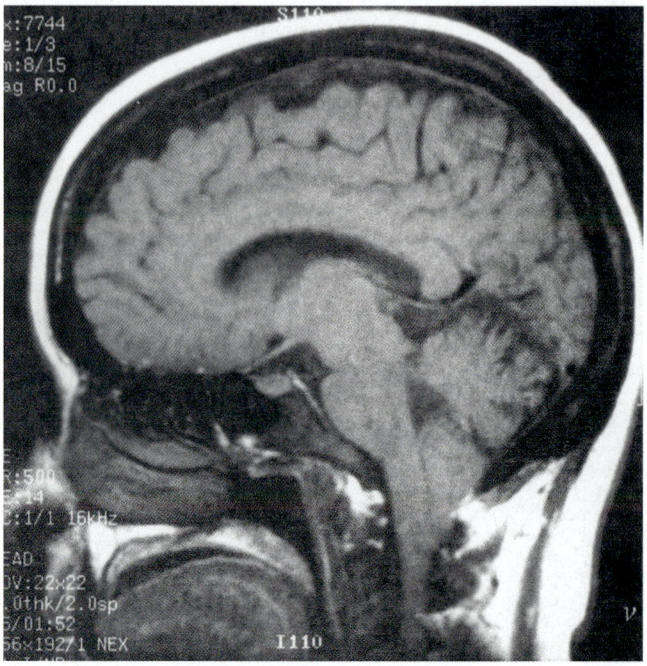

Fig. 12.1 Sagittal magnetic resonance image of a patient with a Chiari I malformation showing the descent of the cerebellar tonsils below the foramen magnum and the classic pointed appearance of the tonsils in this position.

A

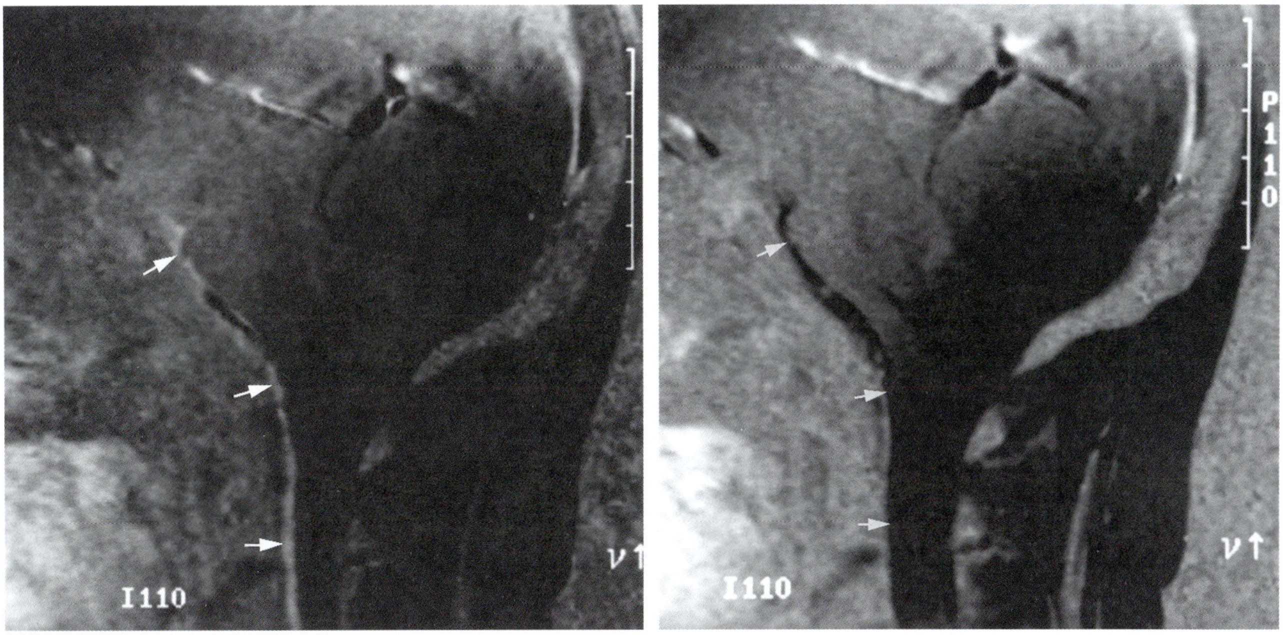

B

Fig. 12.2 Cine magnetic resonance image of a patient with a Chiari I malformation showing the failure of cerebrospinal fluid flow posterior to the hindbrain herniation. This test demonstrates the disconnection of the pressure wave across the foramen magnum, isolating the cortical subarachnoid space from the spinal subarachnoid space. The presence of fluid, which is **(A)** white anteriorly (*arrows*) and **(B)** black during diastole (*arrows*), indicates to-and-fro flow anteriorly but not posteriorly.

to rule out the presence of a tumor or other congenital anomaly.

Cine MRI has gained popularity for the preoperative evaluation of patients. Some evidence suggests that patients with normal CSF flow are more prone to recurrent symptoms after surgery.[8] Current studies do not support the use of this imaging modality alone as an indicator of which patients will respond well to decompression; rather, it is appropriate as an adjunct for decision making. Postoperatively, failure to reestablish CSF flow at the foramen magnum in a persistently symptomatic patient is an indicator that full decompression has not been achieved.

Conditions Associated with the Chiari I Malformation

Four conditions are associated with Chiari I malformations. The first is hydrocephalus. Although it is difficult, if not impossible, to distinguish whether hydrocephalus caused a hindbrain hernia or a hindbrain hernia caused hydrocephalus, this form of Chiari I malformation was the subject of Chiari's original studies.[1,2] Second, cephalocranial disproportion exists when the skull is nondistensible and the growing brain cannot be contained in it. It occurs in craniosynostosis syndromes, such as Crouzon and Pfeiffer syndromes, in which venous hypertension related to jugular foramen stenosis may play a role.[9] There is also a close association between true lambdoid craniosynostosis and a hindbrain hernia in the context of syndromic craniosynostosis.[10] It is seen in patients with synostosis and microcephaly secondary to early treatment of hydrocephalus, with resultant secondary closure of multiple sutures.[11] Third, abnormally low intraspinal pressure has been reported to lead to chronic herniation of the cerebellar tonsil after lumboperitoneal shunting as a result of sacral meningoceles and in the condition known as spontaneous intracranial hypotension, which is presumed to be caused by the spontaneous rupture of a perineural cyst.[6,11–14] Finally, craniovertebral junction (CVJ) abnormalities with crowding and compression of structures at the skull base are discussed in more detail in the section on the management of Chiari malformation associated with basilar invagination. As reported by Aquilina and colleagues[15] in a study of children receiving cranial radiation, growth of the clivus was intimately associated with tonsillar descent. Clival growth was arrested during and immediately after radiation, during which time the tonsillar descent worsened. Subsequently, the posterior fossa enlarged as clival growth returned to normal and the Chiari malformation improved.

Clinical Syndromes

Numerous clinical syndromes are associated with the Chiari I malformation, and the radiological appearance characteristic of the Chiari I malformation may be observed as an apparently incidental finding in patients undergoing MRI examinations for other reasons. In very young children, the presentation can be uncontrollable screaming, occasionally with retropulsion of the head as in opisthotonos. It is not uncommon for children under the age of 6 years to present with oropharyngeal dysfunction.[16] In severe cases, slow feeding, drooling, snoring, and even apnea and stridor can herald a symptomatic Chiari malformation. In older children and adults, the most common complaint is severe suboccipital headache. Clumsiness and unsteadiness are often reported, but true ataxia is rarely documented.

Classic presentations for the Chiari I malformation include severe headaches associated with a Valsalva maneuver and a distinctive neuro-ophthalmologic syndrome. Patients complain of not being on the floor or of the floor coming up to them. They are found to have downbeat nystagmus, which is characteristic of this condition.

Surgical Principles

The goals of surgery are to remove the compression from the brainstem and reestablish normal patterns of CSF flow. As an adjunct to surgery, it is our policy to monitor somatosensory evoked potentials (SSEPs). In one case, the disappearance of the SSEP during positioning of a patient led to the diagnosis of a previously unrecognized occipitocervical instability. Repositioning led to return of function, and a fusion was performed in association with decompression.

The patient is placed in a head holder in a slightly flexed position. We tend to use a 1-cm wide clipper to remove hair on either side of the incision to facilitate closure. The hair is prepared with povidone-iodine scrub. Next, iodine gel is applied to the hair to facilitate its staying in position after it is combed. A midline incision is made from the inion to the midcervical spine and carried down to the fascia.

At this point, the fascial planes are used as a guide and the foramen magnum is exposed. A subperiosteal dissection of one laminar arch below the intended level of laminectomy is performed, and the periosteum is removed from the occipital bone at least 5 cm up from the foramen magnum. Exposure is maximized by the use of "fish hooks" in the muscle attached to the Leyla bars (Aesculap, San Francisco, CA) on either side. This process not only pulls the muscle apart but pulls the skin down and leaves the surgeon without the normal deep hole frequently seen in such surgical procedures (**Fig. 12.3**).

Next, the rostral extension of the ligamentum flavum and epidural fat is removed, exposing the dura from C1 to the foramen magnum. An up-angled curette is used to disconnect the dura from the undersurface of the foramen magnum. The rim of the foramen magnum is removed to a distance of 1.5 to 2.0 cm. How the rim is removed depends primarily on the patient's age. In children, the bone is usually removed with a Kerrison rongeur. In adolescents and adults, removing the rim is quite difficult because of the thickness of the bone in that location and the difficult angle at which the operating surgeon must work. In such cases, the Midas Rex (Midas Rex Pneumatic Tools, Inc., Fort Worth, TX) instrument is used. An AM8 attachment (a cutting bur) is used to thin the bone 1.5 to 2 cm down to the dura, and the remaining bone is removed with a curette or Kerrison rongeurs. Alternatively, the footplate attachment is used to turn a craniotomy flap. If the footplate is used, care must be taken in the midline to remain extradural where a large keel can occur.

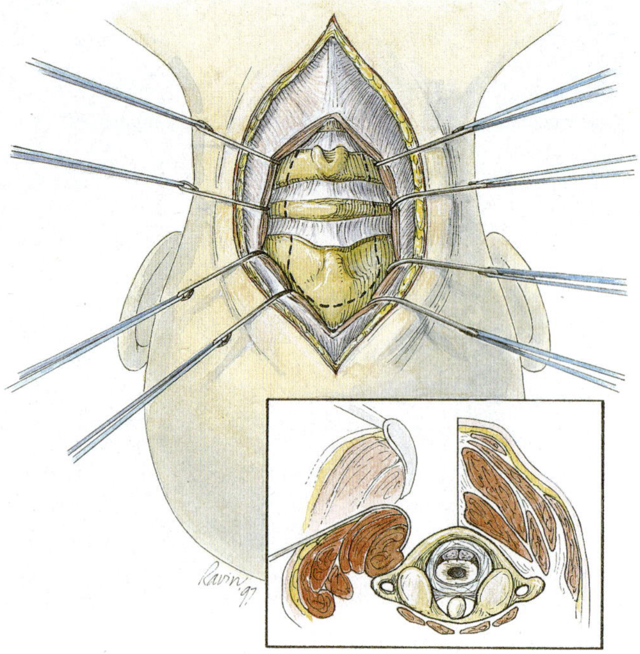

Fig. 12.3 Using fish hooks attached to rubber bands and thus to bars on either side of the patient creates muscle retraction that is down and out as opposed to up and out when standard cerebellar retractors (*ghosted in insert*) are used. The hole is much shallower, allowing greater freedom of movement during a Chiari decompression. *Dotted lines* indicate bone to be removed. (Reprinted with permission from Barrow Neurological Institute.)

The posterior arch of C1 and, if necessary, the laminae and spinous process of C2 are removed with the ligamentum flavum using a combination of Leksell and Kerrison rongeurs. Meticulous hemostasis is essential so that minimal, if any, blood is spilled into the subarachnoid space after the dura is opened. The surgical gutters on either side of the exposure are lined with Cottonoids (DuPuy, Raynham, MA) to help control minor amounts of residual tissue ooze. Surgifoam hemostatic agent can also be applied.

Another controversial step in Chiari management is the need to open the dura. Zamel and colleagues reported that the most significant improvement in brainstem auditory evoked potentials occurred during bony decompression, without significant additional improvement upon dural opening.[17] Many practitioners consider the presence of syringomyelia to be an absolute indication for dural opening. It is also widely held that arachnoid obstruction of the outlet of the fourth ventricle must be released. Conversely, others open the dura only with no disruption of the arachnoid to prevent future scarring.[18]

A 4–0 braided nylon dural stitch is used to tent the dura for opening in the midline, and the dura mater is opened using a no. 11 or 15 blade. The opening should be well below the foramen magnum and should extend caudally to the lowest point of the dural opening. After a small opening is made in the dura, we prefer to use a no. 12 blade to complete the opening. This blade, which has the appearance of a scimitar, allows complete control of the opening, as all movements of the blade are up, out of the wound, and away from the central nervous system (CNS) (**Fig. 12.4**).

This approach to opening the dura is desirable because of the potential risk of severe bleeding when the dura of the posterior fossa is opened. In normal patients, a "circular sinus" exists at the level of the foramen magnum. Dural sinuses are collections of flowing blood between the leaves of the dura. These sinuses do not occur within the spinal dura, but their size and location in the posterior fossa vary greatly, especially in small children. This point is extremely important in the discussion of the Chiari II malformation. If the surgeon opens one of these sinuses directly over the dura, it is likely that only one wall of the sinus will be opened. Consequently, it becomes very difficult to stop the bleeding, and significant blood loss can occur even in a small and relatively unimportant circular sinus. In this situation, use of monopolar or bipolar cauterization often leads to continual expansion of the hole, and the rate of bleeding increases and makes control more difficult. However, if the dura is opened with the no. 12 blade from the cervical dura to the cranial dura, both leaves of the dura are opened simultaneously. In this situation, bleeding can be controlled simply by putting an instrument under the dura and lifting upward, compressing the two leaves of the dura together. At this point, definitive hemostasis can be obtained by coagulating the two leaves, thus sealing them together. When the sinus is so large that it is difficult to execute this technique, titanium clips can be applied to assure the seal. To minimize artifact on postoperative imaging studies, we use 4–0 braided nylon sutures to sew the dural leaves together and then remove the titanium clips.

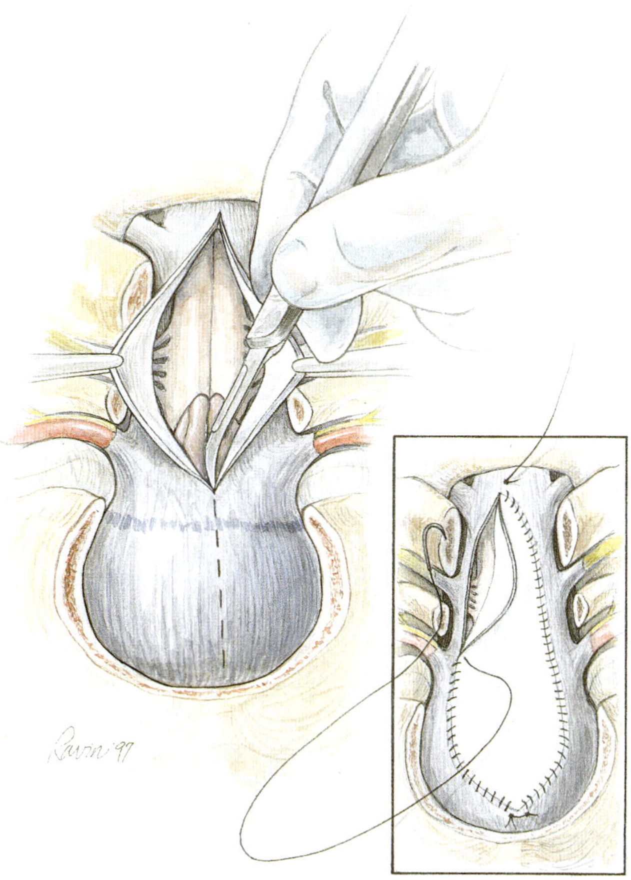

Fig. 12.4 The use of the no. 12 blade is demonstrated. Because the cutting surface is drawn up and away from the central nervous system tissue, the risk of injury is minimized. *Inset* shows dural closure with patch graft. (Reprinted with permission from Barrow Neurological Institute.)

Because the presumed pathophysiology of the symptomatic Chiari I malformation relates to the isolation of the intracranial pressure compartment from the intraspinal pressure compartment, one of the goals of this surgical procedure is to reestablish normal CSF dynamics at the CVJ. For this reason, we believe that part of the surgical approach to this anomaly involves assuring that the foramen of Magendie is patent. Using the microscope, the surgeon either retracts upward or removes a small portion of the lower tip of the cerebellar vermis with bipolar cauterization. A veil, which is typically present, must be opened to visualize the porcelain white floor of the fourth ventricle.

This opening into the fourth ventricle is one of the controversial points in this surgical procedure. Some neurosurgeons believe that this step is unnecessary unless hydrocephalus or syringomyelia is present. It is difficult to prove or disprove this point. We perform this step primarily for theoretical reasons, believing that it does not add to the morbidity of the procedure. Another group of neurosurgeons advocates that the opening into the fourth ventricle be assured using a stent, usually a piece of shunt tubing.[19] However, we believe that these stents become a nidus for scar formation, almost always occluding with time and potentially leading to postoperative tethering of the brainstem.

The most controversial aspect of this procedure, with the possible exception of surgical indications, is the method for closure. Williams[20] and Krieger and colleagues[21] believe that the dura should be left widely open. However, most neurosurgeons believe that the dura should be closed with a patch graft to create a large CSF space around the cervicomedullary junction. Choice of material is also controversial. Available materials include autologous fascia, Durasis porcine graft (Cook Biotech, West Lafayette, IN), and Durepair synthetic material (Medtronic, Inc., Minneapolis, MN). Both the Durasis and Durepair require soaking in irrigation for at least 30 minutes to prevent chemical meningitis.

Autologous material can be obtained from the pericranium, contiguous fascia of the paracervical musculature, or fascia lata of the thigh. The use of the paracervical musculature leads to more postoperative discomfort and occasionally leads to a troublesome pseudomeningocele related to the difficulty in

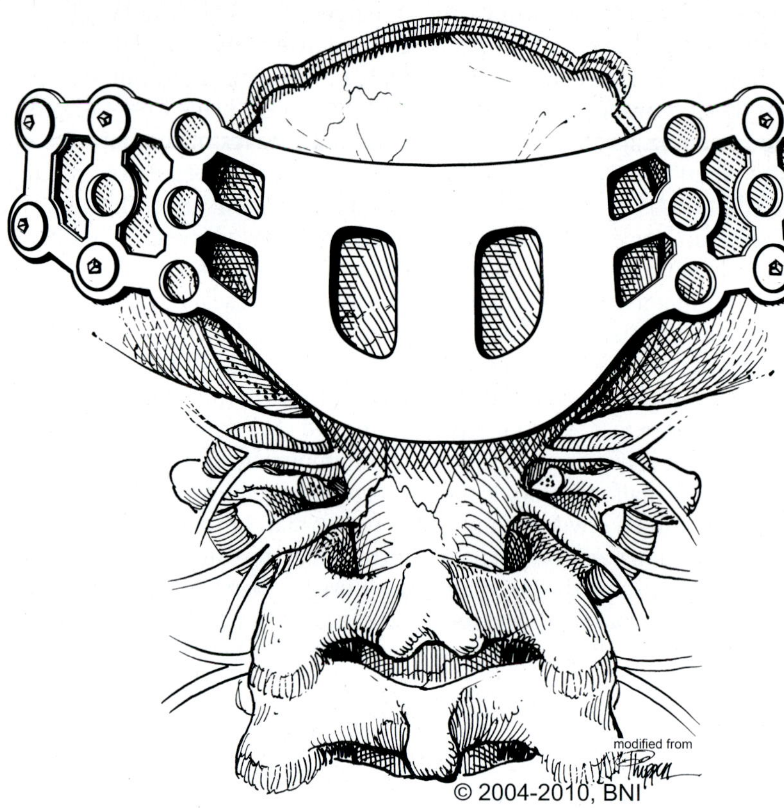

Fig. 12.5 A titanium plate, produced by Codman (Raynham, MA), spans the craniectomy defect. The availability of multiple screw holes bilaterally allows for custom fitting depending on the patient's anatomy and the extent of the bony opening. The dural graft is then "tented" up to the plate with a central suture. (Reprinted with permission from Barrow Neurological Institute.)

creating a watertight seal. Use of fascia lata results in an unsightly scar. At this time we are using pericranium, which can be harvested with only a minor increase in the size of the incision and has handling properties more similar to dura. The graft can be sewn in place with absorbable or nonabsorbable suture (**Fig. 12.4**).

After the graft is sewn in place, its integrity should be checked by having the anesthesiologist perform several Valsalva maneuvers. To prevent the graft from scarring to the underlying tonsils, a titanium plate has been developed to span just above the previous foramen magnum (**Fig. 12.5**). The Codman Chiari plate (Codman Corp., Raynham, MA) is attached with screws bilaterally, and a stitch is placed in the center of the graft to tent it up to the plate. This maneuver re-creates the CSF space dorsal to the tonsils. The deep cervical musculature is then closed, and the fascia is closed with absorbable suture. The integrity of the fascial closure is essential in preventing pseudomeningocele. The remainder of the closure is routine.

Postoperatively, there is no need for cervical immobilization, although the patient will be quite uncomfortable and will require a significant level of analgesia for a few days. We tend to use frequent small doses of intravenous morphine sulfate, which may be supplemented with muscle relaxants in adolescents and adults.

Chiari I Malformation with Syringomyelia

Patients who harbor syringomyelia as a result of a Chiari malformation have many of the same signs and symptoms as those who have only the hindbrain hernia. They also have the symptom and sign complexes typically associated with syringomyelia. Symptoms include burning pain in the shoulders or hands, shock-like pains into the hands or down the back (Lhermitte sign), clumsiness, and poor balance. The most severe cases also exhibit progressive weakness in the arms and legs. The classic neurological sign is a cape-like pattern of sensory loss, the so-called "hanging" distribution of sensory loss. More commonly, patients exhibit various degrees of weakness, scoliosis, and spasticity and show a greater sensory loss in the hands than in the legs or trunk. The finding of syringomyelia during an evaluation of scoliosis, without other complaints, may be a relatively common presentation of this rare condition in adolescents. Some patients may be truly asymptomatic from the perspective of the neurological examination. However, in this situation, deterioration can be so subtle that surgical intervention is probably warranted.

The pathophysiology of syringomyelia in the context of the Chiari I malformation is extremely controversial and, for the most part, outside the scope of this review. As reviewed by Oi and colleagues,[22] this condition is probably analogous to hydrocephalus, except that it occurs within the spinal cord (central canal = ventriculus terminale) rather than within the ventricles of the brain. Based on several clinical and laboratory studies, the disconnection of the intracranial and spinal segments of pressure waves plays a role. That this pressure is pulsatile almost certainly adds energy to the distorting effect of the blockages that occur.[23]

Successful management of syringomyelia in the context of the Chiari I malformation depends on the reestablishment of normal flow patterns of CSF around the upper spinal cord out of the fourth ventricle. The central canal enters the fourth ventricle at the level of the obex, and it is essential to normalize the pressure between the central canal and the spinal subarachnoid space. The required operation is identical to that described previously for the management of the Chiari I malformation alone. From this operation alone, the syringomyelia will resolve, even when no clear-cut connection can be established among the syrinx, central canal, and fourth ventricle.[24] Imaging studies obtained immediately after surgical intervention frequently show residual syringomyelia, even if the patient has improved. Scans obtained 3 to 6 months later almost always reveal marked resolution of the syringomyelia.

If the patient's symptoms are not relieved by the procedure and the postoperative imaging study is not improved, we suggest that an electrocardiogram-gated MRI study of CSF flow be performed to rule out a technical reason that could be addressed by a second exploration of the CVJ. If no such reason is found, it may be necessary to attack the syrinx directly. Since we have been using occipital decompression as the definitive management of syringomyelia, we have not had a patient whose syringomyelia failed to respond.

How to manage syringomyelia by direct surgical maneuver is also controversial. Until recently, syringosubarachnoid shunts have been advocated. Our experience with this form of therapy has not led us to be enthusiastic about it, and neither is the most recent neurosurgical literature.[25,26] The incidences of shunt failure and failure to resolve the syringomyelia are high. We have found a relatively high incidence of symptomatic postoperative tethering in these patients.[25] In this condition, patients experience severe pain upon movement and slow deterioration in neurological function. Before this condition was recognized, radiology reports were said to show only postoperative changes. Careful review of these studies, especially in the axial projection, clearly showed that the area of the myelotomy was densely adherent to the overlying dura. Surgical exploration showed that the stent for the syringosubarachnoid shunt had served as a nidus leading at that point to the fusion of the CNS to the dura.

Shunting of the syrinx to the peritoneal cavity or pleura is more effective in the management of refractory syringomyelia.[26] Because the pleura is easy to access in this situation, because it is a low pressure system, and because the amount of CSF that must be drained is minimal, we prefer to use this space for our syrinx shunts. To date, we have used this technique to treat only syringomyelia associated with the Chiari II malformation, which is discussed later.

The patient is placed prone on an operating table and supported on a frame or rolls, depending on the patient's size and the proposed level of the myelotomy. A single-level myelotomy is performed where the spinal cord is thinnest. It is best if the level chosen is below the brachial plexus outflow, but this option may not be possible for cervical syrinxes. The location of the myelotomy on the spinal cord is also controversial. Some surgeons advocate performing the myelotomy where the spinal cord is thinnest,[13] which is usually at the dorsal nerve root entry zone. In the one case in which the spinal cord was entered at that location, severe dysesthetic pain localized to that nerve root resulted, and we do not advocate the approach. The authors prefer to perform a midline myelotomy ~1 cm long. An Edwards-Barbaro "T" shunt (Heyer-Schulte NeuroCare, Pleasant Prairie, WI) is then placed within the syrinx cavity, with arms aimed both caudad and cephalad (**Fig. 12.6**). A small area of the pia at the edge of the myelotomy is thickened using the bipolar coagulation device. A 6–0 monofilament nylon suture is then used to attach the shunt tubing to the spinal cord. The dura is closed in the usual fashion.

Attention is turned to the distal end of the shunt. Tunneling is performed in the usual manner, and no valve is used. A transverse incision is made over a rib that is palpable below the scapula. With the cutting current, the muscle and fascia are taken down through the periosteum to the bone. Subperiosteally, the dissection proceeds to the space between the ribs. At this point, the parietal pleura can be identified with the lung sliding below it. With the anesthesiologist applying positive pressure, the distal end of the shunt is placed in the pleural space. As the lung remains hyperinflated, the overlying muscles are closed to create a watertight seal, and routine ventilation is reestablished. Irrigation is performed, and the wound is closed as is the laminectomy wound. A postoperative radiograph, which usually shows a small incidental pneumothorax, is obtained. Occasionally, a symptomatic pneumothorax is seen and a chest tube is required. In the case of ventriculopleural shunts, intermittent thoracenteses may be needed for a short period because of the large volume of CSF in the pleural cavity. Thoracenteses is rarely, if ever, needed with syringopleural shunts because of the small volume of CSF produced daily by this space.

Chiari I Malformation with Associated Basilar Invagination

Basilar invagination, particularly when it is from congenital abnormalities of the skull base and upper cervical spine, is often accompanied by hindbrain herniation or the Chiari I malformation. In this instance, the hindbrain hernia is probably from crowding of the foramen magnum

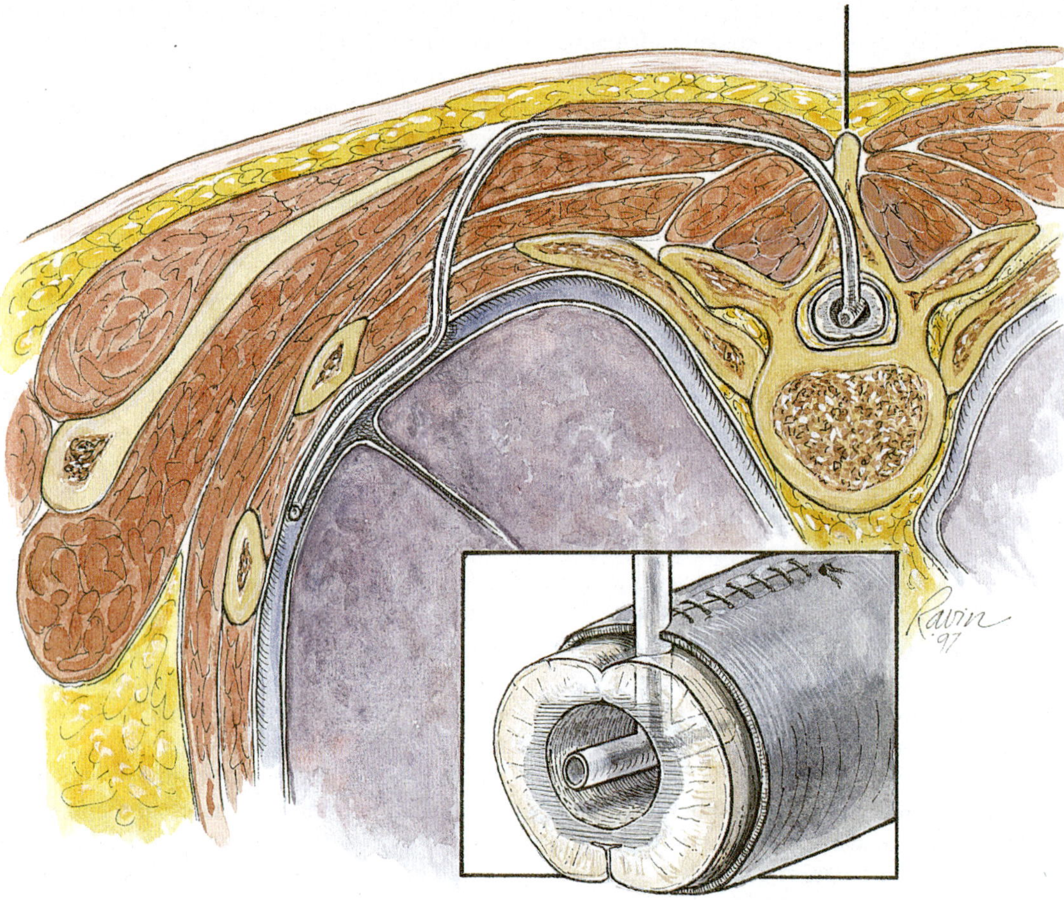

Fig. 12.6 Illustration of the placement of a syringopleural shunt. A midline myelotomy is performed over one segment, and a T-shunt is placed into the syrinx cavity (*inset*). Tubing is then tunneled to the posterior chest wall where it can be inserted into the pleural cavity. (Reprinted with permission from Barrow Neurological Institute.)

caused by the indentation of the brainstem. In our series of children and adolescents at the Barrow Neurological Institute, all patients with coexistent Chiari I malformation and basilar invagination could be managed via a primarily posterior approach using posterior occipitocervical decompression combined with intraoperative reduction in extension and distraction and occipitocervical fusion using a bent titanium rod.[27] In their large series of abnormalities of the CVJ, Menezes and Ryken[28] have stated that most, if not all, children with basilar invagination begin with a reducible lesion. However, pannus develops over time, creating an irreducible anterior compression. They recommend that when basilar invagination and hindbrain hernia coexist, the first step should be a transoral removal of the odontoid process followed by posterior decompression and fusion.[28] Using our technique in seven children, we have needed to perform delayed transoral odontoidectomy in three children who subtly deteriorated 1 to 4 years after the initial procedure. Because posterior fusion does not arrest growth of the anterior skull base, careful follow-up through puberty is recommended to prevent worsening ventral compression.

Pain, the most compelling symptom in this condition, is particularly severe when a Valsalva maneuver is performed. Spasticity, swallowing difficulty, sleep apnea, and lower cranial nerve disturbances are also part of the clinical condition of many of these patients. It seems that several of these patients have had their Chiari I malformation treated without the importance of the anterior bony abnormalities being recognized. This failure inevitably leads to subsequent deterioration, and failure of Chiari decompression to relieve symptoms or subsequent worsening should lead to another MRI study to search for subtle anterior brainstem compression.

Thorough preoperative evaluation of the CNS as well as the bony anatomy of the CVJ is essential in the preoperative assessment of these individuals. We recommend that thin-section computed tomography (CT) scanning with three-dimensional reconstruction be performed as well as plain radiography with flexion and extension views. MRI is mandatory, but magnetic resonance angiography to view the course of the vertebral arteries and/or flexion and extension MRI also may prove useful.

The procedure itself is performed using fluoroscopic guidance and utilizes intraoperative monitoring of SSEPs and brainstem evoked potentials. After anesthesia has been induced and baseline recordings of the evoked potentials have been obtained, the patient is placed in a halo ring and jacket for turning and positioning. The patient is then turned prone on a frame. The back of the halo vest is removed, and the halo ring is attached to the operating table as a head holder. Except in children under 3 years of age, the standard Chiari I operation described previously is performed. In very young children, the reduction itself is sufficient to decompress the brainstem, and it is seldom necessary to open the dura. At this point, Songer cables (Danek Medical, Inc., Memphis, TN; AcroMed, Cleveland, OH) are placed under the lamina of the next two caudal vertebrae (usually C3 and C4). Two or three holes are drilled in the skull ~1 cm from the newly enlarged foramen magnum, and Songer cables are passed epidurally to exit the drilled holes (**Fig. 12.7**). One member of the surgical team breaks scrub and releases the halo ring from the remainder of the vest and the operating table. Reduction is accomplished by applying distraction and extension forces simultaneously and with fluoroscopic and evoked potential monitoring (**Fig. 12.8**). This maneuver brings the cranial and cervical sublaminar wires closer together. A custom-bent threaded titanium rod is then positioned, and Songer cables are tightened and crimped (**Fig. 12.9**). On one occasion while we performed this maneuver, the SSEPs changed and the degree of reduction was compromised. However, the patient did well and has not required a transoral odontoidectomy. At this point in the procedure, bone grafts are applied for long-term fusion. These grafts are obtained from the iliac crest in older children and adults and from the adjacent skull in small children.

With advances in stereotactic navigation and spinal surgery, screw and rod constructs are becoming more feasible to use in the pediatric population. Existing adult constructs have been modified, and new pediatric constructs have been developed.[8,16] Evaluation of the size of C2 pedicles and pars interarticularis, C1 lateral masses, and occipital condyles are crucial to patient selection. As always, care must be taken to avoid the vertebral artery during screw placement.

Chiari II Malformation

The Chiari II malformation is truly malformative in that it occurs early in gestational age and is associated with rather widespread abnormalities of the CNS, including a universal

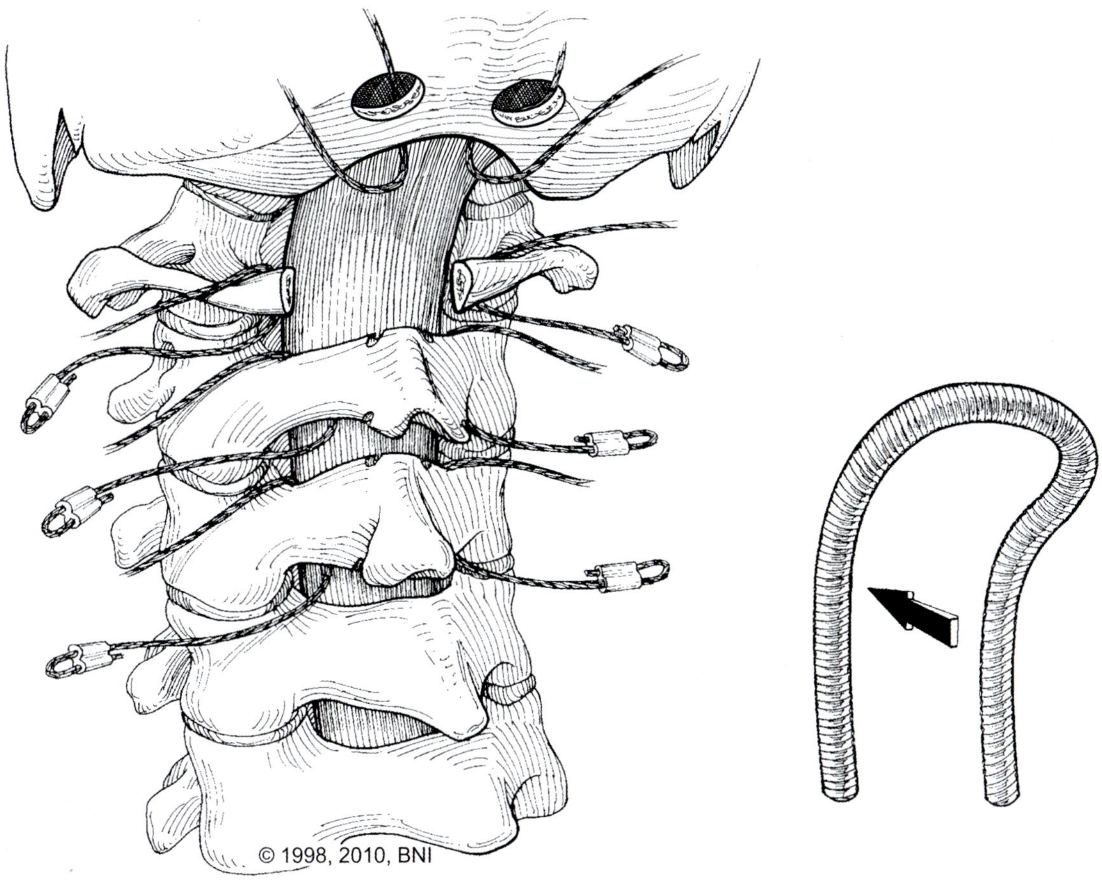

Fig. 12.7 Occipitocervical fusion. A specifically fashioned, threaded, titanium pin is wired to the skull and the laminae of the upper cervical vertebrae using sublaminar wires. (Reprinted with permission from Barrow Neurological Institute.)

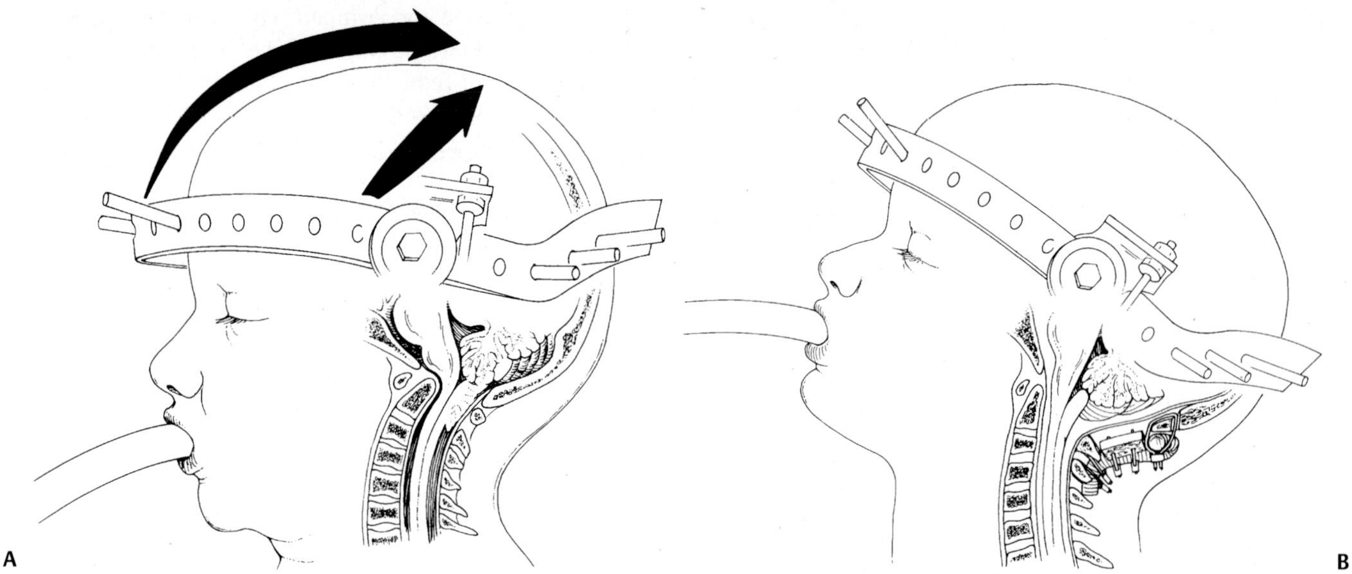

Fig. 12.8 Illustration of the reduction of the craniocervical malalignment in a child with a basilar invagination causing the Chiari I malformation. The head is **(A)** extended and distracted, after which the cables are **(B)** tightened and crimped. (Reprinted with permission from Barrow Neurological Institute.)

association with spina bifida cystica. Many theories concerning the embryology and pathogenesis of this condition have been proposed. McLone and Knapper postulated that the malformation results from the in utero loss of the distending force of CSF, which is lost through the open neural tube defect. This theory is the most plausible and explains most, if not all, of the associated findings.[29] As opposed to the Chiari I malformation in which the cerebellar tonsils are the herniating mass, in the Chiari II malformation, the medulla itself is the lowest brain structure in the cervical spinal canal. It is bent over on itself (medullary kink) and seems to drag the cerebellar vermis with it. The choroid plexus of the fourth ventricle is everted onto the surface of the medulla. In this situation, the posterior fossa is quite small, the midbrain is distorted (beaked), and the tentorium is incompetent and arranged in a vertical configuration. Of vital importance from a surgical perspective is that the torcula and transverse sinuses often can be found at or below the foramen magnum. Failure to recognize these relationships has resulted in fatal exsanguination.

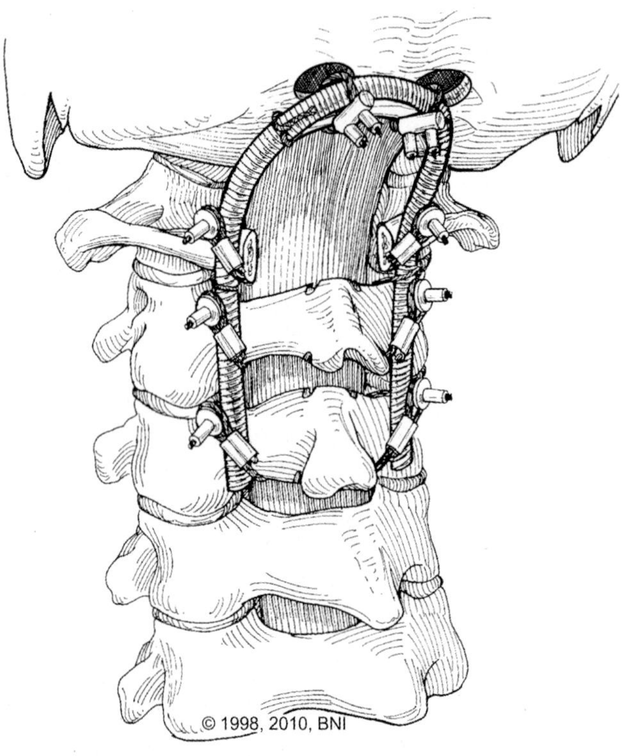

Fig. 12.9 Final appearance of threaded T2 pin construct before placement of autologous bone graft from the occiput to C2. (Reprinted with permission from Barrow Neurological Institute.)

Although the Chiari II malformation is present to a greater or lesser degree in all patients with spina bifida cystica, it becomes symptomatic and requires treatment only in a small percentage of cases. Three distinct clinical syndromes are associated with this condition and occur at three different times in the child's life. The first and most tragic of these is in the delivery room with the child struggling to breathe. Immediate intervention and intubation are required. Neonates who survive do so with the need for a tracheostomy, gastrostomy, and respirator. Surgical decompression of the Chiari malformation is unlikely to change the outcome. Postmortem studies of these infants have shown severe disorganization of brainstem structures and the absence of the nuclei of cranial nerves IX and X.[30]

In the infantile presentation of the symptomatic Chiari II malformation (Chiari crisis), patients initially seem to do well and breathe normally early on. The back repair is accomplished and most, if not all, have received a shunt. They present to their pediatricians or the emergency room with croup. Typically, their stridor can be heard across the room. Urgent intubation is usually necessary. If the stridor is mild, the infants drool and cannot swallow. In these patients, the first step after intubation is to prove that the shunt is working. If the ventricles are large, the shunt should be tested manometrically or by open surgical exploration. This condition represents a clear-cut indication for the Chiari II decompression, which is described later.

The final clinical syndrome associated with the Chiari II malformation is the late childhood type of presentation. These older children or adolescents have had some of the symptoms attributable to the Chiari II malformation for most of their lives, including slow eating, intolerance of certain food textures, and snoring. They present late and somewhat insidiously with progressively severe posterior neck pain that is ameliorated by retroflexion of the head and pain, numbness, or weakness of the hands. Strength testing almost always shows loss of grip strength relative to age-matched controls. Griebel and colleagues have shown significant increases in upper extremity strength and function after Chiari II decompression.[19] Although this condition and the condition described previously are due to the malformation, there are no radiographic clues about who will and who will not develop these problems. One unanswered question then becomes whether decompression should be offered to children with spina bifida and unexpected hand and arm weakness without other symptoms. Two patients treated at our institution with hand function so weak that it interfered with functions such as feeding and dressing were treated with decompression. The improvement in their hand function was excellent.

The operation required to treat problems related to the Chiari II malformation is somewhat different from that used for the Chiari I malformation. Although the posterior fossa is small in this condition, the foramen magnum is quite large. All of the structures to be decompressed reside in the cervical canal. Although not all pediatric neurosurgeons agree, we strongly believe that, except in the most unusual circumstances, no bone needs to be removed from the rim of the foramen magnum and all of the decompression should be done in the cervical region. The operations performed for the infantile form of the disease and the one performed for the late childhood form are identical, but operative findings vary greatly. The opening for this operation is identical to that for the Chiari I procedure except that the number of cervical laminae exposed and removed is greater. It is essential to extend the operation far enough caudally to identify the caudal end of the brainstem. On occasion, a laminectomy down to C7 has been required. The laminectomy should be limited, and great care should be exercised not to expose or damage the facet joints. Despite the great theoretical risk of postlaminectomy kyphosis with multiple level cervical laminectomies, the senior author (HLR) has seen this complication only once, occurring in a child with an extremely large head.

After the laminectomy has been performed with the number of segments determined by the lowest position of the medulla as seen on preoperative MRI, the dura is opened in a caudal to rostral direction as described. This point is extremely important because the venous structure that is likely to be encountered is not the circular sinus but the torcula. When the dura is opened, the degree of arachnoidal thickening (scarring) can be dramatic. The pathophysiology of this problem in small children is truly compressive, whereas in adolescents the problem does not appear to be compressive at all. Rather, the cervical spinal cord and lower brainstem seem to be firmly fused to the dura by dense bands of adherent arachnoiditis. We believe that the surgeon should use the microscope to lyse these bands to untether the brainstem.

The next step in the procedure involves opening the fourth ventricle. The anatomy in this region is extremely unusual, and this step requires complete understanding of the unique relationships that occur here (**Fig. 12.10**). The critical step is identification of the choroid plexus, which is everted from the fourth ventricle. While the choroid plexus lies on the surface of the medulla, it can be modified by its chronic encasement in scar tissue as to make its identification extremely difficult. After microscopic dissection of the scar tissue, which is almost always most dense in the area of the choroid plexus, the choroid should be identifiable. If it is still unclear, attention should be directed to the cerebellar vermis. Once this structure is identified, it can be followed down until it too is encased in scar tissue. At this point, the cerebellar vermis can be resected in a rostral to caudal direction until the choroid plexus is identified. The remnants of the foramen of Magendie lie immediately deep to this confluence and can be entered here with safety. As long as the pristine white surface of the fourth ventricle is seen, the hole is large enough.

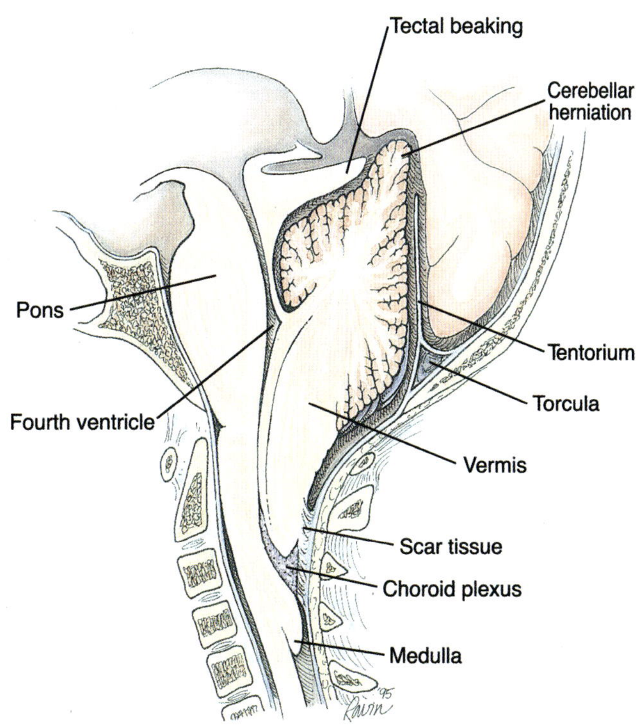

Fig. 12.10 Illustration of the surgical anatomy of the Chiari II malformation showing a low-lying torcula and a medullary kink that is displaced more caudally than the cerebellar vermis. (Reprinted with permission from Barrow Neurological Institute.)

The closures for a Chiari II "decompression" and a Chiari I decompression are essentially the same. It should be reemphasized that meticulous attention to a watertight closure of the dural patch is extremely important, particularly if the donor site for the patch graft is the cervical musculature.

Outside the newborn period, the results of surgery for the Chiari II malformation are very successful. Improvement in cranial nerve function can be expected in a significant majority of infants. Hand strength should increase, and suboccipital headaches should improve in almost all adolescent patients whose shunt function has been idealized as part of the selection process. Based on long-term follow-up, postoperative deformity has occurred in only one patient whose care was made extremely difficult by a very large head.

Conclusion

Although the management of Chiari I and Chiari II malformations differs in the amount and location of bone to be removed, they are the same in terms of the surgical principles involved. In each case, the goals of surgery are to relieve brainstem compression from the bony and dural constrictions caused by the herniation to establish normalized CSF flow across the foramen magnum and to obtain a watertight dural closure.

References

1. Chiari H. Ueber Veränderungen des Kleinhirns infolge von Hydrocephalie des Grosshirns. Dtsch Med Wochenschr 1891;17:1172–1175
2. Chiari H. Über Veränderungen des Kleinhirns, des Pons und der Medulla Oblongata infolge von congenitaler Hydrocephalie des Grosshirns. Denkschriften Der Kais Akad Wiss Math-Naturw 1896;63:71–115
3. Cleland J. Contribution to the study of spina bifida, encephalocele, and anencephalus. J Anat Physiol 1883;17(Pt 3):257–292
4. Schwalbe E, Gredig M. Über Entwicklungsstörungen des Kleinhirns, Hirnstamms und Halsmarks bei Spina bifida. (Arnold'sche und Chiari'sche Missbildung). Beitr Pathol Anat 1907;40:132–194
5. Carmel PW, Markesbery WR. Early descriptions of the Arnold-Chiari malformation. The contribution of John Cleland. J Neurosurg 1972;37(5):543–547
6. Kasner SE, Rosenfeld J, Farber RE. Spontaneous intracranial hypotension: headache with a reversible Arnold-Chiari malformation. Headache 1995;35(9):557–559
7. Girard N, Lasjaunias P, Taylor W. Reversible tonsillar prolapse in vein of Galen aneurysmal malformations: report of eight cases and pathophysiological hypothesis. Childs Nerv Syst 1994;10(3):141–147
8. McGirt MJ, Attenello FJ, Atiba A, et al. Symptom recurrence after suboccipital decompression for pediatric Chiari I malformation: analysis of 256 consecutive cases. Childs Nerv Syst 2008;24(11):1333–1339
9. Francis PM, Beals S, Rekate HL, Pittman HW, Manwaring K, Reiff J. Chronic tonsillar herniation and Crouzon's syndrome. Pediatr Neurosurg 1992;18(4):202–206
10. Cinalli G, Renier D, Sebag G, Sainte-Rose C, Arnaud E, Pierre-Kahn A. [Chiari "malformation" in Crouzon syndrome]. Arch Pediatr 1996;3(5):433–439
11. Hoffman HJ, Tucker WS. Cephalocranial disproportion. A complication of the treatment of hydrocephalus in children. Childs Brain 1976;2(3):167–176
12. Chumas PD, Armstrong DC, Drake JM, et al. Tonsillar herniation: the rule rather than the exception after lumboperitoneal shunting in the pediatric population. J Neurosurg 1993;78(4):568–573
13. Chumas PD, Kulkarni AV, Drake JM, Hoffman HJ, Humphreys RP, Rutka JT. Lumboperitoneal shunting: a retrospective study in the pediatric population. Neurosurgery 1993;32(3):376–383, discussion 383
14. Tsonidas C, Karahalios DG, Rekate HL, Chiari I. Malformation in association with sacral defects and sacral meningoceles. Neurol Psychiatr (Bucur) 1991;12(Suppl 1):74–77
15. Aquilina K, Merchant TE, Boop FA, Sanford RA. Chiari I malformation after cranial radiation therapy in childhood: a dynamic process associated with changes in clival growth. Childs Nerv Syst 2009;25(11):1429–1436
16. Greenlee JD, Donovan KA, Hasan DM, Menezes AH. Chiari I malformation in the very young child: the spectrum of presentations and experience in 31 children under age 6 years. Pediatrics 2002;110(6):1212–1219
17. Zamel K, Galloway G, Kosnik EJ, Raslan M, Adeli A. Intraoperative neurophysiologic monitoring in 80 patients with Chiari I malformation: role of duraplasty. J Clin Neurophysiol 2009;26(2):70–75
18. Perrini P, Benedetto N, Tenenbaum R, Di Lorenzo N. Extra-arachnoidal cranio-cervical decompression for syringomyelia associated with Chiari I malformation in adults: technique assessment. Acta Neurochir (Wien) 2007;149(10):1015–1022, discussion 1022–1023
19. Griebel ML, Oakes J, Worley G. The Chiari malformation associated with myelomeningoceles. In: Rekate HL, ed. Comprehensive Management of Spina Bifida. Boca Raton, FL: CRC Press; 1991:83–89
20. Williams B. A critical appraisal of posterior fossa surgery for communicating syringomyelia. Brain 1978;101(2):223–250
21. Krieger MD, McComb JG, Levy ML. Toward a simpler surgical management of Chiari I malformation in a pediatric population. Pediatr Neurosurg 1999;30(3):113–121
22. Oi S, Kudo H, Yamada H, et al. Hydromyelic hydrocephalus. Correlation of hydromyelia with various stages of hydrocephalus in postshunt isolated compartments. J Neurosurg 1991;74(3): 371–379
23. Oldfield EH, Muraszko K, Shawker TH, Patronas NJ. Pathophysiology of syringomyelia associated with Chiari I malformation of the cerebellar tonsils. Implications for diagnosis and treatment. J Neurosurg 1994;80(1):3–15
24. Batzdorf U. Chiari I malformation with syringomyelia. Evaluation of surgical therapy by magnetic resonance imaging. J Neurosurg 1988;68(5):726–730
25. Smith KA, Rekate HL. Delayed postoperative tethering of the cervical spinal cord. J Neurosurg 1994;81(2):196–201
26. Lesoin F, Petit H, Thomas CE III, Viaud C, Baleriaux D, Jomin M. Use of the syringoperitoneal shunt in the treatment of syringomyelia. Surg Neurol 1986;25(2):131–136
27. Apostolides PJ, Dickman CA, Golfinos JG, Papadopoulos SM, Sonntag VK. Threaded steinmann pin fusion of the craniovertebral junction. Spine 1996;21(14):1630–1637
28. Menezes AH, Ryken TC, Brockmeyer DL. Abnormalities of the craniocervical junction. In: McLone DG, ed. Pediatric Neurosurgery: Surgery of the Developing Nervous System. 4th ed. Philadelphia, PA: WB Saunders; 2001:400–422
29. McLone DG, Knepper PA. The cause of Chiari II malformation: a unified theory. Pediatr Neurosci 1989;15(1):1–12
30. Gilbert JN, Jones KL, Rorke LB, Chernoff GF, James HE. Central nervous system anomalies associated with meningomyelocele, hydrocephalus, and the Arnold-Chiari malformation: reappraisal of theories regarding the pathogenesis of posterior neural tube closure defects. Neurosurgery 1986;18(5):559–564

13 Management of Intramedullary Lesions of the Cervicomedullary Junction and High Cervical Spinal Cord

Jonathan H. Lustgarten and Paul C. McCormick

In the microsurgical era, it has become increasingly clear that surgical excision is the treatment of choice for most intramedullary tumors.[1–9] Current microsurgical techniques allow a cure or long-term remission to be achieved with acceptable neurological morbidity for the benign lesions that constitute the majority of intramedullary tumors. There has been some reluctance to pursue similarly aggressive surgical treatment of intramedullary lesions when they affect the high cervical cord and/or the cervicomedullary junction. The localization of critical neurological function related to respiration and airway protection in this region of the neuraxis has led to a less aggressive approach toward such lesions. In this chapter, we review the available information on intramedullary lesions of the high cervical spinal cord and cervicomedullary junction.

Critical to this discussion is the recent availability of magnetic resonance imaging (MRI) data that has contributed enormously to understanding the biological behavior of various lesions arising in this junctional region. Relatively few reports focus specifically on lesions in this location, but several basic concepts have emerged. First, glial tumors of the high cervical cord and cervicomedullary junction behave more like spinal cord gliomas than traditional "brainstem gliomas," although the latter term represents a heterogeneous group of entities with variable biological behaviors. Second, high cervical and cervicomedullary ependymomas and well-circumscribed astrocytomas in this region are amenable to surgical resection with good results if appropriate perioperative management, particularly of airway and respiratory function, is employed. Finally, for these lesions, extent of resection correlates with long-term outcome, and radiation treatment is inappropriate as a primary modality of therapy. For the less common diffusely infiltrative or malignant lesion, aggressive surgical therapy offers little benefit and the priority is solely on preserving neurological function. Radiation treatment is often used in this setting but is of questionable benefit, and the prognosis for malignant lesions is poor regardless of the therapeutic strategy selected. Anatomical concepts that may explain observed biological behaviors are reviewed.

Anatomical Considerations

The reluctance to offer aggressive surgical treatments to patients harboring high cervical or cervicomedullary lesions often stems from concern regarding neural control of critical respiratory functions and airway protection. Certainly the literature and anecdotal experience on the treatment of these lesions report postoperative compromise of these critical functions, as well as examples of quadriplegia.[2,4,10,11] Anatomical structures that can be involved include the brainstem nuclei related to lower cranial nerves, such as the dorsal motor nucleus of the vagus and the nucleus ambiguus. Also theoretically at risk are cells whose efferents maintain regular and independent respiration. The *dorsal respiratory group* is an aggregation of neurons located in the dorsomedial medulla just ventrolateral to the solitary tract. The *ventral respiratory group* is a longer longitudinally oriented column of cells associated with the retrofascial nucleus, the nucleus ambiguus, and the nucleus retroambigualis. Neurons of the ventral respiratory group have descending input to the phrenic motoneurons. The phrenic motor columns are bilaterally organized in longitudinally oriented columns of cells in the ventromedial aspect of the ventral horn with inspiratory neurons concentrated laterally and expiratory cells concentrated ventrally.[12]

The surgical approach reviewed here emphasizes a dorsal approach in the midline between the posterior columns and extirpation working from within the tumor with very gentle technique and minimal cauterization to spare surrounding neural elements. Approach through the floor of the fourth ventricle transgresses the minimum possible amount of neural tissue. It is not possible to monitor fully all critical functions theoretically at risk during these procedures. The key to successful aggressive surgical treatment of lesions in this location is to apply the techniques to lesions selected appropriately and not attempt radical resection of malignant lesions or benign but infiltrative lesions devoid of a surgical plane.

Favorable surgical outcomes also require judicious application of techniques and strategies for managing airway, swallowing, and respiratory problems and the identification of patients at particular risk. In our experience, preoperative compromise of function is a better predictor of perioperative difficulty than are radiographic criteria, such as size or location of tumor. Anecdotal evidence from our series suggests that the resilience of the high cervical spinal cord is surprising. In several cases, enormous tumors spanning to the ventral pia and splitting and laterally displacing spinal cord tissue have been fully resected—patients had excellent postoperative function. In some cases, postoperative MRI demonstrates a markedly thinned, ribbon-like cervical cord only a fraction of the normal width of the spinal cord in patients with complete or excellent neurological function (**Fig. 13.1**).

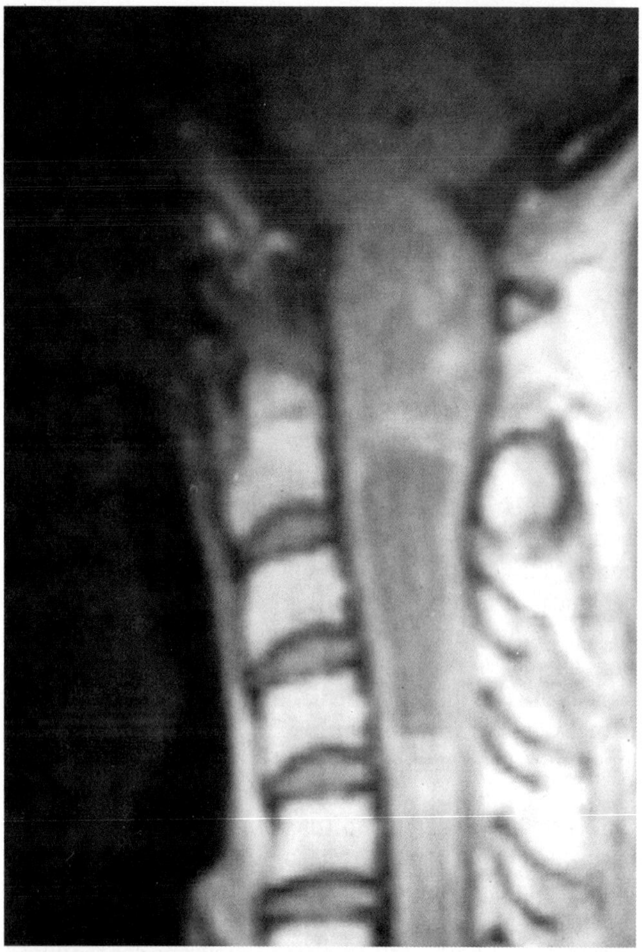

A

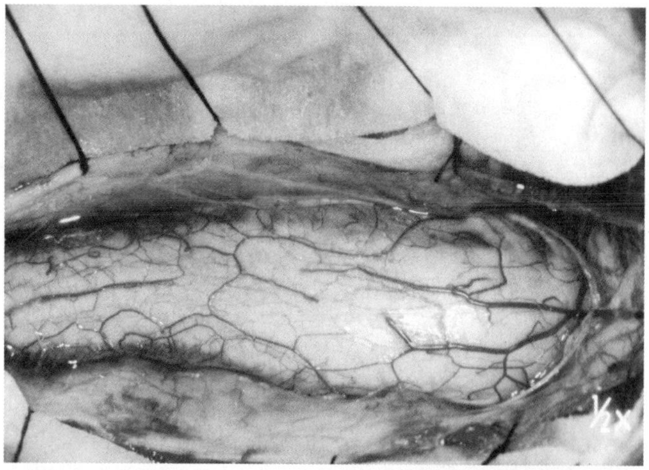

B

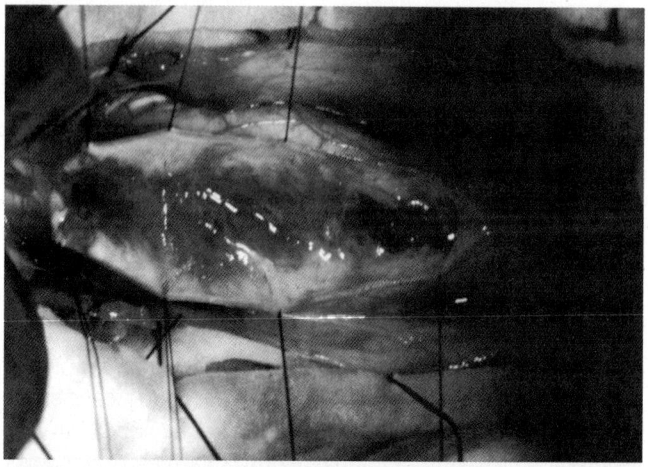

C

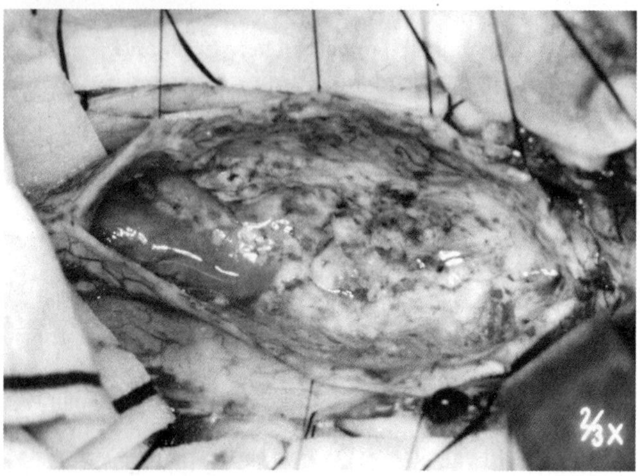

D

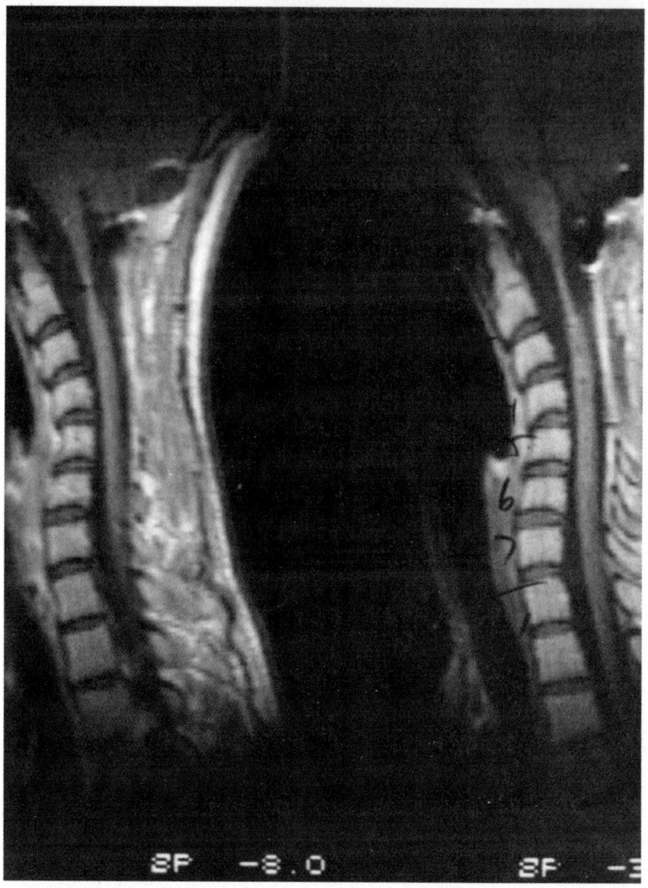

E

Fig. 13.1 **(A)** Sagittal contrast-enhanced magnetic resonance image (MRI) shows a minimally enhancing intramedullary mass of the cervicomedullary junction. **(B)** Intraoperative photograph demonstrates spinal cord enlargement of the cervicomedullary junction. **(C)** Operative photograph following a midline myelotomy demonstrates the typical smooth glistening appearance of a benign intramedullary ependymoma. Note the pial traction sutures. **(D)** Intraoperative photograph following gross total resection of the tumor. **(E)** Follow-up MRI demonstrates no tumor recurrence. Despite the thin, ribbon-like nature of the spinal cord, this patient has had a satisfactory clinical outcome with independent ambulation and adequate fine motor control of both hands.

The approach outlined reflects our belief that high cervical and cervicomedullary lesions behave biologically, in most cases, more as intramedullary spinal cord tumors than as infiltrating brainstem gliomas. In general, gliomas of the brainstem are remarkable for their poor prognosis. Their typical course is steady progression to death in fewer than 2 years. In the past, these gliomas were viewed as uniformly "malignant" from a clinical standpoint in that their location rendered them inoperable. With the advent of MRI, it has become apparent that neoplasms involving the brainstem are heterogeneous and that certain subcategories may offer a different prognosis.[13,14]

Analysis of the growth patterns and categories of these neoplasms based on their MRI appearance has enhanced our understanding of the lesions and the relationship between rostrally disposed cervical cord tumors and brainstem gliomas. Epstein and Wisoff originally described 20 intra-axial neoplasms of the cervicomedullary junction that they believed shared characteristics of low-grade spinal cord gliomas and brainstem gliomas.[4] They found these lesions to be more amenable to surgical treatment than typical brainstem gliomas. Epstein and Farmer refined this concept through further experience in the MRI era.[13] They observed four stereotyped growth patterns in 88 patients harboring brainstem gliomas. One category included cervicomedullary tumors (44 cases). These were lesions whose caudal portion was anatomically identical to an intramedullary tumor and whose rostral extension was, in general, limited at the caudal medulla. Further rostral extension occurred by posterior bulging at the obex, sometimes resulting in frank rupture into the fourth ventricle.

Pathology of High Cervical and Cervicomedullary Lesions

The spectrum of intramedullary lesions encountered in the high cervical cord and cervicomedullary junction is similar to that seen in the rest of the spinal cord.[6] Tumors of glial cell origin account for more than 80% of the lesions seen in both the pediatric and adult populations. Most common are the astrocytomas and ependymomas. Anaplastic astrocytomas are less frequent, as are other glial neoplasms, including gangliogliomas, oligodendrogliomas, and subependymomas. Hemangiomas represent ~10% of the lesions in this location.[2] Metastatic involvement of the high cervical cord and cervicomedullary junction is uncommon, just as it is in the rest of the spinal cord. Lung and breast are the most common locations for primary tumors.

A variety of other uncommon lesions also can be seen in this area, including cavernous malformations, inclusion tumors and cysts, lipomas, intramedullary nerve sheath tumors, and melanocytomas. Nontumorous lesions in the spinal cord that can be mistaken for neoplasm can also occur in the high cervical cord and cervicomedullary junction. These lesions include inflammatory or demyelinating conditions, such as plaques associated with multiple sclerosis, sarcoidosis, viral or parainfectious myelitis, and paraneoplastic inflammatory lesions. These lesions can be grouped under the heading *transverse myelitis*. Relatively rapid progression over hours to days is most typical of these lesions, although demyelinating lesions may be chronically progressive or relapsing and remitting. Plaques of multiple sclerosis tend to be focal, homogeneous areas of enhancement in the white matter, whereas parainfectious myelitides tend to be patchy or infiltrative and involve several segments. In general, a rapid course and significant neurological deficit in the absence of significant mass effect suggest an inflammatory lesion. Slow-growing benign glial tumors tend to displace or slowly infiltrate functional spinal cord tissue so that quite impressive masses may be seen in patients who demonstrate surprising preservation of cord and brainstem function.[6] The differential diagnosis of mass lesions in the spinal cord and cervicomedullary junction includes tuberculoma and bacterial abscess.

Clinical Presentation of High Cervical and Cervicomedullary Tumors

In the adult population, the clinical presentation of these intramedullary lesions usually involves the spine rather than the brainstem. Pain is the most common initial complaint, usually localized to the neck or shoulder. Dysesthesias and paresthesias are also common early symptoms. Other less common complaints include numbness or sensory loss, paravertebral tightness, gait disturbance, and hand incoordination. Bulbar symptoms are unusual and usually the result of a rostral polar cyst extending into the brainstem. Due to the slow growth rate of most of these tumors, the sensitivity of contemporary imaging modalities, especially MRI, and the widespread availability and use of imaging, patients harboring intramedullary tumors are increasingly diagnosed with minimal or no symptoms and no neurological deficit. These features of clinical presentation of high cervical lesions echo previous observations made regarding the clinical features of intramedullary spinal cord lesions in general. The shorter clinical course of more malignant lesions is well known.[1,2,5] Pain as the most common presenting symptom, usually localized to the level of involvement and not clearly radicular in nature, is typical of spinal cord tumors at various levels. In general, objective neurological deficit is present at the time of presentation. A large mass associated with relatively mild deficits suggests a benign lesion. Smaller masses that are proportionally more symptomatic may be seen with malignant pathology. The presence of an enhancing area associated with minimal mass effect but significant neurological deficit, especially one that has developed rapidly, must raise a suspicion of an inflammatory rather than a neoplastic lesion. With the advent of MRI, many lesions are being diagnosed at earlier stages with minimal or no objective deficit in some cases.

Diagnostic Evaluation

The importance of early diagnosis and treatment of intramedullary tumors has been stressed and holds true for intramedullary lesions afflicting the upper cervical cord and medulla.[5,6] The functional result after surgical treatment of intramedullary lesions at any level is directly related to the patient's preoperative neurological status. Operative morbidity is increased, and the potential for functional recovery is lessened proportional to the degree of neurological disability present before surgery. Long-standing and significant deficits are unlikely to recover following surgical excision.[1,2] All intramedullary lesions can cause significant functional deficits related to compromise of ascending and descending long tracts. Other manifestations are related to segmental gray matter involvement. In the case of high cervical and cervicomedullary tumors, this segmental involvement can compromise critical life functions related to swallowing, protection of the airway, and respiratory control.[4] Patients who present with significant compromise of these neurological functions before surgical treatment have a poor prognosis. Exacerbation of these types of deficits after surgery has implications not only for neurological function but for survival. As such, preoperative neurological examination is an important predictor of outcome after surgical therapy for high cervical intramedullary tumors. We have utilized a four-grade clinical/functional classification scheme to evaluate patients harboring intramedullary lesions (**Table 13.1**).[7] This scheme does not explicitly include parameters related to bulbar function, but it is still prognostically useful in characterizing patients whose intramedullary lesion is in the upper cervical cord.

As for all intramedullary lesions, MRI is clearly the diagnostic modality of choice for high cervical and cervicomedullary lesions and has completely supplanted the use of computed tomography myelography.[5] The sagittal images of the cervicomedullary junction afforded by MRI allow accurate preoperative evaluation of the full extent of the lesion and are invaluable in guiding the surgical approach. In addition, the possibility of hydrocephalus can be evaluated, when clinically indicated, with cranial MRI. Most intramedullary tumors are isointense or hypointense with respect to the surrounding spinal cord on T1-weighted images. Spinal cord enlargement may be the only suggestion of tumor on an unenhanced T1-weighted image. T2-weighted images are quite sensitive and tend to demonstrate hyperintensity associated with lesions regardless of pathological type. It may be easier to delineate tumor from polar cysts on the T1-weighted images, however.

Typically, ependymomas are relatively more circumscribed and symmetrically located within the spinal cord than astrocytomas. They usually enhance uniformly. Polar cysts are frequently associated with ependymomas, particularly in the high cervical region (**Fig. 13.2**). The presence of cysts or necrotic areas within an ependymoma may lead to a more heterogeneous or more subtle pattern of enhancement, making their differentiation from astrocytomas difficult.

Astrocytomas vary in their MRI appearance. They often are less circumscribed as a result of irregular tumor margins. Enhancement patterns range from minimal to patchy to uniform. Cysts and areas of necrosis occur in these tumors as well. Despite these characteristic patterns, in our experience it has not been possible to differentiate astrocytomas from ependymomas with certainty. In cases demonstrating the classic well-circumscribed, centrally located enhancing lesion with polar cysts, it is often possible to diagnose the ependymoma correctly based on the preoperative study. Such a diagnosis is possible less often for astrocytomas. However, making this distinction

Table 13.1 Four-Grade Clinical/Functional Classification Scheme

I	Neurologically normal; mild focal deficit not significantly affecting function of involved limb; mild spasticity or reflex abnormality; normal gait
II	Presence of sensorimotor deficit affecting function of involved limb; mild to moderate gait difficulty; severe pain or dysesthetic syndrome impairing patient's quality of life; still functions and ambulates independently
III	More severe neurological deficit; requires cane/brace for ambulation or significant bilateral upper extremity impairment; may or may not function independently
IV	Severe deficit; requires wheelchair or cane/brace with bilateral upper extremity impairment; usually not independent

Source: McCormick PC, Torres R, Post KD, et al. Intramedullary ependymoma of the spinal cord. J Neurosurg 1990;72:523–532. Reprinted with permission from *Journal of Neurosurgery*.

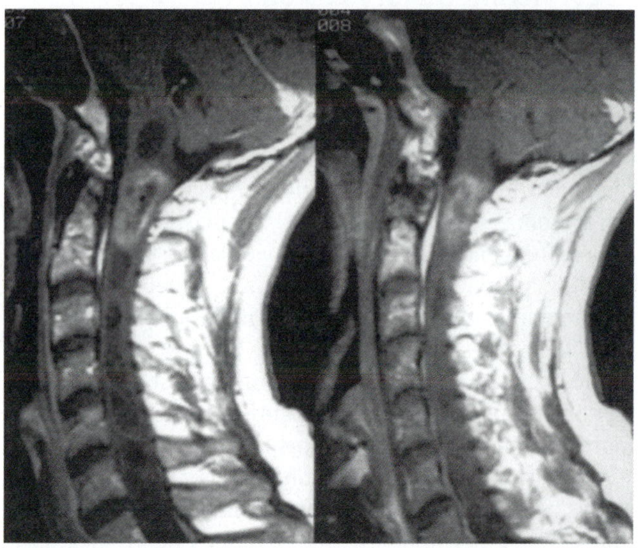

Fig. 13.2 T1-weighted gadolinium-enhanced magnetic resonance image shows heterogeneous contrast uptake of a cervicomedullary ependymoma. Note the polar cyst above and below the solid tumor component.

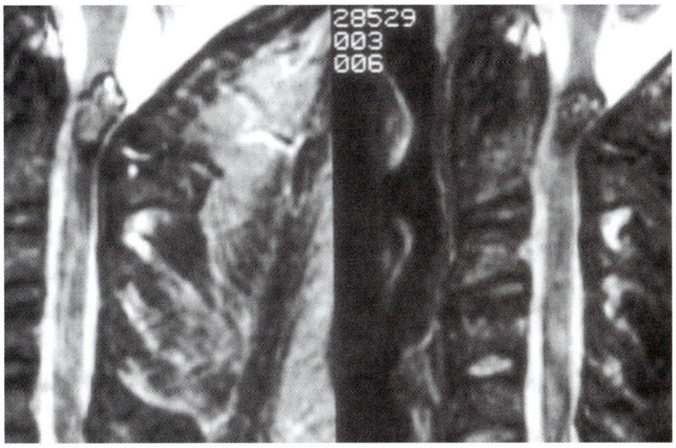

Fig. 13.3 Sagittal magnetic resonance image demonstrates typical heterogeneous core of mixed signal intensity surrounded by a hypointense hemosiderin ring consistent with a diagnosis of a cavernous malformation.

preoperatively is not critical because proper surgical treatment requires full exposure of the rostrocaudal extent of the tumor in almost all cases.

Hemangioblastomas typically are focal and brightly enhancing and may be associated with flow voids. The hallmark finding is marked spinal cord edema, especially notable on T2-weighted images that may extend over many segments through the spinal cord and involve most of the spinal cord. The MRI characteristics of cavernous malformations within the spinal cord have been well described. The hallmark of this lesion is a hyperintense lesion with a surrounding hypointense rim due to hemosiderin deposition in the periphery of the lesion (**Fig. 13.3**).

Regardless of the pathology of the lesion, MRI permits the precise anatomical delineation of the rostrocaudal extent of the lesion to allow for preoperative planning of the exposure. In our series, approximately one-third of the astrocytomas arising in the high cervical region extended above the level of the foramen magnum, requiring suboccipital craniectomy in addition to cervical laminectomy for adequate operative exposure. This approach was required somewhat more frequently for ependymomas. In general, we have found, as have others, that most tumors in this location do not extend above the obex.[4,10]

Surgical Treatment

Most neurosurgeons adhere to the view that microsurgical excision is the mainstay of treatment for most intramedullary tumors. Is a similarly aggressive posture appropriate for those intramedullary lesions located in the upper cervical cord or cervicomedullary junction? Our philosophy in handling these lesions is based on the idea that the biological behavior of tumors arising in the upper cervical cord is similar to that of intramedullary tumors at more caudal locations, even when these tumors extend above the foramen magnum. Therefore, the surgical approach is essentially the same for these lesions as for the lower intramedullary tumors.[5–7] The preoperative plan is dictated by the MRI appearance of the lesion. In almost all cases, the surgery is planned to allow a complete removal of the lesion. The exception is in cases where it is obvious from the MRI appearance that one is dealing with a diffusely infiltrative process that is not amenable to surgical removal (**Fig. 13.4**). MRI clearly demonstrates marked widening and expansion of the spinal cord extending above the foramen magnum and obex. Involvement of the caudal brainstem is diffuse and patchy and strongly suggests an infiltrative process that is not amenable to surgical excision. This lesion is manifesting malignant or diffusely infiltrative behavior. We believe these radiographic features enable the surgeon to determine before surgery that the goal of an operation is to obtain a biopsy. The goal in such a case is preservation of neurological function rather than aggressive resection. Such tumors represent a distinct minority of high cervical and cervicomedullary tumors.

In most cases, the tumor is more circumscribed or focal. In this situation, the surgeon should assume that the lesion is benign and potentially resectable and proceed accordingly. Surgical techniques employed in removal of high cervical and cervicomedullary intramedullary tumors are those utilized for removal of caudally located lesions, with minor modifications specific to this junctional region. The prone position is preferred because it allows two surgeons to operate together, facing one another, using the operating microscope with a bridge attachment. Significant risk of air embolism is also avoided. Before anesthesia is induced, intermittent compression stockings are used to prevent deep venous thrombosis of the lower extremities. Perioperative

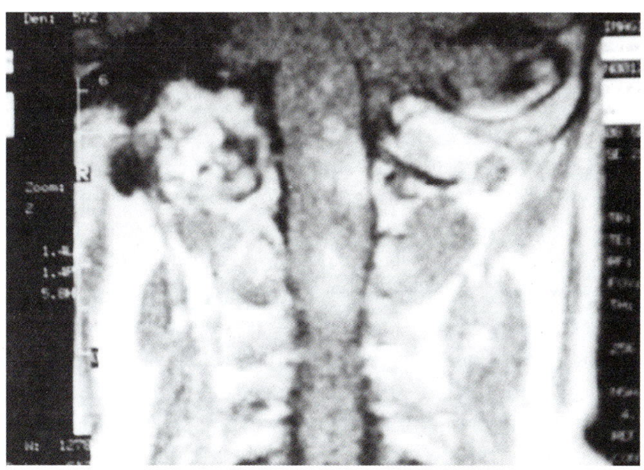

Fig. 13.4 T1-weighted contrast-enhanced coronal magnetic resonance image shows diffuse enlargement with patchy enhancement clearly indicative of an infiltrative tumor. At surgery, only a subtotal removal was accomplished. No apparent tumor mass was identified. The histology demonstrated a diffusely infiltrative astrocytoma.

steroids and broad-spectrum antibiotics are administered. Typically, somatosensory evoked potentials and motor evoked potentials are monitored, although we have not found them useful in guiding surgical resection.

The patient is positioned prone in rigid three-point skull fixation. When the patient is turned, great care is taken to maintain the neck in a neutral position. An attempt is made to place the involved segments of the spinal cord roughly parallel to the floor while the head is elevated above the level of the heart. At times, attaining this position involves placing the table in a reverse Trendelenburg position or extending the table at the waist level while gently flexing and elevating the patient's neck (military prone). The latter maneuver should be done cautiously, avoiding hyperflexion and compromise of cranial venous outflow. If evoked potentials are being monitored, baseline potentials are obtained after the patient has been turned but before the operation begins.

The incision and exposure are planned to span the entire rostrocaudal extent of the tumor and provide access to permit the surgeon to operate comfortably at the poles of the lesion. The exposure should not be minimized if doing so causes the surgeon to struggle at the extremes of the lesion. However, it is unnecessary to fully expose polar cysts as long as the extent of solid tumor is accessible. A midline incision and subperiosteal retraction of the paraspinal musculature are performed. If the lesion extends to the foramen magnum or above, a suboccipital craniectomy or craniotomy is performed with appropriate extension of the midline incision.

At the caudal extreme, a laminectomy is performed one level below the lowest spinal cord segment involved with the tumor as seen on the preoperative images. Laminectomies below C1-C2 include only the medial facet joint. During the bony exposure, the surgeon must remain mindful of the critical degree of compression of neural structures and the tenuous nature of residual neurological function in the spinal cord in many of these cases. Meticulous hemostasis of the paraspinal musculature and epidural venous bleeding is obtained before the dura is opened to prevent blood from pooling in the dependent operative field during the microdissection. Large Cottonoid (DuPuy, Raynham, MA) "wall offs" and oxidized cellulose provide this efficiently. Some surgeons have found intraoperative ultrasound to be critical for localizing the extent of the tumor and the intratumoral or polar cysts at this point in the procedure or during the tumor removal.[1,4,10] Enthusiasts of intraoperative ultrasound find that it facilitates aggressive tumor removal. In our experience, the preoperative MRIs, availability of surgical landmarks at the craniovertebral junction, and the microsurgical appearance of these lesions permit adequate orientation—the ultrasound has not been necessary or particularly helpful in their removal.

The dural opening is performed in the midline and frequently extended rostrally in a "Y" configuration above the level of the foramen magnum. Dural venous lakes in this region are clipped rather than coagulated to avoid shrinking the dura excessively. Preferably, the arachnoid is left intact during the durotomy to protect underlying vessels. Under magnification, the arachnoid is opened in the midline with a small blade.

A midline myelotomy is performed in almost all cases. The location of the midline can be gauged by splitting the distance between the dorsal root entry zones on either side. Recently, intraoperative monitoring techniques have been used to identify the posterior midline.[15] Entry through the dorsal root entry zone can be considered in those rare cases when the tumor is markedly eccentric in its location, especially if it has a surface presentation. Typically, the myelotomy is begun at the area of maximal spinal cord swelling and extended rostrally and caudally to encompass the full extent of the tumor. The pia and crossing microvessels are cauterized gently in the midline, and the midline pia is incised with a fine blade. The myelotomy is deepened by gently spreading the posterior columns using a round blade or microforceps and microdissectors. Identification of the radial array of penetrating pial vessels on the medial surfaces of the posterior columns confirms that a midline orientation has been maintained. This orientation minimizes damage to the posterior columns. When the tumor extends into the medulla, rostral exposure may require separation and retraction of the cerebellar tonsils, with opening of the fourth ventricle. Self-retaining table-mounted retractors are used to maintain gentle cerebellar retraction. Tumors extending into the medulla may require extension of the myelotomy in the area where the tumor comes closest to the surface of the area postrema or floor of the fourth ventricle.[4] Once the tumor is encountered, the myelotomy is lengthened to expose the entire rostrocaudal extent of the dorsal tumor surface.

Pial traction sutures (6–0) are used as the myelotomy is developed to provide countertraction and to increase exposure, facilitating development of the lateral planes of the tumor. Usually, an internal decompression is performed to allow development of the lateral planes of the lesion without exerting undue pressure on surrounding neural tissue. An en bloc resection of large tumors may risk significant trauma to the surrounding spinal cord. In tumors that offer a surgical plane, the plane is developed initially on both sides of the tumor, decompressing internally as necessary. Inadequate myelotomy and scarring from prior radiation therapy or surgery can interfere with the development of satisfactory dissection planes.

Typically, ependymomas are sharply demarcated from the surrounding spinal cord and have a smooth reddish-gray glistening surface (**Fig. 13.1**). Crossing blood vessels may be noted on their surface. Benign astrocytomas have different degrees of circumscription; a significant percentage of these in the adult have infiltrative lesions without a clear tumor mass. At the other extreme are lesions with well-developed pseudoplanes that resemble an ependymoma. The difference in color between tumor and spinal cord may serve as a guide during their removal, and the judgment and experience of the surgeon play an important role.

The use of traction on the tumor and gentle countertraction on the spinal cord are fundamental to the dissection technique, particularly for ependymomas. The former can be provided by the operating assistant, and the latter is aided by the pial traction sutures. Polar cysts facilitate the dissection of the tumor when present, and the gliotic walls of these cysts need not be disturbed. The ventral interface may be the most difficult to discern, and effective countertraction is less feasible during this part of the dissection. These lesions may span the entire anteroposterior axis of the spinal cord. The pia often can be visualized at the ventral surface of the spinal cord as the dissection proceeds. Feeding vessels from the anterior spinal artery are also encountered here and must be coagulated cautiously and divided without injuring the anterior spinal artery.

Additional technical adjuncts that facilitate dissection include irrigating bipolar cauterization, which should be used at low levels and minimized. Our experience using ultrasonic aspiration of intramedullary tumors has been favorable, and we find this technique useful for the internal decompression of these lesions. The surgical laser is used by some surgeons to perform the myelotomy, remove the tumor layer by layer, and vaporize the last fragments of tumor adjoining the normal spinal cord.[1,4] At the conclusion of tumor removal, final hemostasis is obtained with warm saline or oxidized cotton. The pial traction sutures are removed to allow the spinal cord to assume its normal position. The myelotomy is not sutured closed. Dural closure usually is done primarily, although an autologous fascial graft or dural substitute can be utilized. Adequate room at closure is thought to prevent tethering of the spinal cord to the dura, a potential source of delayed morbidity. Particular care must be paid to the closure in patients previously operated or irradiated to prevent cerebrospinal fluid (CSF) fistulas. At times, rotation flaps are used.

Determination of the resectability of an intramedullary lesion at any level of the spinal cord is best determined by direct intraoperative inspection of the tumor–spinal cord interface under magnification. An adequate myelotomy and exposure of the lesion are requisite. Neither preoperative MRI nor intraoperative frozen sections can supplant the judgment of the surgeon. Frozen section analysis is useful but cannot be taken in isolation to determine surgical aggressiveness. It is our experience that most ependymomas of the spinal cord, including those afflicting the cervicomedullary junction, can be fully removed and generally cured by microsurgical removal.[7] A frozen section diagnosis of ependymoma by an experienced neuropathologist combined with a tumor not offering an obvious surgical plane should prompt a thorough search for such a plane. Facing a frozen section diagnosis of astrocytoma, the surgeon must still seek to identify a plane of dissection because some of these tumors are well circumscribed. It is our bias that aggressive removal is correlated with more favorable outcomes, including long-term tumor control in many cases. For lesions that demonstrate astrocytic pathology but are without a surgical plane (i.e., diffusely infiltrative astrocytomas), the priority is preservation of neurological function and not aggressive removal.

The role of surgery in the treatment of malignant intramedullary tumors is limited. Removal of intramedullary metastases is associated with significant palliation but is of no therapeutic benefit for primary malignant spinal cord neoplasms. The aggressive removal of highly anaplastic or glioblastomatous spinal cord lesions at the cervicomedullary junction or elsewhere is associated with morbidity. The finding on frozen section of an obvious malignancy signals the end of the operation, although some authors have reported a correlation between extent of removal and tumor control in patients harboring malignant intramedullary astrocytomas.[16]

Hemangioblastomas account for ~5 to 10% of intramedullary tumors. These lesions are associated with von Hippel Lindau syndrome in 15 to 25% of cases. They typically have a pial attachment and are sharply circumscribed.[5,8] Most are dorsally or dorsolaterally located. These lesions are highly vascular, and internal decompression is not recommended. The key to removal of these lesions is to initially circumferentially detach the tumor at its pial margin (**Fig. 13.5**). As the lesion is rolled out of the spinal cord, the surface of the lesion can be cauterized to shrink it and facilitate its removal.

Inclusion tumors and cysts such as lipomas, dermoid, and epidermoid cysts rarely occur in an intramedullary location.[17] Experience elsewhere in the spinal cord suggests that their interface with normal spinal cord tissue may be obscure in some areas, preventing gross total removal. Small remnants may be left behind and pose only a small risk of recurrence. Lipomas are the most common dysembryogenic lesion. They result from inclusion of mesenchymal cells and are not truly neoplastic. They account for 1% of intramedullary tumors but were not encountered in our series of high cervical lesions. At caudal levels, they have been treated with judicious subtotal internal decompression with satisfactory results (**Fig. 13.6**).[6]

Postoperative Management

In most respects the postoperative management of patients undergoing resection of high cervical and cervicomedullary lesions is similar to routine management of any intramedullary tumor. Perioperative steroids are tapered gradually. Early mobilization is useful to prevent iatrogenic complications, and the spinal column is not destabilized by the approach outlined. Special aspects of management for patients harboring rostrally located tumors pertain to respiratory function, airway protection, and swallowing. Special precautions are undertaken more on the basis of the degree of preoperative functional compromise rather than the radiographic or anatomical features of the lesion. It is normal to assume that a preoperative deficit will be transiently exacerbated by surgery. Posterior column function is also typically compromised temporarily by the approach. Patients demonstrating significant bulbar compromise, such as swallowing dysfunction or a history of aspiration pneumonia, prophylactically remain intubated postoperatively and undergo careful assessment of airway protective function before extubation. Prolonged intubation, tracheostomy, and feeding tube placement may rarely be required. Support from pulmonary and otolaryngological colleagues is important. Diaphragmatic ultrasound, phrenic nerve conduction studies, and swallowing studies are used as indicated to evaluate and manage perioperative difficulties specific to operating in this region.

Awareness of these potential complications allows the surgeon to minimize morbidity from removal of high

A

B

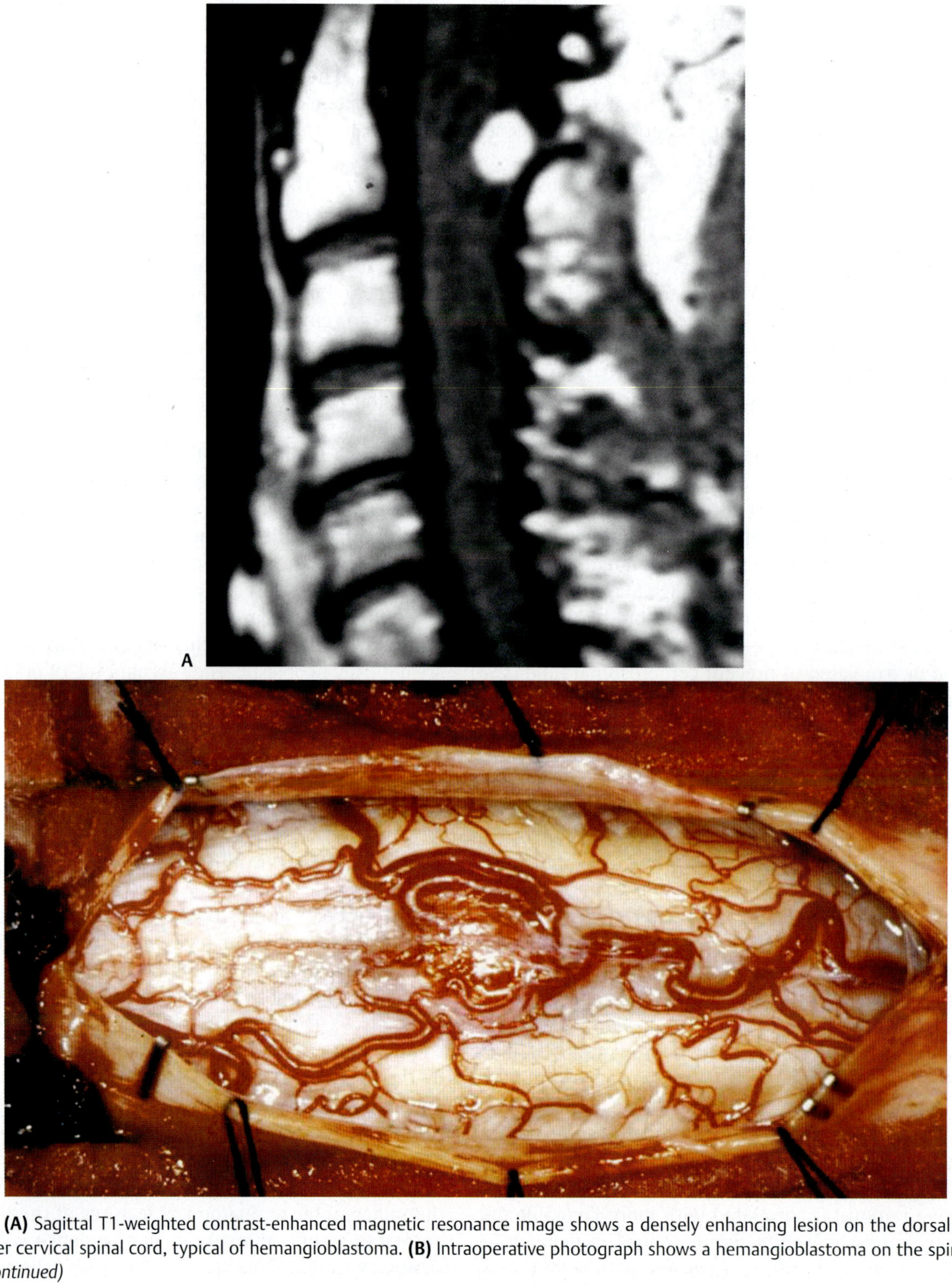

Fig. 13.5 **(A)** Sagittal T1-weighted contrast-enhanced magnetic resonance image shows a densely enhancing lesion on the dorsal surface of the upper cervical spinal cord, typical of hemangioblastoma. **(B)** Intraoperative photograph shows a hemangioblastoma on the spinal cord surface. *(continued)*

cervical and cervicomedullary lesions. CSF leaks and meningitis can complicate intramedullary surgery at any level of the spinal cord, and treatment is individualized. Frequently, lumbar CSF drainage arrests the leak. Posterior fossa syndrome, characterized by fever and meningismus but sterile CSF, can be encountered after the removal of cervicomedullary tumors that require a suboccipital exposure. This syndrome responds to steroid therapy. We have encountered hydrocephalus after the removal of high cervical or cervicomedullary lesions in two patients.

Structural complications related to spinal stability are unusual. In general, we perform a laminectomy wide enough to obtain adequate intradural exposure, but significant removal of facet joints is not required. This issue is not present at the O-C1/C1-C2 level, where the facet joints are ventrally located. We have encountered several cases of reversal of the normal cervical lordosis, but in no patient has overt clinical or radiographic instability occurred. Spinal stability is a more significant consideration in pediatric patients. Osteoplastic laminotomy is recommended for

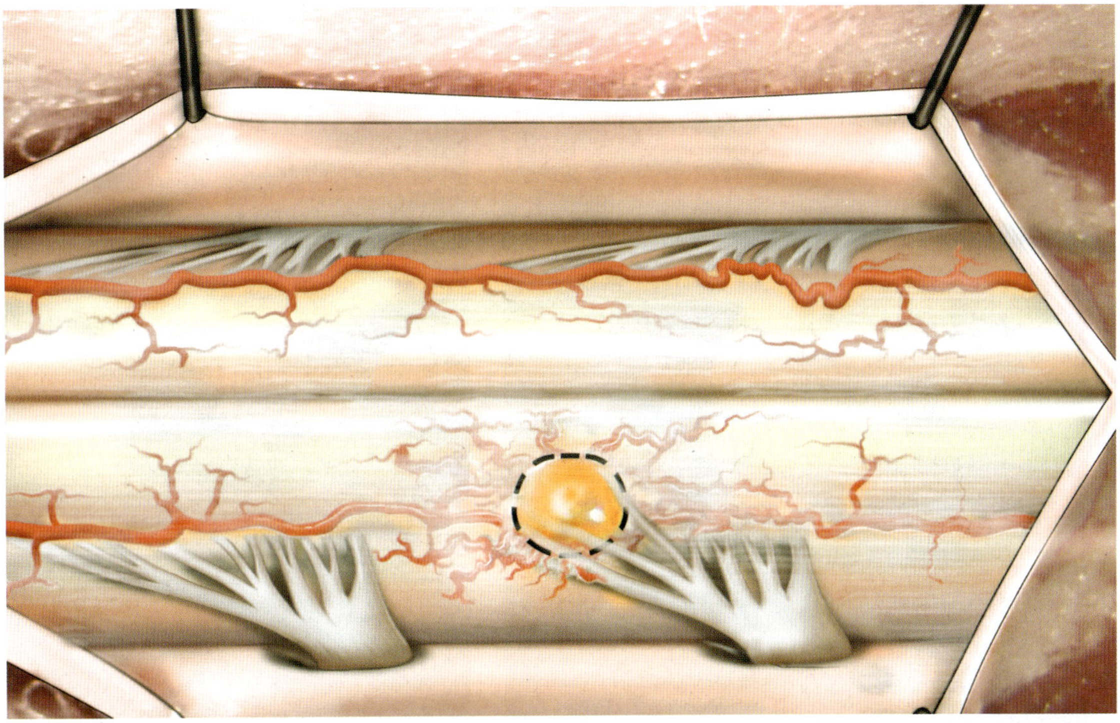

C

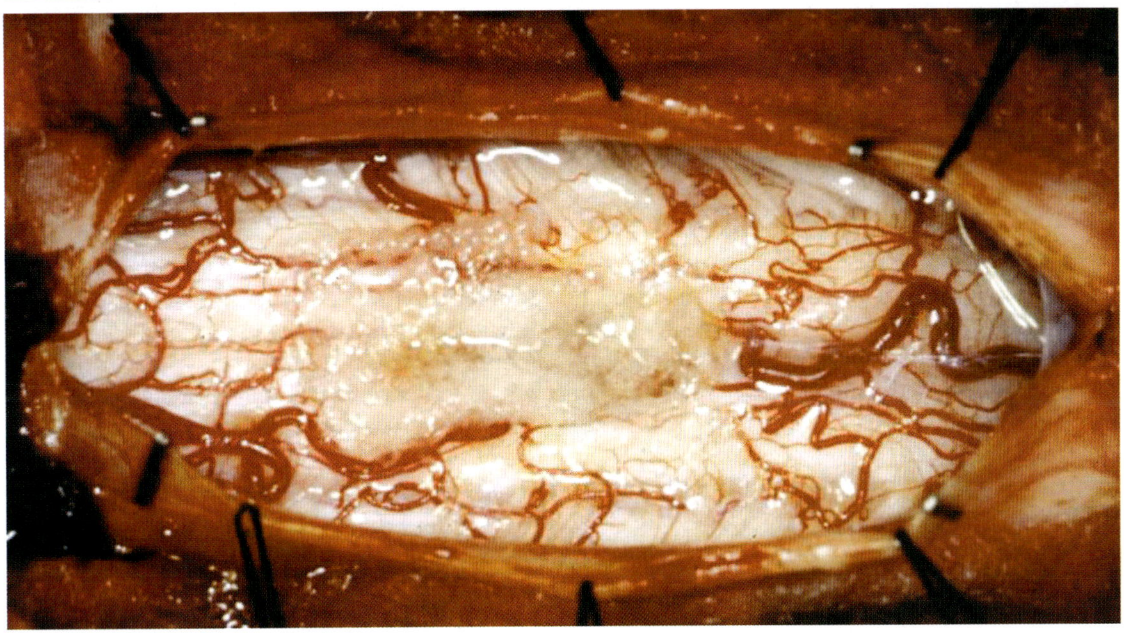

D

Fig. 13.5 *(continued)* **(C)** Drawing demonstrates circumferential detachment of pial origin of tumor. **(D)** Intraoperative photograph shows complete tumor removal.

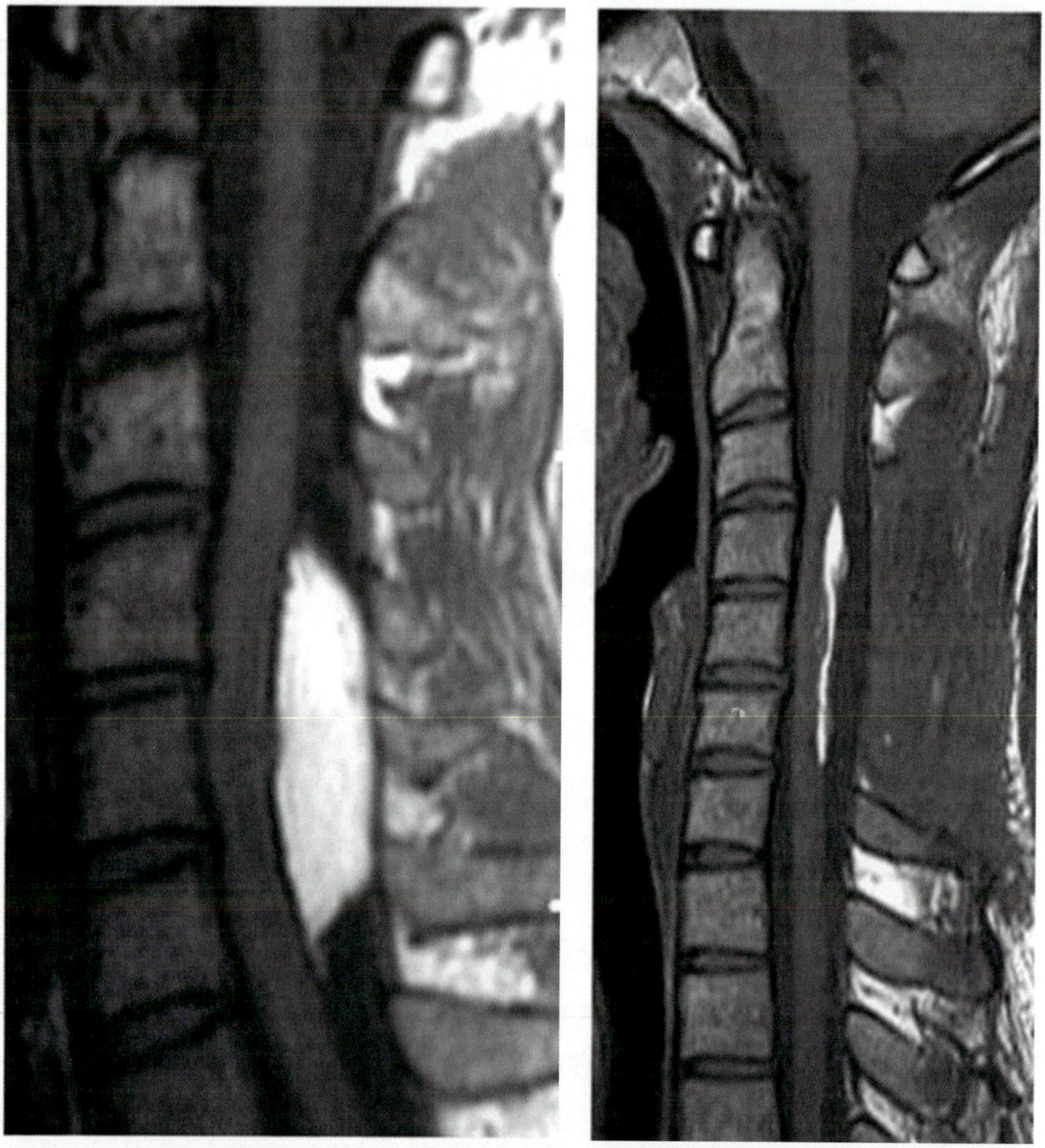

A B

Fig. 13.6 **(A)** Sagittal T1-weighted cervical preoperative magnetic resonance image (MRI) shows a hyperintense lesion on the dorsal aspect of the cervical spinal cord consistent with spinal cord lipoma. **(B)** Postoperative MRI shows radical subtotal removal.

children undergoing surgery for intramedullary tumors.[4,18] Evolution of a postoperative deformity in children relates to several factors and is more likely in patients younger than 3 years of age and in those patients with a significant preoperative deformity or neurological deficit. We prefer simple laminectomy in most adult cases.

Surgical Complications

The immediate results of surgical treatment are best viewed in light of preoperative neurological status. The long-term results of surgery are dependent on histology. In general, preservation rather than restoration of neurological function is the rule following intramedullary surgery.[6] This rule holds true for cervicomedullary lesions as well. Patients with significant or longstanding deficits rarely improve and are more likely to worsen following surgery.[1,2,5,19] Therefore, the greatest clinical benefit and least surgical risk are obtained when surgery is performed on patients who are only minimally symptomatic. Again, the importance of early diagnosis and treatment is underscored. Fortunately, most patients present with mild or moderate neurological deficit (grade I or II). In the immediate postoperative period, one-third of ependymoma patients and 45% of astrocytoma patients worsened by one grade. Most patients note sensory loss acutely after surgery. The degree of subjective change may be more marked than the objective deficit. Loss of position sense may be prominent, and dysesthesias can occur. Sensory changes tend to improve with time, although not always to their preoperative level. Gait problems in the postoperative period are often related to altered position sense and improve significantly in time as well. Early postoperative morbidity specific to the high cervical and cervicomedullary region has been alluded to previously. It typically relates to airway protection, swallowing, and respiratory function. Problems can be minimized by aggressive medical management and a high level of alertness. In general, these problems are manageable and have not prohibited definitive surgical treatment of high cervical intramedullary pathology when indicated.

The surgical outcome in terms of degree of resection, clinical outcome at long-term follow-up, and tumor control is best viewed in terms of specific histologies. Ependymomas are usually managed by gross total resection. The mean clinical grade at long-term follow-up is similar to the preoperative grade. Annual MRIs and clinical surveillance are performed for several years to monitor for tumor recurrence. About 5 to 10% of patients will have recurrence of tumor, usually many years after the initial resection. It is well established that gross total resection of intramedullary spinal cord ependymomas provides a cure or long-term control better than subtotal removal with or without radiation.[1–3,7,20–22] There is no evidence demonstrating therapeutic benefit of prophylactic radiation following gross total removal. Furthermore, experienced groups have shown that ependymomas not previously irradiated or operated on are susceptible to gross total removal in almost all cases. Our experience with these lesions in the high cervical and cervicomedullary region suggests that the same principles apply here, and a similarly aggressive surgical philosophy is indicated. These lesions are amenable to long-term control or surgical cure, as are more caudally disposed ependymomas. Nonetheless, long-term radiographic follow-up is indicated, and reoperation is probably the treatment of choice for recurrence. We do not believe there is a role for radiation in the management of most benign ependymomas. Studies that continue to advocate it are flawed by small numbers, inadequate control groups, and inadequate surgical treatment.[20–23] Radiation should be viewed as salvage therapy for the rare aggressive benign lesion that cannot be totally removed, the rare malignant ependymoma, or for CSF dissemination.

The benefit derived from surgical treatment of high cervical and cervicomedullary astrocytomas is unclear. Although many astrocytomas are well circumscribed, nearly all show some degree of infiltration at their margin with the spinal cord. Thus, with few exceptions, these tumors cannot be safely histologically cured with surgery. Furthermore, the relationship between the extent of removal and disease-free survival is not clear. Thus, we tend to take a more conservative approach to tumor resection and remove them in an "inside out" manner until the distinction between the tumor and surrounding spinal cord is no longer clear.

The results of operative treatment of high cervical and cervicomedullary astrocytomas do not differ dramatically from similar data that exist for intramedullary astrocytomas at other levels of the spinal cord. In general, this literature is flawed by small series without controls or standardized treatment protocols. Cooper found no correlation between extent of resection and outcome in adult patients with astrocytomas.[1] He nonetheless advocated extensive debulking when technically feasible. Stronger correlations were noted between degree of resection and event-free survival (and overall survival) in the series of Rossitch and colleagues,[24] Sandler and colleagues,[25] and Reimer and Onofrio and colleagues.[26] Cristante and Herrmann concluded that aggressive resections were no more attended by higher morbidity than were less aggressive surgeries and were probably beneficial when feasible.[2] The data are unclear whether the degree of resection was an independent variable or it reflected the relatively benign biological behavior of lesions that were circumscribed enough to permit aggressive resection, for example. In reviewing the literature on spinal cord astrocytomas, we concluded that radical removal prolongs event-free survival in some patients but in others probably has little effect. In essence, the biological behavior of that particular tumor is the critical variable, more so than surgical treatment.[5,6] Our data on high cervical and cervicomedullary lesions led us to the same basic conclusion for this subcategory of intramedullary astrocytomas. For well-circumscribed benign lesions, aggressive surgical management affords the best possible outcome: long-term control and preservation of good neurological function. Given that these tumors are usually operated on in patients who manifest progressive neurological symptoms, surgical therapy evidently has a major positive impact on natural history. However, when the tumor is diffusely infiltrative or malignant, very little is accomplished, and significant risk is incurred by operating aggressively.

Conclusion

Tumors of the upper cervical spinal cord and cervicomedullary junction behave biologically more like intramedullary spinal cord tumors than like infiltrating brainstem tumors. In almost all cases, the ependymomas are well demarcated and amenable to gross total removal and long-term control or cure with preservation of neurological function. Some astrocytomas are well circumscribed and can be aggressively removed. When feasible, surgical treatment offers a significant chance of long-term control of disease. Preoperative diagnosis and planning are based on MRI as the definitive study. The determination regarding the resectability of these lesions is best made by the surgeon by direct intraoperative inspection of the tumor/spinal cord interface. Refined surgical techniques and aggressive postoperative management targeted at avoiding the specific hazards of operating at this critical region in the neuraxis are essential for obtaining acceptable results. Malignant lesions or low-grade lesions that violate the relative barriers at the cervicomedullary junction and diffusely infiltrate do not benefit from aggressive surgical treatment.

References

1. Cooper PR. Outcome after operative treatment of intramedullary spinal cord tumors in adults: intermediate and long-term results in 51 patients. Neurosurgery 1989;25(6):855–859
2. Cristante L, Herrmann HD. Surgical management of intramedullary spinal cord tumors: functional outcome and sources of morbidity. Neurosurgery 1994;35(1):69–74, discussion 74–76
3. Epstein FJ, Farmer JP, Freed D. Adult intramedullary spinal cord ependymomas: the result of surgery in 38 patients. J Neurosurg 1993;79(2):204–209
4. Epstein F, Wisoff J. Intra-axial tumors of the cervicomedullary junction. J Neurosurg 1987;67(4):483–487
5. McCormick PC. Intramedullary tumors of the spinal cord. In: Menezes AH, Sonntag VKH, et al, eds. Principles of Spinal Surgery. New York, NY: McGraw Hill; 1996:1355–1370
6. McCormick PC, Stein BM. Spinal cord tumors in adults. In: Youmans JR, ed. Neurological Surgery. 4th ed. Vol 4. Philadelphia, PA: WB Saunders Company; 1996:3102–3122
7. McCormick PC, Torres R, Post KD, Stein BM. Intramedullary ependymoma of the spinal cord. J Neurosurg 1990;72(4):523–532
8. Mandigo CE, Ogden AT, Angevine PD, McCormick PC. Operative management of spinal hemangioblastoma. Neurosurgery 2009;65(6):1166–1177
9. Garcés-Ambrossi GL, McGirt MJ, Mehta VA, et al. Factors associated with progression-free survival and long-term neurological outcome after resection of intramedullary spinal cord tumors: analysis of 101 consecutive cases. J Neurosurg Spine 2009;11(5):591–599
10. Robertson PL, Allen JC, Abbott IR, Miller DC, Fidel J, Epstein FJ. Cervicomedullary tumors in children: a distinct subset of brainstem gliomas. Neurology 1994;44(10):1798–1803
11. Abbott R, Shiminski-Maher T, Wisoff JH, Epstein FJ. Intrinsic tumors of the medulla: surgical complications. Pediatr Neurosurg 1991–1992;17(5):239–244
12. Epstein FJ, Farmer JP. Brain-stem glioma growth patterns. J Neurosurg 1993;78(3):408–412
13. Hoffman HJ, Becker L, Craven MA. A clinically and pathologically distinct group of benign brain stem gliomas. Neurosurgery 1980;7(3):243–248
14. Yanni DS, Ulkatan S, Deletis V, Barrenechea IJ, Sen C, Perin NI. Utility of neurophysiological monitoring using dorsal column mapping in intramedullary spinal cord surgery. J Neurosurg Spine 2010;12(6):623–628
15. McGirt MJ, Goldstein IM, Chaichana KL, Tobias ME, Kothbauer KF, Jallo GI. Extent of surgical resection of malignant astrocytomas of the spinal cord: outcome analysis of 35 patients. Neurosurgery 2008;63(1):55–60, discussion 60–61
16. Ogden AT, Khandji AG, McCormick PC, Kaiser MG. Intramedullary inclusion cysts of the cervicothoracic junction. Report of two cases in adults and review of the literature. J Neurosurg Spine 2007;7(2):236–242
17. Raimondi AJ, Gutierrez FA, Di Rocco CD. Laminotomy and total reconstruction of the posterior spinal arch for spinal canal surgery in childhood. J Neurosurg 1976;45(5):555–560
18. Guidetti B, Mercuri S, Vagnozzi R. Long-term results of the surgical treatment of 129 intramedullary spinal gliomas. J Neurosurg 1981;54(3):323–330
19. Di Marco A, Griso C, Pradella R, Campostrini F, Garusi GF. Postoperative management of primary spinal cord ependymomas. Acta Oncol 1988;27(4):371–375
20. Garcia DM. Primary spinal cord tumors treated with surgery and postoperative irradiation. Int J Radiat Oncol Biol Phys 1985;11(11):1933–1939
21. Whitaker SJ, Bessell EM, Ashley SE, Bloom HJ, Bell BA, Brada M. Postoperative radiotherapy in the management of spinal cord ependymoma. J Neurosurg 1991;74(5):720–728
22. Clover LL, Hazuka MB, Kinzie JJ. Spinal cord ependymomas treated with surgery and radiation therapy. A review of 11 cases. Am J Clin Oncol 1993;16(4):350–353
23. Reimer R, Onofrio BM. Astrocytomas of the spinal cord in children and adolescents. J Neurosurg 1985;63(5):669–675
24. Rossitch E Jr, Zeidman SM, Burger PC, et al. Clinical and pathological analysis of spinal cord astrocytomas in children. Neurosurgery 1990;27(2):193–196
25. Sandler HM, Papadopoulos SM, Thornton AF Jr, Ross DA. Spinal cord astrocytomas: results of therapy. Neurosurgery 1992;30(4):490–493
26. Berger AJ. Control of breathing. In: Murray JF, Nadel JA, eds. Textbook of Respiratory Medicine. Philadelphia, PA: WB Saunders; 1988:199

14 Management of Vertebral Artery Dissections and Vascular Insufficiency

C. Benjamin Newman, Yin C. Hu, Cameron G. McDougall, and Felipe C. Albuquerque

Approximately 80% of strokes are ischemic in origin, of which as many as 25% involve the vertebrobasilar system.[1] The vertebrobasilar system is composed of the vertebral arteries (VAs) and the basilar artery, and it typically supplies blood to the brainstem, cerebellum, thalamus, and occipital and posterior temporal lobes. Outcomes of posterior circulation transient ischemic attacks (TIAs), or stroke, depend on the location of the lesion. Medically refractory, symptomatic atherosclerotic disease of the vertebrobasilar system is associated with a 5 to 11% risk of stroke at 1 year[2,3]; TIAs related to extracranial vertebrobasilar system disease are associated with a 30% risk of stroke at 5 years.[4–6] Patients with symptomatic intracranial atherosclerosis have a 1-year stroke risk of 11% in the subserved vascular territory.[7] If the stenosis is greater than 70%, the risk of stroke increases to 19%. The Warfarin-Aspirin Symptomatic Intracranial Disease (WASID) trial demonstrated that aspirin is not inferior to warfarin in terms of risk reduction for recurrent stroke in patients with symptomatic intracranial disease.[3] In their large posterior circulation registry, Caplan and colleagues reported that 22% of patients with a vertebrobasilar TIA or stroke had a poor functional outcome at 30 days.[8] Thrombosis of the basilar artery is associated with an extremely poor prognosis, with death or dependence in as many as 80% of cases.[9]

Vertebrobasilar insufficiency, the clinical syndrome caused by impaired perfusion of the vertebrobasilar system, is characterized by dizziness, ataxia, discoordination, visual disturbances, and sensorimotor deficits. These symptoms can easily be dismissed as nonspecific; consequently, vertebrobasilar insufficiency is underrecognized and frequently misdiagnosed.[10]

Surgical treatment options for atherosclerosis of the VA include vessel transection distal to the occlusive lesion and reimplantation into the ipsilateral carotid or subclavian artery or an endarterectomy of the VA. Surgical access to the VA, particularly the ostium, is difficult, and the complication rate associated with surgical management is 10 to 20%.[5,11,12] The relatively high complication rates of surgical treatments for occlusive disease of the vertebrobasilar system, coupled with the failure of medical therapy to reduce the risk of stroke in select groups of patients, has led to strong interest in the development of endovascular treatment modalities for this disease.

Initial attempts at revascularization of the VAs involved the application of technology developed for the coronary arterial system. Fundamental differences in the vascular anatomy between the vertebrobasilar system and the coronary system (i.e., increased tortuosity of the VAs) necessitated the modification of coronary microcatheters, angioplasty balloons, and stents for use in the vertebrobasilar system. Indeed, the lessons learned in interventional cardiology in the management of atherosclerotic disease of the coronary arteries ultimately proved applicable to the intracranial circulation, including the vertebrobasilar system.

Percutaneous transluminal angioplasty (PTA) has been used successfully in the treatment of peripheral and coronary arterial disease since its initial description by Dotter and Junkins in 1964.[13] Intracranial angioplasty was first described by Sundt and colleagues who successfully employed the technique to treat severe basilar artery stenosis causing progressive symptoms despite maximal medical therapy.[14] The technique was then repeated with mixed results and was initially associated with what many investigators deemed as an unacceptably high procedural complication rate.[15–17] Major complications from intracranial angioplasty include vasospasm, arterial trauma, vessel perforation, and embolic stroke. Increased complication rates for intracranial angioplasty and stenting compared with the coronary system probably reflect the relative fragility of the intracranial vessels and the potential for substantial neurological morbidity from even tiny foci of ischemia, especially brain tissue supplied by brainstem perforators.

Initially, coronary angioplasty balloons were used off-label to perform intracranial PTA alone. As in the coronary arterial system, angioplasty alone in the VA for the treatment of atherosclerotic disease has a very high restenosis rate, approaching 100% in some series.[18] As balloon-mounted stents became the mainstay of the endoluminal treatment of coronary artery disease, these devices were adopted for the treatment of intracranial atherosclerotic disease. Technological modifications were necessary to allow navigation of the more tortuous intracranial circulation with more flexible catheters and improved stent delivery systems. Initial attempts at treatment of intracranial atherosclerotic disease with stenting resulted in acceptable periprocedural rates of morbidity and mortality but with relatively high rates of technical failure. Angioplasty as a standalone, initial treatment modality for atheromatous disease of the VA has therefore largely been abandoned. However, angioplasty alone may be performed for in-stent stenosis when the pathoetiology is presumed to be intimal hyperplasia rather than progression of atherosclerotic disease.

Approximately 30% of patients who experience strokes involving the vertebrobasilar circulation have a lesion in the V1 segment of the VA.[19] The contrast between the relatively easy endovascular access to the VA ostium and the high morbidity rate associated with an open surgical exposure has led to an interest in stenting high-grade lesions.

As in the coronary stenting experience, the application of drug-eluting stents (DESs) for the treatment of occlusive disease of the VA origin reduces rates of restenosis as has been shown in numerous studies. DESs are not currently employed in the intracranial circulation. Restenosis rates for bare metal stents for symptomatic intracranial and extracranial stenosis have been reported at 35%.[20] In the coronary system, that DES significantly reduced restenosis rates from 30% to 4 to 8% at a 9-month follow-up[21,22] prompted interest in applying DES to the cerebrovascular arteries. In the setting of VA origin stenosis, Ogilvy and colleagues compared DES (sirolimus and paclitaxel-eluting) with bare metal stents.[23] For individuals with >60% symptomatic or >70% asymptomatic VA origin stenosis and an occluded or hypoplastic contralateral VA or significant carotid occlusion, DES reduced angiographic restenosis rates from 38% (9/24) to 17% (2/12). Twenty-nine percent (7/24) of people in the bare metal stenting group required angioplasty for in-stent stenosis, whereas no patients in the DES arm required angioplasty.[23] Although long-term follow-up is needed, these and other preliminary data suggest that it may be reasonable to expect similar reductions in in-stent stenosis in the vertebrobasilar system as have been experienced in the coronary system. Placement of a DES in the setting of in-stent stenosis after placement of a bare metal stent has been reported as an effective treatment.[24]

Although no reports of arterial toxicity have been reported with DES in the cerebrovascular system, reports of delayed hypersensitivity resulting in late thrombosis have been reported in coronary vessels.[25] The optimal duration of treatment with antiplatelet agents after implantation of DES has not been established. Our practice is to continue dual antiplatelet therapy, which is individually tailored based on platelet inhibition assays. Angiography is typically performed 3 months after stent placement. If no evidence of in-stent stenosis is seen, the patient is continued on a single antiplatelet agent indefinitely, unless there is a contraindication.

Vertebral Artery Dissection

VA dissection is an important cause of ischemic stroke in young and middle-aged adults. VA dissections are typically classified as either traumatic or spontaneous. VA injury is also encountered during cervical spine surgery, particularly when instrumentation is employed. The rate of VA injury, either dissection or occlusion, is highest for posterior atlantoaxial instrumented fusion (transarticular or Harms screw fixation). The rate of VA injury is ~4% per screw.[26]

The true incidence of VA dissection is difficult to ascertain because many such patients are asymptomatic or minimally symptomatic and never diagnosed. The V3 segment, the most common site for a dissection, accounts for 65% of all VA dissections. As many as 15% of VA dissections involve the intradural segment. Most dissections of the intradural VA represent intracranial extension of an extradural dissection. Two-thirds of patients with intradural VA dissection are male.[27] After the V3 segment, the second most common location for a VA dissection is in the proximal (V1) segment of the vessel.

Most patients present with stroke, occipital headache or neck pain, or both. Risk factors for VA dissection include trauma, hypertension, smoking, and fibromuscular dysplasia. Traumatic VA dissection has been reported with chiropractic manipulation,[28] yoga,[29] and rapid head turning.[30] Although its natural history is not well understood, spontaneous VA dissection is also recognized as an important cause of stroke. Prognosis for both etiologies is generally thought to be good.[31] Compared with spontaneous dissections, traumatic dissections are thought to be associated with an increased likelihood of causing persistent neurological symptoms.[32]

The incidental discovery of a VA dissection is increasing with the widespread availability of high-resolution, noninvasive imaging such as magnetic resonance angiography (MRA) and computed tomographic angiography (CTA). Many trauma centers have implemented screening protocols that have resulted in the recognition of an increased number of cases of asymptomatic VA dissection, particularly in the setting of blunt force neck trauma. Aggressive screening and individualized treatment protocols for these lesions have failed to demonstrate a survival benefit or improved patient outcomes.[33] Patients with suspected flexion injuries or those who present with ischemic symptoms referable to the VA should undergo noninvasive evaluation at a minimum.[34]

At our institution, suspected VA dissections are initially evaluated with high-quality CTA or MRA of the cervical spine and brain. We believe that the risk of stroke is highest immediately after the development of the dissection flap, at the moment when the highly thrombogenic subintimal is exposed to circulating platelets. The risk of stroke persists for some time after the initial insult, gradually decreasing over the ensuing hours to days. We believe that late strokes (i.e., >24 hours after the event) are related to turbulent flow within the false lumen or to dehiscence of platelet aggregation from the subintimal layer.

Extradural Vertebral Artery Dissections

Most extradural VA dissections can be managed with medical therapy, usually consisting of antiplatelet agents. In the acute setting immediately after VA dissection, thromboembolic phenomena are usually implicated as the cause of a neurological deficit, if present. If indicated, these strokes can be managed with intravenous recombinant tissue-plasminogen activator (r-tPA); if contraindicated, endovascular revascularization (e.g., intraarterial thrombolysis or mechanical thrombectomy) may be considered. Occasionally, revascularization of an acutely dissected or occluded artery may be revascularized by stenting and angioplasty.

Symptomatic extradural VA dissection should prompt consideration of endovascular intervention when intracranial emboli are present or when VA asymmetry is noted. If left untreated, acute vertebrobasilar occlusion is associated with an exceptionally high morbidity rate. Several investigators have reported the substantial benefit associated with prompt recanalization of acute vertebrobasilar thrombosis.[35,36]

In general, endovascular treatment for VA dissection should be considered in patients who are experiencing thromboembolic sequelae and in whom the integrity of the contralateral vessel is uncertain (e.g., atresia, stenosis, or occlusion), in patients in whom augmented flow through the collateral vessels is undesirable (i.e., posterior communicating artery or contralateral VA aneurysms), in patients who experience persistent thromboembolic symptoms despite maximal medical therapy, in patients who demonstrate progressive enlargement of a pseudoaneurysm, or in patients who are symptomatic from the mass effect caused by a pseudoaneurysm.

When a vessel is completely occluded, the potential for distal embolization after blood flow is restored must be considered. If the segment of occluded vessel is thought to be long and the associated clot burden is high, a careful evaluation of the risks and benefits of reopening the diseased vessel should be undertaken before intervention.

Occasionally, iatrogenic injury to the VA is seen during surgery of the craniovertebral junction. The rate of VA compromise associated with contemporary atlantoaxial fusion techniques is ~4% per screw.[26] Although the mechanism for iatrogenic injury to the VA after surgery is different than that involved with traumatic or spontaneous VA dissection, the same rationale for endovascular intervention should be applied. If implanted hardware has compromised vessel integrity, endovascular options for revascularization are limited. Frequently, vessel sacrifice to minimize the chance of thromboembolism is the only recourse. When a penetrating injury to the VA is recognized, careful evaluation for arteriovenous shunting is needed. Our practice is to occlude the fistulous point, which generally implies vessel sacrifice.

Intradural Vertebral Artery Dissections

The management of an intradural dissection depends on the initiating event. A dissecting VA aneurysm presenting with subarachnoid hemorrhage is a completely different clinical entity than a traumatic or spontaneous VA dissection. A discussion of the subtypes and management of dissecting VA aneurysms is beyond the scope of this chapter.

A consensus for the optimal treatment of an intradural VA dissection is lacking. The relative fragility of the intradural vessels and the devastating consequences of intracranial hemorrhage have led many investigators to adopt a more aggressive approach to the management of these lesions. In the absence of hemorrhage or vessel wall dysmorphology (e.g., aneurysm, dolichoectasia), patients who present with ischemia secondary to an intradural VA dissection can reasonably be treated with medical therapy as a first-line therapy.

Intervention should be considered for patients who experience persistent or worsening symptoms attributable to ischemia related to the VA dissection, for cases where mass effect from vessel dilation (pseudoaneurysm, aneurysm) is compressing or endangering neural structures, for cases where enlargement of vessel wall abnormalities is observed, or for cases with limited blood flow related to VA dissection when the competency of the collateral vessels is uncertain. (**Fig. 14.1**)

Traditionally, endovascular management of intradural VA dissection consisted of vessel sacrifice. Technological advances in intracranial stents have increased interest in techniques for managing intradural VA dissection while maintaining vessel patency.

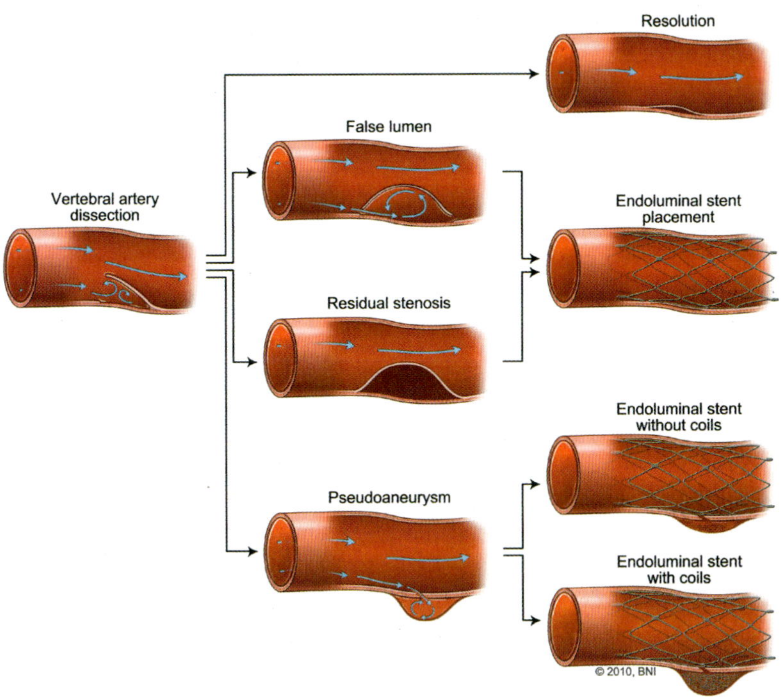

Fig. 14.1 Illustrated diagram demonstrating the progressive stages and various possible outcomes of an acute vascular dissection. In some patients, vascular dissections heal naturally without additional intervention. In patients where a false lumen or an acute or delayed residual stenosis significantly limits antegrade flow or causes neurological symptoms, an endoluminal stent can be placed to dilate over the stenotic region. In cases where patients present with pseudoaneurysms, an endoluminal stent with or without coiling can be performed, depending on the size of the pseudoaneurysm. Delayed coiling can be performed if the pseudoaneurysm persists at follow-up after endoluminal stenting. (Reprinted with permission from Barrow Neurological Institute.)

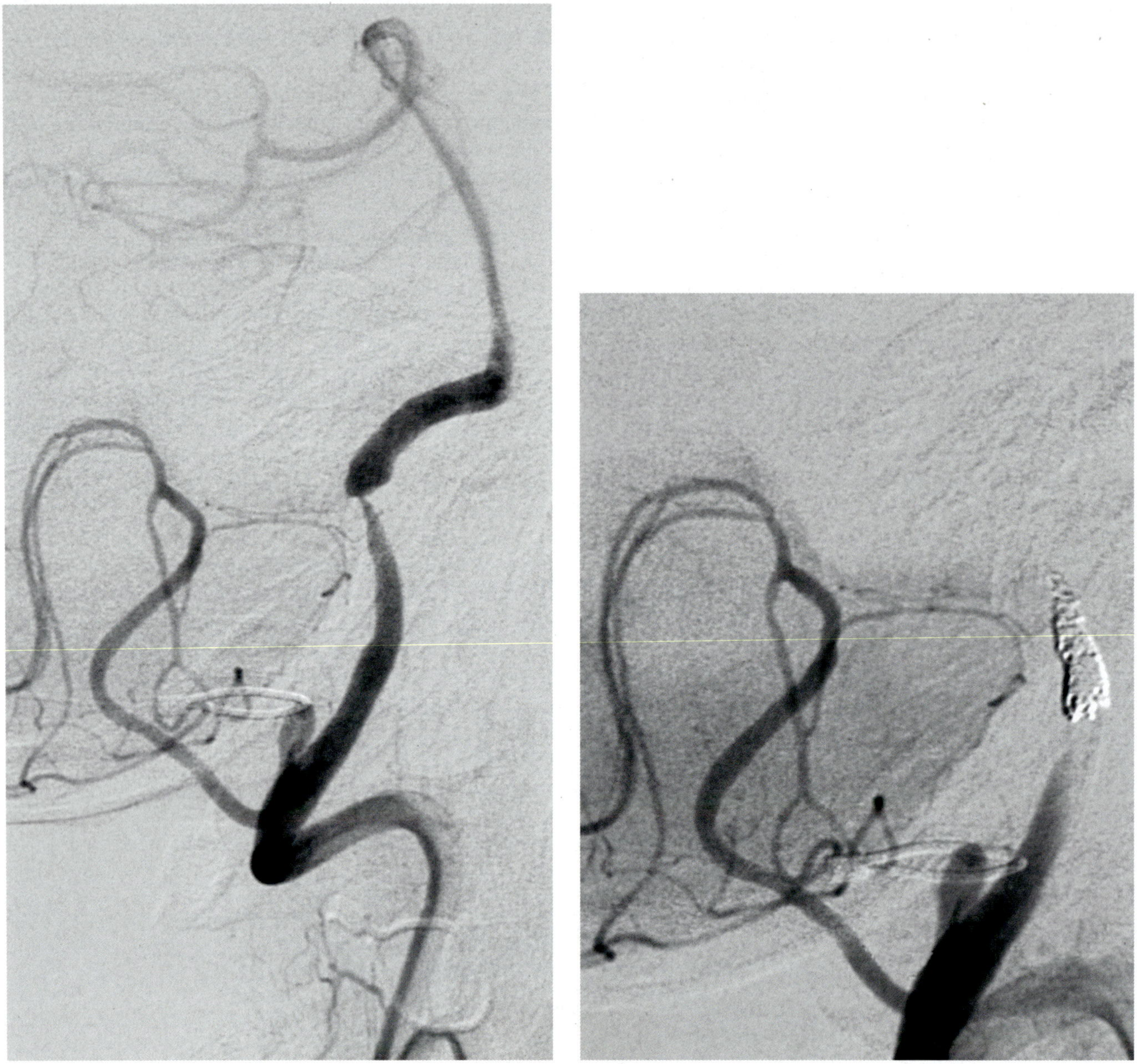

A B

Fig. 14.2 **(A)** Left vertebral artery (VA) angiogram, lateral projection, in a 64-year-old man with a spontaneous VA dissection. He demonstrated a patent contralateral VA as well as clinical and radiographic manifestations of posterior fossa thromboemboli. The treatment for this flow-limiting dissection was VA sacrifice with detachable platinum coils. **(B)** Left VA angiogram, lateral projection, after coil occlusion of the dissected vessel. Unfortunately, after the procedure, this patient suffered a 1-mm medullary infarction, which we believe was due to occlusion of a perforating vessel arising from the occluded segment. However, embolism from the dissection itself cannot be excluded. The infarction resulted in dysphonia and dysphagia. (Reprinted with permission from Barrow Neurological Institute.)

For patients with a competent contralateral VA who demonstrate a flow-limiting dissection and/or persistent clinical sequelae of thromboemboli, vessel sacrifice may be considered as an alternative to stent placement (**Fig. 14.2A**). In patients in whom vessel sacrifice is considered, it is essential to evaluate the remaining vessels to ensure that adequate collaterals exist. It is important to remember that brainstem and medullary perforators exist along the V4 segment and that a stroke can occur if a long segment of this vessel is occluded (**Fig. 14.2B**).

Vertebral Artery Stenting: Technical Comments

At our institution, several standard procedural protocols are used for endovascular revascularization of cranial ischemic pathologies. All patients undergoing angioplasty and stenting as an elective procedure are given dual antiplatelet therapy for 3 days consisting of aspirin (325–350 mg/d orally) and either ticlopidine (250 mg orally twice a day; Ticlid,

Roche Pharmaceuticals, Nutley, NJ) or clopidogrel (75 mg/d orally; Plavix, Bristol-Myers Squibb/Sanofi Pharmaceuticals, New York, NY). In urgent situations requiring endovascular intervention, patients are given a loading dose of aspirin (650 mg) and clopidogrel (450 mg). Intraprocedural functional assays are tested to verify individual responsiveness to aspirin, clopidogrel, and abciximab, and doses of dual antiplatelet regimen may be readjusted after the procedure. The dual antiplatelet regimen is maintained until follow-up angiography (3–6 months), at which time clopidogrel is discontinued if no in-stent restenosis is demonstrated. Unless contraindicated, aspirin is continued indefinitely.

Intraoperative neurophysiological monitoring (somatosensory evoked potentials and electroencephalography) is used throughout the procedure. Arterial access is typically achieved through the common femoral artery. In rare instances, other arterial sites such as transradial, transbrachial, or direct carotid puncture are required. Heparinization is instituted with the goal of achieving an activated coagulation time (ACT) between 250 and 300 seconds after arterial access is obtained. The dosage of heparin is continued throughout the procedure to maintain the ACT in the target range. All interventions are performed through a 6-French system guide catheter.

Intracranial Stenting: Technical Comments

All patients are placed under general anesthesia for PTA of intracranial stenoses using the Wingspan system (**Fig. 14.3**). After conventional catheter-based angiography (**Fig. 14.4**) is performed, a microcatheter is navigated across the target lesion over a 0.014-inch guidewire. The microcatheter is then exchanged over a 0.014-inch exchange microguidewire for a Gateway angioplasty balloon and advanced across the stenotic lesion. The balloon diameter and length are sized to 80% of the normal parent vessel diameter and matched with

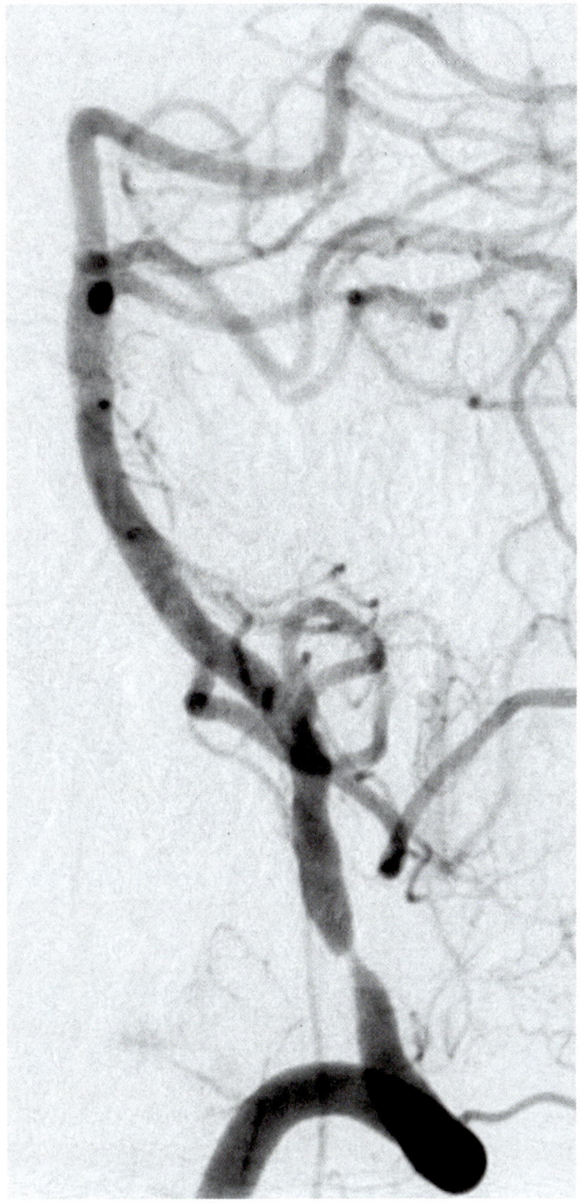

Fig. 14.4 Right vertebral artery (VA) injection, lateral projection, demonstrating a high-grade stenosis at the V3-V4 junction. This patient was experiencing clinical manifestations of vertebrobasilar insufficiency with an incompetent contralateral VA. (Reprinted with permission from Barrow Neurological Institute.)

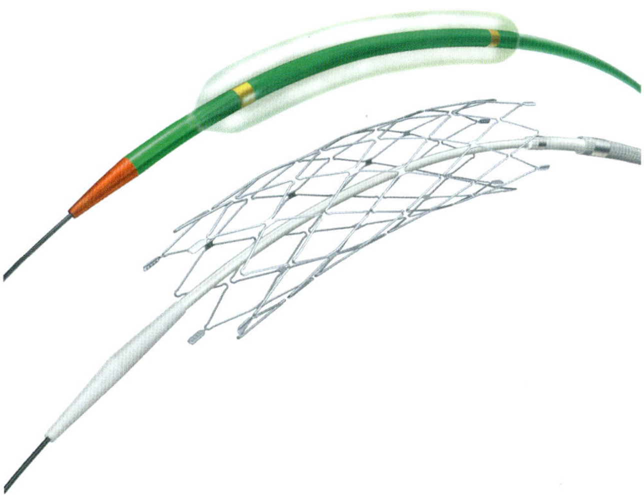

Fig. 14.3 Gateway balloon and wingspan stent. (Reprinted with permission from Boston Scientific.)

the length of the lesion, respectively. Angioplasty is typically performed with slow, graded inflation of the balloon to a pressure of between 6 and 12 atm for ~120 seconds. The balloon is inflated and deflated under direct, continuous fluoroscopic visualization. After angioplasty, the balloon is removed and conventional angiography is repeated.

Next, the Wingspan delivery system is prepared and advanced over the exchange wire across the target lesion. The stent diameter is sized to exceed the diameter of the normal parent vessel by 0.5 to 1.0 mm. The length of the stent is selected to equal or exceed the length of the angioplasty balloon. Ideally, the length of the stent should cover the entire

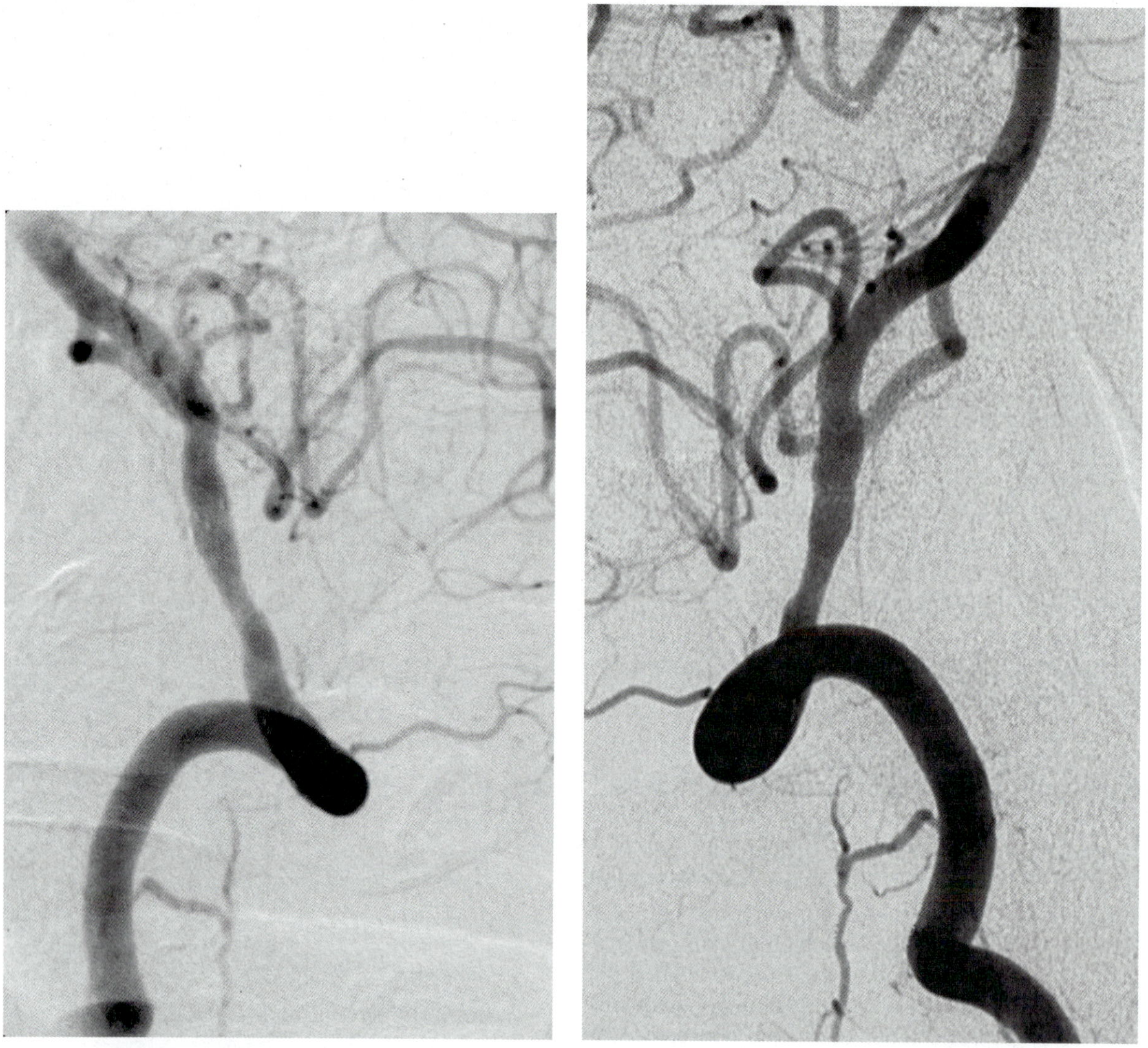

A

B

Fig. 14.5 **(A)** Right vertebral artery (VA) high-magnification angiogram, lateral projection, after stent deployment. The mild degree of residual in-stent stenosis persisted after poststent angioplasty. **(B)** Right VA angiogram, lateral projection, after stent placement at the 5-year follow-up examination of the patient shown in Figs. 14.2 and 14.3A. The image was obtained on newer equipment, which accounts for the different left-to-right orientation of the distal vessels. (Reprinted with permission from Barrow Neurological Institute.)

diseased segment. Care should be taken to place the proximal end of the stent in a position that will not complicate future endovascular access across the stented segment. The diameter of the stenotic lesion is measured using biplanar angiography and compared with a reference diameter of the normal vessel (usually proximal to the lesion), according to the technique used in the WASID study.[7] Angiography is performed after the stent is deployed (**Fig. 14.5**). Poststenting angioplasty may be required if residual stenosis is present. Heparinization is usually neither reversed nor continued postoperatively.

■ Vertebral Artery Origin Stenting: Technical Comments

In contrast to intracranial stenting, VA origin stenting is usually performed under conscious sedation. Conventional catheter-based angiography is performed to visualize the entire course of the VA as well as the intracranial vasculature of the posterior circulation. Typically, noninvasive imaging is adequate for assessment of the contralateral vessel, which may obviate the need for angiography of the nontargeted side.

With the guide catheter positioned near the origin of the VA, angiographic runs are obtained to determine the angles that best delineate the stenotic segment. The working angle is frequently the contralateral obliquity (i.e., right anterior oblique for left VA origin) and is used during follow-up angiography to provide a comparative standard (**Fig. 14.6A**).

Next, a 300-cm, 0.014-inch wire is directed across the lesion. If the degree of stenosis is not prohibitive, a balloon-mounted coronary angioplasty stent is advanced primarily across the target area. Otherwise, prestenting angioplasty may be undertaken by advancing a small-diameter,

Gateway percutaneous angioplasty balloon catheter (Boston Scientific, Natick, MA) over the wire across the area of stenosis. At our institution, we have used three types of stents: hand-mounted, balloon-expandable; self-expanding; and premounted balloon-expandable. Hand-mounted stents were used early in our experience. We transitioned to premounted balloon-expandable stents as they became available. Self-expanding systems are rarely used but may be considered when simultaneous stenting of the subclavian artery is required. Poststenting angioplasty with a noncompliant balloon may be employed when a self-expanding stent is used or when unsatisfactory residual stenosis is present after the stent is placed. Poststenting angiography of the target lesion (**Fig. 14.6B**) and the intracranial vessels is performed to assess for iatrogenic injury to the vessel or distal branch vessel occlusion. Heparinization is usually neither reversed nor continued postprocedurally.

Conclusion

In the past two decades, the armamentarium of endovascular management options for chronic and acute occlusive VA disease has expanded substantially. As new technology

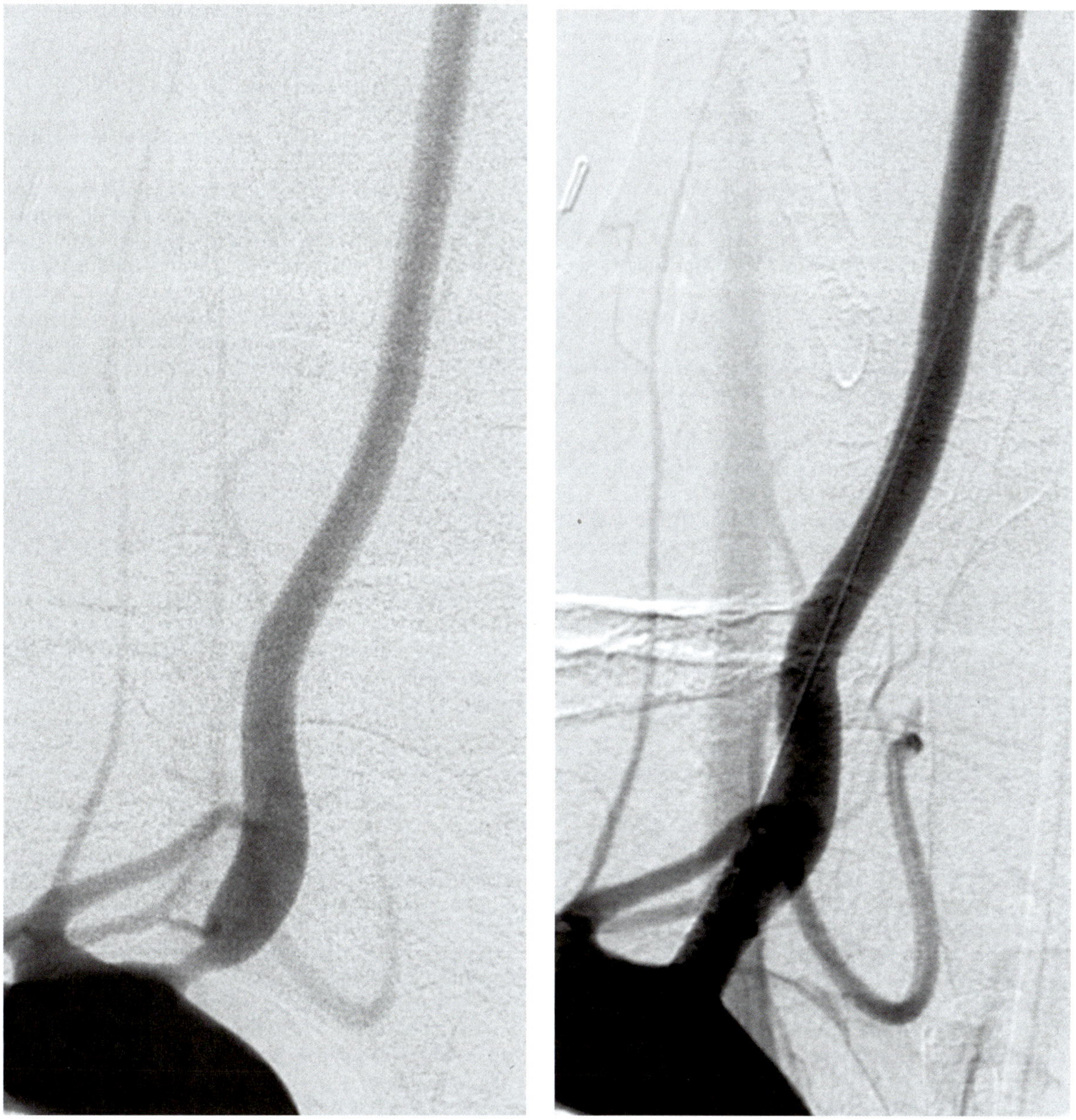

A B

Fig. 14.6 **(A)** Right subclavian artery angiogram, left anterior oblique (LAO) projection, demonstrating a high-grade stenosis of the right V1 segment. **(B)** Right subclavian artery angiogram, LAO projection, demonstrating resolution of the vertebral artery origin stenosis after a Taxus paclitaxel-eluting stent was placed. (Reprinted with permission from Barrow Neurological Institute.)

becomes available and the drive toward minimally invasive procedures as a means of improving patient outcomes advances, we expect this trend to continue. The practicing neurointerventionalist must remain vigilant and aware of emerging data as the indications for treatment of VA pathology are elucidated through clinical investigation.

References

1. Savitz SI, Caplan LR. Vertebrobasilar disease. N Engl J Med 2005; 352(25):2618–2626
2. Ausman JI, Diaz FG, Sadasivan B, Dujovny M. Intracranial vertebral endarterectomy. Neurosurgery 1990;26(3):465–471
3. Chimowitz MI, Lynn MJ, Howlett-Smith H, et al; Warfarin-Aspirin Symptomatic Intracranial Disease Trial Investigators. Comparison of warfarin and aspirin for symptomatic intracranial arterial stenosis. N Engl J Med 2005;352(13):1305–1316
4. Crawley F, Brown MM. Percutaneous transluminal angioplasty and stenting for vertebral artery stenosis. Cochrane Database Syst Rev 2000;(2):CD000516
5. Imparato AM. Vertebral arterial reconstruction: a nineteen-year experience. J Vasc Surg 1985;2(4):626–634
6. Spetzler RF, Hadley MN, Martin NA, Hopkins LN, Carter LP, Budny J. Vertebrobasilar insufficiency. Part 1: Microsurgical treatment of extracranial vertebrobasilar disease. J Neurosurg 1987;66(5): 648–661
7. Kasner SE, Chimowitz MI, Lynn MJ, et al; Warfarin Aspirin Symptomatic Intracranial Disease Trial Investigators. Predictors of ischemic stroke in the territory of a symptomatic intracranial arterial stenosis. Circulation 2006;113(4):555–563
8. Caplan LR, Wityk RJ, Glass TA, et al. New England Medical Center Posterior Circulation registry. Ann Neurol 2004;56(3):389–398
9. Levy EI, Horowitz MB, Koebbe CJ, et al. Transluminal stent-assisted angioplasty of the intracranial vertebrobasilar system for medically refractory, posterior circulation ischemia: early results. Neurosurgery 2001;48(6):1215–1221, discussion 1221–1223
10. Wehman JC, Hanel RA, Guidot CA, Guterman LR, Hopkins LN. Atherosclerotic occlusive extracranial vertebral artery disease: indications for intervention, endovascular techniques, short-term and long-term results. J Interv Cardiol 2004;17(4):219–232
11. Berguer R. Long-term Results of Vertebral Artery Reconstruction. Norwalk, CT: Appleton and Lange; 1993
12. Koskas F, Kieffer E, Rancurel G, Bahnini A, Ruotolo C, Illuminati G. Direct transposition of the distal cervical vertebral artery into the internal carotid artery. Ann Vasc Surg 1995;9(6):515–524
13. Dotter CT, Judkins MP. Transluminal treatment of arteriorsclerotic obstruction. Description of a new technique and a preliminary report of its application. Circulation 1964;30:654–670
14. Sundt TM Jr, Smith HC, Campbell JK, Vlietstra RE, Cucchiara RF, Stanson AW. Transluminal angioplasty for basilar artery stenosis. Mayo Clin Proc 1980;55(11):673–680
15. Alazzaz A, Thornton J, Aletich VA, Debrun GM, Ausman JI, Charbel F. Intracranial percutaneous transluminal angioplasty for arteriosclerotic stenosis. Arch Neurol 2000;57(11):1625–1630
16. Higashida RT, Tsai FY, Halbach VV, Dowd CF, Hieshima GB. Cerebral percutaneous transluminal angioplasty. Heart Dis Stroke 1993;2(6):497–502
17. Takis C, Kwan ES, Pessin MS, Jacobs DH, Caplan LR. Intracranial angioplasty: experience and complications. AJNR Am J Neuroradiol 1997;18(9):1661–1668
18. Randoux B, Marro B, Koskas F, Chiras J, Dormont D, Marsault C. Proximal great vessels of aortic arch: comparison of three-dimensional gadolinium-enhanced MR angiography and digital subtraction angiography. Radiology 2003;229(3):697–702
19. Wityk RJ, Chang HM, Rosengart A, et al. Proximal extracranial vertebral artery disease in the New England Medical Center Posterior Circulation Registry. Arch Neurol 1998;55(4):470–478
20. SSYLVIA Study Investigators. Stenting of Symptomatic Atherosclerotic Lesions in the Vertebral or Intracranial Arteries (SSYLVIA): study results. Stroke 2004;35(6):1388–1392
21. Moses JW, Leon MB, Popma JJ, et al; SIRIUS Investigators. Sirolimus-eluting stents versus standard stents in patients with stenosis in a native coronary artery. N Engl J Med 2003;349(14):1315–1323
22. Stone GW, Ellis SG, Cox DA, et al; TAXUS-IV Investigators. A polymer-based, paclitaxel-eluting stent in patients with coronary artery disease. N Engl J Med 2004;350(3):221–231
23. Ogilvy CS, Yang X, Natarajan SK, et al. Restenosis rates following vertebral artery origin stenting: does stent type make a difference? J Invasive Cardiol 2010;22(3):119–124
24. Karameshev A, Schroth G, Mordasini P, et al. Long-term outcome of symptomatic severe ostial vertebral artery stenosis (OVAS). Neuroradiology 2010;52(5):371–379
25. Virmani R, Guagliumi G, Farb A, et al. Localized hypersensitivity and late coronary thrombosis secondary to a sirolimus-eluting stent: should we be cautious? Circulation 2004;109(6):701–705
26. Aryan HE, Newman CB, Nottmeier EW, Acosta FL Jr, Wang VY, Ames CP. Stabilization of the atlantoaxial complex via C-1 lateral mass and C-2 pedicle screw fixation in a multicenter clinical experience in 102 patients: modification of the Harms and Goel techniques. J Neurosurg Spine 2008;8(3):222–229
27. Yamaura A, Ono J, Hirai S. Clinical picture of intracranial non-traumatic dissecting aneurysm. Neuropathology 2000;20(1): 85–90
28. Lee KP, Carlini WG, McCormick GF, Albers GW. Neurologic complications following chiropractic manipulation: a survey of California neurologists. Neurology 1995;45(6):1213–1215
29. Russell WR. Yoga and vertebral arteries. BMJ 1972;1(5801):685
30. Traflet RF, Babaria AR, Bell RD, et al. Vertebral artery dissection after rapid head turning. AJNR Am J Neuroradiol 1989;10(3): 650–651
31. Touzé E, Gauvrit JY, Moulin T, Meder JF, Bracard S, Mas JL; Multicenter Survey on Natural History of Cervical Artery Dissection. Risk of stroke and recurrent dissection after a cervical artery dissection: a multicenter study. Neurology 2003;61(10):1347–1351
32. Ast G, Woimant F, Georges B, Laurian C, Haguenau M. Spontaneous dissection of the internal carotid artery in 68 patients. Eur J Med 1993;2(8):466–472
33. Berne JD, Norwood SH. Blunt vertebral artery injuries in the era of computed tomographic angiographic screening: incidence and outcomes from 8,292 patients. J Trauma 2009;67(6):1333–1338
34. Giacobetti FB, Vaccaro AR, Bos-Giacobetti MA, et al. Vertebral artery occlusion associated with cervical spine trauma. A prospective analysis. Spine (Phila Pa 1976) 1997;22(2):188–192
35. Arnold M, Nedeltchev K, Schroth G, et al. Clinical and radiological predictors of recanalisation and outcome of 40 patients with acute basilar artery occlusion treated with intra-arterial thrombolysis. J Neurol Neurosurg Psychiatry 2004;75(6):857–862
36. Brandt T, von Kummer R, Müller-Küppers M, Hacke W. Thrombolytic therapy of acute basilar artery occlusion. Variables affecting recanalization and outcome. Stroke 1996;27(5):875–881

15 Arteriovenous Malformations of the Craniovertebral Junction: Spinal and Posterior Fossa AVMs

Louis J. Kim, Joshua W. Osbun, B. Gregory Thompson, and Robert F. Spetzler

Important advances in the understanding and treatment of cranial and spinal vascular malformations have occurred in the past decade. Treatment planning for a cranial arteriovenous malformation (AVM) has become more complex because radiosurgery—a somewhat less risky but less efficacious alternative than surgery—has become a viable alternative for selected deep AVMs of the posterior fossa, such as intrinsic brainstem AVMs. Great advances have been made in endovascular surgery and embolization techniques, allowing for multidisciplinary treatment of what were once inoperable lesions. Fundamentally new observations regarding the anatomical and pathophysiological nature of spinal AVMs have allowed for their reclassification and now enable clinicians to provide safer and more effective treatment through a similar multidisciplinary approach.

Location is a paramount issue in the management of AVMs of the craniospinal axis. The location of a given AVM—intradural or extradural, pial or intramedullary, residing in noneloquent brain or in critical deep nuclei in the brainstem or cerebellum—largely determines the natural history and surgical risk associated with the AVM and often whether treatment is necessary, possible, or recommended. This review clarifies AVMs of the craniovertebral junction (CVJ) by location (cervical or posterior fossa) to discuss their natural history, diagnostic evaluation, and treatment indications with surgical, endovascular, and radiosurgical management.

Classification of Spinal AVMs

The classification of spinal AVMs has evolved with and been limited by the technology available to study them. Before the advent of selective spinal angiography, all spinal vascular malformations were attributed to venous lesions situated on the surface of the spinal cord. In 1914, Dr. Charles Elsberg of New York performed the first successful operation on a spinal AVM.[1] Elsberg excised a 2-cm segment of an abnormal dilated spinal vein as it penetrated the dura of the T9 spinal nerve root. Postoperatively, the patient improved and made a complete neurological recovery 3 months after surgery.

In the 1960s, selective spinal angiography demonstrated the precise radiographic anatomy of spinal AVMs and led to a new classification based on their vascular anatomy and pattern of blood flow rather than on postmortem pathology.[2] Thereafter, spinal AVMs were classified radiographically into three categories. Type I AVMs (single-coiled vessel) were thought to comprise 80 to 85% of all spinal AVMs. Type II (glomus) and type III (juvenile) AVMs accounted for 15 to 20% of the lesions. In all three types, the nidus was believed to lie within the spinal cord or pia mater. In 1977, Kendall and Logue demonstrated that the single-coiled vessel spinal AVM (type I) was the result of an arteriovenous (AV) fistula at the level of the dural sleeve of a spinal nerve root.[3] After undergoing simple surgical excision of the fistula without surgical stripping of the single-coiled vessel, the patients uniformly improved or stabilized.

Kendall and Logue's work resulted in a revised classification scheme for spinal AVMs.[4] Based on differences in origin, epidemiology, anatomy, pathophysiology, and clinical presentation, three categories of spinal vascular malformations were recognized: (1) spinal-dural AV fistulae arising at the nerve root dural sleeve (radiculomedullary AV fistulae), (2) intradural vascular malformations (glomus, juvenile, or perimedullary), and (3) cavernous malformations of the spinal cord. Intradural vascular malformations are further classified into three subgroups: type II or glomus AVMs, type III or juvenile AVMs, and type IV or direct perimedullary AV fistulae. This classification continues to serve as the classic view of spinal AVMs.

The past decade has brought many advances in three-dimensional (3D) imaging technology and, as such, several groups have called for a reappraisal of the classification of spinal AVMs.[5–8] Although other classification systems have been proposed, the classic type I to IV nomenclature persists throughout the literature. In 2002, Spetzler and colleagues initially proposed a modification to the classic classification system based on anatomical location and pathophysiological factors.[7] The system divided spinal AVMs based on anatomical descriptors, such as extradural or intradural, extramedullary or intramedullary, and ventral or dorsal. From this work, a new classification proposed by Kim and Spetzler evolved.[5] The new classification system is important because it not only divides lesions based on anatomical location but makes an important distinction between AV fistulae and AVMs, which carry separate classifications of natural history, pathophysiology, treatment, and prognosis. Their classification scheme divides vascular lesions of the spinal cord into six categories: (1) extradural AV fistulae, (2) intradural dorsal AV fistulae, (3) intradural ventral AV fistulae, (4) extradural–intradural AVMs, (5) intramedullary AVMs, and (6) conus medullaris AVMs. Full descriptions of each of these lesions are provided in this chapter.

Anatomy

The correct interpretation of diagnostic studies and clinical evaluation and management of the various subtypes of spinal AVMs require a precise understanding of spinal vascular anatomy. Planning and implementation of surgical and nonsurgical treatments must be based on a clear understanding of venous and arterial anatomy.

Arterial Anatomy

The spinal cord is supplied by variably collateralized anterior and posterior arterial systems (**Fig. 15.1**).[9] The anterior distribution arises from the anterior spinal artery, extends the entire length of the spinal cord in the anterior median fissure, and supplies the anterior two-thirds of the spinal cord. The posterior system, an arterial network of collaterals between two posterior arteries, supplies the posterior third of the spinal cord. The anterior arterial system supplies the anterior horns, corticospinal tract, and spinothalamic tracts. The posterior arterial system supplies a smaller portion of the corticospinal tracts and the entire dorsal columns. Both arterial systems receive blood from medullary arteries, one of the three terminal branches of intercostal arteries.

During the first 6 months of gestation, paired medullary arteries supply the anterior and posterior arteries at each segmental level of the spine. By birth, however, most of the medullary arteries involute. In adults, only 6 to 10 medullary arteries remain to supply the entire spinal cord.[9] In the cervical region, these medullary arteries are derived from terminal branches of intervertebral arteries (a branch of the posterior spinal ramus of the segmental arteries, which in turn are derived from the vertebral and branches of the subclavian arteries). In addition to the medullary arteries, which supply only the spinal cord, there are two other important terminal branches of the intervertebral

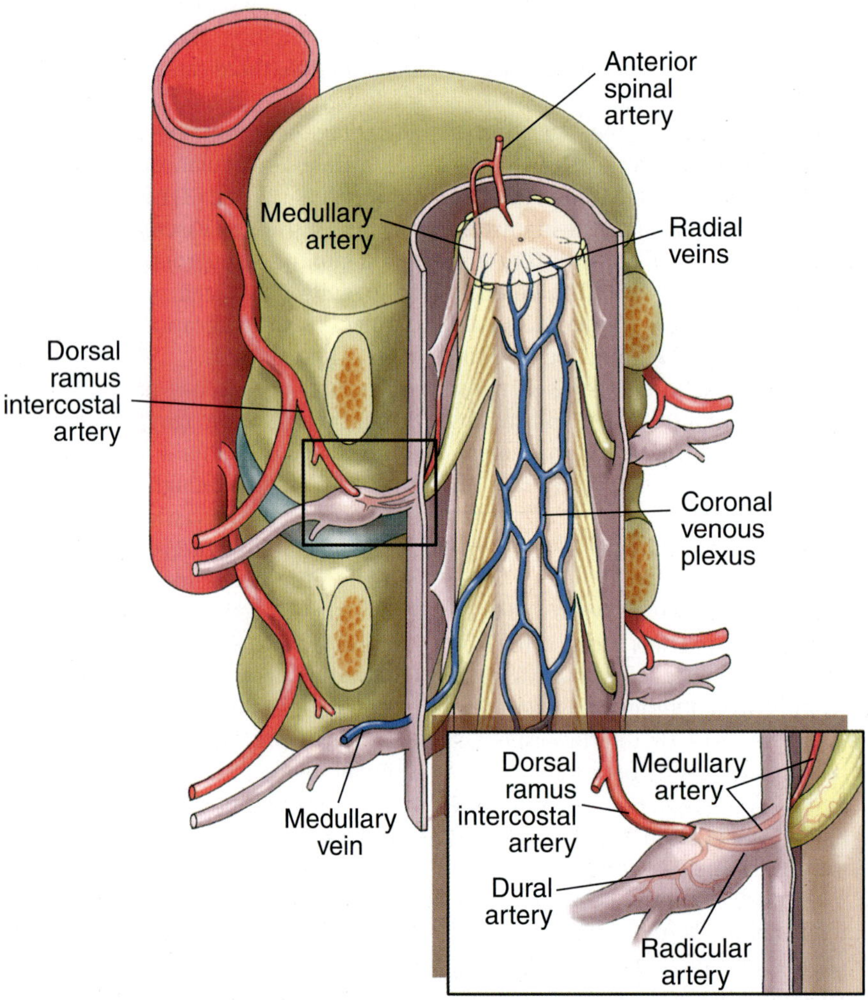

Fig. 15.1 Arterial and venous anatomy of the spinal cord. At each segmental level of the spinal cord, the intercostal artery divides into a dural and radicular branch. At some levels, the intercostal artery gives off a medullary artery that joins an anterior or posterior spinal artery to supply the spinal cord. Radial veins drain the spinal cord to the coronal venous plexus. (Reprinted with permission from Barrow Neurological Institute.)

arteries—the radicular and dural arteries. Unlike the medullary artery, radicular arteries, which supply the nerve root, and dural arteries, which supply the nerve root sleeves surrounding spinal dura, persist at each segmental level on both sides (**Fig. 15.1**).

Venous Anatomy

The venous system of the spinal cord is composed of two radially arranged vascular networks (**Fig. 15.1**). The sulcal veins lie in the anterior median fissure and empty into the anterior median spinal vein. The radial veins lie in the dorsal and anterolateral regions of the spinal cord and drain centrifugally into the pial coronal venous plexus. Both the anterior median spinal vein and the coronal venous plexus are drained by medullary vein through the dura to the epidural (Batson) venous plexus. Like the medullary arteries, medullary veins are not present at each segmental level and penetrate the dura in the region of the nerve root.

Pathophysiology

Extradural Arteriovenous Fistulae

Extradural AV fistulae are known as epidural fistulae under the classic nomenclature based on the work of Kendall and Logue. These lesions arise from an anomalous connection between an extradural artery (usually a radicular artery branch) and an epidural venous plexus (**Fig. 15.2**). Increased flow under arterial pressure to the epidural venous system can result in venous hypertension and engorgement of the plexus. The mass effect of the engorged venous plexus causes compression of the spinal cord and nerve roots, often resulting in myelopathy and radiculopathy (**Fig. 15.3**).

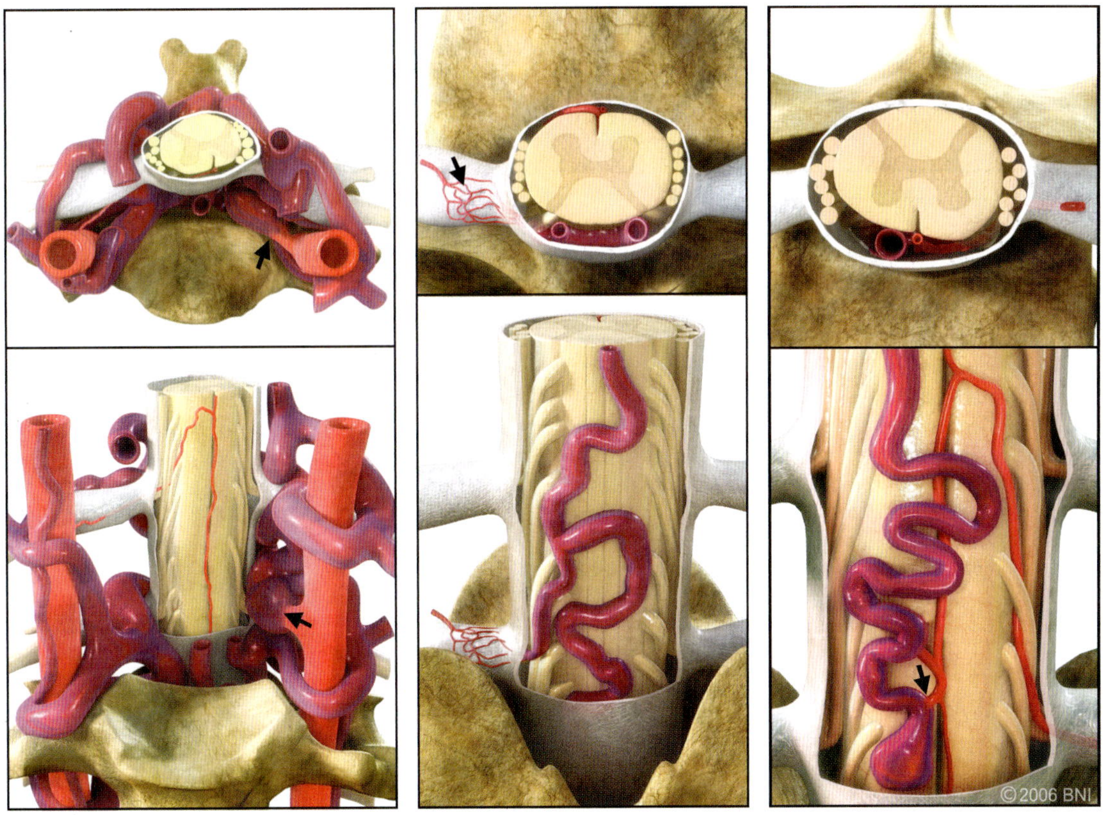

A B C

Fig. 15.2 **(A) Top**, axial and **(B) bottom**, anterior views, demonstrating an extradural arteriovenous fistula (AVF) along a perforating branch of the left vertebral artery (*arrows*) and engorgement of the epidural veins, producing symptomatic mass effect on adjacent nerve roots and spinal cord. **(B) Top**, axial illustration of an intradural dorsal AVF demonstrating an abnormal radicular feeding artery along the nerve root on the right. The glomerular network of tiny branches (*arrow*) coalesces at the site of the fistula along the dural root sleeve. **(B) Bottom**, illustration of the posterior view demonstrating the dilatation of the coronal venous plexus. In addition to venous outflow obstruction (not shown), arterialization of these veins produces venous hypertension. Focal disruption of the point of the fistula by endovascular or microsurgical methods will obliterate the lesion. **(C) Top**, axial illustration demonstrating an intradural ventral AVF, a midline lesion derived from a fistulous connection between the anterior spinal artery and coronal venous plexus. **(C) Bottom**, illustration of the anterior view demonstrating the fistula (*arrow*) along the anteroinferior aspect of the spinal cord. Proximal and distal to this type A lesion, the course of the anterior spinal artery is normal. (*continued*)

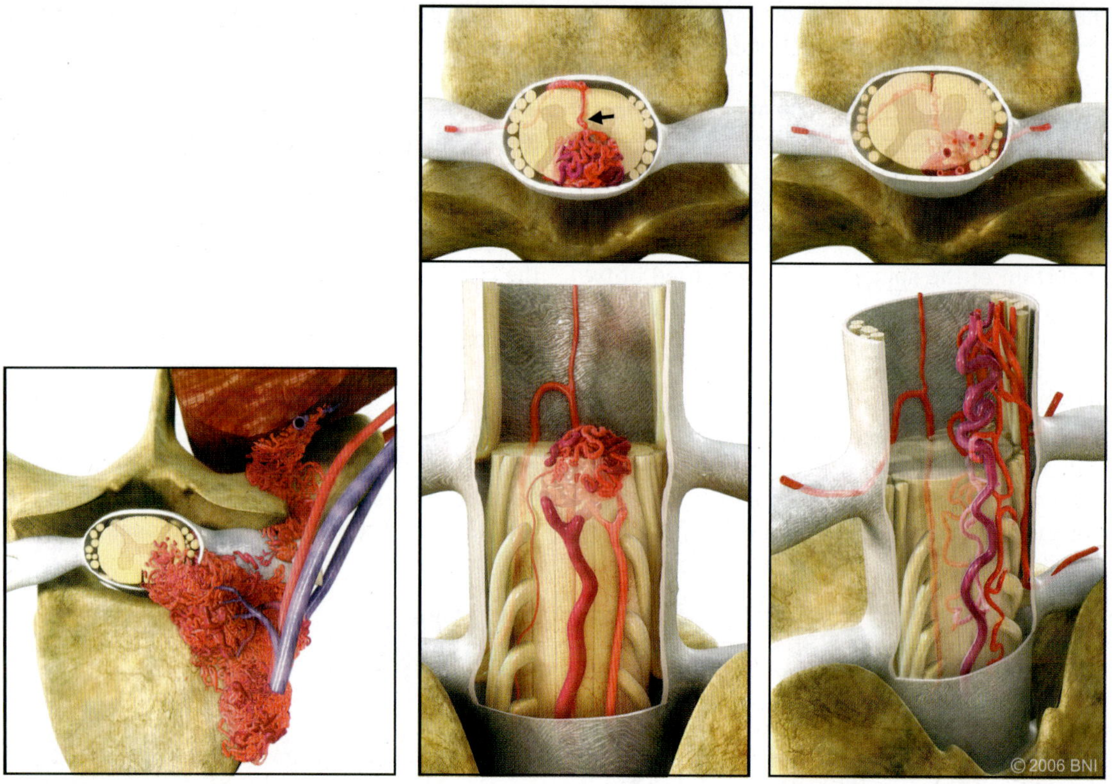

D E F

Fig. 15.2 *(continued)* **(D)** Axial illustration demonstrating an extradural–intradural arteriovenous malformation (AVM). These treacherous lesions can encompass soft tissues, bone, spinal canal, spinal cord, and spinal nerve roots along an entire spinal level. Considerable involvement of multiple structures makes these entities extremely difficult to treat. Although cures have been reported, the primary goal of treatment is usually palliative. **(E) Top**, axial illustration demonstrating a compact intramedullary AVM. In this figure, an arterial feeder from the anterior spinal artery is identified (*arrow*). Note the discrete, compact mass of the AVM. **(E) Bottom**, posterior view demonstrating additional feeding branches from the posterior spinal artery and reemphasizing the compact nature of this type of spinal AVM. Portions of the AVM are evident along the surface of the spinal cord. Surgical resection is the mainstay of treatment. Preoperative embolization is reserved for select cases only. **(F) Top**, axial illustration demonstrating a diffuse intramedullary AVM with areas of intervening neural tissue between the intraparenchymal loops of AVM. Portions of the AVM also course along the pial surface and subarachnoid space. **(F) Bottom**, illustration of the oblique posterior view demonstrating the loops of the AVM coursing in and out of the spinal cord. Normal neural tissue is evident between intraparenchymal portions of the AVM. This view accentuates the diffuse character of these lesions. (Reprinted with permission from Barrow Neurological Institute.)

Intradural Dorsal Arteriovenous Fistulae

These lesions correlate with the type I AV fistulae of previous nomenclature and involve a radicular artery with an abnormal communication to the venous system of the spinal cord along the dural sleeve of the nerve root (**Fig. 15.2**). Its low-flow shunt system results in venous hypertension with engorgement, elongation, and tortuosity of the venous system, thereby causing local mass effect with concomitant myelopathy and propensity for hemorrhage. These fistulae are believed to result initially from venous outflow obstruction, which presumably contributes to fistula formation via arterialization of the venous plexus. A medullary vein is usually the sole venous outflow from the fistula and carries the shunted arterial blood in a retrograde fashion (opposite the normal direction of venous flow) along the coronal venous plexus. The absence of other regional venous drainage creates venous engorgement and venous hypertension. The diversion of blood under high pressure by the arterialized medullary vein into the coronal venous plexus results in further venous dilatation. Because the intrathecal venous system has no valves, the varicocele-like radial and sulcal veins transmit venous hypertension to the spinal cord, producing venous congestion and myelopathy. Although intradural dorsal AV fistulae are truly rare in the cervical spine, similar direct dural AV fistulae at the skull base have been found to drain arterialized venous blood through the coronal venous plexus at the foramen magnum, resulting in the stereotypical engorged spinal venous system and myelopathy (**Figs. 15.4** and **15.5**).[10]

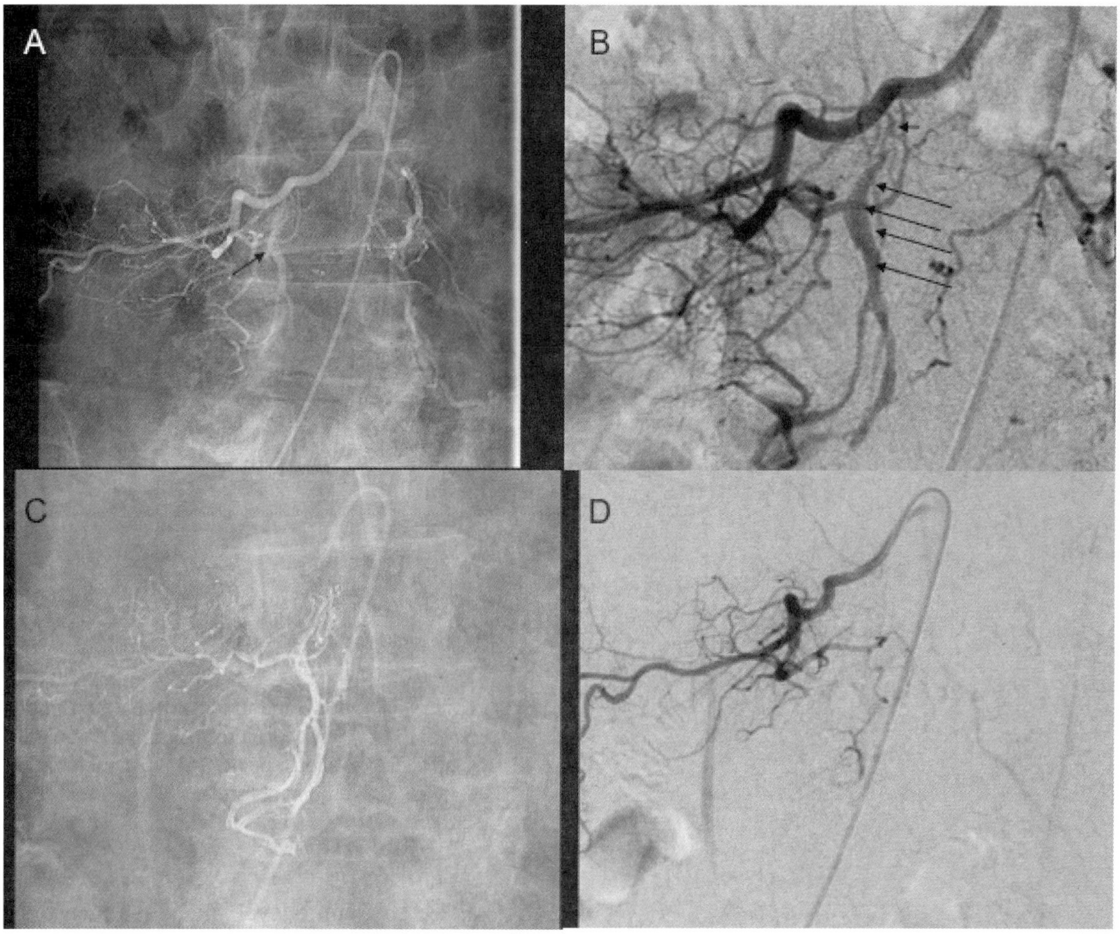

Fig. 15.3 A 65-year-old man with a history of a lumbar discectomy and progressive right lower extremity weakness. **(A)** Spinal angiogram at right L3 demonstrates an extradural dorsal fistula draining into the epidural venous system. The lateral location of the venous drainage is demarcated by arrows. **(B)** The fistulous point (*short arrow*) and venous pouch (*long arrows*) are shown. **(C)** Onyx cast in fistula and venous pouch after patient underwent embolization with Onyx. **(D)** Postembolization angiogram demonstrates obliteration of lesion.

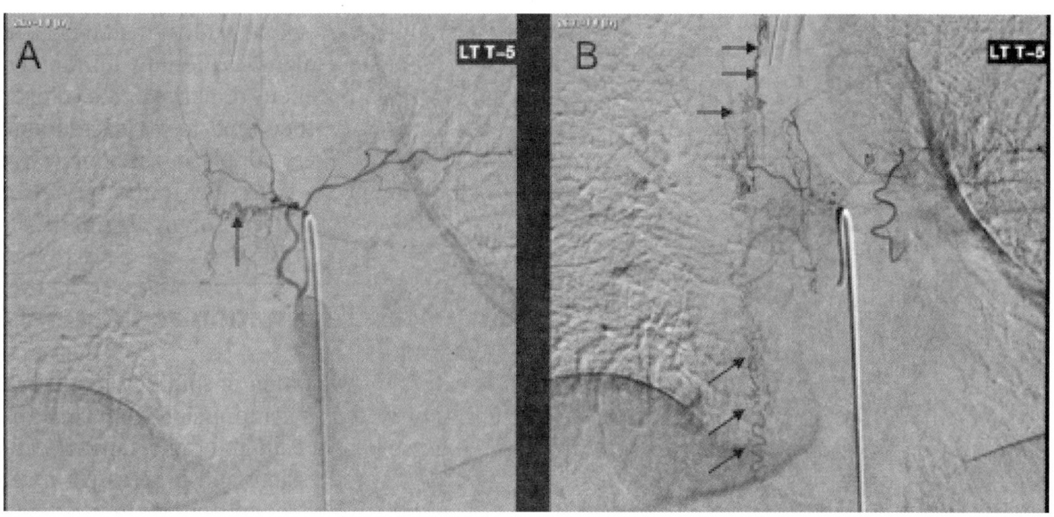

Fig. 15.4 Intradural dorsal arteriovenous fistula in a 45-year-old man presenting with progressive bilateral lower extremity weakness, paresthesias, and urinary retention. **(A)** Left T5 injection demonstrating a dorsal intradural arteriovenous fistula with arrow at fistulous point. **(B)** Venous phase of same angiogram demonstrating dilated coronal venous plexus and sluggish venous outflow (*arrows*) of the fistula.

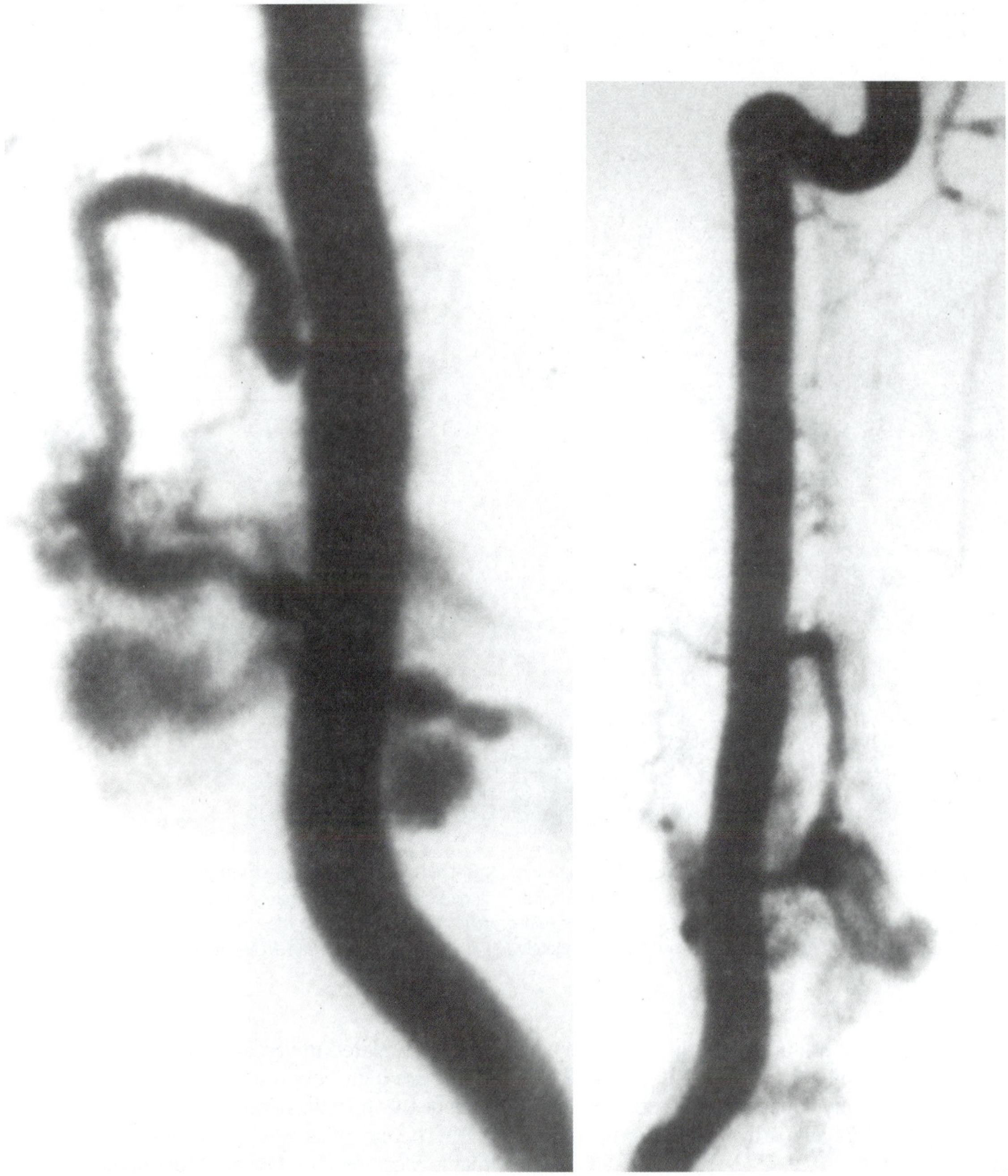

C

D

Fig. 15.6 *(continued)* **(C) (D)**

AVM (type I)—experienced no subsequent neurological progression.[17,18]

Spinal dural fistulae represent a different category of epidemiology and natural history. These lesions tend to present in the fifth and sixth decades of life and have a male predominance.[19,20] However, lesions are seen in the pediatric population. Rodesch and colleagues reported the results of a small series of intradural spinal fistulae and found hemorrhage to be the presenting symptom in 44.8% of adults and 70% of children.[21] Narvid and colleagues determined that 52% presented with lower extremity weakness, 30% with paresthesias, 24% with back pain, and 6% with urinary retention.[20] The study made no distinction between progressive and acute presentation. Foix-Alajouanine syndrome historically has been known as a necrotic myelopathy caused by progressive spinal cord venous thrombosis. Such endomesovasculitis was originally believed to be due to a poorly characterized spinal vascular lesion but, based on the original authors description of progressive myelopathy and their histological findings, this syndrome is likely due to what we now know as intradural dorsal AV fistulae.[22]

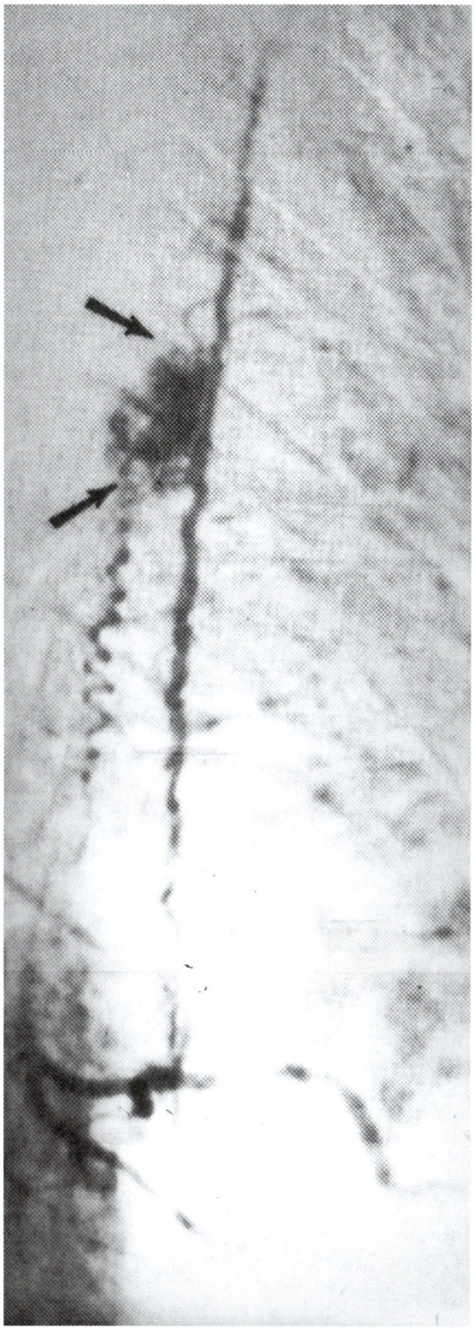

Fig. 15.7 Selective spinal arteriography of a type II (glomus) cervical arteriovenous malformation showing a dense nidus of blood vessels (*arrows*) confined to a short segment of the cervical spinal cord. The lesion is situated in the anterior half of the spinal cord and is supplied by branches of the anterior spinal artery.

Diagnostic Evaluation

Effective management of spinal AVMs depends on precise radiographic evaluation to define the anatomy of the lesion so that the appropriate intervention may be selected. Imaging evaluation has two components: screening studies for the initial evaluation of patients with acute or progressive radiculomyelopathy and vascular imaging studies for diagnostic confirmation and anatomical definition of the lesion for surgical planning.

The evaluation of progressive radiculomyelopathy includes plain radiography of the spine, magnetic resonance imaging (MRI), computed tomography (CT), and myelography. These studies are used to direct the choice of further investigations.

Because it is less invasive and usually more informative, MRI has replaced myelography as the initial diagnostic procedure of choice in patients with progressive myelopathy.[23–25] MRI in patients with spinal AVMs may demonstrate abnormal vessels in the subarachnoid space (**Fig. 15.8**), the nidus of an intramedullary AVM, or changes

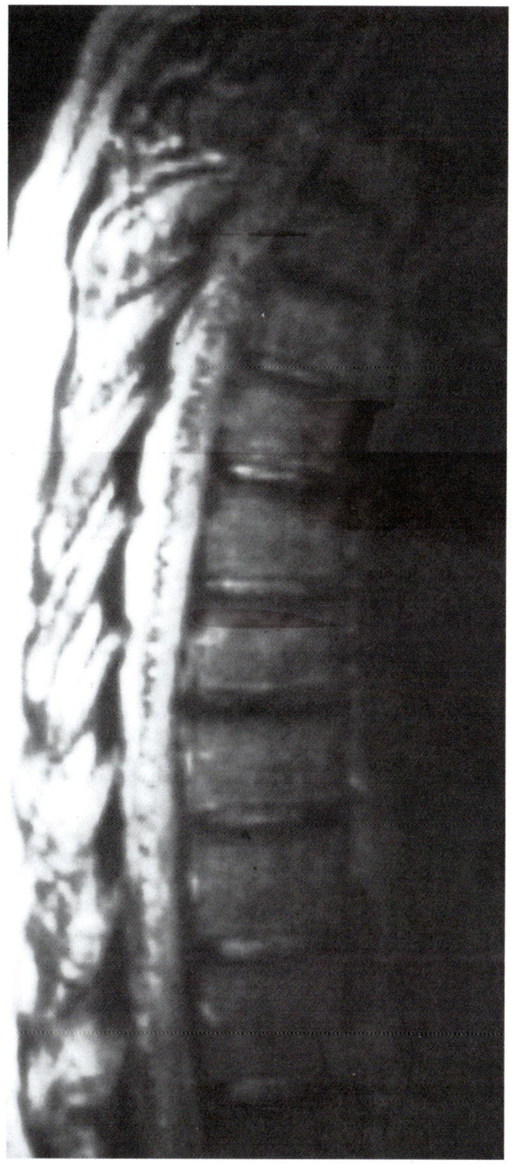

Fig. 15.8 Magnetic resonance image of type I spinal dural arteriovenous fistula demonstrates abnormal, dilated, and tortuous vessels in the subarachnoid space.

in the spinal cord produced by venous congestion, infarction, or hemorrhage.[23] MRI often provides the initial diagnosis of an AVM and readily distinguishes between intramedullary and perimedullary AVMs and AV fistulae.

Due to the excess blood flow in the coronal venous plexus in patients with spinal AVMs, T1- and T2-weighted images often demonstrate a serpentine pattern of blood flow in the subarachnoid space. This "flow-void" signal is derived from dilated tortuous vessels of the arterialized coronal venous plexus or from an enlarged artery feeding an intramedullary AVM of the spinal cord. Tortuous, dilated, arterialized pial veins (varicoceles) of the coronal venous plexus may exert mass effect and compress the spinal cord, producing a scalloped appearance on sagittal T1-weighted images. T2-weighted images and short TI-inversion recovery sequences may demonstrate increased signal intensity within the spinal cord, representing spinal cord edema or hematoma. The enlarged coronal venous plexus often is most prominent posteriorly and may be seen more clearly on axial images.

T1-weighted images of intramedullary spinal AVMs usually demonstrate a focal flow-void signal with local expansion of the spinal cord, suggesting an intramedullary lesion. Axial and sagittal images localize the intramedullary position of an AV nidus. This information is particularly useful for high cervical AVMs, which often are located more dorsally than AVMs occurring in more caudal regions of the spinal cord. Subacute hemorrhage appears as increased signal intensity on T1-weighted images, whereas associated aneurysms or venous varices may be recognized as a globular region of flow void. After an AV fistula has been interrupted or embolized, occlusion of the nidus or venous varices can be confirmed by the absence of the flow-void signal on T2-weighted images.

More recently, magnetic resonance angiography (MRA) has become a powerful diagnostic tool for viewing spinal AVMs.[23,24] A standard 3D contrast-enhanced MRA uses time-of-flight sequences with phase contrast and pre- and postgadolinium contrast along with conventional coils to produce a 3D rendering of the spinal vessels. Repetition time values are typically 20 to 50 ms, and acquisition times are quite long. Usually only the largest arteries and veins are demonstrated in normal spinal vascular anatomy, but vessel dilatations may be easily detected in the case of an AVM or fistula. Fast 3D contrast-enhanced MRA uses high-performance coils and rapid gradient pulse sequences to achieve lower repetition time values in the 10-ms range and much faster scan acquisition times (often less than 1 min).[24] This technique can produce high-quality images and detect vessels of smaller diameter.[26]

Multirow-detector CT angiography has also become a powerful imaging tool when spinal AVM or fistula is suspected.[27–29] This modality involves obtaining phase-injected contrast images on a helical CT with a 16-row detector, using slices from 0.5 to 1 mm. Postcomputer processing of source images can produce a maximum intensity projection sequence that demonstrates the spinal vascular anatomy in 3D. A few small studies have reported that this technique easily demonstrates stigmata of spinal AVMs and fistulae, such as arterialized vessels. However, delineating between AVMs and intradural and extradural fistulae is very difficult.[29]

Although MRI often provides sufficient evidence of an AVM to require subsequent spinal angiography, it may be normal or show only nonspecific changes in patients with type I or type IV spinal AV fistulae. Hence, patients with an unexplained progressive myelopathy in addition to normal MRI require additional diagnostic evaluation with myelography.

Myelography was once the most sensitive diagnostic screening tool for spinal AVMs but has been replaced by the gold standard of MRI and MRA. A technically well-done myelogram reliably demonstrates abnormal vascularity in the subarachnoid space for all types of spinal AVMs and can be very helpful in patients who are unable to undergo MRI. Therefore, a technically proficient myelogram that fails to demonstrate abnormal vessels obviates the need for subsequent spinal angiography. However, once the diagnosis of spinal AVM has been confirmed with MRI or myelography, spinal angiography is necessary to define the vascular supply and the precise anatomical location of the nidus of the AVM.[30,31]

Spinal angiography remains the gold standard for confirmatory diagnosis and for delineating the exact angioarchitecture needed for operative and endovascular treatment (**Fig. 15.9**). Modern spinal angiography involves the use of biplanar flat panel detectors with digital subtraction and roadmapping capabilities. In addition to standard angiographic runs, this technology allows for 3D digital subtraction angiography to be performed for 3D roadmaps of the lesion's angioarchitecture. CT and CT angiography can be obtained in the angiography suite for additional information on soft tissues and bony anatomy surrounding the lesion. The Phillips XperCT system (Phillips Medical Systems, Eindhoven, The Netherlands) combines 3D digital subtraction spinal angiography with 3D CT on a single machine for this purpose (**Figs. 15.6, 15.9,** and **15.10**).

Management of Spinal Arteriovenous Malformations

Current treatment strategy of spinal vascular lesions involves a multidisciplinary approach to management based on size, location, and precise angioarchitecture. This approach may involve endovascular obliteration, surgical ligation, or combined treatment. The ideal treatment of spinal AVM is to obliterate the nidus of the AVM permanently without compromising the blood supply to the spinal cord. Whether this goal is feasible depends on the type, size, and location of the intradural vascular malformation. Preservation of neurological function and prevention of iatrogenic injury are decidedly more difficult to achieve with large

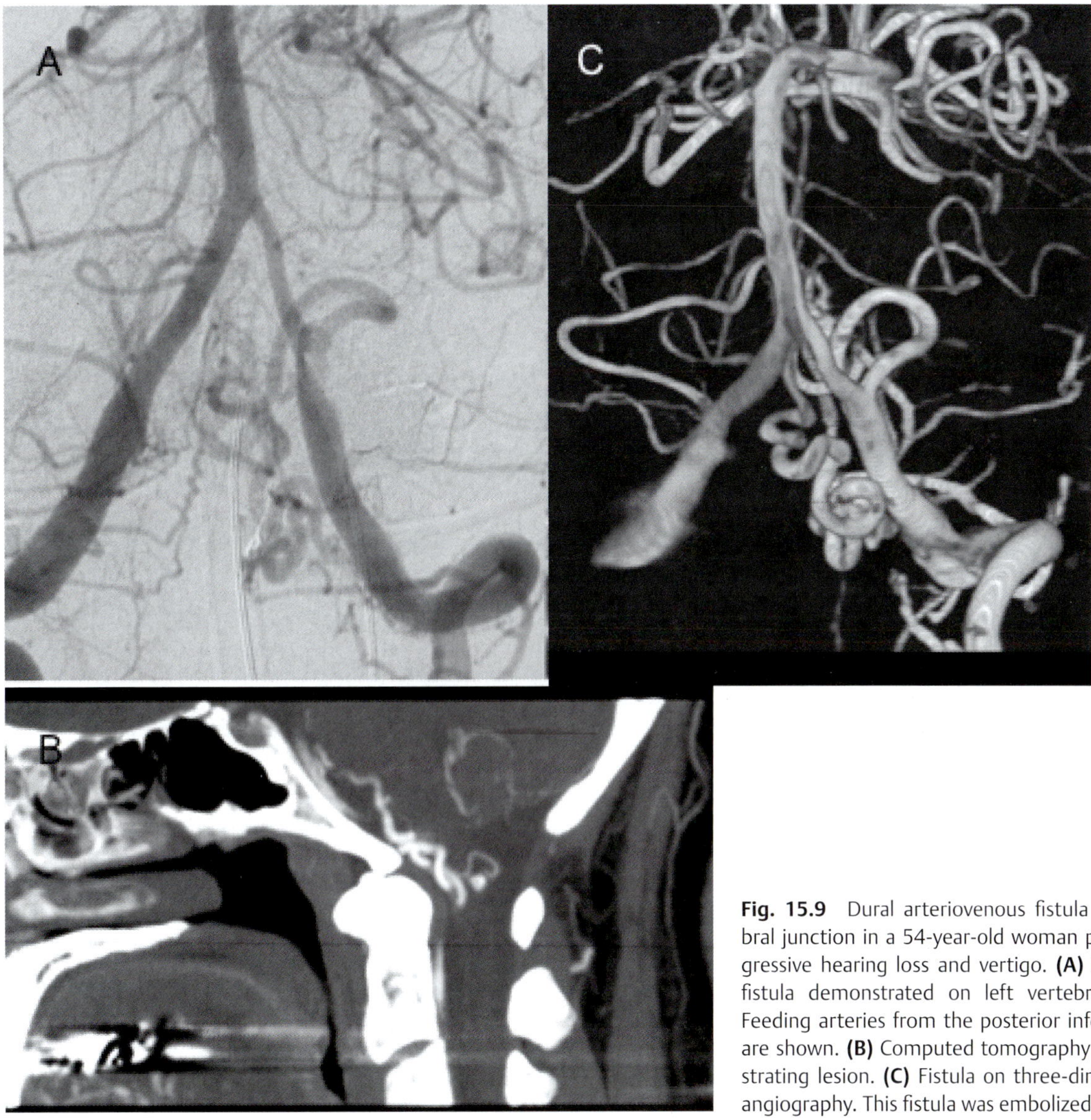

Fig. 15.9 Dural arteriovenous fistula of the craniovertebral junction in a 54-year-old woman presenting with progressive hearing loss and vertigo. **(A)** Dural arteriovenous fistula demonstrated on left vertebral artery injection. Feeding arteries from the posterior inferior cerebral artery are shown. **(B)** Computed tomography angiogram demonstrating lesion. **(C)** Fistula on three-dimensional rotational angiography. This fistula was embolized using Onyx.

lesions located in the ventral aspect of the thoracic or lumbar segment of the spinal cord and those associated with a complex blood supply, particularly if fed from the ventral surface of the spinal cord.

Endovascular Management of Spinal Arteriovenous Malformations

Endovascular treatment of spinal vascular lesions was developed as a natural extension and refinement of spinal angiography. Until recent years, embolization before surgical excision was often used as an adjuvant therapy in lesions that could be excised with an acceptable risk. Although complete embolic occlusion of the AVM nidus was the initial goal of endovascular treatment, angiographic occlusion did not ensure anatomical elimination of the AVM, and occlusion of the nidus was not permanent in all patients.[32,33] In the past decade, several improvements in imaging technology and embolic agents have vastly improved the success of endovascular treatment. More recent literature suggests successful obliteration of spinal AVMs in 25 to 100% of cases with endovascular management.[20,34–36]

Originally, glues such as polyvinyl alcohol and n-butyl 2-cyanoacrylate (NBCA) were used as embolic agents. These agents have historically been associated with high rates of fistula and AVM recanalization and recurrence, leading ultimately to symptom recurrence and surgery.[32]

Onyx (ev3, Inc., Irvine, CA), an ethylene vinyl alcohol copolymer suspended in a dimethyl sulfoxide solvent, has shown great promise in the endovascular treatment of spinal cord AVMs and AV fistulae and has demonstrated great success in treating intracranial AVMs and AV fistulae (**Figs. 15.3** and **15.5**).[37–41] A few small studies have described its success in treating spinal counterparts. Corkill and colleagues reported their experience with Onyx embolization of spinal AVMs in 17 patients, demonstrating complete angiographic

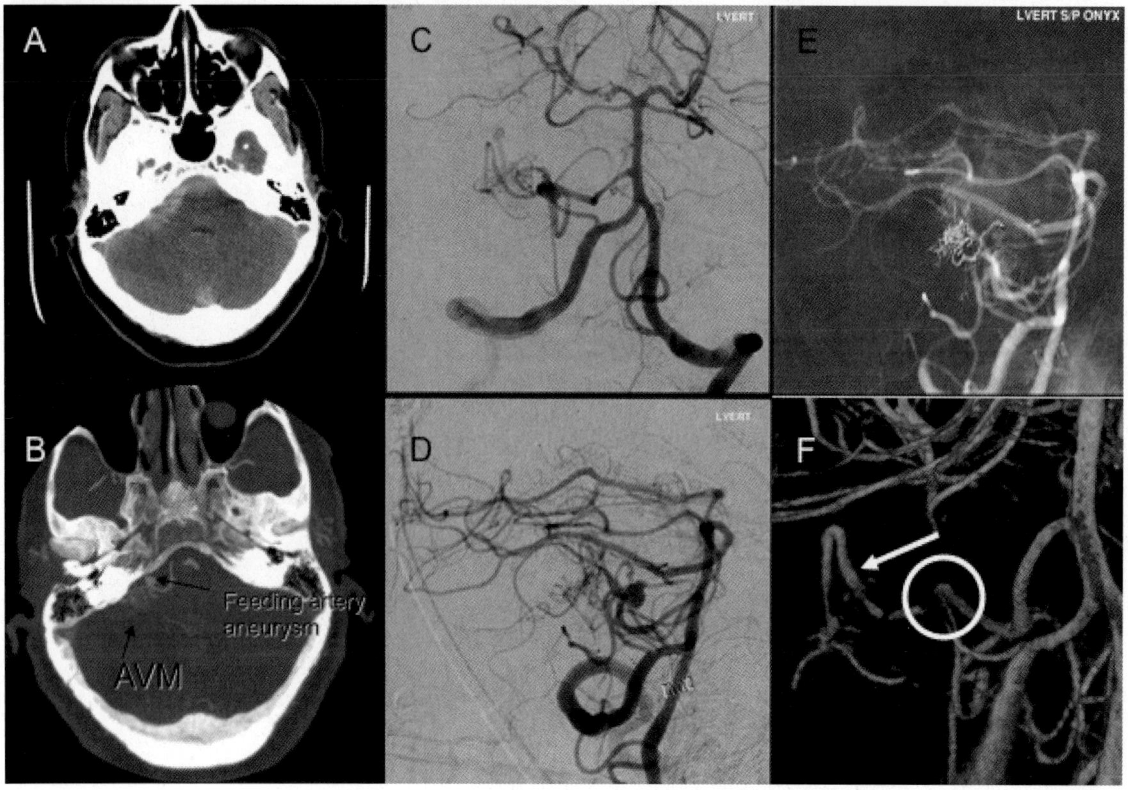

Fig. 15.10 A 59-year-old woman presenting with subarachnoid hemorrhage. **(A)** Noncontrast computed tomography demonstrates subarachnoid hemorrhage. **(B)** Computed tomography angiogram demonstrates an arteriovenous malformation (*AVM*) in the posterior fossa and a flow-related aneurysm involving the anterior inferior cerebellar artery (AICA) as the feeding vessel. **(C)** Left vertebral artery injection anteroposterior view demonstrates the AVM fed by AICA and two flow-related aneurysms. **(D)** Lateral view demonstrating the AVM and flow-related aneurysms. **(E)** Angiogram postcurative Onyx embolization of AVM. Note reflux of embolisate into the ruptured aneurysm dome, partially securing the lesion. The small residual aneurysm was obliterated with coils. **(F)** Three-dimensional rotational angiogram demonstrating that the en passage vessel is preserved (*white arrow*) and the aneurysm and AVM are obliterated (*white circle*).

obliteration in 37.5%, subtotal obliteration with minimal remnant in 31.25%, and partial obliteration in 31.25%.[42] Moreover, 82% of patients showed significant neurological improvement at a mean follow-up of 24.3 months, regardless of angiographic result. Warakaulle initially presented two patients with spinal AV fistulae who received initial angiographic obliteration with Onyx, one of which ultimately recanalized.[43] Nogueira and colleagues demonstrated complete angiographic cure in a series of three patients with lumbar spinal AV fistulae.

A few key technical aspects seem to determine the success of endovascular treatment of spinal vascular malformations. For the treatment of spinal fistulae, the embolic material must not only occlude and obliterate the feeding artery but must reach and pass the nidus of the fistula to occlude the proximal segment of the draining vein.[44,45] Often this feat is accomplished by slow continuous injection of the embolic agent until it reaches the draining vein, with the microcatheter positioned as close to the fistula as possible. Excessive reflux into proximal vascular structures and subsequent embolic complications can be avoided by pausing the injection for 30 to 120 seconds.[46] Another useful technique is to begin embolization with Onyx-34, a higher viscosity type, and then switching to Onyx-18 viscosity, forming a viscous proximal plug to minimize the amount of reflex proximal to the catheter tip. We advocate catheter positions distal to anterior spinal artery feeders/collaterals to eliminate the risk of untoward target embolization and to avoid inadvertent reflux of the dimethyl sulfoxide solvent. For intramedullary AVMs, injection of an embolic agent, such as NBCA or Onyx, into the nidus often results in the most successful treatment. Occlusion of the proximal feeding artery alone usually fails due to recanalization via collaterals. Coils or glue may be used to treat perinodal aneurysms. Reduction of the nidus should be the primary goal over complete angiographic obliteration because partial treatment has been shown to produce good clinical results as evidenced by the series from Corkill and colleagues. Regardless of the embolic agent or endovascular treatment strategy, any intervention should be performed under general anesthesia with the use of neuromonitoring. The use of periprocedural somatosensory evoked potentials (SSEPs) and motor evoked potentials (MEPs) can aid in reducing and eliminating procedural morbidities related to reflux of embolic material or hemorrhage.[47]

In summary, endovascular management of spinal vascular malformations has become an increasingly important treatment modality. New advances in imaging technology and embolic agents have allowed for endovascular cure and improvement of clinical outcomes in a disease once considered to be treatable only by surgery. If endovascular surgery alone is unable to fully treat the vascular lesion, it will at least provide a valuable adjuvant to surgical treatment. The modern era uses a combined multidisciplinary approach to treating this disease in which endovascular and open microsurgery are often used together to treat a patient.

Surgical Management of Spinal Arteriovenous Malformations

The general principles that apply to surgical selection and management of cervical spinal AVMs are the same that apply to all intradural AVMs. Surgery should be attempted only after meticulous examination with selective spinal angiography of the vascular anatomy of the lesion and adjacent spinal cord. Typically, surgical intervention is reserved for symptomatic patients. Asymptomatic lesions that are discovered incidentally are usually followed without operative intervention.

After an acute subarachnoid or intramedullary hemorrhage, operative intervention should be delayed 4 to 6 weeks to permit clot lysis and absorption. We treat patients prophylactically with high doses of perioperative steroids based on the North American Spinal Cord Injury Study protocol.

Use of an operating microscope and appropriate microsurgical armamentarium is mandatory. The operative exposure should extend at least one level above and below the nidus of the AVM. If a type II AVM is not eccentric, the dura is opened in the midline and the arachnoid is preserved. However, a longitudinal myelotomy should be performed over the dorsal root entry zone for small, dorsal, eccentric lesions. If no vessels adhere to the arachnoid, arachnoidal traction sutures are applied. Meticulous hemostasis is crucial to avoid undue neurological injury and to maintain optimal visualization of the lesion. The preoperative angiographic anatomy must be carefully correlated with the intraoperative findings to identify and confirm the major feeding and draining vessels. Because an AVM and normal spinal cord tissue may share a common arterial supply, differentiating AVM feeders from the normal anterior spinal artery supply is critical for successful surgical resection. As with all AVMs, the arterial feeders should be resected before the venous drainage.

Use of a low bipolar setting, meticulous maintenance of clean fine bipolar tips, and continuous saline irrigation during bipolar cauterization prevent undue injury from heat and maintain optimal visualization. Intraoperative use of a directional color-flow Doppler probe can help to localize the intramedullary nidus (particularly for ventral intramedullary lesions) and to distinguish efferent and afferent vessels. Intraoperative indocyanine green can help identify inflow and outflow vessels prior to dissection, and intraoperative catheter-based angiography is routinely used to confirm complete resection. SSEP and MEP monitoring throughout the procedure is often useful as well. Metallic clips are avoided to prevent loss of resolution on postoperative MRI. The malformation is dissected circumferentially along the gliotic plane. As a distinct cleavage plane is developed along the gliotic tissue, the dorsal portion of the spinal cord may be retracted laterally with fine pial sutures to facilitate dissection of the deeper portions of the AVM. Meticulous hemostasis must be ensured before closure.

Although intramedullary or type II spinal AVMs are compact, lack interspersed neural elements, and tend to have a single arterial feeding vessel, their operative treatment typically is more difficult and their outcomes less satisfactory than those of intradural dorsal AV fistulae. Particularly when lesions occur in the low cervical and high thoracic region, the so-called arterial border zone of the spinal cord, there is greater risk for operative morbidity. Operative risk is also greater if a relatively large lesion is situated entirely within the spinal cord parenchyma and in the anterior half of the spinal cord. These lesions can sometimes be treated effectively with multistaged partial embolization and elimination of high-risk features, such as feeding artery and intranidal aneurysms.

Classification of Arteriovenous Malformations of the Posterior Fossa

AVMs of the posterior fossa are relatively uncommon, representing only 10 to 20% of all intracranial parenchymal AVMs.[48–52] We prefer to classify AVMs of the posterior fossa according to their size, presence of deep venous drainage, and proximity to vital structures (eloquent brain), such as deep cerebellar or brainstem nuclei. Perhaps the simplest classification is whether these lesions are situated in the brainstem or cerebellum, whereas AVMs often have been considered together because of their common infratentorial location and proximity in the posterior fossa. Nonetheless, they each have a distinct clinical presentation and natural history. Cerebellar malformations are four to five times as prevalent as brainstem AVMs.[48,50,52] Fortunately, they pose fewer technical difficulties for excision and thus have an inherently lower operative risk. The diagnostic evaluation, particularly with high-resolution MRI and cerebral angiography, is critical for treatment planning because the surgical risk is distinctly different for brainstem and cerebellar AVMs.

Like that of their supratentorial counterparts, risk assessment for treatment of posterior fossa AVMs is greatly aided by classification using the Spetzler-Martin grading system.[53] Typically, posterior fossa AVMs range between 1 and 3 cm; less commonly, they range between 3 and 6 cm. Posterior fossa AVMs greater than 6 cm are decidedly rare, although several holohemispheric lesions have been commonly reported. Lesions with venous drainage into the Galenic system through the precentral cerebellar or deep brainstem veins are considered to have deep drainage. Lesions that drain into the transverse-sigmoid-jugular system are considered to have superficial venous drainage. AVMs of eloquence are those in deep cerebellar or brainstem nuclei or adjacent to them. AVMs involving only the cerebellar hemisphere are considered noneloquent. Therefore, the prognostic value of preoperative MRI is extremely high. Although they may be extensive, purely cerebellar lesions can be treated successfully. However, even moderately sized (3–6 cm) brainstem AVMs can be Spetzler-Martin grade VI lesions that are inoperable.

Pathophysiology

AVMs are congenital and likely reflect an error in embryogenesis during the first 2 to 3 months of embryonic life. The etiology of these lesions is incompletely understood but thought to represent a persistence of primitive AV communications, which are normally replaced by an intervening network of capillaries and small vessels. These primitive AV vessels shunt arterial blood into the venous system, and abnormal hemodynamic conditions result. Not typically exposed to arterial pressures, the venous system enlarges, and ectasia and aneurysmal changes develop.

As an AVM matures, it typically assumes a wedge-shaped form, with its apex directed toward the ventricular system (**Fig. 15.11**). This configuration likely is attributable to the presence of extremely fine transcerebral veins that course through white matter in the hemispheres following myelinated fibers from the cerebral cortex to the deep white matter tracts and the subependymal venous system.

Because the high-resistance arteriolar system is either absent or abnormal, it is postulated that AVMs are incapable of regulating cerebral blood flow normally. Therefore, AVMs may act as sumps of cerebral blood flow to surrounding tissues, resulting in neurological deficit from cerebral vascular steal. Large, high-flow AVMs tend to be fed by low-pressure arteries.[54,55] Typically, larger AVMs tend to present with neurological deficits or seizures, whereas smaller AVMs seem to present with hemorrhage.[30,56–60]

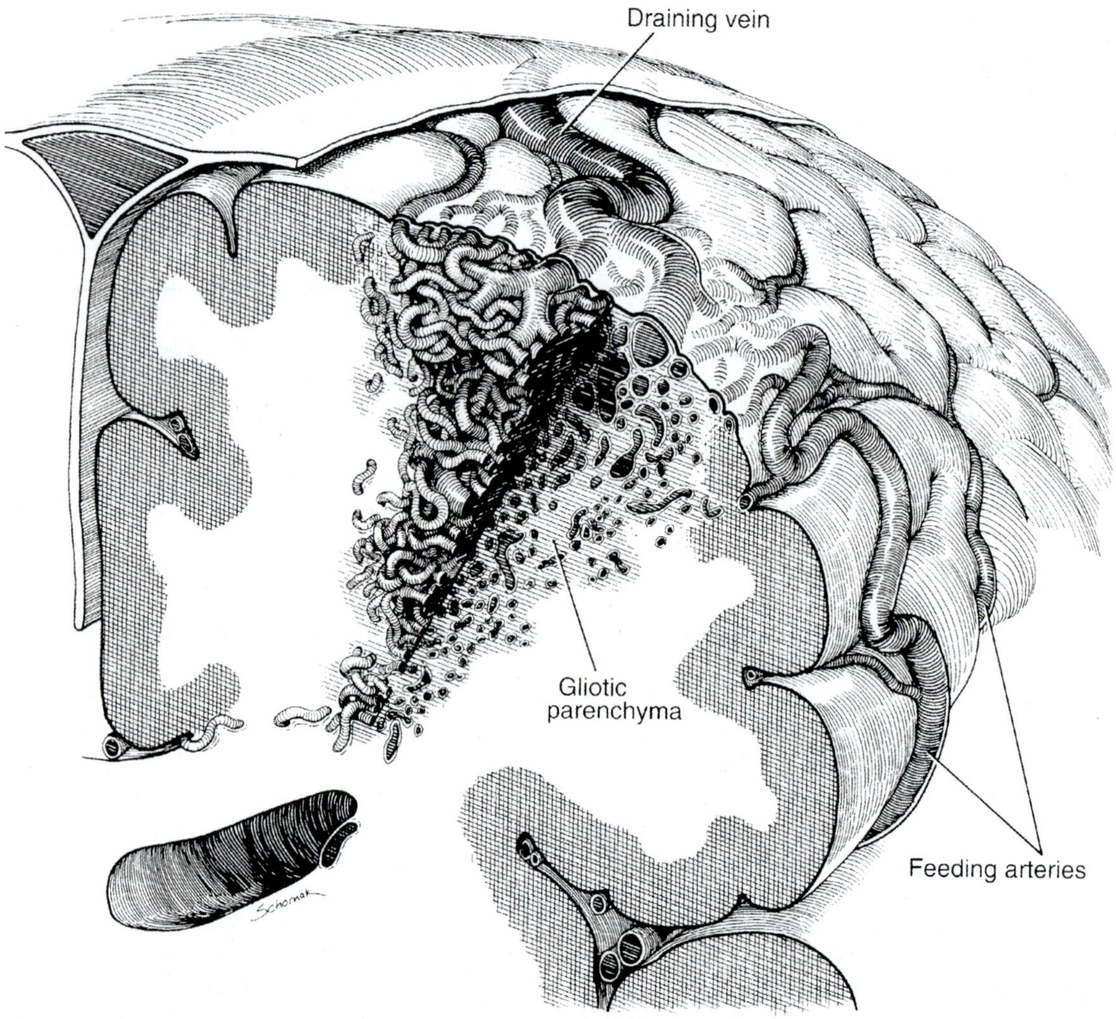

Fig. 15.11 Schematic representation of a typical wedge-shaped arteriovenous malformation with its apex directed to the ventricular system. (Reprinted with permission from Barrow Neurological Institute.)

Large AVMs that exhibit symptoms of chronic cerebral steal from surrounding cerebral tissue may impair the brain's autoregulatory capacity. The underlying pathophysiology may be explained as follows. To be adequately perfused next to the sump effect of a large AVM, the nutrient vessels of the adjacent brain must be chronically dilated, acting as a low-resistance system. After an AVM has been resected, the chronically ischemic normal arterial tree is abruptly exposed to much greater perfusion pressure, but the adjacent brain may have lost its ability to autoregulate this blood flow appropriately. The increased hydrostatic pressure on the chronically dilated capillaries could cause significant edema and hemorrhage due to capillary breakthrough. Spetzler and colleagues termed this clinical picture "normal perfusion pressure breakthrough syndrome" and observed a similar hyperperfusion syndrome after carotid endarterectomy.[61]

Clinical Presentation

Historically, AVMs of the posterior fossa were thought to have a higher propensity to hemorrhage than their supratentorial counterparts.[30,50–52,56,62–67] Most AVMs of the brainstem and cerebellum come to clinical attention after hemorrhage rather than seizure. A meta-analysis of six of the larger surgical series performed by Arnaout and colleagues demonstrated that 84% of patients with posterior fossa AVMs presented with hemorrhage.[30] In addition, recent observational studies have demonstrated that posterior fossa AVMs hemorrhage at nearly twice the rate of supratentorial lesions.[67,68] Attention has also been directed at the relative paucity of other provocative symptoms, such as headache and epilepsy, with posterior fossa malformations. Headache, progressive neurological deficit unassociated with hemorrhage, and ischemia from cerebral steal have been reported in only 15 to 22% of patients, with headache accounting for 10% of the patients. Cranial neuropathies, such as hemifacial spasm or trigeminal neuralgia, have rarely been reported.

Natural History

As previously stated, the natural history of posterior fossa AVMs was thought to entail a higher risk of hemorrhage than that of supratentorial vascular malformations. Arnaout and colleagues' metaanalysis of surgical and observational studies demonstrated a hemorrhage rate at presentation of 72 to 92% of posterior fossa AVMs compared with 35 to 54% of supratentorial AVMs.[30] Whether these statistics reflect a higher bleeding rate for posterior fossa AVMs than for supratentorial AVMs or a lower rate of headache and seizures with lesions in the posterior fossa is unknown. Several series have reported data regarding the annual hemorrhage risk of intracranial AVMs. The consensus of these reports seems to be an annual risk in the range of 1.5 to 4% per year for all intracranial AVMs.[31,49,51,56,63,69]

Some reports suggest that posterior fossa AVMs have a higher rate of rupture compared with intracranial AVMs as a whole. In a recent series by Hernesniemi and colleagues, infratentorial AVMs had an annual rupture rate of 11.6% per year in the first 5 years after presentation.[63] Kelly and colleagues reported the hemorrhage rate of posterior fossa AVMs to be 8.4 to 9.4% per year.[64] Several reports have demonstrated that the risk of rehemorrhage in the first year is 6 to 15%.[30,51,69,70] Classically, Batjer and Samson concluded that each hemorrhage is associated with a 15% risk of mortality and a 30% permanent morbidity rate.[50]

Several series have been published in the literature regarding the natural history of intracranial AVMs. Han and colleagues studied the natural history of high-grade AVMs in the Spetzler-Martin IV and V class.[35] Their series followed the natural history of 73 AVMs, with 56 grade IV patients and 17 grade V patients, and determined the annual rupture risk to be 1.5% per year. This rate is significantly lower than the previously quoted 2 to 4% per year for all AVMs. The group speculated that this difference was due to the lower perfusion pressure of larger AVMs compared with smaller lesions.[71,72] Jayarman and colleagues reported a similar series on the natural history of grade IV and grade V AVMs with 61 patients and conversely found an overall hemorrhage rate of 10.4% per year.[73] This result was not only much higher than the standard 2 to 4% per year hemorrhage risk but much higher than Han and colleagues' results. Jayarman's group argues that the difference in results stems from the manner in which Han's group reported the hemorrhage risk, namely as a lifetime hemorrhage risk from birth rather than the standard risk from presentation. In response, Jayarman's group performed a second analysis of their data adjusted for hemorrhage risk since birth and found an annual risk of 2.08%, similar to the data presented by Han and colleagues.

Diagnostic Evaluation

Because most posterior fossa AVMs present acutely with hemorrhage, the initial diagnostic test is usually CT. Although CT confirms the presence of subarachnoid and/or intraparenchymal hemorrhage, it may not identify the cause of the hemorrhage. Even when CT demonstrates the presence of an AVM, the possible coexistence of a second vascular lesion (e.g., intracranial aneurysm) must be considered. The addition of CT angiography to an initial noncontrast CT can aid the diagnosis of a vascular lesion causing hemorrhage with a fast and noninvasive test. For patients presenting with seizures, magnetic resonance may demonstrate a large region of flow voids on T2-weighted images consistent with the presence of an AVM. Whether a patient's AVM is discovered by hemorrhage, seizure, or incidentally, magnetic resonance is essential for defining the exact location and size of the AVM in relation to eloquent cortex. Both 3D multidetector CT angiography and 3D MRA are becoming powerful tools for establishing the diagnosis and angioarchitecture of intracranial AVMs.

Cerebral angiography remains the gold standard for the diagnosis and evaluation of the angioarchitecture of AVMs and should be employed whenever a hemorrhage is suspicious for AVM rupture. Venous and/or arterial aneurysms have been associated with AVMs of the posterior fossa with a frequency approaching 30%. Thus, angiography is essential to evaluate the cerebrovascular system for associated vascular lesions and as a preoperative tool to assess and even determine the definitive treatment of these lesions. Therefore, high-resolution angiography with biplanar flat panel detectors, 3D digital subtraction, and roadmapping technology is mandatory for posterior circulation and internal carotid arteries, from which 10% of AVMs of the posterior fossa are fed.

Angiography is essential for the surgeon to develop a 3D conceptualization of the location of the AVM. An accurate determination of the location, number, and size of the feeding arterial branches and the number and position of draining veins is vital for surgical planning. In patients who present with hemorrhage, it is usually best to delay surgical treatment unless they are in extremis because of a posterior fossa clot or the source of hemorrhage is due to an unsecured feeding artery or intranidal aneurysm. Angiography in the acute phase after a hemorrhage may fail to demonstrate the entire angiographic nidus or feeders of an AVM because a coexisting hematoma can compress, obscure, or distort the angiographic nidus. Another angiographic study after the acute phase has passed typically provides a more comprehensive picture of the relevant pathological anatomy. Therefore, if possible, definitive surgical therapy of the AVM should be deferred 6 to 8 weeks after a hemorrhage to allow parenchymal swelling to decrease and the hematoma to liquefy.

However, a small subpopulation of patients will present with life-threatening intraparenchymal hematomas that require immediate surgical decompression. The surgical goal for these patients should be evacuation of the hematoma and relief of mass effect with no attempt to disturb or remove the AVM. Patients undergoing evacuation of a hematoma can subsequently be managed medically until there is clinical and radiographic evidence of resolution of the initial hemorrhage. As the patient becomes medically stable, definitive radiographic studies can be performed as required.

Treatment of Posterior Fossa Arteriovenous Malformations

Currently, multidisciplinary approach to the treatment of AVMs is undertaken. After the exact size, location, and angioarchitecture of an AVM are delineated, treatment options may include conservative observation, microsurgical resection, endovascular embolization, radiosurgery, or a combination of multiple modalities. Treatment modalities are dependent on patient presentation, age, and comorbidities as well as radiographic and angiographic features of the AVM, such as size, location, patterns of arterial feeding and venous drainage, and presence of perinodal and flow-related aneurysms.

Surgical Management of Posterior Fossa Arteriovenous Malformations

The general principles of surgical management of posterior fossa AVMs are no different from those applied to the more common supratentorial AVMs. A balanced anesthetic technique is used, with attention to maintenance of normotension, oxygen saturation, and avoidance of hyperglycemia. Patients may be placed in the lateral, park bench, prone, or Concord positions. Typically, the sitting position is avoided due to the risks of air embolus and the surgeon becoming fatigued during lengthy operations. In general, we prefer a wide exposure for AVMs and find it greatly advantageous for access to the arterial supply and venous drainage of these lesions. Preoperative ventriculostomy placement and intraoperative early draining of cerebrospinal fluid provide necessary cerebellar relaxation prior to microdissection in the deep corridors of the posterior fossa.

The first goal of the AVM microsurgical dissection is isolation and interruption of all afferent arterial supply. Draining veins are meticulously preserved until the AVM is completely bereft of its arterial supply. Circumferential dissection of the periphery of the malformation is a basic tenet of surgical removal regardless of location. Significant small-vessel bleeding signifies inadvertent entry into the AVM nidus and requires redirection of the microdissection outside of the nidus. This correctable surgical error is more common in diffuse or racemose AVMs. Careful attention to hemostasis in the periependymal area is necessary due to the friable consistency of perforating veins to the ventricular system. In areas where loops of the AVM have penetrated the brainstem parenchyma, it is best to cauterize and truncate these vessels at the pial margin rather than dissect into the brainstem itself. Immediate postoperative or intraoperative angiography is recommended to rule out the possibility of residual AVM.

Surgical Treatment Outcome

To evaluate the predictive utility of the grading system, Spetzler and colleagues reported a retrospective series of 100 patients in whom the correlation between AVM and the incidence of minor and major neurological deficits was remarkably consistent.[53] An additional 100 patients were treated at UCLA Medical Center from 1986 to 1992.[74] Of 13 grade I patients treated, none developed new minor or major neurological deficits. Only 6% of 30 grade II patients developed minor or major deficits. Thirteen percent of grade III patients developed minor deficits, and 3% developed major deficits. Of the patients with grade IV and grade V AVMs, 39 and 41% developed minor and major deficits, respectively. Only one grade V patient died. These findings, along with similar results discussed by Heros and colleagues, suggest that the Spetzler-Martin grading system is effective in predicting the risk of neurological impairment after surgical treatment.[75–77] Therefore, treatment risk must be compared with a patient's natural history, which is the likely outcome for patients treated nonoperatively.

Endovascular Management of Posterior Fossa Arteriovenous Malformations

Although microsurgical resection remains the preferred treatment of AVMs in surgically accessible locations, endovascular management is beginning to play a larger role in the treatment of these lesions. Preoperative embolization of AVMs has been a mainstay adjuvant treatment to surgical resection.[78] Single or multiple sessions of endovascular treatment have also been used as an adjuvant to radiosurgery,[78–82] and AVM cures in selected cases with Onyx embolization are well reported in the literature (**Fig. 15.10**).[39,78,83]

Onyx is quickly replacing the use of other embolic materials as the treatment of choice.[39,78,84] Hauck and colleagues recently evaluated the efficacy of Onyx as a preoperative embolic agent before microsurgical resection and radiosurgery.[78] On average, AVM size was reduced from 3.71 to 3.06 cm after embolization, and total AVM volume was reduced by an average of 75%. The group was able to achieve complete angiographic obliteration in 10% of AVMs that were embolized. Natarajan and colleagues experienced a similar 74.1% volumetric reduction with preoperative embolization.[39]

Endovascular embolization of AVMs is not without potential complications. Taylor and colleagues published a series of 339 embolizations with polyvinyl alcohol (PVA), NBCA, coils, and Onyx and reported a 6.5% morbidity rate of permanent neurological deficits and 1.2% mortality rate per procedure.[85] Similarly, Kim and colleagues reported an 8.6% rate of permanent morbidity or mortality per procedure in a study of 508 vessel embolizations using PVA, NBCA, or detachable coils.[86] PVA has largely been abandoned for greater safety and efficacy rates of NBCA and Onyx. Onyx and NBCA have recently been shown to have equivalent safety and efficacy profiles in a multicenter randomized controlled trial.[84]

Radiosurgery

Stereotactic radiosurgery takes the form of Gamma Knife (Elekta, Stockholm, Sweden), particle beam radiation, and linear accelerator systems and must be considered as a treatment option for AVMs. Particularly for intraparenchymal AVMs situated entirely in the brainstem or deep nuclei, radiosurgery is a reasonable alternative. It remains most appropriate for smaller lesions less than 3 cm. However, except for purely brainstem AVMs, these small lesions tend to be the best candidates for microsurgery. Several reports have concluded that lower AVM volume, fewer draining veins, younger age, superficial location, and radiation doses of up to 20 Gy have the best outcome for radiosurgery.[87–89] Radiosurgery is often used as an adjuvant to embolization once embolization has reduced lesion volume and made it more amenable to radiosurgery.

Some of the best outcomes have been reported by Friedman and Bova, who attained a 2-year obliteration rate of 91% for a subset of lesions they considered most favorable for radiosurgery.[90,91] More recently, the same group reported that 49% of patients have complete obliteration with no neurological deficits after a single treatment in all AVM subtypes.[89] However, the hemorrhage rate during the first year after radiosurgery (7.7 per year) is almost double the rate of hemorrhage of untreated AVMs.[90]

Somewhat compromised by the use of AVM volume rather than AVM diameter, studies published by Lunsford and colleagues reported that the 2-year obliteration rate of small lesions approached 80%.[92] Maruyama and colleagues reported good success with treating brainstem AVMs, demonstrating complete angiographic obliteration in 66% of patients with a 7% rate of neurological complications.[93]

In treatment planning, surgeons must consider individual patient characteristics such as age, general medical condition, vocation and avocation, and psychological factors. For example, the lifetime risk of hemorrhage for a 21-year-old patient with a grade III AVM is about five times greater than that of a 75-year-old patient with the same lesion. Hence, as a more aggressive attempt to treat the lesion, surgery may be warranted when the lifetime risk of death or disability is high. Treatment, if any, offered to a 75-year-old patient should be associated with a low risk as the patient's lifetime risk of hemorrhage is low.

Conclusion

AVMs of the posterior circulation remain relatively uncommon, accounting for 10 to 20% of intradural cranial AVMs. Small posterior fossa AVMs tend to present with hemorrhage, whereas larger AVMs often present with headache and symptoms of mass effect. The natural history of these lesions is arguably worse than that of supratentorial AVMs, which are thought to entail a 2 to 4% annual risk of hemorrhage. Diagnostic evaluation should include not only the gold standard angiography but MRI as well to clearly delineate whether deep cerebellar or brainstem nuclei are involved with the lesion.

Surgical management of posterior fossa AVMs is determined in large part by their precise anatomical location. Lesions involving brainstem nuclei typically are poor operative candidates and may be treated more appropriately with stereotactic radiosurgery. Endovascular embolization is a useful surgical adjunct, but one must keep in mind that the 5 to 10% morbidity rate must be added to the surgical risk in analysis of the risk-benefit ratio.

Posterior fossa AVMs remain one of the most daunting, technically challenging lesions in neurosurgery today. Successful management of these lesions requires a precise understanding of the location and vascular anatomical characteristics of the AVM in question. To estimate the surgical risk, we grade AVMs according to size, presence of a deep vascular component, and relationship to vital deep nuclei of the cerebellum and brainstem.

References

1. Elsberg C. Diagnosis and Treatment of Surgical Diseases of the Spinal Cord and Its Membranes. Philadelphia, PA: WB Saunders; 1916
2. Di Chiro G, Doppman J, Ommaya AK. Selective arteriography of arteriovenous aneurysms of spinal cord. Radiology 1967;88(6):1065–1077
3. Andres RH, Barth A, Guzman R, et al. Endovascular and surgical treatment of spinal dural arteriovenous fistulas. Neuroradiology 2008;50(10):869–876
4. Kendall BE, Logue V. Spinal epidural angiomatous malformations draining into intrathecal veins. Neuroradiology 1977;13(4):181–189
5. Kim LJ, Spetzler RF. Classification and surgical management of spinal arteriovenous lesions: arteriovenous fistulae and arteriovenous malformations. Neurosurgery 2006;59(5, Suppl 3):S195–S201, discussion S3–S13
6. Rodesch G, Hurth M, Alvarez H, Tadié M, Lasjaunias P. Classification of spinal cord arteriovenous shunts: proposal for a reappraisal—the Bicêtre experience with 155 consecutive patients treated between 1981 and 1999. Neurosurgery 2002;51(2):374–379, discussion 379–380
7. Spetzler RF, Detwiler PW, Riina HA, Porter RW. Modified classification of spinal cord vascular lesions. J Neurosurg 2002;96(2, Suppl):145–156
8. Zozulya YP, Slin'ko EI, Al-Qashqish II. Spinal arteriovenous malformations: new classification and surgical treatment. Neurosurg Focus 2006;20(5):E7
9. Gillilan LA. The arterial blood supply of the human spinal cord. J Comp Neurol 1958;110(1):75–103
10. Mitsuhashi Y, Aurboonyawat T, Pereira VM, et al. Dural arteriovenous fistulas draining into the petrosal vein or bridging vein of the medulla: possible homologs of spinal dural arteriovenous fistulas. Clinical article. J Neurosurg 2009;111(5):889–899
11. Anson JA, Spetzler RF. Classification of spinal arteriovenous malformations and implications for treatment. BNI Q 1992;8:2–8
12. da Costa L, Dehdashti AR, terBrugge KG. Spinal cord vascular shunts: spinal cord vascular malformations and dural arteriovenous fistulas. Neurosurg Focus 2009;26(1):E6
13. Houdart E, Redondo A, Saint-Maurice JP, Merland JJ. Natural history of an incidentally discovered spinal dural arteriovenous fistula. Neurology 2001;57(4):742–743
14. Klopper HB, Surdell DL, Thorell WE. Type I spinal dural arteriovenous fistulas: historical review and illustrative case. Neurosurg Focus 2009;26(1):E3
15. Rodesch G, Hurth M, Alvarez H, Tadie M, Lasjaunias P. Spinal cord intradural arteriovenous fistulae: anatomic, clinical, and therapeutic considerations in a series of 32 consecutive patients seen between 1981 and 2000 with emphasis on endovascular therapy. Neurosurgery 2005;57(5):973–983, discussion 973–983
16. Rosenblum B, Oldfield EH, Doppman JL, Di Chiro G. Spinal arteriovenous malformations: a comparison of dural arteriovenous fistulas and intradural AVM's in 81 patients. J Neurosurg 1987;67(6):795–802
17. Aminoff MJ, Logue V. Clinical features of spinal vascular malformations. Brain 1974;97(1):197–210
18. Aminoff MJ, Logue V. The prognosis of patients with spinal vascular malformations. Brain 1974;97(1):211–218
19. Lad SP, Santarelli JG, Patil CG, Steinberg GK, Boakye M. National trends in spinal arteriovenous malformations. Neurosurg Focus 2009;26(1):1–5
20. Narvid J, Hetts SW, Larsen D, et al. Spinal dural arteriovenous fistulae: clinical features and long-term results. Neurosurgery 2008;62(1):159–166, discussion 166–167
21. Rodesch G, Hurth M, Alvarez H, Ducot B, Tadie M, Lasjaunias P. Angio-architecture of spinal cord arteriovenous shunts at presentation. Clinical correlations in adults and children. The Bicêtre experience on 155 consecutive patients seen between 1981-1999. Acta Neurochir (Wien) 2004;146(3):217–226, discussion 226–227
22. Ferrell AS, Tubbs RS, Acakpo-Satchivi L, Deveikis JP, Harrigan MR. Legacy and current understanding of the often-misunderstood Foix-Alajouanine syndrome. Historical vignette. J Neurosurg 2009;111(5):902–906
23. Eddleman CS, Jeong H, Cashen TA, et al. Advanced noninvasive imaging of spinal vascular malformations. Neurosurg Focus 2009;26(1):E9
24. Pattany PM, Saraf-Lavi E, Bowen BC. MR angiography of the spine and spinal cord. Top Magn Reson Imaging 2003;14(6):444–460
25. Saraf-Lavi E, Bowen BC, Quencer RM, et al. Detection of spinal dural arteriovenous fistulae with MR imaging and contrast-enhanced MR angiography: sensitivity, specificity, and prediction of vertebral level. AJNR Am J Neuroradiol 2002;23(5):858–867
26. Mull M, Nijenhuis RJ, Backes WH, Krings T, Wilmink JT, Thron A. Value and limitations of contrast-enhanced MR angiography in spinal arteriovenous malformations and dural arteriovenous fistulas. AJNR Am J Neuroradiol 2007;28(7):1249–1258
27. Lai PH, Weng MJ, Lee KW, Pan HB. Multidetector CT angiography in diagnosing type I and type IVA spinal vascular malformations. AJNR Am J Neuroradiol 2006;27(4):813–817
28. Yamaguchi S, Eguchi K, Kiura Y, et al. Multi-detector-row CT angiography as a preoperative evaluation for spinal arteriovenous fistulae. Neurosurg Rev 2007;30(4):321–326, discussion 327
29. Yamaguchi S, Nagayama T, Eguchi K, Takeda M, Arita K, Kurisu K. Accuracy and pitfalls of multidetector-row computed tomography in detecting spinal dural arteriovenous fistulas. J Neurosurg Spine 2010;12(3):243–248
30. Arnaout OM, Gross BA, Eddleman CS, Bendok BR, Getch CC, Batjer HH. Posterior fossa arteriovenous malformations. Neurosurg Focus 2009;26(5):E12
31. Crawford PM, West CR, Chadwick DW, Shaw MD. Arteriovenous malformations of the brain: natural history in unoperated patients. J Neurol Neurosurg Psychiatry 1986;49(1):1–10
32. Hall WA, Oldfield EH, Doppman JL. Recanalization of spinal arteriovenous malformations following embolization. J Neurosurg 1989;70(5):714–720
33. Riché MC, Melki JP, Merland JJ. Embolization of spinal cord vascular malformations via the anterior spinal artery. AJNR Am J Neuroradiol 1983;4(3):378–381
34. Eskandar EN, Borges LF, Budzik RF Jr, Putman CM, Ogilvy CS. Spinal dural arteriovenous fistulas: experience with endovascular and surgical therapy. J Neurosurg 2002;96(2, Suppl):162–167
35. Guillevin R, Vallee JN, Cormier E, Lo D, Dormont D, Chiras J. N-butyl 2-cyanoacrylate embolization of spinal dural arteriovenous fistulae: CT evaluation, technical features, and outcome prognosis in 26 cases. AJNR Am J Neuroradiol 2005;26(4):929–935
36. Rodesch G, Hurth M, Alvarez H, David P, Tadie M, Lasjaunias P. Embolization of spinal cord arteriovenous shunts: morphological and clinical follow-up and results—review of 69 consecutive cases. Neurosurgery 2003;53(1):40–49, discussion 49–50
37. Carlson AP, Taylor CL, Yonas H. Treatment of dural arteriovenous fistula using ethylene vinyl alcohol (Onyx) arterial embolization as the primary modality: short-term results. J Neurosurg 2007;107(6):1120–1125
38. Katsaridis V, Papagiannaki C, Aimar E. Curative embolization of cerebral arteriovenous malformations (AVMs) with Onyx in 101 patients. Neuroradiology 2008;50(7):589–597

39. Natarajan SK, Ghodke B, Britz GW, Born DE, Sekhar LN. Multimodality treatment of brain arteriovenous malformations with microsurgery after embolization with Onyx: single-center experience and technical nuances. Neurosurgery 2008;62(6):1213–1225, discussion 1225–1226
40. Panagiotopoulos V, Gizewski E, Asgari S, Regel J, Forsting M, Wanke I. Embolization of intracranial arteriovenous malformations with ethylene-vinyl alcohol copolymer (Onyx). AJNR Am J Neuroradiol 2009;30(1):99–106
41. Velat GJ, Reavey-Cantwell JF, Sistrom C, et al. Comparison of N-butyl cyanoacrylate and Onyx for the embolization of intracranial arteriovenous malformations: analysis of fluoroscopy and procedure times. Neurosurgery 2008;63(1, Suppl 1):ONS73–ONS78, discussion ONS78–ONS80
42. Corkill RA, Mitsos AP, Molyneux AJ. Embolization of spinal intramedullary arteriovenous malformations using the liquid embolic agent, Onyx: a single-center experience in a series of 17 patients. J Neurosurg Spine 2007;7(5):478–485
43. Warakaulle DR, Aviv RI, Niemann D, Molyneux AJ, Byrne JV, Teddy P. Embolisation of spinal dural arteriovenous fistulae with Onyx. Neuroradiology 2003;45(2):110–112
44. Krings T, Thron AK, Geibprasert S, et al. Endovascular management of spinal vascular malformations. Neurosurg Rev 2010;33(1):1–9
45. Sivakumar W, Zada G, Yashar P, Giannotta SL, Teitelbaum G, Larsen DW. Endovascular management of spinal dural arteriovenous fistulas. A review. Neurosurg Focus 2009;26(5):E15
46. Nogueira RG, Dabus G, Rabinov JD, Ogilvy CS, Hirsch JA, Pryor JC. Onyx embolization for the treatment of spinal dural arteriovenous fistulae: initial experience with long-term follow-up. Technical case report. Neurosurgery 2009;64(1):E197–E198, discussion E198
47. Berenstein A, Young W, Ransohoff J, Benjamin V, Merkin H. Somatosensory evoked potentials during spinal angiography and therapeutic transvascular embolization. J Neurosurg 1984;60(4): 777–785
48. Arnaout OM, Gross BA, Eddleman CS, Bendok BR, Getch CC, Batjer HH. Posterior fossa arteriovenous malformations. Neurosurg Focus 2009;26(5):E12
49. Batjer H, Samson D. Arteriovenous malformations of the posterior fossa: clinical presentation, diagnostic evaluation and surgical treatment. Neurosurg Rev 1986;9(4):287–296
50. Batjer H, Samson D. Arteriovenous malformations of the posterior fossa. Clinical presentation, diagnostic evaluation, and surgical treatment. J Neurosurg 1986;64(6):849–856
51. da Costa L, Wallace MC, Ter Brugge KG, O'Kelly C, Willinsky RA, Tymianski M. The natural history and predictive features of hemorrhage from brain arteriovenous malformations. Stroke 2009; 40(1):100–105
52. Drake CG, Friedman AH, Peerless SJ. Posterior fossa arteriovenous malformations. J Neurosurg 1986;64(1):1–10
53. Spetzler RF, Martin NA. A proposed grading system for arteriovenous malformations. J Neurosurg 1986;65(4):476–483
54. Fults D, Kelly DL Jr. Natural history of arteriovenous malformations of the brain: a clinical study. Neurosurgery 1984;15(5):658–662
55. Nornes H, Grip A. Hemodynamic aspects of cerebral arteriovenous malformations. J Neurosurg 1980;53(4):456–464
56. Brown RD Jr, Flemming KD, Meyer FB, Cloft HJ, Pollock BE, Link ML. Natural history, evaluation, and management of intracranial vascular malformations. Mayo Clin Proc 2005;80(2):269–281
57. Fleetwood IG, Marcellus ML, Levy RP, Marks MP, Steinberg GK. Deep arteriovenous malformations of the basal ganglia and thalamus: natural history. J Neurosurg 2003;98(4):747–750
58. Fleetwood IG, Steinberg GK. Arteriovenous malformations. Lancet 2002;359(9309):863–873
59. Han PP, Ponce FA, Spetzler RF. Intention-to-treat analysis of Spetzler-Martin grades IV and V arteriovenous malformations: natural history and treatment paradigm. J Neurosurg 2003;98(1):3–7
60. Lawton MT; UCSF Brain Arteriovenous Malformation Study Project. Spetzler-Martin Grade III arteriovenous malformations: surgical results and a modification of the grading scale. Neurosurgery 2003;52(4):740–748, discussion 748–749
61. Spetzler RF, Wilson CB, Weinstein P, Mehdorn M, Townsend J, Telles D. Normal perfusion pressure breakthrough theory. Clin Neurosurg 1978;25:651–672
62. da Costa L, Thines L, Dehdashti AR, et al. Management and clinical outcome of posterior fossa arteriovenous malformations: report on a single-centre 15-year experience. J Neurol Neurosurg Psychiatry 2009;80(4):376–379
63. Hernesniemi JA, Dashti R, Juvela S, Väärt K, Niemelä M, Laakso A. Natural history of brain arteriovenous malformations: a long-term follow-up study of risk of hemorrhage in 238 patients. Neurosurgery 2008;63(5):823–829, discussion 829–831
64. Kelly ME, Guzman R, Sinclair J, et al. Multimodality treatment of posterior fossa arteriovenous malformations. J Neurosurg 2008;108(6):1152–1161
65. Ondra SL, Troupp H, George ED, Schwab K. The natural history of symptomatic arteriovenous malformations of the brain: a 24-year follow-up assessment. J Neurosurg 1990;73(3):387–391
66. Perret G, Nishioka H. Report on the cooperative study of intracranial aneurysms and subarachnoid hemorrhage. Section VI. Arteriovenous malformations. An analysis of 545 cases of cranio-cerebral arteriovenous malformations and fistulae reported to the cooperative study. J Neurosurg 1966;25(4):467–490
67. Stefani MA, Porter PJ, terBrugge KG, Montanera W, Willinsky RA, Wallace MC. Angioarchitectural factors present in brain arteriovenous malformations associated with hemorrhagic presentation. Stroke 2002;33(4):920–924
68. Khaw AV, Mohr JP, Sciacca RR, et al. Association of infratentorial brain arteriovenous malformations with hemorrhage at initial presentation. Stroke 2004;35(3):660–663
69. Graf CJ, Perret GE, Torner JC. Bleeding from cerebral arteriovenous malformations as part of their natural history. J Neurosurg 1983;58(3):331–337
70. Yamada S, Takagi Y, Nozaki K, Kikuta K, Hashimoto N. Risk factors for subsequent hemorrhage in patients with cerebral arteriovenous malformations. J Neurosurg 2007;107(5):965–972
71. Duong DH, Young WL, Vang MC, et al. Feeding artery pressure and venous drainage pattern are primary determinants of hemorrhage from cerebral arteriovenous malformations. Stroke 1998;29(6):1167–1176
72. Miyasaka Y, Kurata A, Irikura K, Tanaka R, Fujii K. The influence of vascular pressure and angiographic characteristics on haemorrhage from arteriovenous malformations. Acta Neurochir (Wien) 2000;142(1):39–43
73. Jayaraman MV, Marcellus ML, Do HM, et al. Hemorrhage rate in patients with Spetzler-Martin grades IV and V arteriovenous malformations: is treatment justified? Stroke 2007;38(2):325–329
74. Martin NA, Vinters HV. Arteriovenous malformations. In: Carter LP, Spetzler RF, eds. Neurovascular Surgery. New York, NY: McGraw-Hill;1995:875–904
75. Heros RC. Spetzler-Martin grades IV and V arteriovenous malformations. J Neurosurg 2003;98(1):1–2, discussion 2
76. Heros RC, Korosue K, Diebold PM. Surgical excision of cerebral arteriovenous malformations: late results. Neurosurgery 1990; 26(4):570–577, discussion 577–578
77. Nussbaum ES, Heros RC, Camarata PJ. Surgical treatment of intracranial arteriovenous malformations with an analysis of cost-effectiveness. Clin Neurosurg 1995;42:348–369

78. Hauck EF, Welch BG, White JA, Purdy PD, Pride LG, Samson D. Preoperative embolization of cerebral arteriovenous malformations with Onyx. AJNR Am J Neuroradiol 2009;30(3):492–495
79. Gobin YP, Laurent A, Merienne L, et al. Treatment of brain arteriovenous malformations by embolization and radiosurgery. J Neurosurg 1996;85(1):19–28
80. Henkes H, Nahser HC, Berg-Dammer E, Weber W, Lange S, Kühne D. Endovascular therapy of brain AVMs prior to radiosurgery. Neurol Res 1998;20(6):479–492
81. Sirin S, Kondziolka D, Niranjan A, Flickinger JC, Maitz AH, Lunsford LD. Prospective staged volume radiosurgery for large arteriovenous malformations: indications and outcomes in otherwise untreatable patients. Neurosurgery 2008;62(Suppl 2):744–754
82. Starke RM, Komotar RJ, Otten ML, et al. Adjuvant embolization with N-butyl cyanoacrylate in the treatment of cerebral arteriovenous malformations: outcomes, complications, and predictors of neurologic deficits. Stroke 2009;40(8):2783–2790
83. Maimon S, Strauss I, Frolov V, Margalit N, Ram Z. Brain arteriovenous malformation treatment using a combination of Onyx and a new detachable tip microcatheter, SONIC: short-term results. AJNR Am J Neuroradiol 2010;31(5):947–954
84. Loh Y, Duckwiler GR; Onyx Trial Investigators. A prospective, multicenter, randomized trial of the Onyx liquid embolic system and N-butyl cyanoacrylate embolization of cerebral arteriovenous malformations. Clinical article. J Neurosurg 2010;113(4):733–741
85. Taylor CL, Dutton K, Rappard G, et al. Complications of preoperative embolization of cerebral arteriovenous malformations. J Neurosurg 2004;100(5):810–812
86. Kim LJ, Albuquerque FC, Spetzler RF, McDougall CG. Postembolization neurological deficits in cerebral arteriovenous malformations: stratification by arteriovenous malformation grade. Neurosurgery 2006;59(1):53–59, discussion 53–59
87. Friedman WA, Bova FJ, Bollampally S, Bradshaw P. Analysis of factors predictive of success or complications in arteriovenous malformation radiosurgery. Neurosurgery 2003;52(2):296–307, discussion 307–308
88. Pollock BE, Gorman DA, Coffey RJ. Patient outcomes after arteriovenous malformation radiosurgical management: results based on a 5- to 14-year follow-up study. Neurosurgery 2003;52(6):1291–1296, discussion 1296–1297
89. Raffa SJ, Chi YY, Bova FJ, Friedman WA. Validation of the radiosurgery-based arteriovenous malformation score in a large linear accelerator radiosurgery experience. J Neurosurg 2009;111(4):832–839
90. Friedman WA, Bova FJ. Linear accelerator radiosurgery for arteriovenous malformations. J Neurosurg 1992;77(6):832–841
91. Friedman WA, Bova FJ, Mendenhall WM. Linear accelerator radiosurgery for arteriovenous malformations: the relationship of size to outcome. J Neurosurg 1995;82(2):180–189
92. Lunsford LD, Kondziolka D, Bissonette DJ, Maitz AH, Flickinger JC. Stereotactic radiosurgery of brain vascular malformations. Neurosurg Clin N Am 1992;3(1):79–98
93. Maruyama K, Kondziolka D, Niranjan A, Flickinger JC, Lunsford LD. Stereotactic radiosurgery for brainstem arteriovenous malformations: factors affecting outcome. J Neurosurg 2004;100(3):407–413

16 Aneurysms of the Craniovertebral Junction

Joseph M. Zabramski, David J. Fiorella, and Wendy C. Gaza

The craniovertebral junction (CVJ) is an intricate anatomical region with transitions not only in bony anatomy but in neural and vascular tissue as well. In this transitional zone, arterial histologic changes occur including the loss of the external elastic lamina and a thinning of the muscularis layer. Additionally, as these arteries traverse the dura, they immediately undergo a serpiginous course, causing a disruption of laminar blood flow. It is perhaps this combination of features that causes aneurysms of the CVJ to be second in frequency only to those of the basilar tip in the posterior intracranial circulation.

Aneurysms of the CVJ consist of lesions that arise from the vertebral artery, the posterior inferior cerebellar artery (PICA), and the vertebrobasilar junction. About 75% of these aneurysms occur near the origin of the PICA.[1–5] They occur more often on the left, probably because this artery is frequently the dominant vertebral artery. As with most cerebral aneurysms, lesions of the CVJ are more common in women than men. Due to the complex anatomical configuration of the arteries involved and to the intimate association between vascular and neural tissue at the CVJ, it is imperative that any comprehensive examination of this topic start with the basic vascular anatomy of the region.

Vascular Anatomy of the Vertebral Arteries

Classically, the vertebral artery originates as the first and largest branch off the subclavian artery on each side (**Fig. 16.1A**). In rare cases, it arises directly from the aorta or the external carotid artery. The vertebral artery ascends behind the anterior scalene muscle to enter the foramen transversarium at C6 ~90% of the time. It continues vertically through these transverse foramina passing anteriorly to the exiting nerve roots. After traversing the foramen at C2, the artery curves laterally to reach the foramen of C1 (**Fig. 16.1B**). The vertebral artery then travels posteromedially around the superior articular process of the atlas and into the sulcus arteriosus in the lamina of C1. Next the artery pierces the atlantooccipital membrane and dura while traveling superiorly and ventrally through the foramen magnum. It continues rostrally around the lower medulla, anterior to the most superior dentate ligament and ventral to the lower cranial nerves. From this point, the two vertebral arteries continue superiorly a variable distance along the clivus, before joining to form the basilar artery (**Table 16.1**).

Throughout its course, the vertebral artery supplies numerous spinal and muscular branches. Its two major arterial branches are the anterior spinal artery and the PICA (**Fig. 16.2**). The anterior spinal artery usually originates just distal to the PICA and proximal to the vertebrobasilar junction.[6] It usually runs inferiorly and medially to form a common trunk with the opposite anterior spinal artery and continues caudally in the ventral median fissure of the spinal cord.

The PICA usually arises from the posterior or lateral side of the vertebral artery at a point 13 to 16 mm proximal to the basilar artery origin (**Fig. 16.3**).[6] Based on data from several large angiographic series, the origin of the artery is caudal to the foramen magnum in 18% of the specimens, at its level in 4%, and above the foramen in 57%. In the remainder of cases, the origin cannot be clearly identified.[6,7] The diameter of the PICA measures ~2 mm at its origin (range, 0.5 to 3.4 mm), whereas the diameter of the parent vertebral artery is approximately twice that.[8] PICA may be absent or hypoplastic 15 to 20% of the time, and in this case the anterior inferior cerebellar artery (AICA) usually will supply the territory, although the contralateral PICA may also contribute.[7,9] In 2% or fewer cases, the PICA arises as a duplicate artery.

Although the course of the PICA is highly variable, Lister and colleagues,[8] Rhoton,[10] and others[6,11,12] have divided the artery into five general segments (**Table 16.2** and **Fig. 16.3**). The short anterior medullary segment traveling around the anterior surface at the medulla is followed by the lateral medullary segment, which includes the first half of the caudal loop of the artery and ends at the approximate origin of cranial nerves IX, X, and XI. The caudal loop of the artery may dip below the level of the foramen magnum in ~35% of cases. This position, therefore, cannot be used as a sign of tonsillar herniation. The tonsillomedullary or posterior medullary segment of the artery continues as the ascending portion of the loop and reaches the upper surface of the cerebellar tonsil. It passes behind or posterior to the rootlets of the lower cranial nerves. The telovelotonsillar segment continues over the superior aspect of the tonsil creating a cranial loop. At this apex, a branch artery is given off to the choroid plexus of the fourth ventricle, creating the "choroidal point." This point serves as an important diagnostic landmark because of its constant relationship to the fourth ventricle. The artery continues caudally in the retrotonsillar fissure and usually branches into medial and lateral hemispheric or cortical segments.

Perforating arterial branches to the medulla commonly arise from the proximal three segments of PICA. Perforators may be seen from the anterior segment in more than 50% of specimens, from the lateral segment in more than 70%, and

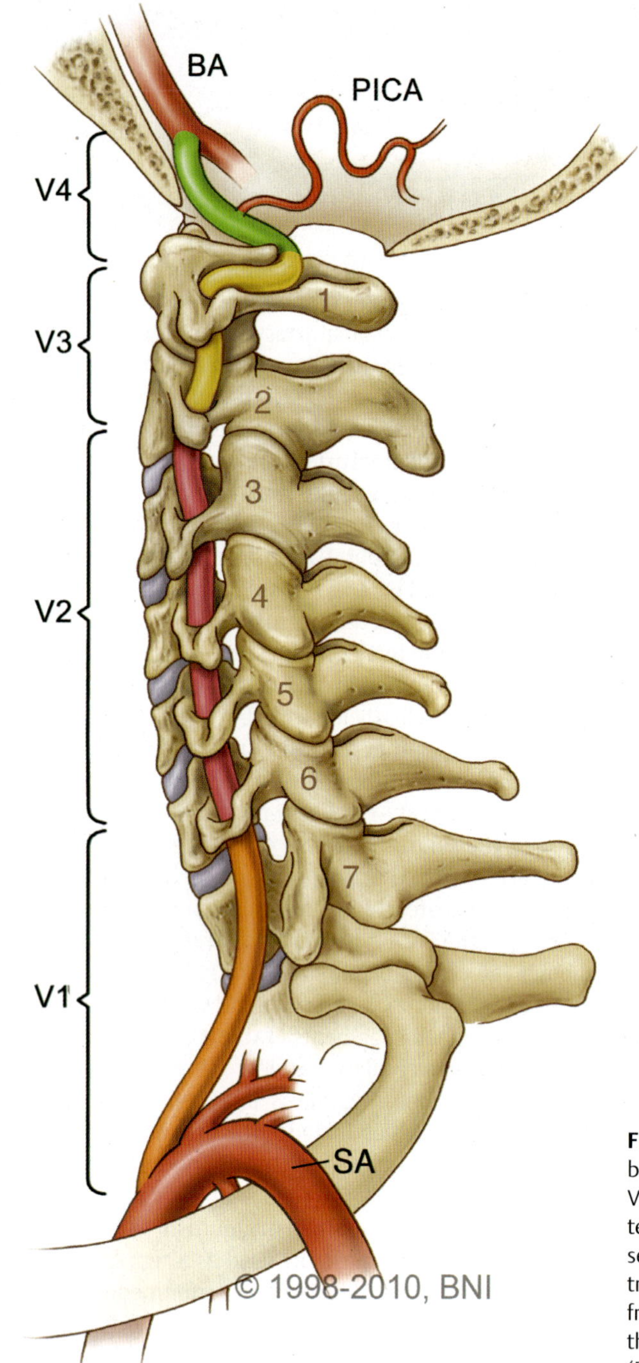

A

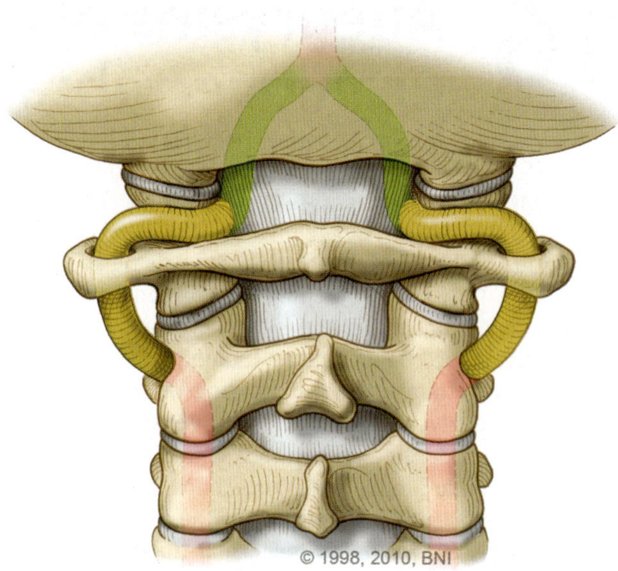

B

Fig. 16.1 **(A)** Lateral and **(B)** posterior views of the course of the vertebral artery. The vertebral artery is commonly divided into four segments: V1 segment (*orange*), which extends from the origin at the subclavian artery until it enters the vertebral transverse foramen—usually at C6; V2 segment (*red*), the portion of the artery passing through the vertebral transverse foramen from C6 to C2; V3 segment (*yellow*), which extends from the exit of the C2 foramen to the point where the artery pierces the dura; and the V4 segment (*green*), or intradural portion of the artery. (Reprinted with permission from Barrow Neurological Institute.)

Table 16.1 The Four Segments of the Vertebral Artery

Segment	Anatomy
V1	From vertebral artery origin to entrance in foramen transversarium
V2	Within foramen transversarium up to C2
V3	From C2 to dural penetration
V4	Intradural course of vertebral artery

from the tonsillomedullary segment in more than 75%.[5,8] These arterioles have a diameter of 0.4 mm or less and may be quite numerous.

Vascular Anatomy of the Basilar Artery

At the level of the pontomedullary sulcus, the vertebral arteries join to form the basilar artery trunk. Traveling within the prepontine cistern, the artery courses superiorly between the sixth cranial nerves before arching slightly posteriorly

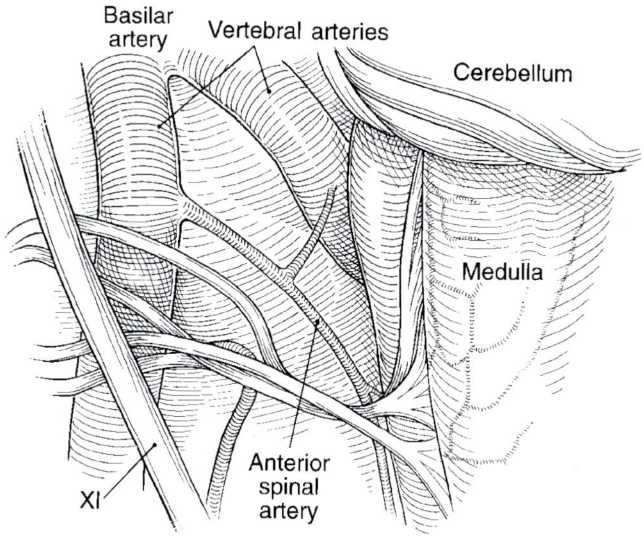

A

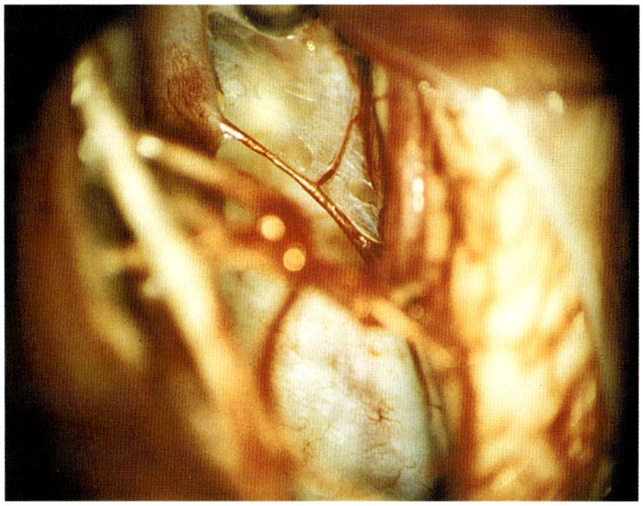

B

Fig. 16.2 **(A)** Illustration and **(B)** intraoperative photograph of the microscopic anatomy of the intradural vertebral artery show a rare view of the branches joining to form the anterior spinal artery. The anterior spinal artery continues distal to the brainstem. Both vertebral arteries and their junction are seen. (Illustration used with permission from Barrow Neurological Institute.)

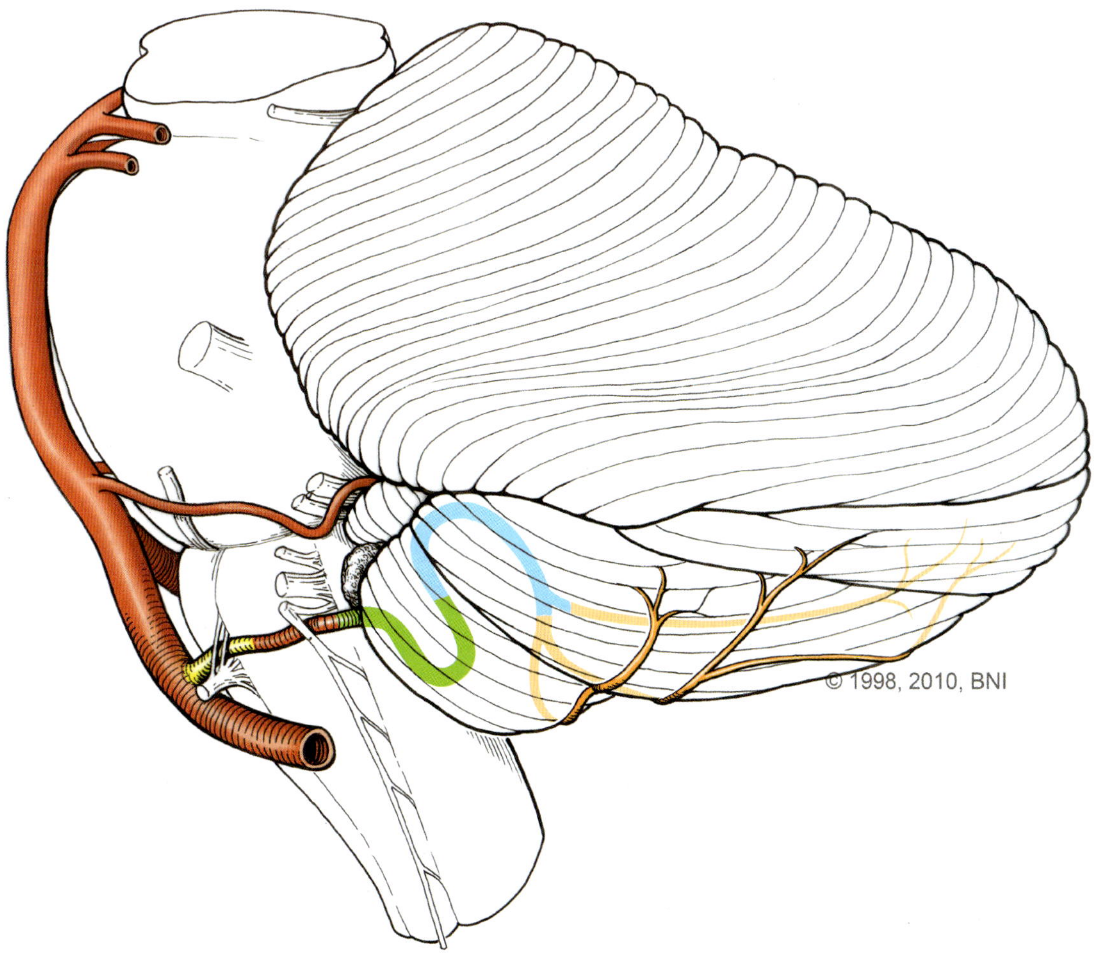

Fig. 16.3 The course of the posterior inferior cerebellar artery (PICA) is illustrated. Although quite variable in its course, PICA is usually divided into five segments: (1) the anterior medullary segment (*yellow*), (2) the lateral medullary segment (*red*), (3) the caudal loop (*green*), (4) the tonsillomedullary segment (*blue*), and (5) the telovelotonsillar segment (*orange*). The telovelotonsillar segment courses over the superior aspect of the cerebellar tonsil creating a loop. At its apex a branch exits to the choroid plexus of the fourth ventricle. The origin of this branch is called the "choroidal point" and serves as an important angiographic landmark for the position of the fourth ventricle. (Reprinted with permission from Barrow Neurological Institute.)

Table 16.2 The Five Segments of the Posterior Inferior Cerebellar Artery

Segment	Anatomy
Anterior medullary	From PICA origin to olive
Lateral medullary	From olive to origin of CN IX–XI
Tonsillomedullary	From origin of CN IX–XI to midtonsil of cerebellum
Telovelotonsillar	From midtonsil to retrotonsillar fissure
Cortical (hemispheric)	Through fissure to cerebellar hemispheres

Abbreviations: CN, cranial nerve; PICA, posterior inferior cerebellar artery.

after entering the interpeduncular cistern close to its termination. The trunk has an average length of 32 mm and diameter of 3 to 4 mm.[13] The artery often dilates rostrally by 0.3 to 0.8 mm. Only 25 to 50% of cases demonstrate a straight arterial course for the basilar artery.[14] The remainder assume an S-shaped configuration, which is especially prominent in older patients and those with extensive atherosclerotic disease. In this latter group, the diameter of the artery is also frequently enlarged. Fenestrations are relatively common in the basilar trunk, most often in its lower half. The incidence of this anomaly appears to be between 1 and 5% of cases.[15] In one report of 59 vertebrobasilar junction aneurysms, 21 (35.5%) arose in a fenestration of the proximal basilar artery.[15]

Considerable variation occurs in the level of the basilar artery at both its origin and termination. Normally situated at the lower end of the pons, the basilar origin may be several millimeters above or 1.5 cm below this level. Alternatively, the upper termination varies depending on the patient's age, clival configuration, and vessel integrity. In 51% of the specimens, the basilar artery terminates at the level of the posterior clinoid process (or dorsum sellae), whereas in 30% it is above and in 19% it is below this level.[6] In infants, the basilar bifurcation typically is located well above the posterior clinoid process. The basilar artery gives rise to various branches including numerous paramedian, short, and long circumflex pontine rami, as well as the anterior/inferior and superior cerebellar arteries. The basilar artery terminates into the bilateral P1 segments of the posterior cerebral artery. Lang found an average of 6.2 perforators per dissection (mean diameter, 0.3 mm).[14] On average, there were two arteries at each paramedian, short, and long circumflex location. The territory irrigated by these rami includes the pontine tegmentum, the middle cerebral peduncle, and the adjacent cranial nerves.

AICA most often arises from the proximal third of the basilar artery (52 to 75%). In 16 to 41% of the specimens, it branches off the middle third of the parent vessel. This artery is most often single but may be multiple in as many as 26% of specimens.[14] It is rarely absent (2 to 7%). The artery has been divided into premeatal, meatal, and postmeatal segments. The initial arterial course is downward and lateral with angles of ~45 degrees. AICA gives rise to several recurrent perforating arteries. The first two perforators most often arise from the premeatal segment. The internal auditory artery is rarely duplicated and passes immediately into the internal auditory canal to supply the nerve roots and ear sensory organs. Most commonly, it is ventral and medial to the nerves. AICA divides into a medial and lateral branch within the cerebellopontine angle in close relation to cranial nerves VII and VIII. The lateral branch curls around the flocculus and into the horizontal fissure. Here hemispheric branches anastomose with those of PICA and the superior cerebellar artery. The medial branch travels inferomedially, supplying primarily the biventral lobule, as does PICA. The size of AICA is inversely related to the size of PICA. In ~8% of cases, PICA itself may arise from the basilar artery.[14]

Like aneurysms in other locations, those at the CVJ follow the three basic anatomical principles of formation defined by Rhoton.[10] First, intracranial saccular aneurysms arise at branch points off a parent artery, either at the site of a side branch or at a bifurcation of the parent artery. For CVJ lesions, those arising at the PICA–vertebral artery branch and those arising at the vertebrobasilar junction (**Fig. 16.4**) illustrate both aspects of this

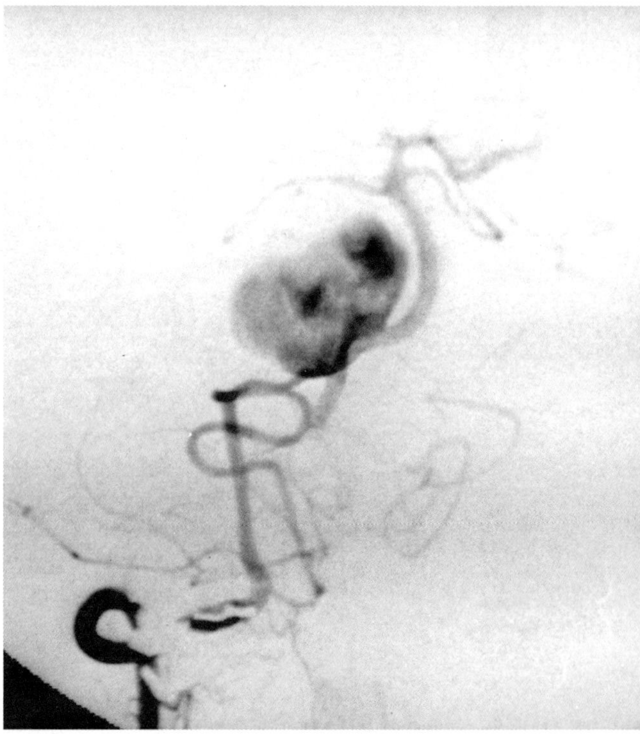

A

Fig. 16.4 A giant vertebrobasilar junction aneurysm demonstrates Rhoton's first principle of aneurysm formation. **(A)** Right vertebral artery injection shows the aneurysm dome with the basilar artery pushed medially and to the left. *(continued)*

Fig. 16.4 *(continued)* **(B)** Left vertebral artery injection. **(C)** Oblique vertebral injection demonstrates the mass of the lesion. **(D)** Lateral and **(E)** anteroposterior postoperative angiograms show the aneurysm to be well clipped and the surrounding vessels to be patent.

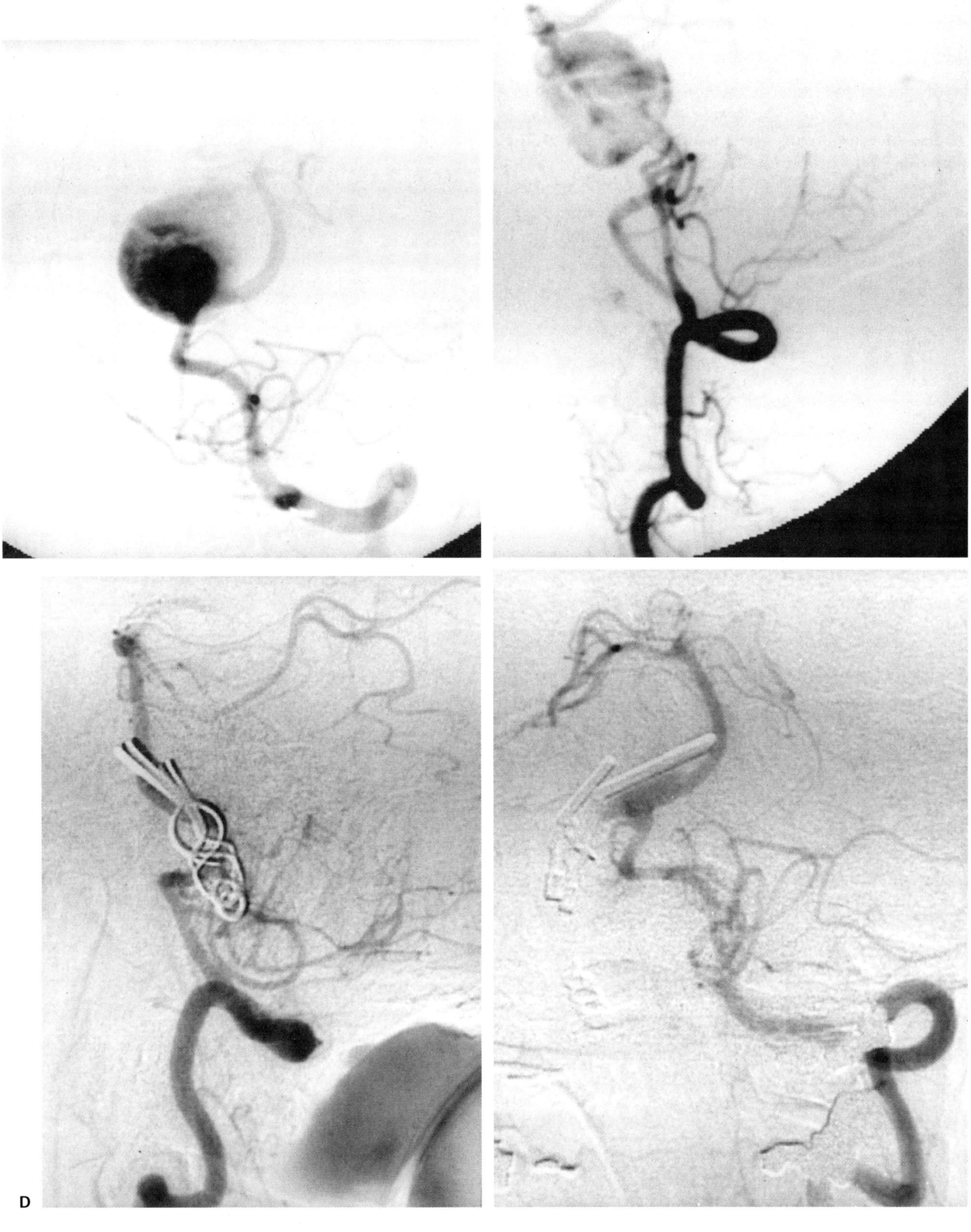

B C D E

principle, respectively. The second tenet suggests that saccular aneurysms tend to occur at curves or loops in arteries due to local hemodynamic stresses in these regions from directional changes in flow. Aneurysms that arise in the peripheral segments of PICA demonstrate this principle by occurring most commonly at either the cranial or caudal loops of PICA (**Fig. 16.5**).[11,16,17] The association of saccular aneurysms occurring in relation to a fenestrated basilar artery also may typify this point.[15,18,19] Third, an aneurysm, and more specifically its dome, points in the direction of blood flow irrespective of the accompanying side branch or curve associated with it. Prime examples of this tenet are aneurysms arising at the origin of PICA (**Fig. 16.6**). This lesion often occurs such that the rostral half of the PICA origin is involved as part of the aneurysm neck, with the dome most often pointing superiorly, a position that corresponds with the direction of blood flow in the parent artery.

Additionally, the CVJ harbors a disproportionately high number of dissecting aneurysms.[20] Dissecting aneurysms most often involve the intracranial V4 portion of the vertebral artery (**Fig. 16.7**).[21,22] As with saccular aneurysms, these pathological lesions tend to congregate around the PICA–vertebral artery junction.[23] It is hypothesized that the dissection itself is the main cause of fusiform aneurysmal formation. Other factors such as atherosclerotic plaques, fibromuscular dysplasia, or collagen vascular disease can also contribute to dissecting/fusiform aneurysm formation. The V4 segment of the vertebral artery is also exposed to sheer forces from head movement as it passes through the dura. This stress point is associated with tapering of the tunica media and adventitia, making this location more vulnerable to spontaneous dissection. When the dissection occurs between the internal elastic lamina and the tunica media, the lumen narrows, producing ischemic symptoms. When the dissection occurs between the tunica media and the adventitia, subarachnoid hemorrhage (SAH) results. SAHs from dissecting aneurysms are of concern as they are associated with considerably higher rates of early recurrent

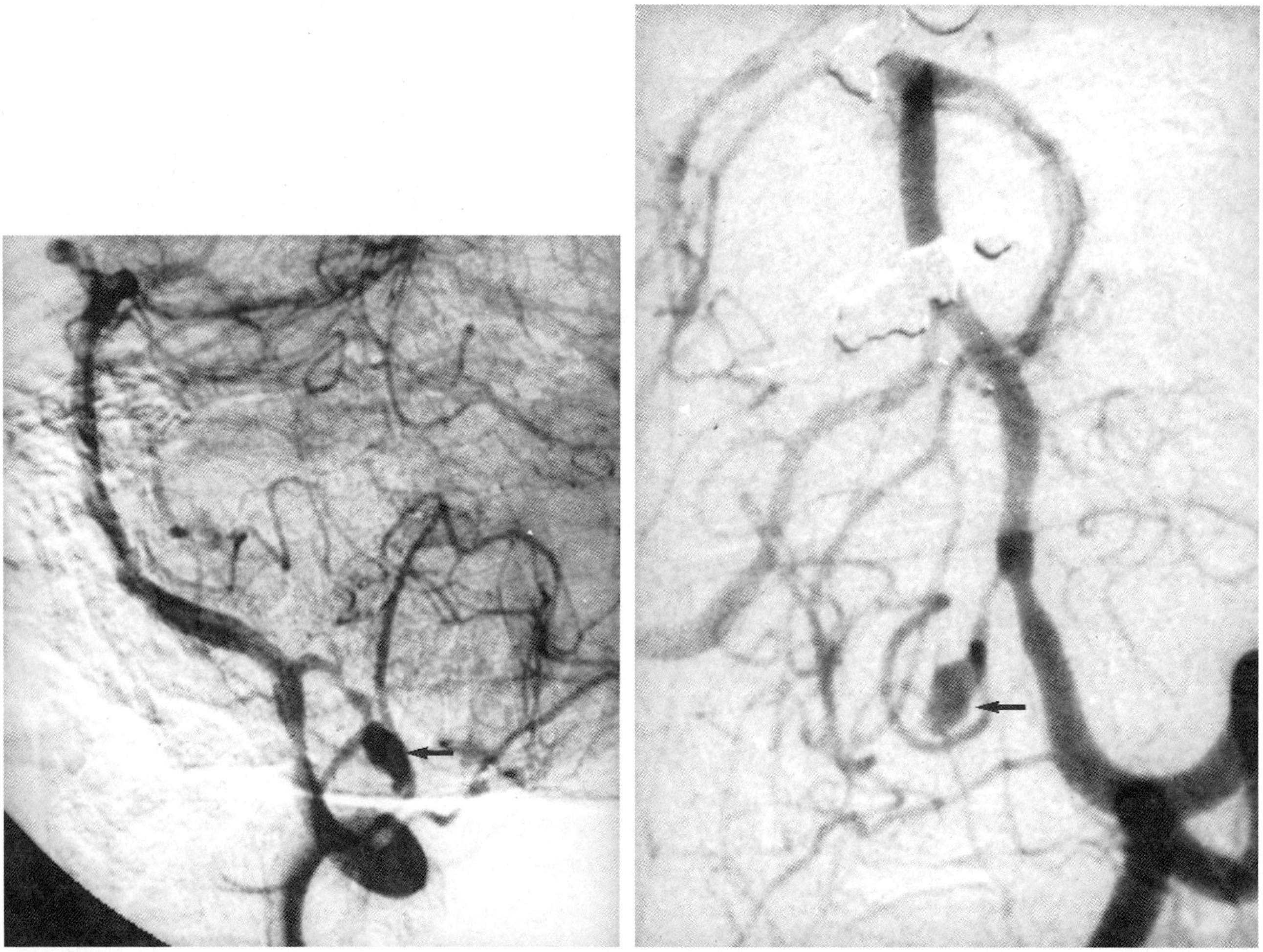
A B

Fig. 16.5 The posterior inferior cerebellar artery (PICA) aneurysm arises along the caudal loop of the artery, as suggested by the second tenet of aneurysm formation. **(A)** Lateral projection. **(B)** Submental vertex view of the aneurysm (*arrows*) off the caudal loop of PICA.

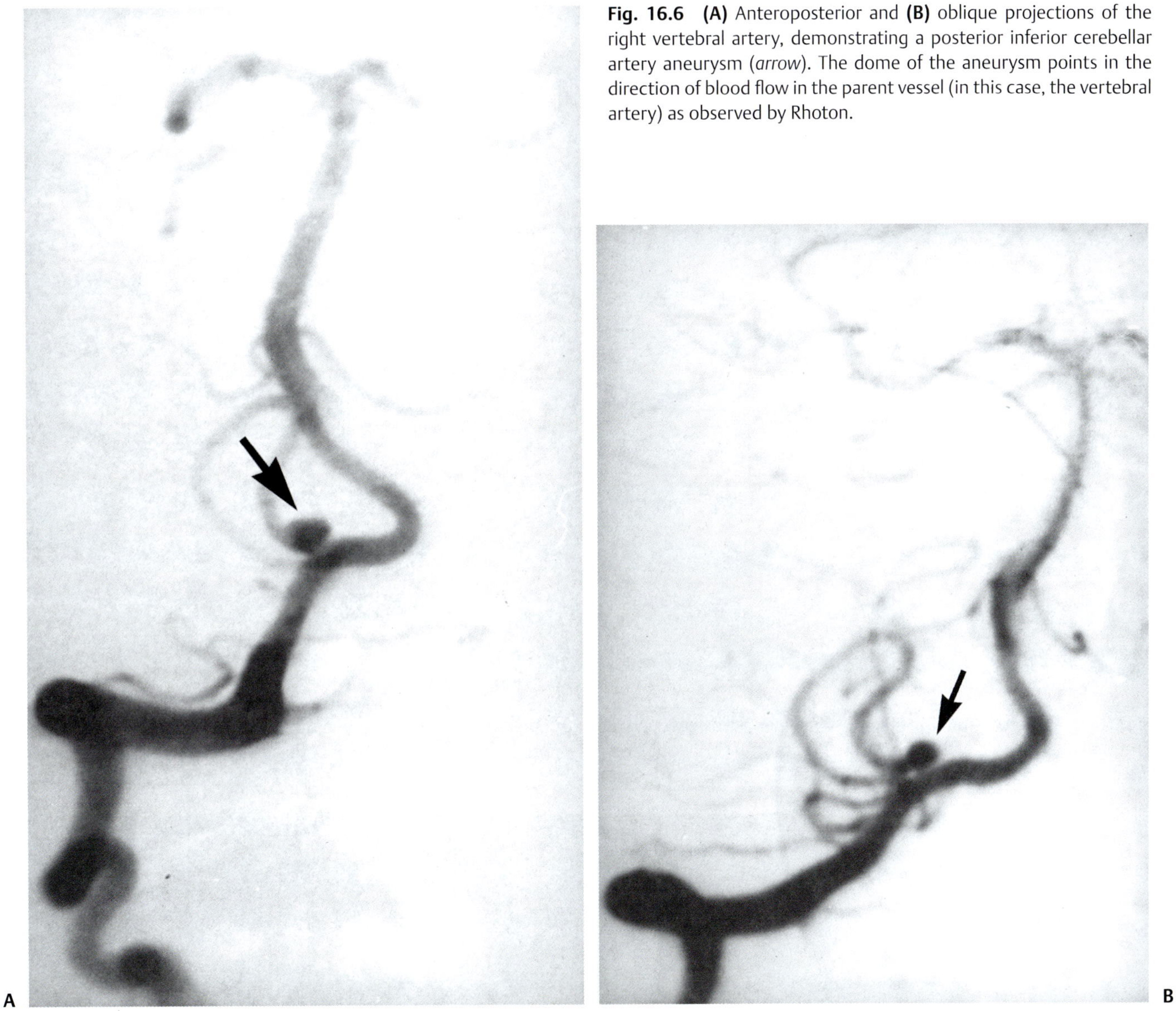

Fig. 16.6 **(A)** Anteroposterior and **(B)** oblique projections of the right vertebral artery, demonstrating a posterior inferior cerebellar artery aneurysm (*arrow*). The dome of the aneurysm points in the direction of blood flow in the parent vessel (in this case, the vertebral artery) as observed by Rhoton.

hemorrhage. Immediate attention and treatment are therefore indicated.[2,25,32,33] Traumatic aneurysms of the CVJ are rare[26] and should be treated like traumatic aneurysms elsewhere.

Clinical and Radiographic Features

Aneurysms of the CVJ represent ~3 to 5% of all intracranial aneurysms and 20 to 25% of posterior fossa aneurysms. Although aneurysms in general tend to be more common in women,[2,11,16,24,27] recent studies have suggested that dissecting and fusiform aneurysms are an exception and may be more common in men.[2,25]

SAH is the most common presentation of aneurysms of the CVJ, occurring in about two-thirds of cases. Although the age at onset is quite variable, patients tend to be in their fifth or sixth decade of life at presentation. Myriad clinical presentations are possible depending on the distribution of subarachnoid blood and/or the presence of mass effect from the aneurysm. Among these are cranial nerve deficits,[28] long tract signs, ischemic events, ataxia, hydrocephalus, seizures,[29] Horner syndrome,[25] vertigo,[23] Wallenberg syndrome, decreased mentation including loss of consciousness, and cardiopulmonary arrest.[29] Of those who present with cranial nerve palsies, cranial nerve complex of IX, X, and XI and cranial nerve VI are affected about equally for proximal aneurysms, whereas lesions of the basilar trunk most often cause cranial nerve VI palsy.[3,11,16,27] Furthermore, unusual anatomical presentations in these locations are possible, including paraplegia and contralateral crural monoparesis.[30,31]

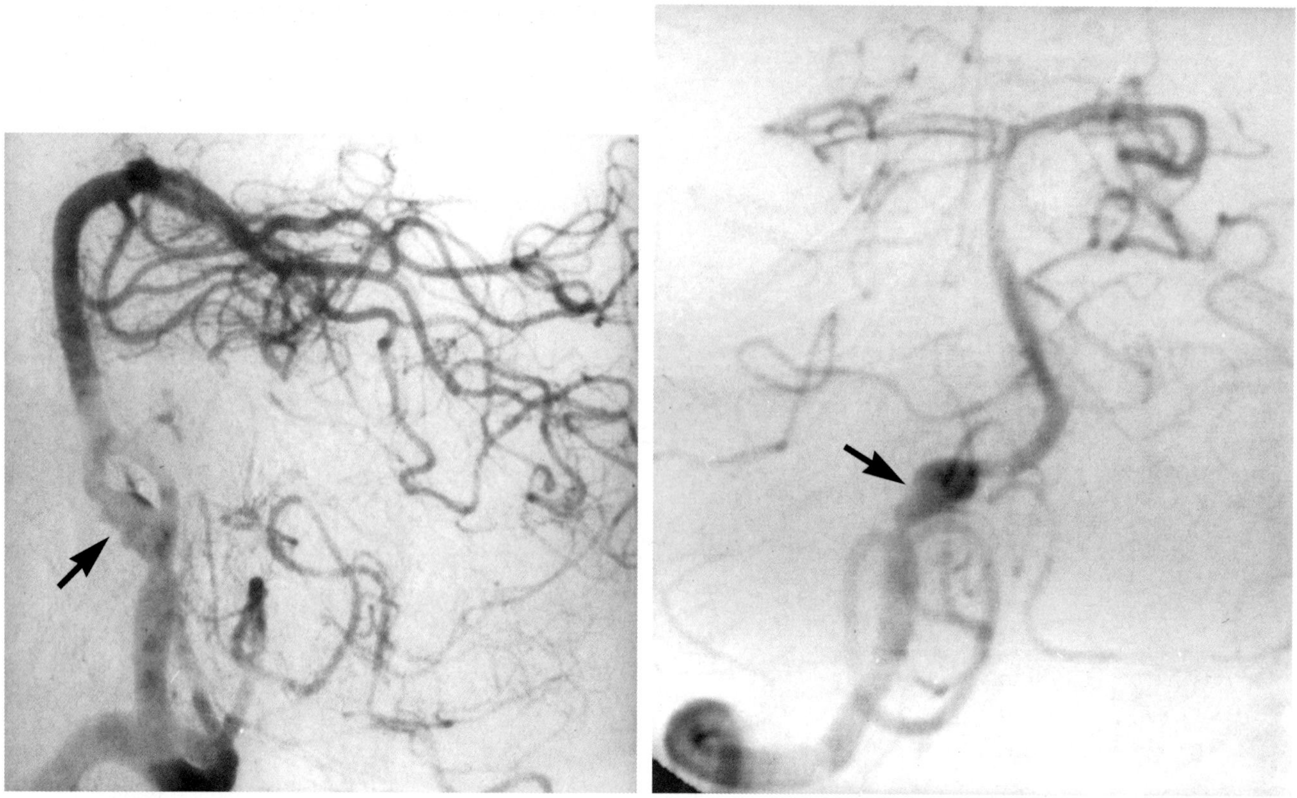

A B

Fig. 16.7 **(A)** Lateral and **(B)** anteroposterior views of a dissecting right vertebral artery aneurysm that occurred after a motor vehicle accident. The patient presented with a subarachnoid hemorrhage 1 week after the accident. The dilated segment of the artery (*arrow*) is the result of the dissection extending into the adventitial layer.

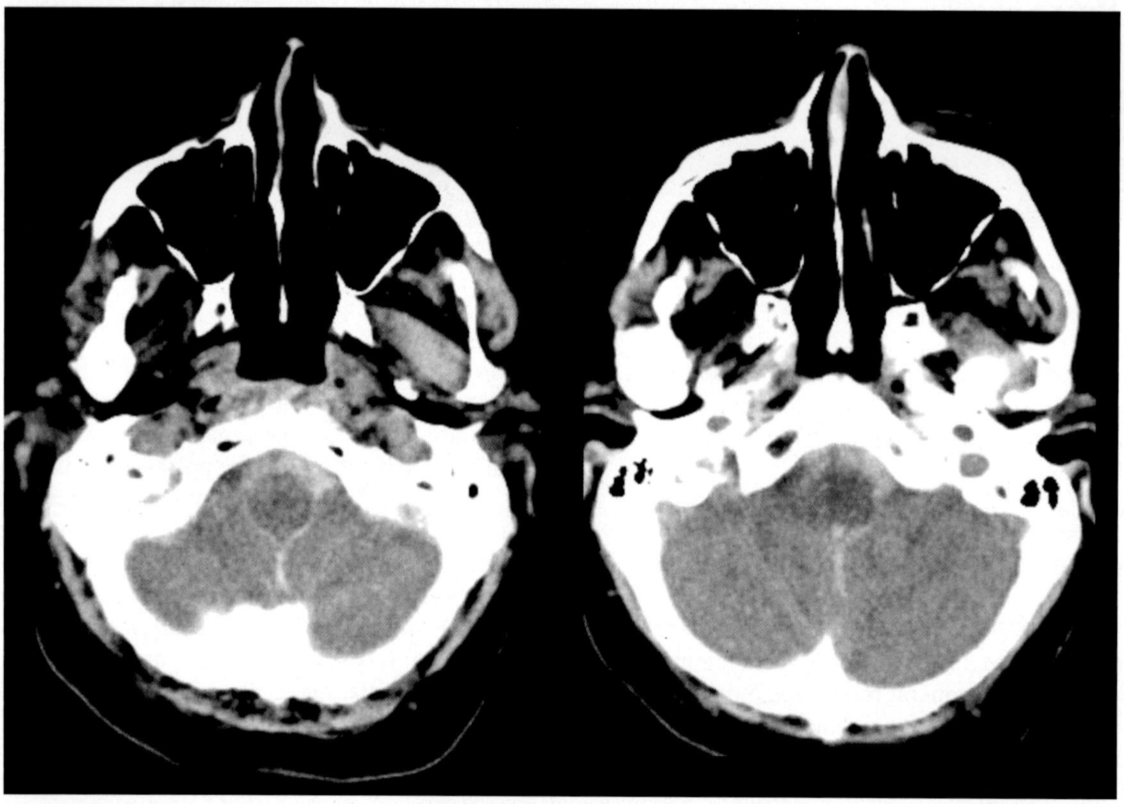

A

Fig. 16.8 **(A)** Axial computed tomography (CT) scan images of the head without contrast demonstrate subarachnoid hemorrhage lateralizing to the left side at the level of the medulla. *(continued)*

Radiographic Imaging

Once the history and physical examination of the patient are completed, the first diagnostic study of importance is head computed tomography (CT). With modern CT techniques, SAH can be diagnosed in <95% of patients. In most patients, the thickest layer of blood will be in the cerebellomedullary and cerebellopontine cisterns (**Fig. 16.8**). SAH with intraventricular hemorrhage (IVH) has been reported in 40 to 85% of patients.[2,11,27] IVH alone occurs in <25% of patients with these aneurysms, whereas SAH associated with IVH in only the fourth ventricle is almost diagnostic of vertebral artery and PICA aneurysms.[34,35] In these cases, blood

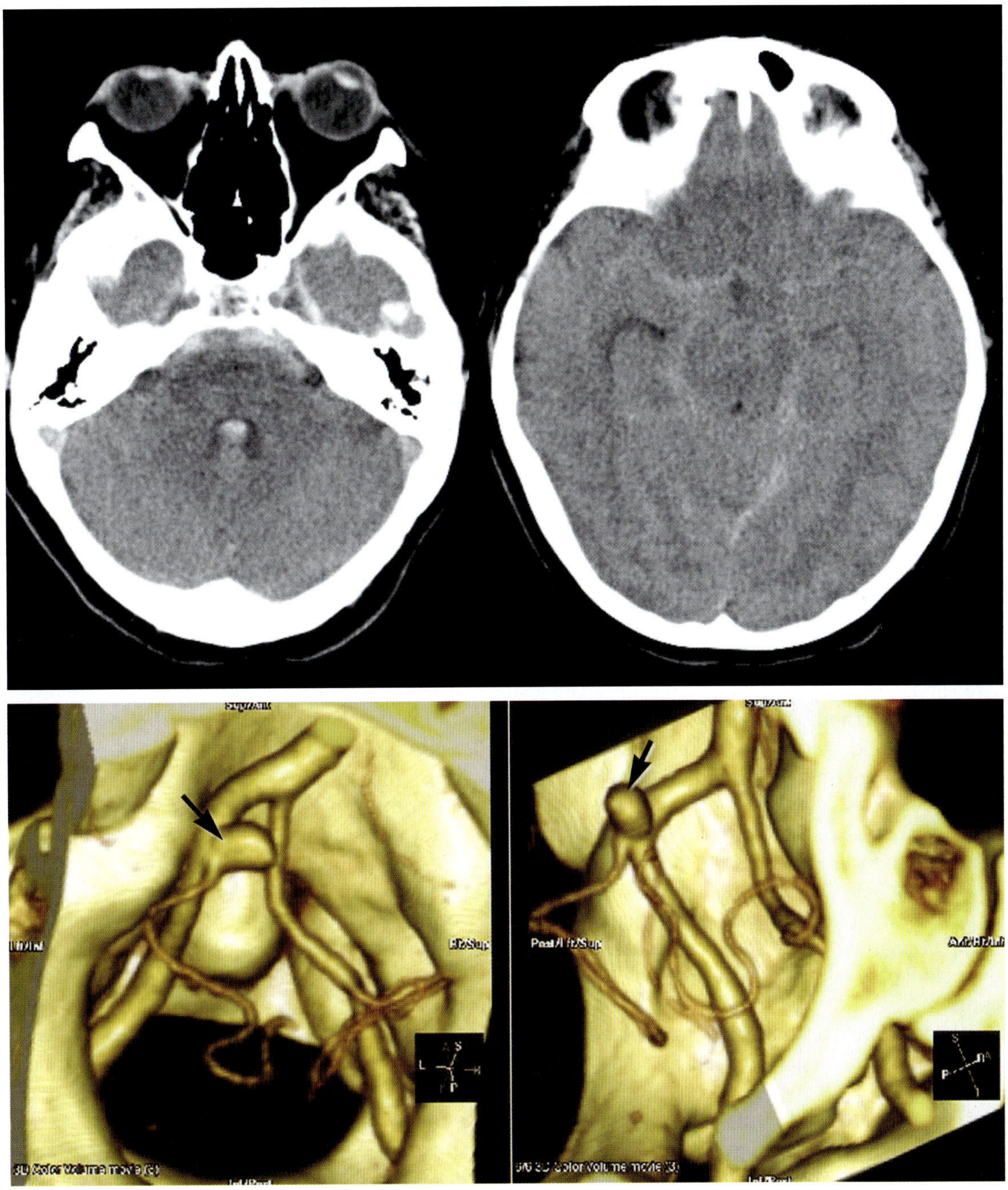

B

C

Fig. 16.8 *(continued)* **(B)** Additional sections from the same CT study reveal a more diffuse pattern of subarachnoid blood at the level of the pons and midbrain, as well the presence of blood within the fourth ventricle (*arrow*). **(C)** Volumetric three-dimensional reconstructions from the CT angiogram demonstrate a 5-mm aneurysm arising from the origin of posterior inferior cerebellar artery (*arrows*) on the left side as the source of this patient's hemorrhage. (Reprinted with permission from Barrow Neurological Institute.)

enters the ventricular system through either the foramen of Luschka or Magendie.[36–38] Hydrocephalus is a common consequence of this pathology, occurring in 29 to 50% of cases.[2,16,27,36]

If the basic head CT scan is negative, but the history or physical examination is suggestive of SAH, lumbar puncture is the next appropriate diagnostic choice. In the patient with SAH confirmed by lumbar puncture or head CT, four-vessel (bilateral carotid and vertebral arteries) cerebral angiography is warranted.[39] The four-vessel study should include both vertebral arteries. Alternatively, CT angiography (CTA) may be used for screening such patients. At the Barrow Neurological Institute (BNI), CTA has replaced conventional angiography as the initial choice for evaluation of patients with SAH, with angiographic evaluation reserved for those cases in which the CTA is negative or technically inadequate. CTA has the advantage of being quick and relatively easy to perform. Specialized software packages, combined with the development of high-speed multislice spiral CT scanners, have improved image quality to the point where it has begun to approach that of conventional digital subtraction techniques (**Fig. 16.8C**).

Conventional angiography remains an integral component of the assessment of these aneurysms. Angiography definitively delineates between the anatomy of the aneurysm and regional parent arteries and is often necessary to determine the feasibility of endovascular treatment. With modern angiographic equipment, selective vessel catheterization provides direct visualization of larger perforators and is also useful for evaluating the collateral blood supply when temporary or permanent vessel occlusion is being considered in the management of an aneurysm. The addition of three-dimensional (3D) rotational angiography with reconstructed images is useful in obtaining optimized endovascular working angles and/or surgical windows. Magnetic resonance imaging (MRI) and magnetic resonance angiography (MRA) can complement both CTA and conventional angiography in selected circumstances—particularly for large and giant aneurysms, that contain large volumes of thrombus and are associated with regional mass effect or parenchymal edema. MRI also provides detailed anatomical information about the relationship of the aneurysm to the brainstem and cranial nerves. In some cases, bony artifact caused by the skull base at the CVJ may present a limitation to CT imaging.

Dissecting and fusiform lesions are characterized by the *string sign* and the *pearl and string sign*.[21,40] These morphologies result from the irregular stenosis of the vessel lumen, which occurs after subintimal dissection and the development of an intramural hematoma. Very rarely, conventional angiography can demonstrate an intimal flap or retention of contrast medium within the vessel wall persisting into the venous phase.[41] In the absence of these latter two specific findings, the diagnosis of a "dissecting aneurysm" by angiography alone is tenuous. These diagnoses should be entertained cautiously because arterial vasospasm as a result of SAH may have a similar angiographic appearance.

Differentiating atherosclerotic ectasia from a true "dissecting" or "fusiform" aneurysm by angiography may be difficult but is suggested when a diffusely dilated vessel is associated with vessel tortuosity and elongation in the setting of advanced atheromatous disease. MRI can be useful with both dissecting and atherosclerotic aneurysms. A double lumen, characteristic of a dissecting aneurysm, may occasionally be seen on MRI when findings on conventional angiography are equivocal. Rarely, a linear abnormality is noted and recognized as an intimal flap (**Fig. 16.9**).[23,42] In instances that suggest a second lumen, the true lumen is most often hypointense while the false lumen is hyperintense on T1-weighted MRI.

Endovascular Approach to Craniovertebral Junction Aneurysms

Multiple techniques have been employed in the treatment of CVJ aneurysms and may be largely governed by mode of presentation. Stenting tends to be avoided if possible in the setting of acute SAH because these patients will require pharmacological platelet inhibition after the procedure. Conventional aneurysm coiling or balloon-assisted coiling techniques are typically employed to secure these lesions. We find it useful to utilize a balloon catheter while performing endovascular therapy not only for coil stabilization but also to achieve flow control in the case of intraoperative rupture. During these situations, a proximal balloon inflation may be a life-saving measure. Additionally, when severe angiographic vasospasm is identified at the time of treatment, intra-arterial nicardipine or gentle angioplasty can be performed during the same setting.

In unruptured CVJ aneurysms several new endovascular treatment options are available, and more devices are anticipated to become available in the near future. These new devices include intravascular self-expanding stents (currently commercially available) and flow diverters (currently investigational devices in the United States). These devices have been increasingly utilized for the treatment of more complex intracranial aneurysms. Flow-diverting devices function to reconstruct the parent vessel lumen and direct flow away from the aneurysm (**Fig. 16.10**). In some cases, fusiform aneurysms that are not amenable to either classic endovascular or surgical treatment have been successfully treated with these flow-diverting constructs. During the preliminary case experience, flow-diverting constructs have been shown to preserve the patency of small regional perforators arising from the parent vessel while at the same time achieving occlusion of the aneurysm.

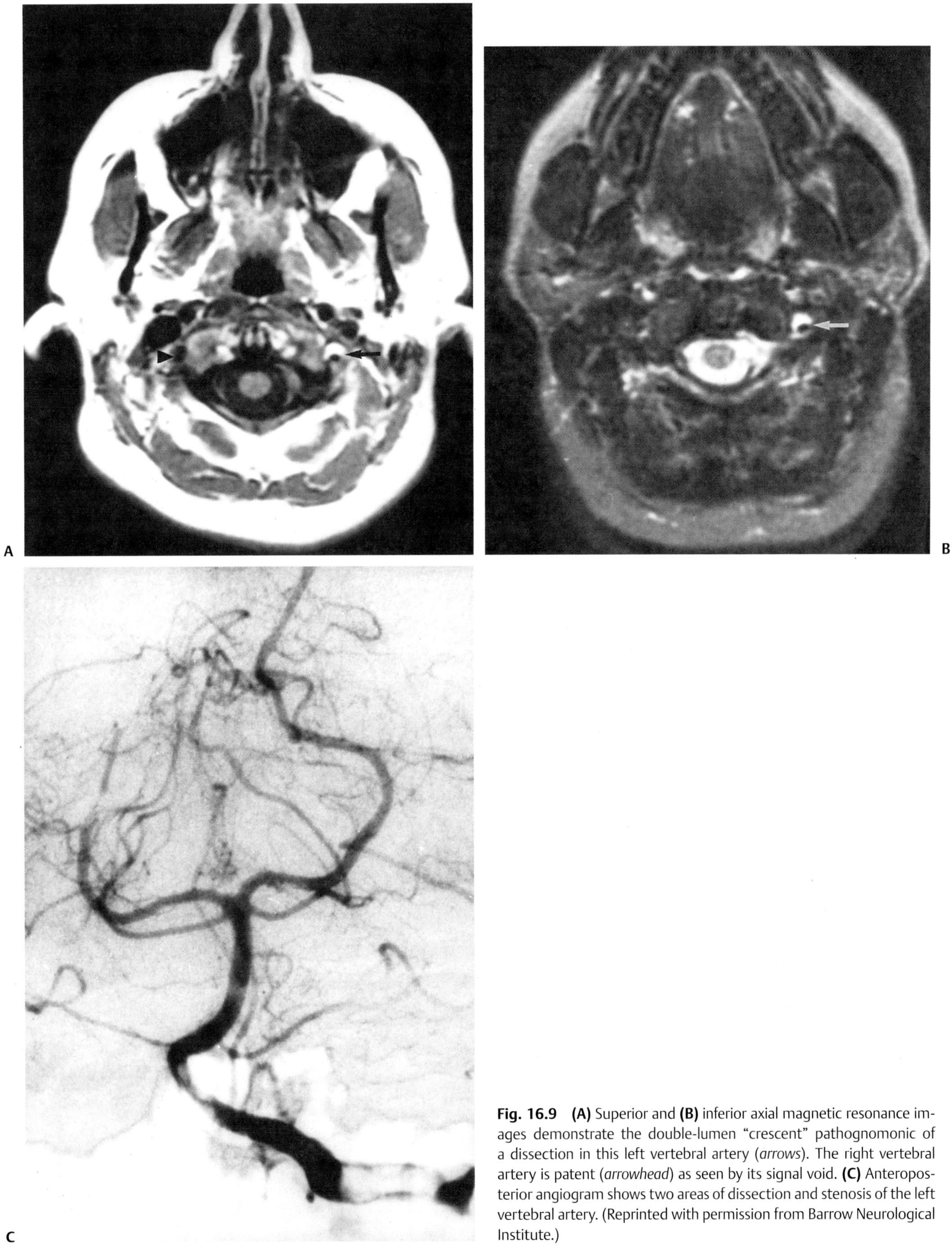

Fig. 16.9 **(A)** Superior and **(B)** inferior axial magnetic resonance images demonstrate the double-lumen "crescent" pathognomonic of a dissection in this left vertebral artery (*arrows*). The right vertebral artery is patent (*arrowhead*) as seen by its signal void. **(C)** Anteroposterior angiogram shows two areas of dissection and stenosis of the left vertebral artery. (Reprinted with permission from Barrow Neurological Institute.)

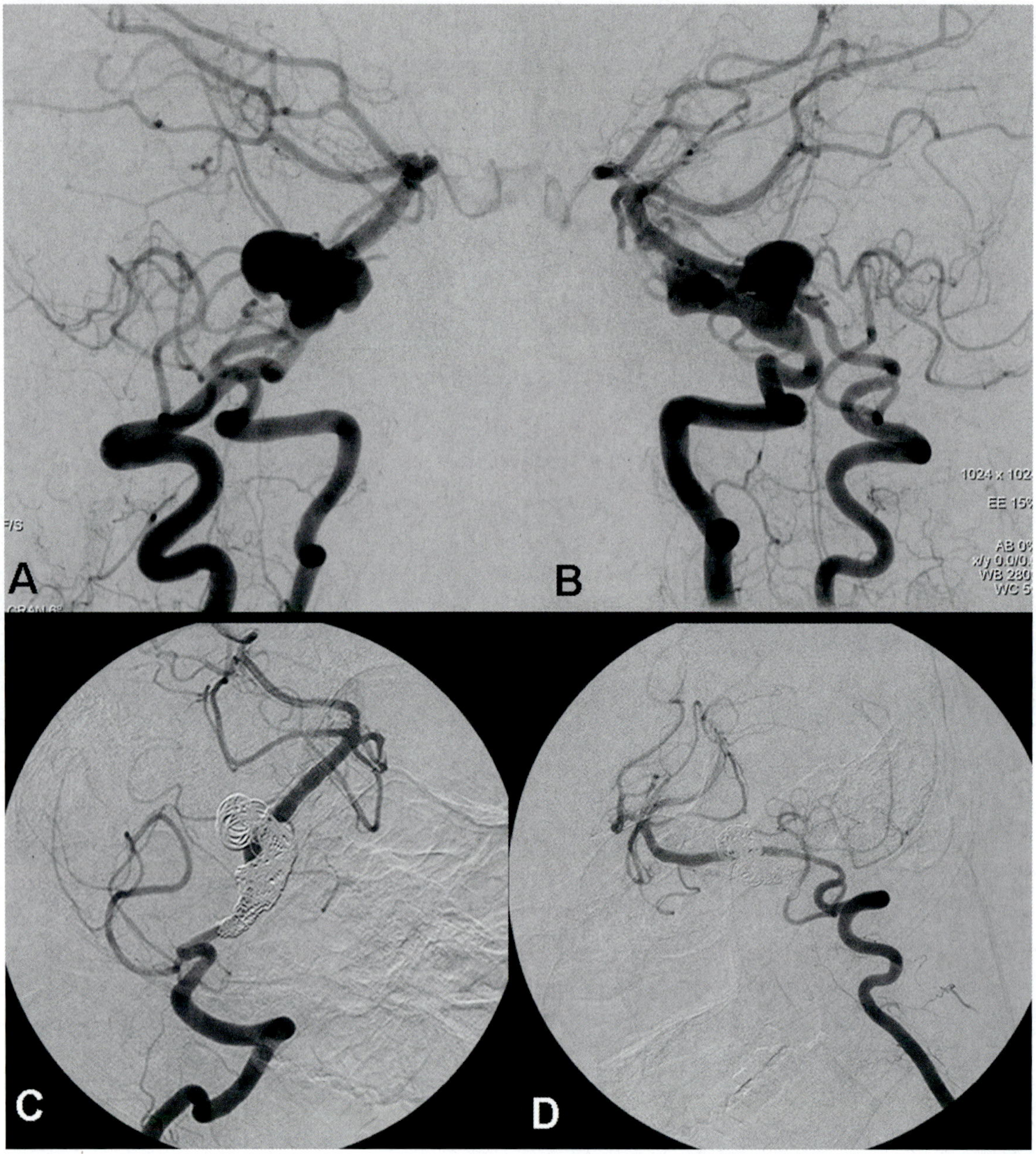

Fig. 16.10 Vertebral artery angiography in a young patient with a giant fusiform aneurysm. Subtracted images in the working angles **(A,B)** for endovascular treatment show the irregularly lobulated aneurysm incorporating the entire vertebrobasilar (VB) junction and progressing into the proximal basilar trunk. Reconstruction of the left vertebral artery, VB junction, and basilar trunk was achieved with a flow-diverting construct followed by deconstruction of the right vertebral artery and VB junction with coils. Images from a 6-month angiographic follow-up **(C,D)** show the aneurysm to be angiographically cured and the VB system to be anatomically reconstructed.

The Barrow Neurological Institute Experience with Aneurysms of the Craniovertebral Junction

Over the 34-month interval from April 2007 through January 2010, 1102 aneurysms were treated at the BNI, including 898 in the anterior circulation and 204 in the posterior circulation. As a percentage of posterior circulation aneurysms, there were a total of 68 (33%) involving the CVJ. Among the CVJ aneurysms, PICA was the most common location, accounting for 32 cases, followed by 25 lesions involving the V4 segment of the vertebral artery, and 11 at the vertebrobasilar junction (**Table 16.3**). Management of these lesions was divided equally between surgery (49%) and endovascular (51%) treatments.

Table 16.3 Barrow Neurological Institute Patient Data Regarding Posterior Circulation Aneurysm Location

Aneurysm Location	No. of Lesions
P1-P2 junction	1
Basilar tip	104
Superior cerebellar artery	11
Basilar trunk	16
AICA	4
Vertebrobasilar junction	11
PICA	32
Vertebral artery	25
Saccular	(15)
Dissecting	(10)
Total	204

Abbreviations: AICA, anterior inferior cerebellar artery; PICA, posterior inferior cerebellar artery.

Various direct surgical approaches have been reported for aneurysms of the CVJ.[3,4,43–46] For aneurysms located on cortical or hemispheric branches of PICA, a suboccipital craniotomy adequately exposes the lesion and allows proximal control of the parent vessel. Lesions of the tonsillomedullary and telovelotonsillar segment of the PICA or at the initial segment of the intradural portion of the vertebral artery probably can be clipped safely via a lateral suboccipital craniotomy or retromastoid approach. Early in our experience several such aneurysms were treated in this fashion. Since then, however, we have found the far-lateral approach[47,48] to be optimum for accessing most aneurysms of the CVJ, excluding cortically placed lesions as noted and those of the upper basilar trunk. The far-lateral technique provides a very flat and direct surgical approach to the cerebellopontine/cerebellomedullary angle and to the brainstem itself. It also has the advantage of providing proximal control of the vertebral artery just before it penetrates the dura (V3 segment). The flat approach is obtained by combining removal of the ipsilateral arch of C1, the inferior rim of the foramen magnum, and one-third to one-half of the occipital-C1 condyle. This surgical route allows a view of the anterior and lateral aspects of the inferior brainstem, upper cervical spinal cord, and the associated neurovascular structures and cranial nerves (IX to XII). The far-lateral exposure also provides excellent access to the upper vertebral artery, vertebrobasilar junction, and the lower basilar artery aneurysms located along the lower one-half of the clivus (**Fig. 16.11**). The great advantage of this approach is the exquisite exposure achieved through bony resection rather than brain retraction.

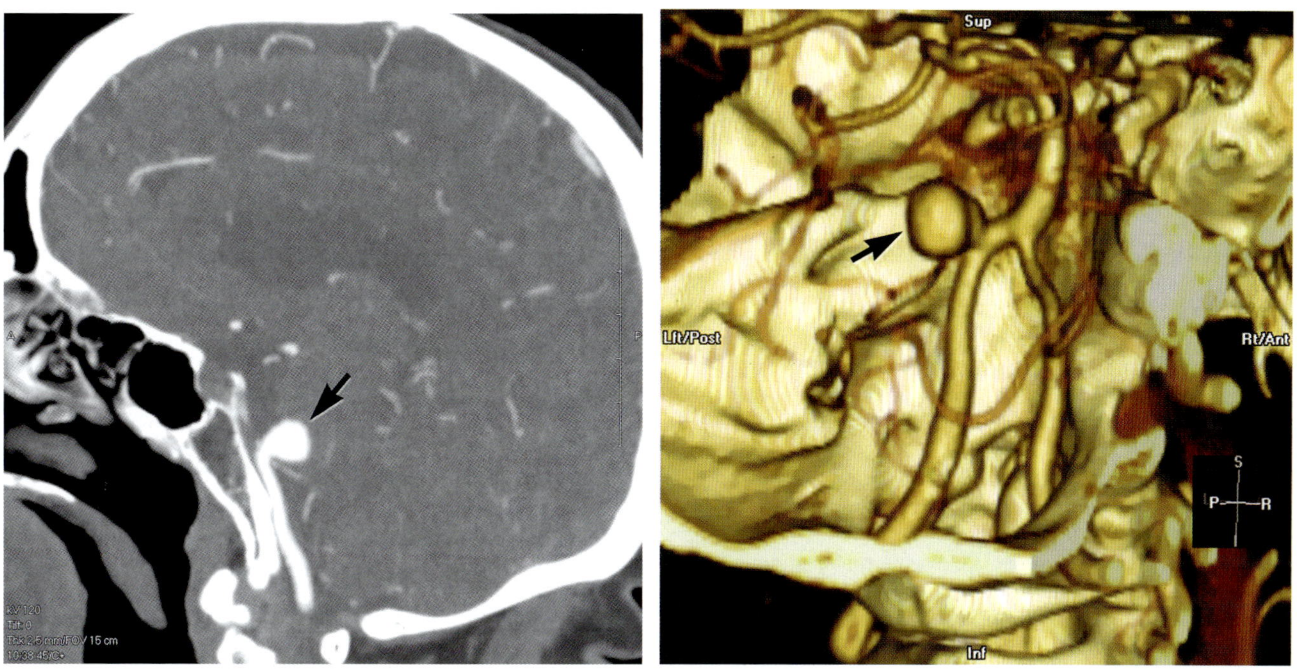

A B

Fig. 16.11 **(A)** Sagittal reconstruction from a computed tomography (CT) angiogram demonstrating a 1-cm aneurysm arising from the origin of posterior inferior cerebellar artery (*arrow*) in a 61-year-old woman with sudden onset of severe headache. Note the high location of the aneurysm, just above the midpoint of the clivus. **(B)** A three-dimensional (3D) reconstruction from the same CT angiogram shows that the aneurysm lies just proximal to the vertebrobasilar junction at about the level of the internal auditory meatus. The aneurysm was clipped uneventfully through a retrosigmoid far-lateral approach. *(continued)*

C

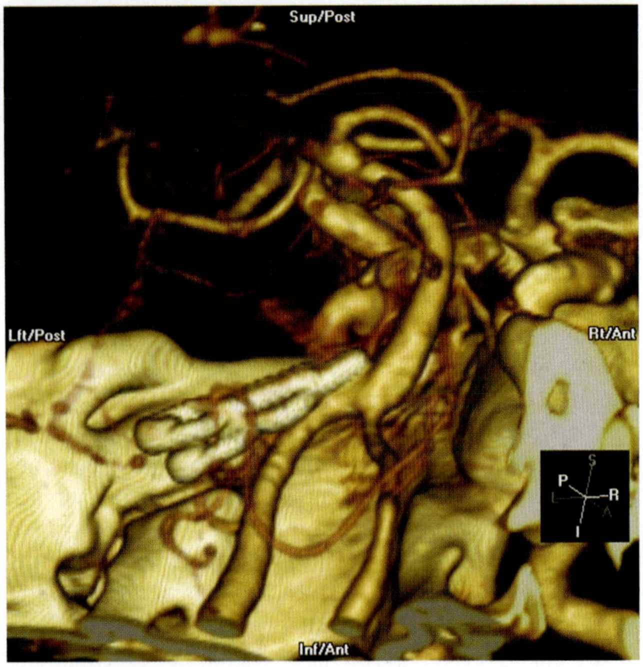

Fig. 16.11 *(continued)* **(C)** A 3D reconstruction from the postoperative CT angiogram demonstrates good clipping of the aneurysm and no compromise of the parent vessels. (Reprinted with permission from Barrow Neurological Institute.)

In the BNI series of CVJ aneurysms, a suboccipital craniotomy was utilized in three cases involving unusual distal aneurysms of PICA. The far-lateral approach was used in the remaining 65 cases (95%).

Conclusion

The CVJ is an intricate anatomical region with transitions in bony structures and in neural and vascular tissues. The histological changes in the vasculature combined with the local hemodynamic stress of blood flow in the region may account for the relatively large number of aneurysms in this location. Most of these lesions occur at the major branch point, the vertebral artery–PICA origin, and most patients present with SAH. Although SAH can be devastating, up to 70% of patients may be neurologically intact upon initial examination. Radiological evaluation, especially CT angiography, is essential in quickly confirming the diagnosis of ruptured aneurysm and in planning definitive treatment. A thorough knowledge of the surrounding anatomy is crucial in this region, because the neural and vascular relationships are quite complex.

References

1. Yonas H, Dujovny M. "True" traumatic aneurysm of the intracranial internal carotid artery: case report. Neurosurgery 1980;7(5):499–502
2. Andoh T, Shirakami S, Nakashima T, et al. Clinical analysis of a series of vertebral aneurysm cases. Neurosurgery 1992;31(6): 987–993, discussion 993
3. Ausman JI, Sadasivan B. Aneurysms. Posterior inferior cerebellar artery-vertebral artery aneurysms. In: Apuzzo MLJ, ed. Brain Surgery. New York, NY: Churchill Livingstone; 1993:1879–1894
4. Batjer HH, Kopitnik TA, Purdy PD, et al. Vertebral and PICA aneurysms. In: Carter LP, Spetzler RF, Hamilton MG, eds. Neurovascular Surgery. New York, NY: McGraw Hill; 1995:763–776
5. Weir B. Aneurysms Affecting the Nervous System. Baltimore, MD: Williams & Wilkins; 1987:335–336
6. Huber P, Bosse G. Cerebral Angiography. 2nd ed. Stuttgart, Germany: Georg Thieme Verlag; 1982:142–143, 152–156
7. Margolis MT, Newton TH. The posterior inferior cerebellar artery. In: Newton TH, Potts DG, eds. Radiology of the Skull and Brain. St. Louis, MO: C.V. Mosby; 1974:1710–1774
8. Lister JR, Rhoton AL Jr, Matsushima T, Peace DA. Microsurgical anatomy of the posterior inferior cerebellar artery. Neurosurgery 1982;10(2):170–199
9. Hlavin ML, Takaoka Y, Smith AS. A "PICA communicating artery" aneurysm: case report. Neurosurgery 1991;29(6):926–929
10. Rhoton AL Jr. Anatomy of saccular aneurysms. Surg Neurol 1980;14(1):59–66
11. Hudgins RJ, Day AL, Quisling RG, Rhoton AL Jr, Sypert GW, Garcia-Bengochea F. Aneurysms of the posterior inferior cerebellar artery. A clinical and anatomical analysis. J Neurosurg 1983;58(3): 381–387
12. Tanaka A, Kimura M, Yoshinaga S, Tomonaga M. Extracranial aneurysm of the posterior inferior cerebellar artery: case report. Neurosurgery 1993;33(4):742–744, discussion 744–745
13. Saeki N, Rhoton AL Jr. Microsurgical anatomy of the upper basilar artery and the posterior circle of Willis. J Neurosurg 1977;46(5): 563–578
14. Lang J. Skull Base and Related Structures. Atlas of Clinical Anatomy. Stuttgart, Germany: Schattauer; 1995:255–257
15. Campos J, Fox AJ, Viñuela F, et al. Saccular aneurysms in basilar artery fenestration. AJNR Am J Neuroradiol 1987;8(2):233–236
16. Lee KS, Gower DJ, Branch CL Jr, Kelly DL Jr, McWhorter JM, Bell WO. Surgical repair of aneurysms of the posterior inferior cerebellar artery—a clinical series. Surg Neurol 1989;31(2):85–91
17. Nishizaki T, Tamaki N, Nishida Y, Fujita K, Matsumoto S. Aneurysms of the distal posterior inferior cerebellar artery: experience with three cases and review of the literature. Neurosurgery 1985; 16(6):829–832
18. Crivelli G, Bianchi M, Dario A, Dorizzi A. Saccular aneurysm associated with proximal basilar artery fenestration. Case report. J Neurosurg Sci 1993;37(1):29–34
19. Hoshimaru M, Hashimoto N, Kikuchi H, Kamijyo Y, Kang Y, Namura S. Aneurysm of the fenestrated basilar artery: report of two cases. Surg Neurol 1992;37(5):406–409
20. Pritz MB. Evaluation and treatment of aneurysms of the vertebral artery: different strategies for different lesions. Neurosurgery 1991;29(2):247–256
21. Caplan LR, Baquis GD, Pessin MS, et al. Dissection of the intracranial vertebral artery. Neurology 1988;38(6):868–877
22. Sasaki O, Ogawa H, Koike T, Koizumi T, Tanaka R. A clinicopathological study of dissecting aneurysms of the intracranial vertebral artery. J Neurosurg 1991;75(6):874–882
23. Nagahiro S, Goto S, Yoshioka S, Ushio Y. Dissecting aneurysm of the posterior inferior cerebellar artery: case report. Neurosurgery 1993;33(4):739–741, discussion 741–742
24. Yamaura A. Diagnosis and treatment of vertebral aneurysms. J Neurosurg 1988;69(3):345–349

25. Yamaura A, Watanabe Y, Saeki N. Dissecting aneurysms of the intracranial vertebral artery. J Neurosurg 1990;72(2):183–188
26. Morard M, de Tribolet N. Traumatic aneurysm of the posterior inferior cerebellar artery: case report. Neurosurgery 1991;29(3): 438–441
27. Salcman M, Rigamonti D, Numaguchi Y, Sadato N. Aneurysms of the posterior inferior cerebellar artery-vertebral artery complex: variations on a theme. Neurosurgery 1990;27(1):12–20, discussion 20–21
28. Hedera P, Friedland RP. Duane's syndrome with giant aneurysm of the vertebral basilar arterial junction. J Clin Neuroophthalmol 1993;13(4):271–274
29. Ruelle A, Cavazzani P, Andrioli G. Extracranial posterior inferior cerebellar artery aneurysm causing isolated intraventricular hemorrhage: a case report. Neurosurgery 1988;23(6):774–777
30. Ferrante L, Acqui M, Mastronardi L, Celli P, Lunardi P, Fortuna A. Posterior inferior cerebellar artery (PICA) aneurysm presenting with SAH and contralateral crural monoparesis: a case report. Surg Neurol 1992;38(1):43–45
31. Kashiwagi S, Tsuchida E, Shiroyama Y, Ito H, Yamashita T. Paraplegia due to a ruptured aneurysm of the distal posterior inferior cerebellar artery. J Neurol Neurosurg Psychiatry 1992;55(9):836–837
32. Aoki N, Sakai T. Rebleeding from intracranial dissecting aneurysm in the vertebral artery. Stroke 1990;21(11):1628–1631
33. Kitanaka C, Tanaka J, Kuwahara M, et al. Nonsurgical treatment of unruptured intracranial vertebral artery dissection with serial follow-up angiography. J Neurosurg 1994;80(4):667–674
34. Pinto AN, Ferro JM, Canhão P, Campos J. How often is a perimesencephalic subarachnoid haemorrhage CT pattern caused by ruptured aneurysms? Acta Neurochir (Wien) 1993;124(2-4):79–81
35. Rinkel GJE, Wijdicks EFM, Vermeulen M, et al. Nonaneurysmal perimesencephalic subarachnoid hemorrhage: CT and MR patterns that differ from aneurysmal rupture. AJNR Am J Neuroradiol 1991;12(5):829–834
36. Kayama T, Sugawara T, Sakurai Y, Ogawa A, Onuma T, Yoshimoto T. Early CT features of ruptured cerebral aneurysms of the posterior cranial fossa. Acta Neurochir (Wien) 1991;108(1-2):34–39
37. Shapiro SA, Campbell RL, Scully T. Hemorrhagic dilation of the fourth ventricle: an ominous predictor. J Neurosurg 1994;80(5):805–809
38. Yeh H-S, Tomsick TA, Tew JM Jr. Intraventricular hemorrhage due to aneurysms of the distal posterior inferior cerebellar artery. Report of three cases. J Neurosurg 1985;62(5):772–775
39. Pelz DM, Viñuela F, Fox AJ, Drake CG. Vertebrobasilar occlusion therapy of giant aneurysms. Significance of angiographic morphology of the posterior communicating arteries. J Neurosurg 1984;60(3):560–565
40. Endo S, Nishijima M, Nomura H, Takaku A, Okada E. A pathological study of intracranial posterior circulation dissecting aneurysms with subarachnoid hemorrhage: report of three autopsied cases and review of the literature. Neurosurgery 1993;33(4):732–738
41. Mizutani T, Aruga T. "Dolichoectatic" intracranial vertebrobasilar dissecting aneurysm. Neurosurgery 1992;31(4):765–773, discussion 773
42. Hosoda K, Fujita S, Kawaguchi T, et al. Spontaneous dissecting aneurysms of the basilar artery presenting with a subarachnoid hemorrhage. Report of two cases. J Neurosurg 1991;75(4):628–633
43. Mizoi K, Yoshimoto T, Takahashi A, Ogawa A. Direct clipping of basilar trunk aneurysms using temporary balloon occlusion. J Neurosurg 1994;80(2):230–236
44. Steinberg GK, Drake CG, Peerless SJ. Deliberate basilar or vertebral artery occlusion in the treatment of intracranial aneurysms. Immediate results and long-term outcome in 201 patients. J Neurosurg 1993;79(2):161–173
45. Drake CG. The treatment of aneurysms of the posterior circulation. Clin Neurosurg 1979;26:96–144
46. Yamaura A, Ise H, Makino H. Radiometric study on posterior inferior cerebellar aneurysms with special reference to accessibility by the lateral suboccipital approach. Neurol Med Chir (Tokyo) 1981;21(7):721–733
47. Heros RC. Lateral suboccipital approach for vertebral and vertebrobasilar artery lesions. J Neurosurg 1986;64(4):559–562
48. Spetzler RF, Grahm TW. The far-lateral approach to the inferior clivus and the upper cervical region: technical note. BNI Q 1990; 6(4):35–38

17 Cavernous Malformations of the Cervicomedullary Junction

Joseph M. Zabramski, John R. Robinson, Jr., and Robert F. Spetzler

Cavernous malformations are low-flow, hemorrhagic vascular lesions that affect 0.4 to 0.5% of the population. Because they are "angiographically occult" and poorly visualized by computed tomography (CT), they were once considered rare. With the introduction of magnetic resonance imaging (MRI), the importance of these lesions as a surgically treatable cause of seizures and neurological impairment has been well documented. For the most part, the excision of cavernous malformations is not difficult; however, the location of a specific lesion may raise a significant risk for perioperative complications. This risk is particularly true for lesions that involve the craniovertebral junction (CVJ).

This chapter reviews the epidemiology, presentation, and management of cavernous malformations with a particular emphasis on the surgical decision making for lesions located at the CVJ. As elsewhere in this text, the term CVJ is used to refer to the posterior fossa and upper cervical spine. Other chapters describe the technical details of the specific surgical approaches to this region.

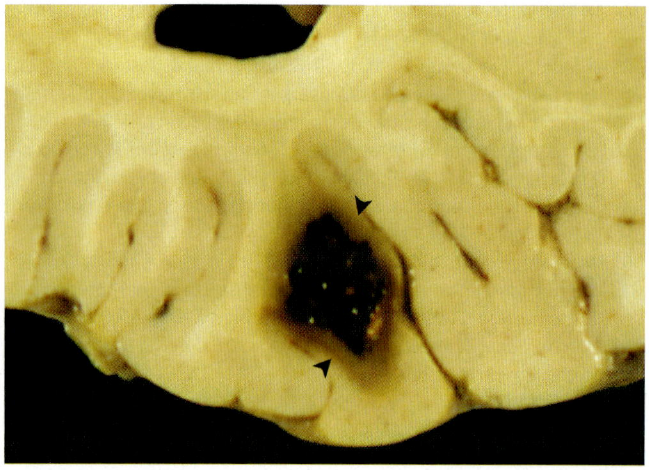

Fig. 17.1 Gross pathologic specimen demonstrating the typical appearance of a cavernous malformation. Hemosiderin from recurrent episodes of intralesional hemorrhage and thrombosis accumulates by diapedesis in macrophages and glia around these lesions, producing a characteristic brown or dark yellow-stained border that surrounds the mass (*arrowheads*). (From Zabramski JM, Spetzler RF. Cavernous malformations. In: Aminoff M, Daroff R, eds. Encyclopedia of the Neurological Sciences. San Diego, CA: Academic Press; 2003:532–538. Reprinted with permission from Elsevier.)

Pathology

Grossly, cavernous malformations are well-defined dark red or purple, mulberry-like masses, surrounded by a characteristic brown or dark yellow-stained, gliotic border (**Fig. 17.1**). They may range from a few millimeters to several centimeters in size. In one study in which dimensions were measured by MRI, the average lesion was 1.7 cm in diameter, with a range of 3 mm to 4 cm.[1] There was no significant difference in the size of lesions in the supra- and infratentorial compartments, but posterior fossa lesions were more commonly symptomatic, particularly when located in the lower brain stem.

Microscopically, cavernous malformations are characterized by a complex of markedly dilated vascular channels (caverns) arranged in a back-to-back pattern with little or no intervening brain parenchyma (**Fig. 17.2**).[2–7] A loose collagenous matrix may separate the channels at the periphery. The dilated channels frequently contain thrombus of various ages and degrees of organization. Histologically, the vascular channels are thin-walled and lined by a single layer of vascular endothelium. The walls contain no elastin or smooth muscle and characteristically have no basement membrane (**Fig. 17.2**).[8] The lack of a supporting matrix for the vascular structures appears to make the lesions susceptible to repeated episodes of focal intralesional hemorrhage and thrombosis. Focal areas of calcification are also relatively common and may be visualized on CT.

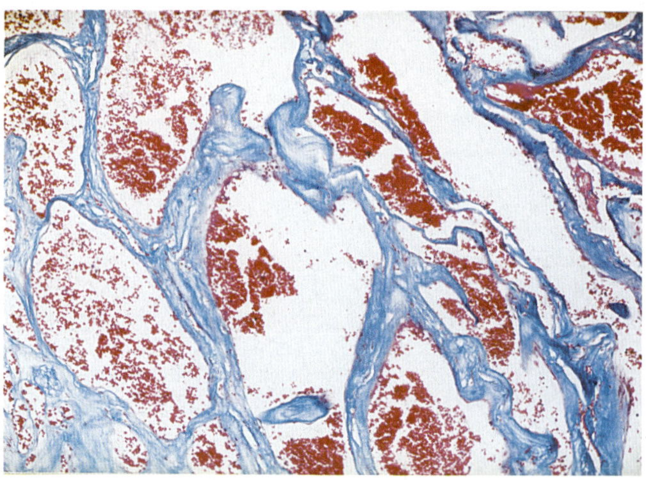

Fig. 17.2 Masson's trichrome stain of a characteristic cavernous malformation. Note the back-to-back vessel arrangement of markedly dilated capillary vessels (caverns) that compose the lesion. The vessel walls are lined by a single layer of vascular endothelium with an abundance of collagen (*blue stain*) and an absence of elastin (*black stain*) or a basement membrane.

Epidemiology

Cavernous malformations account for 5 to 10% of all central nervous system (CNS) vascular malformations.[7,9] In surgical series they are the second most common vascular malformation, outnumbered only by arteriovenous malformations (AVMs). Cavernous malformations have been reported from almost all corners of the world, although the incidence may be slightly lower in African and Asian cultures.

The overall incidence of cavernous malformations in the general population is estimated to be between 0.4 and 0.5%. In two large reviews of nonselected autopsies cases, Sawar and McCormick[9] reported an incidence of 0.4% in 4069 patients, whereas Otten and colleagues[10] reported 0.53% in a series of 24,535 cases. These results closely agree with those from two large MRI reviews: Del Curling and colleagues[11] cited an incidence of 0.39% in a series of 8131 patients undergoing MRI, whereas Robinson and colleagues[1] found a 0.47% incidence in their review of 14,035 sequential MRIs. These findings were recently confirmed by Vernooij and colleagues[12] in a study describing the incidental findings on brain MRI in the general population: The authors reported the results of MRI studies in 2000 adult patients over the age of 45 (mean 63.3 years) and found that 0.4% of this population had incidental cavernous malformations. Although various authors have reported a slight male or female preponderance for cavernous malformations, overall both sexes appear to be affected equally.[13]

Cavernous malformations are distributed throughout the CNS in rough relationship to the volume of the various compartments; 70 to 80% occur supratentorially, 10 to 20% are in the posterior fossa, and 5 to 10% are in the spine.[14–21] In the posterior fossa, the lesion preferentially involves the pons and cerebellum. **Table 17.1** lists the distribution of cavernous malformations at the CVJ in 142 patients from the three largest available series.[14,22,23]

Cavernous malformations occur in two forms: spontaneous and familial. The spontaneous form occurs as isolated cases and is characterized by the presence of a single lesion, whereas the familial form is characterized by multiple lesions and an autosomal dominant mode of inheritance. Multiple lesions and a family history of seizures are nearly pathognomonic for the familial form of cavernous malformations. With careful screening we find that more than 80% of patients with three or more lesions have a history consistent with the familial form of this disease.[22] Indeed, many individuals with multiple lesions but lacking a clear family history have been shown to harbor a de novo germline mutation.[24–27]

Table 17.1 Distribution of 142 Cavernous Malformations Involving the Craniovertebral Junction

Location	No. of Lesions (%)
Pons	56 (39)
Pontomedullary	10 (7)
Medulla	23 (16)
Cerebellum	49 (35)
Cervicomedullary	4 (3)

The introduction of MRI, with the resulting ability to readily detect cavernous malformations, combined with an explosion of genetic technology provided the tools necessary to identify the genetic mutations that cause these lesions. The onset of cavernous malformations occurs either sporadically or in an inherited autosomal dominant form due to mutations in one of three genes, *CCM1*/KRIT1,[28,29] *CCM2*/malcavernin,[24,30] or *CCM3*/PDCD10.[25] Based on available data, at least two of these loci (CCM1 and CCM2) appear to be involved in the regulation of β_1 integrin signal transduction, which plays a crucial role in the regulation of cell adhesion and migration during angiogenesis. The third locus (CCM3) involves an apoptotic pathway. The role of the latter gene in angiogenesis and the formation of cavernous malformations remains to be investigated.

Diagnosis

Prior to the introduction of modern imaging techniques, cavernous malformations were considered rare curiosities. In 1976 Voigt and Yasagil[31] described their experience with one case and reviewed the world literature, finding only 126 reported cases. Because cavernous malformations are low-flow, capillary lesions, angiography is of little use in their diagnosis.[32] Occasionally, larger lesions will produce some degree of mass effect or late-phase venous pooling. For the most part, however, these lesions are not visualized by angiography and in the pre-CT/MRI era were commonly referred to as “angiographically occult AVMs,” or “thrombosed AVMs.”

Although CT scanning was a significant advance in neuroimaging, it lacked the sensitivity and specificity necessary to be diagnostic for cavernous malformations. The averaged, mixed-tissue density of many cavernous malformations is almost identical to that of the normal brain on CT. In addition, mass effect, contrast enhancement, and edema, which are the key diagnostic features on CT for other pathologies, are not characteristic of cavernous malformations. In general, CT identifies only ~50% of the lesions demonstrated by MRI studies.[33] Nevertheless, CT is a useful screening test in patients presenting with the new onset or exacerbation of focal neurological deficits, as it is exquisitely sensitive to acute blood and may identify new episodes of hemorrhage.

MRI is the study of choice for the diagnosis of cavernous malformations. It is both highly sensitive and selective. The characteristic MRI appearance is considered nearly pathognomonic. To provide some idea of the impact of MRI on the recognition of this disease, we reviewed the MEDLINE database and found only five articles published on cavernous malformations during the first 10 years of the CT era (1976 to 1985), compared with 110 articles

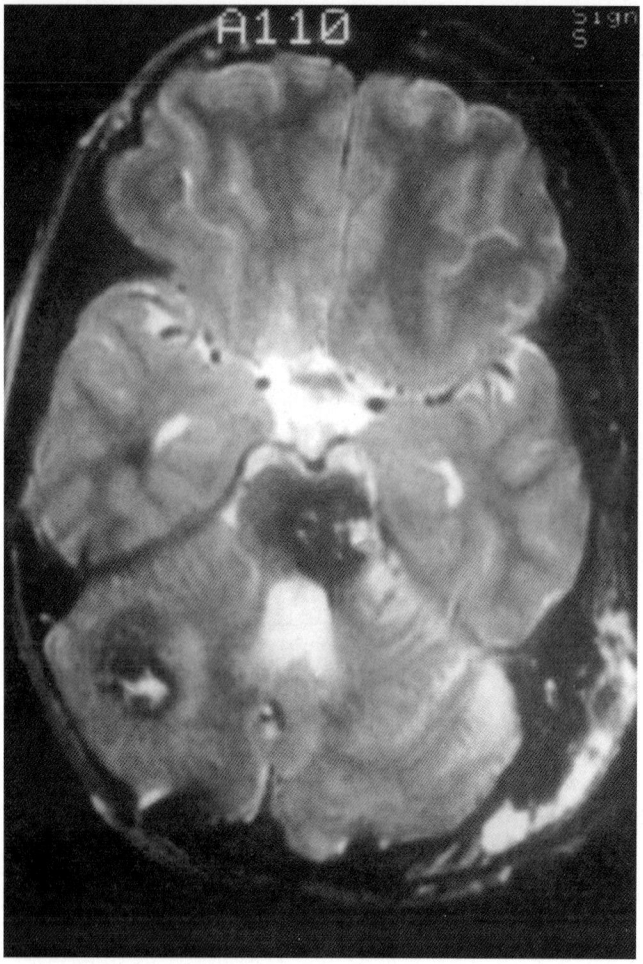

A

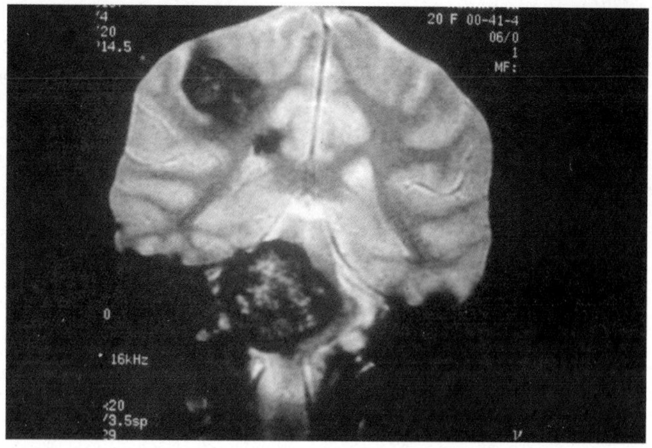

B

Fig. 17.3 The classic magnetic resonance imaging appearance of cavernous malformations is demonstrated on these heavily T2-weighted **(A)** spin echo and **(B)** gradient echo images in this patient with the familial form of the disease. The lesions typically contain a variegated core of mixed signal intensity produced by the presence of hemorrhage and thrombus of widely differing ages and degrees of organization. The core of the lesion is surrounded by a ring of low signal intensity that is characteristic of chronic hemorrhage, produced by the deposition of iron and hemosiderin in the surrounding tissue (Fig 17.1). **(B)** This metallic artifact is significantly greater on gradient echo images.

during the subsequent 10 years when MRI became generally available (1986 to 1995).

The classic appearance of cavernous malformations on MRI—that of a mass with a core of mixed signal intensity on T1- and T2-weighted spin echo images surrounded by a ring of low signal intensity—is most apparent on heavily T2-weighted spin echo and gradient echo images (**Fig. 17.3**). This halo of signal loss is diagnostic for remote hemorrhage and is a result of magnetic field distortions produced by the deposition of hemosiderin in the tissue adjacent to the cavernous malformation. Signal loss and distortion are minimized on heavily T1-weighted images, which are recommended for surgical planning.

Despite their size, the lesions produce little mass effect on the surrounding brain (**Fig. 17.3A**). Extensive edema is rare, and there is little or no contrast enhancement after the administration of gadolinium. Lesions containing a large component of hyperacute hemorrhage may appear dark on both T1- and T2-weighted MRI but are readily identified by CT. Subacute hemorrhage may produce areas of high or low signal intensity depending on its age and stage of resorption (**Table 17.2**).

Other lesions with a propensity for hemorrhage may occasionally masquerade as cavernous malformations. The presence of extensive edema in the surrounding tissue should bring the diagnosis of cavernous malformation

Table 17.2 Changes in Imaging Characteristics of Hemorrhage with Time

Diagnostic Study	Acute (1–2 days)	Subacute Early (1–2 weeks)	Subacute Late (1–2 months)	Chronic (>6 months)
CT	+ +	±	–	–
T1-weighted MRI	–	+ +	+ +	–
T2-weighted MRI	–	+ +	±	– (+ halo)

Abbreviations: CT, computed tomography; MRI, magnetic resonance imaging; +, hyperintense to surrounding brain; –, hypointense to surrounding brain; ±, mixed intensity; + halo, a ring of low signal intensity surrounding the core of the lesion.

into question. Repeat imaging after a short period of observation (2 to 3 weeks) will resolve the issue in difficult cases. Mixed forms of vascular malformations, containing cavernous malformations in combination with an AVM or other vascular malformations, may be suggested by CT or MRI findings.[2] The addition of angiography is helpful in such cases.

When other lesions are found in association with cavernous malformations, they are most commonly venous malformations. Venous malformations, also called developmental venous anomalies (DVAs), are benign vascular lesions found in ~2% of the population. They are identified in association with cavernous malformations in 20 to 30% of cases.[2,18,34] On angiography, venous malformations are readily visualized as radial collections of multiple small veins draining into a large central trunk to produce a characteristic *caput medusa* pattern (**Fig. 17.4**). On CT and MRI, the large central draining vein can frequently be recognized as a linear-enhancing flow void (**Fig. 17.4**). It is critical to understand that these lesions provide the normal venous drainage of the surrounding brain. Larger branches must be carefully preserved. Their sacrifice, particularly of the central draining vein, may lead to venous infarction with associated swelling, hemorrhage, and even death.

Presentation

Cavernous malformations appear to grow and to produce symptoms as a result of recurrent episodes of intralesional hemorrhage and thrombosis. More rarely, they present with extralesional hemorrhage. These episodes are asymptomatic until the lesion reaches a critical size that irritates or compresses adjacent structures.

Headache is a relatively common but nonspecific symptom in patients with cavernous malformations. It is present in approximately one-third of patients regardless of whether lesions are supra- or infratentorial, or whether there is evidence of acute hemorrhage.[1,11,18,22] The mechanism by which these lesions produce headache is unknown. Significant mass effect and the obstruction of cerebrospinal fluid (CSF) pathways are rare, and hemorrhage rarely reaches pial surfaces. Whatever the etiology, headache is the complaint that initiates the diagnostic evaluation in a significant number of patients.

Although seizures are the most common presenting symptom when lesions are located supratentorially, focal neurological deficits predominate when lesions involve the CVJ. Combinations of long tract signs and cranial nerve deficits vary, depending on the exact location of the lesion and its

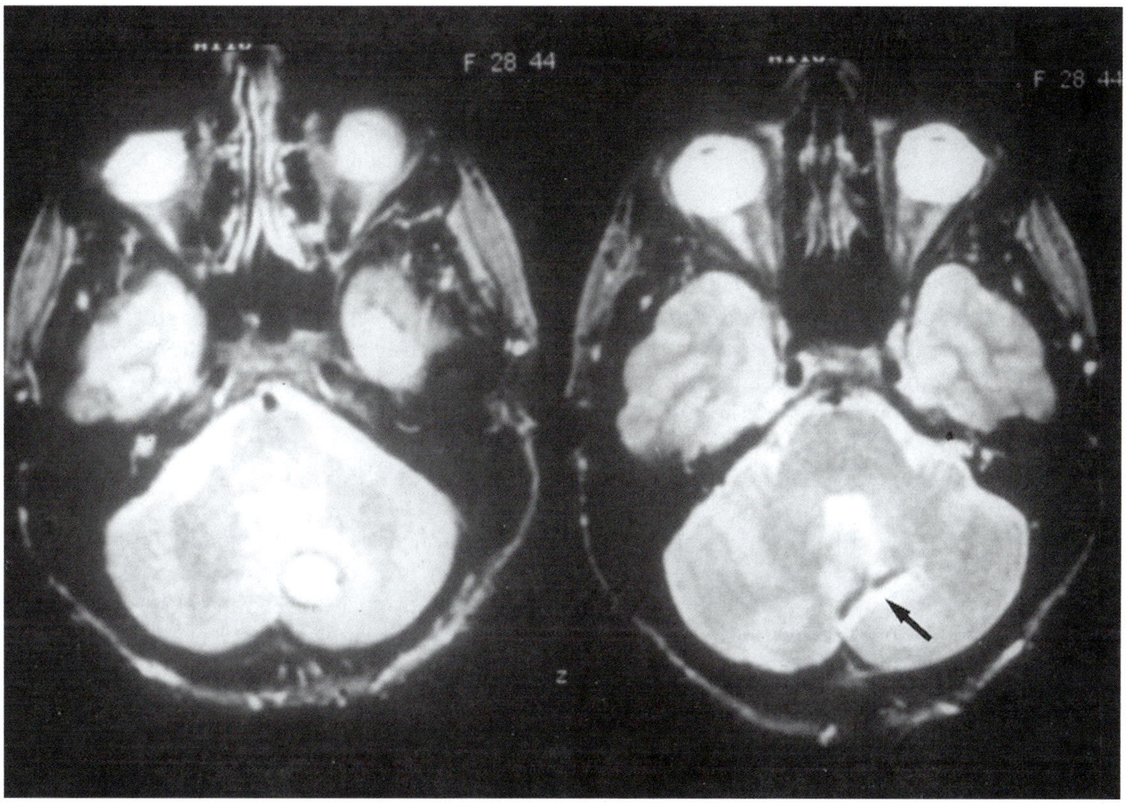

A B

Fig. 17.4 This 52-year-old woman had a long history of headache. An exacerbation of her normal headache pattern led to this magnetic resonance imaging (MRI) study. The MRI findings are consistent with subacute hemorrhage from a cavernous malformation in the left cerebellum. The conversion of hemoglobin to methemoglobin in subacute hemorrhage produces a bright signal on both **(A,B)** the heavily T2-weighted spin echo images and **(C,D)** T1-weighted images. *(continued)*

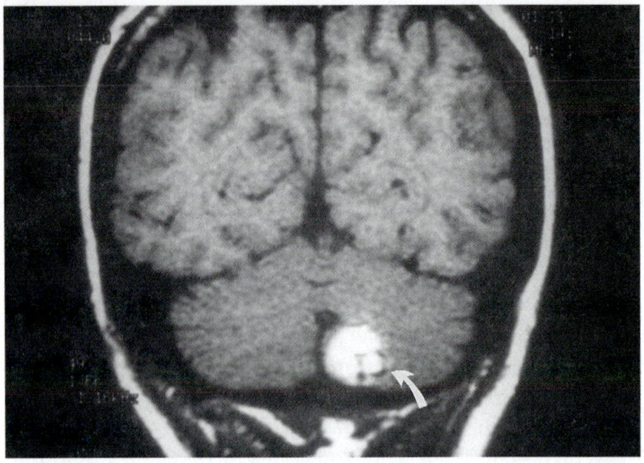

C

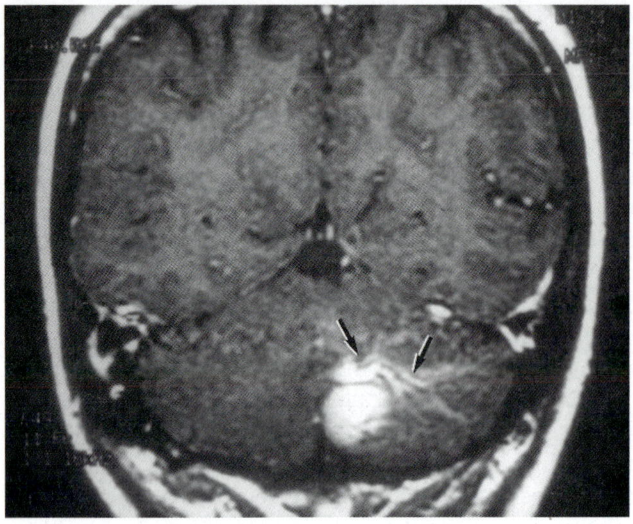

D

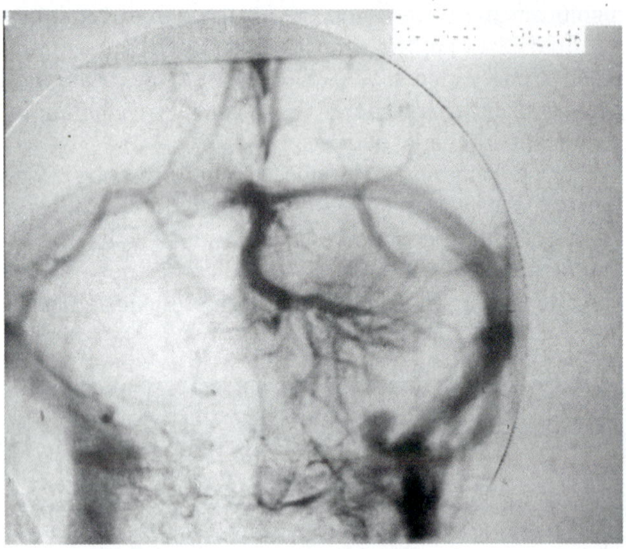

E

Fig. 17.4 *(continued)* (**C**, *curved arrow*) The source of the hemorrhage, a small cavernous malformation, is best seen on the nonenhanced T1-weighted coronal image. **(B)** Note the linear flow void immediately adjacent to the lesion (*arrow*) on the T2-weighted axial image; **(E)** this finding is characteristic for a venous malformation and is confirmed by subsequent catheter angiography. **(D)** The venous malformation is also apparent on the gadolinium-enhanced coronal, T1-weighted image draped over the superior aspect of the hemorrhage (*straight arrows*). It is important to recognize that the venous malformation is not the source of the hemorrhage in this case. Resection or obliteration of the venous malformation, which drains most of the left cerebellar hemisphere, would result in massive venous infarction. The surgical approach chosen for this lesion must allow resection of the cavernous malformation while avoiding injury to the associated venous malformation.

size. The most common presentation (**Table 17.3**) is acute onset of oculomotor motor dysfunction (47%), followed by ataxia/dizziness (37%), sensory disturbances (30%), headache (30%), and motor weakness or spasticity (28%).[18]

The development of symptoms in patients with hemorrhage from cavernous malformations of the CVJ is characteristically acute and maximal at onset. Neurological deficits from the first symptomatic episode of hemorrhage tend to resolve completely as the hemorrhage is organized and absorbed, whereas recurrent hemorrhages are likely to be associated with progressively more severe deficits and an increased risk of permanent neurological impairment. Before the advent of MRI, this stuttering clinical course was frequently mistaken for multiple sclerosis, particularly when lesions involved the lower brainstem.

Table 17.3 Symptom Profile of 62 Cavernous Malformations Involving the Cervicomedullary Junction

Symptom	Number
Ocular motility	47
Ataxia	37
Sensory deficits	31
Headache	31
Motor deficits	28
Facial pain and hyperesthesia	26

Natural History

The natural history of cavernous malformations has become a topic of increasing interest as physicians struggle with management decisions, particularly in patients with minimally symptomatic or deeply seated lesions of the CVJ. The decision of whether to proceed with operative intervention should be based on a clear understanding of the risks of the surgical procedure compared with those of the natural history of the disease.

Numerous studies have been published on the natural history of cavernous malformations. Hemorrhage rates vary widely from series to series depending on the authors' definition of hemorrhage and the population being studied. Not surprisingly, hemorrhage rates tend to be higher in surgical series,

Table 17.4 Methods of Calculating Hemorrhage Rates

Method	Retrospective (assume present from birth)	Prospective (from time from first identification)
Rate per lesion	Retrospective per lesion	Prospective per lesion
Rate per patient	Retrospective per patient	Prospective per patient

as patients with symptomatic lesions are more likely to be referred for neurosurgical intervention. The literature is further complicated by the use of four different methods of calculating hemorrhage rates including retrospective and prospective methods—either of which can be reported as risk of hemorrhage per patient or as risk of hemorrhage per lesion (**Table 17.4**).

The retrospective method assumes that all lesions have been present from birth. Using this assumption, Del Curling and colleagues[11] calculated a symptomatic hemorrhage rate of 0.25% per patient per year. Kondziolka and colleagues[35] reported a rate of 1.3% per patient per year, and Kim and colleagues[36] calculated a rate of 2.3% per patient per year (1.4% per lesion per year). This method of calculation, which depends on the patient's recall to define episodes of hemorrhage and assumes that all lesions are present from birth, is likely to underestimate the actual risk of significant bleeding. Once considered congenital in origin, there is increasing evidence that new lesions may appear de novo in both the sporadic and familial forms of the disease.[22,37,38]

Another confounding factor is the highly variable nature of these lesions. Zabramski and colleagues[22] classified cavernous malformations into four subtypes based on MRI characteristics (**Table 17.5**). These authors and others have found that the risk of hemorrhage appears greatest for type I and type II lesions, which are more likely to be symptomatic.[1,39–43] Most clinical and surgical series are heavily biased toward these two subtypes of lesions, which are readily identified on MRI studies and are frequently symptomatic. These uncertainties emphasize the need to rely on prospective data for the natural history in these patients.

Robinson and colleagues[1] prospectively followed a group of 57 patients with serial clinical examinations and MRI studies for a mean of 26 months and found a risk of symptomatic hemorrhage of 0.7% per lesion per year. Kondziolka and colleagues[35] reported a slightly higher hemorrhage rate of 2.6% per year but noted that the risk of hemorrhage was strongly related to clinical presentation. They prospectively followed 122 patients for a mean of 34 months and found that the hemorrhage rate was significantly lower in patients who presented with incidental lesions: 0.6% per year ($n = 61$) compared with 4.5% per year in those with a history of previous symptomatic hemorrhage ($n = 61$). Aiba and colleagues[39] followed 110 patients with cavernous malformations for a mean of 4.5 years and reported a 0% hemorrhage rate for patients with incidental lesions.

In general, the natural history of cavernous malformations involving the brainstem and the upper cervical cord at the CVJ parallels that of lesions elsewhere in the CNS. However, because of eloquence of the surrounding structures, episodes of hemorrhage (even from relatively small hemorrhages) are much more likely to be symptomatic. A conservative estimate, based on the assumption that lesions are present from birth to first

Table 17.5 Magnetic Resonance Imaging Classification of Cavernous Malformations

Lesion Type	MRI Signal Characteristic	Pathological Characteristics
Type I_A	T1: hyperintense focus of hemorrhage T2: hyper- or hypointense focus of hemorrhage extending through at least one wall of the hypointense rim that surrounds the lesion (Figs. 17.3 and 17.4) Focal edema* may be present (Fig. 17.8)	"Overt" extralesional focus of hemorrhage extending outside the lesion capsule
Type I_B	T1: hyperintense focus of hemorrhage T2: hyper- or hypointense focus of hemorrhage surrounded by a hypointense rim (Fig. 17.5)	Subacute focus of intralesional hemorrhage
Type II	T1: reticulated mixed signal core T2: reticulated mixed signal core surrounded by a hypointense rim (Fig. 17.1 and Fig. 17.2, *straight arrows*)	Loculated areas of hemorrhage and thrombosis of various ages surrounded by gliotic, hemosiderin-stained brain; in large lesions, areas of calcification may be seen
Type III	T1: iso- or hypointense T2: hypointense, with hypointense rim that magnifies the size of lesion GE: hypointense with greater magnification than T2 (Fig. 17.9)	Chronic resolved hemorrhage with hemosiderin staining within and around the lesion
Type IV	T1: poorly seen or not visualized at all T2: poorly seen or not visualized at all GE: punctate hypointense lesions (Fig. 17.9)	Two lesions in the category have been pathologically documented to be telangiectasias

* Focal edema may surround the extralesional portion of hemorrhage in type I_A lesions.

Abbreviations: T1 and T2, T1- and T2-weighted magnetic resonance images, respectively; GE, gradient echo sequences; MRI, magnetic resonance imaging.

Source: Adapted from Feiz-Efran I, Zabramski JM, Kim LJ, Klopfenstein, JD. Natural history of cavernous malformations of the central nervous system. In: Lanzino G, Spetzler RF, eds. Cavernous Malformations of the Brain and Spinal Cord. New York, NY: Thieme Medical Publishers; 2008:3–10.

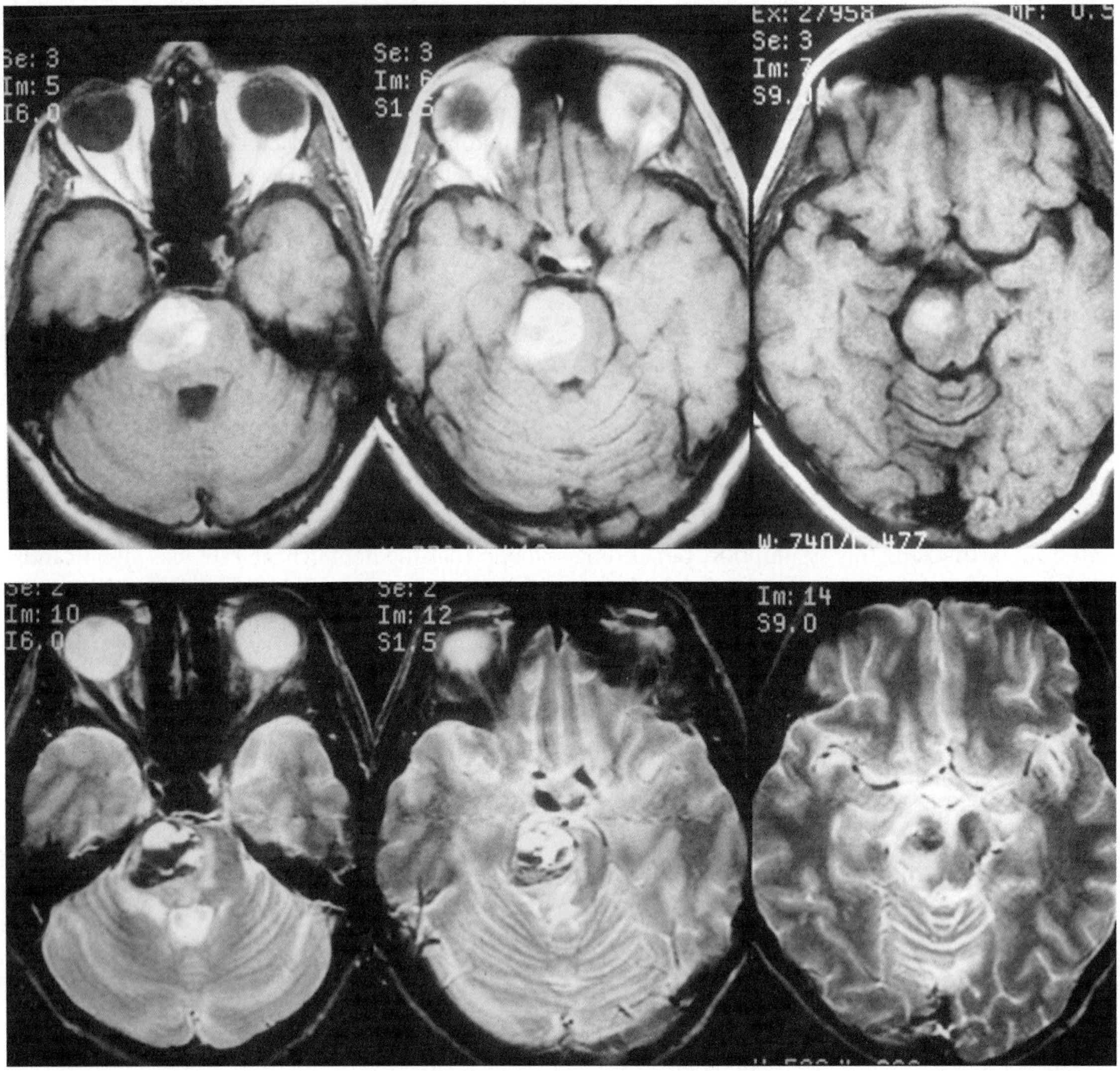

A

B

Fig. 17.5 Magnetic resonance imaging (MRI) in a 34-year-old woman with a 1-week history of sudden onset of left-sided weakness and sensory loss demonstrates findings consistent with a large subacute hemorrhage from a pontine cavernous malformation. Note that the bulk of the subacute hemorrhage—areas of high signal intensity on **(A)** T1-weighted and **(B)** T2-weighted images—lies outside the normal confines of the lesion capsule (ring of low signal intensity) on **(B)** the T2-weighted images. This pattern and the presence of edema on **(B)** the T2-weighted images are consistent with "gross," or extralesional hemorrhage, and are associated with a high risk of recurrent symptomatic bleeding. The area of recent subacute hemorrhage reaches the pial surface on the ventral pons and provides a safe path for surgical excision of the lesion. The hematoma and associated cavernous malformation were removed via an orbitozygomatic approach without complications, and the patient was discharged home in good condition 1 week after surgery. The patient has been symptom-free with no evidence of recurrent hemorrhage or residual lesion during 2 years of follow-up. *(continued)*

symptom, places the risk of symptomatic hemorrhage in the range of 2.5 to 6.8% per year (mean, 4.5% per lesion-year).[35,44–48] This estimate is similar to the 2% per year risk reported by Mathiesen and colleagues[49] in a group of 11 patients with asymptomatic brainstem cavernous malformations who were followed prospectively for a mean of 4 years. For patients who present with a history of previous symptomatic hemorrhage, the risk of rebleeding ranges from 5.1 to 60% (mean, 28.7% per lesion-year),[35,44–47,50] with higher rates reported for those presenting with evidence of recent hemorrhage on MRI.[42,47]

Hemorrhage rates appear to be particularly high in patients who present with acute/subacute bleeding episodes that violate the lesion capsule, producing a so-called "overt," extralesional hemorrhage (type I_A lesion, **Table 17.5**; **Fig. 17.5A,B**) into the surrounding brain. Aiba and colleagues[39] followed 62 such patients for a mean of 3.12 years and noted a risk of recurrent symptomatic hemorrhage of 22.3% per lesion-year. Barker and colleagues[42] reported a similar experience with 141 patients selected for intervention who presented with "overt" hemorrhages. In this series, 63 patients experienced a second hemorrhage before treatment. Hemorrhages clustered around the initial event, with a rehemorrhage rate of 25.2% per year for the first 28 months. Comparable rates of rebleeding have been

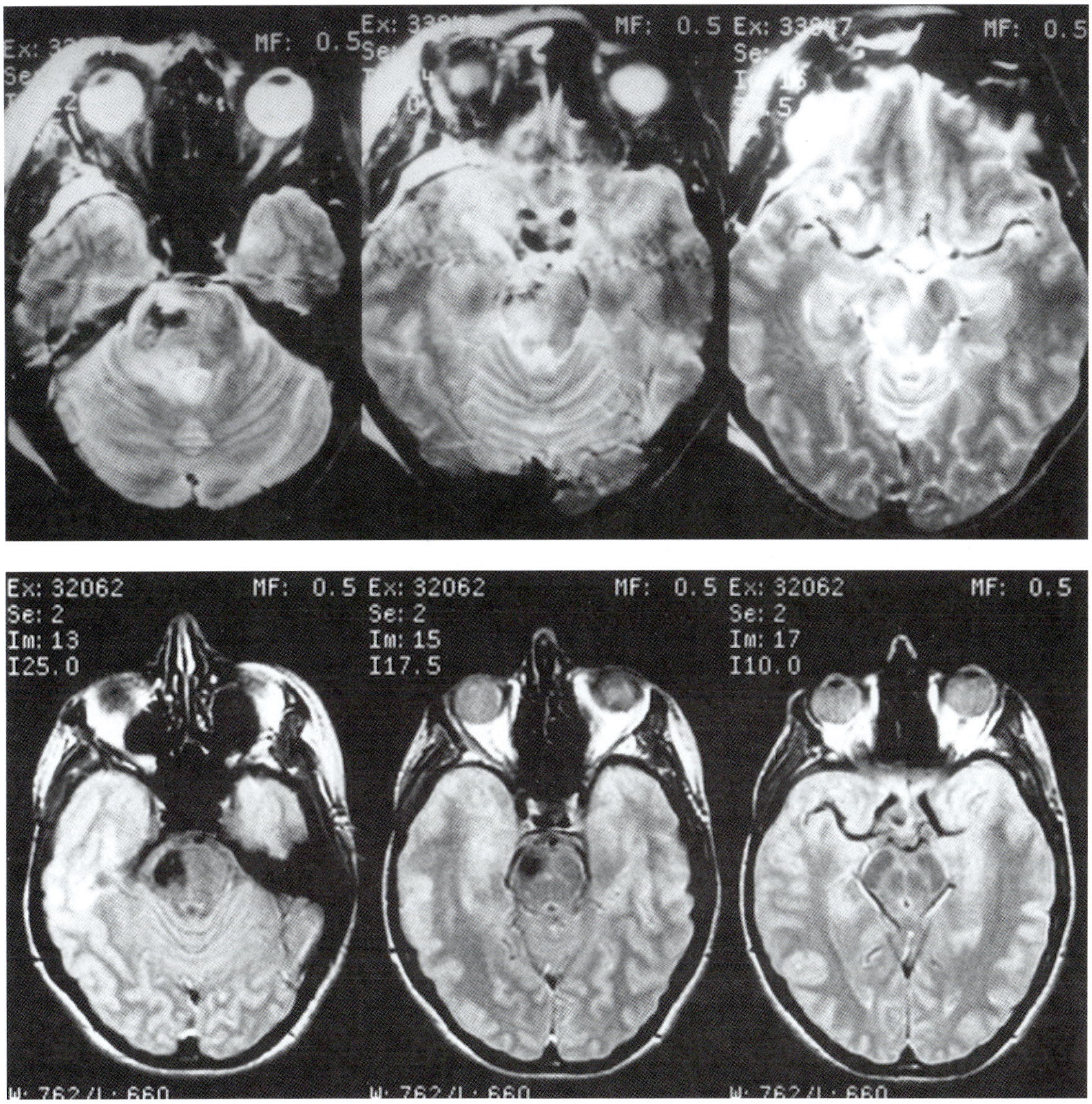

C

D

Fig. 17.5 *(continued)* **(C)** The difficulty in interpreting early postoperative MRI studies is demonstrated by the T2-weighted, spin echo images obtained on the second day after surgery in this patient; edema and blood in the surgical bed produce an image readily confused with residual cavernous malformations. **(D)** The repeat MRI 6 months after surgery reveals only the characteristic low signal signature of hemosiderin associated with chronic resolved hemorrhage on T2-weighted, spin echo images. The absence of any high signal intensity areas within this region on this delayed image confirms the complete resection of the cavernous malformation.

reported following incomplete resection of cavernous malformations, presumably due to interruption of the lesion capsule, stressing the importance of complete resection during the initial surgical procedure.[42,44,50,51]

Management

The surgical management of patients with cavernous malformations, particularly those of the CVJ, must be carefully individualized. Factors affecting the decision of whether to recommend operative resection should include the patient's history, general medical and neurological status, associated findings, and the exact location of the lesion in relation to other CNS structures.[18,23,35,44,52,53] When combined together into an appropriate algorithm, these factors can help guide the surgeon in recommending treatment (**Fig. 17.6**).

As discussed in the previous section, the natural history of asymptomatic cavernous malformations is typically benign. Incidental lesions and those diagnosed during evaluation for nonspecific symptoms such as headache have a low risk of symptomatic hemorrhage—in the range of 0.5 to 1% per year for cerebellar lesions and 2 to 4% per year for those located in the brainstem and spinal cord.

In patients with incidental, asymptomatic CVJ lesions, the best option appears to be observation. Cavernous malformations in such patients are often identified when MRI is

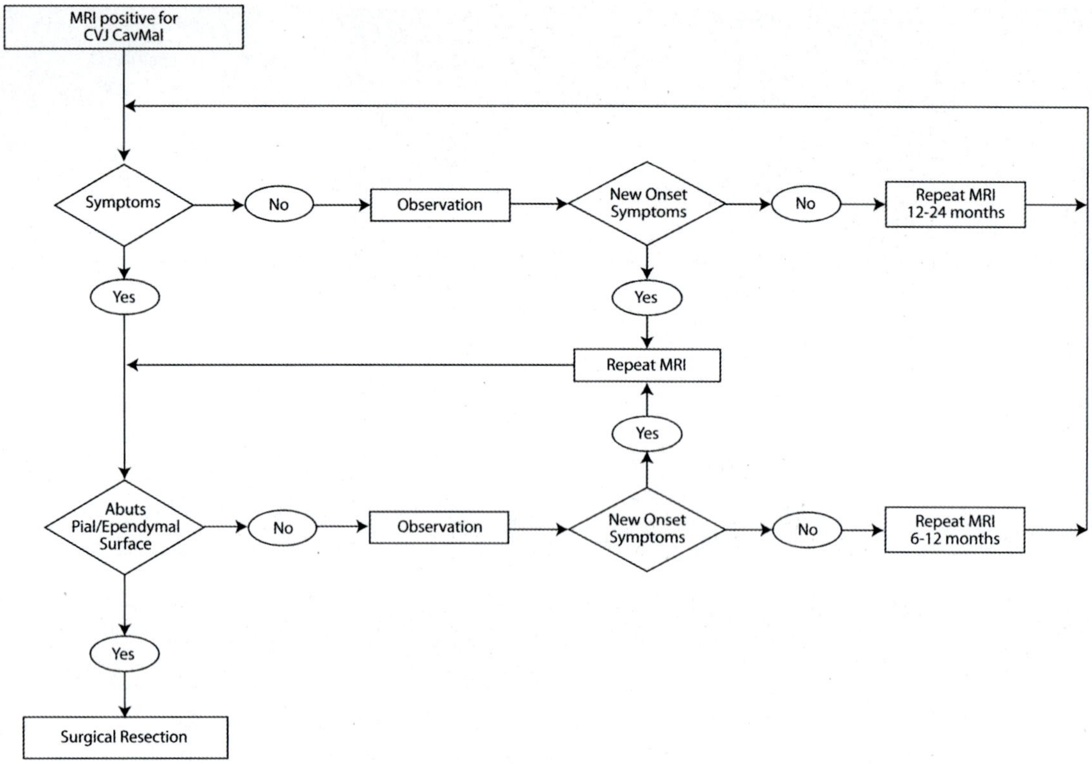

Fig. 17.6 General treatment algorithm for the management of brainstem cavernous malformations. Although surgery is generally reserved for symptomatic lesions, occasional patients present with large minimally symptomatic/asymptomatic lesions that are potential candidates for resection. (Reprinted with permission from Barrow Neurological Institute.)

performed to evaluate headaches or other unrelated problems. Incidental lesions also may be identified in patients being screened for the familial form of the disease. The authors do not consider simple headaches alone as an indication for the removal of these lesions. Patients who are not surgical candidates should be followed with MRI. Our protocol is to evaluate patients with MRI at 1- to 2-year intervals unless there is an exacerbation, or a new onset, of symptoms.

In symptomatic CVJ cavernous malformations, the clinical course, size, and location of the lesion become the important considerations in whether or not to recommend surgery. Often patients are referred for evaluation only after all symptoms from a minor episode of hemorrhage have resolved. In such cases, we will frequently recommend nonoperative management if the lesion is small ($\leq$1 cm) and has caused no symptoms prior to the presenting event. Indications for surgery include a history of multiple symptomatic hemorrhages, MRI characteristics consistent with acute hemorrhage, or an "overt," extralesional hemorrhage (type I and type II lesions; **Table 17.5**), and a location that allows surgical exposure without transgressing normal tissue.[1,11,18,45,52,54] In general, resection of a cavernous malformation of the brainstem should not be considered if the lesion fails to come within 1 to 2 mm of a surgically accessible pial or ependymal surface (**Fig. 17.7**). The greater tolerance of the cerebellum to surgical manipulation allows a more aggressive approach to the management of lesions in this area. As a rule, we prefer to excise all symptomatic cerebellar lesions.

Surgical Considerations

The decision of whether to recommend surgery for any CVJ lesion must include a thoughtful assessment of the operative risks. For cavernous malformations located in the lower brainstem and CVJ, the risks are markedly increased. Early postoperative morbidity for brainstem lesions is high, ranging from 29 to 67% in larger surgical series. Fortunately, many complications are transient and resolve or improve. In a recent review of the literature on brainstem cavernous malformations, Gross and colleagues[55] noted that across 35 publications (316 patients), long-term outcome was improved in 71%, the same in 19%, and worse in 10%, with a mortality rate of 1.9%.

Porter and colleagues[45] reviewed the Barrow Neurological Institute (BNI) experience with 100 patients harboring brainstem cavernous malformations. Altogether, the 100 patients harbored 103 brainstem lesions: 39 in the pons, 16 in the midbrain, 16 in the medulla, 15 in the pontomesencephalic junction, 10 in the pontomedullary junction, and 2 in the midbrain–thalamic region, and 5 lesions involved more than two brainstem levels. Eight-six patients underwent surgical resection of their lesions. In the immediate

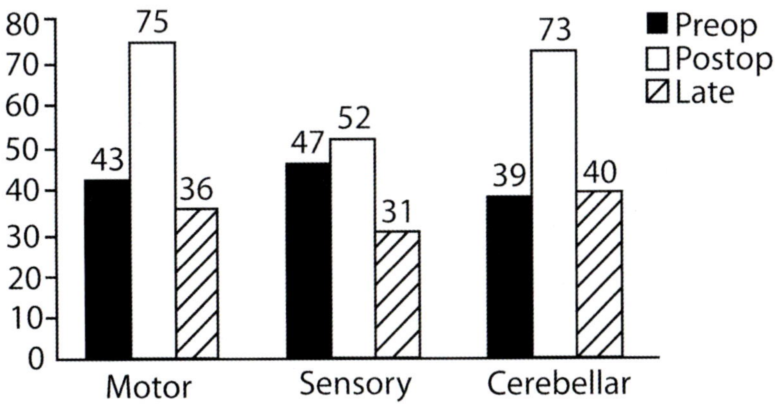

Fig. 17.7 Bar graph illustrating the surgical outcome in a series of 86 patients from the authors' institution who underwent resection of brainstem cavernous malformations.[45] Increased deficits were common in the early postoperative period (mean 7 days); however, the majority of patients improved on delayed follow-up (mean 35 months). Two patients were lost to follow-up, and nine died. (Reprinted with permission from Barrow Neurological Institute.)

postoperative period, 58% of patients had new or worsened neurological deficits; 28 patients (33%) had one or more new cranial nerve deficits; new-onset weakness was observed in 25 patients (29%); and cerebellar findings were observed in 26 (30%). Combinations of deficits were common (**Fig. 17.7**). At late follow-up (mean of 35 months), most patients had improved; permanent postoperative deficits were documented in 10 of the 86 patients (12%). There were three deaths in the early postoperative period, creating a 30-day surgical mortality rate of 3.5%.

The management of cavernous malformations involving the floor of the fourth ventricle requires additional comment. Although long-term outcome is usually good, early postoperative deficits are often significant. Transient internuclear ophthalmoplegia and deficits involving the sixth and seventh cranial nerves are frequent. The need for transient tracheostomy, feeding tube, or both can be expected in 13 to 20% of these patients, and the possibility of sudden death related to Ondine's curse needs to be kept in mind.[45] In the BNI series reported by Porter and colleagues,[45] 2 of 14 patients (14%) with cavernous malformations excised through the floor of the fourth ventricle died of unexplained cardiopulmonary arrest (one at 5 days and the other 2 weeks after surgery), and two patients (both with lesions beneath the facial colliculus) were worse at long-term follow-up. Ferroli and colleagues also noted increased deficits in this group. They reported that 36% of their patients with fourth ventricle lesions were worse at long-term follow-up.[50] Respect for the floor of the fourth ventricle is crucial, with surgical resection considered only for symptomatic lesions that clearly abut the ependymal surface.

MRI is the study of choice for surgical planning. Heavily T1-weighted MRIs should be used to determine whether the lesion approaches a pial or ependymal surface and for stereotactic location. T1-weighted images are the most anatomically accurate and least prone to artifact. In contrast, T2-weighted and gradient echo images tend to significantly overestimate the size of these lesions and may give the false impression that a cavernous malformation approaches a pial/ependymal surface when, in fact, it does not.

The choice of surgical approach for resection of a cavernous malformation should minimize trauma to normal tissue. A good technique for defining the best or "ideal" approach to a lesion is the simple two-point method (**Fig. 17.8**).[56] The line of this "ideal" approach should allow access to the center of the mass while passing through a point in the lesion that comes closest to the pial or ependymal surface of the brain or spinal cord. The approach defined by this two-point method is then modified, taking into account the

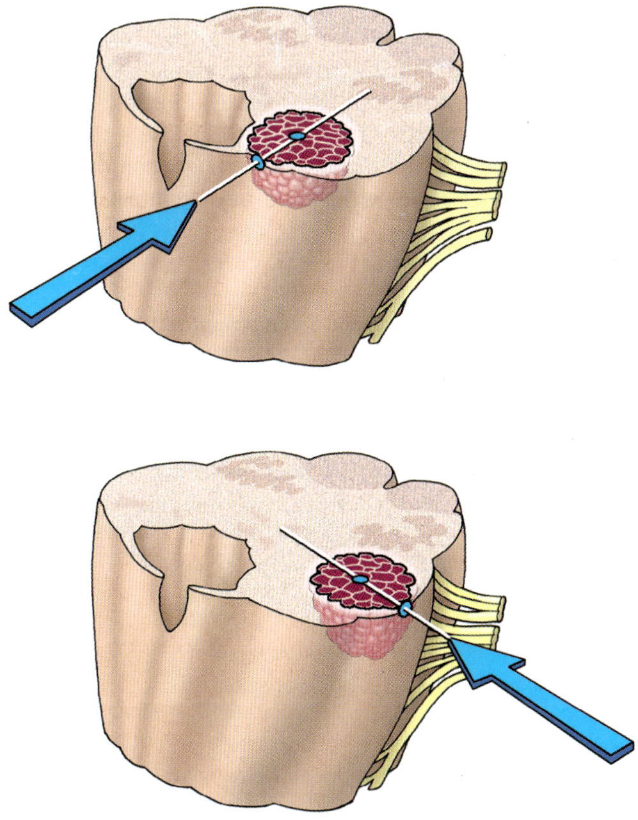

Fig. 17.8 Diagram of the two-point method for selecting a surgical approach to vascular malformations of the posterior fossa and brainstem. Note the two points used to define the line for the best surgical approach: the center of the lesion and the pial/ependymal contact point. (Reprinted with permission from Barrow Neurological Institute.)

risks of neurological impairment. For example, a far-lateral retrolabyrinthine approach would be used in a patient with intact hearing, even though a translabyrinthine approach might provide a more ideal exposure. We routinely use a frameless stereotactic system to help localize the lesion for surgical resection.

Familiarity with the various posterior fossa and skull base approaches is key in planning the resection of these lesions. The authors' recommended approach to cavernous malformations at various brainstem locations is listed in **Table 17.6**. We believe that the translabyrinthine and transcochlear exposures are rarely indicated in these patients. A retrolabyrinthine approach, combined with a far-lateral exposure if needed, is sufficient for the vast majority of anteriorly and anterolaterally situated cerebellopontine angle lesions. The details of the surgical approaches to this region are covered elsewhere in this text, in the chapters devoted to surgical techniques.

In our experience and that of others, surgery should be performed early after hemorrhage, as soon as the patient's condition has stabilized. Resection is easier in the acute or subacute stage after hemorrhage, before the hematoma resolves, leaving in its place a dense gliotic capsule. Surgical resection of cavernous malformations is performed using routine microsurgical techniques. Because the lesions are low-flow, hemostasis is readily maintained. In larger lesions, the center can be resected, allowing the walls to collapse in and minimizing trauma to the adjacent brain. Microsurgical instruments, particularly multiple sizes of round knifes, are useful for freeing the capsule of the lesion. The hemosiderin-stained junction between the lesion and the normal brainstem should be left intact, and the capsule of the malformation should be used as the plane of dissection.

Care should be taken to avoid damage to any large venous channels associated with the lesion. When a venous malformation is identified in association with a cavernous malformation, the operative approach should be modified to allow resection of the cavernous malformation without interruption of the main trunk of the venous malformation. If the main trunk is damaged, or coagulated, venous infarction of the brainstem or cerebellum may result in devastating consequences.

After the malformation has been removed, the lesion cavity should be carefully inspected for any remnants. Partial resection of cavernous malformations appears to be associated with a higher risk of hemorrhage and relatively rapid recurrence of symptoms. The risk of symptomatic recurrence may be as high as 25% per year.[39] Early postoperative MRI to check for residual lesion can be difficult to interpret.

Delayed imaging at 3 to 6 months is recommended to rule out residual cavernous malformation and at 12 to 24 months to check for recurrence. This policy of delayed MRI after surgical excision developed after several negative surgical re-explorations at our institution. MRI soon after surgery (2 to 3 days) had demonstrated areas of mixed signal intensity suggestive of residual lesion (**Fig. 17.5C**). At surgery, this appearance was found to be the result of a mixture of blood and CSF within the lesion cavity that slowly resolved over several months. It is important to note that the ring of low signal intensity, which is secondary to hemosiderin deposition, remains indefinitely around the surgical cavity (**Fig. 17.5D**).

Table 17.6 Lesion Location and Surgical Approach Preference

Brainstem Segment	Surgical Approach
Midbrain	
Cerebral peduncle	Orbitozygomatic
Tectum or posterolateral midbrain	Supracerebellar-infratentorial
Midbrain–thalamic	Supracerebellar-infratentorial
Pontomesencephalic junction	Supracerebellar-infratentorial
Pons	
Cerebellopontine angle	Retrosigmoid
Lateral/anterior basis pontis	Retrosigmoid or supracerebellar-infratentorial
Floor of fourth ventricle	Suboccipital
Middle cerebellar peduncle (medial)	Suboccipital-telovelar
Middle cerebellar peduncle (lateral)	Retrosigmoid
Pontomedullary junction	Retrosigmoid or far-lateral
Medulla and cervicomedullary junction	Suboccipital or far-lateral

Radiosurgery

The indications for stereotactic radiosurgery in the management of cavernous malformations remain controversial. In a recent editorial, Steiner and colleagues[57] thoughtfully reviewed the radiosurgery literature available through January 2010 and concluded that "the 20 year-old debate remains unresolved." They noted that although there is some evidence from retrospective studies that radiosurgery may reduce the risk of rebleeding, treatment has also been associated with a significant risk of complications. If all 15 studies reporting the results of radiosurgery for cavernous malformations are considered, treatment-related complications occurred in 19% of cases, and about one-half of the complications were permanent.[58–72]

Another major issue contributing to the ongoing debate regarding the effectiveness of radiosurgery for this indication is the absence of radiologically demonstrated improvements after treatment. Unlike AVMs, in which gradual obliteration of the lesion is the rule, cavernous malformations rarely show improvement after radiosurgery. In fact, the only changes typically seen are adverse effects related to radiation-induced injury in the surrounding brain, resolution of a prior hemorrhage, or an occasional new hemorrhage.[73] The

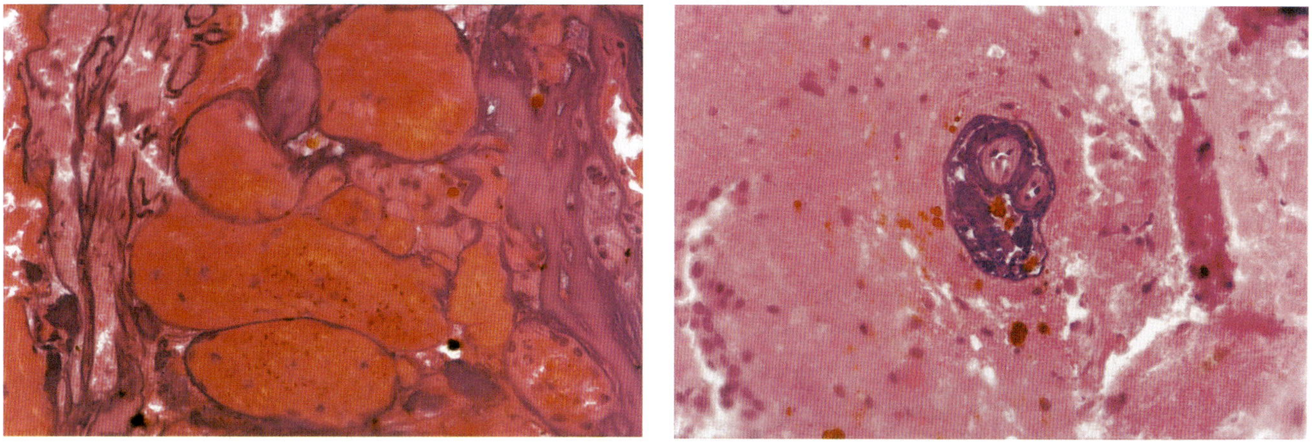

A B

Fig. 17.9 **(A)** Hematoxylin and eosin–stained photomicrograph of a cavernous malformation treated with radiation therapy 10 years prior to its excision for repeated hemorrhage. Note the absence of radiation changes. The cavernous channels within the lesion appear normal with no evidence of endothelial hypertrophy. **(B)** In contrast, extensive radiation changes are noted in the vessels of the normal brain surrounding the cavernous malformation, including endothelial hypertrophy, marked thickening of the muscularis layer, and extravascular sclerosis.

beneficial effect of radiosurgery is limited to a reported reduction in the risk of recurrent bleeding soon after symptomatic hemorrhage; however, it is well recognized that there is a persistent risk of hemorrhage of 1 to 2% per year even years after radiosurgery treatment. Opponents of radiosurgery argue that this persistent risk of hemorrhage is evidence that cavernous malformations are resistant to radiation.

The rationale for the use of radiosurgery and other forms of ionizing radiation for the treatment of cavernous malformations is based on its success in the obliteration of small AVMs. However, there are fundamental differences in the structure of AVMs and cavernous malformations that alter the response to radiation. Unlike AVMs, the vascular channels of cavernous malformations are lined by a single layer of vascular endothelium with no associated basement membrane or smooth muscle cells. Radiation effects on these latter components of the vessel walls are believed to account for a large portion of the narrowing and obliteration of AVM vessels. Pathological examination of a cavernous malformation resected at the authors' institution 10 years after treatment with 5000 rads of focal radiation revealed no significant endothelial cell damage (**Fig. 17.9**), whereas in the normal brain surrounding the lesion there was evidence of vessel obliteration secondary to marked endothelial hyperplasia and hypertrophy. These findings provide additional support for the argument above that suggests that cavernous malformations are resistant to radiation treatment.

Until a prospective, randomized trial is available, radiosurgery cannot be recommended for these lesions.

Conclusion

Management of CNS cavernous malformations should consider the natural history of the lesions and the risks of any proposed treatment. Most lesions grow and produce symptoms as a result of repeated episodes of intralesional hemorrhage and thrombosis. For cavernous malformations of the CVJ, these intralesional hemorrhages tend to be asymptomatic until the lesion reaches a critical size and irritates or compresses adjacent neurological structures. For patients with incidental lesions, the risk of symptomatic hemorrhage is no more than 2 to 4% per year. Once a lesion has become symptomatic, the risk of recurrent symptomatic hemorrhage increases. Recurrent intralesional hemorrhages tend to produce small stepwise increases in deficits. In patients presenting with evidence of "gross" hemorrhage outside the lesion capsule, the risks of repeat hemorrhage may be as high as 25 to 30% per year.

Surgical risks are related to the exact location of the lesion and are highest for lesions that involve the lower brainstem, particularly the floor of the fourth ventricle, and are least for those that involve the cerebellar hemispheres. Overall, mortality and permanent morbidity rates related to the surgical resection of brainstem lesions are in the range of 10 to 15%.

Surgical resection is recommended for all patients with recurrent or persistent symptoms from lesions within 1 to 2 mm of a pial/ependymal surface. When symptoms have resolved observation should be considered, particularly for small lesions (<1 cm) and those in difficult surgical locations. The treatment algorithm in **Fig. 17.6** summarizes these recommendations. A more aggressive approach can be considered for cerebellar lesions, as the surgical risks are considerably less.

Regardless of the location of the lesion, care should be taken to avoid injury to the venous anomalies that are frequently associated with cavernous malformations. If a venous malformation and cavernous malformation are present together in a patient with symptomatic hemorrhage, the cavernous malformations should be resected and the venous malformation should be left intact.

References

1. Robinson JR, Awad IA, Little JR. Natural history of the cavernous angioma. J Neurosurg 1991;75(5):709–714
2. Awad IA, Robinson JR Jr, Mohanty S, Estes ML. Mixed vascular malformations of the brain: clinical and pathogenetic considerations. Neurosurgery 1993;33(2):179–188, discussion 188
3. Robinson JR Jr, Awad IA, Masaryk TJ, Estes ML. Pathological heterogeneity of angiographically occult vascular malformations of the brain. Neurosurgery 1993;33(4):547–554, discussion 554–555
4. Jellinger K. Vascular malformations of the central nervous system: a morphological overview. Neurosurg Rev 1986;9(3):177–216
5. Rigamonti D, Spetzler RF. Cerebral vascular malformations. BNI Q 1987;3(3):18–28
6. Russell DS, Rubinstein LJ. Pathology of Tumors of the Nervous System. 4th ed. Baltimore, MD: Williams & Wilkins; 1977
7. McCormick WF. Pathology of vascular malformations of the brain. In: Wilson CB, Stein BM, eds. Intracranial Arteriovenous Malformations. Baltimore, MD: Williams & Wilkins; 1984:44–63
8. Robinson JR Jr, Awad IA, Zhou P, Barna BP, Estes ML. Expression of basement membrane and endothelial cell adhesion molecules in vascular malformations of the brain: preliminary observations and working hypothesis. Neurol Res 1995;17(1):49–58
9. Sarwar M, McCormick WF. Intracerebral venous angioma. Case report and review. Arch Neurol 1978;35(5):323–325
10. Otten P, Pizzolato GP, Rilliet B, Berney J. [131 cases of cavernous angioma (cavernomas) of the CNS, discovered by retrospective analysis of 24,535 autopsies]. Neurochirurgie 1989;35(2):82–83, 128–131
11. Del Curling O Jr, Kelly DL Jr, Elster AD, Craven TE. An analysis of the natural history of cavernous angiomas. J Neurosurg 1991;75(5):702–708
12. Vernooij MW, Ikram MA, Tanghe HL, et al. Incidental findings on brain MRI in the general population. N Engl J Med 2007;357(18):1821–1828
13. Zabramski JM, Feiz-Erfan I. Natural history of cavernous malformations. In: Winn HR, ed. Youmans Neurological Surgery. 6th ed. Philadelphia, PA: Elsevier; 2010
14. Hsu FPK, Rigamonti D, Huhn SL. Epidemiology of cavernous malformations. In: Awad IA, Barrow DL, ed. Cavernous Malformations. Park Ridge, IL: American Association of Neurological Surgeons; 1993:13–23
15. Acciarri N, Padovani R, Pozzati E, Gaist G, Manetto V. Spinal cavernous angioma: a rare cause of subarachnoid hemorrhage. Surg Neurol 1992;37(6):453–456
16. Mehdorn HM, Stolke D. Cervical intramedullary cavernous angioma with MRI-proven haemorrhages. J Neurol 1991;238(8):420–426
17. Scott RM. Brain stem cavernous angiomas in children. Pediatr Neurosurg 1990-1991;16(6):281–286
18. Zabramski JM, Kawaguchi S, Spetzler RF. Management of brainstem cavernous malformations. Contemp Neurosurg 1994;16(11):1–5
19. McCormick WF, Hardman JM, Boulter TR. Vascular malformations ("angiomas") of the brain, with special reference to those occurring in the posterior fossa. J Neurosurg 1968;28(3):241–251
20. Fahlbusch R, Strauss C, Huk W, Röckelein G, Kömpf D, Ruprecht KW. Surgical removal of pontomesencephalic cavernous hemangiomas. Neurosurgery 1990;26(3):449–456, discussion 456–457
21. Itoh J, Usui K. Cavernous angioma in the fourth ventricular floor—case report. Neurol Med Chir (Tokyo) 1991;31(2):100–103
22. Zabramski JM, Wascher TM, Spetzler RF, et al. The natural history of familial cavernous malformations: results of an ongoing study. J Neurosurg 1994;80(3):422–432
23. Amin-Hanjani S, Ogilvy CS, Ojemann RG, Crowell RM. Risks of surgical management for cavernous malformations of the nervous system. Neurosurgery 1998;42(6):1220–1227, discussion 1227–1228
24. Liquori CL, Berg MJ, Siegel AM, et al. Mutations in a gene encoding a novel protein containing a phosphotyrosine-binding domain cause type 2 cerebral cavernous malformations. Am J Hum Genet 2003;73(6):1459–1464
25. Bergametti F, Denier C, Labauge P, et al; Société Française de Neurochirurgie. Mutations within the programmed cell death 10 gene cause cerebral cavernous malformations. Am J Hum Genet 2005;76(1):42–51
26. Liquori CL, Berg MJ, Squitieri F, et al. Low frequency of PDCD10 mutations in a panel of CCM3 probands: potential for a fourth CCM locus. Hum Mutat 2006;27(1):118
27. Davenport WJ, Siegel AM, Dichgans J, et al. CCM1 gene mutations in families segregating cerebral cavernous malformations. Neurology 2001;56(4):540–543
28. Laberge-le Couteulx S, Jung HH, Labauge P, et al. Truncating mutations in CCM1, encoding KRIT1, cause hereditary cavernous angiomas. Nat Genet 1999;23(2):189–193
29. Sahoo T, Johnson EW, Thomas JW, et al. Mutations in the gene encoding KRIT1, a Krev-1/rap1a binding protein, cause cerebral cavernous malformations (CCM1). Hum Mol Genet 1999;8(12):2325–2333
30. Denier C, Goutagny S, Labauge P, et al; Société Française de Neurochirurgie. Mutations within the MGC4607 gene cause cerebral cavernous malformations. Am J Hum Genet 2004;74(2):326–337
31. Voigt K, Yaşargil MG. Cerebral cavernous haemangiomas or cavernomas. Incidence, pathology, localization, diagnosis, clinical features and treatment. Review of the literature and report of an unusual case. Neurochirurgia (Stuttg) 1976;19(2):59–68
32. Little JR, Awad IA, Jones SC, Ebrahim ZY. Vascular pressures and cortical blood flow in cavernous angioma of the brain. J Neurosurg 1990;73(4):555–559
33. Rigamonti D, Drayer BP, Johnson PC, Hadley MN, Zabramski J, Spetzler RF. The MRI appearance of cavernous malformations (angiomas). J Neurosurg 1987;67(4):518–524
34. Rigamonti D, Spetzler RF. The association of venous and cavernous malformations. Report of four cases and discussion of the pathophysiological, diagnostic, and therapeutic implications. Acta Neurochir (Wien) 1988;92(1-4):100–105
35. Kondziolka D, Lunsford LD, Kestle JR. The natural history of cerebral cavernous malformations. J Neurosurg 1995;83(5):820–824
36. Kim DS, Park YG, Choi JU, Chung SS, Lee KC. An analysis of the natural history of cavernous malformations. Surg Neurol 1997;48(1):9–17, discussion 17–18
37. Labauge P, Laberge S, Brunereau L, Levy C, Tournier-Lasserve E. Hereditary cerebral cavernous angiomas: clinical and genetic features in 57 French families. Société Française de Neurochirurgie. Lancet 1998;352(9144):1892–1897
38. Zabramski JM, Henn JS, Coons S. Pathology of cerebral vascular malformations. Neurosurg Clin N Am 1999;10(3):395–410
39. Aiba T, Tanaka R, Koike T, Kameyama S, Takeda N, Komata T. Natural history of intracranial cavernous malformations. J Neurosurg 1995;83(1):56–59
40. Labauge P, Brunereau L, Laberge S, Houtteville JP. Prospective follow-up of 33 asymptomatic patients with familial cerebral cavernous malformations. Neurology 2001;57(10):1825–1828
41. Labauge P, Brunereau L, Lévy C, Laberge S, Houtteville JP. The natural history of familial cerebral cavernomas: a retrospective MRI study of 40 patients. Neuroradiology 2000;42(5):327–332
42. Barker FG II, Amin-Hanjani S, Butler WE, et al. Temporal clustering of hemorrhages from untreated cavernous malformations of the central nervous system. Neurosurgery 2001;49(1):15–24, discussion 24–25
43. Yoon PH, Kim DI, Jeon P, Ryu YH, Hwang GJ, Park SJ. Cerebral cavernous malformations: serial magnetic resonance imaging findings in patients with and without gamma knife surgery. Neurol Med Chir (Tokyo) 1998;38(Suppl):255–261

44. Fritschi JA, Reulen HJ, Spetzler RF, Zabramski JM. Cavernous malformations of the brain stem. A review of 139 cases. Acta Neurochir (Wien) 1994;130(1-4):35–46
45. Porter RW, Detwiler PW, Spetzler RF, et al. Cavernous malformations of the brainstem: experience with 100 patients. J Neurosurg 1999;90(1):50–58
46. Kupersmith MJ, Kalish H, Epstein F, et al. Natural history of brainstem cavernous malformations. Neurosurgery 2001;48(1):47–53, discussion 53–54
47. Sandalcioglu IE, Wiedemayer H, Secer S, Asgari S, Stolke D. Surgical removal of brain stem cavernous malformations: surgical indications, technical considerations, and results. J Neurol Neurosurg Psychiatry 2002;72(3):351–355
48. Wang CC, Liu A, Zhang JT, Sun B, Zhao YL. Surgical management of brain-stem cavernous malformations: report of 137 cases. Surg Neurol 2003;59(6):444–454, discussion 454
49. Mathiesen T, Edner G, Kihlström L. Deep and brainstem cavernomas: a consecutive 8-year series. J Neurosurg 2003;99(1):31–37
50. Ferroli P, Sinisi M, Franzini A, Giombini S, Solero CL, Broggi G. Brainstem cavernomas: long-term results of microsurgical resection in 52 patients. Neurosurgery 2005;56(6):1203–1212, discussion 1212–1214
51. Jain KK, Robertson E. Recurrence of an excised cavernous hemangioma in the opposite cerebral hemisphere. Case report. J Neurosurg 1970;33(4):453–456
52. Robinson JR Jr, Awad IA, Magdinec M, Paranandi L. Factors predisposing to clinical disability in patients with cavernous malformations of the brain. Neurosurgery 1993;32(5):730–735, discussion 735–736
53. Zimmerman RS, Spetzler RF, Lee KS, Zabramski JM, Hargraves RW. Cavernous malformations of the brain stem. J Neurosurg 1991;75(1):32–39
54. Rigamonti D. Natural history of cavernous malformations, capillary malformations (telangiectases), and venous malformations. In: Barrow DL, ed. Intracranial Vascular Malformations. Park Ridge, IL: The American Association of Neurological Surgeons; 1990:45–51
55. Gross BA, Batjer HH, Awad IA, Bendok BR. Brainstem cavernous malformations. Neurosurgery 2009;64(5):E805–E818, discussion E818
56. Brown AP, Thompson BG, Spetzler RF. The two-point method: evaluating brain stem lesions. BNI Q 1996;12(1):20–24
57. Steiner L, Karlsson B, Yen CP, et al. Radiosurgery in cavernous malformations: anatomy of a controversy. J Neurosurg 2010;113(1):16–21
58. Amin-Hanjani S, Ogilvy CS, Candia GJ, Lyons S, Chapman PH. Stereotactic radiosurgery for cavernous malformations: Kjellberg's experience with proton beam therapy in 98 cases at the Harvard Cyclotron. Neurosurgery 1998;42(6):1229–1236, discussion 1236–1238
59. Chang SD, Levy RP, Adler JR Jr, Martin DP, Krakovitz PR, Steinberg GK. Stereotactic radiosurgery of angiographically occult vascular malformations: 14-year experience. Neurosurgery 1998;43(2):213–220, discussion 220–221
60. Hasegawa T, McInerney J, Kondziolka D, Lee JY, Flickinger JC, Lunsford LD. Long-term results after stereotactic radiosurgery for patients with cavernous malformations. Neurosurgery 2002;50(6):1190–1197, discussion 1197–1198
61. Huang YC, Tseng CK, Chang CN, Wei KC, Liao CC, Hsu PW. LINAC radiosurgery for intracranial cavernous malformation: 10-year experience. Clin Neurol Neurosurg 2006;108(8):750–756
62. Karlsson B, Kihlström L, Lindquist C, Ericson K, Steiner L. Radiosurgery for cavernous malformations. J Neurosurg 1998;88(2):293–297
63. Kida Y, Kobayashi T, Tanaka T. Treatment of symptomatic AOVMs with radiosurgery. Acta Neurochir Suppl (Wien) 1995;63:68–72
64. Kim DG, Choe WJ, Paek SH, Chung HT, Kim IH, Han DH. Radiosurgery of intracranial cavernous malformations. Acta Neurochir (Wien) 2002;144(9):869–878, discussion 878
65. Kim MS, Pyo SY, Jeong YG, Lee SI, Jung YT, Sim JH. Gamma knife surgery for intracranial cavernous hemangioma. J Neurosurg 2005;102(Suppl):102–106
66. Liscák R, Vladyka V, Simonová G, Vymazal J, Novotny J Jr. Gamma knife surgery of brain cavernous hemangiomas. J Neurosurg 2005;102(Suppl):207–213
67. Liu KD, Chung WY, Wu HM, et al. Gamma knife surgery for cavernous hemangiomas: an analysis of 125 patients. J Neurosurg 2005;102(Suppl):81–86
68. Mitchell P, Hodgson TJ, Seaman S, Kemeny AA, Forster DM. Stereotactic radiosurgery and the risk of haemorrhage from cavernous malformations. Br J Neurosurg 2000;14(2):96–100
69. Pollock BE, Garces YI, Stafford SL, Foote RL, Schomberg PJ, Link MJ. Stereotactic radiosurgery for cavernous malformations. J Neurosurg 2000;93(6):987–991
70. Stea RA, Schicker L, King GA, Winfield JA. Stereotactic linear radiosurgery for cavernous angiomas. Stereotact Funct Neurosurg 1994;63(1-4):255–265
71. Tsien C, Souhami L, Sadikot A, et al. Stereotactic radiosurgery in the management of angiographically occult vascular malformations. Int J Radiat Oncol Biol Phys 2001;50(1):133–138
72. Zhang N, Pan L, Wang BJ, Wang EM, Dai JZ, Cai PW. Gamma knife radiosurgery for cavernous hemangiomas. J Neurosurg 2000;93(Suppl 3):74–77
73. Blamek S, Boba M, Larysz D, et al. The incidence of imaging abnormalities after stereotactic radiosurgery for cerebral arteriovenous and cavernous malformations. Acta Neurochir Suppl (Wien) 2010;106:187–190

18 Radiosurgical Management of Lesions of the Craniovertebral Junction

Alia Hdeib and Andrew E. Sloan

Tumors of the craniovertebral junction (CVJ) pose a challenge for the clinician because their anatomical location makes them difficult to access. Treatment, both surgical and nonsurgical, can be associated with significant morbidity from injury to surrounding neurovascular structures as well as from biomechanical instability at the CVJ.[1,2] The main goals of treatment of cranial base tumors of the CVJ are relief of neurological symptoms, eradication of tumor progression and recurrence, and preservation of structural stability.[2] Ideally, these objectives should be achieved with the least degree of morbidity allowed by the treatment modality, which can be difficult for pathology in this area given the local anatomy. Stereotactic radiosurgery (SRS) has become a popular treatment method for numerous neurological conditions, both as adjuvant and primary therapy. For many lesions of the CVJ, SRS offers a means of safe treatment for local control of skull base lesions that are not easily surgically curable.

Numerous radiosurgical delivery systems are available, including cobalt-60 (i.e., Gamma Knife) and linear accelerator (LINAC) based systems. Some systems typically require frame placement and are primarily used for single fraction radiosurgery, whereas others can be used in a frameless fashion to deliver up to five fractions of SRS or for additional fractions in intensity modulated radiation therapy (IMRT) mode. For some radioresistant tumors, proton beam therapy is an emerging treatment modality. This chapter reviews the experience, safety, and efficacy of these radiosurgical delivery systems for various lesions of the CVJ.

Historical Aspects and General Principles of Radiosurgery

The history of radiosurgery dates back to the 1950s in Stockholm, Sweden, where Lars Leksell developed a means of precise delivery of a single high dose of radiation capable of noninvasive destruction of deep tissue in the cranium.[3] As it evolved, SRS became particularly useful for lesions not easily accessible or safely amenable to open surgical intervention. Today the indications for radiosurgery have evolved to more complex patient treatment algorithms.

Radiosurgery was first performed with the first Gamma Knife unit (Elekta, Stockholm, Sweden) in the 1960s in Sweden.[3] The Gamma Knife used a cobalt-60 source to produce gamma rays that converge on a central point that represents the pathology of interest. In this unit, the head is rigidly fixed in a collimator helmet, with the target lesion more or less in the center of the helmet. Unlike radio**therapy**, which is typically practiced by radiation oncologists, radio**surgery** is surgical in intent and relies on spatial accuracy and precision with the goal of ablation of a precise target by utilizing a sharp dose fall-off to spare adjacent normal tissue.[4] Conversely, radio**therapy** relies on the "four Rs" of reoxygenation, reassortment, repopulation, and repair to slow neoplastic growth in a generalized region of the brain while minimizing damage to surrounding brain based on the principles of dosimetry.[5] Essentially, radiosurgery is surgery for which the surgeon utilizes ionizing radiation rather than mechanical energy (via the edge of a scalpel blade) to remove or destroy tumor with surgical precision. As Leksell noted:

> The term stereotactic radio**surgery** has been used deliberately to stress the fact that this combination of mechanically directed instruments and modern radiation physics is still **surgery**, albeit using another physical agent in place of the knife or radiofrequency heat lesion... The Gamma Unit merely represents a change in the type of energy used... the same condition may be treated best in one patient with microsurgery and in another by stereota[ctic surgery]... The simplicity of using the Gamma Unit makes this integration possible... Someone competent in both techniques is best fitted to decide where the boundaries between the two methods should lie.[3]
>
> Because radiosurgery is used as a surgical tool, SRS is typically performed by a multidisciplinary team comprised of a neurosurgeon, a radiation oncologist, a radiation physicist, and a radiology technician.

The Gamma Knife uses a 192–201 photon cobalt-60 source delivery system that emits gamma ray photons as high-energy beams. These beams converge on a central target point, which is the only location where enough energy is produced to promote tissue destruction through absorption of radiation. Tissue destruction generally occurs over weeks to months.[6] Typically, the goal of radiosurgery using the Gamma Knife is to construct a treatment plan that exposes the entire lesion to the prescription dose of radiation at the 50% isodose line while keeping the dose to brainstem and other critical structures below tolerated levels. Numerous reports have detailed the use of the Gamma Knife for treatment of the CVJ.[1,7,8]

In the 1980s, neurosurgeons and radiation oncologists began modifying linear accelerators to perform radiosurgery for cranial lesions, including those of the CVJ.[9,10] While there are some differences in technique and custom, including the practice of treating lesions at the 70 to 90% isodose line rather than the 50% isodose line, the general principles of radiosurgery using LINAC systems are the same as those for Gamma Knife. An additional advantage is that various LINAC systems developed bite blocks to allow radiosurgery without a head frame.[11] However, concerns about the precision and reproducibility of this approach somewhat limited their widespread utilization, particularly for lesions near critical structures such as the brainstem and the optic nerve.

The CyberKnife SRS system (Accuray Inc., Sunnyvale, CA), developed by neurosurgeon John Adler, is a LINAC-based system with an integrated industrial robot that compensates for the lack of precision and reproducibility inherent in the frameless devices and for the potential for patient movement.[12–14] This compensation is achieved by incorporating a real-time imaging system to check for changes from planning or "ideal" position, which then allows the robot to adjust the beam in compensation.[12–14] An orthogonal pair of X-ray cameras takes images seconds before beams are delivered at each nodal position by a dynamic robot-mounted LINAC with six degrees of freedom. These images are then reconstructed into a digitally reconstructed radiograph (DRR) that compares them to the ideal or planning position at the time of planning and adjusts for variations in *x*, *y*, and *z* coordinates as well as *pitch*, *yaw*, and *roll*. The robotic arm then makes the required adjustments to target the radiation beams to the lesion with a spatial accuracy of 1.1 mm.[15] BrainLAB (Westchester, IL), in cooperation with Varian Medical Systems, has developed a gantry-mounted LINAC system called Novalis Tx that utilizes DRR to similarly target and track movement of the cranium and spine.[16] Finally, TomoTherapy (Accuray Inc.) incorporates an axial computed tomography scanner into a gantry-based LINAC system to image and compensate for changes in position of the cranium and spine.[17] Numerous reports have detailed the efficacy of these devices for the treatment of lesions of the CVJ.[18–22]

Although frame-based radiosurgical technologies, including Gamma Knife and many LINAC-based systems, are limited to the treatment of lesions of the cranium and high cervical spine, the CyberKnife and Novalis systems are also capable of radiation delivery with high accuracy to lesions throughout the spine.[14,23] These developments have enabled routine radiosurgical treatment of CVJ lesions that extend into the lower cervical spine. In addition, this frameless technology allows for fractionation of radiation, which is difficult to do with frame-based systems because of the morbidity of frame placement and because even slight changes in positioning/repositioning of the frame might account for major changes in the treatment plan. More recently, several of the frame-based platforms have developed bite blocks to allow fractionation using conventional platforms.

The radiobiology of radio**surgery** also differs somewhat from conventional radio**therapy**. Radiotherapy relies on delivery of radiation over large intracranial volumes that include normal brain structures. Fractionation is employed because normal brain repairs damage between fractions to a greater extent than do tumor cells.[4] Conversely, radiosurgery delivers the entire dose of radiation in one to five fractions, and these small numbers of high-dose fractions provide approximately three times the biological effectiveness of fractionated conventional treatment.[4] However, dose inhomogeneity is a noted part of Gamma Knife treatment in which the center of a target receives more radiation than the periphery.[6] In general, SRS is limited for tumors less than 3.5 cm in size because treatment of larger volumes may minimize the precision of radiosurgery and increasing the fall-off can put surrounding normal tissues at risk of receiving high radiation doses.

However, like conventional radiotherapy, radiosurgery, whether a single fraction or up to five fractions, is typically delivered on an outpatient basis. On the day of treatment, a rigid stereotactic head frame, mouthpiece, or mask is placed, helping to stabilize the target and eliminate subcentimeter patient movement. In addition, the frame provides exact coordinates for target and treatment plan localization. Before placement, patients are appropriately medicated. In frame-based radiosurgery, the frame is attached to the skull via pins inserted on the frame: two frontal and two occipital. This procedure is performed by a neurosurgeon, usually with the administration of local anesthetic and mild sedation. Sometimes a bite block is used as a substitute for frame placement, particularly when fractionated stereotactic radiosurgery (FxSRS) is contemplated. After frame placement, image acquisition is performed.

Radiosurgery is comprised of two stages: planning and delivery. Planning for radiosurgery cases involves a combined effort between a neurosurgeon, radiation oncologist, and medical physicist. In general, the images are transferred to treatment planning software and the quality of the images is reviewed, which can be done by the physicist or one of the clinicians. If the quality is accurate, the images are co-registered with the frame or whatever non–frame-based reference system will be used. Co-registration is generally done by the neurosurgeon, often with support of the medical physicist. Finally, the target lesion as well as the critical anatomical or functional regions to avoid are contoured by the neurosurgeon with the treatment planning system software (**Fig. 18.1**). Various collimator sizes that correspond to the diameter of the beam are available (4, 8, 14, and 18 mm for Gamma Knife). In addition, the beam can be more precisely "shaped" using various other approaches unique to each treatment platform. Examples include hybrid collimators in the new Gamma Knife Perfection, the adjustable IRIS used in the CyberKnife system, and the beam-shaping software, which employs mini microleaf collimators used by BrainLAB and Varian. Typically, to maximize conformality and minimize dose to surrounding normal structures, multiple versions of the plan are made as the plan gets more refined. The net effect is a highly conformal treatment plan that precisely demarcates the lesion to be treated. The radiation oncologist and neurosurgeon then choose a treatment dose based on conformality, treatment effect on surrounding normal structures, and radiation sensitivity of the pathology being treated.

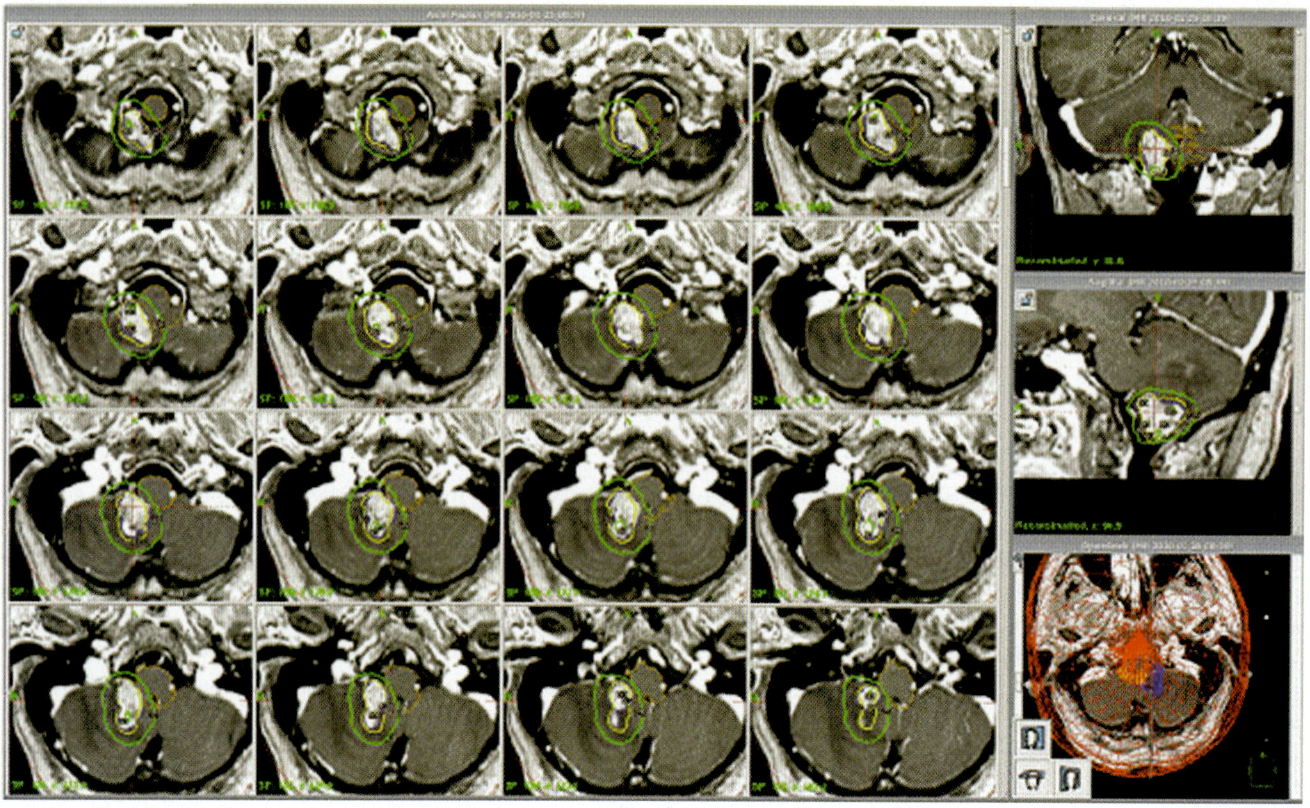

Fig. 18.1 Treatment planning for a breast cancer metastasis to the brain. The patient received 12 Gy to the 50% isodose line.

The goal of radiosurgery is control of the tumor rather than the complete elimination that might be achieved with conventional surgery. Thus, treatment selection is critical. Large tumors in accessible locations or those associated with clinical symptoms are preferentially treated surgically; smaller tumors and those in less accessible locations as well as those in older, more debilitated patients are often treated with radiosurgery with the goal of tumor control rather than tumor elimination.

It has been increasingly recognized that tumor biology is also relevant to radiosurgical treatment. Malignant tumors require higher radiation doses, whereas benign tumors require less. As treatment volume increases, the dose delivered is lowered to prevent adverse reactions to the surrounding normal tissues. Different dose regimens are used for specific tumors, and data are often extrapolated from the experiences previously reported in the literature. Dose-volume histograms should be carefully examined to determine whether the dose planning is safe, and the conformality of the treatment plan should also be carefully reviewed.[6] Although most patients are safely treated with radiosurgery, it is important to note that radiosurgery is not without risk. Adverse effects include skin reactions, tissue swelling, and severe radiation necrosis. Radiation necrosis is generally due to the surrounding normal brain reacting to the death of tumor cells, and some necrosis of normal tissue surrounding previously irradiated tumors can also be responsible for this phenomenon.[6,24] Radiation necrosis is usually noted 6 to 24 months after initial radiation.[24] Treatment is generally conservative with corticosteroids, but some patients with significant symptoms may require surgical resection of the areas of radiation necrosis. Recent studies suggest that hyperbaric oxygen, anticoagulation, and/or bevacizumab may be efficacious in the treatment of radiation necrosis, but these methods remain controversial.[25] The risk of developing radiation reactions is dose-volume dependent and related to the dose of normal rather than abnormal tissues.

Although planning SRS treatment shares many commonalities across platforms, treatment may vary with the platform selected. Gamma Knife requires a stereotactic frame, which fits precisely in a helmet containing the collimators. The helmet and patient are then rolled into the Gamma Knife unit where the cobalt-60 sources sit, and the frame is moved around in the helmet to align the various "shots" that have been planned for the tumor. In the most recent versions, these movements are performed robotically by moving the frame itself (Version 4C) or moving the entire treatment couch (Perfection). In contrast, LINAC systems utilize photons produced by accelerating electrons along a linear path that collide with a tungsten target plate producing 6-MV X-rays for treatment.[10] Unlike the

Table 18.1 Treatment Delivery Platforms

Platform	Description	Practice Application	Special Features
Elekta Leksell Gamma Knife (Stockholm, Sweden)	192–201 cobalt-60 sources arranged in a hemispherical pattern Frame-based	SRS	Hybrid collimator in the new Leksell Gamma Knife Perfection System; new bite block
Elekta Synergy (Stockholm, Sweden)	LINAC-based, multileaf collimator, high-resolution beam shaping Conformal arc	IMRT	3D X-ray volume imaging during treatment delivery
Varian/BrainLAB Novalis Tx (Westchester, IL)	Powerful LINAC–6–20 MV High-definition multileaf collimator for beam shaping	SRS IMRT	RapidArc SRS with faster treatment time
Radionics Xknife (Integra, Plainsboro, NJ)	LINAC-based multileaf collimator Frameless and frame-based	SRS SRT IMRT	Relocatable head ring (noninvasive) for fractionated SRT
Accuray CyberKnife (Sunnyvale, CA)	LINAC-based Continual image guidance and robotic arm mobility	SRS SRT IMRT	Frameless system Full-body radiosurgery Respiratory tracking system, bony anatomy tracking
TomoTherapy (Accuray, Sunnyvale, CA)	LINAC LINAC with built-in CT	SRS SRT IMRT	Identifies and compensates for changes in position of the cranium and spine
Varian Proton Beam Therapy (Palo Alto, CA)	Proton-based charged particle therapy	SRS	Delivery of higher doses, Bragg peak effect

Abbreviations: 3D, three-dimensional; CT, computed tomography; LINAC, linear accelerator; SRS, stereotactic radiosurgery; SRT, stereotactic radiotherapy; IMRT, intensity modulated radiation therapy.

Gamma Knife in which radiation sources are stationary, LINAC systems typically move in a rotational arc around the patient's head and the bed changes positions, which changes the gantry and delivery angles and results in numerous noncoplanar arcs around the patient's head.[26] Lastly, the CyberKnife utilizes a smaller LINAC mounted on an industrial robot arm that tracks the patient's movements in a near real-time fashion and "paints" the tumor with ionizing beams in a noncoplanar fashion from one of the 400 nodal points in its firing range with six degrees of freedom.[12]

In some of the more advanced systems, such as BrainLAB/Varian and CyberKnife, mini-multileaf collimators can be used to shape the radiation beam for optimal conformality. Increasingly, LINAC systems allow for use of bite blocks and masks, resulting in reproducible positioning and immobilization, which also allows for dose fractionation. Thus, many LINAC platforms are capable of FxSRS as well as fractionated image-guided radiotherapy, unlike frame-based systems, which are used primarily for single fraction SRS.[4] Currently available treatment platforms are presented in **Table 18.1** for comparison.

Stereotactic Radiosurgery for Lesions of the Craniovertebral Junction

Tumors of the foramen magnum pose a challenge for invasive surgical treatment because they are difficult to access and intervention is associated with high morbidity, usually due to cranial nerve palsies as well as vascular and brainstem injury. Radiosurgery provides an attractive treatment option for these tumors, both as an adjunct to microsurgical resection, in the case of residual or recurrent tumor, and as an alternative option (e.g., for elderly patients with comorbidities).[1] However, the use of frame-based platforms such as the Gamma Knife has historically been limited anatomically by the foramen magnum and CVJ. Modifications to frame placement to allow for treatment of these low-lying tumors have been described, and several manufacturers have designed modifications to their platforms to accommodate this challenge.[27] LINAC-based designs have been less subject to these limitations, and recent versions have enabled these devices to treat tumors extending lower than the foramen and to compensate for cervical spine movements.

Although radiosurgery for lesions of the CVJ is not as well described as for lesions in other locations, the safety and efficacy for radiosurgery for various types of axial and extra-axial cranial tumors is starting to be better delineated in the literature.[28,29] Dosimetry and tumor control have been defined for intra-axial tumors (e.g., gliomas, metastases) and extra-axial tumors (e.g., meningiomas, schwannomas, and neurofibromas) in various regions of the brain. The data can be extrapolated, and similar dosimetry and radiosurgery principles can be applied to neoplasms of the same type, even when they occur at the CVJ (**Figs. 18.2** and **18.3**). The main distinction in this location is that care must be given to surrounding critical structures, including the brainstem and cranial nerves.

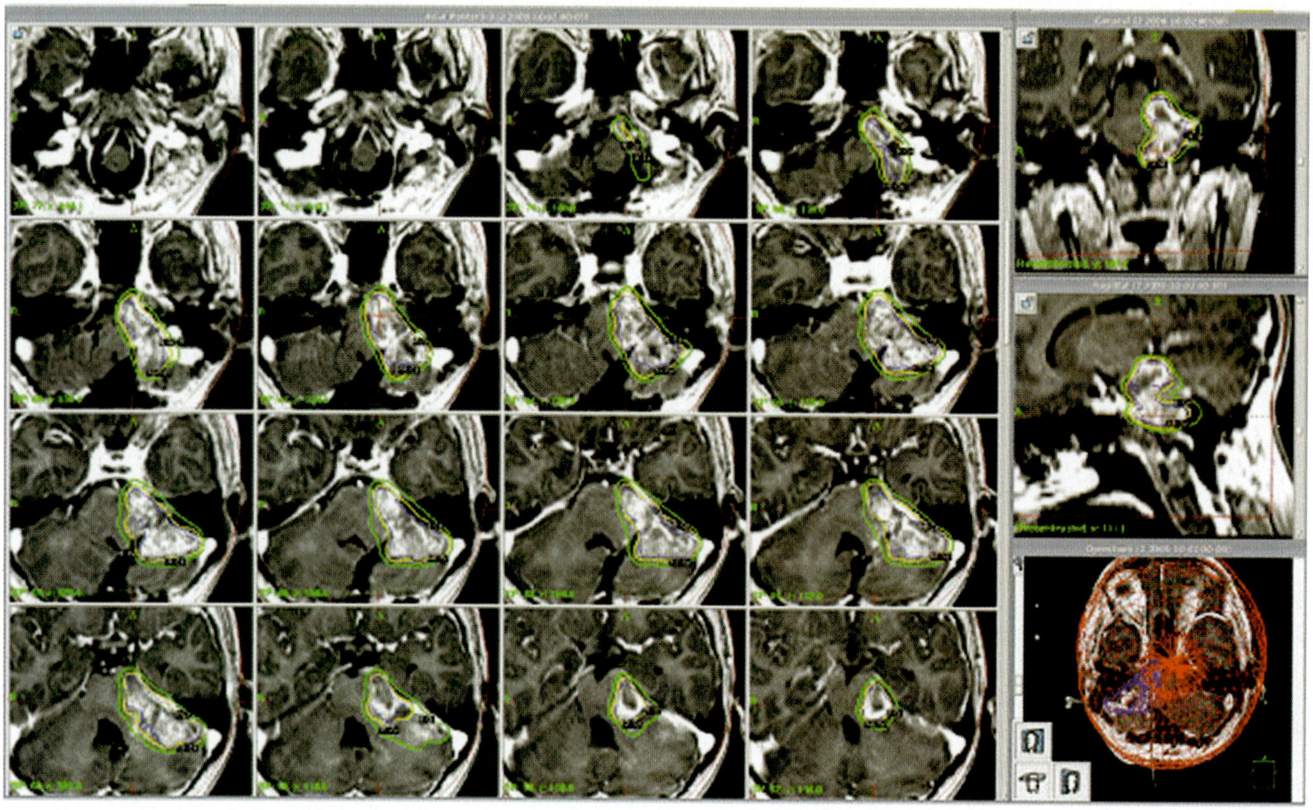

Fig. 18.2 Treatment planning for a residual ependymoma. The patient received 10 Gy to the 50% isodose line.

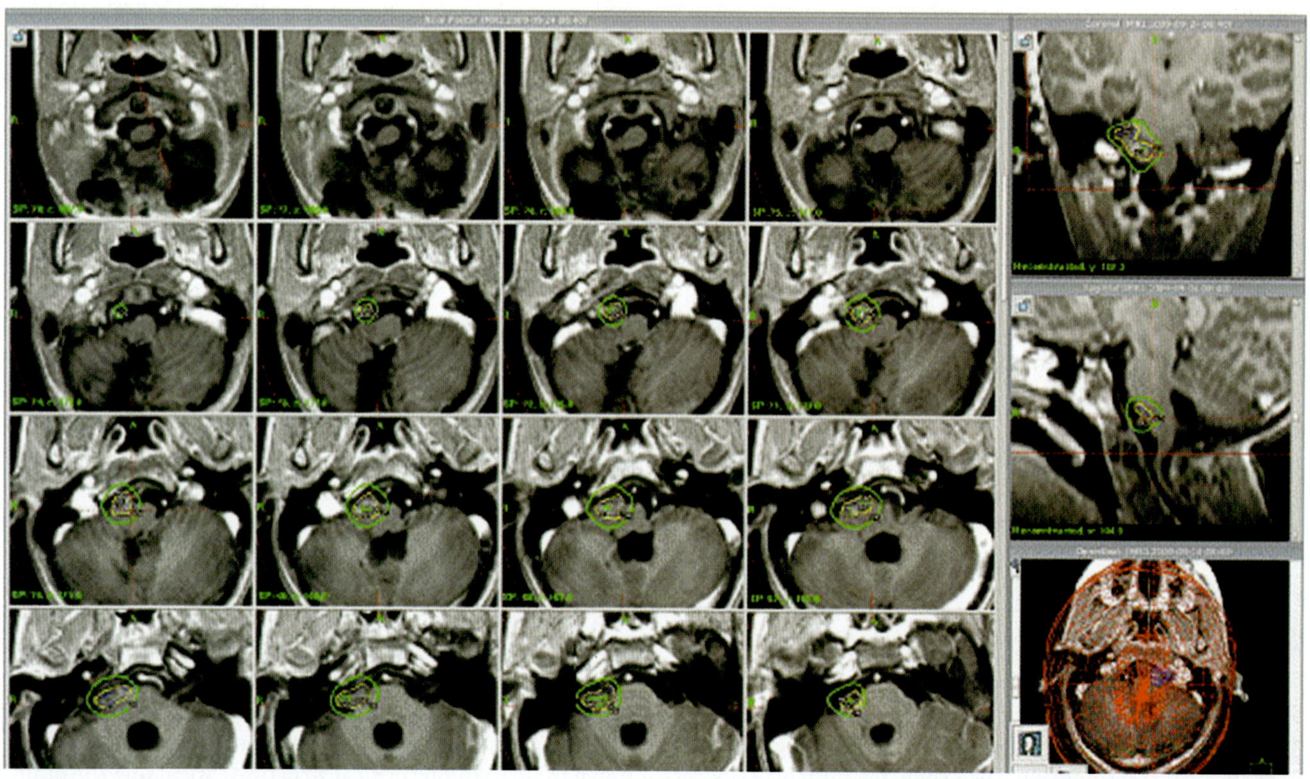

Fig. 18.3 Treatment planning for a pediatric patient with a recurrent ependymoma. The patient was treated with 12 Gy to the 50% isodose line.

Stereotactic Radiosurgery for Neoplasms

Recently, Cheshier and colleagues reported their experience with frameless radiosurgery treatment of foramen magnum lesions, demonstrating that this type of treatment is an effective option for these tumors.[19] Thirty-five patients with lesions either directly at the foramen magnum or spanning the CVJ, including benign and malignant tumors (meningiomas, schwannomas, neurofibromas, hemangioblastomas, ependymomas, astrocytomas, chordomas, chondrosarcomas, and metastases), underwent radiosurgical treatment. Twenty-three percent of patients were asymptomatic at the time of treatment, whereas 77% had referable signs and symptoms, most commonly cranial nerve XII dysfunction. The size of the lesions determined the fractionation schedule, with a mean of 1.8 sessions (range of 1–5 sessions). The mean dose was 19 gray (Gy). Radiographic follow-up was achieved in 66% of patients and, of these, 39% showed stabilization of their tumor size, 43% had a decrease in their tumors, and 17% showed an increase. Data on 69% of patients were analyzed in terms of symptom relief, with 75% of those patients having their symptoms stabilized or improved and 25% showing continued clinical worsening. Mortality was reported as 31% in this series, with eight deaths due to the primary disease although not directly related to the radiosurgical treatment, and three deaths due to intercurrent illness. Side effects were reported in the 11% range and included one patient with temporary emesis after treatment, one case of cystic tumor enlargement 2 months after treatment, and two patients with radiation necrosis 1.5 to 2.5 years after treatment.[19]

Other investigators describe their institutional experience with SRS for posterior fossa meningiomas. Nicolato and colleagues reported on a series of 57 patients with 62 posterior fossa meningiomas who were treated with Gamma Knife radiosurgery.[30] Of these, 26 were in the foramen/jugular/petrous bone area, 23 were petroclival, 6 were in the cerebellum, and 1 was solely confined to the foramen magnum region. Fifty-five percent of tumors showed tumor reduction, 40% remained stable, and 5% progressed. Several prognostic factors were also analyzed, and the only factor to statistically significantly influence efficacy for control of tumor progression was the histological tumor grade. Transient side effects were noted in 6.5% due to postradiosurgery edema. Four mortalities were reported—two from tumor progression and two from unrelated causes (**Fig. 18.4**).

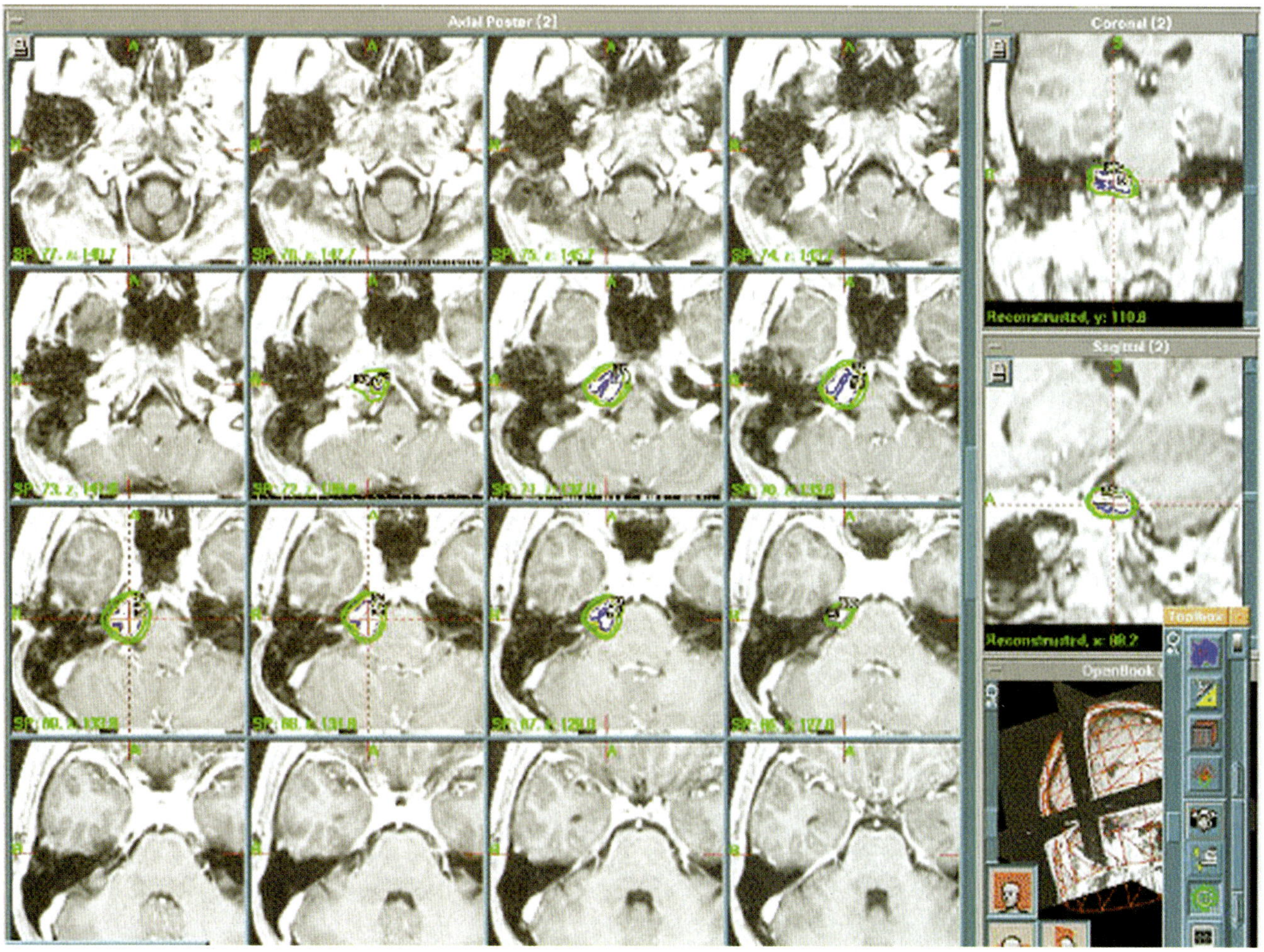

Fig. 18.4 Treatment planning for a right petroclival meningioma. The patient received 12 Gy to the 50% isodose line.

Muthukumar and colleagues published their experience with treatment of anterior foramen magnum meningiomas.[1] In their series, five patients aged 73 to 84 years with foramen magnum meningiomas underwent SRS. Three patients had radiosurgery treatment as an alternative to microsurgery, and the remaining two underwent SRS as an adjuvant to surgery. Median tumor volume was 10.5 mL, with dose ranges from 10 to 16 Gy to the tumor margin. Multiple isocenters were required (mean of 4.4 isocenters) given the irregular morphology of these tumors along the clivus. Follow-up ranged from 1 to 5 years (mean 3 years), with one mortality due to an unrelated disease process. This series showed that in 20% of patients reduction in tumor volume was noted, and in the remaining 80% tumor volume growth was arrested (**Fig. 18.5**).[1]

Chordomas and chondrosarcomas of the skull base are notoriously difficult to treat. Total surgical resection often is not achievable and, although these tumors are slow growing, recurrences and local invasion are inevitable. Several groups have described their experience with stereotactic radiosurgical treatment of these lesions. A recent series by Martin and colleagues reported SRS treatment of 28 patients with chordomas and chondrosarcomas as primary or adjuvant management.[31] Average tumor volume was 9.8 mL, with 16 Gy as the median dose to the tumor margin. Results showed that, at 5 years, local tumor control for chondrosarcomas was 80% and 62.9% for chordomas. The same group had also reported promising results in a series from the 1990s of six patients treated with Gamma Knife.[32] No tumor progression was noted in any of the patients; however, mean follow-up was only 22 months.

Hagesawa and colleagues recently reported the results of radiosurgery treatment in 37 patients (48 treated lesions) with chordomas and chondrosarcomas.[33] Mean tumor volume was 20 mL, mean dose to the tumor margin was 14 Gy, and patient follow-up averaged 59 months. The 5-year and 10-year survival rates were 80% and 53%, respectively, for all patients, with 76% and 67% reported for local tumor control rates. The study also found that smaller tumor volume (e.g., <20 mL) correlated with better local disease control. As with previous studies, this series shows that adjuvant SRS is safe and effective in tumor control for the follow-up periods indicated in each study.

Henderson and colleagues evaluated the efficacy and safety of radiosurgery using the CyberKnife platform for chordoma treatment in a series of 18 patients with a total of 24 lesions, mostly as adjuvant treatment.[20] Forty-four percent of the tumors were spinal, 39% were cranial, and 17% were sacral. Mean tumor volume was 128 mL, with a

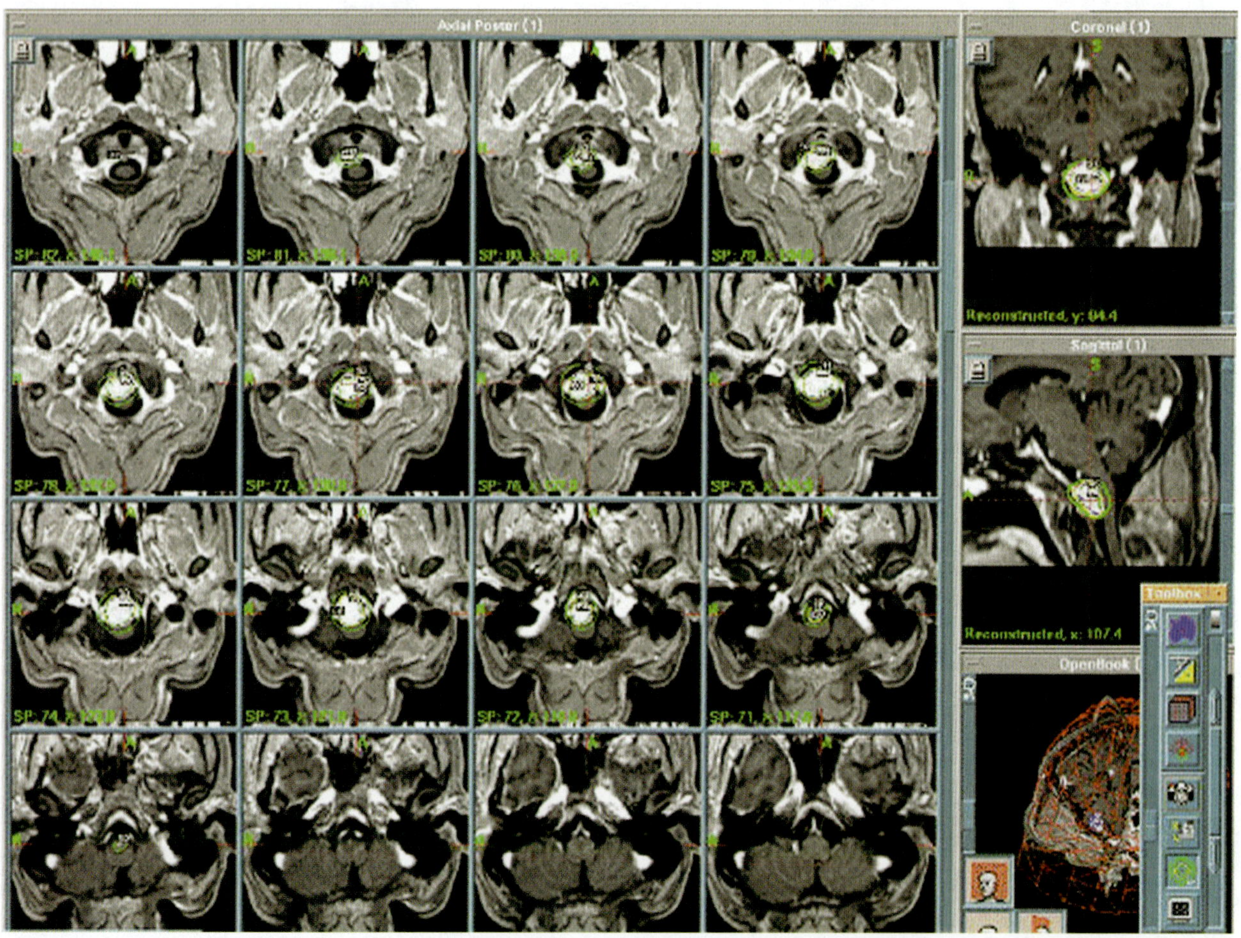

Fig. 18.5 Treatment planning for a meningioma of the anterior foramen magnum. The patient received 10 Gy to the 50% isodose line.

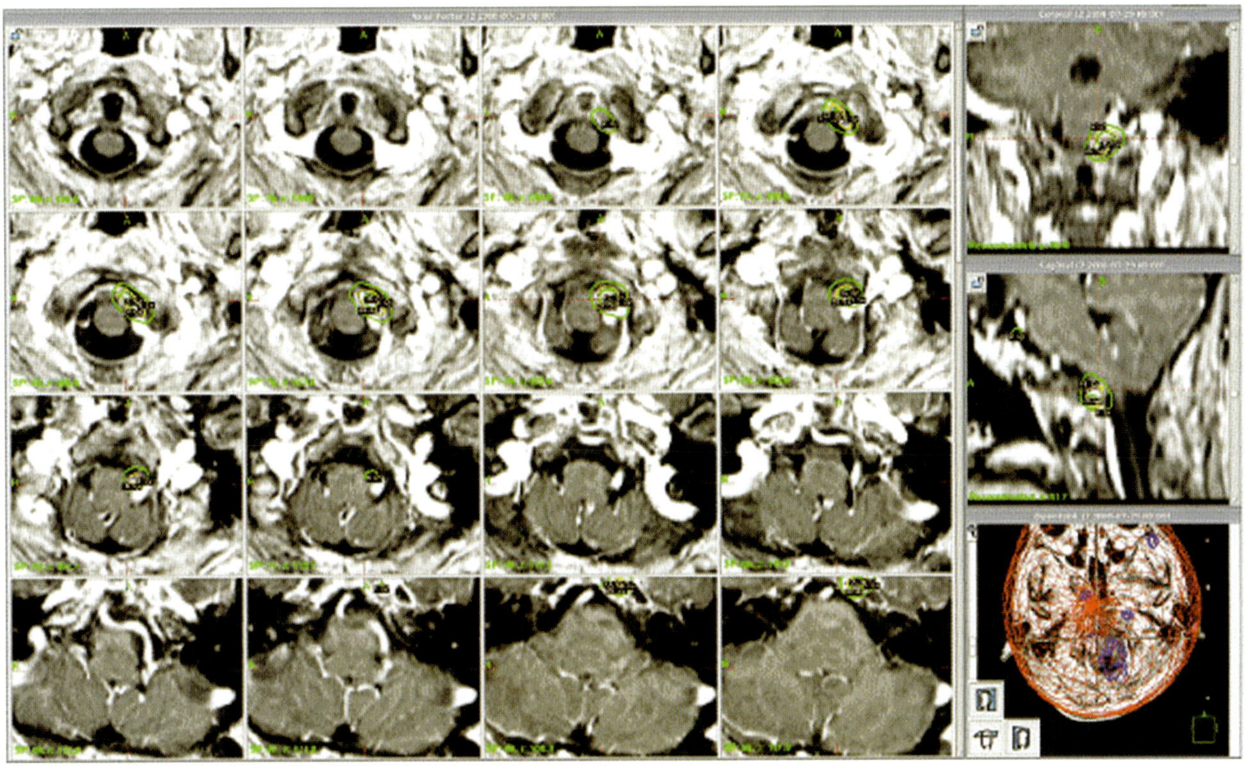

Fig. 18.6 Treatment planning for a chordoma of the clivus, treated with 15 Gy to the 50% isodose line.

median dose of 35 Gy fractionated over five sessions. Median follow-up was 46 months. Seven patients had a recurrence within a median of 10 months, and four patients succumbed to their disease during the study period. Three patients experienced complications, including infection at the previous surgical/radiation site in two patients and decreased vision in one patient. In this series, the local tumor control rate at 65 months was 59.1%, and overall survival was 74.3% with 88.9% disease-specific survival. The authors of the study advocate a regimen of 40 Gy to the tumor volume and an approximate 1-cm margin fractionated over five sessions.

A series from the Mayo Clinic recently reported efficacy of SRS for chordomas and chondrosarcomas and evaluated treatment side effects.[34] Twenty-nine patients (25 with chordomas and 4 with chondrosarcomas) underwent SRS alone or in combination with radiotherapy (19 patients, mean dose 50.4 Gy). Mean age was 45, median tumor volume was 14.4 mL, median dose to the tumor margin was 15 Gy (with maximum median dose of 30 Gy), and follow-up was >4 years. For chordomas, tumor control rates were 87% and 32% at 2 and 5 years, respectively, and all chondrosarcoma patients had good tumor control at follow-up. Three patients died due to tumor progression. In addition, 2% showed worsening of symptoms during the follow-up period. Thirty-four percent had radiation-related complications that included cranial nerve deficits, pituitary dysfunction, and radiation necrosis. Of note, there were no such side effects in patients who underwent SRS alone. The clinic concluded that radiosurgery is a safe adjunct for treatment of these tumors, but radiation complications are more commonly noted when SRS is used in combination with fractionated radiotherapy. Treatment will depend on pathology and difficulty of tumor control (**Fig. 18.6**).

With the advent of new systems and removable head frames, FxSRS has proven feasible and is increasingly viewed as a management option. One series reported an institutional experience with FxSRS treatment of patients with histologically proven chordomas and chondrosarcomas of the skull base and upper cervical region, as an adjunct to surgical resection.[21] Some of the patients had received previous conventional radiation, and one had previous SRS treatment. Doses to the tumor volume ranged from 21 to 43.6 Gy, delivered over three to five sessions. No significant major side effects or toxicities were noted during the treatment and in the immediate follow-up period, although two patients eventually developed radiation-induced myelopathy. Patients were followed for a median of 24 months. Tumor volume reduction was seen in four patients during the study, and one patient had disease recurrence. Care was taken to minimize radiation to surrounding critical structures within acceptable ranges.

As previously noted, it is important to consider that the slow-growing nature of chordomas and chondrosarcomas can confound the perceived efficacy of radiosurgery/radiotherapy treatment of these tumors, especially because progression can occur over several years. Several authors propose a clinical algorithm of surgical resection followed by adjuvant radiation/SRS for local residual disease control for chordomas and chondrosarcomas.[35] Therefore, care must be taken in interpreting control of tumor growth rates in the literature because lack of tumor growth may be due to the indolent nature of these tumors rather than the effect of radiosurgery over the reported follow-up periods.

The feasibility and efficacy of fractionated SRS treatment to spinal lesions have been reported in the literature for a variety of conditions previously considered inoperable.[36,37] The data can be extrapolated to treatment of tumors of the upper cervical cord extending into the CVJ. Other tumors in the region of the foramen magnum have also been treated with radiosurgery. A report of a clival medullary plasmacytoma extending into the foramen magnum showed no adverse effect from SRS treatment, with a complete response 12 months after radiosurgery.[22]

Stereotactic Radiosurgery for Vascular Lesions

Vascular lesions of the CVJ, including arteriovenous malformations and cavernomas, are amenable to SRS treatment. Vascular tumors, such as glomus jugulare tumors, have also been treated with SRS. One reported series described the treatment of 10 patients with glomus jugulare tumors.[38] Eight of the patients had previous surgery, and the remaining two had no prior treatment. Doses to the tumor margin ranged from 12 to 16 Gy, and average tumor volume was 4 mL. Median follow-up was 9.7 months. Eighty percent of lesions showed stabilization of growth at follow-up, and the remaining 20% showed decrease in volume. In addition, symptom relief was achieved in 50% of patients—no worsening was noted. A recent study by Miller and colleagues proposed a new treatment paradigm for glomus jugulare tumors, namely staged Gamma Knife radiosurgery after selective surgical resection.[39] In the series, five patients with glomus tumors and contraindications to extensive surgery underwent an outpatient otologic resection of a portion of their tumor extending into the middle ear and mastoid area. Patients returned 2 to 5 months later for planned radiosurgery to the remainder of the tumor, especially the portion extending into the jugular bulb. Treatment consisted of 15 Gy to the 50% isodose line, with a follow-up of 3 years. All patients were noted to have a preservation or improvement in hearing and resolution of their pulsatile tinnitus and otalgia. One patient had transient facial palsy after surgery but before Gamma Knife. No other complications were noted, and tumor volumes were stable or decreased at follow-up (**Fig. 18.7**).

Proton Beam Radiation for Craniovertebral Junction Tumors

Fractionated high-beam proton radiation has been in clinical use since the 1970s.[40] This treatment modality has not gained popularity in treating many potential neuro-oncologic processes largely due to the high cost of delivery of proton beam treatment. However, proton beam radiation has been used effectively at centers with facilities built to deliver proton beam radiation, particularly for specific tumors such as uveal melanomas, chordomas, and chondrosarcomas of the skull base and upper cervical spine.[40] Doses are generally 10 to 20% greater than the dose regimens that can be safely given with conventional treatments.[40] In comparison to photon-based

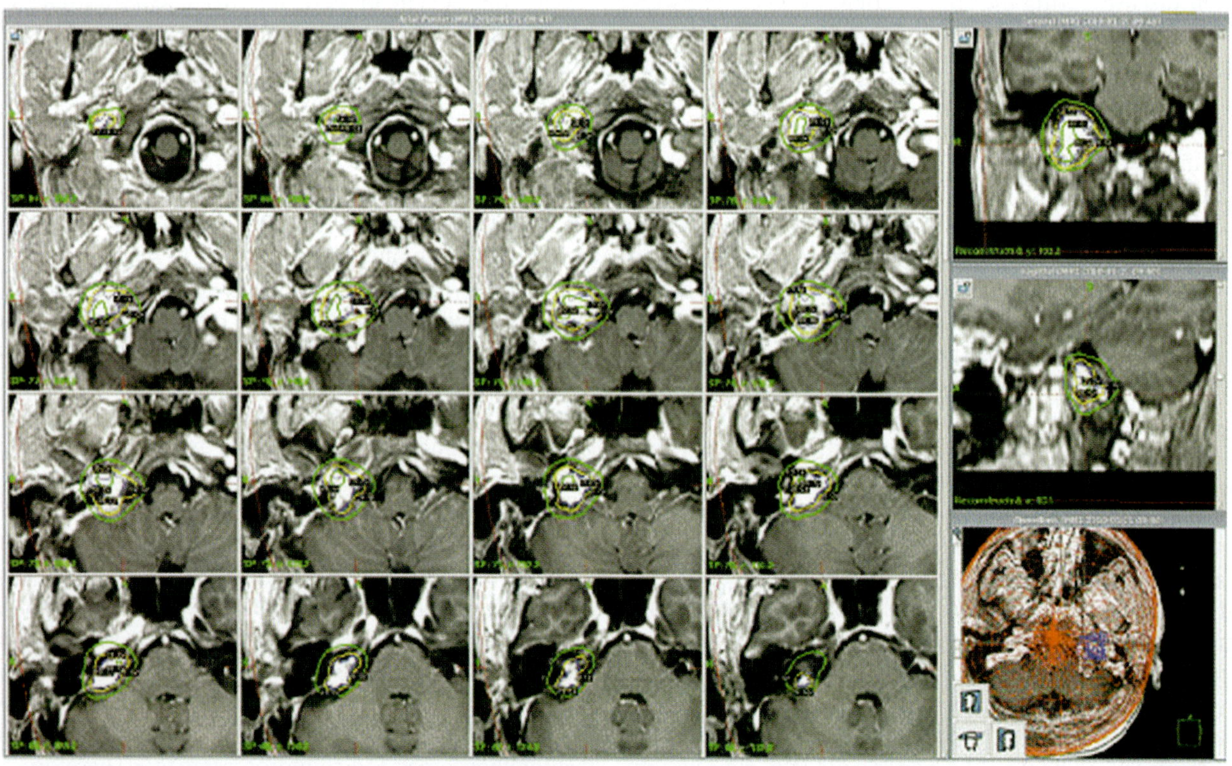

Fig. 18.7 Treatment planning for a glomus jugulare tumor at the right craniovertebral junction, treated with 13 Gy to the 50% isodose line. The patient received 15 Gy to the 50% isodose line.

radiosurgery, proton beam treatment is centered on better target definition and higher dose delivery.

When radiation doses are well localized to tumors, the delivery of protons can be safely achieved, with more control of local disease and less toxic effect on surrounding structures.[41] The rationale for using proton beam radiation is that, unlike photon therapy, high-energy protons abruptly stop in tissues at the end of their range, depositing energy in that volume with better tissue localization and less dose delivery to dose-limited normal tissue.[41] Due to this Bragg peak effect, the range of photon effects in tissues is finite. However, photon effects are exponential; therefore, there is some radiation delivery outside of the target area.[41] Proton beam therapy can provide better distribution of optimal tumor dose when compared with X-ray delivery systems.

Radiation with charged particles is yet another means of delivering high-dose radiation to a specific target while minimizing effects to the surrounding tissue.[42] The goal of proton beam treatment is to achieve higher rates of tumor control compared with conventional SRS.[42] Although theoretically attractive, significant evidence-based clinical efficacy for proton beam treatment use is lacking.[43] A recent review of the literature concluded that there are very few studies that directly compare treatments with charged particles with conventional treatments; therefore, overall efficacy for various oncological processes is difficult to interpret.[44]

To date, the clinical experience in neuro-oncology with proton beam radiation is limited, and few centers have specialized facilities for this type of treatment modality. The modality has been particularly used for the treatment of chordomas and chondrosarcomas, which are historically very radioresistant.[41] Currently there are not enough reports of chordoma and chondrosarcoma treatment with proton beam radiation with large enough numbers and statistical analyses to allow clinicians to draw effective conclusions about the role of this mode of treatment in comparison with conventional radiation, although the series reported in the literature appear promising.[45] For these tumors, quoted local tumor control rates with proton beam therapy are 91% for chondrosarcomas and 65% for chordomas compared with 35% seen with conventional radiation treatment.[41]

Several clinical series report good tumor control and excellent safety profiles for patients with chordomas and chondrosarcomas treated with proton beam radiation.[46] Massachusetts General Hospital's experience with proton beam treatment of chordomas and chondrosarcomas provides some of the extensive clinical series for review of efficacy.[47] Sixty-eight patients with these tumors were treated after surgery with high-dose fractionated proton beam radiation. The follow-up period was at least 17 months, with a median of 34 months. The median dose delivered to the tumors was 69 cobalt gray equivalents (CGE) with a daily dose ranging from 1.8 to 2.1 CGE. No significant adverse effects were reported with acceptable safety profiles. This series showed a 5-year local control of 82% with a disease-free survival rate of 76%.[47]

Another series described the combined use of fractionated proton and photon beam radiation in 44 patients with chordomas and chondrosarcomas.[48] Of the total dose delivered, photons constituted two-thirds and protons the remaining third. Mean follow-up was 30.5 months. The 3-year local control rates reported were 83.1% and 90% for chordomas and chondrosarcomas, respectively, with 3-year survival rates of 91% and 90%, respectively. Eighteen percent of patients showed local tumor control failure. Six deaths were reported—two due to intercurrent disease and four due to tumor effects. Although the number of patients was limited, there is promise regarding local tumor control for patients treated with a combination of radiosurgery and photon beam radiation with acceptable safety profiles.[48]

Conclusion

Lesions of the CVJ present a treatment challenge. Surgical resection, when feasible, can be associated with significant morbidity given the inherent surrounding anatomy of these lesions. Radiosurgery is a safe, efficacious, and minimally invasive option, both as a primary means of addressing CVJ pathology and as an adjunct to surgical resection. Varying types of radiosurgical treatment modalities are available, with some better suited for specific pathologies. The overall management of CVJ lesions depends on the biology of the lesion and the local anatomy, with the goal to optimize outcome in terms of low morbidity and cure or control of the disease process. Radiosurgery has a promising role in optimizing safe and efficacious treatment.

References

1. Muthukumar N, Kondziolka D, Lunsford LD, Flickinger JC. Stereotactic radiosurgery for anterior foramen magnum meningiomas. Surg Neurol 1999;51(3):268–273
2. Desai R, Bruce J. Meningiomas of the cranial base. J Neurooncol 1994;20(3):255–279
3. Leksell L. Stereotactic radiosurgery. J Neurol Neurosurg Psychiatry 1983;46(9):797–803
4. Barnett GH, Linskey ME, Adler JR, et al; American Association of Neurological Surgeons; Congress of Neurological Surgeons Washington Committee Stereotactic Radiosurgery Task Force. Stereotactic radiosurgery—an organized neurosurgery-sanctioned definition. J Neurosurg 2007;106(1):1–5
5. Dewey WC, Bedford JA. Radiobiologic principles. In: Leibel SA, Phillips TL. Textbook of Radiation Oncology. 2nd ed. Philadelphia, PA: WB Saunders; 2004:31–43
6. Yu JS, Luptrawan A, Wallace R, et al. Radiosurgery of intracranial lesions. In: Bernstein M, ed. Neurosurgical Operative Atlas, Neuro-Oncology. 2nd ed. New York, NY: Thieme Medical Publishers, Inc.; 2007:124–130
7. Liscák R, Kollová A, Vladyka V, Simonová G, Novotný J Jr. Gamma knife radiosurgery of skull base meningiomas. Acta Neurochir Suppl (Wien) 2004;91:65–74
8. Kreil W, Luggin J, Fuchs I, Weigl V, Eustacchio S, Papaefthymiou G. Long term experience of gamma knife radiosurgery for benign skull

base meningiomas. J Neurol Neurosurg Psychiatry 2005;76(10): 1425–1430
9. Rahman M, Murad GJ, Bova F, Friedman WA, Mocco J. Stereotactic radiosurgery and the linear accelerator: accelerating electrons in neurosurgery. Neurosurg Focus 2009;27(3):E13
10. Friedman WA. LINAC radiosurgery. Neurosurg Clin N Am 1990;1(4): 991–1008
11. Nath SK, Lawson JD, Wang JZ, et al. Optically-guided frameless linac-based radiosurgery for brain metastases: clinical experience. J Neurooncol 2010;97(1):67–72
12. Adler JR Jr, Chang SD, Murphy MJ, Doty J, Geis P, Hancock SL. The Cyberknife: a frameless robotic system for radiosurgery. Stereotact Funct Neurosurg 1997;69(1-4 Pt 2):124–128
13. Kuo JS, Yu C, Petrovich Z, Apuzzo ML. The CyberKnife stereotactic radiosurgery system: description, installation, and an initial evaluation of use and functionality. Neurosurgery 2008;62(Suppl 2): 785–789
14. Gerszten PC, Burton SA, Ozhasoglu C. CyberKnife radiosurgery for spinal neoplasms. Prog Neurol Surg 2007;20:340–358
15. Chang SD, Main W, Martin DP, Gibbs IC, Heilbrun MP. An analysis of the accuracy of the CyberKnife: a robotic frameless stereotactic radiosurgical system. Neurosurgery 2003;52(1):140–146, discussion 146–147
16. Andrews DW, Bednarz G, Evans JJ, Downes B. A review of 3 current radiosurgery systems. Surg Neurol 2006;66(6):559–564
17. Mackie TR. History of tomotherapy. Phys Med Biol 2006;51(13): R427–R453
18. Mori Y, Hashizume C, Kobayashi T, Shibamoto Y, Kosaki K, Nagai A. Stereotactic radiotherapy using Novalis for skull base metastases developing with cranial nerve symptoms. J Neurooncol 2010; 98(2):213–219
19. Cheshier SH, Hanft SJ, Adler JR, Chang SD. CyberKnife radiosurgery for lesions of the foramen magnum. Technol Cancer Res Treat 2007; 6(4):329–336
20. Henderson FC, McCool K, Seigle J, Jean W, Harter W, Gagnon GJ. Treatment of chordomas with CyberKnife: Georgetown University experience and treatment recommendations. Neurosurgery 2009;64 (2, Suppl):A44–A53
21. Gwak HS, Yoo HJ, Youn SM, et al. Hypofractionated stereotactic radiation therapy for skull base and upper cervical chordoma and chondrosarcoma: preliminary results. Stereotact Funct Neurosurg 2005;83(5-6):233–243
22. Wong ET, Lu XQ, Devulapalli J, Mahadevan A. Cyberknife radiosurgery for basal skull plasmacytoma. J Neuroimaging 2006;16(4):361–363
23. Hara W, Soltys SG, Gibbs IC. CyberKnife robotic radiosurgery system for tumor treatment. Expert Rev Anticancer Ther 2007;7(11): 1507–1515
24. Giglio P, Gilbert MR. Cerebral radiation necrosis. Neurologist 2003; 9(4):180–188
25. Torcuator R, Zuniga R, Mohan YS, et al. Initial experience with bevacizumab treatment for biopsy confirmed cerebral radiation necrosis. J Neurooncol 2009;94(1):63–68
26. Foote KD, William AF, Francis JB, et al. Linear accelerator (LINAC) radiosurgery. In: Fessler RG, Sekhar LN, eds. Atlas of Neurosurgical Techniques, Brain. New York, NY: Thieme Medical Publishers, Inc.; 2006:991–1006
27. Samblas JM, Bustos JC, Gutiérrez-Díaz JA, Donckaster G, Santos M, Ortiz de Urbina DI. Stereotactic radiosurgery of the foramen magnum region and upper neck lesions: technique modification. Neurol Res 1994;16(2):81–82
28. Liscák R, Kollová A, Vladyka V, Simonová G, Novotný J Jr. Gamma knife radiosurgery of skull base meningiomas. Acta Neurochir Suppl (Wien) 2004;91:65–74
29. Kreil W, Luggin J, Fuchs I, Weigl V, Eustacchio S, Papaefthymiou G. Long term experience of gamma knife radiosurgery for benign skull base meningiomas. J Neurol Neurosurg Psychiatry 2005;76(10): 1425–1430
30. Nicolato A, Foroni R, Pellegrino M, et al. Gamma knife radiosurgery in meningiomas of the posterior fossa. Experience with 62 treated lesions. Minim Invasive Neurosurg 2001;44(4):211–217
31. Martin JJ, Niranjan A, Kondziolka D, Flickinger JC, Lozanne KA, Lunsford LD. Radiosurgery for chordomas and chondrosarcomas of the skull base. J Neurosurg 2007;107(4):758–764
32. Kondziolka D, Lunsford LD, Flickinger JC. The role of radiosurgery in the management of chordoma and chondrosarcoma of the cranial base. Neurosurgery 1991;29(1):38–45, discussion 45–46
33. Hasegawa T, Ishii D, Kida Y, Yoshimoto M, Koike J, Iizuka H. Gamma Knife surgery for skull base chordomas and chondrosarcomas. J Neurosurg 2007;107(4):752–757
34. Krishnan S, Foote RL, Brown PD, Pollock BE, Link MJ, Garces YI. Radiosurgery for cranial base chordomas and chondrosarcomas. Neurosurgery 2005;56(4):777–784, discussion 777–784
35. Yoneoka Y, Tsumanuma I, Fukuda M, et al. Cranial base chordoma—long term outcome and review of the literature. Acta Neurochir (Wien) 2008;150(8):773–778, discussion 778
36. Gerszten PC, Ozhasoglu C, Burton SA, et al. Evaluation of CyberKnife frameless real-time image-guided stereotactic radiosurgery for spinal lesions. Stereotact Funct Neurosurg 2003;81 (1-4):84–89
37. Gerszten PC, Ozhasoglu C, Burton SA, et al. CyberKnife frameless single-fraction stereotactic radiosurgery for benign tumors of the spine. Neurosurg Focus 2003;14(5):e16
38. Navarro Martín A, Maitz A, Grills IS, et al. Successful treatment of glomus jugulare tumours with gamma knife radiosurgery: clinical and physical aspects of management and review of the literature. Clin Transl Oncol 2010;12(1):55–62
39. Miller JP, Semaan M, Einstein D, Megerian CA, Maciunas RJ. Staged Gamma Knife radiosurgery after tailored surgical resection: a novel treatment paradigm for glomus jugulare tumors. Stereotact Funct Neurosurg 2009;87(1):31–36
40. Munzenrider JE, Austin-Seymour M, Blitzer PJ, et al. Proton therapy at Harvard. Strahlentherapie 1985;161(12):756–763
41. Loeffler JS, Smith AR, Suit HD. The potential role of proton beams in radiation oncology. Semin Oncol 1997;24(6):686–695
42. Suit H, Urie M. Proton beams in radiation therapy. J Natl Cancer Inst 1992;84(3):155–164
43. Terasawa T, Dvorak T, Ip S, Raman G, Lau J, Trikalinos TA. Systematic review: charged-particle radiation therapy for cancer. Ann Intern Med 2009;151(8):556–565
44. Olsen DR, Bruland OS, Frykholm G, Norderhaug IN. Proton therapy - a systematic review of clinical effectiveness. Radiother Oncol 2007;83(2):123–132
45. Hug EB, Slater JD. Proton radiation therapy for chordomas and chondrosarcomas of the skull base. Neurosurg Clin N Am 2000;11(4): 627–638
46. Suit HD, Goitein M, Munzenrider J, et al. Definitive radiation therapy for chordoma and chondrosarcoma of base of skull and cervical spine. J Neurosurg 1982;56(3):377–385
47. Austin-Seymour M, Munzenrider J, Goitein M, et al. Fractionated proton radiation therapy of chordoma and low-grade chondrosarcoma of the base of the skull. J Neurosurg 1989;70(1):13–17
48. Noël G, Habrand JL, Mammar H, et al. Combination of photon and proton radiation therapy for chordomas and chondrosarcomas of the skull base: the Centre de Protonthérapie D'Orsay experience. Int J Radiat Oncol Biol Phys 2001;51(2):392–398

III Surgical Techniques

19 Brief Overview of Surgical Approaches to the Craniovertebral Junction

Nicholas C. Bambakidis, Robert F. Spetzler, and Curtis A. Dickman

Section III of *Surgery of the Craniovertebral Junction* addresses the surgical approaches that are available for exposing lesions at the craniovertebral junction (CVJ). The next several chapters are devoted to these surgical approaches, attesting to their variety and the difficulty in selecting the optimal approach. This overview introduces the surgical approaches and provides a brief discussion of the surgical decision-making process. Approaches to lesions of the CVJ traverse anatomical regions that are the domains of several surgical subspecialties (neurosurgery, otolaryngology, and plastic/craniofacial surgery), and a multidisciplinary skull base team is therefore mandatory.

The surgical approach is selected to maximize operative exposure and to minimize the associated rate of morbidity. First, the surgeon must determine how much exposure is needed. The specific pathology and size of the lesion are important factors in this determination. For example, a small cavernous malformation in a cerebellar peduncle might be removed completely through the limited exposure of a retrolabyrinthine approach, but a large petroclival meningioma might require the extensive exposure of a combined supratentorial and infratentorial approach. Second, the surgeon must determine from which direction to approach a lesion (**Fig. 19.1**).

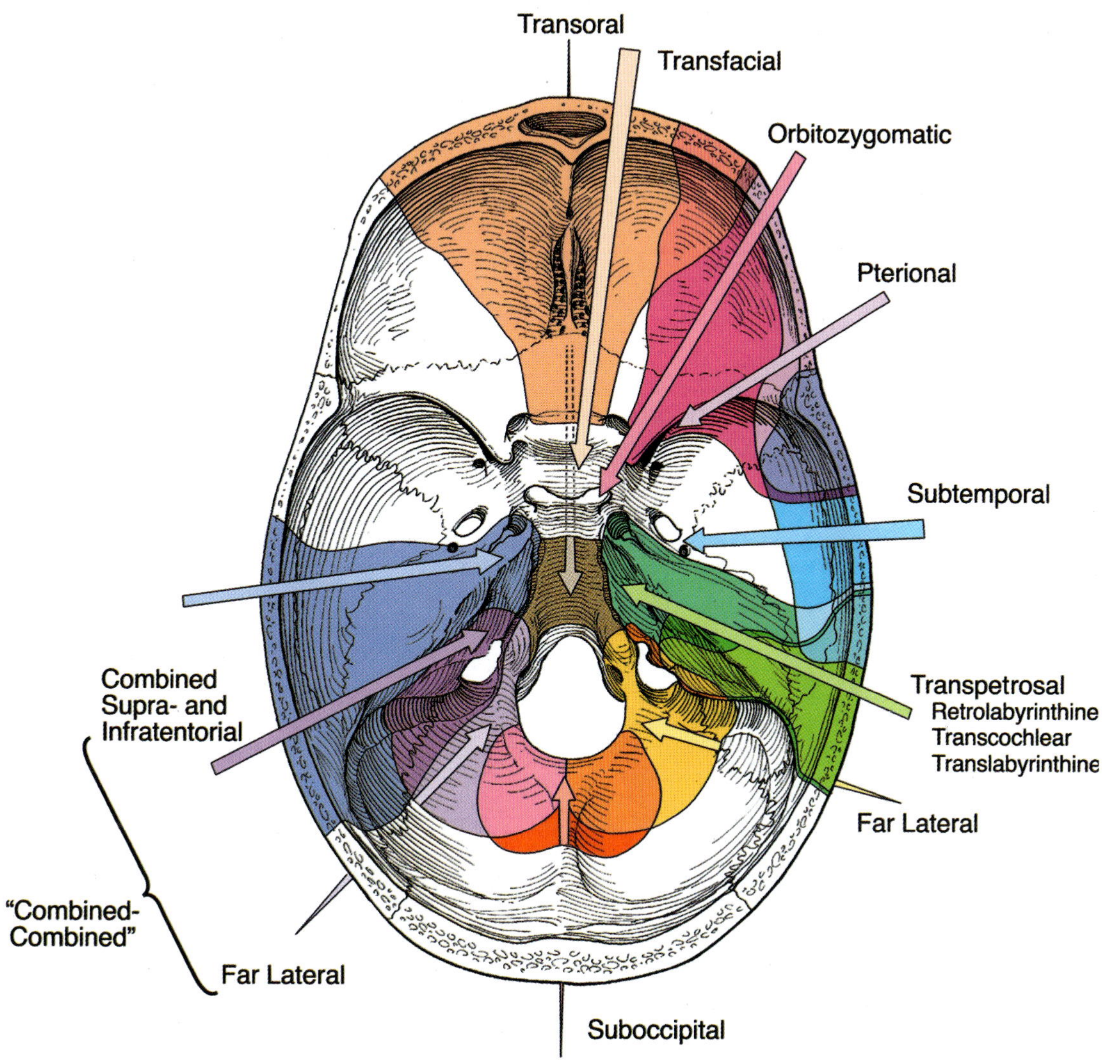

Fig. 19.1 The angles of approach and areas of exposure are shown for some of the surgical approaches to the CVJ. (Reprinted with permission from Spetzler RF, Koos WT, Richling B, Lang J, eds. Color Atlas of Microneurosurgery. Stuttgart, Germany: George Thieme Verlag; 1996.)

When the skull base is considered in the axial plane, the CVJ can be approached from three directions: anteriorly, laterally, and posteriorly. Similarly, when the skull base is considered in the sagittal plane, the CVJ can be approached from three directions: superiorly (transcranial), inferiorly (transcervical), and with a combination of both (**Fig. 19.2**). The location of the lesion and the adjacent anatomy are critical factors in selecting the best angle of approach. In the past decade stereotactic methods of localization have been refined and are invaluable in minimizing surgical morbidity while pinpointing the location of a lesion. These methods are discussed in Chapter 20.

Anterosuperior approaches to the CVJ consist of the transoral (Chapter 21), transoral–transmaxillary (Chapter 22), transoral–translabiomandibular (Chapter 23), and transfacial approaches, which include the transpalatal and transfrontal-nasal-orbital approaches (Chapter 24). Minimally invasive approaches include endoscopic approaches, which may diminish the need for high morbidity exposures (Chapters 25 and 26). The transoral and transfacial approaches are best suited for extradural midline lesions. Attacking intradural pathology through one of these approaches risks contamination with nasopharyngeal organisms, meningitis, and cerebrospinal fluid (CSF) leaks. Consequently, midline intradural lesions are better treated through a lateral approach (i.e., one of the transpetrosal approaches or a far-lateral approach). For extradural pathology, the upward extension of a lesion from the CVJ determines which of these transoral or transfacial approaches to select. Lesions on the inferior clivus can be accessed with a transoral, transpalatal, or transmaxillary approach. Lesions with further upward extension might require a transnasomaxillary approach or, if the middle and anterior cranial fossae are involved, one of the transfrontal-nasal-orbital approaches. Midline lesions that extend inferiorly from the CVJ and that cannot be exposed fully with one of the transoral approaches may require the additional exposure provided by osteotomies of the mandibular rami bilaterally or by a midline exposure, splitting the tongue and

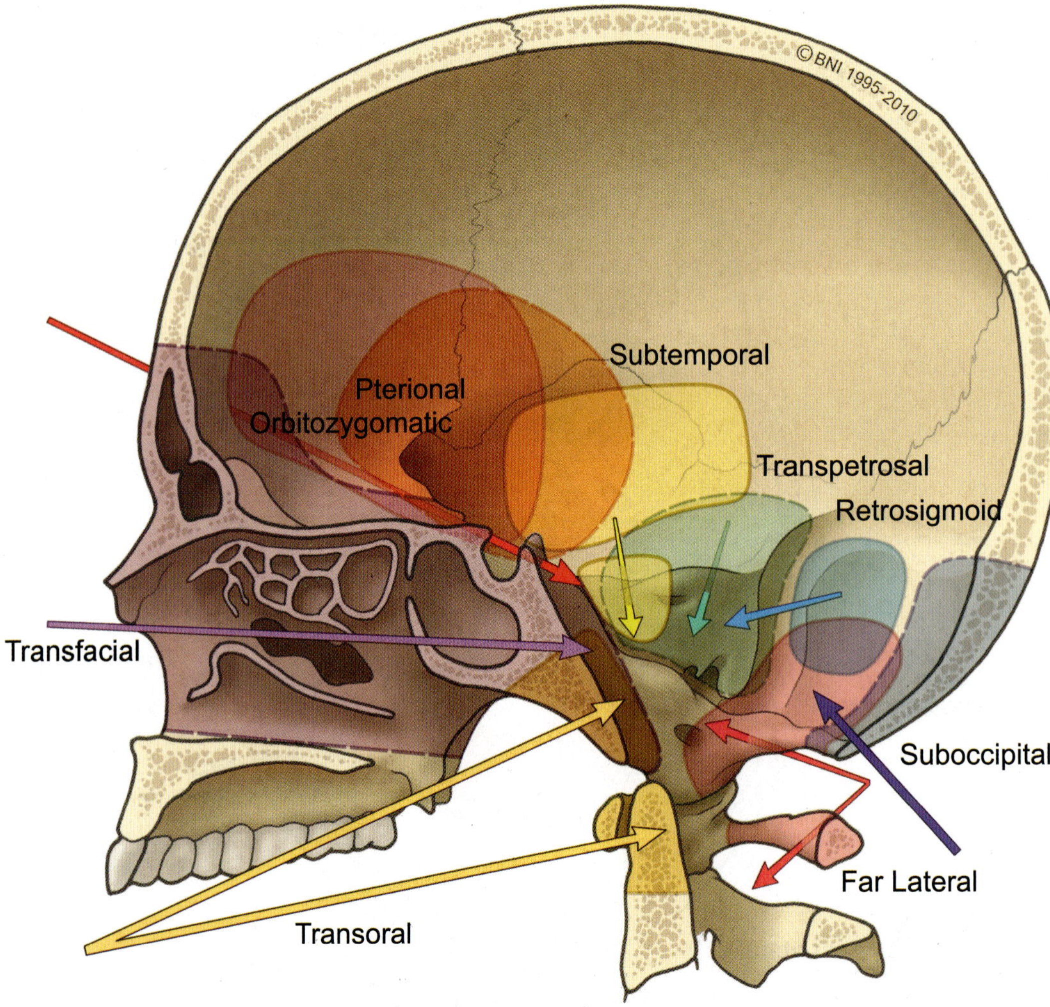

Fig. 19.2 Angles of approach in the sagittal plane. (Reprinted with permission from Barrow Neurological Institute. Bambakidis NC, Safavi-Abbasi S, Spetzler RF. Combined surgical approaches. In: Bambakidis NC, Megerian CA, Spetzler RF, eds. Surgery of the Cerebellopontine Angle. Shelton, CT: BC Decker/PMPH; 2009:79.)

mandible. Lesions that extend inferiorly from the CVJ and off midline might best be exposed through a retropharyngeal or mandibular swing approach.

The lateral approaches to the CVJ consist of the retrosigmoid approach (Chapter 33) and the presigmoid/transpetrosal approaches (Chapter 28). The extended transpetrosal approaches combine a petrosectomy with the standard neurosurgical approaches to increase exposure. For example, a petrosectomy combined with a subtemporal craniotomy adds a supratentorial exposure for lesions that extend superiorly. Similarly, a petrosectomy combined with a far-lateral craniotomy adds exposure of the foramen magnum for lesions that extend inferiorly. These approaches are most appropriate for laterally placed intradural lesions, but extensive bone removal through the transpetrosal approaches can provide access to midline lesions (e.g., aneurysms, chordomas, and meningiomas). These lateral approaches are preferred over anterior approaches for intradural lesions because they avoid the contaminated spaces in the nasopharynx and optimize dural repair, thus minimizing the risk of CSF leakage in the postoperative period.

Because some degree of petrosectomy is required for lateral approaches, the surgeon must estimate the amount of temporal bone resection needed to obtain adequate exposure. This evaluation is balanced with an assessment of the patient's preoperative neurological function—specifically, the function of cranial nerves VII and VIII. When hearing preservation is a goal, temporal bone removal is limited to retrolabyrinthine drilling. However, the exposure is then limited to the cerebellopontine angle. When patients have poor hearing before surgery, translabyrinthine drilling increases exposure to the anterolateral brainstem at the expense of hearing. When large lesions compress the brainstem and produce hearing loss and facial nerve deficits before surgery, transcochlear drilling, which transposes the facial nerve at the expense of transient deficits, is ideal. However, the increase in surgical exposure of the cranial base is traded for increased surgical morbidity, leading to an emphasis on careful selection of aggressive transpetrosal approaches based on these factors. In particular when applied to the management of benign tumors, such as meningiomas, the addition of stereotactic radiosurgical management (Section II, Chapter 18) has affected our treatment algorithm, and the use of transcochlear exposures in such cases has declined significantly.[1,2] With the development of endovascular techniques over the past decade (Chapter 30), treatment of vascular lesions has evolved. Nevertheless, such approaches remain necessary and helpful and should be part of the armamentarium of the experienced skull base surgeon. Examples of approach selection for upper cervical spine pathology are presented in Chapter 29, whereas those for upper cervical vertebral artery pathology are reviewed in Chapter 31.

Posterior approaches to the CVJ consist of the suboccipital approach (Chapter 33) and the far-lateral approach (Chapter 27). Determining which of these two approaches to use depends on whether an inferior exposure is needed below the level of the internal auditory canal and pontine structures to view the distal vertebral artery and inferior clivus. The far-lateral approach provides such additional lateral and inferior exposure; the standard suboccipital approach is adequate for higher and more midline lesions. These two approaches are remarkably versatile and are used to treat a variety of posterior and posterolateral lesions at the CVJ that are discussed in Section II Chapters 12, 15, and 16, including Chiari malformations (Chapter 12), cerebellar and brainstem vascular malformations (Chapter 15), vertebral and vertebrobasilar artery aneurysms (Chapter 16), and jugular foramen tumors (Chapter 32).

References

1. Bambakidis NC, Kakarla UK, Kim LJ, et al. Evolution of surgical approaches in the treatment of petroclival meningiomas: a retrospective review. Neurosurgery 2007;61(5, Suppl 2):202–209, discussion 209–211
2. Bambakidis NC, Safavi-Abbasi S, Spetzler RF. Combined surgical approaches. In: Bambakidis NC, Megerian CA, Spetzler RF, eds. Surgery of the Cerebellopontine Angle. Shelton, CT: BC Decker/PMPH; 2009

20 Stereotactic Methods of Localization and Image-Guided Surgery

Mark P. Garrett, Nicholas C. Bambakidis, and Robert F. Spetzler

Frameless stereotactic neuronavigation is an excellent example of the integration of modern technology into the practice of neurosurgery. Since its initial description by Roberts and colleagues in 1986,[1] the technology has advanced significantly and gained wide acceptance in the field of neurosurgery for both cranial and spinal applications. Neuronavigation assists the surgeon in maintaining spatial orientation and provides real-time information about precise anatomical locations during a procedure. This information allows a neurosurgeon to pursue a surgical objective with greater accuracy while identifying and preserving critical structures. This technology is particularly useful in surgery of the craniovertebral junction (CVJ) because this region contains a high concentration of critical neural and vascular structures.

■ Neuronavigation

The basic principle of neuronavigation is the correlation of a point within the stereotactic space of an operative field with a location on a digital image. Any location within the operative field can be defined as a distance from a reference point along three spatial planes, and this location can be referenced to a particular point on a three-dimensional (3D) image. There are many commercially available neuronavigational systems from companies such as BrainLAB, Medtronic, and Stryker, but we currently use the StealthStation (Medtronic Corporation, Minneapolis, MN) system (**Fig. 20.1**). For cranial cases, this system utilizes a dynamic reference frame mounted on a rigid arm

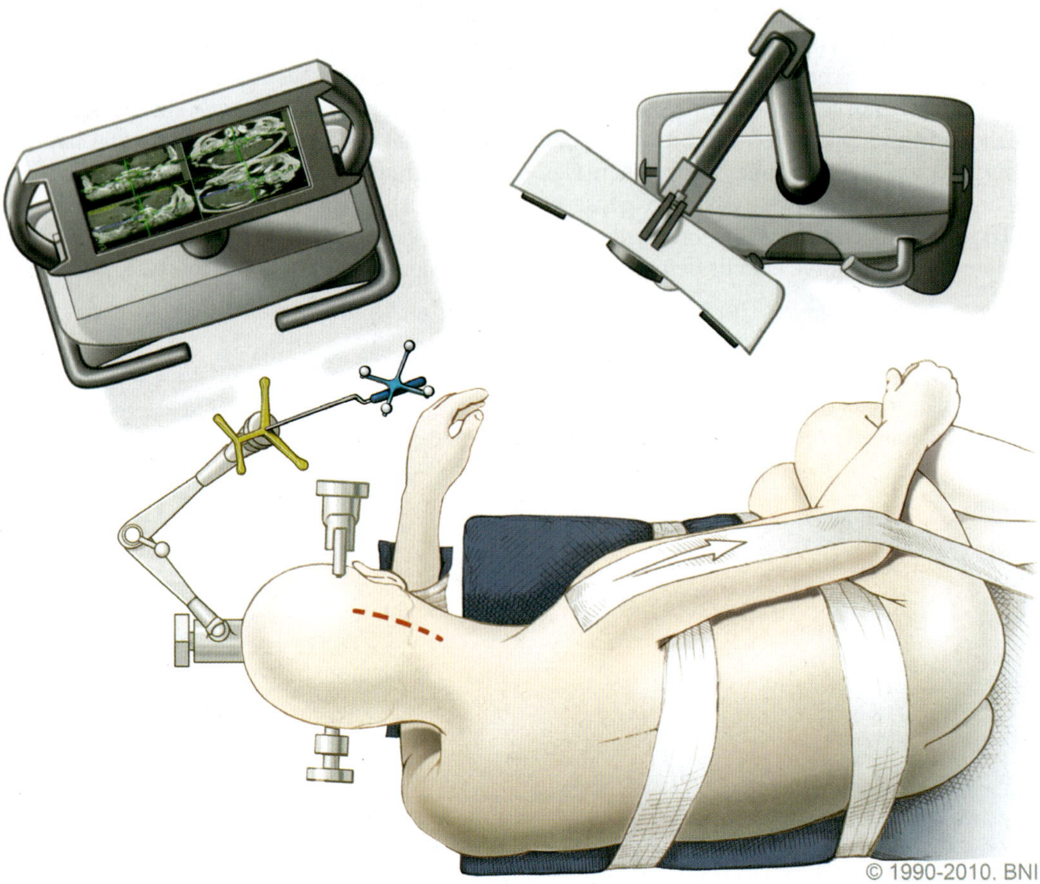

Fig. 20.1 The Medtronic StealthStation (Minneapolis, MN) apparatus when arranged for use in a far-lateral approach. (Reprinted with permission from Barrow Neurological Institute.)

attached to the Mayfield head holder, a stereotactic pointing device, a computer workstation, and mounted infrared cameras. The reference frame and pointing device utilize light-emitting diodes (LEDs) or reflective objects that allow the cameras to localize their relative positions in space. The patients' anatomy must be registered with the wand system by registering the points marked by fiducials placed before imaging or by mapping surface anatomy at surgery. Once the system is registered, the pointing device is placed in a particular location and the corresponding location on the magnetic resonance image (MRI) or computed tomography (CT) scan is displayed on the computer workstation. The microscope also can be mounted with an LED-containing frame that uses the focal point as the tip of the pointing device.

Neuronavigation also can be used to assist with placement of instrumentation during fusion procedures of the upper cervical spine. Because the spine is not a fixed structure like the cranial vault, the use of preoperative imaging for intraoperative navigation is precluded. We use the Iso-C (Siemens, Munich, Germany) system (**Fig. 20.2**), which employs rotational C-arm fluoroscopy and a reference frame attached to the spine near the operative site.[2] The intraoperative C-arm acquires images as it rotates around an isocentric point in space and produces CT-quality images that are immediately registered with the system for neuronavigation.[2] Various spinal instruments mounted with LED frames can be used for real-time navigation as instrumentation is placed.

For the StealthStation system to operate correctly, the camera must have a direct line of sight to the reference frame, but the frame must be positioned in a manner that does not obstruct the surgeon or other equipment. Consequently, the exact configuration and location of each piece of the system must be tailored to a given procedure. For cranial cases, the position of the microscope most often determines the position of the camera and reference frame. For suboccipital approaches with a prone patient, we usually operate from directly above the patient. Doing so allows lateral movements so that various surgical angles can be achieved. The reference frame is placed at or below the patient's shoulder level with the optical camera

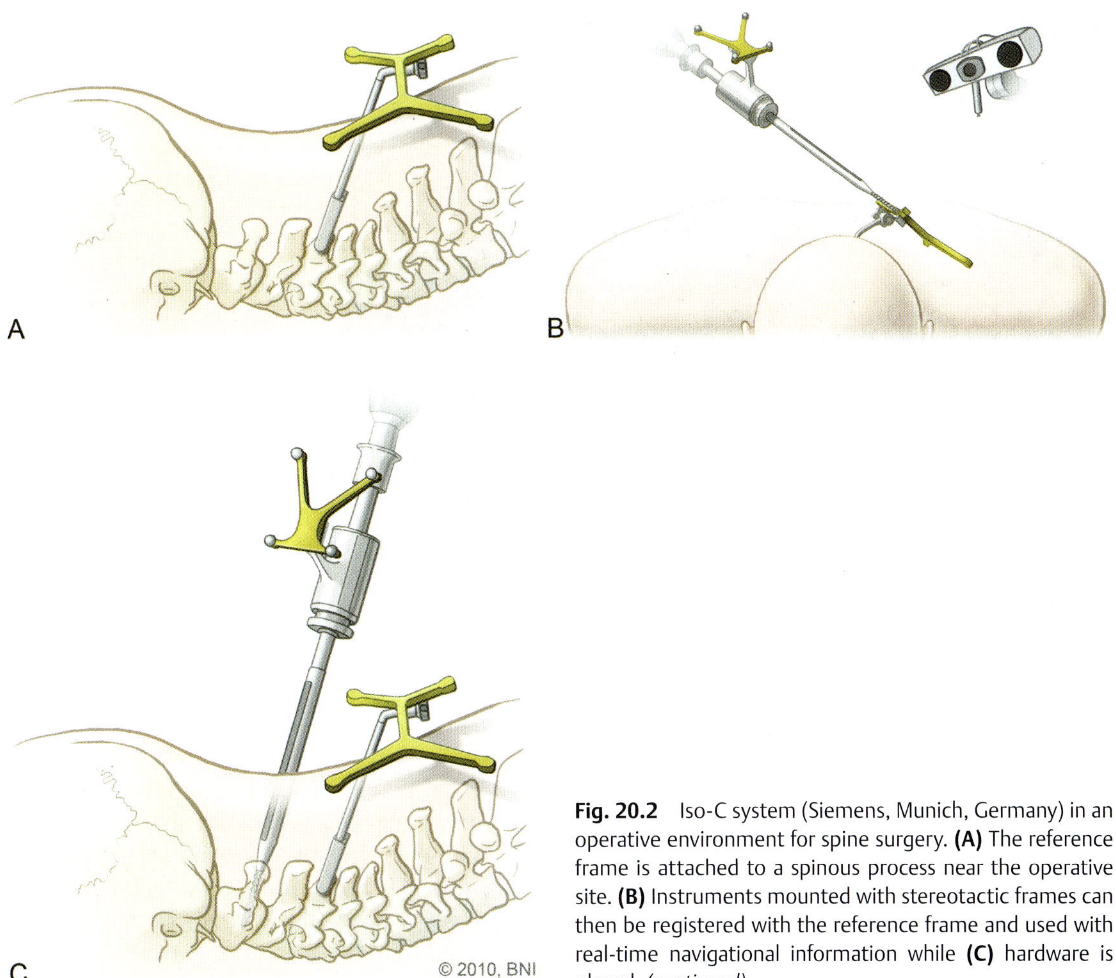

Fig. 20.2 Iso-C system (Siemens, Munich, Germany) in an operative environment for spine surgery. **(A)** The reference frame is attached to a spinous process near the operative site. **(B)** Instruments mounted with stereotactic frames can then be registered with the reference frame and used with real-time navigational information while **(C)** hardware is placed. *(continued)*

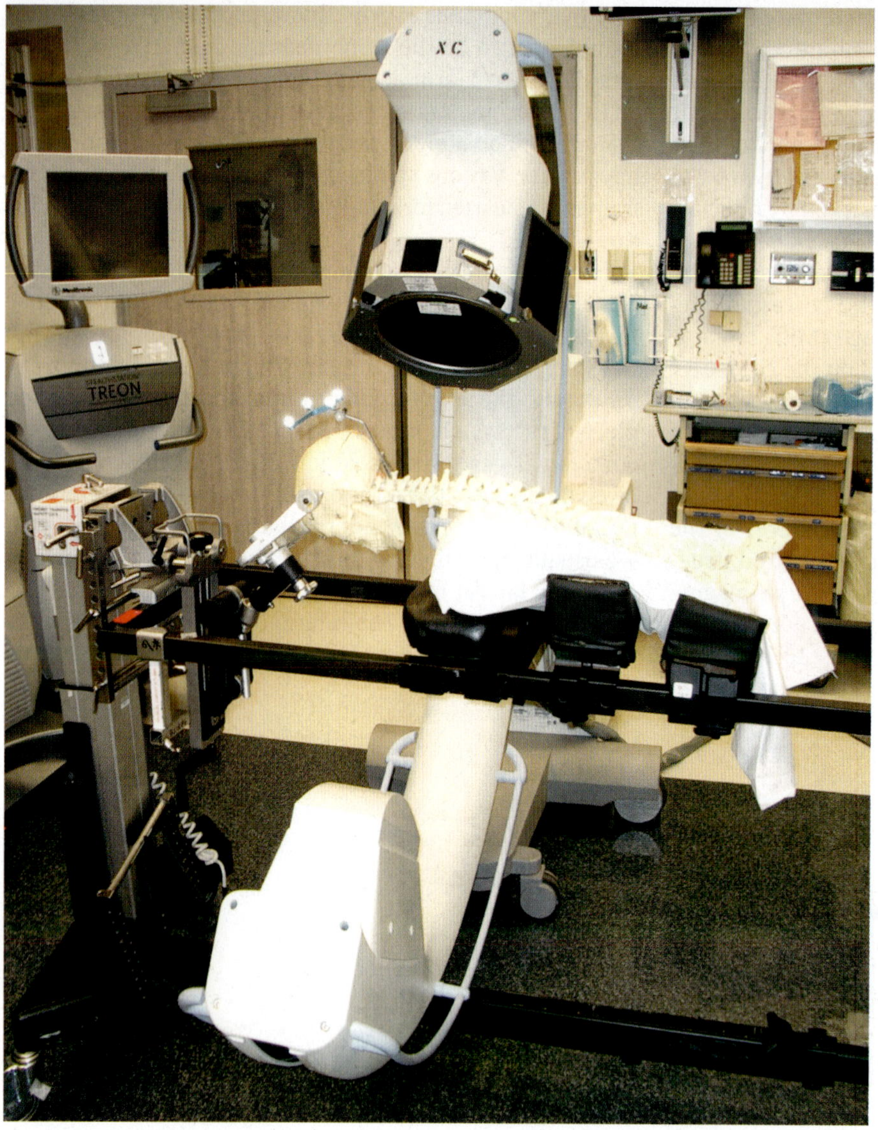

D

Fig. 20.2 *(continued)* **(D)** A photograph of the rotational C-arm that acquires images used to construct the CT-quality images used for navigation. (Reprinted with permission from Barrow Neurological Institute.)

at the patient's feet. For retrosigmoid or far-lateral craniotomies, the patient is usually placed in the park bench or supine position with the surgeon and microscope situated lateral to the patient. To maintain a direct line of sight, the reference frame and camera are positioned on the side opposite the surgeon. For upper cervical spine cases, the camera is often placed at the patient's feet with the reference arc attached to the spine just below the levels of interest.

Utility in Cranial Procedures

The usefulness of neuronavigation is most evident in its application to intracranial surgery. Its use has been widely adopted for intracranial surgery, and we believe that it is particularly useful for approaches to the skull base at the CVJ. The benefit of neuronavigation in skull base surgery is realized during all stages of a craniotomy.

Incision Planning

Once a patient is secured in a Mayfield pin head holder, the Stealth system is registered and used to plan the skin incision. The trajectory to the lesion is visualized, and the incision is placed in a location that ensures that the scalp tissues do not obstruct the surgeon's view. The guidance system also can be used to verify that the patient's position is appropriate and that the surgeon will be able to operate comfortably while achieving the necessary working angles. Using navigation in this manner also ensures the minimum incision length and avoids an excessively large incision related to uncertainty about the exact trajectory needed. A good example of this is the hockey stick incision, which historically has been used for far-lateral approaches to easily identify midline structures and to avoid arterial injury. However, the resulting large myocutaneous flap is associated with a certain level of morbidity and often obstructs surgical views. If a smaller, linear, paramedian incision is made, neuronavigation can assist in the identification and preservation of the vertebral artery during the initial stages of the approach.

Craniotomy

Neuronavigation is particularly helpful when performing a craniotomy of the posterior fossa. Craniotomies in this region often must be placed adjacent to or across the dural sinuses. When neuronavigation is used, the location of a craniotomy can quickly be mapped at the bone surface. The craniotomy can then be opened away from the sinus, or it can be skeletonized if necessary. This method decreases operative time and helps avoid injury to the dural sinus. Just as with the skin incision, neuronavigation allows the smallest possible craniotomy to be made because the trajectory can be verified before drilling proceeds. In this way, neuronavigation is critical when applying the principles of "keyhole surgery" to lesions of the CVJ.[3]

Lesion Resection

Once a craniotomy has been performed, neuronavigation enables the efficient identification of the lesion or anatomical structure of interest. It allows the surgeon to constantly verify the proximity of critical structures (**Fig. 20.3**). It also can be used to estimate the extent of resection during a procedure.

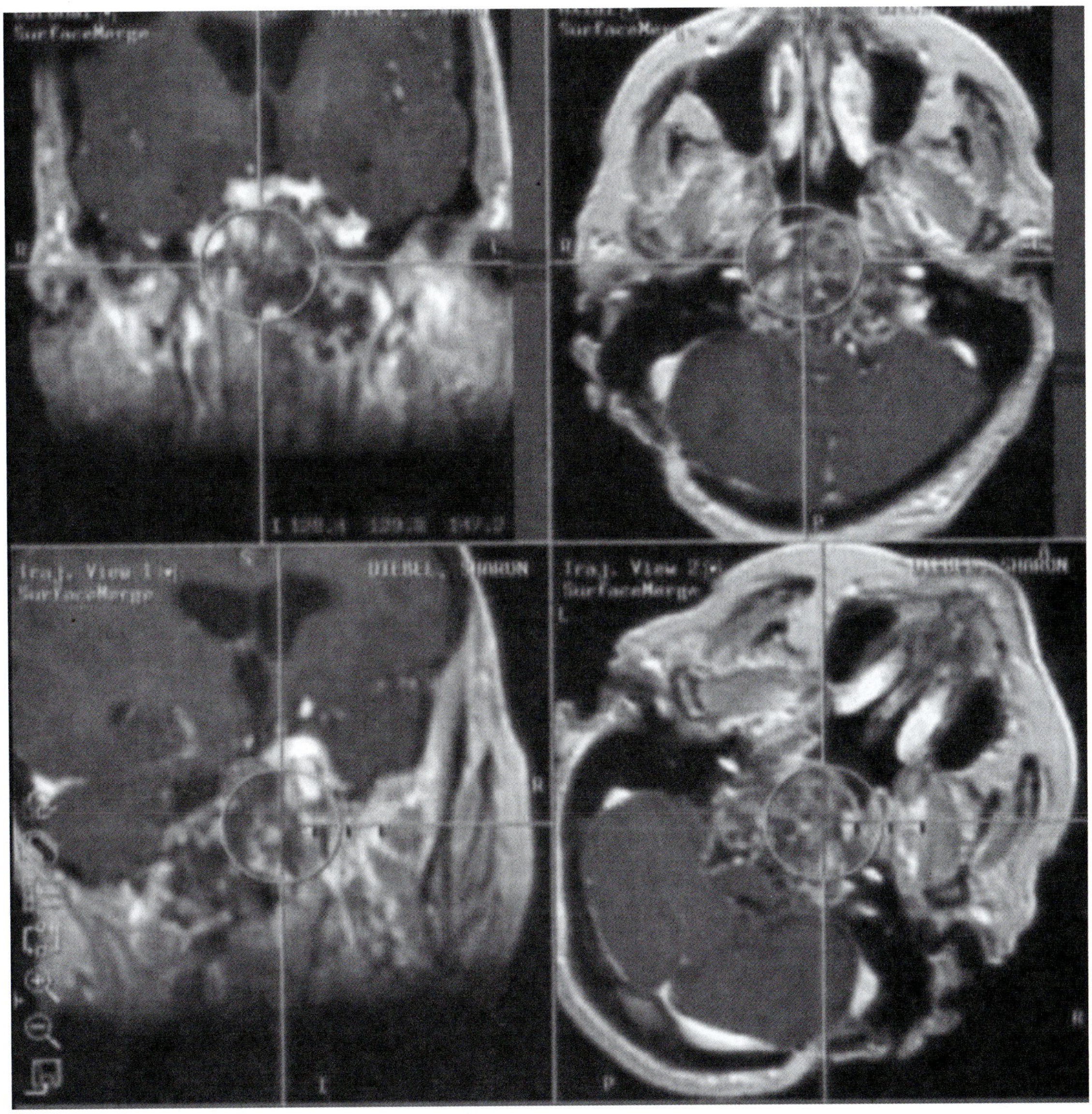

Fig. 20.3 Navigational imaging during the debulking of a large clival chordoma through a retrosigmoidal craniotomy. The navigation allows constant awareness of the proximity of the contralateral carotid artery and brainstem during tumor removal. (Reprinted with permission from Barrow Neurological Institute.)

Intramedullary lesions of the brainstem, such as cavernous malformations, are excellent examples of surgical scenarios where neuronavigation is extremely useful. The following two cases illustrate this point.

Case 1

A 21-year-old woman who was 20 weeks pregnant suffered the acute onset of visual disturbances and gait instability. She was found to have a hemorrhage in the pontomesencephalic region of the brainstem likely from a cavernous malformation. After consultation with the patient, an extreme lateral supracerebellar approach was planned for surgical resection of the lesion. Thin-cut stereotactic MRIs were obtained for use with neuronavigation (**Fig. 20.4A**). Navigation was used to determine the location of the craniotomy to provide an optimal trajectory to the posterolateral aspect of the midbrain and pons. Using navigation, the transverse sinus was efficiently identified and partially exposed to maximize dural retraction (**Fig. 20.4B**). With the aid of navigation, the exact location for entering the brainstem was determined (**Fig. 20.4C**). The cavernous malformation was removed in a piecemeal fashion (**Fig. 20.4D**), and gross total resection was achieved.

Case 2

A 45-year-old man presented with dizziness and hearing loss in the right ear. Imaging demonstrated a presence within the petrous apex of an enhancing mass, which was biopsied and debulked through a right transmastoid approach (**Fig. 20.5**). Navigation was utilized in approaching the lesion and allowed debulking across the level of the clivus to the midline. The final diagnosis was consistent with a plasmacytoma, and the patient's dizziness improved markedly following decompression of the petrous apex.

Utility in Spinal Procedures

Instrumentation of the upper cervical spine is challenging due to the neurovascular structures that must be preserved. Instrumentation often must be placed near the vertebral artery or spinal canal, and its misplacement can have devastating consequences. Many studies have described the benefit of using neuronavigation for instrumentation of the upper cervical spine.[2,4–7] As noted earlier, we use the Iso-C system for intraoperative spinal instrumentation.

One of the primary benefits of using a neuronavigation system for spinal instrumentation is the reduction in the amount of radiation that the surgeon receives. Spinal instrumentation procedures typically require multiple X-rays with the surgeon present to verify the depth and trajectory as the hardware is placed. The Iso-C requires only one series of X-rays, which can be obtained within 90 seconds, during which time the surgeon can step behind a protective lead shield. After the instrumentation is placed, a final CT-quality image can be obtained to evaluate the accuracy of placement before the patient leaves the operating room.

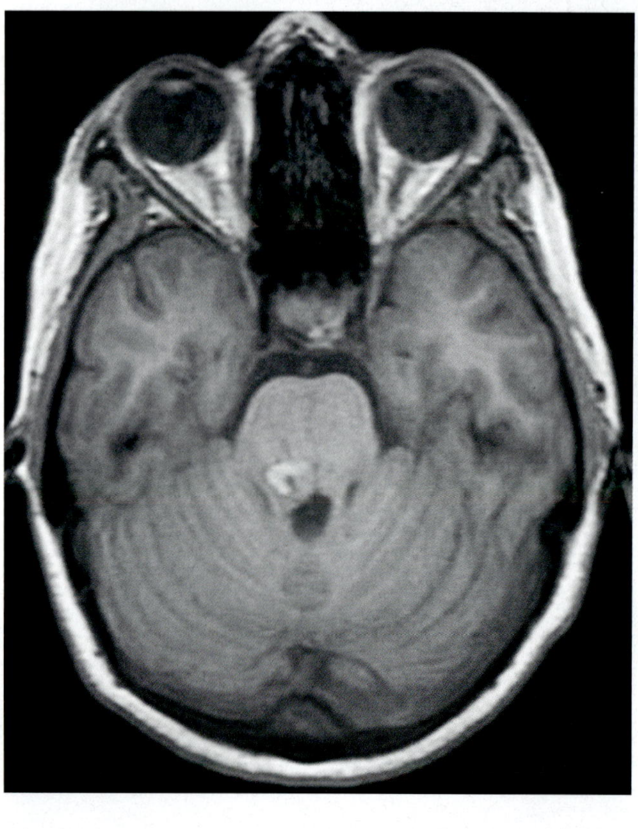

A

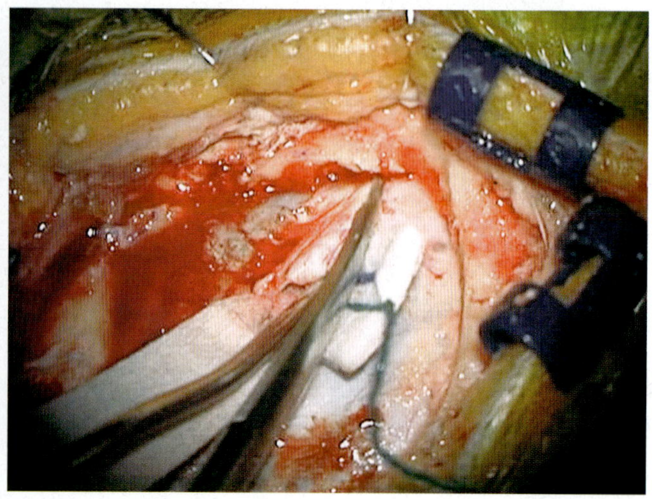

B

Fig. 20.4 **(A)** A thin-cut axial T1-weighted magnetic resonance image reveals hemorrhage in the posterolateral pontomesencephalic region. **(B)** Navigation is used to quickly identify and expose the transverse sinus and safely open the dura. *(continued)*

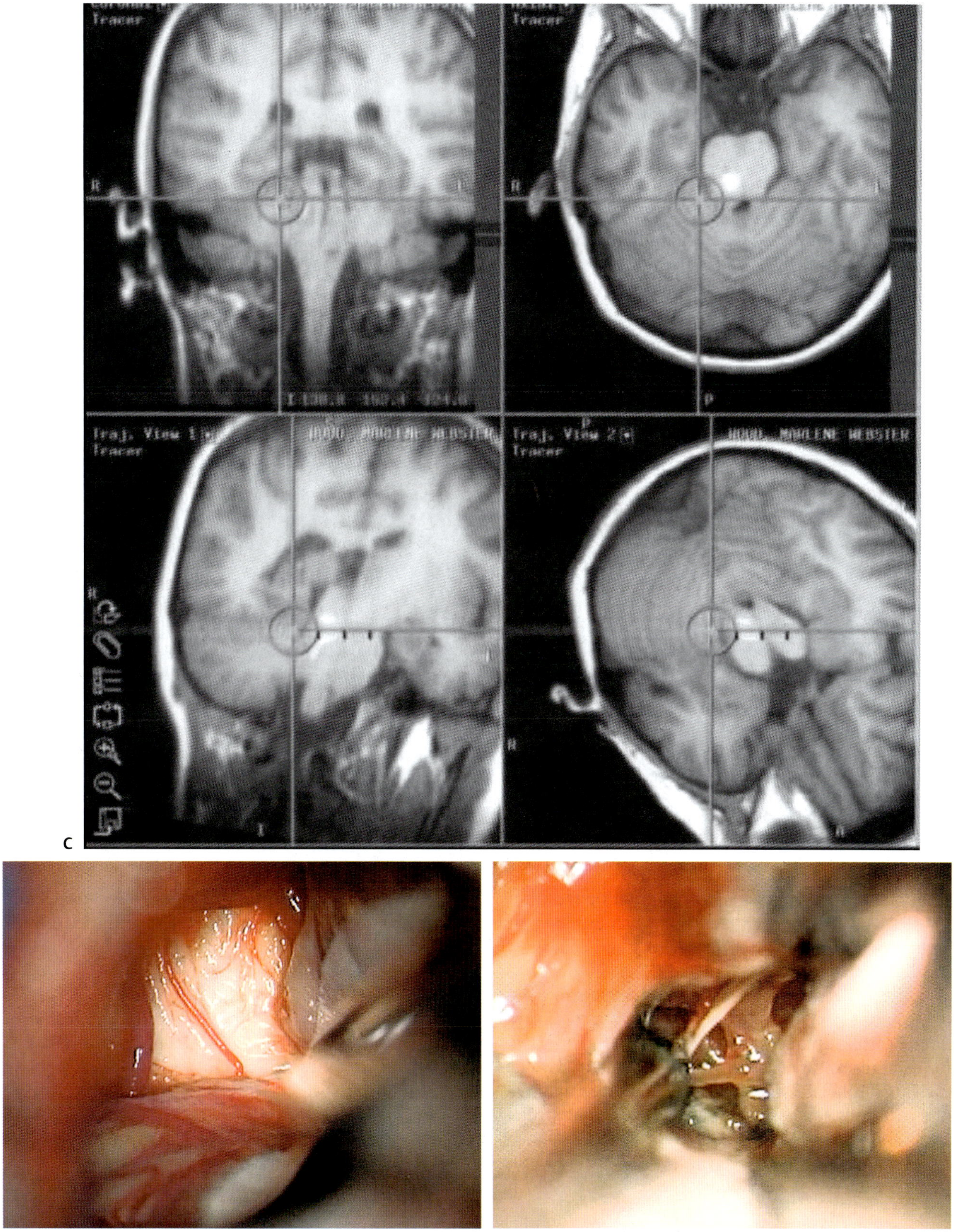

C

D

E

Fig. 20.4 *(continued)* **(C)** Navigational images identify an entry point on the posterior brainstem surface **(D)** that provides the best trajectory to the lesion. **(E)** The cavernous malformation is removed in piecemeal fashion. (Reprinted with permission from Barrow Neurological Institute.)

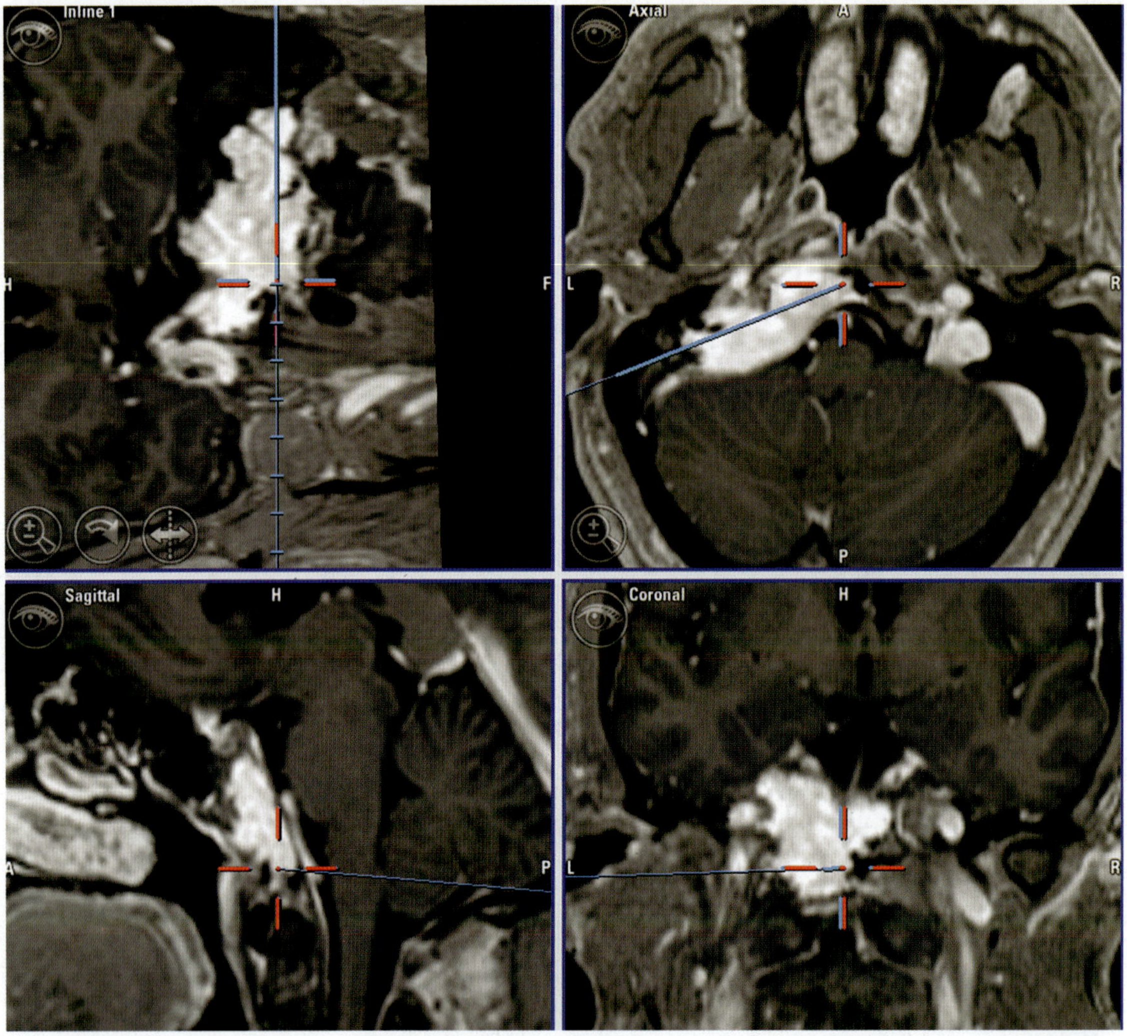

Fig. 20.5 Intraoperative navigation photographs demonstrate the trajectory taken to access a plasmacytoma. The transpetrosal approach to the tumor allows for unimpeded access up through the level of the clivus and midline structures.

Neuronavigation is particularly useful during the placement of C1-C2 transarticular screws, which are long and inserted near the vertebral artery. Acosta and colleagues[6] reported 20 patients who underwent C1-C2 transarticular screw placement with the use of frameless stereotaxy. They had no complications related to injury of the vertebral artery or spinal cord, and they reported that 92% of their screws were "well placed." This article also highlighted that neuronavigation is helpful in patients with abnormal anatomy. Of their 20 cases, four were determined to be anatomically difficult, if not impossible, but surgical navigation allowed the procedure to proceed with success. Navigation can be extremely helpful when a patient's anatomy is distorted by injury, congenital deformity, or other causes.

Odontoid screws also can be inserted with the assistance of neuronavigation. We prefer to use a combination of navigation and lateral fluoroscopy (**Fig. 20.6**). The force required to drill into C2 and to drive the screw can alter its position, shifting it posteriorly along the sagittal plane and introducing error along that plane. For this reason, a simple lateral fluoroscopic view can be checked while navigation is used to verify the accuracy of the depth and trajectory in the coronal plane.

Case 3

A 70-year-old woman fell and was found to have a C2 fracture that required surgical fixation (**Fig. 20.7A**). At the time of presentation, the patient was neurologically intact. She underwent placement of an odontoid screw with the assistance of neuronavigation. Her head was secured in a radiolucent Mayfield head holder, and the reference arm was attached and placed in a position above the patient (**Fig. 20.7B**). A tube and securing arm were used to retract the soft tissues of the neck. The Iso-C system was used to obtain the 3D images, which were then transferred to the workstation for Stealth navigation. Using reference frames attached to the drill and screwdriver, the odontoid screw was placed at the appropriate depth and trajectory (**Fig. 20.7C–E**).

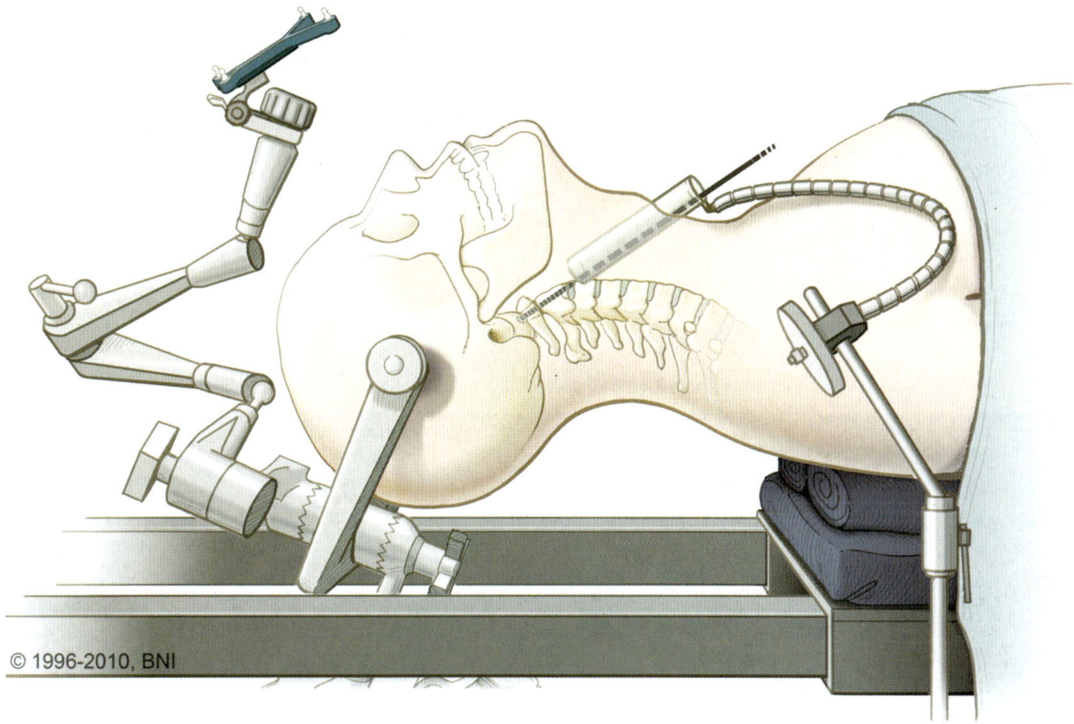

Fig. 20.6 Illustration showing the use of neuronavigation for the placement of an odontoid screw. The reference frame is placed on a rigid arm attached to the Mayfield head holder. (Reprinted with permission from Barrow Neurological Institute.)

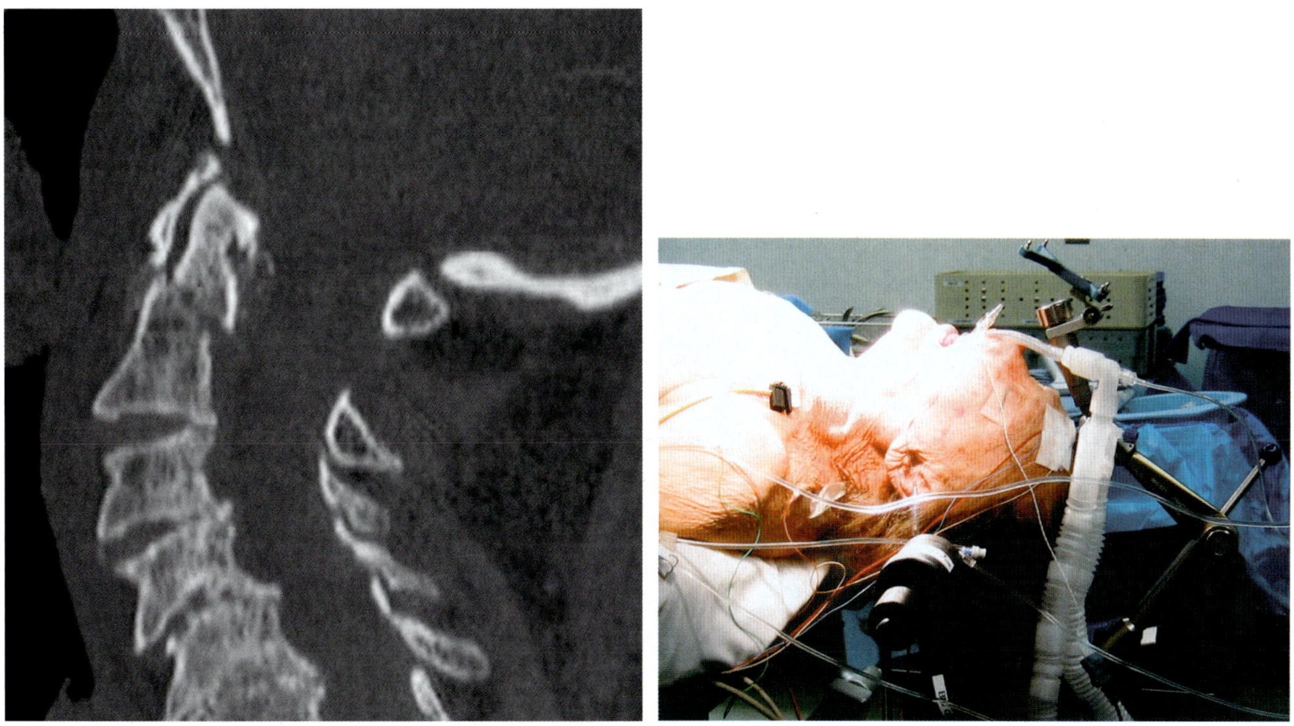

A B

Fig. 20.7 **(A)** Sagittal computed tomography (CT) scan shows a type II odontoid fracture planned for odontoid screw placement. **(B)** The patient's head is secured in the Mayfield head holder, and the reference frame is positioned above the head. *(continued)*

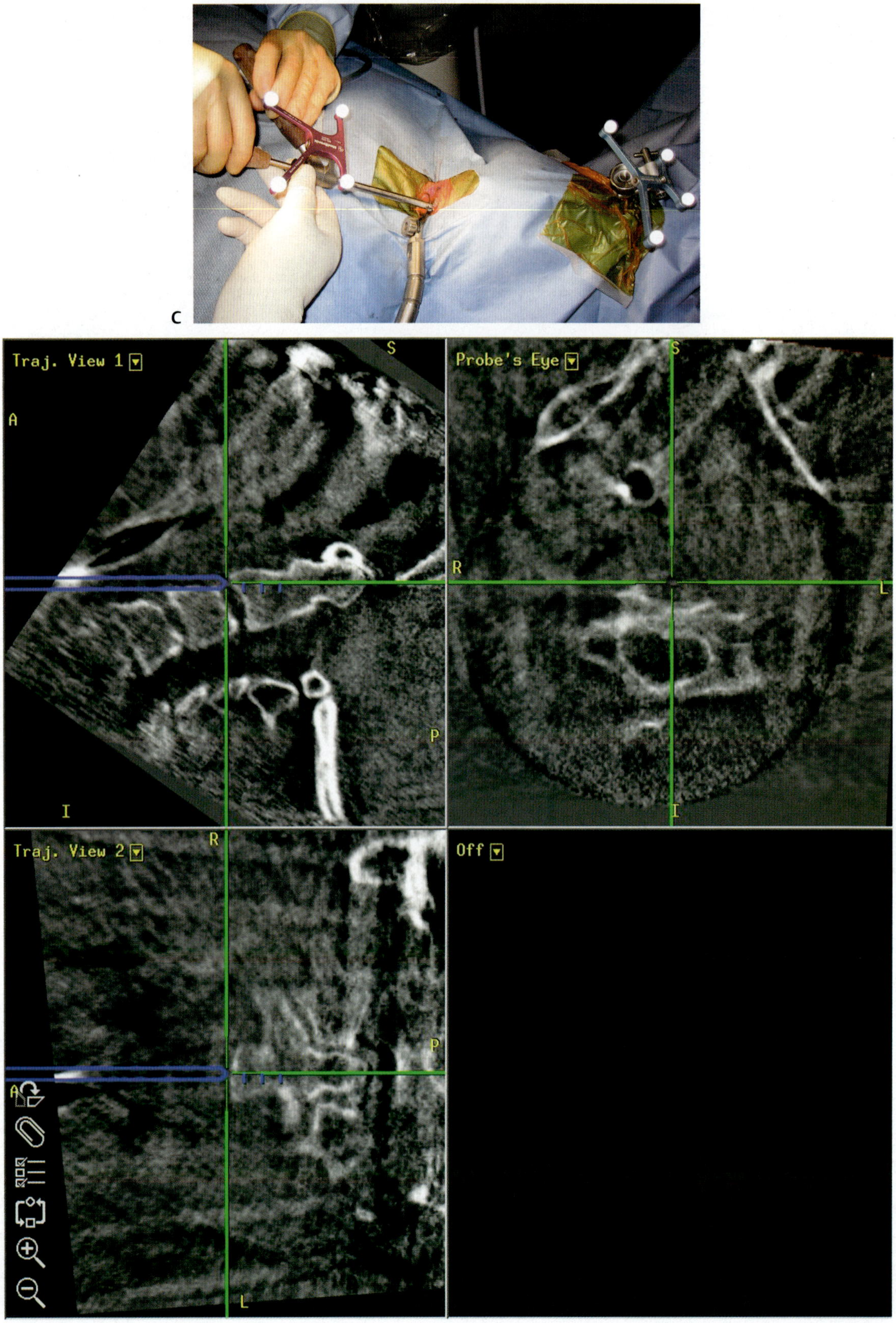

C

D

Fig. 20.7 *(continued)* **(C)** A screwdriver guide mounted with a stereotactic frame is used to place the odontoid screw with **(D)** real-time navigational images. *(continued)*

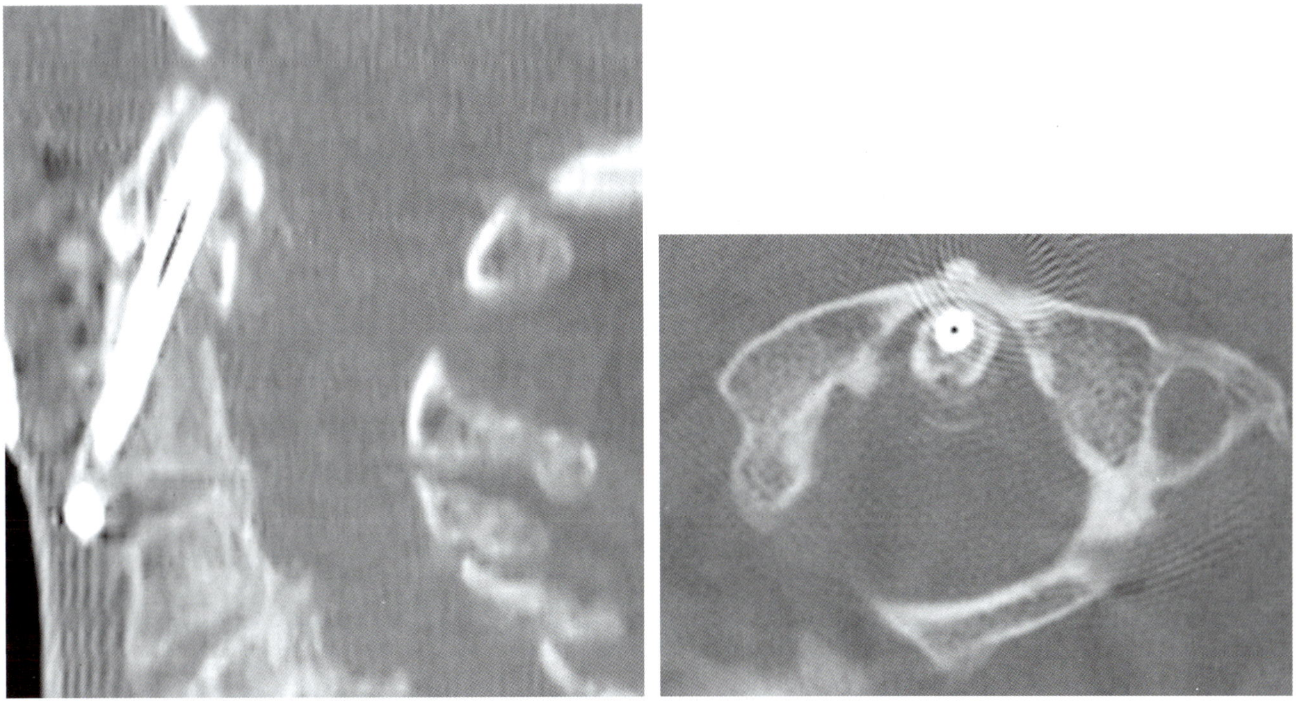

E F

Fig. 20.7 *(continued)* Postoperative **(E)** sagittal and **(F)** axial CT scans confirm successful placement of the odontoid screw. (Reprinted with permission from Barrow Neurological Institute.)

Dangers

Neuronavigation is a useful tool in the neurosurgeon's armamentarium, but it does have limitations. A certain level of technical error is inherent because the system calculates its own position in space as it registers the reference matrix between the navigation and the image space.[8] Although this error should not be ignored completely, modern algorithms have reduced it to an acceptable level. The primary pitfall of neuronavigation is that any shift of the patient's anatomy in relation to the reference frame after it has been registered renders it inaccurate. A classic example is the brain shift that occurs as a tumor is removed. In this sense, neuronavigation should not be considered truly real time, and the surgeon should always account for anatomical changes that occur during the course of a procedure.

A similar issue applies to spinal neuronavigation where the vertebral segments are inherently mobile. This issue is especially problematic during lateral mass instrumentation of the atlas when stereotactic guidance is used. As the necessary pressure is applied to advance the drill, the ring of C1 can rotate, thereby rendering the neuronavigational image inaccurate. Such a shift could place the vertebral artery at high risk as the surgeon would likely have confidence in the information provided by the navigation system. To avoid this problem, the ring of C1 can be secured by the surgeon's assistant on the contralateral side to prevent its movement.

This problem also exists with any shift of the reference frame itself. Typically, the reference frame is well secured to the spinal column or to a mechanical arm for cranial cases. However, inadvertent movements could cause a shift in its position. To identify such shifts, the surgeon, both at the beginning of the case and throughout the case, should verify the navigational image against a known fixed point in the surgical field, such as the skull surface or vertebral bone surface. If the navigation is found to be inaccurate at such a fixed point, it can be re-registered and the operation can proceed.

Conclusion

Neuronavigation is a technological achievement that has helped advance the practice of neurosurgery, including the treatment of pathologies of the CVJ. Some authors believe that neuronavigation is often unnecessary and cite the lack of conclusive evidence that it improves outcome.[9,10] However, we believe that neuronavigation is advantageous in ways that are difficult to measure objectively. The value of the ability to maintain spatial orientation during a procedure should not be underestimated. As the technology continues to improve, the current limitations of stereotactic neuronavigation will certainly be reduced if not eliminated.

References

1. Golfinos JG, Fitzpatrick BC, Smith LR, Spetzler RF. Clinical use of a frameless stereotactic arm: results of 325 cases. J Neurosurg 1995; 83(2):197–205
2. Hott JS, Deshmukh VR, Klopfenstein JD, et al. Intraoperative Iso-C C-arm navigation in craniospinal surgery: the first 60 cases. Neurosurgery 2004;54(5):1131–1136, discussion 1136–1137
3. Lan Q. Clinical application of keyhole techniques in minimally invasive neurosurgery. Chin Med J (Engl) 2006;119(16): 1327–1330
4. Sugimoto Y, Tanaka M, Nakanishi K, et al. Safety of atlantoaxial fusion using laminar and transarticular screws combined with an atlas hook in a patient with unilateral vertebral artery occlusion (case report). Arch Orthop Trauma Surg 2009;129(1):25–27
5. Rajasekaran S, Vidyadhara S, Shetty AP. Intra-operative Iso-C3D navigation for pedicle screw instrumentation of hangman's fracture: a case report. J Orthop Surg (Hong Kong) 2007;15(1):73–77
6. Acosta FL Jr, Quinones-Hinojosa A, Gadkary CA, et al. Frameless stereotactic image-guided C1-C2 transarticular screw fixation for atlantoaxial instability: review of 20 patients. J Spinal Disord Tech 2005;18(5):385–391
7. Börm W, König RW, Albrecht A, Richter HP, Kast E. Percutaneous transarticular atlantoaxial screw fixation using a cannulated screw system and image guidance. Minim Invasive Neurosurg 2004;47(2):111–114
8. Grunert P, Darabi K, Espinosa J, Filippi R. Computer-aided navigation in neurosurgery. Neurosurg Rev 2003;26(2):73–99, discussion 100–101
9. Enchev YP, Popov RV, Romansky KV, Marinov MB, Bussarsky VA. Cranial neuronavigation—a step forward or a step aside in modern neurosurgery. Folia Med (Plovdiv) 2008;50(2):5–10
10. Willems PW, van der Sprenkel JW, Tulleken CA, Viergever MA, Taphoorn MJ. Neuronavigation and surgery of intracerebral tumours. J Neurol 2006;253(9):1123–1136

21 Transoral Approach to the Craniovertebral Junction

Curtis A. Dickman, Robert F. Spetzler, Volker K. H. Sonntag, Nicholas C. Bambakidis, and Paul J. Apostolides

The transoral approach to the craniovertebral junction (CVJ) provides versatile, direct access to extradural midline pathology. This transmucosal approach allows excellent decompression of the ventral medulla and upper cervical spinal cord. In most circumstances, the transoral approach permits access from the inferior third of the clivus to the C3 vertebra. The operative exposure is constrained by the patient's ability to open his or her mouth and by the soft tissue boundaries of the nasopharynx, the oropharynx, the mandible, and the skull base. Although multiple techniques have been described both in the literature and elsewhere in this text,[1–4] in this chapter we discuss our preferred technique, which has proven to be efficacious in a large number of patients.

■ General Considerations

Transoral access to the CVJ can be performed with a simple, uncomplicated approach that involves retracting the soft palate and the tongue without incising these soft tissue structures. Dysphagia, dysphonia, and nasal regurgitation of fluids (velopharyngeal incompetence) can occur after palatal or lingual incisions. Extended transoral exposures include the transmaxillary, transpalatal, transfacial, and transmandibular exposures (**Fig. 21.1**). The extensions of the transoral exposure provide broader access to more extensive pathology and are fully discussed in Chapters 22, 23, and 24. The extended transoral exposures increase the morbidity rates associated with the surgical procedures and, therefore, are reserved for pathology that is more extensive than can be accessed by a simple transoral exposure.

Typically, transoral decompression is indicated for irreducible compressive pathology of the ventral brainstem and spinal cord (**Fig. 21.2**). This was recommended for all cases of ventral compression as the initial procedure of choice. Yet, in many cases of pannus formation in which compression is purely from inflammatory fibrous tissue, a posterior fusion alone may result in resorption of the compressive lesion and neurological improvement.[5–7] In cases where reduction is attempted, as in cranial settling associated with bone softening diseases or rheumatoid arthritis, a magnetic resonance imaging (MRI)-compatible halo ring is best utilized. The vector of the traction should be neutral, or the neck should be extended slightly. For axial traction, weights are applied, beginning with 4 pounds. Slowly and progressively, the weight is increased to a maximum of 10 to 12 pounds. Traction should be applied carefully to avoid distraction, which can cause neurological or vascular injury. Flexion of the neck should be avoided because it can increase the compression associated with cranial settling. The duration of traction should be limited to a few days to avoid decubitus ulcers, venous thrombosis, infections, or other complications associated with prolonged bed rest. As an alternative in selected cases, manual cervical distraction and extension followed by posterior fixation alone may be attempted, particularly in patients with basilar invagination associated with Chiari malformation.[8]

The progress of the reduction is monitored with radiographs. The final decompressive effect of the traction is assessed with MRI. If full reduction can be achieved with traction and no residual compression exists, the patient's instability is treated with posterior occipitocervical fusion.

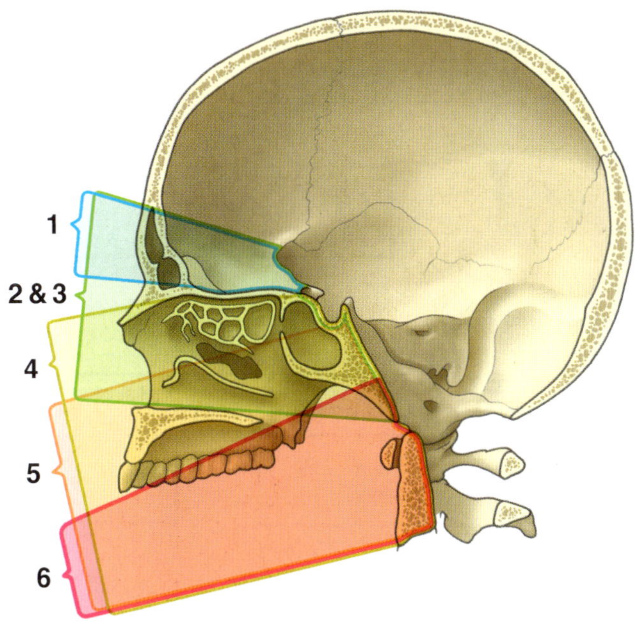

Fig. 21.1 Access to the clivus provided by combined exposures of the skull base and craniovertebral junction: (*1*) frontobasal approach; (*2, 3*) transfrontal, transethmoidal, and transmaxillary approaches; (*4*) transoral approach combined with transmaxillary, transfacial approach; (*5*) transoral approach combined with transmaxillary approach allows access from the upper clivus to the C2-C3 disk space; and (*6*) transoral–transpalatal approach provides access to the middle and lower clivus. The transoral approach alone usually provides access from the lower third of the clivus to the C2-C3 disk space. (Reprinted with permission from Barrow Neurological Institute.)

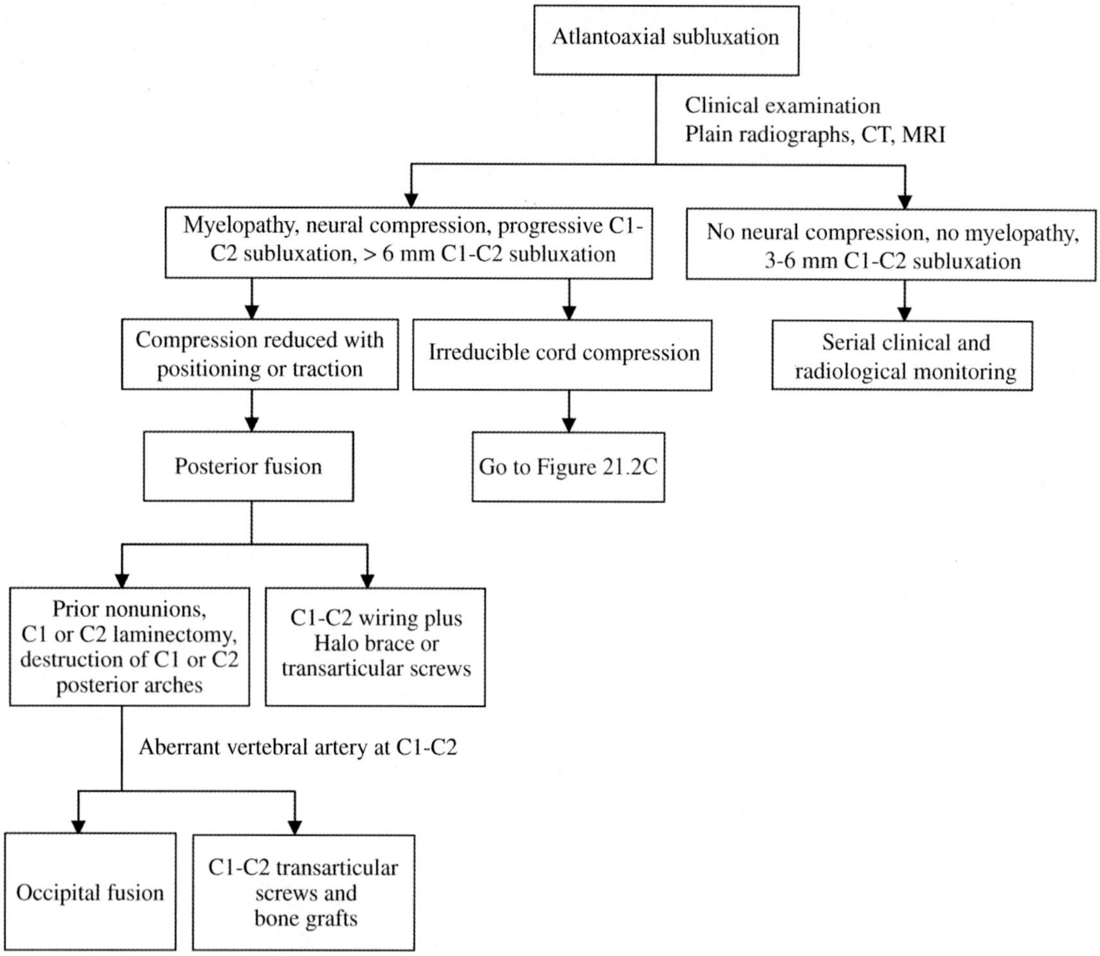

A

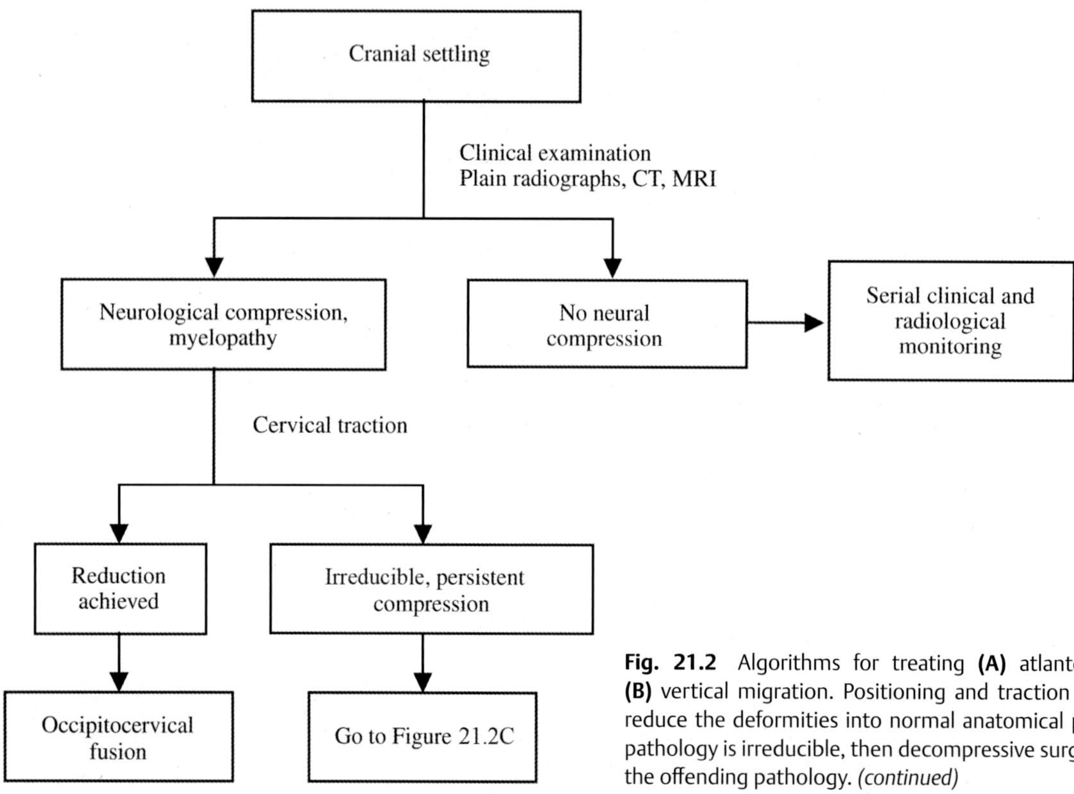

B

Fig. 21.2 Algorithms for treating **(A)** atlantoaxial subluxations and **(B)** vertical migration. Positioning and traction are used to attempt to reduce the deformities into normal anatomical positions. If compressive pathology is irreducible, then decompressive surgery is needed to remove the offending pathology. *(continued)*

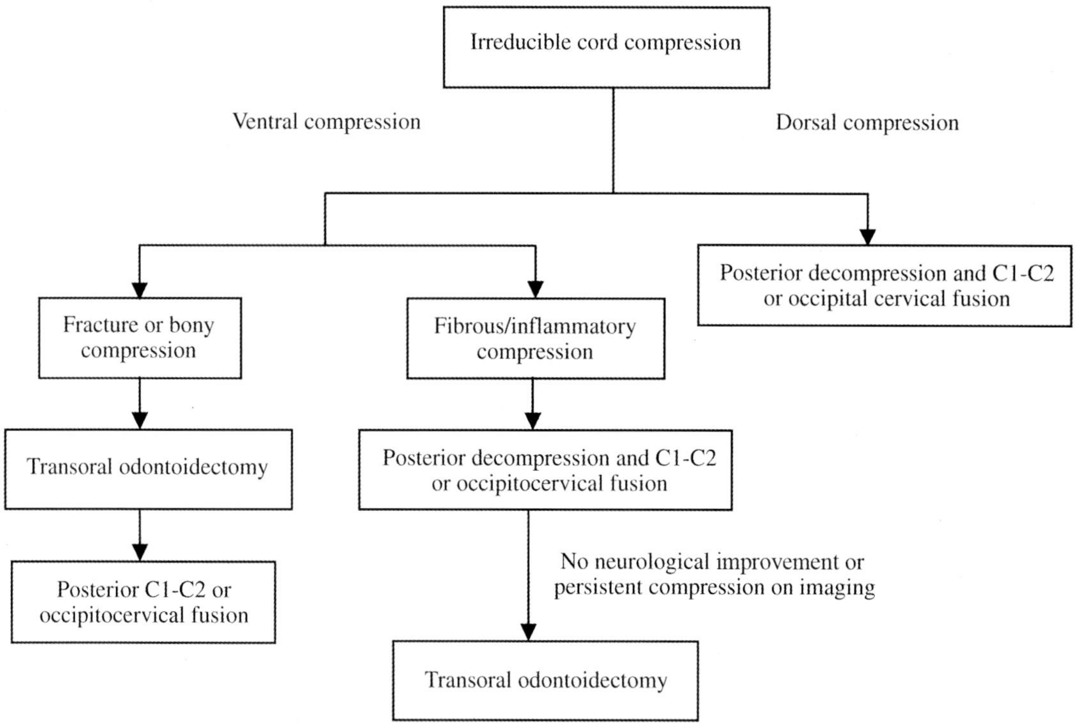

C

Fig. 21.2 *(continued)* This can be done **(C)** either anteriorly or posteriorly, depending on the nature and location of the compressive lesion. The extent of the stabilization procedures to treat the pathological motion depends on the patient's anatomy, the extent of the pathology, and the surfaces available for fixation. (Figs. 21.2A and B reprinted from Dickman CA, Ronderos JF, Sonntag VKH. Stabilization of the craniovertebral junction in rheumatoid arthritis. Part I: Pathophysiology, diagnosis and surgical criteria. Contemp Neurosurg 1995;17[12]:1–6.)

However, if the compressive pathology is irreducible and consists of bony or noninflammatory elements (**Figs. 21.3** and **21.4**), decompression and staged internal fixation are required.

Reduction with traction is attempted primarily in patients with rheumatoid arthritis, infections, neoplasms, and bone softening diseases.[1–3,9–16] Congenital malformations of the CVJ usually are static and cannot be reduced with traction.[13,17,18] Patients with ventral CVJ tumors or infections may require transoral surgery for resection or debridement of their pathology in addition to neural decompression. If instability is associated with the pathology or develops

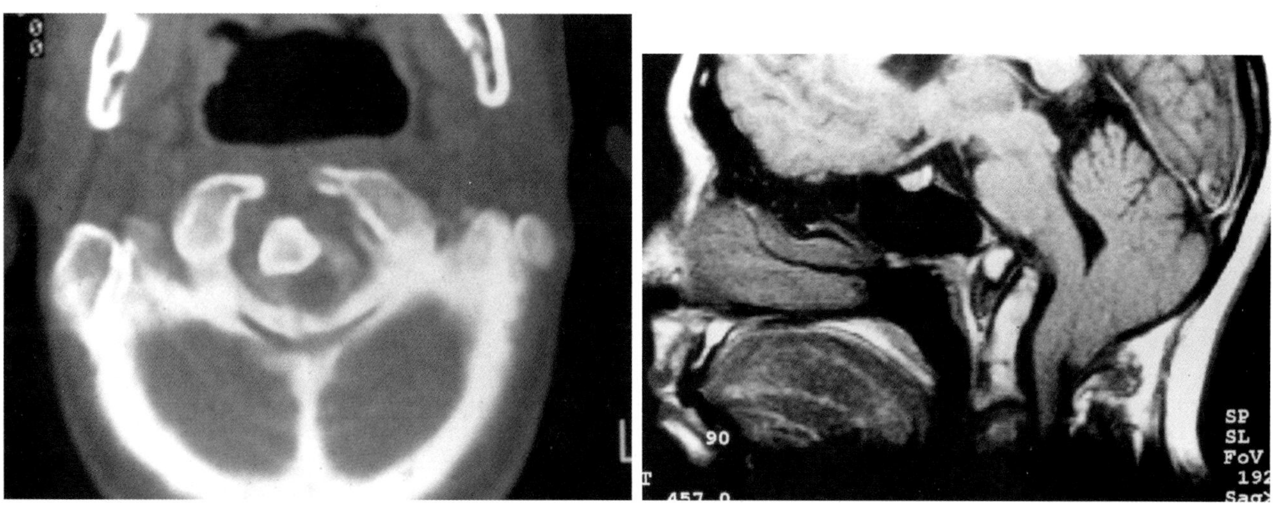

A B

Fig. 21.3 **(A)** Postmyelogram computed tomography scan of an irreducible congenital malformation of the craniovertebral junction. The odontoid process is compressing and distorting the medulla. **(B)** Sagittal magnetic resonance image provides an excellent perspective of the pathoanatomical relationships. This patient has platybasia, failure of segmentation, occipitalization of C1, fusion of C2-C3, compression of the pons and medulla, and a Chiari malformation.

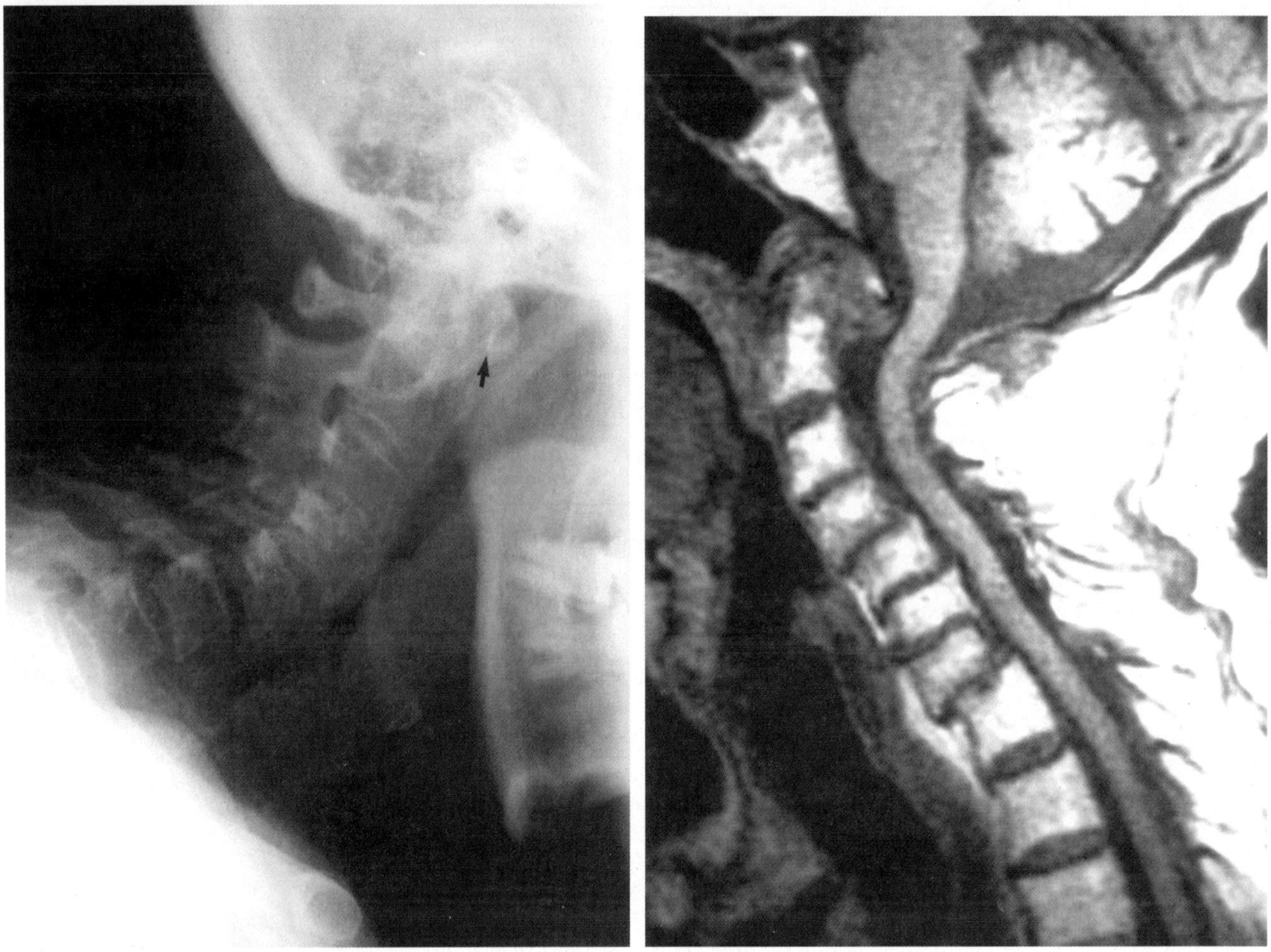

A B

Fig. 21.4 **(A)** Lateral cervical radiograph of a myelopathic patient with rheumatoid arthritis. This patient's deformity was irreducible with traction and neck extension. The anterior arch of C1 (*arrow*) and skull base are displaced ventrally and inferiorly. **(B)** Magnetic resonance image demonstrates the soft tissue pannus, bone erosion, and compression and distortion of the medulla and spinal cord. The lax ligaments in the subaxial spine create a "staircase" effect with the vertebral bodies.

postoperatively, a staged posterior approach is used for occipitocervical or atlantoaxial fixation (**Fig. 21.2**).

Myriad symptoms occur with compression of the CVJ.[1–3,9,10,12,14,15,19,20] These symptoms can be nonspecific and difficult to localize. The diagnosis often is delayed and mistaken for demyelinating diseases or other types of pathology. Ischemic symptoms may develop if the vertebrobasilar system, posterior inferior cerebellar artery, or anterior spinal artery is involved. Compressive symptoms can occur if the lower cranial nerves, brainstem, spinal cord, or cerebellum is involved. Spinal instability can be superimposed on the compression, causing severe neck pain, occipital neuralgia, radicular pain, or worsening neurological symptoms.

Transoral odontoidectomy provides a midline ventral extradural exposure of the CVJ that avoids traction or manipulation of critical anatomical structures such as the cranial nerves, brainstem, spinal cord, or vertebral arteries. In comparison, during the high retropharyngeal approach to the anterior CVJ, the lower cranial nerves are retracted, branches of the external carotid arteries are sacrificed, and the pharynx is mobilized extensively. These maneuvers result in extensive, prolonged dysphagia and can be avoided with the transoral approach. The retropharyngeal approach has the relative advantage of being extramucosal and is better suited for ventral bone grafting or application of anterior screw plate fixation devices because bacterial contamination is avoided.

Transoral surgery is contraindicated if an active nasopharyngeal infection is present or if any vascular structures (i.e., vertebral or basilar arteries) are within or ventral to the lesion. Typically, the transoral approach is inappropriate for intradural pathology because of the risks of meningitis and cerebrospinal fluid (CSF) leakage.[11,20,21] These complications reflect the inability to obtain a watertight dural closure transorally. Patients with compressive pathology posterior or lateral to the spinal cord and brainstem or with reducible anterior compressive lesions can be treated with alternative approaches. They do not need transoral decompression.

■ Operative Technique

Transoral odontoidectomy is performed with simple techniques designed to facilitate the ease and safety of the procedure. Custom-designed instrumentation is used for exposure, retraction, and tissue dissection (**Fig. 21.5**). Self-retaining retractor systems are used. The tongue and endotracheal tube are retracted caudally with a wide-blade retractor, and the soft palate is retracted superiorly with a malleable blade retractor. A tracheostomy is avoided unless severe, preoperative bulbar or respiratory disturbances exist. If possible, a palatal incision is avoided because it can cause nasal regurgitation, dysphagia, and a nasal tone of voice.

Positioning

The patient is positioned supine on the operating table with the head slightly extended. Reverse Trendelenburg positioning of the operating table and neck extension provide the surgeon with direct visualization of the pathology (**Fig. 21.6**). The skull is rigidly fixated with a Mayfield head holder; however, a halo brace can be used if the patient has preoperative spinal instability. The anterior bars of the halo brace can be removed temporarily to allow room for the retractors and to bring the surgeon's hands closer to the patient's mouth. The surgeon is seated at the top of the patient's head. Surgery is enhanced by the precise visualization, magnification, and illumination provided by a binocular surgical microscope. A microscope with a 350-mm or 400-mm lens is used to allow for the depth of the working field.

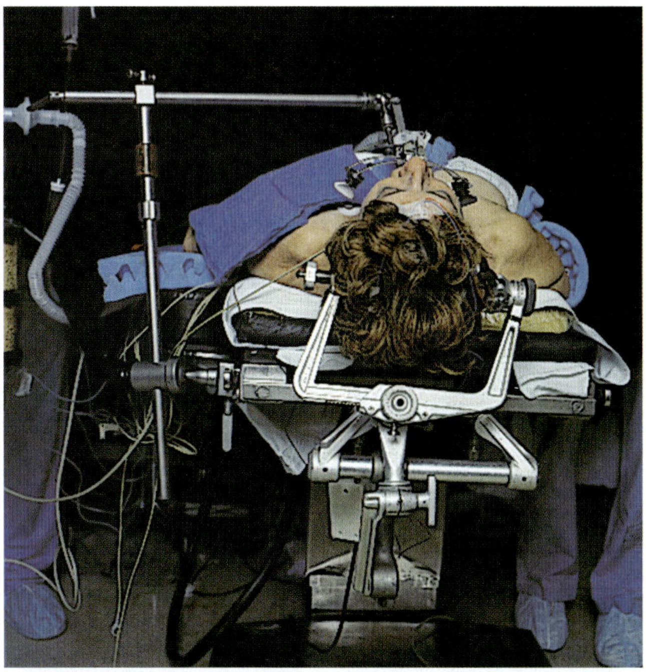

A

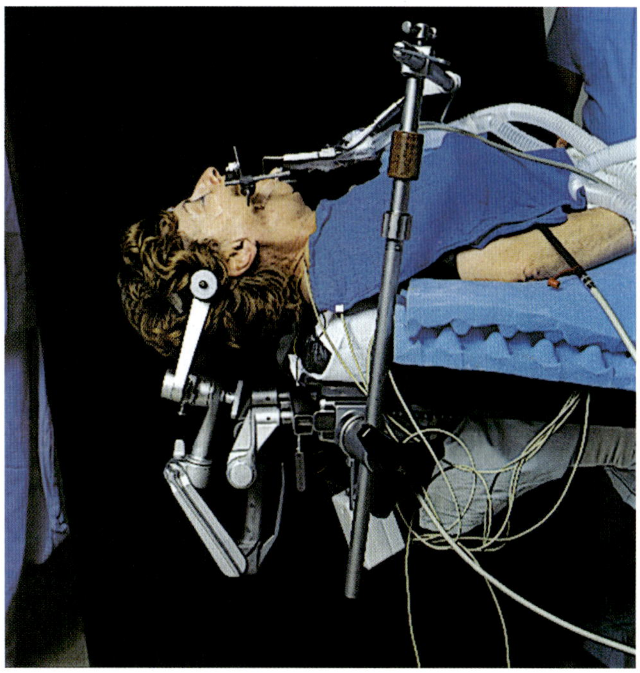

B

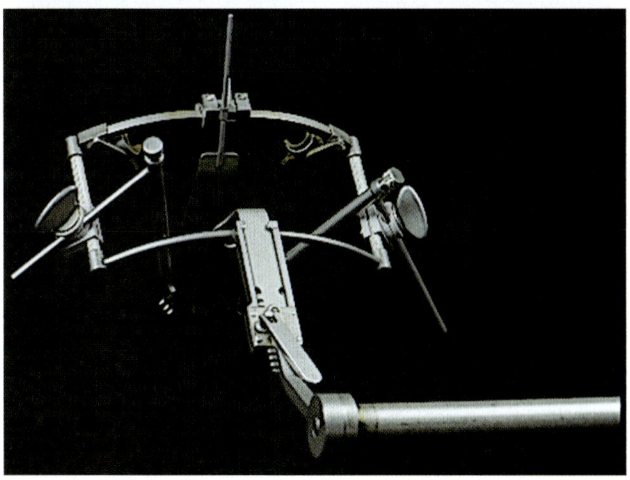

C

Fig. 21.5 Table-mounted, self-retaining transoral retractor system. **(A,B)** The patient's head is slightly extended and fixated with a Mayfield head holder. Cross bars are used to rigidly attach the transoral retractors to the operating table. **(C)** Four adjustable retractors mount to the curved rectangular frame. A malleable blade is used to retract the soft palate and uvula. A caudal rigid blade is used to retract the tongue and the endotracheal tube and to open the mouth widely. Lateral retractors are used for soft tissue exposure. Padded guards protect the teeth.

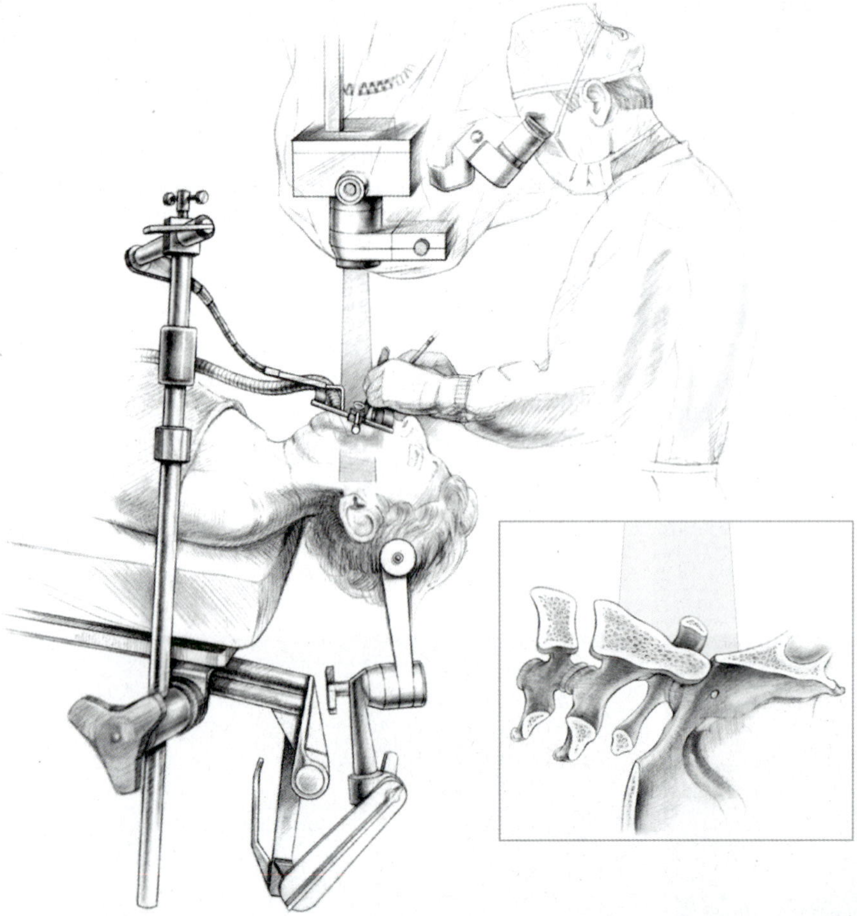

Fig. 21.6 Operative positioning. The patient's head is extended, and the table is tilted to provide the surgeon with a direct line of sight to the lower clivus and upper cervical spine (*inset*). The surgeon is positioned at the top of the patient's head to provide unrestricted hand movement and a comfortable body position. (Reprinted with permission from Barrow Neurological Institute.)

Instrumentation

A table-mounted retractor system is used to facilitate the exposure. The retractor frame is rigidly attached to the operating table with cross bars to prevent the retractors from moving intraoperatively (**Fig. 21.5A,B**). The patient's tongue and the endotracheal tube are retracted caudally by a rigid, adjustable, wide retractor blade. A malleable retractor blade is used to displace the soft palate and the uvula superiorly to provide access to the upper posterior oropharynx. Teeth guards attached to the retractor frame protect the patient's teeth. Adjustable soft tissue retractors are used to retract the pharyngeal tissue flaps laterally (**Fig. 21.7**). This retractor system was developed specifically to facilitate wide exposure of the posterior oropharynx for transoral decompression. After the retractor system is positioned, the patient's tongue should be inspected to ensure that it is not pinched by the teeth to avoid severe necrosis or swelling of the tongue. The oropharynx and the retractors are sterilized with Betadine solution after the retractors have been positioned.

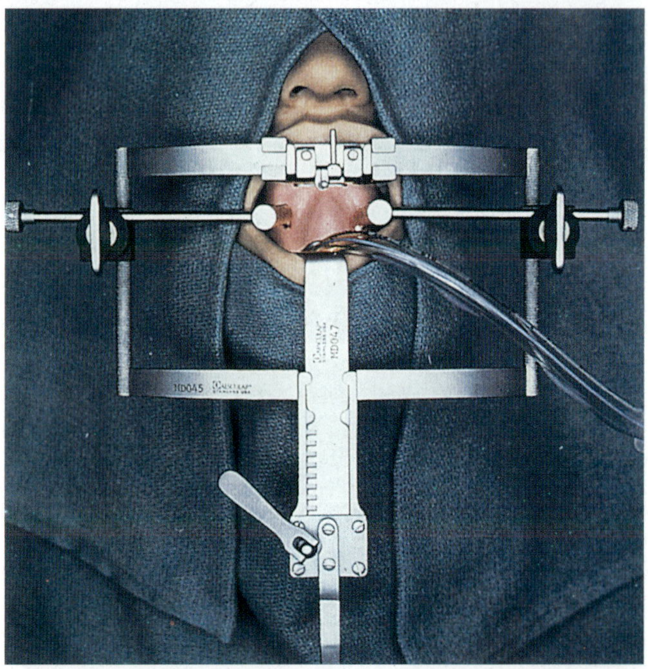

Fig. 21.7 The adjustable retractor provides wide access to the posterior oropharynx. The endotracheal tube and tongue are retracted caudally by a stiff blade that also opens the mouth. Adjustable palatal and pharyngeal retractors mount directly to the frame and are accessible for intraoperative repositioning.

Odontoidectomy

An intraoperative radiograph is obtained to judge the spinal alignment after positioning and to confirm the extent of the cephalad and caudal exposure provided by the

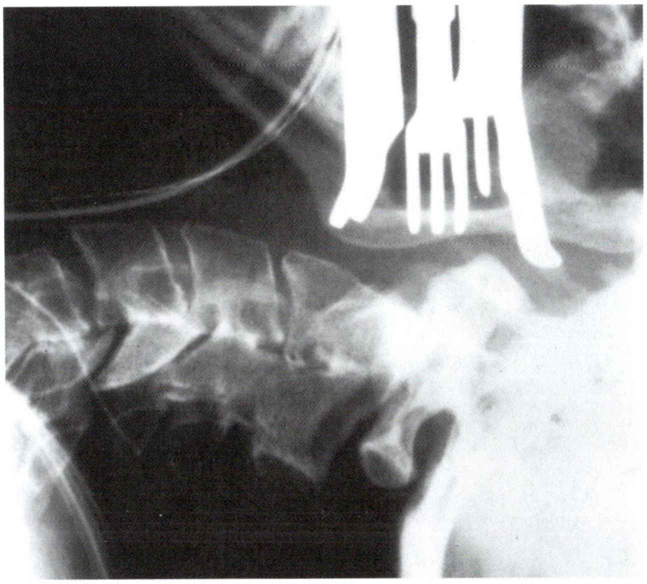

Fig. 21.8 Intraoperative lateral cervical radiograph demonstrates the position of the retractors relative to the patient's pathology and allows assessment of spinal alignment.

retractor system (**Fig. 21.8**). The C1 tubercle is palpated to verify the position of the midline. A linear midline incision is created in the median raphe of the posterior pharyngeal wall and proceeds downward sharply through the mucosa, pharyngeal muscles, and the anterior longitudinal ligament (**Fig. 21.9A**). The layers are not dissected separately but are maintained as a single thick layer for a strong tissue closure. The single-layer tissue flap is elevated from the surface of the spine and clivus to retain continuity of the layers. Monopolar cauterization or a Shaw scalpel can be used to create the incision and simultaneously to obtain hemostasis. Periosteal elevators are used to dissect the anterior longitudinal ligament subperiosteally and to separate the tissue flap from the anterior surfaces of the C1 arch, C2 vertebral body, and inferior clivus. Tooth-bladed retractors are inserted to retract the pharyngeal flaps laterally to maintain a wide exposure (**Fig. 21.9B**).

Curettes and periosteal elevators are used to define the boundaries of the clivus, the base of the odontoid process, and the anterior C1 arch and C2 vertebral body. The inferior rim of the anterior arch of C1 is resected to expose the base of the odontoid process using a high-speed pneumatic drill and a Kerrison rongeur. Osseous dissection is performed with small cutting burrs and diamond burrs. The soft tissue structures are detached with curettes and microsurgical tools. As much of the anterior arch of C1 as possible should be left intact to preserve the structural integrity of the C1 ring. However, enough bone needs to be removed to access the dens adequately. The surgeon can usually work between the clivus and C1 arch to access the tip of the dens while preserving part of the C1 ring.

After the anterior arch of C1 is partially removed, the lateral margins of the odontoid process are defined (**Fig. 21.10A**). The odontoid is removed by transecting it across its base and pulling the centrum and apex of the dens caudally and ventrally away from the cervicomedullary junction (**Fig. 21.10B,C**). The base of the dens is partially transected with a cutting burr; the osteotomy is completed by removing the posterior cortex of the dens with a 1-mm Kerrison rongeur or diamond burr. The dens is grasped with a toothed odontoid rongeur and pulled ventrally and caudally to decompress the neural structures before the ligamentous attachments are cut. The alar and apical ligaments are detached sharply with curved curettes (**Fig. 21.10D**). The odontoid fragment is then completely removed. The dens can also be removed in a piecemeal fashion; however, it is more

A 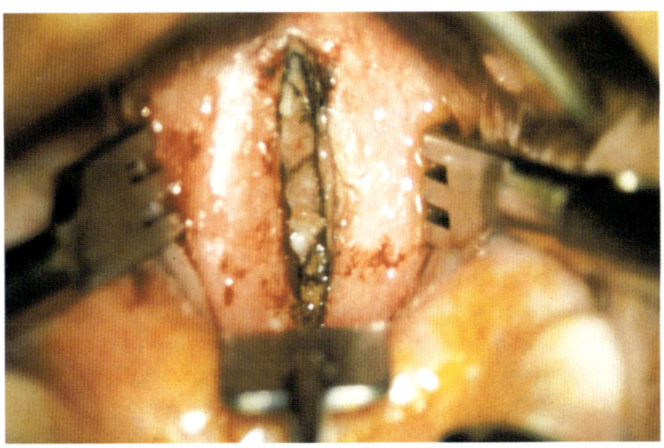 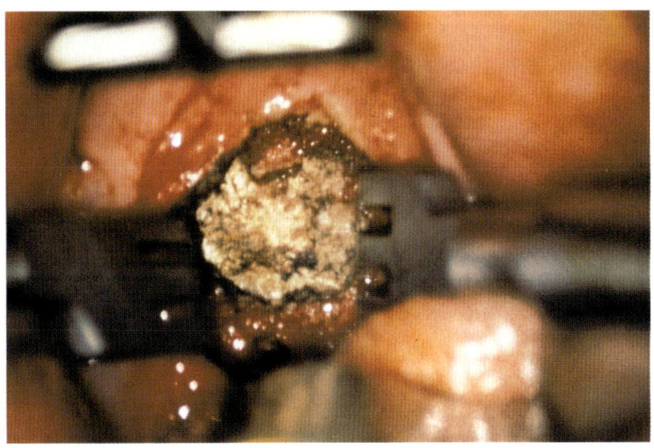 B

Fig. 21.9 Intraoperative photographs of the surgeon's view of the transoral surgical site. The clivus and skull base are oriented at the bottom of the photographs while the tongue and mandible are at the top. **(A)** A midline incision is made through all three layers of the oropharynx, and a single-layer soft tissue flap is elevated from the surface of the spine and clivus. **(B)** Self-retaining retractors are inserted to spread the margins of the incision laterally. The anterior arch of C1 is completely visible within the incision.

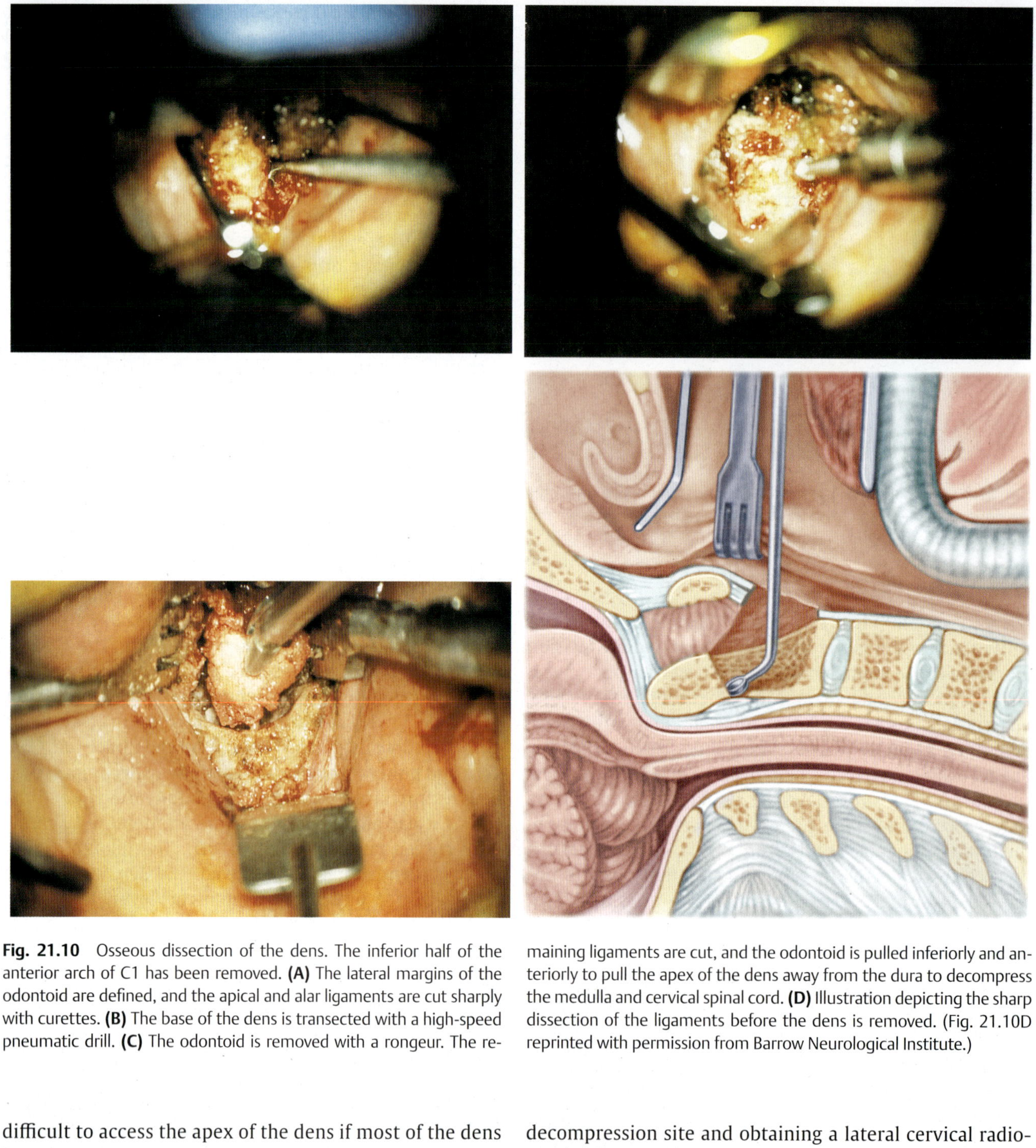

Fig. 21.10 Osseous dissection of the dens. The inferior half of the anterior arch of C1 has been removed. **(A)** The lateral margins of the odontoid are defined, and the apical and alar ligaments are cut sharply with curettes. **(B)** The base of the dens is transected with a high-speed pneumatic drill. **(C)** The odontoid is removed with a rongeur. The remaining ligaments are cut, and the odontoid is pulled inferiorly and anteriorly to pull the apex of the dens away from the dura to decompress the medulla and cervical spinal cord. **(D)** Illustration depicting the sharp dissection of the ligaments before the dens is removed. (Fig. 21.10D reprinted with permission from Barrow Neurological Institute.)

difficult to access the apex of the dens if most of the dens is gone.

Soft tissue pathology often must be resected to obtain adequate decompression of the dura. The transverse ligament and tectorial membrane may need to be removed to visualize the dura and normal pulsation of the thecal sac (**Fig. 21.11**). However, the surgeon must be aware of attenuated dura and ligaments that can adhere to the dura. Meticulous microsurgical techniques are necessary to avoid a CSF leak from inadvertent intradural entry. The boundaries of the decompression can be assessed intraoperatively by placing iodinated contrast material into the decompression site and obtaining a lateral cervical radiograph (**Fig. 21.12**).

Once the brainstem and spinal cord have been decompressed adequately, the wound is irrigated with antibiotic solution and hemostasis is achieved. The wound is closed in a single layer with interrupted or running 2–0 Vicryl suture (Ethicon, Somerville, NJ). The mucosa, pharyngeal muscles, and ligaments are included in the single-layer closure. This single-layer tissue closure is more effective and easier to perform than a multiple-layer closure, which attenuates the tissue layers and weakens the closure. Immediately after the incision is closed, a nasogastric feeding tube is inserted while directly visualizing the oropharyngeal wound to avoid complications from malpositioning the feeding tube. If an intradural procedure was performed or if the dura was opened intraoperatively, a fascial patch is placed directly over the dura and secured with fibrin glue. A lumbar drain is inserted immediately; antibiotic coverage and the lumbar drain are maintained for at least 1 week. Intradural entry is associated with a high risk of postoperative meningitis. Vigilance should be maintained to prevent infectious complications. Immediately after surgery, a cervical orthosis is applied until spinal stability is assessed.

Postoperative Management

Postoperatively, the endotracheal tube is maintained until the patient's tongue swelling subsides. Typically, moderate tongue swelling can be expected after surgery, but it usually subsides within 36 hours. Topical steroids have been applied to the tongue preoperatively to minimize tongue swelling. However, their benefit has not been established. On the first postoperative day, enteral feedings are begun using a nasoduodenal feeding tube. After the first week, patients are advanced from clear liquids to full liquids and then to a soft diet.

In all cases, spinal stability should be assessed immediately after surgery because transoral odontoidectomy is likely to destabilize the CVJ unless a preexisting congenital assimilation or bone fusion is present (**Fig. 21.13**).[13,14] More than 90% of patients with rheumatoid arthritis and half of patients with congenital malformations will become unstable after transoral odontoidectomy.[17,22] Transoral odontoidectomy can have dramatic mechanical effects. It significantly increases the amount of translational and rotational motion in all directions.[22] It also induces tremendous laxity in the atlantoaxial joints. If the CVJ is unstable after surgery, the patient should be immobilized with a cervical orthosis until surgery can be performed for internal fixation.

Ventral bone grafts are seldom placed into the transoral defect because they are associated with a high rate of infection, dislodgement, and reabsorption. Ventral bone grafts provide a compressive strut (**Fig. 21.14**); however, they can become displaced easily, cannot be fixated, and do not restore spinal stability.[19,23,24] If postoperative

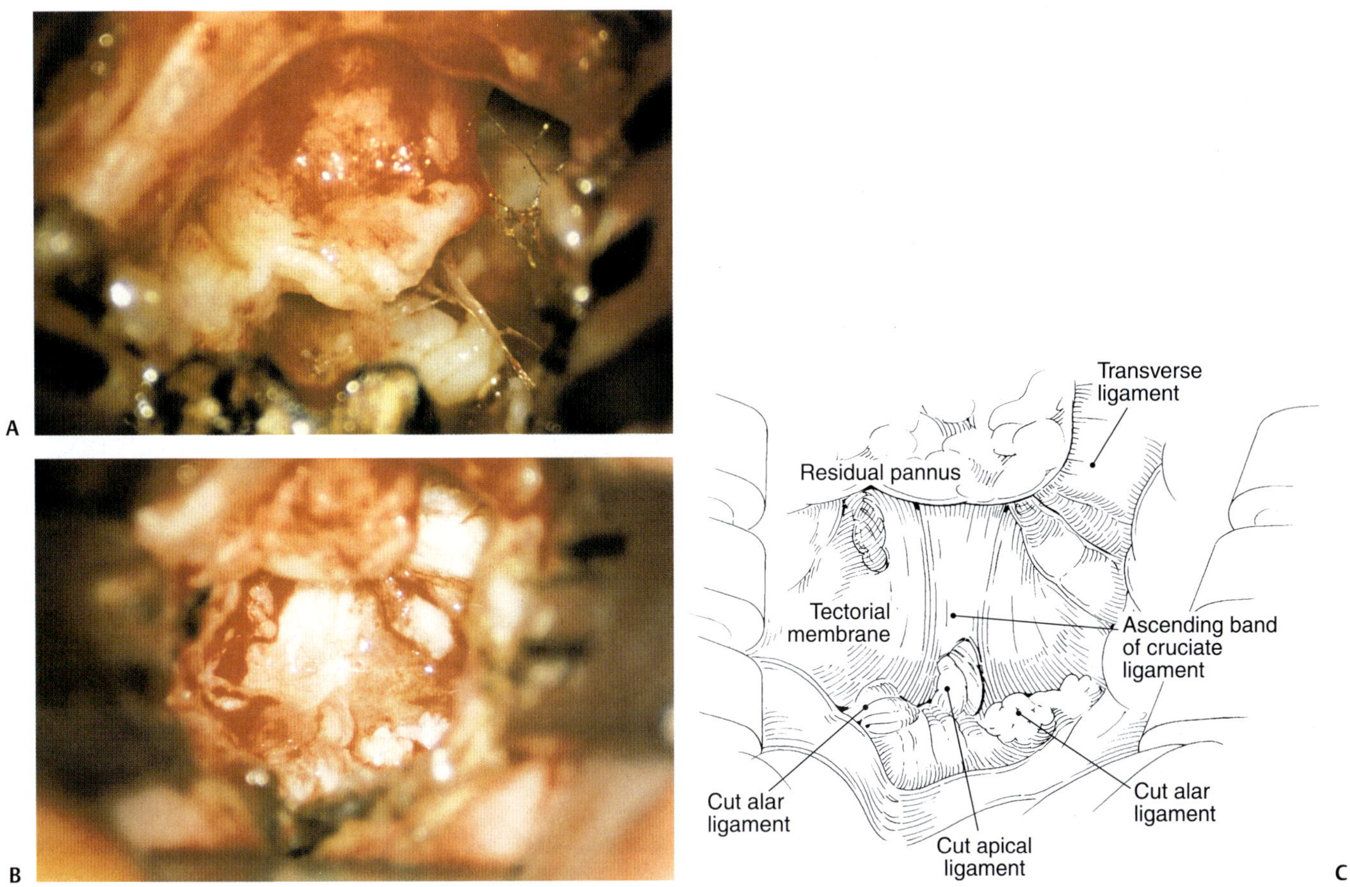

Fig. 21.11 **(A)** Intraoperative photograph of a 62-year-old woman with rheumatoid arthritis and extensive soft tissue pannus compressing the cervicomedullary junction. The odontoid process has been removed, yet extensive mass effect persists from the remaining pannus (*center*). **(B)** Intraoperative photograph and **(C)** illustration showing most of the pannus removed. The transverse atlantal ligament, the ascending band of the cruciate ligament, and the tectorial membrane are revealed. *(continued)*

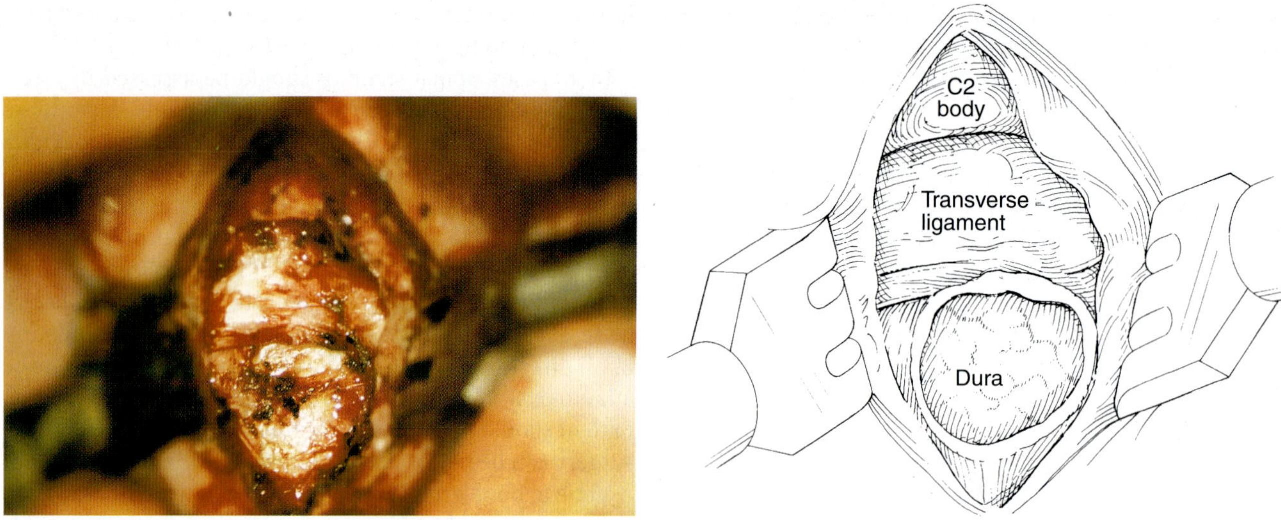

D E

Fig. 21.11 *(continued)* **(D)** Intraoperative photograph and **(E)** illustration showing that the tectorial membrane has been resected last to reveal the dura. Intraoperatively, visible dural pulsations and palpation along the margins verify that decompression is adequate. (Reprinted with permission from Barrow Neurological Institute.)

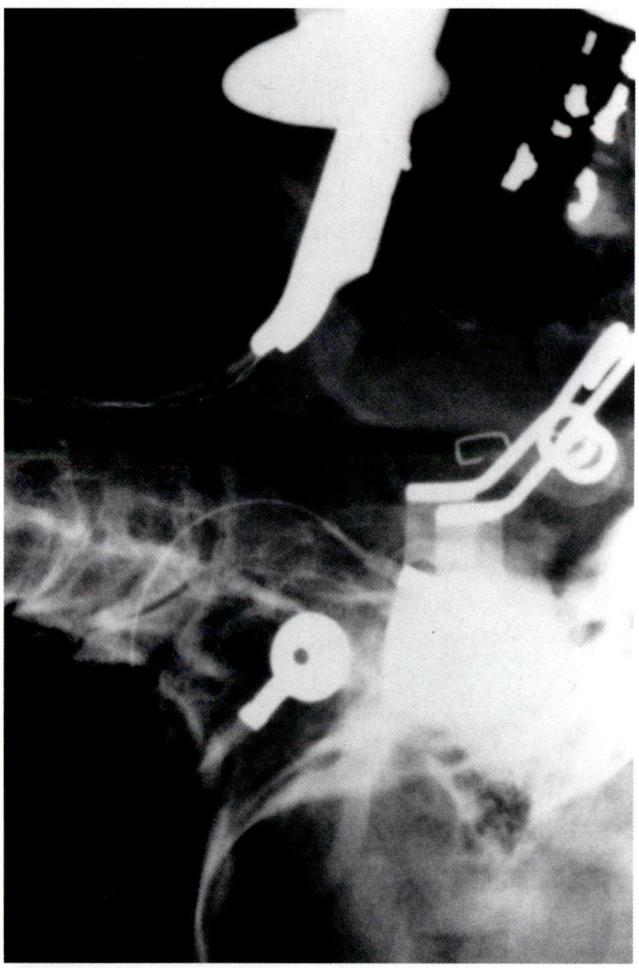

Fig. 21.12 Intraoperative lateral cervical radiograph with contrast media filling the decompression site to verify the cephalad and caudal boundaries of the exposure.

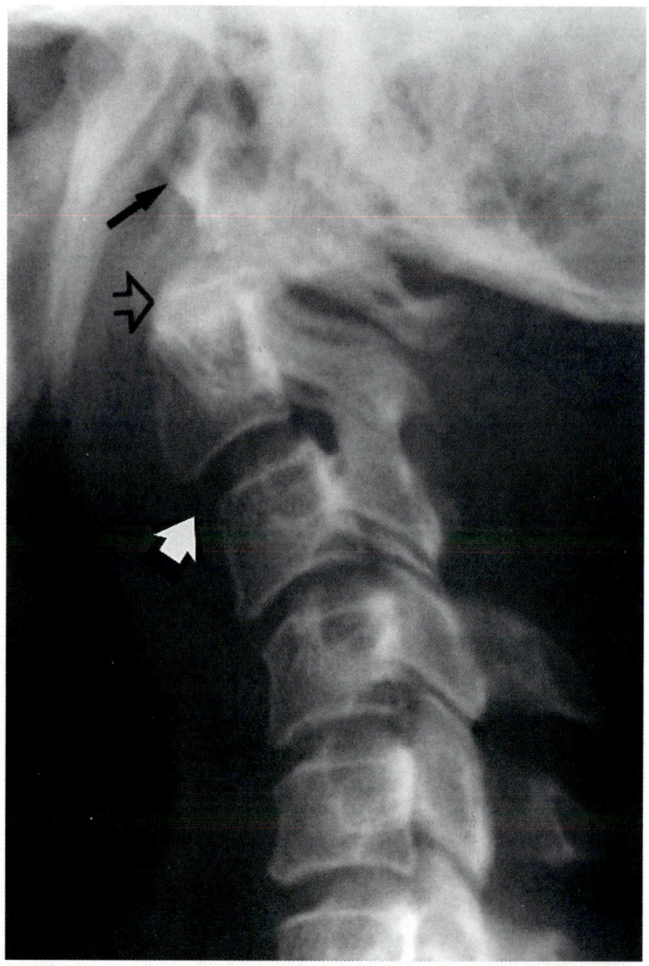

Fig. 21.13 Postoperative lateral cervical radiograph after transoral odontoidectomy demonstrates hypermobility. The C1 arch (*narrow dark arrow*) is displaced posteriorly in relationship to the anterior edge of the C2 body (*open arrow*). Due to rheumatoid involvement, a subluxation is also present at C2-C3 (*solid white arrow*). This patient was stabilized with a posterior occipitocervical fusion that extended from the occiput through C3.

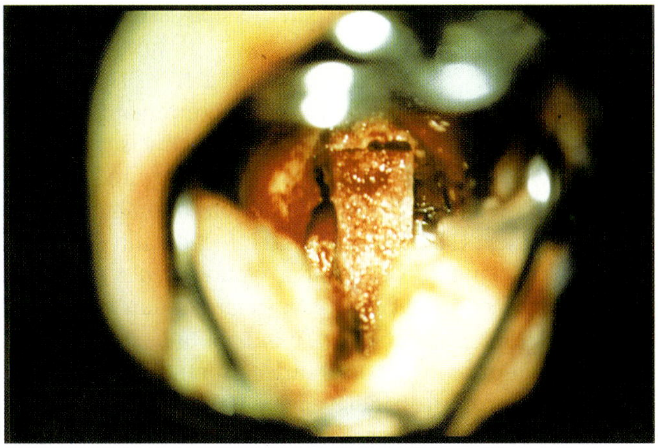

A

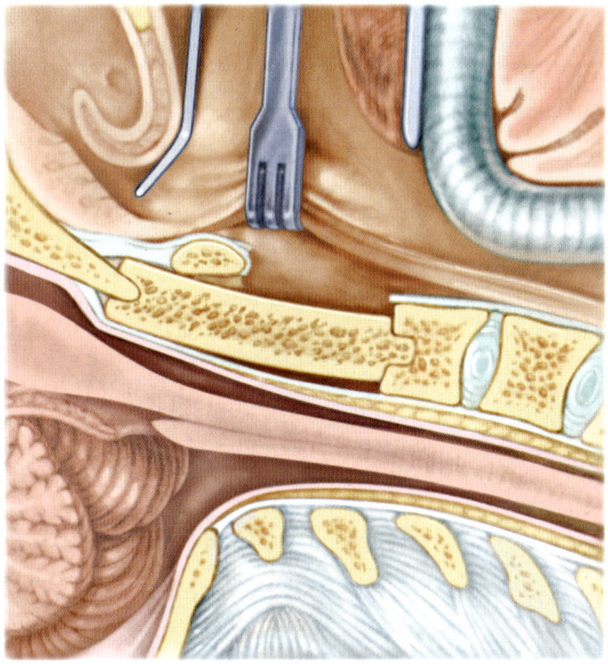

B

Fig. 21.14 **(A)** An autologous iliac crest strut graft was placed transorally and seated between the clivus and C2 to reconstruct the bone defect. **(B)** Illustration of transoral bone graft placed in a lock-and-key fit between the clivus and spine. The graft acts as a spacer and a strut. Posterior fixation is still required when a transoral graft is used. (Fig. 21.14B reprinted with permission from Barrow Neurological Institute.)

instability exists, posterior atlantoaxial or occipitocervical fixation should be performed. Occipitocervical fixation is required when basilar invagination or occipitoatlantal instability occurs, or if C1 and C2 cannot be fixated directly. Atlantoaxial instability is treated with atlantoaxial fixation devices. When possible, we limit the fixation to C1-C2 to preserve normal motion.[17,20,22,23] Although some surgeons advocate immediate posterior fixation of the spine after transoral surgery, we prefer to wait several days to reduce the risk of wound infection in the posterior cervical wound.

Surgical Results

The neurological outcome of patients treated with transoral odontoidectomy is directly related to the severity of their preoperative neurological deficits.[1–4,10,12–15] Ambulatory patients demonstrate the most neurological recovery after surgery. Severely myelopathic patients who are unable to walk before surgery have a poor chance of ambulating afterward. Early detection and early treatment of pathology can facilitate recovery. Once advanced myelopathy develops, function may not be salvageable, although even in nonambulatory patients some improvement may be seen and may warrant aggressive surgical management.[25]

Table 21.1 delineates the authors' surgical experience with 148 patients treated with transoral odontoidectomy. Most of the patients were treated for rheumatoid arthritis, congenital malformations, or chronic dens fractures. A small proportion of patients was treated for extradural tumors, and intradural lesions were rare. Most patients complained of neck pain, incoordination, dysesthesias, and numbness and weakness of arms, legs, or both (**Table 21.2**). On examination, most patients had decreased neck motion and myelopathy. Postoperatively, after transoral decompression, the neurological outcome has been excellent; the neurological function of 79% of the patients improved objectively, and the neurological deficits of 21% stabilized.

Postoperative medical complications were relatively common, primarily because the patients had severe, incapacitating, preoperative neurological deficits and debilitating medical illnesses. The most frequent complications included pneumonia and urinary tract infections.

Table 21.1 Barrow Neurological Institute Experience: Transoral Odontoidectomy 1978–1996

Pathology	No. of Procedures (N = 148)
Nonneoplastic ($n = 130$)	
Rheumatoid arthritis	58
Congenital malformations	37
Chronic dens dislocations	29
Granuloma	4
Bullet wound	2
Extradural tumors ($n = 16$)	
Primary tumors	11
Metastatic neoplasms	5
Intradural lesions ($n = 2$)	
Epidermoid	1
Spinal arteriovenous malformation with pseudoaneurysm	1

Table 21.2 Neurological Signs and Symptoms of Ventral Foramen Magnum Lesions (148 patients)

Neurological Condition	No. (%)	Neurological Condition	No. (%)
Symptoms		Signs	
Neck pain	130 (88)	Decreased neck motion	134 (91)
Incoordination/ clumsiness	125 (84)	Myelopathy	120 (81)
Dysesthesia	122 (82)	Nasal voice	43 (29)
Numbness	122 (82)	Upper extremity atrophy	42 (28)
Arm and leg weakness	113 (76)	Decreased rectal tone	33 (22)
Voice changes	42 (28)	Decreased gag	26 (18)
Urinary incontinence	31 (21)	Lower extremity atrophy	20 (14)
Difficulty swallowing	29 (20)	Uncoordinated swallowing	18 (12)
Apnea	3 (2)	Bilateral sixth nerve palsy	1 (0.7)
Diplopia	1 (0.7)		

Direct operative complications occurred in 14 patients. Three patients (2%) died. One had an intraoperative CSF leak and subsequently developed *Enterobacter* pneumonia, meningitis, and sepsis. The second experienced respiratory arrest after extubation. The third had a transoral–transdural approach for treatment of a C2-C3 spinal arteriovenous malformation and pseudoaneurysm. He developed purulent meningitis without evidence of wound dehiscence and died 16 weeks after surgery from rupture of a new mycotic basilar artery aneurysm.

Seven patients (5%) had a CSF leak at surgery. Four patients had a CSF leak alone, and it was treated satisfactorily with lumbar drainage. Two patients had associated meningitis. One was treated satisfactorily with lumbar drainage and antibiotics; however, the other died of sepsis as described in the preceding paragraph. The remaining patient had an associated wound dehiscence that was treated successfully with reoperation, dural patching, and reclosure of the pharyngeal incision, in addition to lumbar drainage. Two patients (1.4%) had a wound infection and dehiscence, and three patients (2%) had a wound dehiscence alone. There were no direct operative-related neurological injuries. However, one patient who did not undergo a stabilization procedure after transoral decompression developed a brainstem stroke from delayed vertical occipitoatlantal subluxation and bilateral occlusion of the vertebral arteries.

■ Conclusion

Transoral odontoidectomy is an effective surgical method for the direct decompression of irreducible ventral midline extradural compressive pathology of the CVJ. This procedure is facilitated with wide retraction of the mouth and oropharyngeal soft tissue boundaries using specialized retractor systems. Tracheostomy, soft palate incision, and extended exposures are usually unnecessary because they increase the morbidity rates associated with this procedure.

The early signs of ventral foramen magnum compression can be subtle; however, early diagnosis can be achieved with a thorough clinical and neurological examination and high-resolution imaging studies. Early decompressive surgery facilitates neurological recovery by preserving existing neurological function. Once advanced myelopathy has developed, a patient's chances of achieving functional recovery are reduced significantly.

References

1. Crockard HA, Pozo JL, Ransford AO, Stevens JM, Kendall BE, Essigman WK. Transoral decompression and posterior fusion for rheumatoid atlanto-axial subluxation. J Bone Joint Surg Br 1986; 68(3):350–356
2. Menezes AH, VanGilder JC. Transoral-transpharyngeal approach to the anterior craniocervical junction. Ten-year experience with 72 patients. J Neurosurg 1988;69(6):895–903
3. Crockard HA. The transoral approach to the base of the brain and upper cervical cord. Ann R Coll Surg Engl 1985;67(5):321–325
4. Mouchaty H, Perrini P, Conti R, Di Lorenzo N. Craniovertebral junction lesions: our experience with the transoral surgical approach. Eur Spine J 2009;18(1, Suppl 1):13–19
5. Bouchaud-Chabot A, Lioté F. Cervical spine involvement in rheumatoid arthritis. A review. Joint Bone Spine 2002;69(2):141–154
6. Grob D, Schütz U, Plötz G. Occipitocervical fusion in patients with rheumatoid arthritis. Clin Orthop Relat Res 1999;366(366): 46–53
7. Grob D. [Surgical aspects of the cervical spine in rheumatoid arthritis]. Orthopade 2004;33(10):1201–1212, quiz 1213–1214
8. Kim LJ, Rekate HL, Klopfenstein JD, Sonntag VK. Treatment of basilar invagination associated with Chiari I malformations in the pediatric population: cervical reduction and posterior occipitocervical fusion. J Neurosurg 2004;101(2, Suppl):189–195
9. Masferrer R, Hadley MN, Bloomfield S, et al. Transoral microsurgical resection of the odontoid process. BNI Q 1985;1(3):34–40
10. Spetzler RF, Selman WR, Nash CL Jr, Brown RH. Transoral microsurgical odontoid resection and spinal cord monitoring. Spine 1979;4(6):506–510
11. Bonkowski JA, Gibson RD, Snape L. Foramen magnum meningioma: transoral resection with a bone baffle to prevent CSF leakage. Case report. J Neurosurg 1990;72(3):493–496
12. Hadley MN, Spetzler RF, Sonntag VKH. The transoral approach to the superior cervical spine. A review of 53 cases of extradural cervicomedullary compression. J Neurosurg 1989;71(1):16–23
13. Menezes AH, VanGilder JC, Graf CJ, McDonnell DE. Craniocervical abnormalities. A comprehensive surgical approach. J Neurosurg 1980;53(4):444–455
14. Mullan S, Naunton R, Hekmat-Panah J, Vailati G. The use of an anterior approach to ventrally placed tumors in the foramen magnum and vertebral column. J Neurosurg 1966;24(2):536–543

15. Scoville WB, Sherman IJ. Platybasia, report of 10 cases with comments on familial tendency, a special diagnostic sign, and the end results of operation. Ann Surg 1951;133(4):496–502
16. Spetzler RF, Dickman CA, Sonntag VKH. The transoral approach to the anterior cervical spine. Contemp Neurosurg. 1991;13(9):1–6
17. Dickman CA, Locantro J, Fessler RG. The influence of transoral odontoid resection on stability of the craniovertebral junction. J Neurosurg 1992;77(4):525–530
18. Chamberlain WE. Basilar impression (platybasia). A bizarre developmental anomaly of the occipital bone and upper cervical spine with striking and misleading neurologic manifestations. Yale J Biol Med 1939;11(5):487–496
19. Fang D, Leong JCY, Fang HSY. Tuberculosis of the upper cervical spine. J Bone Joint Surg Br 1983;65(1):47–50
20. Yamaura A, Makino H, Isobe K, Takashima T, Nakamura T, Takemiya S. Repair of cerebrospinal fluid fistula following transoral transclival approach to a basilar aneurysm. Technical note. J Neurosurg 1979;50(6):834–838
21. Hadley MN, Martin NA, Spetzler RF, Sonntag VK, Johnson PC. Comparative transoral dural closure techniques: a canine model. Neurosurgery 1988;22(2):392–397
22. Dickman CA, Crawford NR, Brantley AGU, Sonntag VK. Biomechanical effects of transoral odontoidectomy. Neurosurgery 1995;36(6):1146–1152, discussion 1152–1153
23. Dickman CA, Crawford NR, Brantley AGU, et al. In vitro cervical spine biomechanical testing. BNI Q 1993;9(4):17–26
24. Panjabi M, Dvorak J, Duranceau J, et al. Three-dimensional movements of the upper cervical spine. Spine 1988;13(7): 726–730
25. Nannapaneni R, Behari S, Todd NV. Surgical outcome in rheumatoid Ranawat Class IIIb myelopathy. Neurosurgery 2005;56(4): 706–715, discussion 706–715

22 Transoral Approaches to Midline Pathology of the Ventral Skull Base, Craniovertebral Junction, and Upper Cervical Spine

David Choi and Hugh Alan Crockard

The maxim "ventral pathology should be approached ventrally" is usually adhered to by most spinal surgeons throughout the spine, but is frequently forgotten when considering the craniovertebral junction (CVJ). Here, differing opinions are put forward, sometimes with little evidence to support them. There is no doubt that all surgical approaches to this region are technically demanding, require much practice and skill, and are best performed within a suitably specialized multidisciplinary framework. There are particular situations where a lateral approach would be ideal, and equally it is our opinion that there are specific occasions when a direct midline anterior approach through the mouth offers considerable benefits for extradural midline pathologies. The family of transoral procedures should be added to the surgical armamentarium of those who operate at this junctional level.

History

Surgery in the mouth—including dental treatment, nasal passages, and sinuses—has been performed for centuries without significant mortality of infection. Surgery through the nose for pituitary tumors was used by Cushing, but only came into widespread use with the development by Jules Hardy, of Montreal, of dedicated retraction instruments, forceps, and rongeurs and is now considered a standard neurosurgical procedure.[1] Fear of infection is still one of the reasons given for avoiding transoral surgery,[2] but use of specific retraction instrumentation (Crockard instruments; Codman, Raynham, MA) and attention to good technique will minimize this hazard.[3]

The first transoral removal of a bullet lodged in the clivus was described by Kanaval in 1917.[4] It was not until the advent of computed tomography (CT) and magnetic resonance imaging (MRI) in the 1980s that the anatomy of the CVJ was better understood in regular clinical practice, allowing the development of appropriate retractors and, more importantly, the results of surgery could be seen by all and not just the operating surgeon.

In this chapter we lay out the indications and contraindications for ventral approaches as well as describe the variations on the standard transoral approach that we have developed in almost 600 cases over a 30-year period.

Transoral Surgery

The standard or "simple" transoral approach is ideal for midline extradural pathology between the anterior rim of the foramen magnum and C2 vertebra, in particular congenital or acquired bony abnormalities without basilar invagination, infections, and extradural tumors. It is contraindicated for completely intradural tumors, intradural vascular abnormalities, and lateral extradural tumors.

In the 1980s, for improved superior exposure, division of the hard palate or LeFort I osteotomy was tried,[5] but these did not improve visibility sufficiently to warrant the increased risk of complications, particularly nasal regurgitation and midface problems. However, if the LeFort I maxillotomy was combined with a midsagittal division of the hard palate, it was found that the resultant "halves" could be swung laterally, thereby providing a much better field of view.[6]

Superior extension by this so-called "open-door maxillotomy" allows surgery of the upper clivus to the sphenoid sinus and pituitary regions, whereas inferior extension by mandibulotomy and glossotomy permits visualization down to the C4 vertebra.

Table 22.1 shows the numbers of these operations performed over 30 years in our institute.

Further approaches have been developed via the midface degloving transmaxillary approach[7] and the transnasal endoscopic approach.[2] Over time, the choice of approach has often been influenced by changes in the pathologies that have presented to surgeons. For example, 25 years ago we were surrounded by patients with rheumatoid disease and myelopathy from extensive translocation, but now we only

Table 22.1 Numbers of Transoral and Extended Procedures Performed at the National Hospital for Neurology and Neurosurgery Over Three Decades (1980–2009)

Operation	Number
Standard transoral	317
Transoral with palate split	103
Open-door maxillotomy	58
Mandibulotomy	8

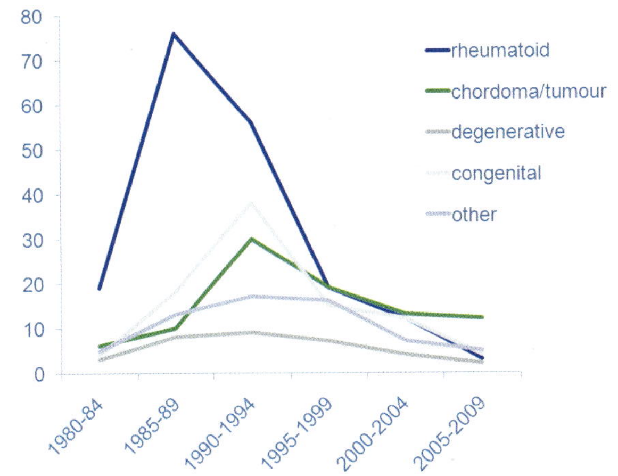

Fig. 22.1 Changes in the numbers of operations performed in the National Hospital for Neurology and Neurosurgery, United Kingdom, over the past three decades, showing a decrease in the number of patients presenting with rheumatoid disease and other pathologies.

see one or two a year in our unit.[8] In contrast, the referral rate for tumors of the CVJ has encouraged us to develop and modify our approach.[3] **Figure 22.1** shows the change in number of operations performed for different pathologies over the past three decades in our unit. The number of transoral operations for chordomas has remained fairly constant, whereas there has been a steady decline for many other pathologies, particularly rheumatoid disease. For all these complex procedures, a team approach in specialized units is essential.

Standard Transoral Surgery

Transoral surgery may be performed with or without division of the soft palate. The approach is suitable for pathology in the midline, between the foramen magnum and the C2-C3 disk space. Division of the soft palate improves superior exposure of the lower third of the clivus. For all transoral procedures, the key to orientation is to identify the midline: from the rostrum of the sphenoid, the anterior tubercle of the lower clivus and the tubercle of the C1 anterior arch, to the midline of C2, which also may have a midline crest or tubercle. If in doubt, lateral fluoroscopy or frameless stereotactic equipment may be used, but is often unnecessary.

Viewed from the anterior, the vertebral arteries circumscribe a hexagonal shape: 9 to 11 mm from the midline they penetrate the dura, 22 to 23 mm from the midline at the C1 foramina transversaria, and 9 to 10 mm at the body of C2. However, within the upper C2 vertebral body, the artery may loop medially before exiting the bone and passing superiorly to the C1 vertebra, and care should therefore be taken not to catch the vertebral artery when drilling in the C2 body. Careful preoperative evaluation with CT scan is important.

Indications for Transoral Surgery

1. In the past, the procedure was used extensively for odontoidectomy and removal of pannus in late-stage rheumatoid disease and neurological symptoms. However this is now much less common largely due to improvements in the medical management of the disease. The operation is now reserved for patients with acutely deteriorating neurology from bone or degenerative soft tissue compression of the cervical cord and in inflammatory or degenerative arthritides.
2. Predominantly midline extradural tumors of the clivus and C1-C2 region, usually chordomas or primary neoplasms.
3. Diagnostic biopsy for midline C1-C2 infections.
4. Although some pathologies such as chordomas may be followed intradurally, we do not recommend this approach for tumors that are fundamentally intradural (but often a far-lateral procedure should be performed in preference[9]).

Contraindications for Transoral Surgery

1. Oral infections.
2. Limited mouth opening (less than 25 mm between the upper and lower teeth in the midline). In the presence of limited opening, extension of the transoral approach can be performed with an "open-door" maxillotomy, or mandibulotomy.
3. If there is a fixed flexion deformity of the cervicothoracic spine, surgical access can be limited by the close proximity of the manubrium and sternum.
4. Tumors extending laterally more than 15 mm from the midline, unless supplementary surgery is planned by an additional lateral approach.

Preoperative Assessment and Anesthesiology

1. Flexion-extension X-rays are useful for assessing the degree of normal and abnormal movement at the craniovertebral junction
2. CT scans and CT angiography are useful for assessing vertebral anatomy and position of the vertebral artery, particularly when involved or displaced by tumor, or in cases of congenital variations in bone anatomy.
3. MRIs define the relationship of the pathology and vertebral arteries to the brainstem and cervical spinal cord.
4. Digital subtractive angiography should be considered for tumors and embolization performed if the feeding vessels are accessible or acquired anomaly.
5. Bacteriological swabs of the nasal and oropharyngeal cavity should be taken. If methicillin-resistant *Staphylococcus aureus* is detected, then preoperative eradication therapy should be given. If another unusual commensal organism is identified, then an

appropriate antibiotic may be prescribed later if a postoperative infection develops subsequently. Usually antibiotics (cefuroxime and metronidazole) are administered with induction of anesthesia and continued during the first 24 hours from the start of surgery. Long-term antibiotics should be avoided unless there is a clinically significant infection, as they may encourage a postoperative infection with resistant bacteria or fungi.

6. Somatosensory evoked potentials (SSEPs) and motor evoked potentials (MEPs) should be recorded pre- and perioperatively, providing real-time information during the operation to alert the surgeon if certain maneuvers are compromising cord function.[10]
7. Fiberoptic nasotracheal intubation is performed in the awake patient or tracheostomy if there is significant preexisting neurological or bulbar dysfunction.[11]
8. A nasogastric tube is used for perioperative gastric emptying and postoperative feeding, which is initiated 4 hours postoperatively.
9. Pulmonary function (vital capacity, arterial blood gases, and oxygen saturation) is assessed preoperatively and followed intraoperatively. A vital capacity of less than 1.2 L is associated with a greater risk of postoperative complications.
10. When there is a high chance of intraoperative cerebrospinal fluid (CSF) leakage, then a lumbar drain may be inserted after the induction of anesthesia and prior to surgery. If the dura is not breached during the operation, then the drain should be removed at the completion of surgery.

Surgical Procedure

Positioning

The patient is positioned supine, with the head fixed in a Mayfield headrest, extended at the CVJ. This extension allows better access to the lower clivus, particularly in the case of limited mouth opening (**Fig. 22.2**). Tilting the table

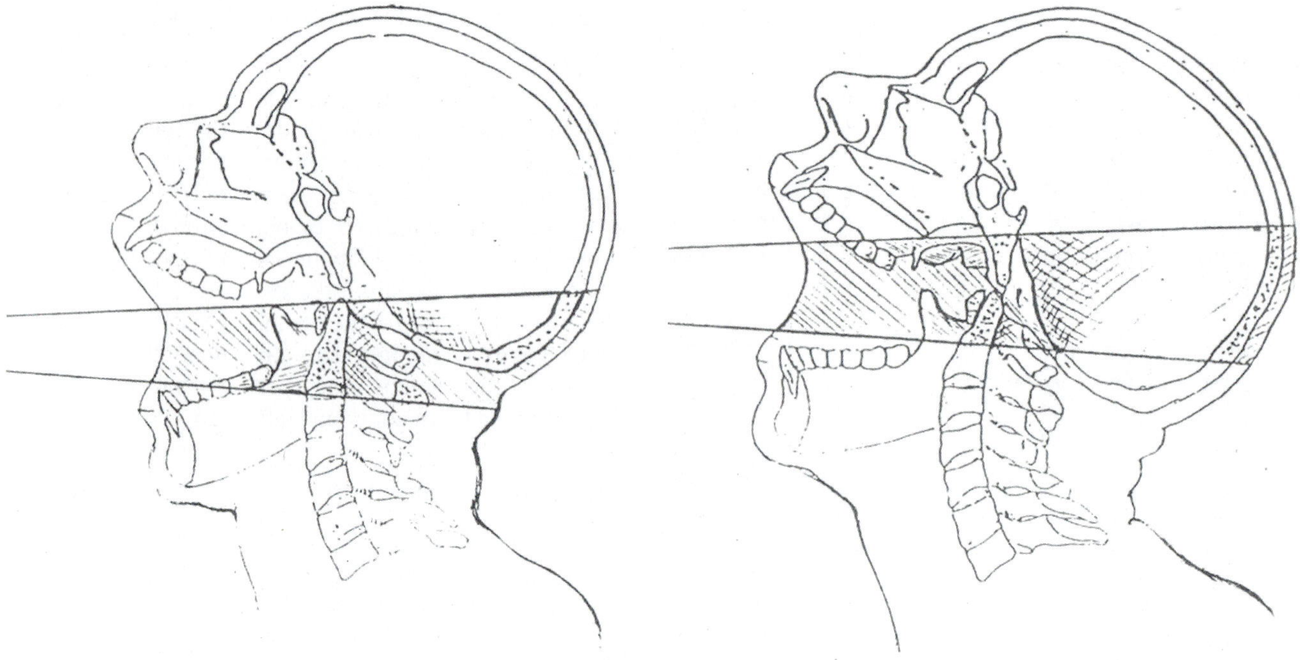

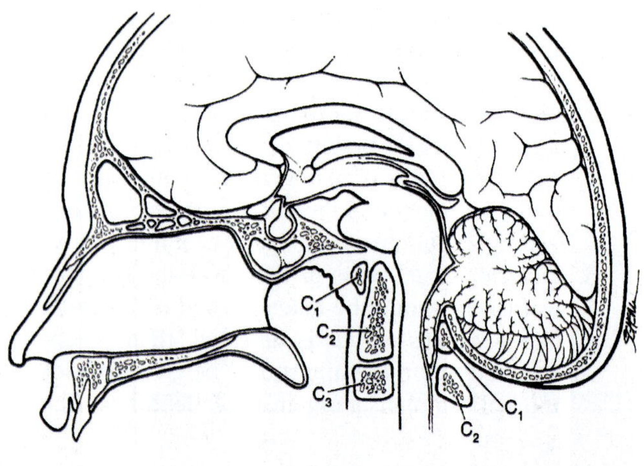

Fig. 22.2 **(A)** Neutral head position. **(B)** Extension of the head affords better access to the clivus. **(C)** However, for severe basilar impression, positioning alone does not usually provide adequate access, and a maxillotomy or endonasal approach should be used.

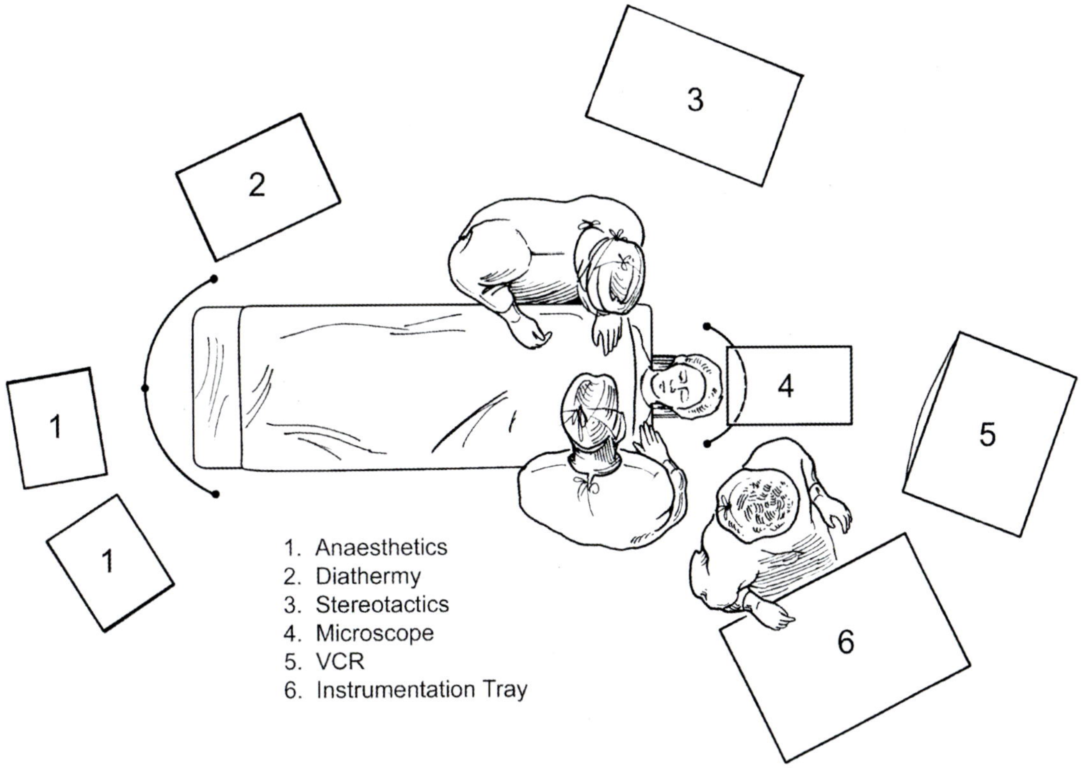

Fig. 22.3 The operating room setup for transoral surgery. Orientation of the surgeon, anesthesiologist, and scrub nurse.

laterally may allow the surgeon to have a better view within the mouth, while keeping the orientation of the patient in a neutral midline sagittal plane. Head rotation by itself on the fully supine body is not advised because this may cause distortion of the anatomy and may also rotate the vertebral arteries into the operative field.

The surgeon stands on the right side of the patient if right-handed, and the opposite side if left-handed, with the anesthetic team at the feet of the patient and the scrub nurse at the head of the patient (**Fig. 22.3**).

Equipment

Use of a dedicated transoral system (Crockard Transoral Instruments, Codman & Shurtleff, Raynham, MA) makes access easier. Newer retractor systems developed for the minimally invasive market have also been used with some success. The traditional equipment includes an oral retractor/tongue depressor, attachable retractors for the soft palate and tubes, a long monopolar diathermy cutting blade, and appropriately long bayoneted instruments. (Additional components are available for performing extended transoral surgery.) Additional necessary equipment includes an operating microscope, a high-speed air drill with different burrs, and a knot pushing device for use during closure of the prevertebral muscles and pharyngeal mucosa.

Procedure

The oropharyngeal cavity is cleaned with an aqueous solution of 0.5% chlorhexidine, although many otolaryngologists do not use preoperative sterilizing solution prior to routine nose and throat surgery, and preoperative cleaning perhaps does not influence the usually low rate of infection. The mouth, tongue, and lips are coated with topical 1% hydrocortisone ointment to minimize postoperative inflammation. The dedicated transoral retractor system is inserted to depress the tongue and open the mouth, while retracting also the soft palate superiorly and the endotracheal and nasogastric tubes laterally. A small bolster, such as a rolled-up towel, is placed between the handle of the retractor and the sternum to allow further exposure below the arch of C1. One percent lidocaine with 1:200,000 adrenaline is injected submucosally at the back of the pharynx, prior to making a vertical incision through the mucosa. Box incisions in the mucosa may also be performed, but a linear incision is easier to close and provides good lateral exposure with the correct use of dedicated retractor systems. The mucosa is retracted with a pharyngeal self-retaining retractor, exposing the deeper muscle layer. These longus colli and longus capitis muscles are elevated from the underlying foramen magnum, C1, and C2 with a Howarth elevator and monopolar diathermy to expose the bone. To remove the odontoid process, the tough apical and alar ligaments must be divided by sharp dissection or diathermy after the drilling has been completed, with care to avoid creating a CSF leak.

For odontoid resection in rheumatoid and degenerative conditions (**Fig. 22.4**), the peg is thinned and disconnected from the C2 body using a high-speed drill, and after division of the apical and alar ligaments, the remaining cortex of peg is removed using the odontoid grasping forceps of the

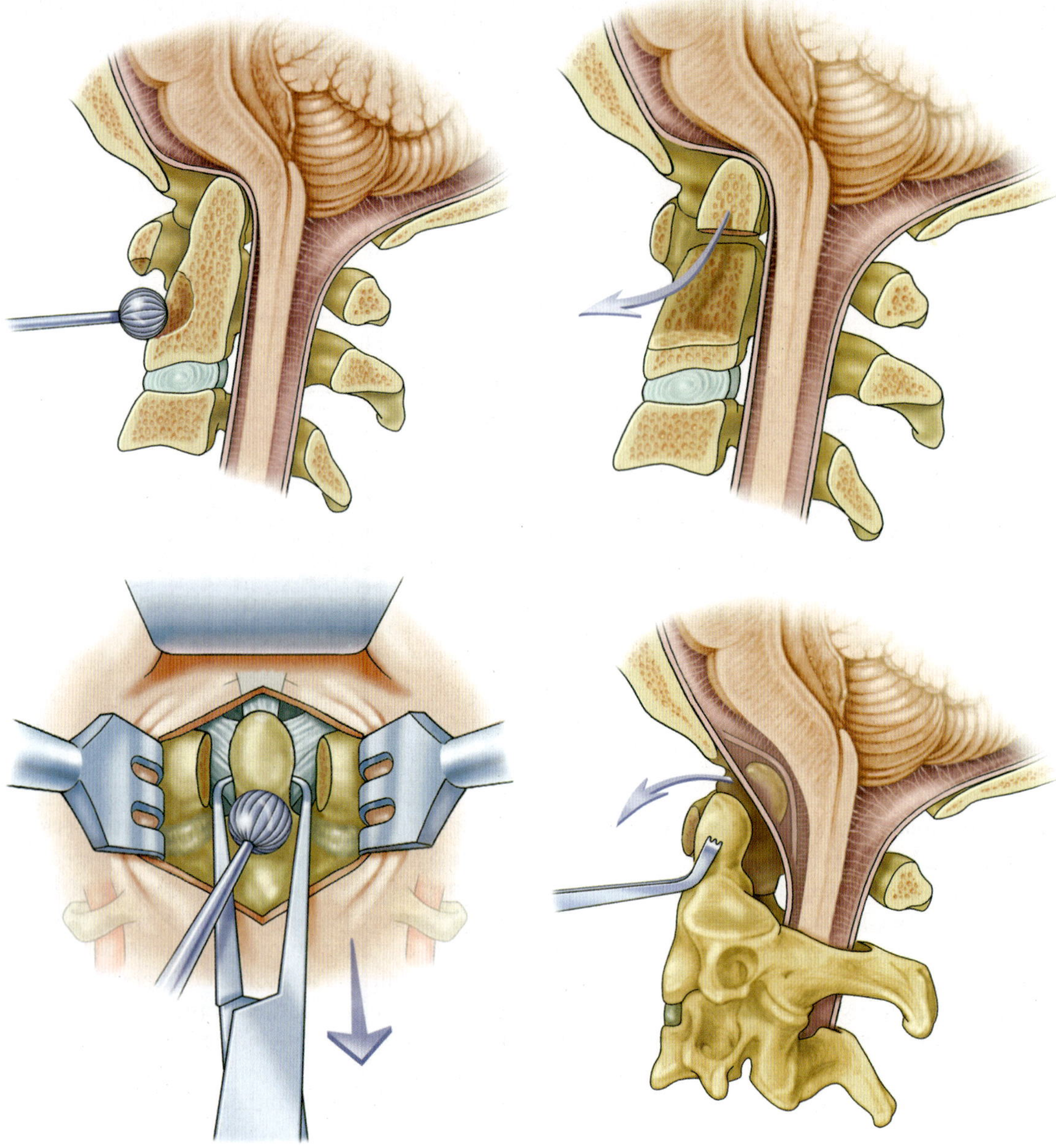

Fig. 22.4 Odontoid resection. **(A,B)** Shelling out the base of the odontoid peg with a high-speed drill. **(C,D)** Extraction of the odontoid peg with division of the apical and alar ligaments (anterior and lateral views). (Reprinted with permission from Barrow Neurological Institute.)

transoral instrument set. In tumors, pituitary rongeurs and curettes may be used together with suction to remove the tumor, or an ultrasonic aspirator can be used if the tumor is firm.

Closure is performed in two layers: The longitudinal prevertebral muscles are closed with interrupted 2–0 Vicryl (Ethicon, Somerville, NJ) or similar absorbable sutures, and the mucosa is closed as a separate layer using inverted 3–0 Vicryl. If there is a small dural defect, it can be closed with DuraGen artificial dura (Integra, LifeSciences Corp., Plainsboro, NJ) and Tisseel fibrin glue (Baxter, Deerfield, IL). Larger dural defects may require fascia lata and fat grafts or flaps of nasopharyngeal mucosa.

Outcome

From our series of 527 operations, mortality was 4.6% within 3 months of surgery. The mortality rate depends on many factors, but the most important predictor of outcome is the degree of preoperative neurological impairment. Rheumatoid patients who are bed-bound or unable to walk due to brainstem and cord compression (Ranawat classification IIIb) have a mortality rate of ~12%, compared with 0% in patients who are relatively independent (Ranawat I). This also applies to other pathological conditions.[12,13]

Complication rates for different types of transoral operations are shown in **Fig. 22.5**. It is important to note that the

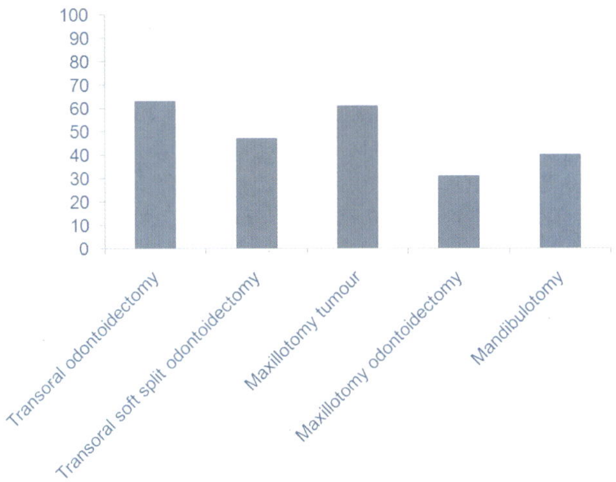

Fig. 22.5 The percentage of patients undergoing surgery who did not have any major or minor complications, for the different extents of transoral surgeries at the National Hospital for Neurology and Neurosurgery, 1980–2010.

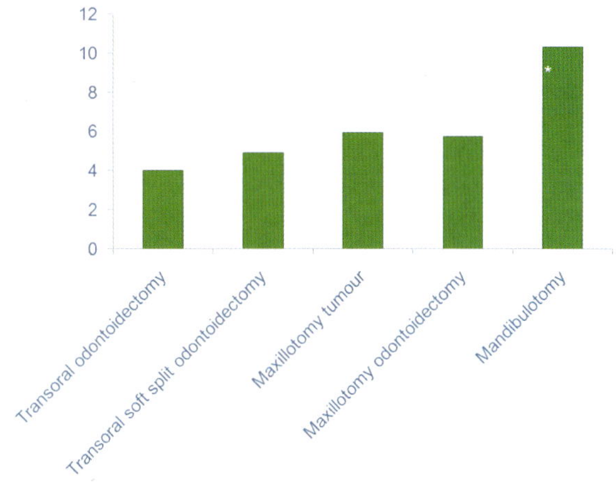

Fig. 22.6 Length of time (hours) in the operating room, from induction of anesthesia to the completion of surgery, for the different types of transoral operations.

infection rate for transoral operations in our experience is similar to lateral and posterolateral approaches, and in our series only 1.5% of patients developed a pharyngeal wound infection.[14–17] The length of operation, determined from the start of anesthesia to the time of exiting the operating room, increases with complexity of surgery, as did the blood loss (**Figs. 22.6** and **22.7**).

Surgical Pitfalls

1. Vascular injuries may occur if there has been rotation of C1 during the positioning of the patient, causing disorientation of the surgeon.
2. To avoid CSF leakage, care should be taken when dissecting the tip of the odontoid process, particularly in cases of vertical translocation, and when dissecting tumors from the dura.
3. Soft tissue swelling may occur due to venous congestion and edema, especially if the tongue or lips are trapped between the retractor and the teeth, which should be avoided. Hydrocortisone ointment should be liberally applied during the procedure and may be continued every 6 hours for 24 hours after surgery.
4. Local infection and wound breakdown. A clean incision in the mucosa should be made, and care should be taken when retracting the mucosa to avoid diathermy or retraction injury, which makes closure difficult at the end of the procedure. Nasogastric feeding should be used for 5 postoperative days to avoid contamination of the wound. Wound healing may be impaired by malignant disease, immunosuppressants, cytotoxic drugs, and steroids.
5. Ensure that the teeth are protected with a custom-made teeth guard, or cover the teeth with a section of silicon tubing over which the retractor may be applied to prevent dental problems. At the end of the procedure, correct occlusion of the teeth should be checked to avoid undetected temporomandibular dislocation, which can sometimes occur during transoral retraction.
6. Regarding craniovertebral instability, consider whether posterior craniocervical fusion is required. Usually degenerative conditions require fixation, whereas tumors in young people may not, because the lateral mass joints and capsules of the CVJ are usually intact and maintain stability. Radiographic stability should be checked immediately postoperatively and at 6 weeks thereafter.

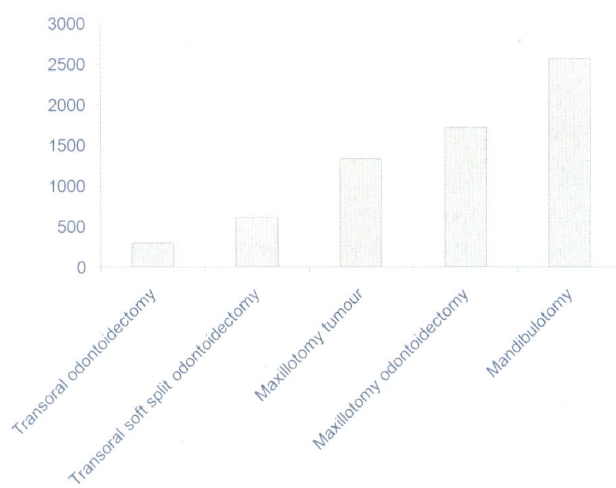

Fig. 22.7 Total blood loss (in milliliters) for the different types of transoral and extended transoral procedures. Blood loss increases with greater complexity of the surgical approach.

Open-door Maxillotomy

The extended maxillotomy ("open-door" variant) provides access to the whole of the sphenoid sinus and clivus from the ethmoids to the lower border of C2 vertebra and was developed in response to the challenges of profound basilar invagination seen in osteogenesis imperfecta and for extensive midline tumors such as chordomas and chondrosarcomas. This approach allows direct exposure of the clivus without obstruction by cranial nerves or vessels and gives better access to ventral midline lesions, especially in the middle and upper thirds of the clivus, compared with lateral and posterior approaches. The approach should be performed with a maxillofacial surgeon to minimize oral and dental complications.

Preoperative Assessment and Anesthesiology

The general principles for standard transoral surgery apply to the extended approaches. In addition, although nasotracheal intubation is the norm for standard transoral surgery, it is our practice to perform an elective tracheostomy for open-door maxillotomy because postoperative airway swelling and delayed extubation may be anticipated with more extensive surgery. An elective percutaneous gastrostomy tube is inserted for perioperative gastric drainage and postoperative feeding, rather than a standard nasogastric tube.

Systemic monitoring is performed by use of an arterial line, a central venous line, Foley catheter, electrocardiography, and a pulse oximeter. If there is a possibility of dural breach, a lumbar spinal drain is inserted for continuous CSF drainage (10–15 mL/hour) and remains in situ for around 5 days after the operation. It may be converted to a lumboperitoneal shunt in cases of persistent CSF leakage.

The patient should be examined for loose or decaying teeth and to evaluate the patient's dental occlusion prior to surgery to ensure perfect reconstruction. In cases of congenital basilar invagination there may also be abnormalities of the bones and teeth, with often fragile maxillae making reconstruction more difficult.

Surgical Procedure

The procedure begins with generous application of 1% hydrocortisone ointment to the lips and oral mucosa to limit tissue swelling. The mucoperiosteum of the nasal septum and maxilla is infiltrated with 1% lidocaine and 1/100,000 units of epinephrine to facilitate dissection. The location of the palatal osteotomy is determined by the location of the septum and teeth. The paramedian osteotomy must avoid the septum yet pass between the two teeth nearest to the midline.

A horizontal mucoperiosteal incision is made above the mucogingival reflection from one maxillary tuberosity to the other (**Fig. 22.8A**). The mucoperiosteum is elevated to expose the nasal floor and septum similar to a sublabial transsphenoidal approach, except that the dissection extends further laterally along the anterior maxilla (**Fig. 22.8B**). Care is taken not to strip too much of the mucoperiosteum because it helps to maintain the vascularity of the maxilla. The cartilaginous septum is detached from the maxilla and vomer at this point and reflected to one side.

The transverse and midline osteotomies are marked on the exposed maxilla, and titanium compression plates are contoured to fit both maxillary buttresses and the prespinal area. The drill holes are made, and the plates are secured before the osteotomies are made (**Fig. 22.8C**). The plates are then removed and carefully marked for replacement. This trial application of the plates ensures precise relocation of the maxilla at the completion of the procedure and avoids malocclusion. An incision is made in the oral mucosa overlying the hard palate osteotomy site and reflected several millimeters. The midline incision is then extended through the full thickness of the soft palate to the base of the uvula.

Taking care to avoid injury to the dental roots, bilateral LeFort I osteotomies are made with an oscillating saw (**Fig. 22.8D,E**). A sagittal aligned oscillating saw is used to make the parasagittal osteotomy, passing along one side of the vomer and between the two incisors nearest to the midline. Finally, the maxillary tuberosities are separated from the pterygoid process with a curved osteotome. At this point, the two halves of the maxilla will be free to swing inferiorly and laterally, providing a wide exposure of the posterior nasopharynx and oropharynx. Blood supply to each maxillary segment is maintained via the soft palate with its remaining connections to the pharynx and the pterygoid muscles.

The free maxillary segments are carefully mobilized, and the Crockard transoral retractor (Codman), with the midfacial osteotomy retractor plate, is inserted. The hard palate retractor is positioned to hold the maxillary segments out of the operative field, completing the exposure of the posterior nasopharynx from the sphenoid sinus to the upper cervical spine (**Fig. 22.8F**).

Before proceeding with the pharyngeal incision, it is helpful to identify the midline (anterior tubercle of atlas) and lateral limits of the exposure (pharyngeal recess). After infiltrating with epinephrine, a midline incision is made in the pharyngeal mucosa. To allow for retraction, the incision should extend well above and below the lesion. The pharyngeal muscles and mucosa are reflected laterally with monopolar electrocauterization and a periosteal dissector. The pharyngeal retractor is then inserted to retain the soft tissue. The sphenoid, clivus, arch of C1, and the body of C2 are exposed as required. The lateral limits of exposure are defined by the lateral walls of the sphenoid sinus, the medial edge of the foramen lacerum, the medial border of the occipital condyle, and the lateral masses of the atlas and axis. These lateral landmarks plus the basion, anterior arch of C1, and the base of the odontoid should be clearly identified before removing any bone.

The osseous dissection is best performed with a high-speed drill and a long match-head burr attachment. Surgery proceeds

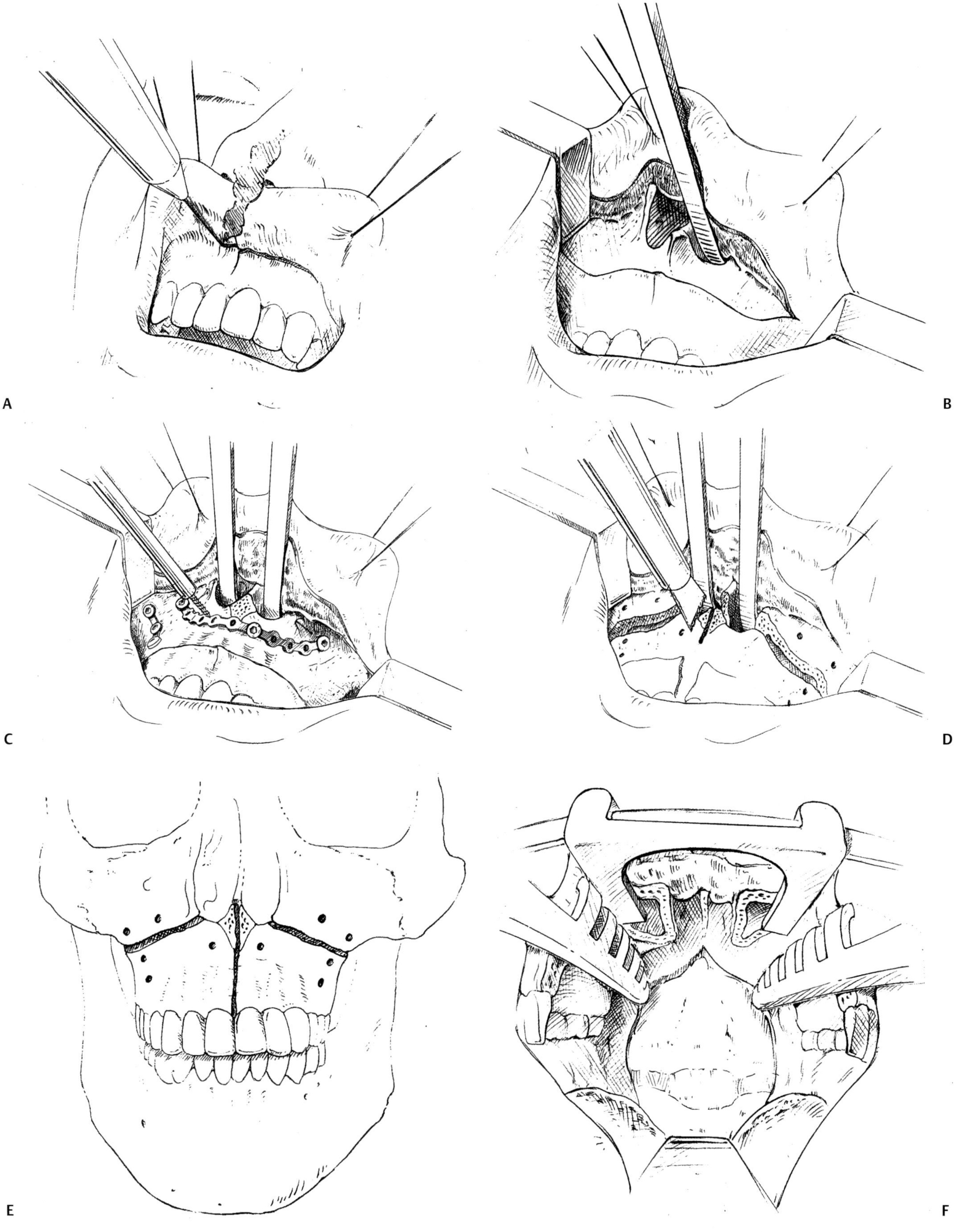

Fig. 22.8 Open-door maxillotomy. **(A)** Sublabial gingival incision. **(B)** Elevation of the periosteum to expose the external nasal apertures. **(C)** Miniplates are shaped and fitted prior to the division of the maxilla to allow accurate reconstruction later. **(D)** Sagittal saw division of the maxilla. **(E)** Schematic diagram showing the position of the osteotomies. **(F)** Exposure provided by open-door maxillotomy. *(continued)*

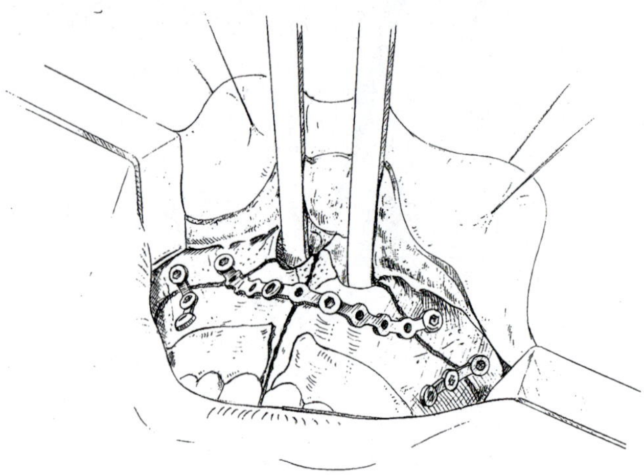

G

Fig. 22.8 *(continued)* **(G)** Reconstruction of the maxillary halves.

from here in a similar fashion to that described for the standard transoral operation. The rostral clivus is quite thick (18 to 22 mm) and can be associated with significant hemorrhage from venous channels. Bone wax and hemostatic agents should be used to limit blood loss.

When this exposure is used for basilar impression, the bony decompression is the crux of the procedure. The decompression should extend as far laterally as possible, recognizing that the invagination, which typically involves all sides of the foramen magnum, cannot be completely decompressed. The goal of this surgery is to remove bone that severely deforms the brainstem. For extradural tumors of this region, bony removal should be tailored to the lesion. A bony margin should be removed if possible around primary bone tumors such as chordomas. Other extradural tumors require sufficient bony dissection to expose the extent of the tumor. Throughout the removal of the clivus and body of C2, the surgeon should keep in mind the relative positions of vital structures such as the hypoglossal nerve and vertebral arteries.

Closure of the posterior pharyngeal wall is similar to the standard transoral operation. The maxillary segments are returned to their appropriate positions and secured with the precontoured plates and the previously drilled holes. The medial plate spans the parasagittal osteotomy and the two lateral plates attach to the maxillary buttresses (**Fig. 22.8G**). It is not necessary to place a plate on the hard palate, nor is it necessary to reapproximate the mucosa over the hard palate. The soft palate should be closed in three layers to reduce the likelihood of a palatal fistula, or at least with two layers of 3–0 absorbable sutures (such as Vicryl) to both the superior and inferior mucosal surfaces of the soft palate. The nasal septum is reconstructed by replacing the vomer and cartilaginous septum and repositioning the nasal mucosa with a speculum. Large-bore nasal cannulae inserted in each nostril will maintain the position of the septum and overlying mucosa until some healing occurs. Each cannula and the anterior septal structures should be secured with a single suture. Finally, the sublabial incision is closed with interrupted Vicryl sutures.

Postoperatively, the nasal stents or packing may be removed after 2 to 3 days. The patient is fed via percutaneous endoscopic gastrostomy (PEG) tube for 5 days, after which oral diet may commence and the tracheostomy may be removed once pharyngeal edema has subsided (usually 2 to 3 days after surgery). If a lumbar drain is utilized, this is usually removed after 5 days.

Mandibulotomy

The transmandibular (median labiomandibulotomy and/or glossotomy) approach is a caudal extension of the standard transoral procedure that affords excellent visualization of the anterior craniovertebral junction as far down as the C3-C4 vertebral bodies. It was developed principally for the following situations:

1. Limited mouth opening due to rheumatoid arthritis in the temporomandibular joint or flexion deformities of the neck.
2. Craniofacial and intraoral anomalies (macroglossia, micrognathia, retrognathia) that limit the space for anterior surgical decompression.
3. Tumor at the CVJ with caudal extension (e.g., C1-C3 chordomas). For such cases the ventral operation is part of a 360-degree approach that includes instrumentation.

Surgical Procedure

A PEG tube is inserted prior to surgery, and a tracheostomy before the mandibulotomy proceeds. The line of incision is marked to start from the midline of the lower lip and to end at the midline of the mylohyoid raphe under the chin to the level of the hyoid bone. In between these midline marks, the line may be taken in a crescentic fashion or "Z" shaped to make it less obvious after healing. In the mouth the mucosal incision extends to the lower buccal sulcus, in front of the mandibular origin of the genioglossus and geniohyoid muscles, and the frenulum of the tongue. The periosteum over the mandible is incised and elevated for 1 cm on either side of the midline to allow room for the osteotomy. This is performed in the midline between the central incisors using an oscillating saw and osteotomes (**Fig. 22.9A**). Care should be taken not to damage the mental cutaneous branches of the mandibular nerve (V3), which are essential for sensation in the lower lip.

Similar to the open-door maxillotomy reconstruction, the one or two mandibular plates are shaped, positioned, and temporarily fixed with screws. After demarcating and drilling the holes, the plate is removed. This initial planning helps to accurately relocate the mandible at the end of the procedure and avoids malocclusion of the teeth.

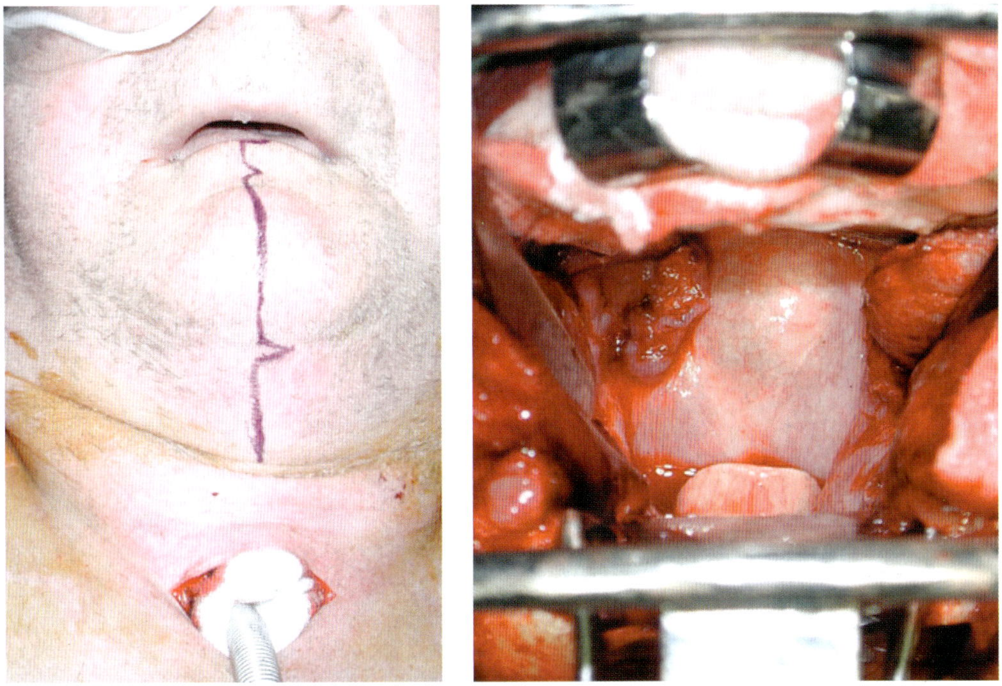

A B

Fig. 22.9 Mandibulotomy: **(A)** skin incision and **(B)** exposure of the posterior pharynx down to the epiglottis, after osteotomy and glossotomy.

In some patients, for example in rheumatoid disease, after mandibulotomy the tongue does not necessarily need to be divided and may be retracted down sufficiently with the standard tongue retractor. However, usually a median glossotomy is required, split in the midline using monopolar cutting diathermy, down to the anterior border of the vallecula and epiglottis (approximately C4 vertebral level). Bleeding is minimized by keeping to the midline of the tongue. Self-retaining retractors are used to push the divided halves of the tongue laterally, exposing the posterior pharyngeal wall from the lower clivus down to the C3-C4 level (**Fig. 22.9B**)

For closure, the mandibular halves are reapproximated and the preshaped plates are used to secure the mandible, paying attention to align the teeth and reestablishing correct dental occlusion. Sometimes the mandible becomes dislocated during the procedure and requires relocation prior to closing. The tongue should be closed in three layers using 3–0 Vicryl sutures to the upper mucosa, muscle layer, and lower mucosa and floor of the mouth. The soft tissues of the lip, chin, and submental region are sutured in anatomical layers.

Midface Degloving Transmaxillary Approach

The upper third of the clivus can be exposed by the midface degloving technique. The operation proceeds in a similar fashion to the open-door maxillotomy by a horizontal mucoperiosteal incision made above the mucogingival reflection on the inner surface of the upper lip. The soft tissues are dissected free from the underlying maxilla to expose the anterior wall of the maxillary sinus, taking care not to damage or stretch the infraorbital neurovascular bundle (**Fig. 22.10A**). The anterior wall of the sinus is marked for plating and then removed and, by opening the medial wall of the sinus, a unilateral window is created to the posterior nasopharynx and ethmoid and sphenoid sinuses (**Fig. 22.10B**). After excision of tumor, the anterior wall of the maxillary sinus is secured with miniplates (**Fig. 22.10C**). This procedure may be considered as an extension of the subgingival transnasal approach to the pituitary fossa, and to a certain extent has become superseded by the transnasal endoscopic approach.

Transnasal Endoscopic Approach

The anterior skull base may be approached with a nasal endoscope, originally developed by functional endoscopic sinus surgeons but now used increasingly for anterior skull base surgery. The endoscope allows good visualization from the sphenoid sinus superiorly to the posterior nasopharynx, inferiorly limited by the plane of the soft palate. There are potential advantages to the endoscopic approach over standard transoral surgery, in particular: faster recovery from surgery and the patient can start a normal diet almost immediately after surgery.[18] **Figure 22.11** shows preoperative and postoperative imaging of a patient who underwent endoscopic resection of recurrent clivus chordoma.

However, there are potential drawbacks of the endoscopic approach also. With a smaller exposure, the working space can become limited, especially when operating on tumors of tough consistency, or with uncontrolled bleeding. It is also not possible to insert anterior instrumentation if this is required. **Figure 22.12** demonstrates a case in which only partial excision of a clival chordoma was possible with endoscopy and completed by a transoral route.

Perhaps the major disadvantage of the endoscopic approach is that of persistent postoperative CSF leakage. Initial reports suggested a high CSF leak rate of 25%.[19] Closure of the dura is difficult using endoscopic instruments and is often a cause of morbidity in these cases. The Kassam group developed inlay-onlay graft techniques for

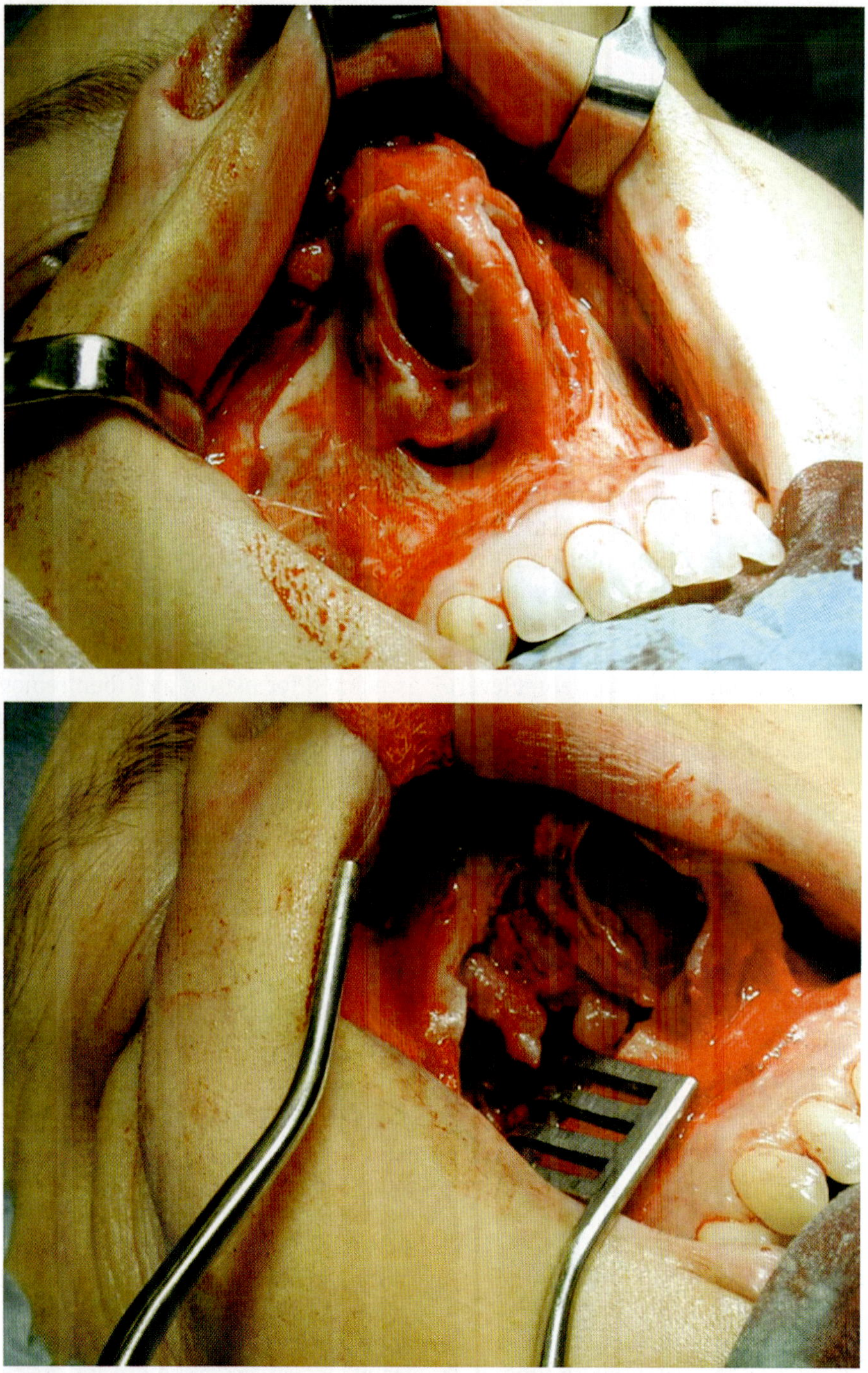

A

B

Fig. 22.10 Midface degloving technique. **(A)** Subperiosteal dissection and facial degloving to expose the external nasal apertures. **(B)** Removal of the anterior wall of the maxillary sinus and exposure of the ethmoid, sphenoid sinuses, and nasopharynx. *(continued)*

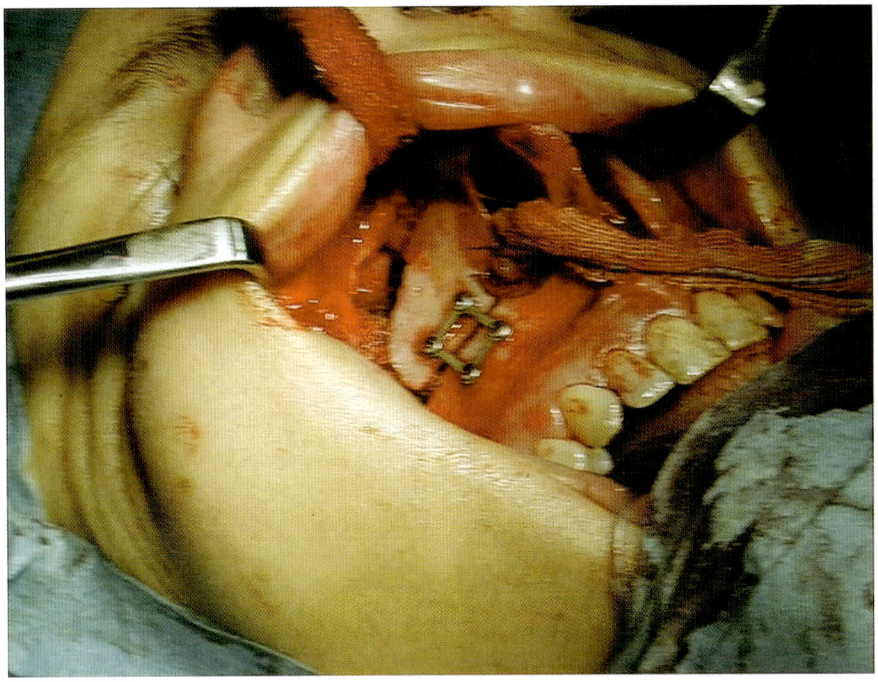

C

Fig. 22.10 *(continued)* **(C)** Replating the anterior wall of the maxillary sinus.

minimizing CSF leakage and, with the regular use of mucosal flaps, reported a much lower CSF leak rate than other groups—a rate of 5%.[20]

Endoscopic approaches are certainly useful to add to the armamentarium of techniques available for operating on the CVJ and are likely to develop further with time. But "one size does not fit all," and endoscopic surgery is not likely to replace open transoral techniques. Rather, an endoscope adds to the available options for solving a particular problem. It will become necessary in the future for surgeons who

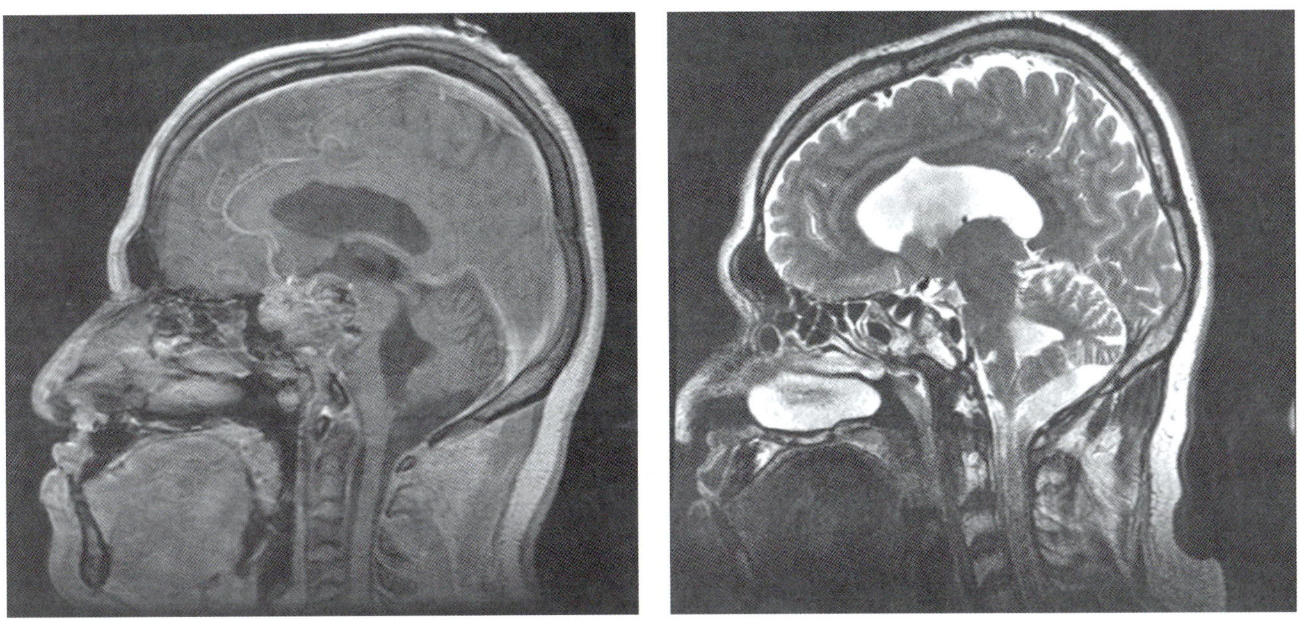

A B

Fig. 22.11 **(A)** Magnetic resonance images of a patient who presented with recurrent clival chordoma 4 years after excision by open-door maxillotomy, involving a difficult 6-month postoperative course in the intensive care unit. **(B)** Successful endoscopic resection of the recurrent tumor, involving a total 9-day hospital stay. Delay in discharge was due to transient diabetes insipidus.

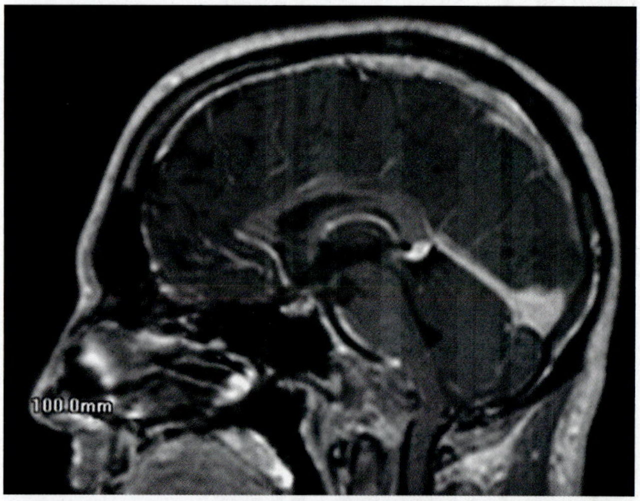

A

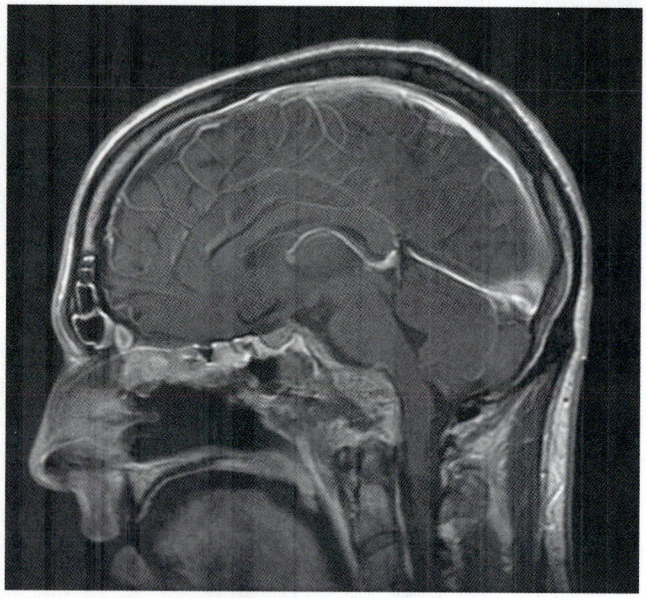
B

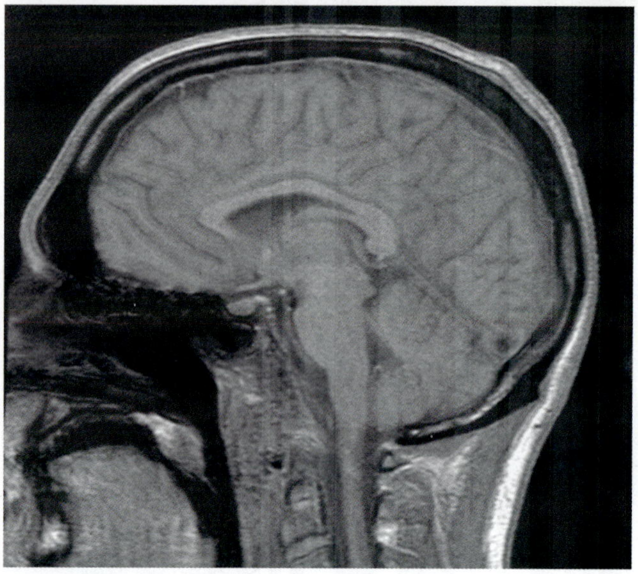
C

Fig. 22.12 **(A)** Preoperative magnetic resonance images of a patient who presented with a clival chordoma and underwent primary endoscopic resection of the tumor, which was difficult due to bleeding and firm consistency of the tumor. **(B)** Postoperative imaging revealed significant residual tumor. **(C)** Successful complete resection of the remaining tumor via standard transoral surgery.

operate at the CVJ to be skilled in both open and endoscopic approaches.

Conclusion

The family of transoral approaches is useful for midline pathology from the sphenoid sinus and clivus down to the C3-C4 disk level. In the past, the main indication for these procedures was neurological compromise from end-stage rheumatoid disease, but now the approach is most commonly used for tumors such as chordomas and chondrosarcomas, and in acute neurological deterioration secondary to degenerative disease and occasionally rheumatoid arthritis. A thorough knowledge of the anatomy and physiology of the CVJ is required, and such surgery should be performed in specialized units with multidisciplinary support from rheumatologists, oncologists, radiologists, and anesthesiologists to minimize complications. Endoscopic approaches are a significant adjunct, but "open" surgery may still be required in many cases.

References

1. Comtois R, Beauregard H, Somma M, Serri O, Aris-Jilwan N, Hardy J. The clinical and endocrine outcome to trans-sphenoidal microsurgery of nonsecreting pituitary adenomas. Cancer 1991;68(4):860–866
2. Baird CJ, Conway JE, Sciubba DM, Prevedello DM, Quiñones-Hinojosa A, Kassam AB. Radiographic and anatomic basis of endoscopic anterior craniocervical decompression: a comparison of endonasal, transoral, and transcervical approaches. Neurosurgery 2009;65(6, Suppl):158–163, discussion 63–64
3. Choi D, Melcher R, Harms J, Crockard A. Outcome of 132 operations in 97 patients with chordomas of the craniocervical junction and upper cervical spine. Neurosurgery 2010;66(1):59–65, discussion 65

4. Crockard HA. The transoral approach to the base of the brain and upper cervical cord. Ann R Coll Surg Engl 1985;67(5):321–325
5. Uttley D, Moore A, Archer DJ. Surgical management of midline skull-base tumors: a new approach. J Neurosurg 1989;71(5 Pt 1): 705–710
6. James D, Crockard HA. Surgical access to the base of skull and upper cervical spine by extended maxillotomy. Neurosurgery 1991;29(3):411–416
7. Maniglia AJ, Phillips DA. Midfacial degloving for the management of nasal, sinus, and skull-base neoplasms. Otolaryngol Clin North Am 1995;28(6):1127–1143
8. Choi D, Casey AT, Crockard HA. Neck problems in rheumatoid arthritis—changing disease patterns, surgical treatments and patients' expectations. Rheumatology (Oxford) 2006;45(10):1183–1184
9. Tuite G, Crockard HA. On the use of lateral surgical approaches to lesions at the craniocervical junction. Neuro-orthopaedics 1995; 17(18):47–56
10. May DM, Jones SJ, Crockard HA. Somatosensory evoked potential monitoring in cervical surgery: identification of pre- and intraoperative risk factors associated with neurological deterioration. J Neurosurg 1996;85(4):566–573
11. Sidhu VS, Whitehead EM, Ainsworth QP, Smith M, Calder I. A technique of awake fibreoptic intubation. Experience in patients with cervical spine disease. Anaesthesia 1993;48(10):910–913
12. Casey AT, Crockard HA, Bland JM, Stevens J, Moskovich R, Ransford A. Predictors of outcome in the quadriparetic nonambulatory myelopathic patient with rheumatoid arthritis: a prospective study of 55 surgically treated Ranawat class IIIb patients. J Neurosurg 1996;85(4):574–581
13. Casey AT, Crockard HA, Stevens J. Vertical translocation. Part II. Outcomes after surgical treatment of rheumatoid cervical myelopathy. J Neurosurg 1997;87(6):863–869
14. Colli B, Al-Mefty O. Chordomas of the craniocervical junction: follow-up review and prognostic factors. J Neurosurg 2001;95(6): 933–943
15. Roberti F, Sekhar LN, Kalavakonda C, Wright DC. Posterior fossa meningiomas: surgical experience in 161 cases. Surg Neurol 2001; 56(1):8–20, discussion 20–21
16. Crockard HA, Cheeseman A, Steel T, et al. A multidisciplinary team approach to skull base chondrosarcomas. J Neurosurg 2001; 95(2):184–189
17. Crockard HA, Steel T, Plowman N, et al. A multidisciplinary team approach to skull base chordomas. J Neurosurg 2001;95(2): 175–183
18. Kassam A, Snyderman CH, Mintz A, Gardner P, Carrau RL. Expanded endonasal approach: the rostrocaudal axis. Part II. Posterior clinoids to the foramen magnum. Neurosurg Focus 2005;19(1):E4
19. Stippler M, Gardner PA, Snyderman CH, Carrau RL, Prevedello DM, Kassam AB. Endoscopic endonasal approach for clival chordomas. Neurosurgery 2009;64(2):268–277, discussion 277–278
20. Hadad G, Bassagasteguy L, Carrau RL, et al. A novel reconstructive technique after endoscopic expanded endonasal approaches: vascular pedicle nasoseptal flap. Laryngoscope 2006;116(10): 1882–1886

23 Transoral–Translabiomandibular Approach to the Craniovertebral Junction

Ivo P. Janecka

The clivus and upper cervical vertebral bodies constitute the craniovertebral junction (CVJ). These anatomical structures at the cranial base are located anterior to the neural axis (**Fig. 23.1**). In general, surgical treatment of lesions located anterior to the neural axis should be accessed through an anterior approach. To do so requires selection of a transfacial approach because of the anteroinferior anatomical relationship of the facial viscerocranium to the cranial base (**Fig. 23.2**).

The advantages of transfacial approaches include the following:

1. Facial anatomy has developed through the embryonic fusion of nasofrontal, maxillary, and mandibular processes. Normally, the fusion takes place in the midline or in the paramedian region, thus logically presenting optimal lines of "separation" of facial units for a surgical approach, permitting the least traumatic displacement.
2. The primary blood supply to the "facial units" is through the external carotid system, which also has a lateral-to-medial direction of flow, thus ensuring viability of displaced surgical units.
3. The midface contains multiple "hollow" anatomical spaces (oronasal cavity, nasopharynx, paranasal sinuses) that facilitate the relative ease of surgical access to the central skull base.
4. Displacement of facial units for an approach to the central cranial base offers much greater tolerance to postoperative surgical swelling, as opposed to similar displacement of the content of the neurocranium.
5. Reestablishment of the normal anatomy, following repositioning of the facial units during the reconstructive phase of surgery, has a high degree of functional as well as aesthetic achievement.

However, transfacial approaches also have certain disadvantages, such as the following:

1. The surgical wound can be contaminated with oropharyngeal bacterial flora.
2. Facial incisions can cause visible scars to develop.
3. The patient may have emotional considerations related to "surgical facial disassembly."
4. Supplementary airway management (postoperative endotracheal intubation, temporary tracheostomy) may be needed.

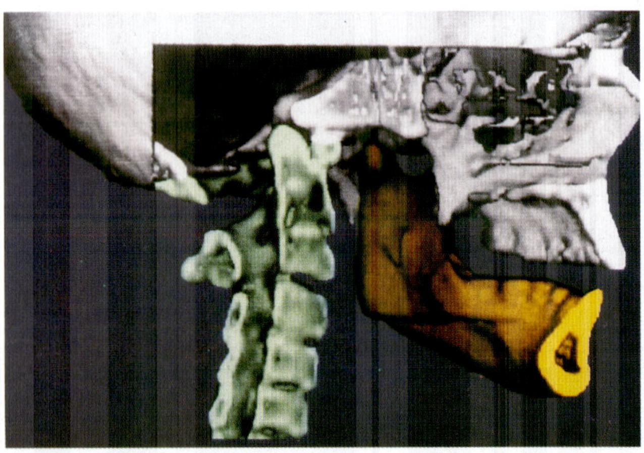

Fig. 23.1 Three-dimensional reconstruction of platybasia with odontoid invagination.

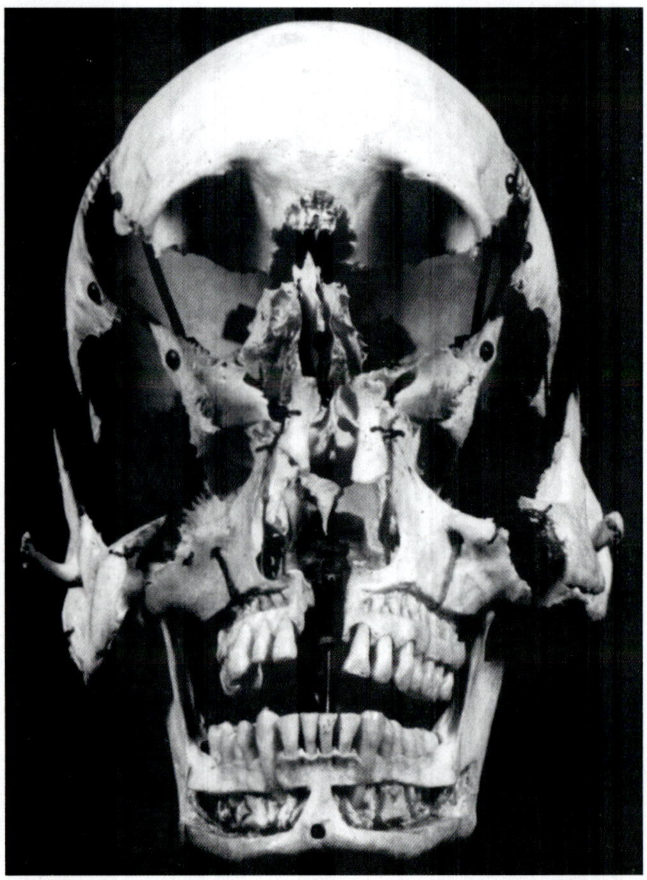

Fig. 23.2 Human skull demonstrating potential skeletal units, which can be displaced for surgical exposure to the skull base.

Patient Selection

To be considered for transfacial/transoral surgery to the CVJ, the patient must have a pathological entity located at the central cranial base that is judged to be best treated with surgery. Such entities would include benign and malignant tumors, as well as congenital and posttraumatic deformities.

Adequate imaging is necessary to define the extent of the pathological process, as well as to show the key neighboring anatomical structures and the potential for their preservation. Appropriate modalities include computed tomography (CT), magnetic resonance imaging (MRI; static and dynamic), and sometimes four-vessel angiography. Numerous questions need to be answered by the imaging studies: the true extent of the lesion, its relationship to the key anatomical structures (e.g., vessels, dura, brainstem, cranial nerves), and the potential expendability of such structures during surgical resection. A patient would not be considered for this type of surgery if the lesion (e.g., lymphoma, most metastatic lesions) is best treated by nonsurgical modalities, or if the oronasopharynx is actively infected.

The timing of surgery is guided by the nature of the pathological process and the urgency for treatment as well as by the patient's overall medical status. In general, malignant processes or impending brainstem compressions are treated expeditiously. Benign tumors and congenital deformities are treated electively.

A biopsy for tissue diagnosis will differentiate the neoplasms into surgical and nonsurgical categories. Patients with malignant tumors for whom transfacial/transoral surgery is not recommended are usually offered radiotherapy and/or chemotherapy. External beam radiotherapy may be supplemented with brachytherapy. Some benign lesions may be followed with scans to assess their growth potential if the surgical treatment has a high likelihood of worsening the patient's deficit.

Transoral approaches create potential risk to the function and aesthetics of the following structures: skin, dentition, facial skeleton, mucosal lining of the upper airway, paranasal sinuses, eustachian tubes, superior constrictor muscles, soft and hard palate, and tongue. From the neurovascular point of view, the locations of the upper cervical and petrous segments of the internal carotid arteries, as well as cranial nerves V3 (especially the lingual nerve) and XII, must be recognized. Furthermore, the vertebral arteries are at potential risk, especially in congenital anomalies of the CVJ with an associated asymmetry. If the vertebral arteries are exposed during surgery, these vessels must be covered with vascularized tissue to prevent the likelihood of subsequent vessel rupture.

The potential postoperative risks are related to the quality of wound healing, involving the dura as well as the wall of the oropharynx. Cerebrospinal fluid (CSF) leakage and/or breakdown of the wound closure are highly undesirable and require intensive treatment.

Preoperative Planning

All patients are given a broad-spectrum antibiotic with Gram-positive and Gram-negative coverage. It is started within 1 hour prior to surgery and continued for ~48 hours postoperatively or until the spinal drain (if used) is removed. Preoperative oral irrigation with a clindamycin solution may be used to reduce microbial flora.

Surgical Technique

Anesthetic Technique

Anesthesia is usually induced with pentobarbital and maintained with enflurane. Oral endotracheal intubation is usually satisfactory (a contoured Raey tube is preferred). In some cases, preliminary tracheostomy is performed. Neurophysiological monitoring includes monitoring of cranial nerve XII (by tongue electromyography) as well as monitoring of brainstem evoked potentials in transdural cases. All patients have arterial as well as central venous pressure lines. Elective hypotension is not used. A precordial stethoscope is used to alert the anesthesiology team to venous air embolism. When dural transgression is anticipated, a spinal drain is inserted.

Patient Positioning

Most patients are positioned supine on the operating table with the head rigidly fixed. An alternative position is a right lateral position (for right-handed surgeons) for a limited midline lesion. The advantage of this position is gravity-dependent drainage away from the immediate surgical field.

Draping

A complete preparation of the face and neck is performed with Betadine, and the oropharynx is irrigated with diluted Betadine solution. This area is then draped. In addition, the lateral thigh is prepared and draped as a fascia lata donor site.

Skin Incisions

Depending on which approach is used, the extent of the incisions varies considerably. For the basic transoral approach, no skin incisions are made. Only the soft palate is retracted with transnasal rubber catheters. This palatal elevation exposes the palpable arch of C1. If significant platybasia is present or the lower one-third of the clivus must be reached, a midline soft palate split is added. An extended transoral approach includes lateral incisions of the palate, the floor of the mouth, and a mandibular osteotomy. In addition, when very wide exposure of the central and paracentral skull base is required, bilateral maxillary osteotomies are performed through additional facial incisions. For the harvesting of the vascularized muscle flap used in reconstruction, a hemicoronal scalp incision is performed to reach the temporalis muscle. When a mandibular split is performed, the lower lip is incised in a paramedian position, and the incision is extended horizontally into the soft tissues of the upper neck.

Splitting of the Soft Palate

The midline of the soft palate and the posterior pharyngeal wall is infiltrated with 0.5% lidocaine viscous with 1:200,000 epinephrine for hemostasis. The soft palate is incised in the midline with a no. 11 scalpel blade, as is the uvula. Care must be taken to avoid injuring the posterior pharyngeal wall with the tip of the no. 11 blade. It is possible to release the levator palati muscle submucosally from its attachment to the hard palate. This maneuver permits more lateral retraction of the bisected soft palate, further increasing the surgical exposure at the CVJ. The soft palate halves are gently retracted laterally with 4–0 Dexon sutures (Covidien, Norwalk, CT) affixed to the perioral frame of the Dingman's mouth gag (**Fig. 23.3**).

Mandibular Split

The lower lip incision is performed in a zigzag fashion to conform to the tension lines of the paracentral lip skin with possible extension horizontally into the upper neck. Mandibular osteotomy is performed just medial to the mental foramen, preserving lower lip sensation. Usually an interdental space is found that is wide enough to permit placement of a reciprocating saw for the osteotomy. This cut is also performed in a step fashion, which then permits more stable reconstructive reapproximation of the bone. Prior to the osteotomy, it is wise to select an appropriate miniplate for ventral fixation, contour it to the mandible, and create

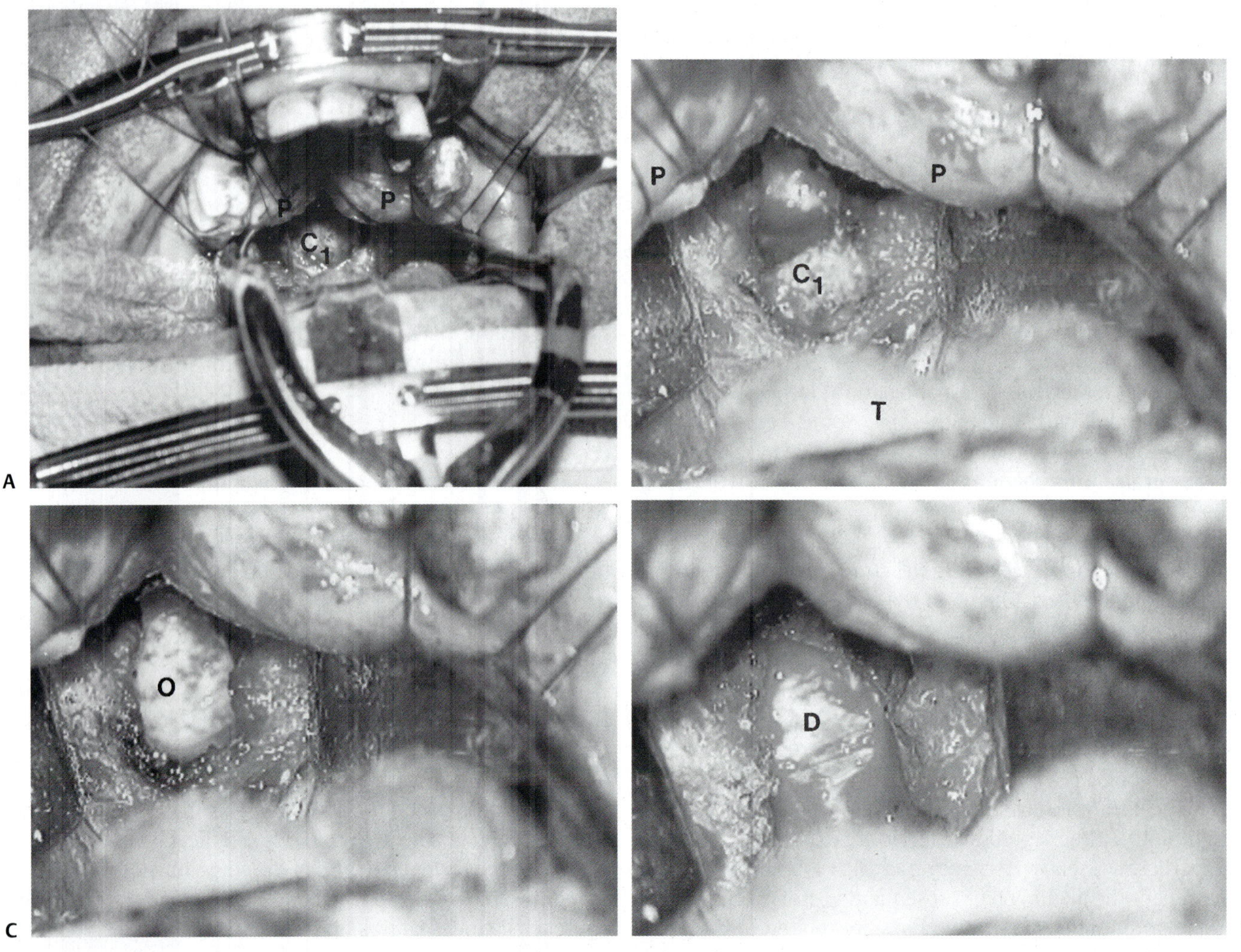

Fig. 23.3 **(A)** View of oral cavity with Dingman's mouth gag, split of soft palate, and self-retaining retractor separating posterior pharyngeal wall. Arch of C1 is in view (*C1*); soft palate (*P*) is split. **(B)** View through the microscope centered on the arch of C1 (*C1*); split soft palate (*P*) is retracted with sutures; tongue (*T*) is seen inferiorly. **(C)** Similar view as in **(B);** the arch of C1 has been removed, and the odontoid is visible (*O*). **(D)** View following removal of odontoid; the dura (*D*) is visible.

drill holes. This strategy assists in the postoperative reestablishment of a normal occlusion (**Fig. 23.4**).

Extended Bilateral Facial Translocation or Midfacial Split

These approaches are used to achieve extensive exposure at the central skull base including the vertebrobasilar junction (**Figs. 23.5** and **23.6**).

Closure Techniques

Following extirpation of the lesion at the cranial base, the dura is repaired or examined for intactness. If a suture repair is performed, fibrin glue is also used to reinforce the dural closure. A separate segment of fascia lata or pericranium may be applied directly to this suture line (**Fig. 23.7**). The soft palate is closed in layers (**Fig. 23.8**).

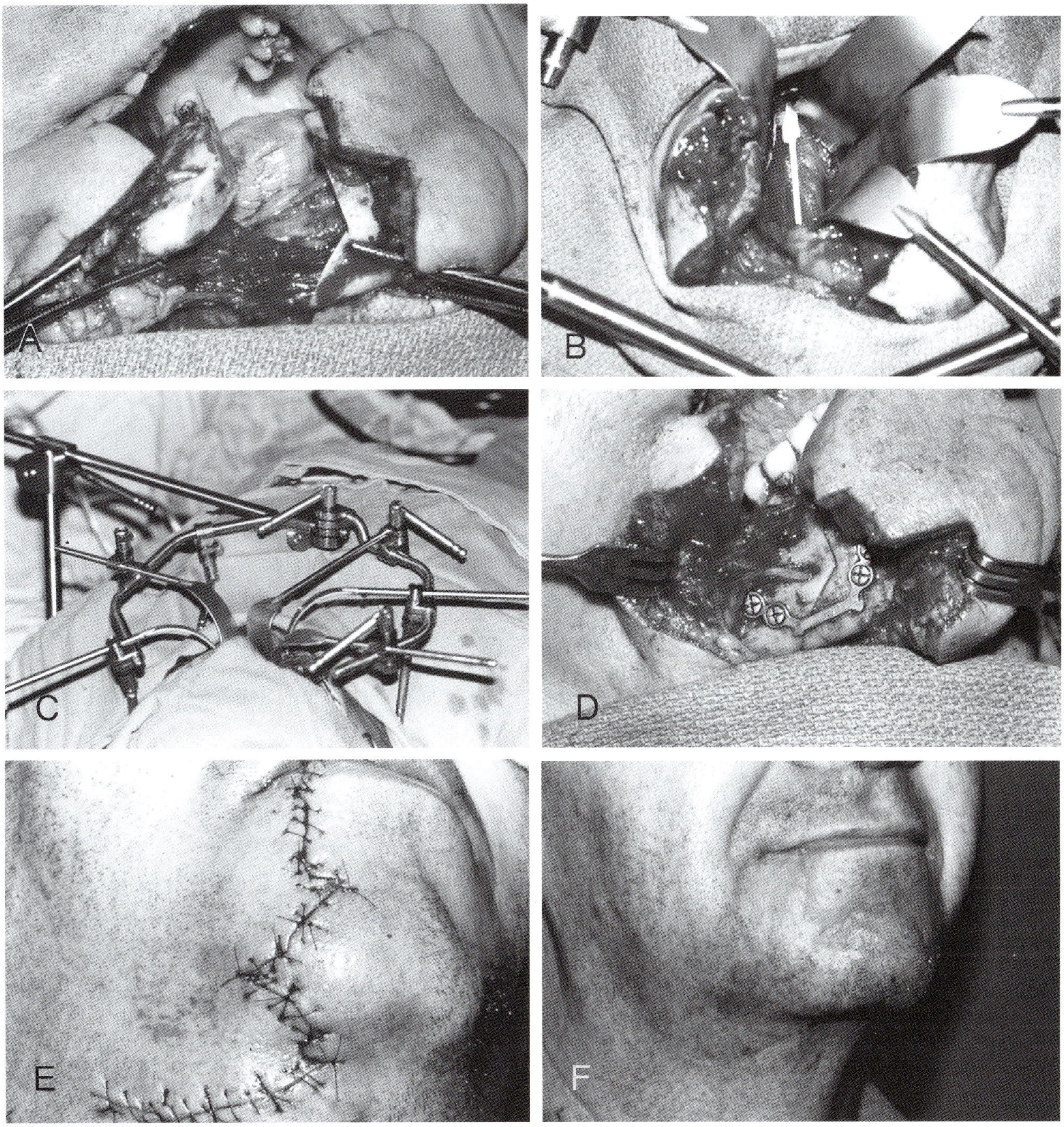

Fig. 23.4 **(A)** Skin incision and right mandibular osteotomy (just in front of the mental nerve). **(B)** Exposure of the craniovertebral junction and the upper cervical spine; arrow denotes the midline. **(C)** The external frame (Omni-tract retractor) used for intraoral exposure. **(D)** Plating of the mandibular osteotomy. **(E)** Skin closure. **(F)** The patient's appearance at 6 months.

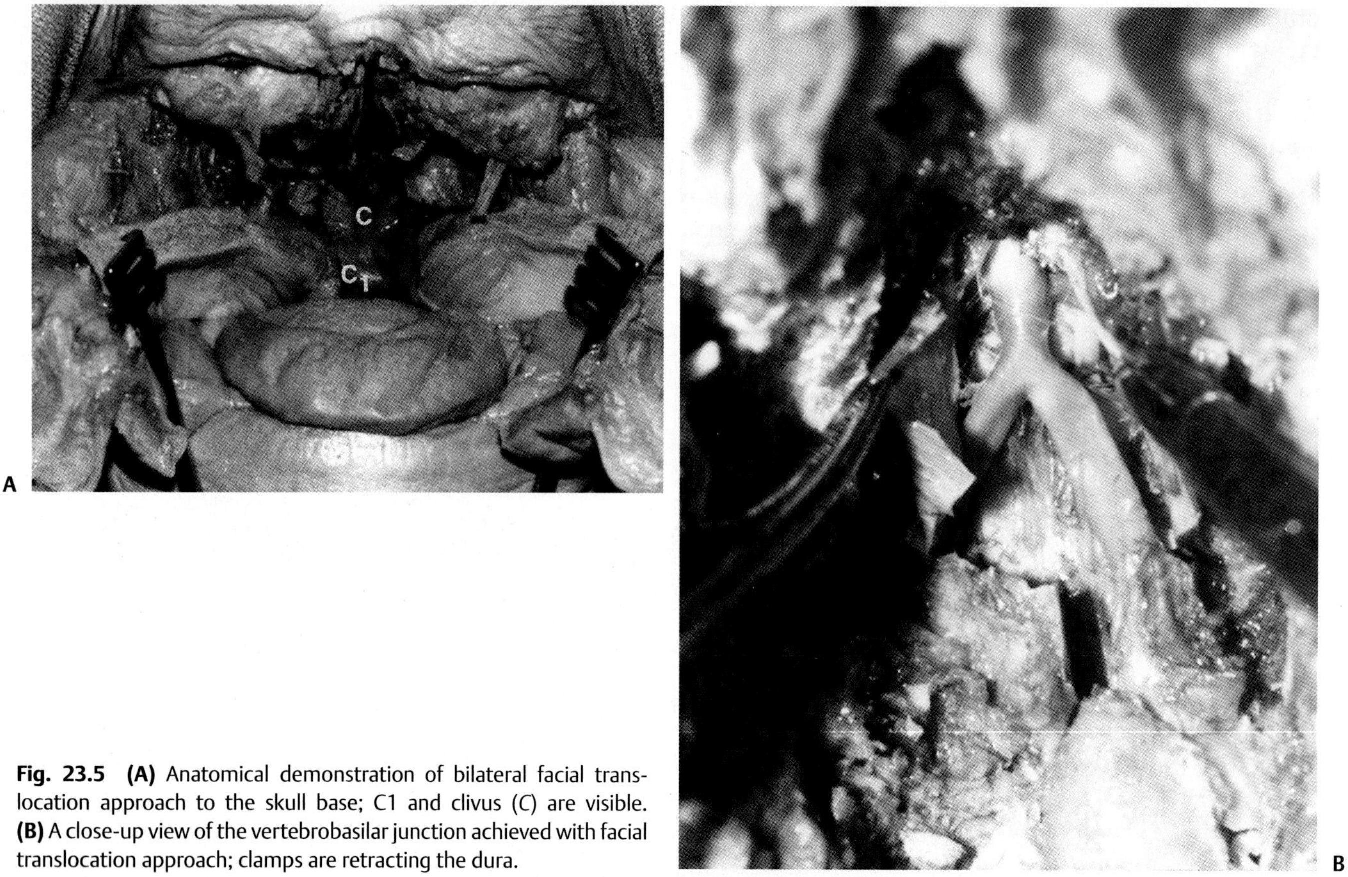

Fig. 23.5 **(A)** Anatomical demonstration of bilateral facial translocation approach to the skull base; C1 and clivus (*C*) are visible. **(B)** A close-up view of the vertebrobasilar junction achieved with facial translocation approach; clamps are retracting the dura.

Following large resection with dural or vessel exposure, an ipsilateral temporalis muscle flap is transferred into the wound from the temporal fossa and laid into the central and paracentral skull base. The attached deep temporalis fascia permits circumferential suturing of this muscle-fascia unit to the surrounding soft and bony tissues under moderate tension, thus preventing postoperative gravity-dependent displacement of the temporalis muscle from its vertical anatomical position to its new horizontal reconstructive position at the central skull base. (The temporal fossa donor defect may be filled with an abdominal fat graft or a preformed polyethylene implant.) The remnant of nasopharyngeal mucosa with the underlining constrictor muscle may then be placed over this temporalis muscle. If pharyngeal mucosa is not available, it is reasonable to leave the temporalis muscle exposed to the nasopharynx. Usually within several weeks, mucosal coverage develops from the periphery of the nasopharynx. It is important, however, to suture the periphery of the muscle to the surrounding structures to ensure support and to seal the surgical site.

The compound vascularized facial segments are repositioned. The dental occlusal plane is reestablished with a prefabricated occlusal splint fashioned preoperatively from the patient's dental models. Osteotomies are stabilized with miniplates. A horizontal lag screw is placed at the region of the nasal spine (above the roots of the central incisor teeth). Posterior craniocervical fusion is performed subsequently if instability occurs.

Specialized Instrumentation

Surgical guidance systems (e.g., ISG wand; ISG Technologies, Mississauga, Ontario, Canada) have been very useful for the rapid identification of anatomy as well as for delineation of the extent of the surgical resection (**Fig. 23.9**).

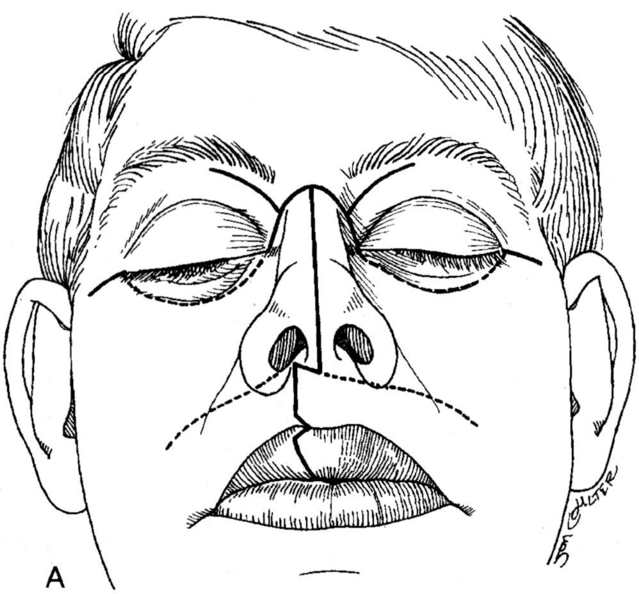

Fig. 23.6 **(A)** Schema of a midfacial split for exposure of the clivus. *(continued)*

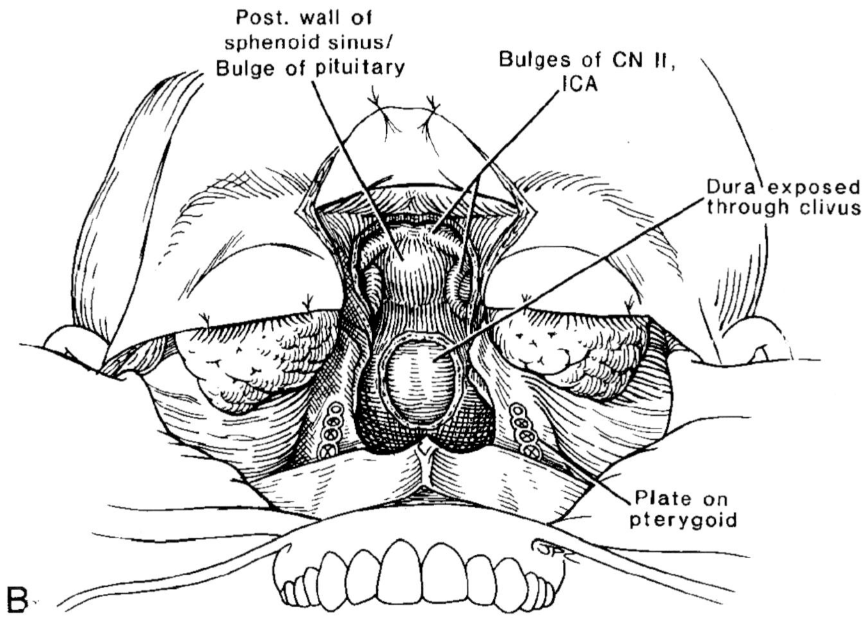

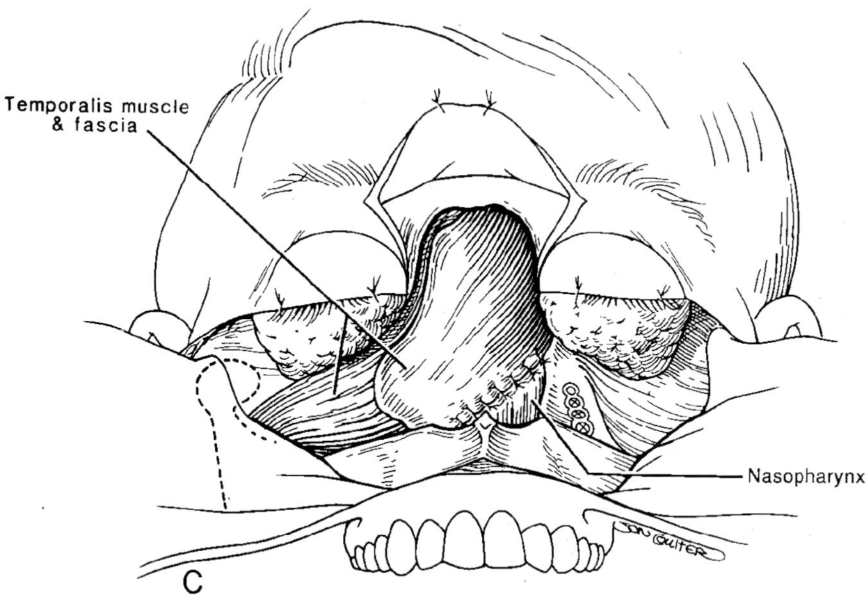

Fig. 23.6 *(continued)* **(B)** Exposure of the central skull base. **(C)** Coverage of the surgical defect with the right temporalis muscle.

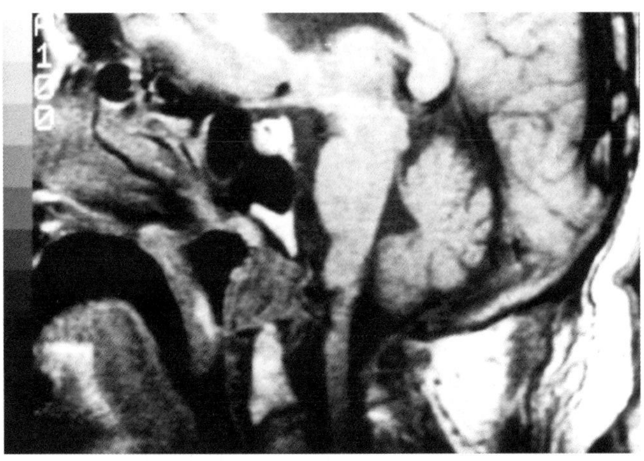

Fig. 23.7 Postoperative lateral magnetic resonance image demonstrating a repair with fascia lata and fibrin glue of the craniovertebral junction.

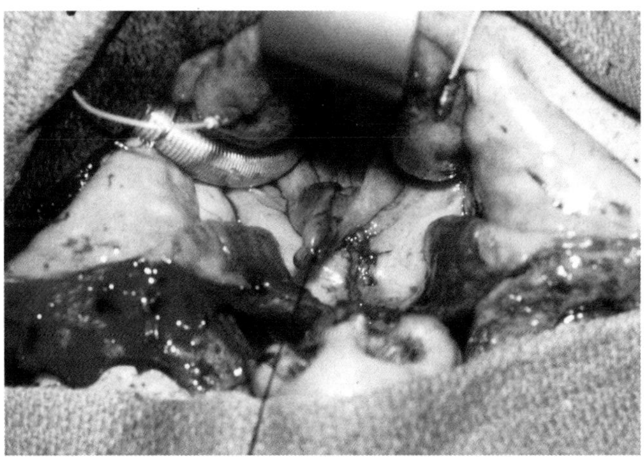

Fig. 23.8 View of the soft palate repair (nasal side; see suture); electromyography electrodes are visible in the tongue.

A Zimmer Micro 100 reciprocating saw (Warsaw, IN) is used to create facial osteotomies. It offers 1-mm-thick blades in short and long versions, ideal for facial osteotomies. For drilling, the Midas Rex system (Midas Rex Pneumatic Tools, Inc., Fort Worth, TX) is used, with straight or angulated hand pieces. It comes with appropriate long attachments suitable for deep central skull base surgery. Cutting as well as diamond burrs are used with suction irrigation. For very soft tumors (e.g., some chordomas and invasive pituitary adenomas), a Cavitron ultrasonic aspirator can be used. For adequate microsurgical visualization, the Zeiss microscope (Carl Zeiss, Thornwood, NY) on a Contraves stand is very useful. Bipolar cautery is essential. An Omni-tract retractor with customized blades as well as a standard Dingman's mouth gag have been found to be very useful for exposing lesions of the central skull base.

Postoperative Management

The adequacy of the airway must be individualized. Some patients are extubated at the completion of skull base surgery or 24 to 48 hours after surgery. For high-risk patients an

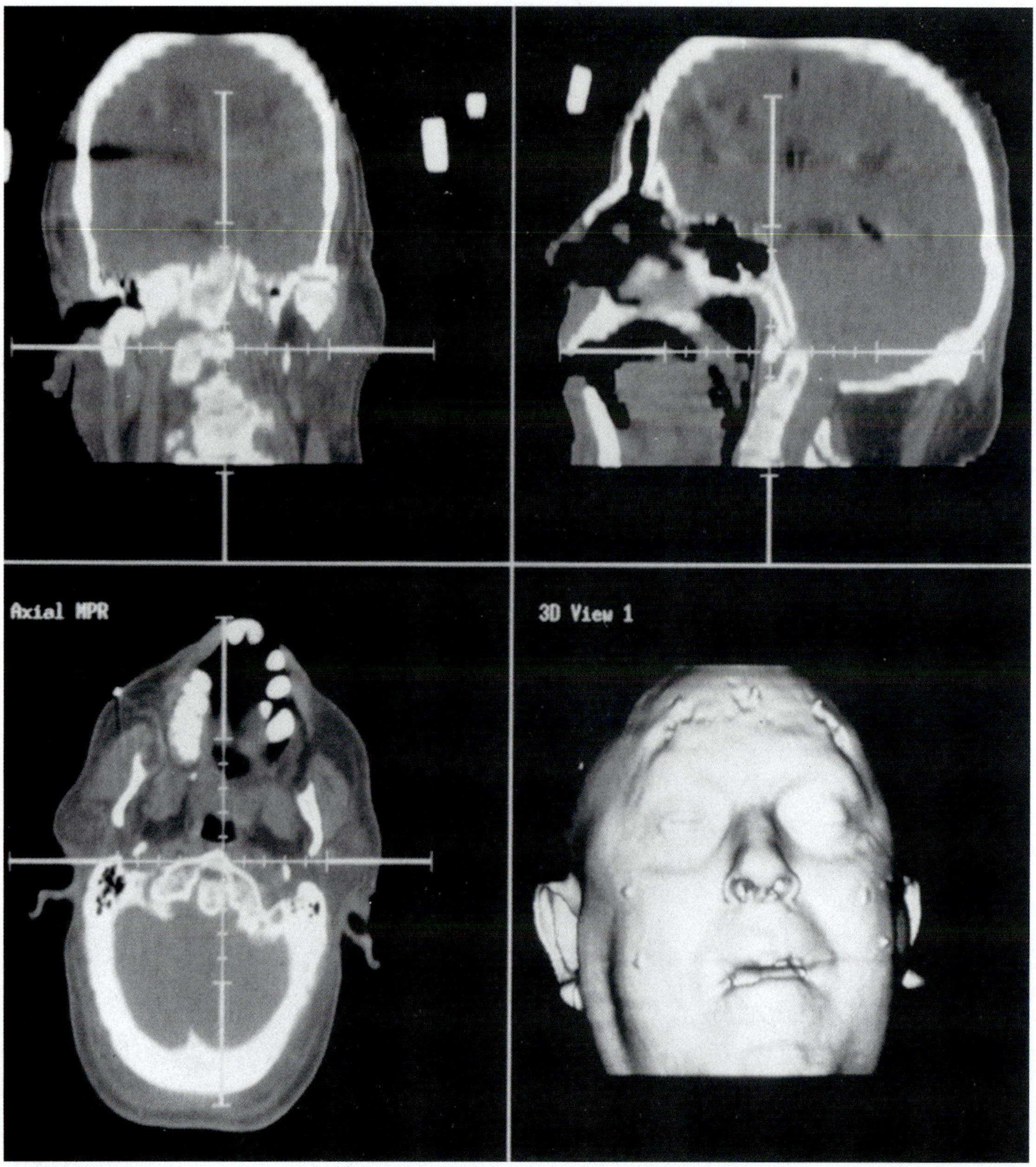

A

Fig. 23.9 **(A)** Computer screen of patient's computed tomography scan with surgical localizer (ISG) centered on the arch of C1. *(continued)*

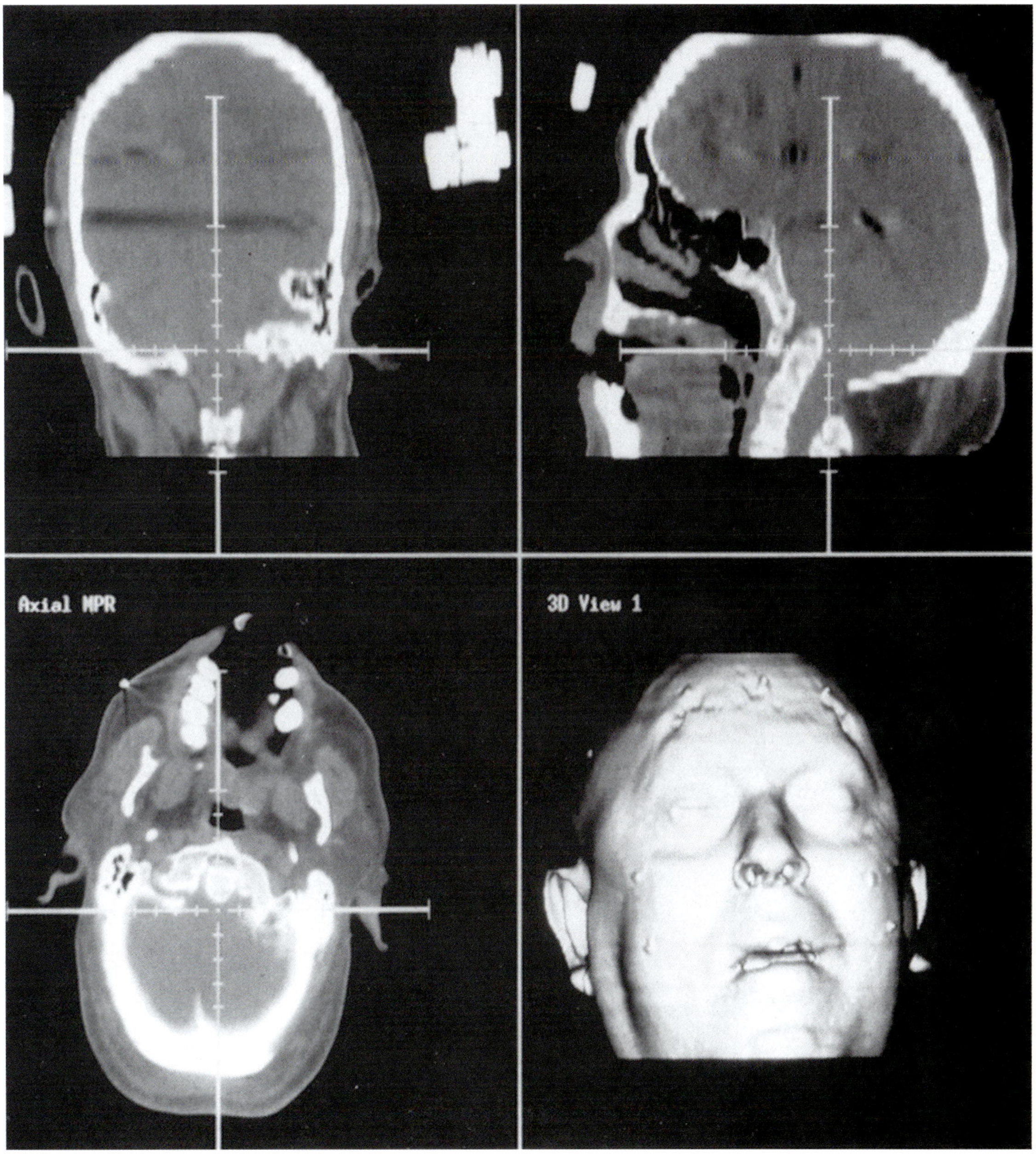

B

Fig. 23.9 *(continued)* **(B)** Localizer centered behind the odontoid, confirming removal of the odontoid.

elective temporary tracheostomy is considered. All suction drains maintain vacuum through a closed system. An external dressing is seldom used. Arterial and central venous pressure lines and the Foley catheter remain in place during the immediate postoperative period. Both lower extremities are covered with intermittent air compression stockings to assist with venous circulation. Once ambulation is resumed, the stockings are removed. The nasogastric tube is connected to low-pressure suction until bowel activity resumes. External tube feeding is continued for 5 to 6 days. Oral intake is then resumed. Antibiotic coverage is usually discontinued after 48 to 72 hours. If a spinal drain is in place, 50 to 75 mL are removed every 8 hours for 2 to 4 days. A CT scan is obtained within the first 24 to 48 hours to ascertain the immediate postoperative changes and the completion of surgical resection. General systemic as well as neurological examinations are continued throughout the postoperative period.

Complications

Complications at the central skull base may be quite hazardous. The major complications tend to fall into three categories: bleeding, infection, and wound healing problems.

Bothersome venous bleeding at the clivus is usually controlled intraoperatively with bone wax or Gelfoam (Baxter,

Table 23.1 Sensitivity in Tissue Assay

Drug	Case 1: Chordoma of clivus	Case 2: Myxoid fibrosarcoma	Case 3: Meningioma, middle and infratemporal fossa	Case 4: Chordoma of clivus	Case 5: Synovial cell sarcoma of upper neck	Case 6: Squamous cell carcinoma, maxilla	Case 7: Neuroendocrine carcinoma, ethmoid sinuses	Case 8: Meningioma, orbit, middle and infratemporal fossae	Case 9: Myxoid fibrosarcoma, orbit, infratemporal fossa, skull base
Bleomycin						X			
Cisplatin	X					X			
Dacarbazine and taxanes								X	
Docetaxel				X		X			
Doxorubicin liposomal									X
Doxorubicin					X				X
Epirubicin									X
Estramustine								X	
Gemcitabine						X			X
Gemcitabine (+ doxorubicin liposomal + high-dose tamoxifen, gemcitabine + ifosfamide [4HI])									X
Gemcitabine + cisplatin		X		X		X			X
Gemcitabine + CP + high-dose tamoxifen				X					
Gemcitabine + melphalan		X							X
Gemcitabine + melphalan + high-dose tamoxifen		X		X	X				
Gemcitabine + melphalan + high-dose tamoxifen	X				X				
Gemcitabine									
Ifosfamide									
Irinotecan + cisplatin						X			
Irinotecan + cisplatin + high-dose tamoxifen						X			
Paclitaxel			X						
Topotecan + cisplatin						X			
Trimetrexate				X					
Vinorelbine + high-dose tamoxifen							X		

Hayward, CA). Arterial bleeding may be encountered from the vertebral arteries as well as from the internal carotid arteries. If arterial injury occurs, repair should be attempted after temporary vascular clips have been applied.

Infection is often the result of the presence of nonvascularized tissue and/or postsurgical "dead space." The transfer of the temporalis muscle flap into the central skull base provides vascularized reconstruction of a large surgical defect to cover the exposed dura and blood vessels. Postoperative CSF leakage with the threat of meningitis is also possible and should be treated aggressively with spinal drainage and/or reoperation. Beta-2-transferrin electrophoresis of suspected fluid is currently the most accurate test to document CSF leakage.

Wound healing problems are more frequent in patients who have had previous surgery and/or radiotherapy and include minor or major tissue necrosis. The extent of local wound care depends on the size and location of the necrosis. When it overlies an essential structure, surgical debridement and vascularized tissue transfer are indicated.

Certain surgical steps lessen the potential for complications. First is the assurance of tissue viability, which requires detailed knowledge of the vascular anatomy, as well as judicial use of electrocoagulation. The use of vascularized muscle transfer (temporalis transfer or microvascular flap) to provide vascularized coverage of the surgical site is the second essential element in lessening the risk of postoperative complications. This step also increases the chances for a seal of the CSF-containing space. When only pharyngeal and/or palatal incisions are used for exposure, a layered closure with mattress sutures is performed.

Additional Considerations

Oncological surgery with clear surgical margins is difficult to achieve at the CVJ; combined treatment modalities may be considered. Tissue assay, performed on a sample of a removed tumor, may offer potential for finding a more specific chemotherapy drug for each patient. In vitro drug testing on tumor cells is in its infancy and still not a perfect predictor of clinical response. However, treatment with assay "positive" drugs is reported to be more strongly associated with clinical response than is treatment with assay "negative" drugs.[1] We have obtained assays on several skull base tumors. Clinical conclusions cannot be drawn yet at this early stage; these findings could be used only as guidance to planning when chemotherapy option needs be considered (**Table 23.1**).

Acknowledgment

This chapter was adapted with permission from Janecka IP. Transfacial approaches to the clivus and upper cervical spine. In: Rengachary SS, ed. Neurosurgical Operative Atlas, Vol. 3. Park Ridge, IL: American Association of Neurological Surgeons; 1993:793–202.

References

1. Weisenthal Cancer Group. Individualized Cancer Treatment. Available at: http://www.weisenthalcancer.com/. Accessed January 21, 2010

24 Transfacial Approaches to the Craniovertebral Junction

Stephen P. Beals and Edward F. Joganic

Lesions of the craniovertebral junction (CVJ) and midline skull base can be accessed through facial routes by application of craniofacial surgical techniques.[1–41] Paul Tessier's well-established principles for correction of congenital anomalies are fundamental[42]: (1) the craniofacial skeleton can be stripped of its periosteum, units osteotomized and repositioned, and the fragments still survive; (2) the eyes can be moved without causing visual loss; and (3) combined intracranial and extracranial exposures can be performed without undue risk of infection. Tessier's principles have proven valuable in allowing removal or retraction of facial skeletal units to access complex lesions of the CVJ and midline skull base.

Single-stage resection with shorter operating times and low morbidity rates are a tribute to these techniques. Direct anterior approaches to the CVJ and midline skull base have several advantages over anterolateral and lateral approaches: (1) the midline plane is relatively avascular; (2) vital neurovascular structures, the temporomandibular joint, and the muscles of mastication are avoided; (3) and wide exposure is possible by degloving, thereby diminishing the need for facial incisions.

Classification of Transfacial Approaches

The anatomical site of lesions of the CVJ and midline skull base guides the level of the transfacial approach. The kyphotic shape of the skull base is perpendicular to the vertical plane of the face and thus requires that lesions that extend anteriorly be accessed from a more superior approach (i.e., through the frontal nasal region), whereas posteriorly located lesions with more superior extension, especially those extending posterior to the sella turcica, be accessed through a more inferior or transmaxillary surgical approach. The most advantageous angle of approach to the lesion is the most important determining factor in selecting the level of transfacial exposure.

We have found it useful to classify transfacial approaches into six levels (**Fig. 24.1** and **Table 24.1**).[1,43] The *transfrontal* (level I) approach yields access to lesions of the anterior cranial fossa. Exposure is achieved by removal of the supraorbital bar (**Fig. 24.2A–C**).

The *transfrontal nasal* (level II) approach is indicated for lesions of the cribriform plate, nasopharynx, frontal and sphenoid sinuses, and tumors of the clivus that exhibit anterior growth. Vertical access to the midline portion of the anterior foramen magnum is possible. Additional exposure is achieved over the level I approach by retaining the nasal and medial orbital wall complex on the supraorbital bar (**Fig. 24.2D–F**).

Larger lesions of the same region can be accessed with the *transfrontal-nasal-orbital* (level III) approach. Greater lateral exposure is obtained by the ability to laterally retract the globes. This lateral retraction is made possible by including the lateral orbital walls and orbital roofs on the fragment (**Fig. 24.2G–I**).

The fragments removed in these three intracranial approaches are variations of the supraorbital bar (**Fig. 24.3**). The subfrontal access achieved by the removal of the supraorbital bar is extended vertically to include the entire midline skull base to the CVJ by retaining the nasal complex and medial orbital walls on the supraorbital bar. Greater horizontal exposure is achieved by adding the lateral orbital walls and orbital roofs to the fragment.

Wider posterior exposure with the level II and III approaches can be achieved with a circumferential cribriform plate osteotomy (**Fig. 24.4**).[44] This osteotomy allows retraction of the cribriform plate. Preservation of the cribriform plate is possible when the region is not involved with tumor. Its preservation also has the advantages of preserving olfaction, diminishing the incidence of cerebrospinal fluid (CSF) leak, and simplifying skull base reconstruction.

The *transnasomaxillary* (level IV) approach provides wide extracranial exposure of the entire midline skull base and CVJ, allowing resection of large nasopharyngeal, paranasal sinus, or clival lesions that extend in any direction. The upper cervical vertebrae are readily accessible through this route for tumors that extend into these regions. Exposure is achieved through a modified Weber-Ferguson incision and a LeFort II osteotomy. The fragment is split at the nasal process on one side and at the palatal midline (**Fig. 24.5A–D**).

Clival and CVJ lesions with superior and inferior extension and moderately sized nasopharyngeal lesions can be accessed via the *transmaxillary* (level V) approach. The exposure is accomplished through a LeFort I osteotomy with or without a palatal split. This exposure provides a good angle of view for clival lesions that extend superiorly behind the sella turcica and for CVJ lesions that extend to the upper cervical vertebrae (**Fig. 24.5E–G**).

The *transpalatal* (level VI) approach provides access to the lower clival and CVJ region for resection of small lesions.

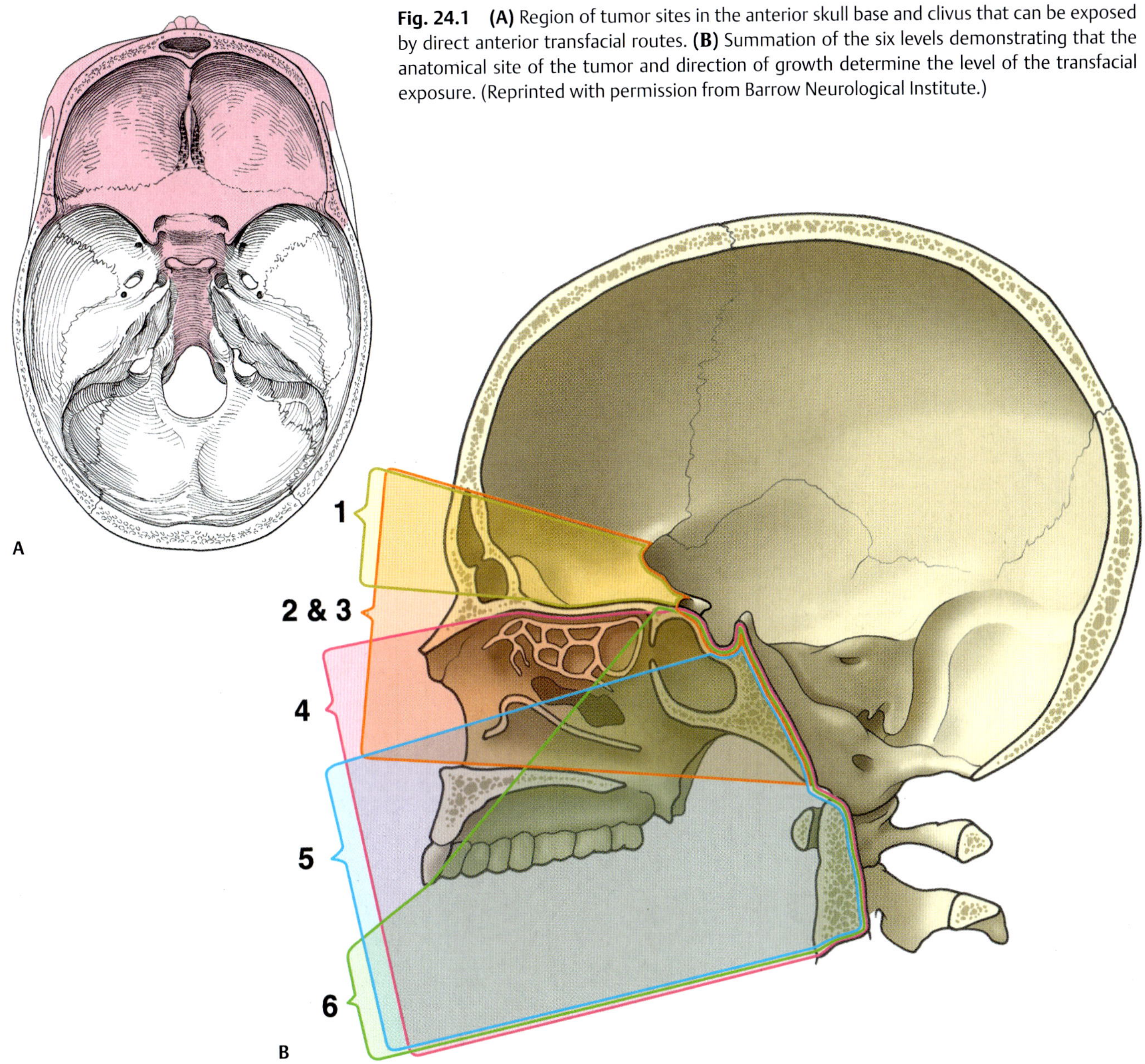

Fig. 24.1 **(A)** Region of tumor sites in the anterior skull base and clivus that can be exposed by direct anterior transfacial routes. **(B)** Summation of the six levels demonstrating that the anatomical site of the tumor and direction of growth determine the level of the transfacial exposure. (Reprinted with permission from Barrow Neurological Institute.)

Table 24.1 Transfacial Approaches to Midline Skull Base: Classification Scheme

Level	Name	Anatomic Sites of Lesions	Figure
I	Transfrontal	Anterior cranial fossa	Figure 24.2A–C
II	Transfrontal nasal	Anterior cranial fossa, nasopharynx, clivus tumors with anterior growth	Figure 24.2D–F
III	Transfrontal-nasal-orbital	Large anterior cranial fossa or nasopharyngeal lesions, clivus tumors with anterior growth	Figures 24.2G–I and 24.13
IV	Transnasomaxillary	Nasopharyngeal lesions; large clivus lesions that extend anteriorly, posteriorly, or inferiorly	Figure 24.5A–D
V	Transmaxillary	Clivus lesions with superior and inferior extensions, small nasopharyngeal lesions	Figures 24.5E–G and 24.13
VI	Transpalatal	Lower clivus region lesions	Figure 24.5H–J

Source: Beals SP, Joganic EF, Hamilton MG, et al. Posterior skull base transfacial approaches. Clin Plast Surg 1995;22(3):491–511. Reprinted with permission from W.B. Saunders Company.

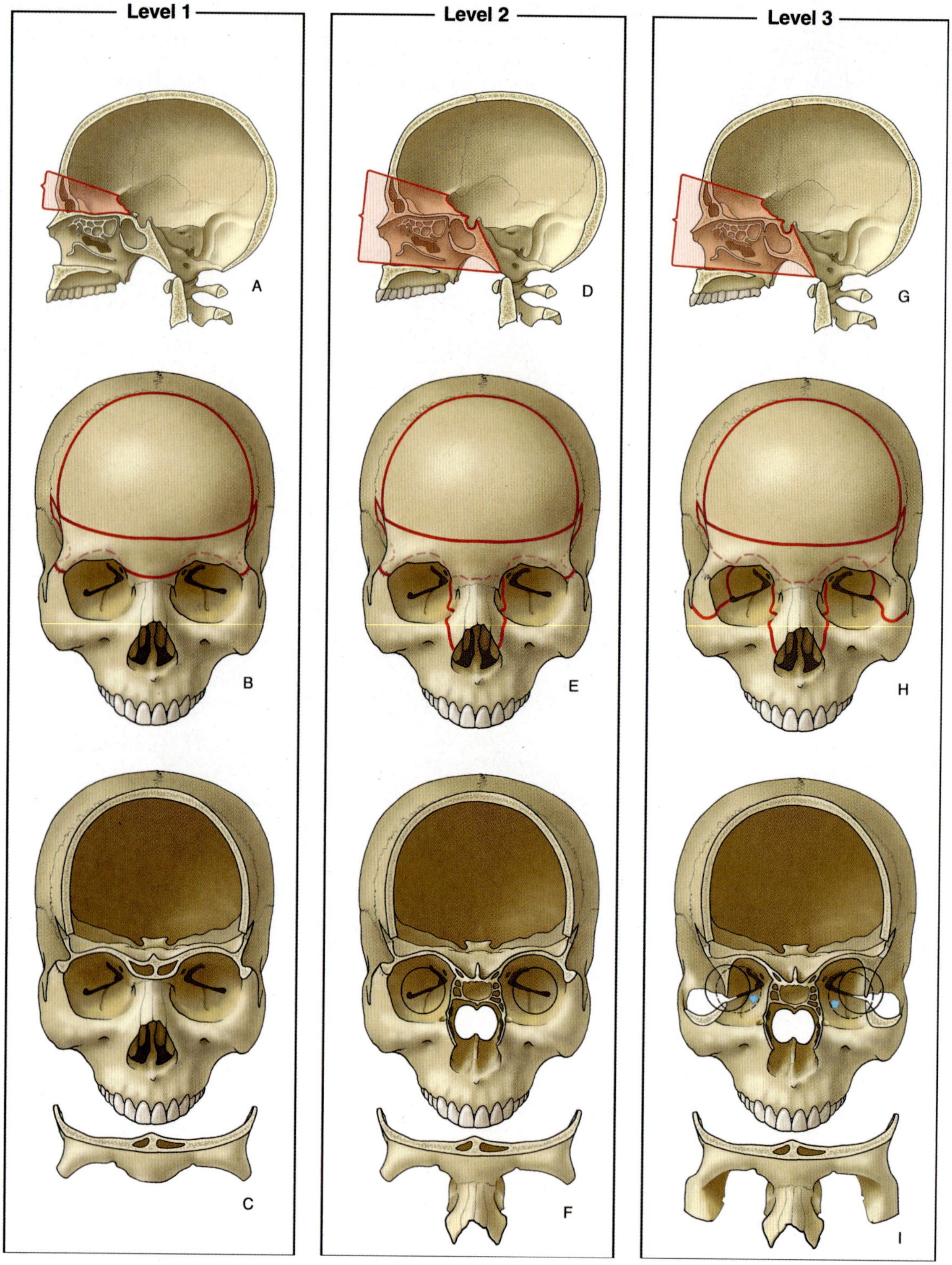

Fig. 24.2 Composite illustration showing the levels of exposure for the three intracranial approaches and the osteotomies required for each. **(A)** Level I transfrontal exposure for anterior cranial fossa. **(B,C)** The level I exposure requires removal of the supraorbital bar. **(D)** Level II transfrontal nasal exposure for anterior approach to the anterior cranial fossa and clivus. **(E,F)** The level II exposure requires removal of the frontonasal fragment. **(G)** Level III transfrontal-nasal-orbital exposure for larger lesions of the anterior cranial fossa, nasopharynx, and clivus. This approach is similar to level II, except that it provides a wider exposure by allowing lateral retraction of the globes (see Fig. 24.2D). **(H,I)** The level III exposure requires inclusion of the lateral orbital walls on the frontonasal fragment (frontal naso-orbital unit). (Reprinted with permission from Barrow Neurological Institute.)

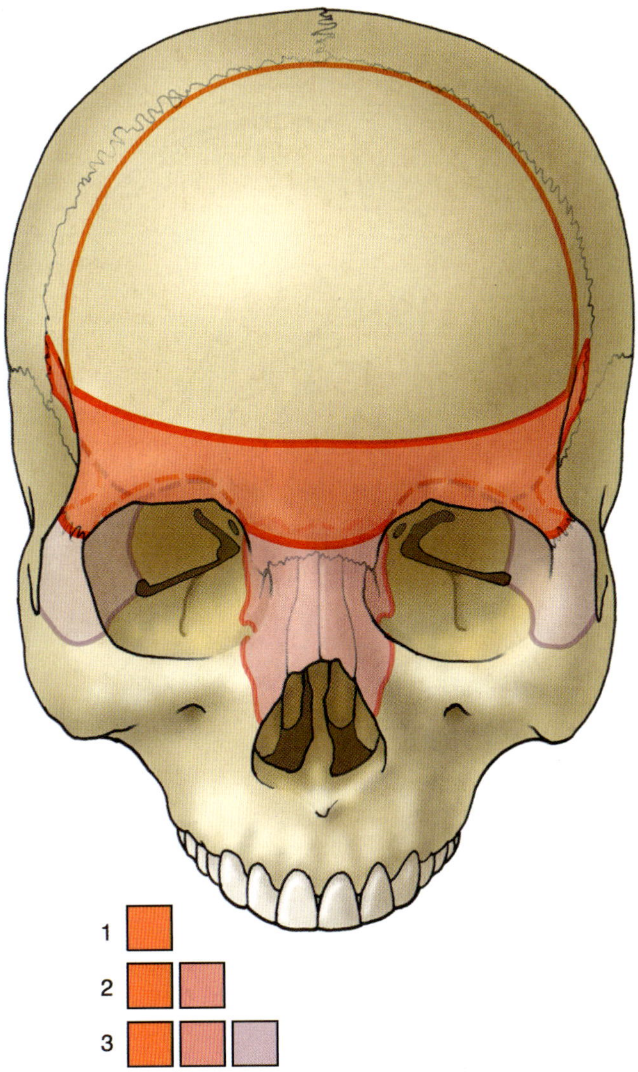

Fig. 24.3 The three intracranial approaches represent variations of the amount of bone resected with the supraorbital bar. The shaded areas indicated by the numbers *1*, *2*, and *3* represent the amount of exposure for levels I, II, and II, respectively. (Reprinted with permission from Barrow Neurological Institute.)

The hard palate is removed and the soft palate is split to provide this exposure (**Fig. 24.5H–J**).

The extracranial approaches are variations of maxillary osteotomies. Increasing exposure is possible as more of the maxilla is removed (**Fig. 24.6**). Although the transnasomaxillary approach provides exposure of the entire midline skull base, the transmaxillary approach provides access to the lower half and the transpalatal approach to the lower third of the skull base. The overlapping exposure shared by these six approaches provides great flexibility. Each can be used in isolation, or the intracranial and extracranial approaches can be combined to allow simultaneous intracranial and extracranial tumor resection.

Technique

Intracranial Approaches

Preoperative Workup

After a thorough understanding of the patient's clinical presentation and deficits related to the tumor, additional workup should include cephalometric X-rays, computed tomography (CT) with true coronal cuts of the orbits, magnetic resonance imaging (MRI), and life-size photographs.

Informed Consent

Counseling is essential to relate the potential risks and complications as well as the expectations and limitations of the procedure. In addition to the risks associated with a craniotomy, these risks include possible alteration of orbital adnexal function, such as alteration of blink dynamics, tear production or drainage, extraocular muscle imbalance, visual loss, and altered globe position within the orbit. The patient can lose olfaction or experience diminished facial sensation, either temporarily or permanently. Furthermore, brow weakness or paralysis is possible, as well as a change in the orbital nasal configuration. The latter is only significant when major soft tissue and skeletal resection is needed to achieve complete removal of the tumor. When temporalis and frontal galeal muscle flaps are utilized, soft tissue contour defects can be noted in the forehead and temporal fossa regions.

Patient Positioning

The patient is positioned on the operating table in the supine position, and general anesthesia is induced utilizing an orotracheal tube. The tube is secured to the lower dentition with a 26-gauge wire to assure a secure airway, as well as to eliminate the need for any tape that could obstruct the surgeon's view of the face. After monitoring lines and intravenous lines are placed, the patient is given prophylactic antibiotics and a lumbar drain is placed, if indicated. If the dura is opened intraoperatively, the lumbar drain reduces the postoperative incidence of CSF leaks and infections. The patient's head is positioned in a Mayfield headholder. A localizing device, such as the StealthStation S7 (Medtronic Navigation, Louisville, Colorado), is useful intraoperatively. The wand is clamped directly on the Mayfield frame and sterilely draped. The pins of the Mayfield skull fixation device are positioned posterior to the ears to allow a posteriorly positioned bicoronal skin incision. After electroencephalographic (EEG) leads are placed and fiduciary reference points for the localizing wand are confirmed, the patient's face and scalp are prepared and draped. Temporary tarsorrhaphy sutures of 5–0 cardiovascular silk are placed in the eyelids to protect the corneas.

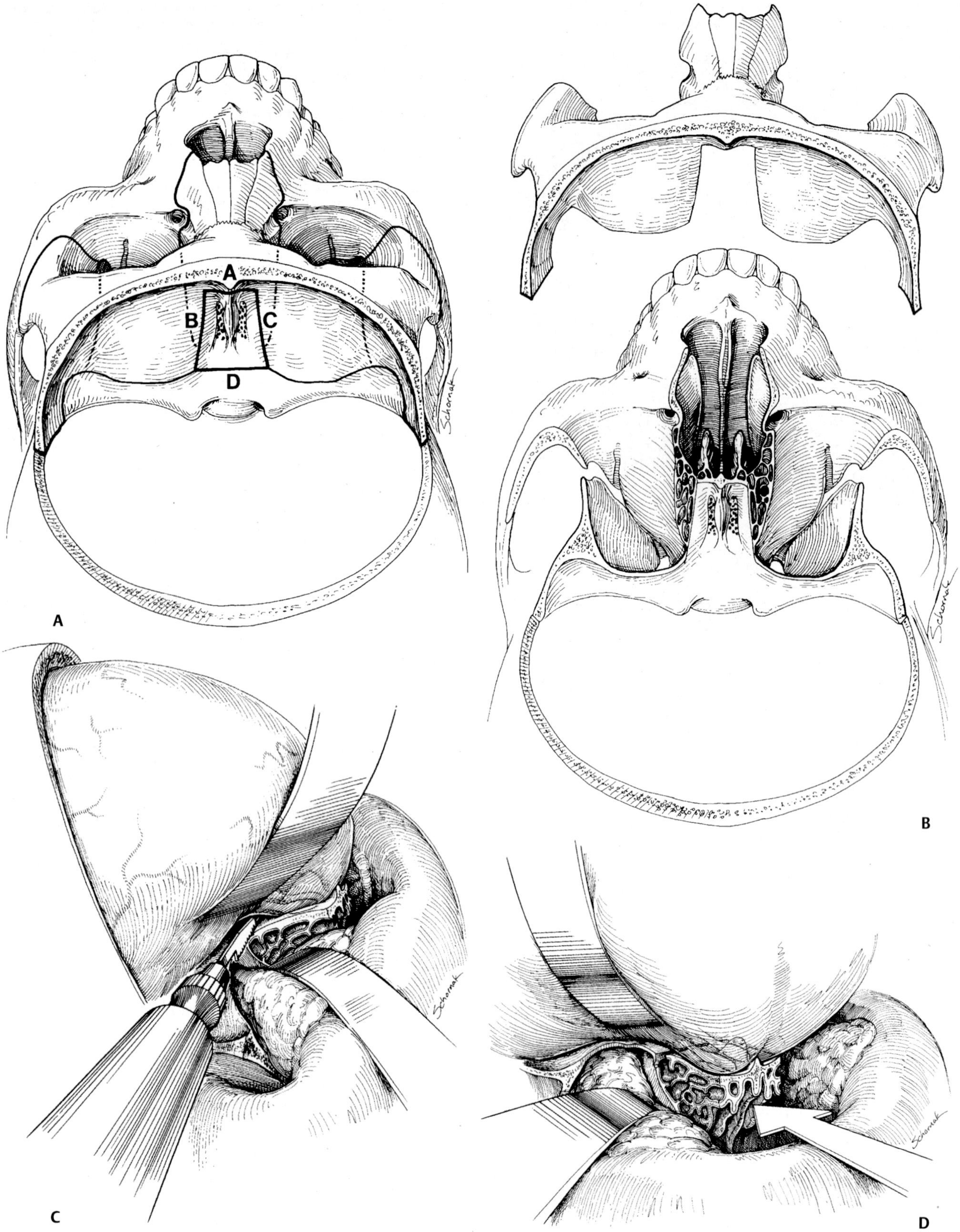

Fig. 24.4 **(A)** Anterior cranial fossa demonstrating the initial circumferential cribriform plate osteotomies. *A*, anterior osteotomy; *B* and *C*, parasagittal osteotomy; *D*, posterior osteotomy through the planum sphenoidale. The additional lines indicate osteotomy cuts for removal of the frontal naso-orbital unit. **(B)** All osteotomy cuts, except for the posterior cut, are performed to allow removal of the frontal naso-orbital unit. **(C)** The final, posterior osteotomy through the planum sphenoidale is performed with appropriate retraction of the frontal lobe dura and paranasal soft tissues. **(D)** After the trabeculae are divided and a generous cuff of mucosa is left intact, the intact cribriform plate unit is released from the skull base.[44] (Reprinted with permission from Barrow Neurological Institute.)

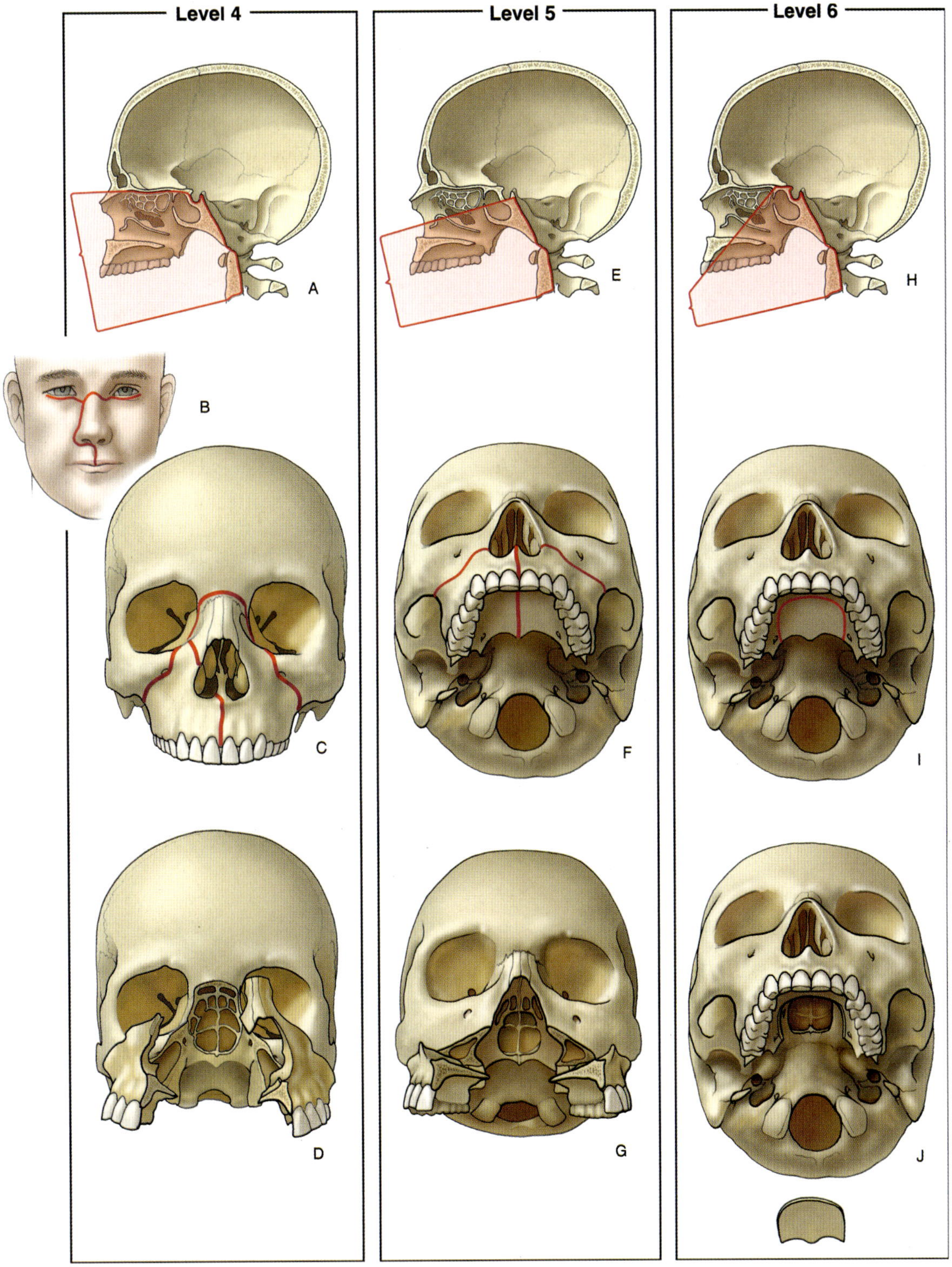

Fig. 24.5 Composite illustration showing the levels of exposure for the three extracranial transfacial approaches and the osteotomies required for each. **(A)** A level IV transnasomaxillary approach yields a wide exposure of the entire central skull base from the radix to the craniocervical junction. A similar degree of exposure can usually be obtained with a combination of the level III and level V exposures. **(B)** Skin incisions for the transnasomaxillary approach. **(C)** The level IV exposure requires a LeFort II osteotomy and then **(D)** splitting of the maxillary fragment. **(E)** A level V transmaxillary approach provides exposure of the clivus and nasopharyngeal area. **(F)** The level V exposure requires a LeFort I osteotomy and **(G)** splitting of the palate for further exposure. **(H)** A level VI transpalatal approach provides access to the lower clivus and upper cervical region. The level VI exposure requires an **(I)** osteotomy and **(J)** removal of the hard palate. (Reprinted with permission from Barrow Neurological Institute.)

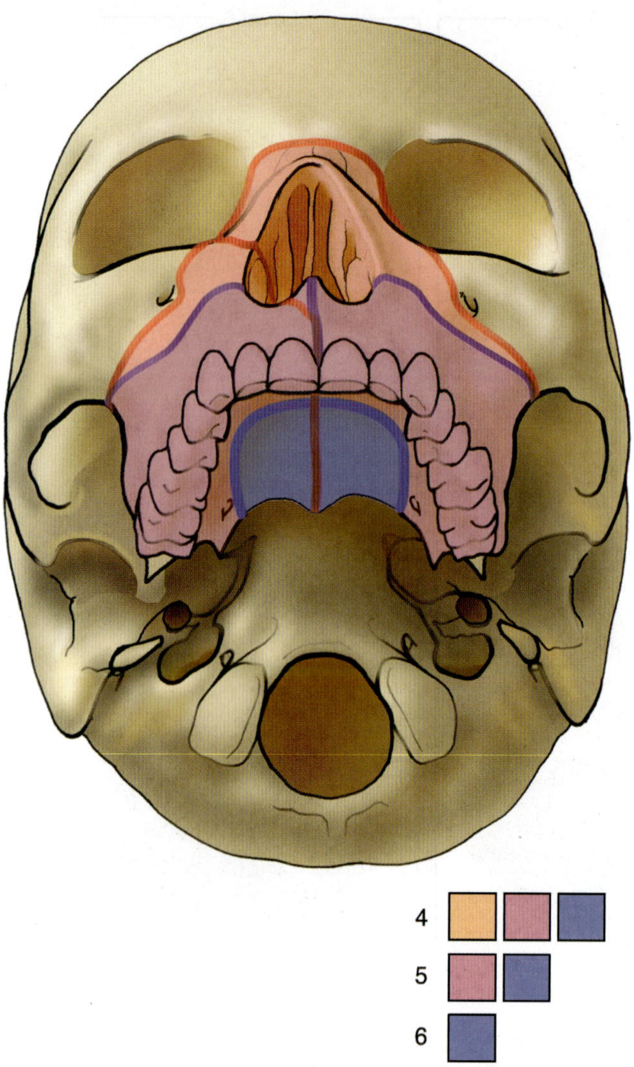

Fig. 24.6 The extracranial approaches provide increasing exposure as more of the maxilla is removed. The shaded areas indicated by the numbers *4*, *5*, and *6* represent the amount of exposure for levels IV, V, and VI, respectively. (Reprinted with permission from Barrow Neurological Institute.)

Incision

The bicoronal incision is positioned in the middle or posterior aspect of the calvarium to preserve adequate length of pericranial and frontal galeal flaps for use in the skull base reconstruction after the tumor resection.

Dissection

The anterior scalp flap is reflected by microneedle dissection,[45] as it is more hemostatic and preserves the important pericranial and temporalis tissues for possible use as flaps. The scalp flap is reflected to the superior orbital rims on either side, then inferiorly into the temporalis region beneath the intermediate temporalis fascia to avoid the innervation of the frontalis muscle. The pericranial flap can be based either anteriorly, preserving its axial blood supply, or laterally on the temporalis muscle. The pericranium is scored against the calvarium at the midline or asymmetrically if it is anticipated that a laterally based pericranial flap of greater length will be needed from one side. The entire pericranium can be mobilized from one temporalis muscle, if needed. Even if the pericranial flap is not needed for skull base reconstruction, its attachment to the temporalis muscles is useful in reattaching the temporalis muscles in their anatomical position in the temporal fossa (**Fig. 24.7**).

For level II and III exposures, the pericranium and temporalis muscles are reflected, the periorbita is stripped 360 degrees, and the periosteum in the region of the nasal process of the maxilla is stripped. Great care is taken to preserve the nasolacrimal ducts. The medial canthal ligaments are detached from the bone or, if desired, a small island of bone, attached to the medial canthal ligament, can be preserved to facilitate reattachment. The upper lateral nasal cartilages are detached from the undersurface of the caudal margin of the nasal bones. The nasal mucosa is dissected from the underside of the nasal bones.

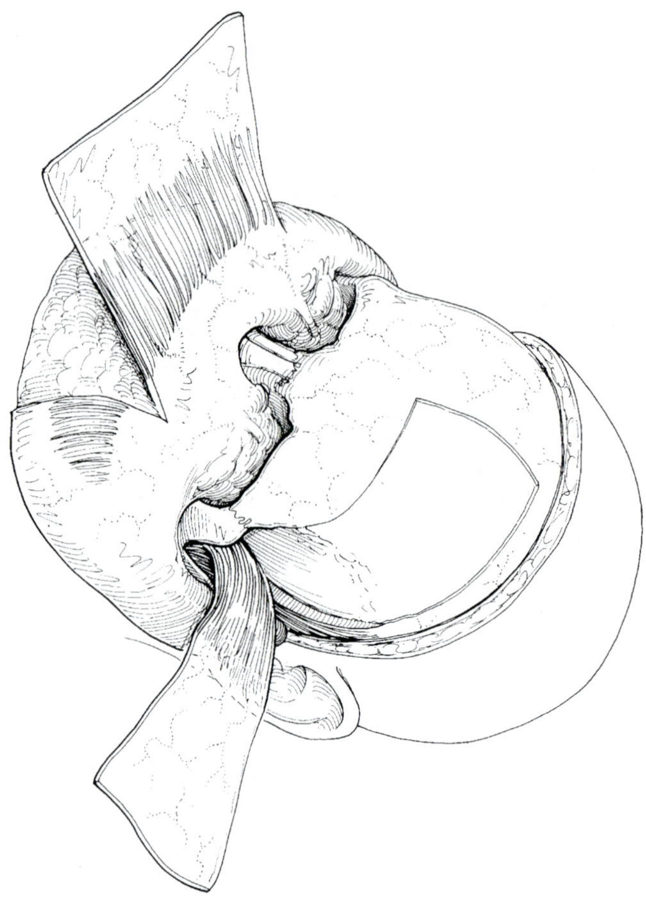

Fig. 24.7 Frontogaleal and pericranial flaps must be preserved during the initial dissection. (Reprinted with permission from Barrow Neurological Institute.)

Bifrontal Craniotomy

The bifrontal craniotomy is performed, and the dura is retracted from the anterior cranial fossa. If the cribriform plate is to be preserved, the posterior margin of the bifrontal craniotomy must be positioned at the level of the coronal suture, and the cranial osteotomy must extend laterally and inferiorly to the skull base in the temporal region. This configuration is necessary to allow the reciprocating saw to be positioned perpendicular to the planum sphenoidale.

Osteotomies

After the soft tissue dissection is completed, a sterilized pencil is used to mark the facial and cranial osteotomy lines. For the transfrontal-nasal-orbital (level III) approach, lines are marked along the lateral orbital walls from the inferior orbital fissures superiorly. The lines continue along the inferior margin of the temporal limbs of the supraorbital bars (**Fig. 24.4B**). The lines are usually positioned ~2 cm posteriorly from the superolateral orbital rim. Lines are also marked from the superior margins of the zygomatic arches to the inferior orbital fissures in the region of the inferolateral orbital floors. Medially, a line is drawn across the nasal process of the maxilla, brought anteriorly and medially to the nasolacrimal ducts, and then positioned posteriorly along the lower aspects of the medial orbital walls to within 1 cm of the optic canals. The line then extends superiorly along the medial orbital wall onto the orbital roof to maintain most of the orbital roof on the fragment. This orbital roof osteotomy extends laterally to intersect with the lines on the lateral orbital walls.

The frontal lobes are retracted gently, and an extradural exposure of the floors of the frontal and middle fossa is performed. Parasagittal osteotomies are planned lateral to each cribriform plate, posteriorly in the region of the planum sphenoidale, and anteriorly in the region of the crista galli. The same lines are placed symmetrically on the opposite side (**Fig. 24.4A**).

Before the osteotomies are made, small plates are bent for passive adaptation across the planned osteotomy sites in the region of the zygomatic arch and lateral orbital wall. Drill holes are placed, and the plates are labeled and set aside.

The osteotomies are then performed in the same order on both sides. Great care is taken to preserve the periorbita and dura, as well as the nasolacrimal duct and nasal mucosa. After the osteotomies are completed with a reciprocating saw, an osteotome is positioned anteriorly and inferiorly through the crista galli osteotomy site to separate the bony septum. The entire single fragment can now be mobilized and removed (**Fig. 24.2G**).

Circumferential Cribriform Plate Osteotomy

When the cribriform plate is not involved with tumor, the cribriform plate can be preserved with a circumferential osteotomy (**Fig. 24.4**). Parasagittal and anterior cuts have already been made in the process of removing the frontal naso-orbital fragment. After the posterior osteotomy is performed, an inferior cut is made, preserving a 1-cm cuff of nasal mucosa and septum. The cribriform plate is thus freed and can be elevated with the dura.

Tumor Resection

The mucosa of the ethmoid sinus as well as the posterior nasal septum can be resected to achieve greater exposure to the region of the tumor. The advantage of the level III approach is that removing the lateral orbital walls permits the globes to be retracted laterally to achieve a wide central interorbital access to the tumor. If the size of the tumor does not require this degree of exposure, the lateral orbital walls can be preserved, removing only the nasal-medial orbital wall complex with the supraorbital bar (level II approach) (**Fig. 24.2D–F**). If the tumor is more localized within the anterior cranial fossa, the supraorbital bar alone can be removed (level I approach) (**Fig. 24.2A–C**).

Resection of soft tissue and the nasal, orbital, and skeletal tissues depends on the pathology and extent of the tumor. This approach is flexible and can be individualized according to the anatomical site of the tumor and its extension, as well as the surgeon's preference.

Reconstruction

After tumor resection, reconstruction is addressed. If needed, the skull base and orbital walls are reconstructed with split cranial grafts. Grafts usually can be harvested from the inner table of the bifrontal bone flap (**Fig. 24.8**). Interosseous fixation with light-gauge wire is appropriate for this region.

Sealing the extracranial and intracranial interfaces is important if the dura has been entered. Depending on the location and size of the defect, regional flaps (such as pericranial, frontogaleal, and temporalis muscle) can be used. The tissue flaps should be inset and secured with sutures after replacing the frontal naso-orbital unit. If the cribriform plate has been sacrificed, it is ideal to place separate tissue flaps on the nasal and intracranial sides of the bone graft. If the level I approach is used, two anteriorly based flaps can be used (frontogaleal, pericranial). One is placed below the supraorbital bar on the nasal side, and the other tissue flap is placed above the bar on the intracranial side. For the level II and III approaches, access beneath the facial skeletal fragment is impossible; therefore, one laterally based tissue flap is preferred. When two tissue flaps are used, both flaps must access the defect between the bifrontal bone flap and frontal naso-orbital fragment. If the cribriform plate is preserved, a single flap is used to cover the osteotomy defect. Either an anteriorly based or laterally based flap can be used. The tissue must be incised to cover all sides of the cribriform plate osteotomy (**Figs. 24.9** and **24.10**).

The frontal naso-orbital unit is rigidly fixed with screw plates, except at the osteotomy through the nasal process of

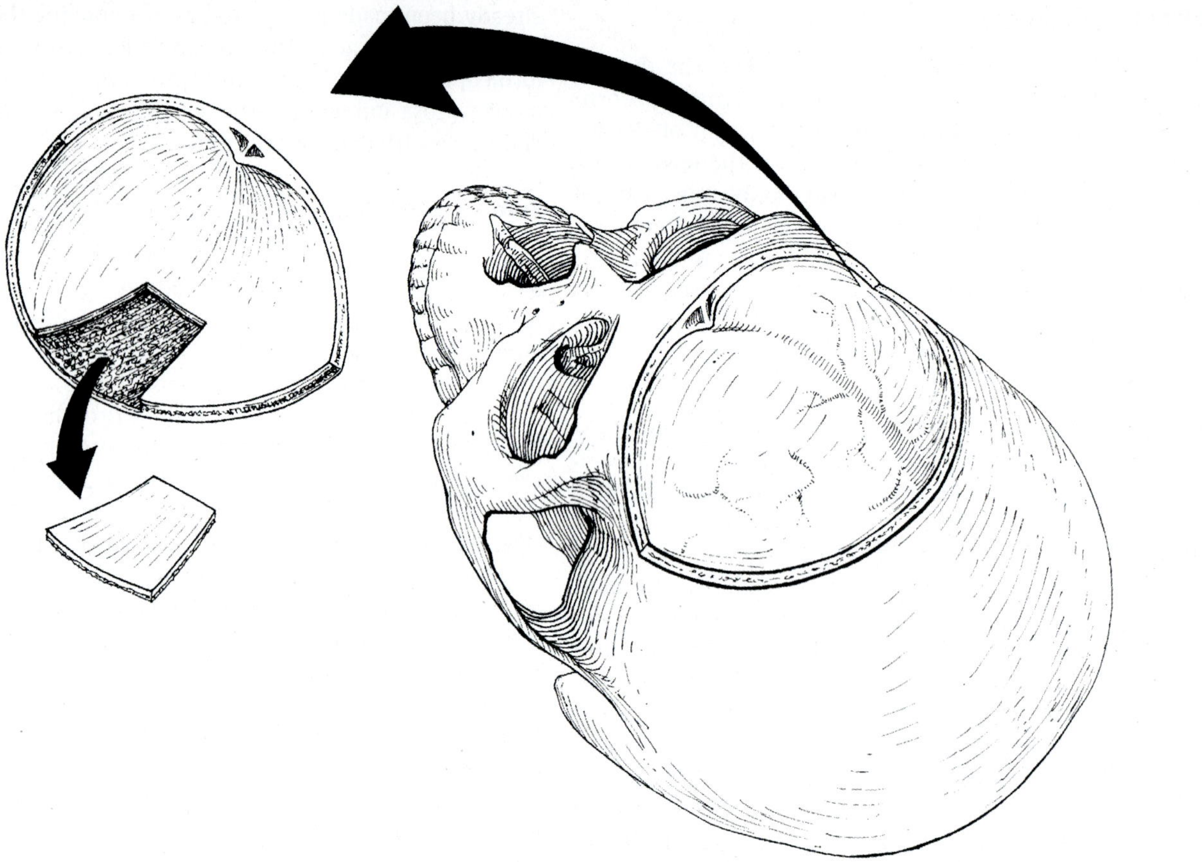

Fig. 24.8 Cranial bone grafts are harvested from the frontal bone for orbital and skull base reconstruction. (Reprinted with permission from Barrow Neurological Institute.)

the maxilla, where light-gauge interosseous wires are utilized. Great care is taken to place small plates in concealed areas so that they will never be visible or palpable. For example, plates are placed in the lateral orbital wall region in the temporal fossa rather than on the lateral or superior orbital rim.

When the cribriform plate has been preserved, it is reattached into its anatomical site with wire fixation. Fibrin glue can be used to seal the flap margins in an effort to obtain a watertight closure. The upper lateral nasal cartilage must be reattached to the caudal margins of the nasal bones to prevent a saddle-nose deformity. This reattachment is accomplished by drilling holes in the bony margin and suturing the cartilages to the bone with nonabsorbable suture.

The medial canthal ligaments are repaired by transnasal wiring. Before the frontal bone is replaced, the frontal sinuses are exenterated in adults. The frontal bone can be reattached with plates or wires. Any unused temporalis muscle or pericranial flaps are directly reattached in their anatomical position, with sutures, to drill holes in the bone. The wounds are irrigated with one-half strength peroxide and one-quarter strength Betadine, followed by Bacitracin solution, and the scalp is closed with galeal and skin sutures.

Extracranial Approaches

Preoperative Workup

For the transnasomaxillary (level IV) and the transmaxillary (level V) approaches, preparation requires life-size photographs including occlusal views, anteroposterior (AP) and lateral cephalometrograms, a Panorex of the mandible, and dental models. An acrylic splint, which has adequate depth to allow the two palatal halves to snap into the splint, is fabricated and obviates the need for arch bars in referencing with the mandibular arch (an orotracheal tube makes this more difficult). The splint also has a palatal cross-piece to assure greater stability of the posterior aspect of the fragments.

Informed Consent

Preoperative counseling with the patient should include explanation of potential risks and complications which, in addition to the usual risks of a major procedure, include possible postoperative malocclusion, which could require secondary surgery or orthodontics for correction, and loss of segment circulation, which could result in an oronasal fistula and abnormal speech. In children, there is a risk of losing the secondary tooth buds.

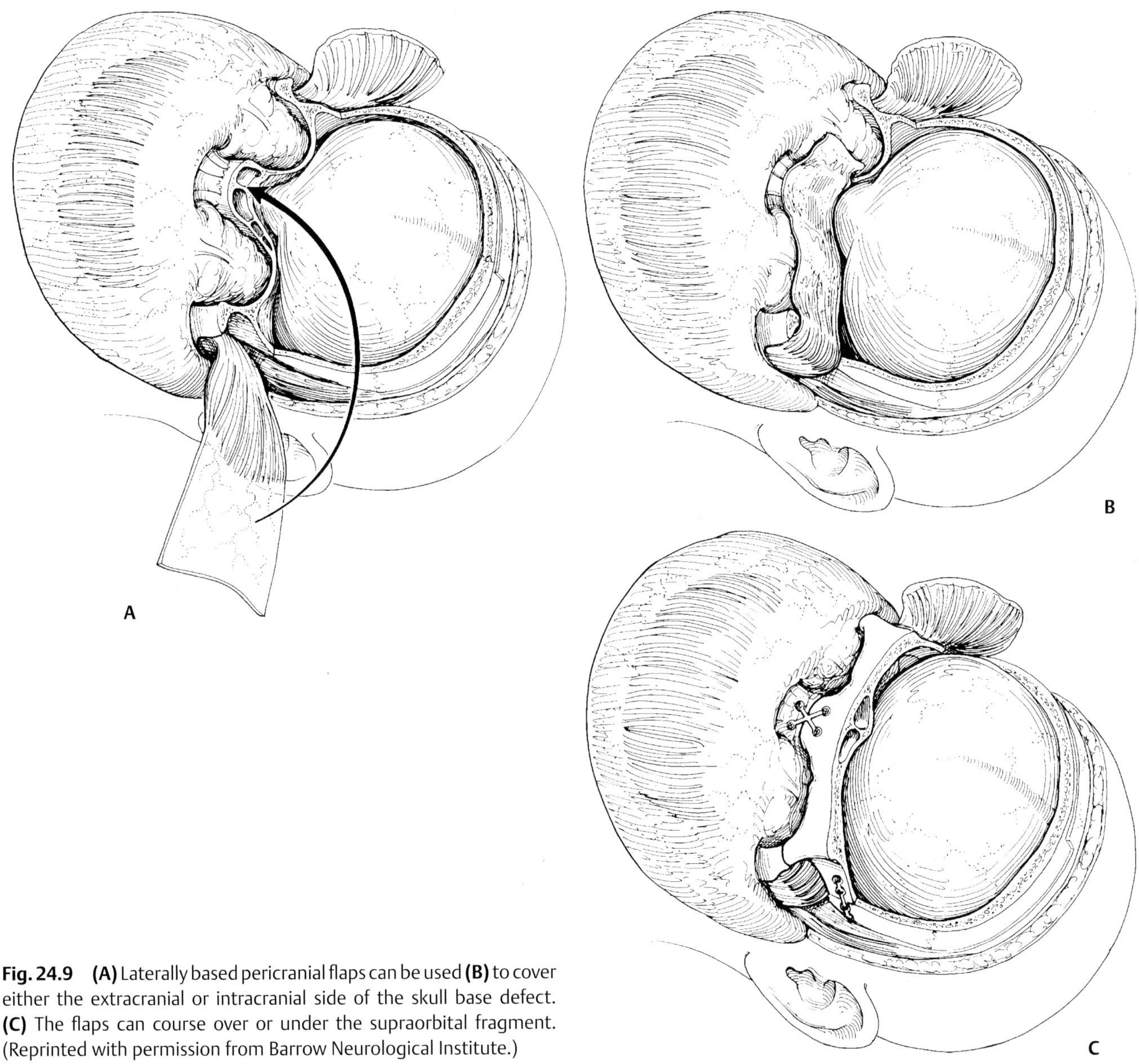

Fig. 24.9 **(A)** Laterally based pericranial flaps can be used **(B)** to cover either the extracranial or intracranial side of the skull base defect. **(C)** The flaps can course over or under the supraorbital fragment. (Reprinted with permission from Barrow Neurological Institute.)

Patient Positioning

The patient is positioned on the operating table in supine position, and general anesthesia is induced utilizing an orotracheal tube. The tube is secured to the lower dentition with a 26-gauge wire to assure a secure airway and to keep any tape from obstructing the surgeon's view of the face. After intravenous lines and monitoring lines are placed, the patient is given prophylactic antibiotics. A lumbar drain is placed, if indicated. The patient's head is fixated with a three-point rigid skull clamp. EEG leads and fiduciary reference points for the localizing wand are confirmed. Temporary tarsorrhaphy sutures of 5–0 cardiovascular silk are placed in the eyelids to protect the corneas. An adrenaline solution is infiltrated into the upper buccal sulcus and mucosa in the anterior maxillary region.

Transnasomaxillary Approach (Level IV) (Fig. 24.5A–D)

Incision and Dissection

The nasomaxillary region is exposed through a modified Weber-Ferguson incision. A bilateral buccal sulcus incision is also made. The periosteum is stripped in preparation for a LeFort II osteotomy. The piriform aperture and orbital and nasal floor are exposed. The nasolacrimal duct and infraorbital nerves are isolated.

Plate Preregistration

Lines are drawn for the LeFort II osteotomy. Plates are contoured for a perfect passive fit to the zygomatic buttress, inferior orbital rims, and radix. Also, a plate adapted to the anterior nasal floor adds stability after the palatal split.

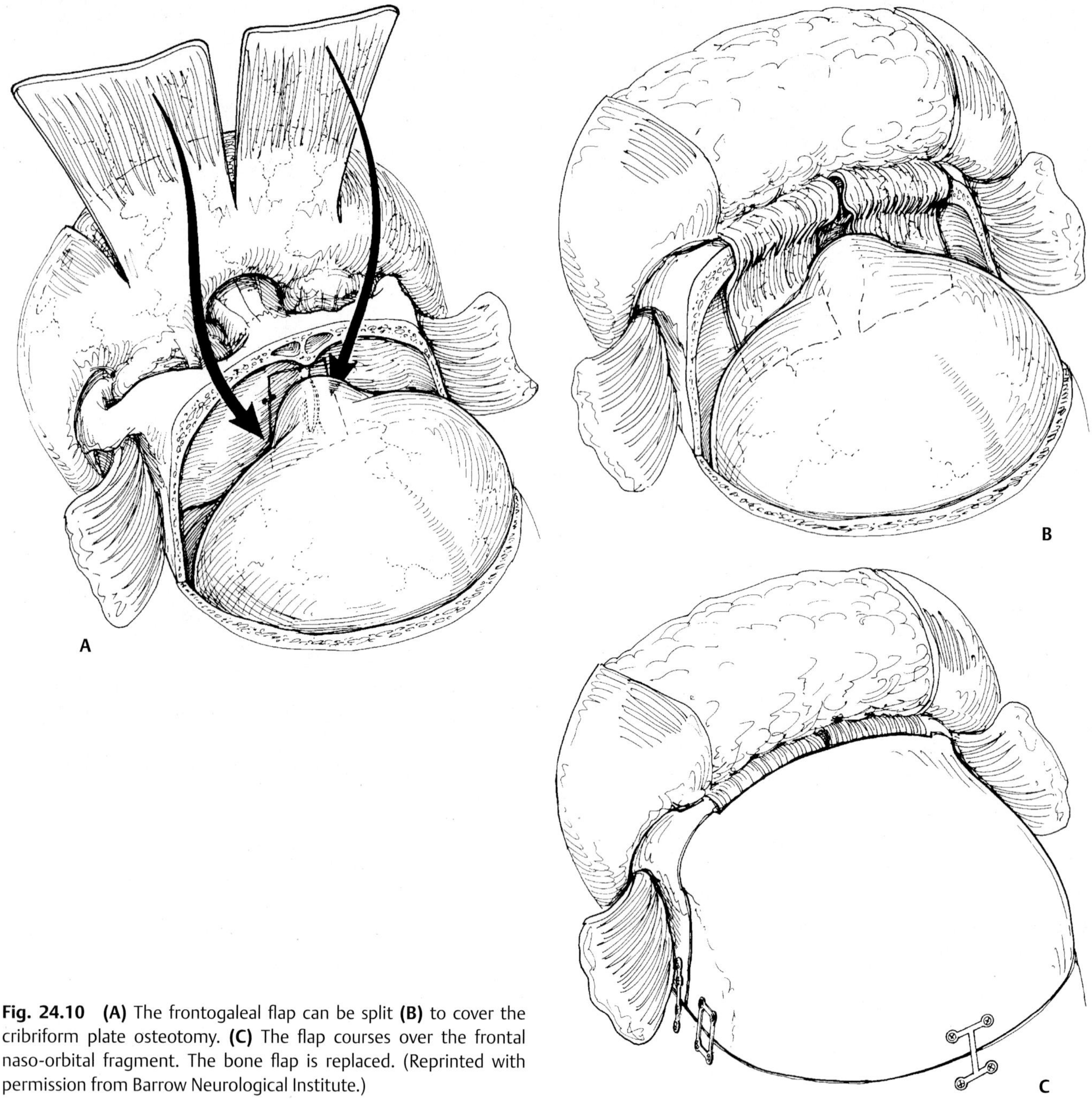

Fig. 24.10 **(A)** The frontogaleal flap can be split **(B)** to cover the cribriform plate osteotomy. **(C)** The flap courses over the frontal naso-orbital fragment. The bone flap is replaced. (Reprinted with permission from Barrow Neurological Institute.)

Screw holes are placed on each side of the osteotomy. The plates are then removed, labeled, and set aside. The screw holes are drilled before the osteotomies are made so that the reassembly with screw plates will allow perfect anatomical alignment.

Osteotomy

The LeFort II osteotomy is performed and the fragment mobilized. The fragment is split at the nasal process of the maxilla and the midline of the hard and soft palates. The fragments can then be retracted as needed to gain exposure for tumor resection. If the exposure is limited by tethering of the nasolacrimal ducts, one or both ducts can be divided and subsequently repaired after inserting tubes into the lumens of the nasolacrimal ducts after tumor resection. If more lateral exposure is needed, the pterygoid plates can be outfractured, resected, or retained on the maxillary fragment.

Defect Reconstruction

After tumor resection, the skull base defect may require reconstruction with a fat graft or bone graft prior to mucosal closure.

Reassembly

The occlusal splint is used to reorient the maxillary fragments. The preregistered plates are applied. The soft palate and oral mucosa are repaired. The facial incisions are closed. If desired, the orotracheal tube can be reinserted into the nose before reassembly by removing the coupler and passing the tubes retrograde through the nostril on one side. The splint is used for 10 to 14 days. A liquid diet is recommended for 4 weeks.

Transmaxillary Approach (Level V) (Fig. 24.5E–G)

Incision and Dissection

An upper buccal sulcus incision is made, leaving a generous cuff of muscle and mucosa on the gingival side. The anterior maxilla is stripped of its periosteum. Periosteum is also stripped posteriorly to the pterygomaxillary suture line, anteriorly to the inferior orbital rims (carefully preserving the infraorbital nerve), and along the piriform aperture. The mucosa is stripped from the piriform aperture, lateral nasal walls, and nasal floor; the anterior nasal spine is exposed. Meticulous hemostasis is needed because any oozing during the tumor resection pools in the neurosurgeon's field of dissection. Hypotensive anesthesia, targeted at a mean arterial pressure of two-thirds of normal, is helpful.

Plate Preregistration

When the dissection of the anterior maxilla is complete, a pencil is used to mark the LeFort I osteotomy site. In children, this osteotomy should be high, positioned at the level of the inferior margin of the infraorbital foramen. In adults, the osteotomy is positioned above the nasal floor parallel to the occlusal plane. Miniplates are then bent to a perfect passive fit along the piriform apertures and zygomatic buttresses bilaterally. Drill holes are placed on each side of the LeFort I osteotomy line, and a screw is placed in one hole on each side of the osteotomy. When each of the four plates has been applied, the plates are removed and labeled.

Osteotomy

A LeFort I osteotomy is performed with a reciprocating saw. The lateral nasal wall and nasal septum are cut with guarded osteotomes, and the pterygomaxillary fissure is separated with a curved osteotome. The LeFort I fragment is down-fractured with finger pressure and mobilized with disimpaction forceps. Depending on the tumor location, the tumor may be visible at this point, and the degree of exposure needed for its removal is reevaluated. Small tumors may require no further maxillary osteotomy to provide adequate exposure for complete resection.

If more exposure is needed, the palate can be split in the midline and the two fragments are retracted laterally.[4] Before splitting the palate, the nasal floor is smoothed along the anterior third of the maxilla so that a screw plate can be easily applied. A straight plate is bent for a passive fit along the anterior nasal floor, and two drill holes are placed and screws are applied. The final two screw holes are placed using a centering device to assure accuracy of subsequent plate reapplication. The plate is removed and set aside. The soft palate is split in the midline. The oral mucosa is cut on the lingual and labial surfaces between the incisor teeth. The reciprocating saw is used to split the hard palate at the midline adjacent to the region of the central incisor roots. A thin osteotome is used to complete the separation of the two fragments. To ensure the ideal circulation to these two fragments, the greater palatine artery is preserved. Even if the artery cannot be preserved due to tumor involvement, there is usually adequate circulation from the remaining soft tissue attachments. Depending on the tumor's location, the vomer, the quadrilateral cartilage, and the inferior turbinates may be partially resected to yield the desired exposure. If adequate lateral exposure is not achieved with maximum fragment retraction, one or both pterygoid plates can be resected.

Some tumors will require a partial or total maxillectomy to achieve a cure. If so, the site of segmentation of the maxillary fragment may be altered.

Defect Reconstruction

The defect is evaluated for reconstruction after the tumor is resected. Sella turcica, sphenoidal, or clival midline defects may be filled with a dermal fat graft or reconstructed with a bone graft before the mucosa is closed.

Reassembly

When tumor resection and reconstruction are completed, the palatal fragments are returned to their anatomical position with the help of the prefabricated splint. If this splint was properly fabricated, arch bars and referencing with the mandibular arch are unnecessary. Referencing with the mandibular arch requires displacing the orotracheal tube to the retromolar region if there is room, or the tube must be repositioned into the nasal cavity. This maneuver usually can be avoided with an appropriately fitted splint and screw plate preregistration. The maxillary fragments are snapped into the splint, and the preregistered plates are retrieved. The first plate is placed across the nasal floor. The first screws are placed in the holes closest to the osteotomy. These screw holes have already been tapped; therefore, a wider screw should be utilized to ensure rigid fixation. Screws are then placed in the adjacent holes. The anatomical repositioning of the fragments should be perfect. A secure muscular mucosal realignment and closure of the soft palate are critical and can be done either before or after the maxillary repositioning, depending on the surgeon's preference. No nasal packing is required.

The splint should be worn for 10 to 14 days. It can be left off the first 3 postoperative days if there is concern about palatal mucosal swelling against the cross-piece. Routine oral care for a LeFort I osteotomy is used. The patient is kept on a liquid diet for 4 weeks, transitioned to a soft diet for 4 weeks, and then returned to a regular diet 8 weeks after surgery.

Transpalatal Approach (Level VI) (Fig. 24.5H–J)

Incision and Dissection

An upper buccal sulcus incision is made, and the nasal floor is exposed. A midline palatal mucosal incision is made, also splitting the soft palate. The oral palatal mucosa may be undercut anteriorly along the junction of the rough and smooth mucoperiosteum to allow wide mobilization of the entire hard palate. The levator muscle is detached from the posterior margins of the hard palate. The osteotomy should be positioned just medial to the greater palatine arteries. If necessary, the arteries can be sacrificed to position the osteotomy laterally.

Osteotomy

The hard palate is cut with a reciprocating saw, extending along the alveolar bone. The remaining attachments to the nasal septum and lateral nasal walls are separated from the labial sulcus incision with guarded osteotomes. The hard palate is removed. Exposure to the clivus is created through the oral and nasal mucosa.

Defect Reconstruction

After tumor resection, the skull base defect may be reconstructed with fat or a bone graft. The hard palate is sometimes thick enough to split, yielding a suitable bone graft for clival reconstruction.

Reassembly

Small two- or three-hole plates are applied to the hard palatal fragment in three locations before anatomical repositioning. Rigid fixation is then completed, taking care to avoid the tooth roots. The palatal mucosa and soft palate are closed and the buccal sulcus incision is closed.

■ Case Illustrations

Case 1

A 16-year-old Caucasian boy presented with nasal obstruction and recurrent epistaxis. Imaging studies revealed the presence of a large angiofibroma that filled the midline interorbital space and extended posterior to the soft palate in the midline (**Fig. 24.11**). A transfrontal-nasal-orbital approach was utilized, and the tumor was resected completely. A circumferential cribriform plate osteotomy was utilized. One year after surgery, the patient had no evidence of recurrence

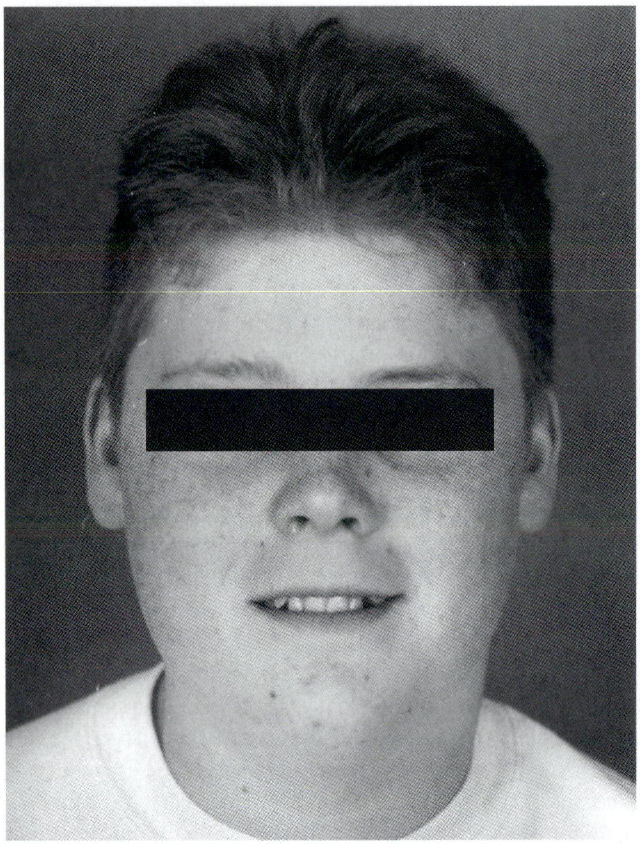
A

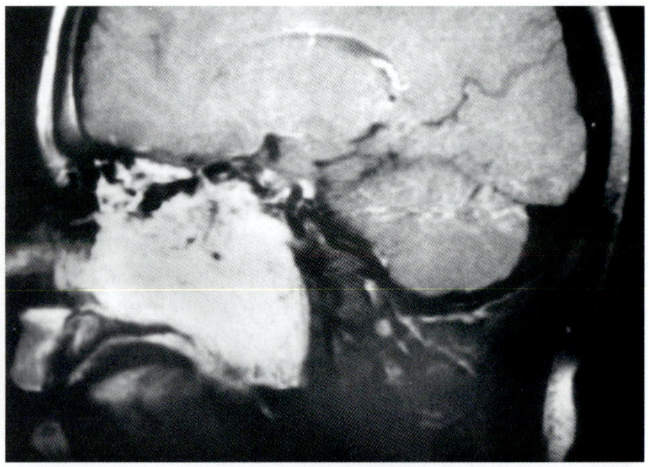
B

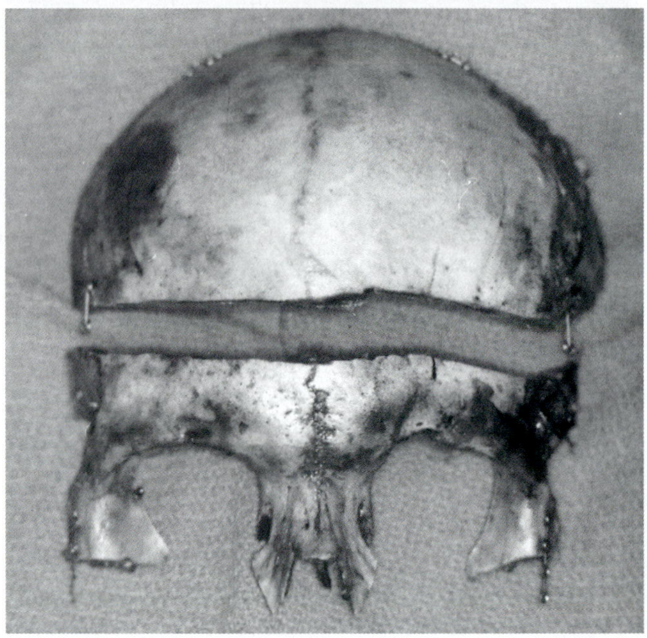
C

Fig. 24.11 **(A)** Preoperative photograph of a 16-year-old boy with an angiofibroma as seen on a **(B)** sagittal magnetic resonance image. He underwent a **(C)** level III exposure for *(continued)*

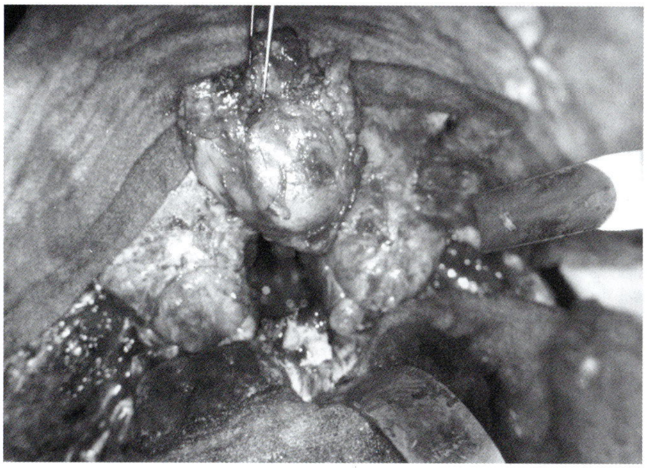

D

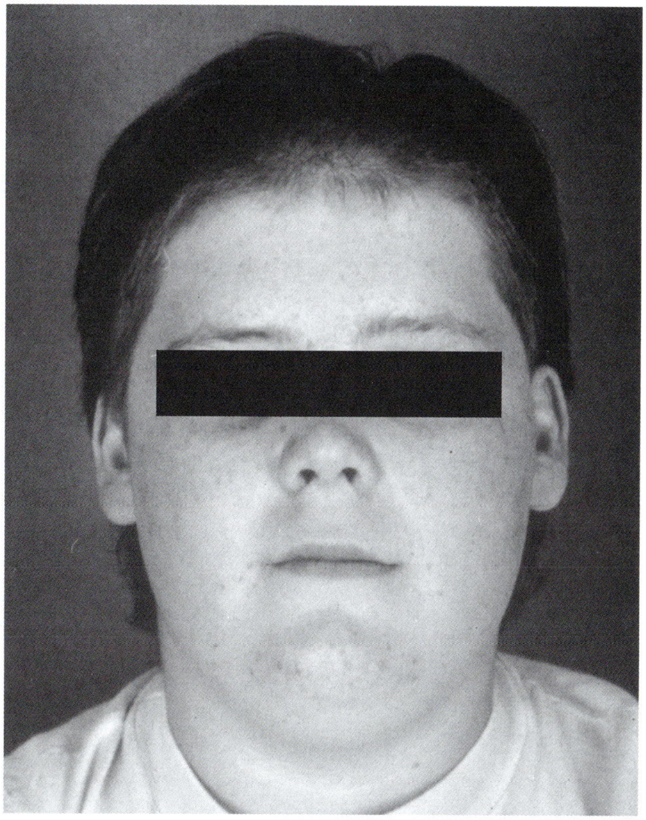

E

Fig. 24.11 *(continued)* **(D)** tumor resection. **(E)** The patient's appearance 3 months after surgery. (Reprinted with permission from Barrow Neurological Institute.)

and had experienced no complications from the exposure. His olfaction was preserved.

Case 2

A 16-year-old Caucasian boy presented with nasal obstruction and severe life-threatening epistaxis. Workup revealed the presence of a very large angiofibroma that extended from the nasopharynx into the midline of the skull base anteriorly. It filled the interorbital region and inferiorly involved the right retromaxillary region (**Fig. 24.12**). Symptoms included loss of olfaction. The patient underwent a combined transfrontal-nasal-orbital (level III) and transmaxillary (level V) approach. The tumor was resected completely. The reassembly restored facial and occlusal integrity. Additionally, a circumferential cribriform plate osteotomy was utilized, and the patient's olfaction returned within 2 weeks of surgery. One year after surgery, there was no evidence of recurrent tumor. Cannulation of the nasolacrimal duct on the right side was required because of persistent epiphora.

Discussion

Combined Surgical Approaches

Any of the intracranial approaches can be combined with the transmaxillary or transpalatal approaches as dictated by the anatomical site of the tumor. The level III (transfrontal-nasal-orbital) and level V (transmaxillary) approaches provide wide exposure of the anterior cranial fossa and midline skull base and are usually preferred over the level IV (transnasomaxillary) approach because a facial incision is avoided (**Fig. 24.13**).

When combined intracranial and extracranial exposures are used, the intracranial approach is performed first. The dural boundaries are defined. The tumor is removed from the region of the vital skull base structures after extracranial exposure is completed. The extracranial approach facilitates resection of any intradural tumor and minimizes the need for brain retraction. Skull base and orbital reconstruction and fragment reassembly are then addressed.

Clinical Pearls

Perfect contouring (passive adaptation) of the fixation screw plates and placing the drill holes before the osteotomies are performed to ensure anatomical reconstruction of the facial skeleton after its disassembly for tumor exposure. It is particularly important to restore exact dental occlusion.

The nasolacrimal duct is vulnerable to injury during disassembly using the transfrontal-nasal-orbital approach and during retraction for tumor resection. If the nasolacrimal duct is excessively stretched or severed, it should be cannulated and repaired to avoid a secondary procedure to correct epiphora.

During reassembly of the frontal naso-orbital fragment, it is essential to reattach the upper lateral cartilages to the

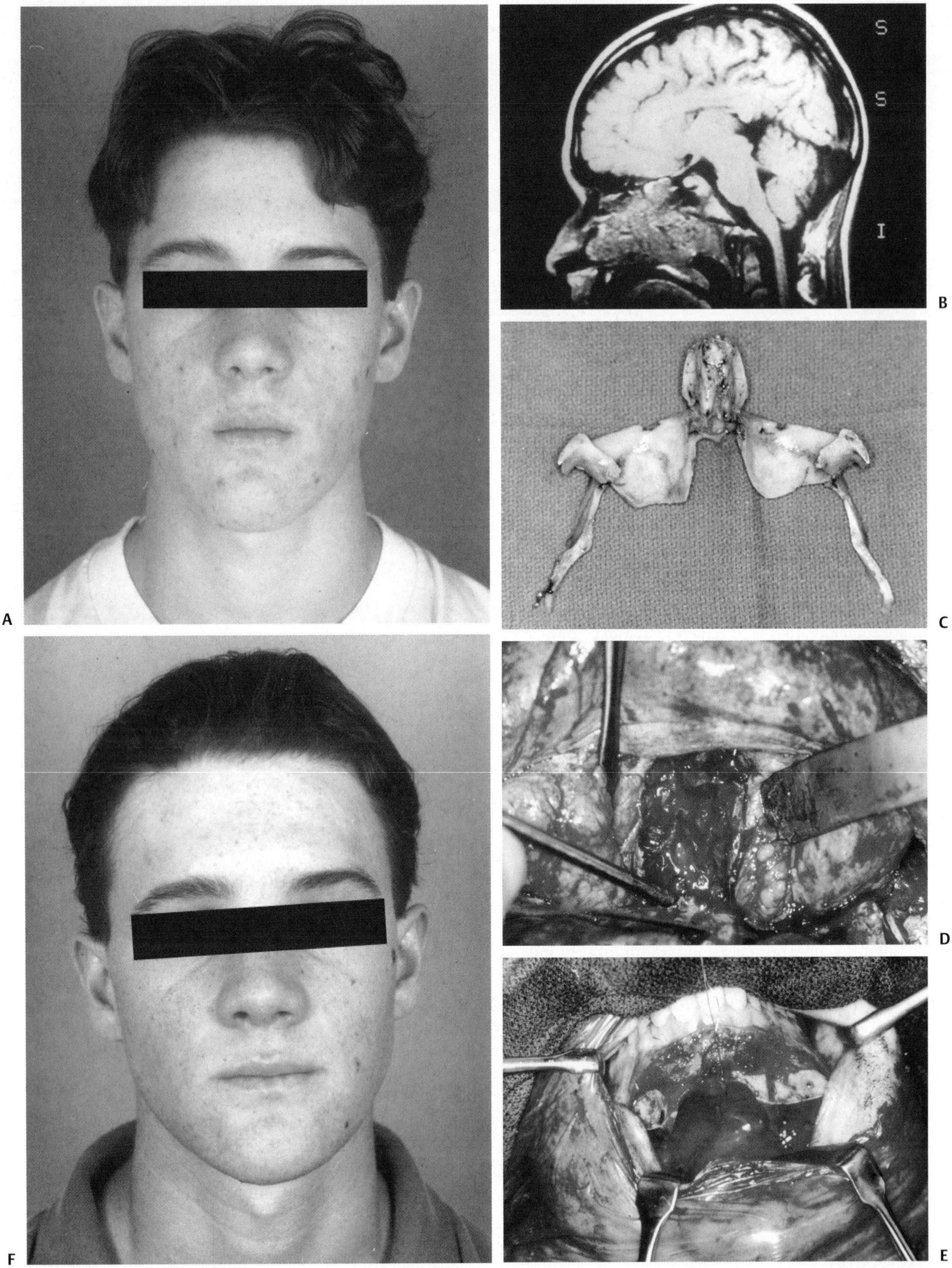

Fig. 24.12 **(A)** Preoperative photograph of a 16-year-old boy with an angiofibroma underwent combined level III and level V approaches with preservation of the cribriform plate. **(B)** A sagittal magnetic resonance image demonstrates the large nasopharyngeal mass. **(C)** Frontal naso-orbital fragment. **(D)** Intraoperative photograph showing exposure of the tumor obtained with the level III approach. The dura of the frontal lobe is at the bottom, and the retractor blade is positioned on the medial aspect of the right globe. **(E)** Intraoperative photograph showing extended exposure of the tumor obtained with the level V approach. **(F)** The patient's appearance 1 year after surgery. (Reprinted with permission from Barrow Neurological Institute.)

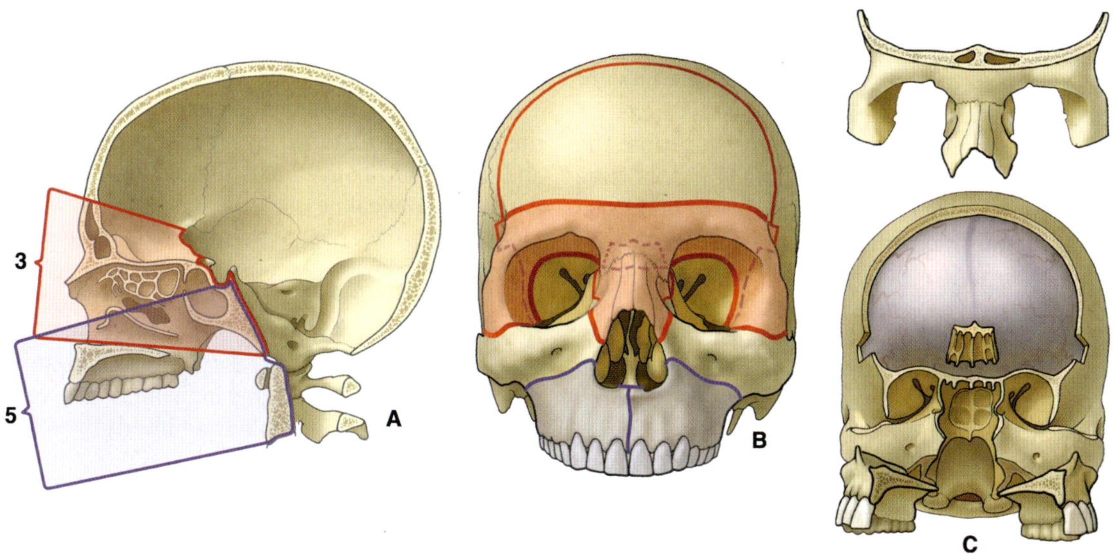

Fig. 24.13 **(A)** Combination of the level III and V approaches provides wide exposure of the anterior skull base and clivus. **(B)** The combination of the two approaches is illustrated **(C)** with preservation of the cribriform plate. (Reprinted with permission from Barrow Neurological Institute.)

nasal bones to be sure that a saddle-nose deformity does not occur. Holes can be drilled in the fragment before the fragment is repositioned, and nonabsorbable sutures should be used to attach the cartilage to the underside of the nasal bone. A deep suture through the septum will cinch the entire unit up against the nasal bones.

The repair of the medial canthal ligaments can be facilitated and greater anatomical accuracy achieved, if transnasal wires are placed through separate drill holes on the frontal naso-orbital fragment. The wires can be placed before the fragment is repositioned to prevent the need to cross wires transnasally after repositioning. These wires can then be passed through the medial canthal ligament with the aid of an 18-gauge needle, which is passed percutaneously above and below the ligament. The wires are then passed retrograde through the needle. After the wires are passed and the needle is withdrawn, a small incision is made between the wires. The wires can be twisted and the medial canthal ligaments pushed down to the dacryon. Fine absorbable sutures are used to close the medial canthal incisions.

To assure adequate flap length of the frontal galeal and pericranial flaps, it is essential to create the bicoronal scalp incision far enough posteriorly. To create a flap that will reach to the lower aspect of the clivus, the incision must at least be level with the preauricular line and preferably 1 to 2 cm posterior.

Intraoperative referencing with a frameless stereotactic navigation tool (i.e., wand) is very helpful when approaching tumors. Vital neurovascular structures in the skull base are often obscured by tumor and are vulnerable to injury when using an anterior approach.

The circumferential cribriform plate osteotomy can be used when the region is not involved with tumor. This osteotomy preserves olfaction, increases exposure, simplifies reconstruction, and reduces the incidence of CSF leaks.

Proper splint fabrication for the transmaxillary surgical approach allows restoration of normal occlusion without the need for arch bars or for changing the tube to the nasotracheal position.

After transfacial access to the CVJ is achieved, the pharyngeal incision is planned. Although a midline incision is often used, an inferiorly based pharyngeal flap has advantages. Parallel incisions are made in the lateral gutters of the oropharynx and extended superiorly, where they are joined in a Gothic window configuration. The musculomucosal flap is elevated at the prevertebral facial plane, and the flap is rolled into the hypopharynx for the duration of the lesion resection.

After resection, the defect is filled with bone or a dermal fat graft, as indicated, and the flap is resutured with absorbable suture. A small radius needle facilitates the suturing.

This approach has the advantages of keeping the suture line away from the defect site and of yielding a watertight closure. The lateral pharyngeal walls are distensible and allow for greater ease of closure without tension.

Avoidance of Complications

Malocclusions, which are very troublesome to patients after surgery, can occur. They can be avoided if proper referencing and plating techniques are utilized. If malocclusion occurs, it can leave long-lasting effects that require either prolonged orthodontic treatment or secondary surgical correction.

Nasolacrimal duct disruption, either partial or complete, can leave a patient with long-lasting epiphora, which may require secondary nasolacrimal duct surgery. If the integrity of the nasolacrimal duct is doubtful at surgery, it should be cannulated at that time.

Palatal fistulae are possible if reapproximation of the palatal mucosa is not meticulous. The risk can be diminished by offsetting the mucosal incision and the midline osteotomy. Closure can be facilitated by mobilizing the mucosa from the edge of the osteotomy ~1 cm in each direction. This mobilization allows greater ease of passage of suture for closure. If a fistula occurs, reoperation for closure is necessary.

The cross-piece on the splint posteriorly can help eliminate yaw from the posterior aspects of the palatal segments, but it can also induce palatal mucosal necrosis if it is placed too tightly against the mucosa. In the process of fabricating the splint, the plaster model can be built up with wax so that there is a small space between the cross-piece and the mucosa.

Velopharyngeal insufficiency is a potential complication of the transmaxillary approaches to the CVJ. The chance of developing this complication is higher if the palate is split (fistula and soft palate scarring) and if the pterygoid plate requires an osteotomy or resection (soft palate paralysis due to nerve injury). It can also develop if the nasopharyngeal posterior wall becomes significantly concave after tumor resection.

If velopharyngeal insufficiency occurs postoperatively, the cause is determined by clinical and speech evaluation and nasal endoscopy. If a fistula exists, it must be repaired. Paralysis or weakness of the levator may resolve spontaneously with speech therapy and sufficient time for complete healing. If the posterior nasopharynx is concave, surgical augmentation may be indicated with autologous tissue. If a pharyngoplasty is indicated, an alternative to the superiorly based flap technique should be considered due to the previous incisions in the pharynx, depending on whether a midline incision or an inferiorly based flap was utilized.

Acknowledgments

We thank Dr. Robert F. Spetzler for his contributions in developing the organization of these transfacial levels and Cheryl Czaplicki for her assistance in preparation of this manuscript.

References

1. Beals SP, Joganic EF. Transfacial exposure of anterior cranial fossa and clival tumors. BNI Q 1992;8(4):2–18
2. Jackson IT, Marsh WR, Bite U, Hide TA. Craniofacial osteotomies to facilitate skull base tumour resection. Br J Plast Surg 1986;39(2):153–160
3. Sataloff RT, Bowman C, Baker SR, Osterholm J. Transfacial resection of intracranial tumor. Am J Otol 1988;9(3):222–228
4. Munro IR. The transfacial approach for tumors of the midline skull base. Abstract. American Association of Plastic Surgeons, 69th Annual Meeting. Hot Springs, VA; 1990
5. Lauritzen C, Vällfors B, Lilja J. Facial disassembly for tumor resection. Scand J Plast Reconstr Surg 1986;20(2):201–206
6. deFries HO, Deeb ZE, Hudkins CP. A transfacial approach to the nasal-paranasal cavities and anterior skull base. Arch Otolaryngol Head Neck Surg 1988;114(7):766–769
7. Panje WR, Dohrmann GJ III, Pitcock JK, et al. The transfacial approach for combined anterior craniofacial tumor ablation. Arch Otolaryngol Head Neck Surg 1989;115(3):301–307
8. Wei WI, Lam KH, Sham JS. New approach to the nasopharynx: the maxillary swing approach. Head Neck 1991;13(3):200–207
9. Belmont JR. The Le Fort I osteotomy approach for nasopharyngeal and nasal fossa tumors. Arch Otolaryngol Head Neck Surg 1988;114(7):751–754
10. Uttley D, Moore A, Archer DJ. Surgical management of midline skull-base tumors: a new approach. J Neurosurg 1989;71(5 Pt 1): 705–710
11. Kawakami K, Yamanouchi Y, Kubota C, Kawamura Y, Matsumura H. An extensive transbasal approach to frontal skull-base tumors. Technical note. J Neurosurg 1991;74(6):1011–1013
12. Blacklock JB, Weber RS, Lee YY, Goepfert H. Transcranial resection of tumors of the paranasal sinuses and nasal cavity. J Neurosurg 1989;71(1):10–15
13. Sandor GK, Charles DA, Lawson VG, Tator CH. Trans oral approach to the nasopharynx and clivus using the Le Fort I osteotomy with midpalatal split. Int J Oral Maxillofac Surg 1990;19(6):352–355
14. Fujitsu K, Saijoh M, Aoki F, et al. Telecanthal approach for meningiomas in the ethmoid and sphenoid sinuses. Neurosurgery 1991;28(5):714–719, discussion 719–720
15. Maran AG. Surgical approaches to the nasopharynx. Clin Otolaryngol Allied Sci 1983;8(6):417–429
16. Haughey BH, Wilson JS, Barber CS. Massive angiofibroma: a surgical approach and adjunctive therapy. Otolaryngol Head Neck Surg 1988;98(6):618–624
17. Spetzler RF, Pappas CT. Management of anterior skull base tumors. Clin Neurosurg 1991;37:490–501
18. Crockard HA. The transmaxillary approach to the clivus. In: Sekhar LN, Janecka IP, eds. Surgery of Cranial Base Tumors. New York, NY: Raven Press; 1993:235–244
19. Jackson IT, Marsh WR, Hide TA. Treatment of tumors involving the anterior cranial fossa. Head Neck Surg 1984;6(5):901–913
20. Persing JA, Jane JA, Levine PA, Cantrell RW. The versatile frontal sinus approach to the floor of the anterior cranial fossa. Technical note. J Neurosurg 1990;72(3):513–516
21. Schramm VL Jr, Myers EN, Maroon JC. Anterior skull base surgery for benign and malignant disease. Laryngoscope 1979;89(7 Pt 1): 1077–1091
22. Sundaresan N, Shah JP. Craniofacial resection for anterior skull base tumors. Head Neck Surg 1988;10(4):219–224
23. Van Buren JM, Ommaya AK, Ketcham AS. Ten years' experience with radical combined craniofacial resection of malignant tumors of the paranasal sinuses. J Neurosurg 1968;28(4):341–350
24. Derome PJ, Bisot A, Monteil JP, et al. Management of cranial chordomas. In: Sekhar LN, Schramm VLJ, eds. Tumors of the Cranial Base: Diagnosis and Treatment. Mount Kisco, NY: Futura Publishing; 1987:607–622
25. Derome PJ. The transbasal approach to tumors invading the base of the skull. In: Schmidek HH, Sweet WH, eds. Operative Neurosurgical Techniques, 2nd ed. Orlando, FL: Grune & Stratton; 1988:619–633
26. Janecka IP, Sen CN, Sekhar LN, Arriaga M. Facial translocation: a new approach to the cranial base. Otolaryngol Head Neck Surg 1990;103(3):413–419

27. Price JC. The midfacial degloving approach to the central skull-base. Ear Nose Throat J 1986;65(4):174–180
28. Mann WJ, Gilsbach J, Seeger W, Flöel H. Use of a malar bone graft to augment skull-base access. Arch Otolaryngol 1985;111(1):30–33
29. Millar HS, Petty PG, Wilson WF, Hueston JT. A combined intracranial and facial approach for excision and repair of cancer of the ethmoid sinuses. Aust N Z J Surg 1973;43(2):179–183
30. Sundaresan N. Craniofacial resection for paranasal sinus tumors. Indian J Cancer 1994;16:74–79
31. Shah JP, Galicich JH. Surgical approach to carcinoma of the nasal cavity and paranasal sinuses with extension to the base of the skull. Clin Bull 1978;8(2):61–66
32. Kaplan MJ, Jane JA, Park TS, Cantrell RW. Supraorbital rim approach to the anterior skull base. Laryngoscope 1984;94(9):1137–1139
33. Sekhar LN, Janecka IP, Jones NF. Subtemporal-infratemporal and basal subfrontal approach to extensive cranial base tumours. Acta Neurochir (Wien) 1988;92(1-4):83–92
34. Cocke EW Jr, Robertson JH, Robertson JT, Crook JP Jr. The extended maxillotomy and subtotal maxillectomy for excision of skull base tumors. Arch Otolaryngol Head Neck Surg 1990;116(1):92–104
35. Lewis WJ, Richter HA, Jabourian Z. Craniofacial resection for large tumors of the paranasal sinuses. Ear Nose Throat J 1989;68(7):539–547
36. Ketcham AS, Van Buren JM. Tumors of the paranasal sinuses: a therapeutic challenge. Am J Surg 1985;150(4):406–413
37. Brown AM, Lavery KM, Millar BG. The transfacial approach to the postnasal space and retromaxillary structures. Br J Oral Maxillofac Surg 1991;29(4):230–236
38. Wood GD, Stell PM. The Le Fort I osteotomy as an approach to the nasopharynx. Clin Otolaryngol Allied Sci 1984;9(1):59–61
39. Kennedy DW, Papel ID, Holliday M. Transpalatal approach to the skull base. Ear Nose Throat J 1986;65(3):125, 127–133
40. Weissler MC. Transoral approaches to the skull base. Ear Nose Throat J 1991;70(9):587–592
41. James D, Crockard HA. Surgical access to the base of skull and upper cervical spine by extended maxillotomy. Neurosurgery 1991;29(3):411–416
42. Tessier P, Guiot G, Rougerie J, Delbet JP, Pastoriza J. [Cranio-naso-orbito-facial osteotomies. Hypertelorism]. [French] Ann Chir Plast 1967;12(2):103–118
43. Beals SP, Hamilton MG, Joganic EF, et al. Classification of transfacial approaches in the treatment of tumors of the anterior skull base and clivus. Plast Surg Forum 1993;16:211–213
44. Spetzler RF, Herman JM, Beals S, Joganic E, Milligan J. Preservation of olfaction in anterior craniofacial approaches. J Neurosurg 1993;79(1):48–52
45. Farnworth TK, Beals SP, Manwaring KH, Trepeta RW. Comparison of skin necrosis in rats by using a new microneedle electrocautery, standard-size needle electrocautery, and the Shaw hemostatic scalpel. Ann Plast Surg 1993;31(2):164–167

25 Posterior Neuroendoscopic Applications at the Craniovertebral Junction

Andrew S. Little, Pankaj A. Gore, Charles Teo, and Peter Nakaji

Neuroendoscopy has been applied to diverse pathologies at the craniovertebral junction (CVJ). The endoscope provides a view that is complementary and in some ways superior to that of a microscope. It provides a high-magnification, panoramic view of the operative field and the ability to look around neurovascular structures that obstruct the view through the microscope. Endoscopy can be applied to anterior approaches (e.g., transnasal and transoral), midline posterior approaches (e.g., suboccipital), and posterolateral approaches (e.g., far-lateral and retrosigmoid) either as the sole source of visualization or as an adjunct to standard microsurgical techniques. In this chapter we consider the CVJ as the region from the pineal gland caudally to the second cervical vertebrae. We discuss the basics of neuroendoscopy, review the instrumentation and setup, describe the advantages and limitations of endoscopy compared with standard microscopy, and present its application to lesions near the CVJ approached from posterior and posterolateral corridors. Anterior approaches to the skull base are addressed in a separate chapter.

Neuroendoscopy Basics and Terminology

The endoscope can be used at the CVJ in three different manners. The most common application is the use of the endoscope to assist microsurgical procedures as a supplemental method of visualization in the same operative corridor. This is called *endoscopic-assisted* neurosurgery.[1] Using the endoscope in this way permits inspection of resection cavities to assess for tumor remnants or to identify compressive vessels in patients with trigeminal neuralgia.[2] The second type of application of the endoscope at the CVJ is termed *endoscopic* neurosurgery. In endoscopic neurosurgery, the endoscope provides the only source of visualization, and the instruments are passed through the endoscope's working ports. This technique is used to fenestrate arachnoid cysts and for third ventriculostomy. When the endoscope is used as the only source of visualization and the instruments are passed alongside the endoscope, the technique is called *endoscopic-controlled*. Endoscopic Chiari decompression and endonasal endoscopic surgery are performed in this manner.

A system for endoscopic-assisted work at the CVJ consists of a 0-degree and 30-degree rigid endoscope, a fiberoptic light source, a video camera, a digital recorder with video and still image–capture functionalities, and a video monitor. The 0-degree endoscope provides excellent in-line visualization and a panoramic view at high magnification. The 30-degree endoscope supplements the 0-degree scope by allowing the surgeon to look around obstructing neurovascular structures that might otherwise be hidden from the microscopic view. For example, a 30-degree endoscope is used to look at the shoulder and axilla of the trigeminal nerve to inspect for compressive vessels, to assess for tumor remnants, or to identify neurovascular structures before tumor removal. Endoscopes of 70 degrees are available, but we avoid their use because they provide limited straight-ahead visualization, which places neurovascular structures at risk during insertion and manipulation of the endoscope. We prefer to use pistol-grip style endoscopes because they are well balanced, the surgeon's hand is removed from the operative field, and their image resolution is excellent. The digital recorder, light source, and monitor should be housed in a mobile tower that can be repositioned in the theater depending on the surgeon's preference. The use of additional monitors, often attached to the ceiling on mobile booms, further improves the surgeon's ability to maintain ergonomics. Standard microsurgical instruments can be employed along with the endoscope. A variety of angled dissecting instruments allows the surgeon maximum use of the view provided by the endoscope. Every attempt should be made to use usual microsurgical technique, including sharp bimanual dissection, while using the endoscope. Doing so may require the adjunctive use of a holding arm or a good assistant to free the surgeon's hands.

Anatomical Considerations for Neuroendoscopy at the Craniovertebral Junction

The posterior fossa presents the surgeon with a variety of challenges because it is a relatively tight space, the operative targets are often deeply located, and the cranial nerves provide both tethers and barriers to dissection that must be manipulated with caution to prevent functional deficits. However, the anatomy of the posterior fossa also presents opportunities. A relatively small opening in the retrosigmoid or far-lateral region provides extensive access up and down the cerebellopontine region. Drainage of spinal fluid often creates adequate room. Furthermore, the pathology itself may create space, such as in the case of a large acoustic neuroma or epidermoid tumor. Space must be developed to pass the endoscope safely into the posterior fossa, and care must be taken not to allow the endoscope itself to compress the brain.

Avoidance of Complications in Neuroendoscopy

There are several important caveats to using endoscopy near the CVJ. Because of the tight working space with numerous critical neurovascular structures, familiarization with basic endoscopy technique is essential. Surgeons wishing to develop endoscopy skills are encouraged to practice in a laboratory setting because of the steep learning curve. Practice with a cadaver allows the surgeon to become familiar with the endoscopic equipment and to learn about the pitfalls and technical challenges of working with new instrumentation.

Most complications occur because of deviation from two principles. The greatest risk of endoscopy is the operator becoming disoriented. Because of endoscope construction, the camera can rotate separately from the endoscope. The operator must maintain orientation of the camera regardless of the orientation of the scope. Orientation of the image can be easily verified by viewing an object with writing on it and adjusting the camera as necessary. The second principle is that structures outside the field of view are at risk for injury by the endoscope's shaft and instruments. As the endoscope is passed into the operative field, the neural and vascular structures that are within the visual field are easily avoided. However, after the endoscope passes these structures, they are no longer visible and lateral movements of the endoscope present risks to the cranial nerves. When instruments are inserted, they should be placed in a parallel trajectory along with the endoscope, trailing slightly to enable visualization of their tip. If the endoscopic view needs to be changed, the scope should be removed by withdrawing it straight backward. Its orientation is then confirmed, redirected, and reintroduced in a straight line toward the target. One way to limit complications resulting from the shaft of the endoscope is to have the assistant visualize the endoscope and adjacent critical structures through the operative microscope as the endoscope is being used.

Applications of Neuroendoscopy

Tumors

Acoustic Neuromas and Epidermoid Tumors

Neuroendoscopy is a powerful tool for tumor surgery near the CVJ because of its abilities to look around corners and to provide a panoramic operative view. Acoustic neuroma surgery is a good illustration of the application of neuroendoscopy to tumor surgery (**Fig. 25.1**). We have found endoscopy useful for the early identification of the facial nerve before tumor removal and for detecting residual tumor in the internal auditory canal (IAC). Drilling of the internal acoustic meatus can open temporal bone air cells. If the air cells are not sealed adequately, patients may develop spinal fluid rhinorrhea. One disadvantage of microsurgery is that some air cell violations may not be detected because they are hidden from the line-of-sight. Valtonen and colleagues demonstrated that angled endoscopes provided superior visualization of the IAC and permitted better closures.[3] Postoperative rhinorrhea declined to 0 of 24 patients with endoscopy compared with 7 of 38 patients without endoscopy. Endoscopy combined with neuronavigation also may allow a more complete and accurate drilling of the IAC. Pillai and colleagues performed a cadaveric study using the retrosigmoid exposure coupling these two techniques and were able to drill the posterior IAC completely without violating the bony labyrinth.[4]

Neuroendoscopy also may improve the extent of tumor resection. One common site of residual tumor is within the fundus of the IAC. Wackym and colleagues reviewed their experience with 68 patients treated primarily through a retrosigmoid approach.[5] Their impression was that neuroendoscopy detected residual tumor in the IAC in 11 cases that were not detected with light microscopy. They also noted improved detection of open air cells.

Epidermoids are also good targets for endoscopy because they are soft and suctionable tumors that insinuate themselves in hard-to-visualize spaces. Angled endoscopy is useful for detecting tumor remnants and cystic contents outside the field of view. Because of their suctionable nature, the remnants can be removed safely with angled suction using a one-handed technique.

In our experience, the application of endoscopy to tumor surgery involves several key considerations. A thorough understanding of the limitations of endoscopy allows the surgeon to maximize its advantages safely. For example, although it may improve visualization, endoscopy does not abrogate the need for thorough drilling of the IAC in acoustic neuroma surgery. Without sufficient bony exposure, tumor in the fundus is not accessible even with angled instrumentation. Furthermore, direct tumor suctioning instead of careful microdissection can inadvertently traumatize the facial nerve by aspirating it into the suction device. In endoscopic-assisted work, the surgeon often holds the endoscope in one hand and a suction device or dissector in the other. Therefore, the surgeon is functionally one-handed, making it difficult to complete fine microdissection of tumor from the facial nerve. When used this way, the primary use of the endoscope is to identify tumor remnants, and then using standard microscopy with a two-handed technique, to remove the tumor. Where possible, a two-handed technique with the endoscope is preferred if the microscopic view is inadequate.

For any endoscope-assisted work in the posterior fossa, standard endoscope-handling principles should be followed to reduce risk maximally. The endoscope should be directed in and out in straight lines. When the direction of an angled endoscope is altered, it should be removed from the head, re-angled, and re-directed. Back-and-forth swinging movements within the operative field should be avoided because of the risk of injury to neurovascular structures. The shaft can conflict with critical anatomy any time the endoscope is beyond a nerve or vessel and the structure is therefore out

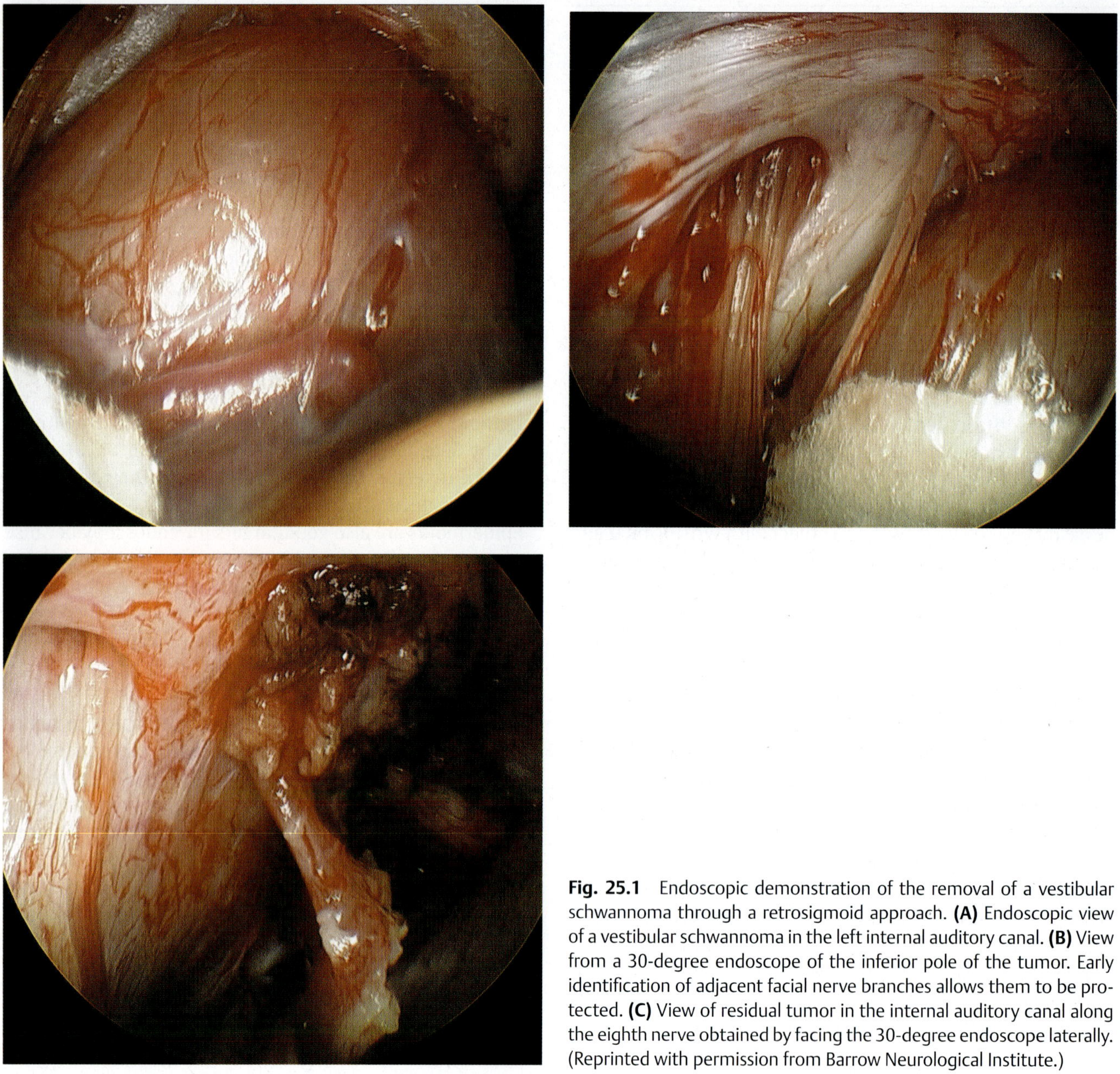

Fig. 25.1 Endoscopic demonstration of the removal of a vestibular schwannoma through a retrosigmoid approach. **(A)** Endoscopic view of a vestibular schwannoma in the left internal auditory canal. **(B)** View from a 30-degree endoscope of the inferior pole of the tumor. Early identification of adjacent facial nerve branches allows them to be protected. **(C)** View of residual tumor in the internal auditory canal along the eighth nerve obtained by facing the 30-degree endoscope laterally. (Reprinted with permission from Barrow Neurological Institute.)

of view. The cranial nerves (CNs) at risk primarily include CN V superiorly, the CN VII–VIII complex centrally, and the CN IX–XI complex inferiorly.

Disorders of Spinal Fluid Dynamics

Endoscopic Third Ventriculostomy

The best-established role for neuroendoscopy is the treatment of hydrocephalus caused by obstructive masses of the posterior fossa. Endoscopic third ventriculostomy (ETV) has an excellent technical success rate (90%) and good long-term patency.[6] In patients older than 2 years of age who underwent ETV for a diverse set of primary pathologies, the senior author found that 84% of stomas were patent at 1 year and 58 to 78% were patent at 5 years, depending on the patient's age. ETV is very effective in pediatric patients with fourth ventricular tumors. Tamburrini and colleagues reviewed 30 patients with persistent ventriculomegaly after tumor resection and reported a 90% success rate.[7] Third ventriculostomy also can be performed in conjunction with biopsy of pineal masses. Yamini and colleagues described six cases where biopsy and ETV were performed in the same sitting and proposed that it was a reasonable initial management paradigm.[8] In our experience, this procedure requires two burr holes and two different operative trajectories to avoid lacerating the brain with the endoscope.

The most common complications are wound infection (5%), intraoperative bleeding that stops spontaneously with irrigation (2%), and a delayed need for shunting. Fortunately, basilar artery injury is rare (0.5%).[6] There is a theoretical risk of cognitive difficulties from injury to the columns of the fornix or mammillary bodies and diabetes insipidus from injury to the hypothalamus or infundibulum. Factors associated with poor ETV patency include age under 2 years, history of arachnoidal scarring such as may occur in bacterial meningitis, and inadequate size of fenestration (<5 mm).

The operative technique for performing a third ventriculostomy involves making a precoronal burr hole ~3 cm off midline, usually on the right side. Placement of a peel-away sheath into the lateral ventricle through which the endoscope is placed is optional. Stereotactic guidance helps identify the correct in-line trajectory through the foramen of Monro to avoid manipulation of the fornix. If image guidance is unavailable, the ventricle should be tapped with a brain needle before the endoscope or peel-away sheath is introduced. We use a 30-degree endoscope to inspect the ventricular anatomy. There are several techniques for creating the perforation in the tuber cinereum. We favor a blunt technique using the tip of the endoscope to breach the membrane with the bezel looking posteriorly toward the basilar artery. Others use a Fogarty balloon or a closed grasper passed through a working channel. The stoma in the floor of the third ventricle is made about one-half to two-thirds of the distance from the infundibular recess to the mamillary bodies. We score the tuber cinereum with the tip of the endoscope to confirm the entry point is appropriate before making the final perforation. After making the perforation, we continue by placing the endoscope into the prepontine cistern to ensure perforation of the membrane of Liliequist and open cerebrospinal fluid pathways. Although the technical success rate of creating a perforation is high, the endoscopist should abort the procedure when the ventricular anatomy is distorted or unfavorable. For example, some patients have a thickened floor from prior infection or hemorrhage that is difficult to perforate.

Chiari Type I Malformations

One application of endoscopic-controlled neurosurgery is in the treatment of Chiari type I malformations. Several preliminary reports described its technical feasibility.[9,10] In brief, the endoscope is used as the sole source of visualization, replacing the operating microscope. By using 30-degree endoscope and angled instrumentation, surgeons can make a small midline incision and still achieve an adequate decompression. Di reported the outcome of 26 pediatric patients who underwent endoscopically assisted suboccipital decompression and cervical laminectomies.[9] Most patients also underwent intradural exploration. Symptomatic improvement was noted in 24 of the 26 patients. One patient developed meningitis. The author suggests that the endoscopic technique is well tolerated and may result in shorter hospital stays and improved pain control. In our experience, the main disadvantages of the endoscopic technique are difficulty sewing in a patch graft for dural expansion and assuring an adequate bony opening. Regardless of the operative technique chosen, the guiding principle is to achieve sufficient dural expansion to restore spinal fluid flow.

Other Spinal Fluid Circulation Disorders

Case reports and small series have also described the application of neuroendoscopy to less common causes of disrupted spinal fluid dynamics at the CVJ, such as membranous aqueductal obstruction and primary obstruction of the fourth ventricular outlet foramina. Aqueductoplasty for membranous aqueductal obstruction can be achieved through a supratentorial approach with a precoronal burr hole or through a suboccipital approach through the foramen of Magendie and fourth ventricle.[11–13] The ideal candidate for a suboccipital approach has a short-segment obstruction located nearer the fourth ventricle. The indications for inferior aqueductoplasty rather than third ventriculostomy are when the basilar artery lies near the floor of the third ventricle, when the distance between the infundibular recess and mammillary bodies is small, and when the foramen of Monro is stenotic.

The suboccipital approach is performed using a 2-cm midline neck incision along the trajectory of the fourth ventricle and aqueduct. After a small suboccipital craniectomy, a rigid ventriculoscope is passed through the foramen of Magendie into the fourth ventricle and aqueduct. Often, the membranous veil responsible for the obstruction can be opened with the tip of the endoscope. In a series of 9 patients, Sansone and colleagues reported 2 patients with transient ocular movement difficulties from manipulation of the periaqueductal brain tissue during the fenestration.[12] Gawish and colleagues reported one case of diplopia in 5 patients.[11]

Primary fourth ventricular obstruction is a rare entity thought to be caused by basilar inflammatory processes or congenital disorders like Chiari malformation. There are a few reports of treatment using neuroendoscopy. We usually prefer to treat these patients with third ventriculostomy, which is a safe and established procedure. However, others have tried direct endoscopic fenestration of the obstruction. Longatti and colleagues inspected the fourth ventricle through a supratentorial-transaqueductal route in 10 patients and performed magendieplasty in 1 patient.[14] The other 9 patients were treated with ETV. They discovered occasional inflammation around the foramen of Magendie and Luschka in their series.

Trigeminal Neuralgia and Hemifacial Spasm

Trigeminal Neuralgia

Because of its enhanced visualization, neuroendoscopy has made a significant contribution to improving microvascular decompression surgery for trigeminal neuralgia. The failure rate for microvascular decompression for trigeminal neuralgia is reported to be 5 to 40%.[15] One explanation for this is failure to identify a neurovascular conflict that may be hidden from view of the microscope. With better magnification and angled scopes, neuroendoscopy can supplement microsurgery by identifying compressive vessels that may be hidden from view.

There are two ways to apply the endoscope in this setting. We advocate a standard microvascular decompression through a high keyhole retrosigmoid craniotomy supplemented with endoscopy to assess for neurovascular conflicts on the back side of the root entry zone and brainstem. A 30-degree endoscope is inserted with the bezel pointed medially to view the backside of the nerve and the brainstem. It can then be turned with the bezel pointed superiorly to inspect the nerve from below. Once the compressive vessels have been identified, the decompression is performed using standard microsurgery. Teo and colleagues reported 114 patients with trigeminal neuralgia and identified a neurovascular conflict in 8% of patients with endoscopy where the operating microscope failed to reveal a compressive vessel.[2] Jarrahy and colleagues noted that 27% of the compressive vessels identified in their series could only be detected with endoscopy.[16]

In endoscopic-assisted applications through a retrosigmoid exposure, we position the patient supine with the head turned and the neck in midline flexion and lateral extension. After a keyhole craniotomy is performed and the nerve is dissected, the endoscope is inserted under direct visualization. The surgeon stands in the usual position for microscopic work, and the microscope is raised to accommodate the endoscope shaft. The tower containing the digital recorder and monitor is positioned as if the patient were looking at it.

The second method for applying endoscopy in trigeminal neuralgia is through a fully endoscopic approach. Kabil and colleagues described 255 patients with trigeminal neuralgia treated between 1999 and 2004[17]: 93% of their patients were pain-free at 3 years. Their work demonstrates that a fully endoscopic approach is technically feasible and results in excellent postoperative pain control. Although fully endoscopic technique is reasonable, our experience suggests that it does not significantly decrease the size of the craniotomy, operative time, or morbidity. Furthermore, by continuing to use standard microscopy, one can visualize the endoscope as it is being inserted into the field, thus avoiding injury to the facial nerve complex. Ultimately, the goals of the procedure are the same whether it is performed with microsurgery or endoscopy: to successfully identify all compressive vessels and to treat them.

Hemifacial Spasm

Neuroendoscopy has also been successfully applied to hemifacial spasm because the typical compressive vessel is on the anterocaudal aspect of the root entry zone, which may be difficult to visualize with standard microscopy. After performing a low retrosigmoid craniotomy, we use a 30-degree endoscope with the bezel directed medially. Badr-el-Dine and colleagues reported 80 patients who underwent endoscopically assisted microvascular decompression and noted that 90% had substantial relief of symptoms at 1 year.[18] Applying neuroendoscopy allows the surgeon to limit the cerebellar retraction and manipulation of the facial nerve complex that otherwise would be needed to visualize the root entry zone completely.

Pineal Approaches

There are a large number of possible approaches to pineal region tumors, including stereotactic needle biopsy, open anterior interhemispheric transcallosal craniotomy, posterior interhemispheric transtentorial subsplenial craniotomy, and supracerebellar infratentorial craniotomy. Endoscopic approaches to this region can usually be divided into two groups. One is the anterior endoscopic transventricular route, which is primarily used for tumor biopsy, often in conjunction with ETV, to treat associated obstructive hydrocephalus. The other is the supracerebellar infratentorial endoscope-assisted or endoscope-controlled approach for pineal tumor biopsy or removal. The anterior transventricular endoscopic route has gradually come into favor for many pineal region tumors as part of a multimodality treatment paradigm. Because many tumors in the pineal region will respond to chemotherapy and radiation, simple biopsy may be adequate. The germinoma is the classic example of this sort of tumor. The disadvantages of this strategy are that it requires transiting the frontal lobe, that the incision is often forward of the hairline, that a separate opening and trajectory are often necessary to perform third ventriculostomy, and that there is little opportunity to perform more than simple biopsy using the ventriculoscope (**Fig. 25.2**).

The posterior supracerebellar infratentorial endoscopic approach, another viable option for approaching pineal tumors, has not yet become popular. Some authors have dismissed it because of the need for retraction to develop working space for the endoscope and because of the risk of injury to the large veins between the cerebellum and the tentorium and vein of Galen complex. When approached in the same way as microsurgery, these objections are valid. However, this approach has intrinsic appeal for neuroendoscopy in that there is a large potential space between the tentorium and cerebellum that can allow access to the pineal region without transiting brain or nerves. The keys to making this approach work are (1) use of the sitting position (**Fig. 25.3**) to allow the cerebellum to fall away from the tentorium without retraction, (2) use of lumbar drainage, and (3) an off-midline opening that allows the surgeon to work to the side of the vermis, rather than having to work over the top of it. The opening should be made wide enough to admit the endoscope as well as a suction and dissecting instrument or microscissor. Typically an opening 1.5-cm high and 2-cm wide located just below the transverse sinus centered ~2 cm off midline suffices (**Fig. 25.4**).

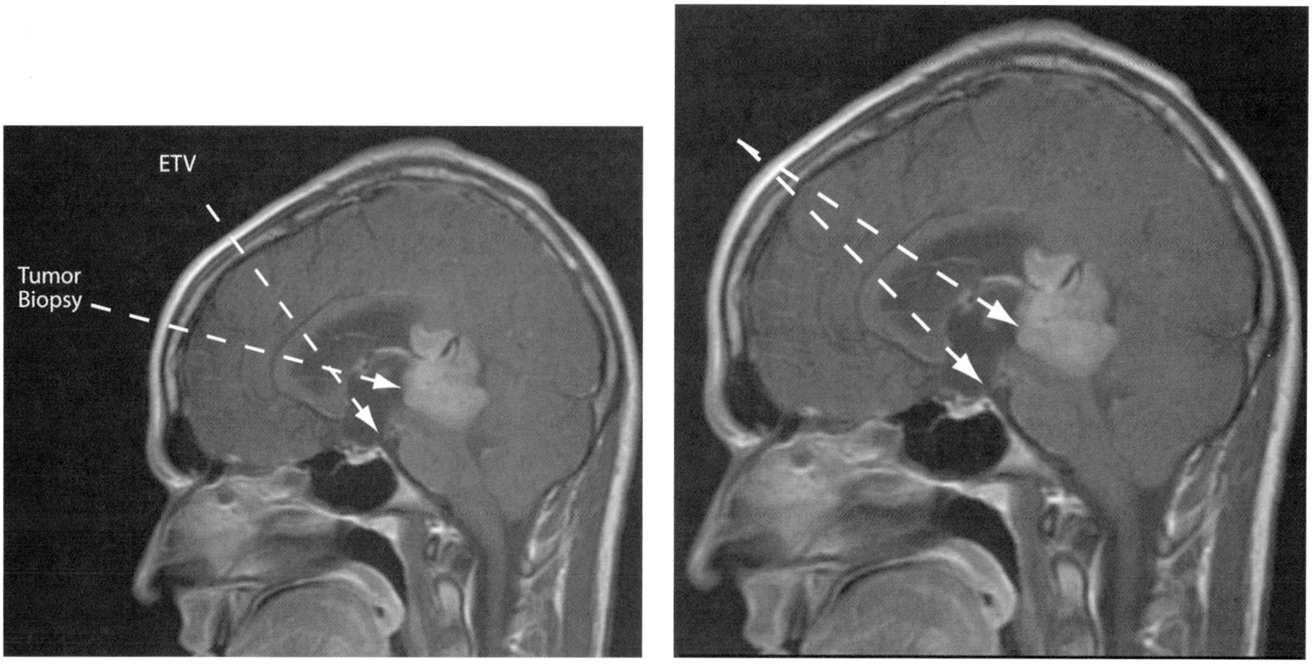

A B

Fig. 25.2 Separate endoscopic trajectories for biopsy of pineal region mass and endoscopic third ventriculostomy (ETV). **(A)** The ideal trajectories for ETV and pineal tumor biopsy are usually far enough apart that separate openings are needed for each if a rigid endoscope is used. **(B)** When the foramen of Monro is large, a single opening may suffice. (Reprinted with permission from Barrow Neurological Institute.)

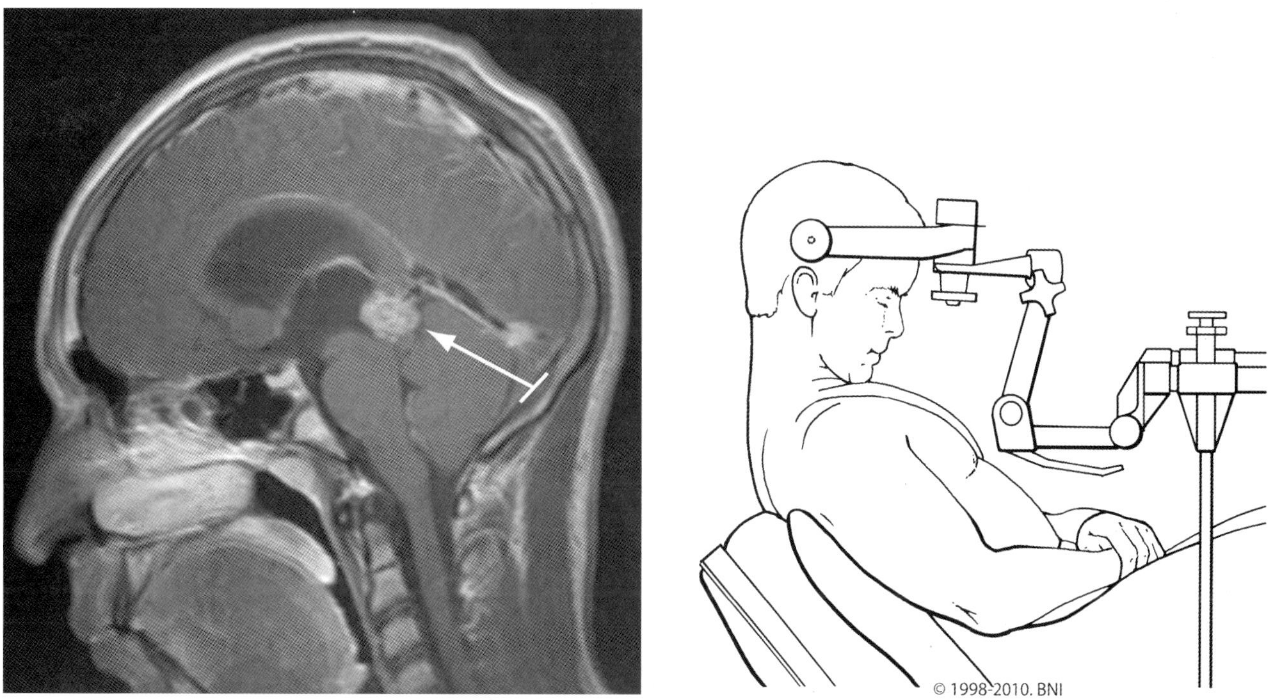

A B

Fig. 25.3 **(A)** The sitting position allows the cerebellum to fall away from the tentorium, creating a potential space between the cerebellum and tentorium. **(B)** The chin should be tucked and the cushions low enough not to obstruct the hands holding the endoscope. (Reprinted with permission from Barrow Neurological Institute.)

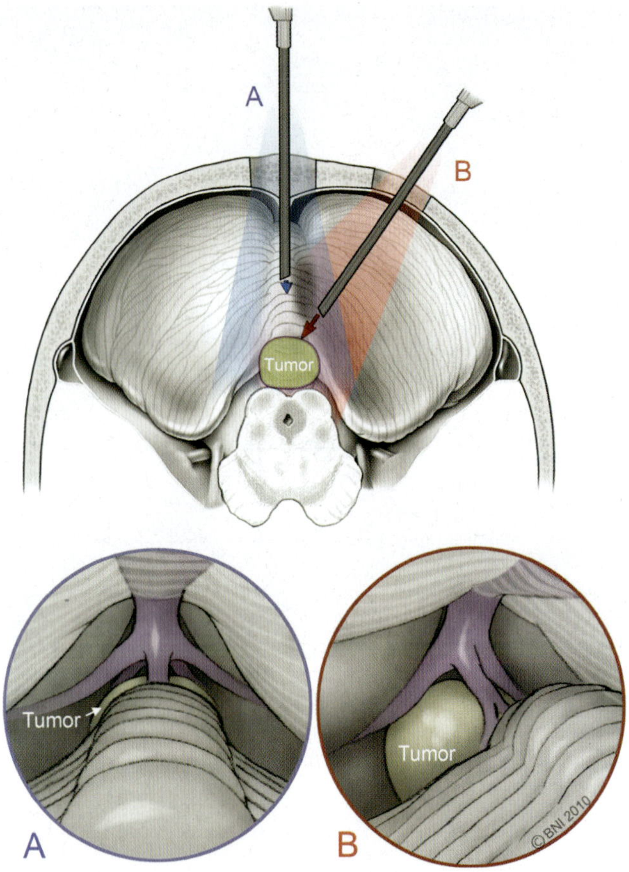

Fig. 25.4 **(A)** The traditional posterior supracerebellar infratentorial approach is not ideal for endoscopy because the vermis has a tendency to obscure the view of the tumor and the entire pineal region under the vein of Galen. **(B)** The off-midline approach provides a better trajectory and still allows access to both sides using the angled endoscope and instruments.

■ Conclusion

Neuroendoscopy applications to the CVJ are numerous. Because of the improved image quality, neuroendoscopes are intriguing as both adjuncts to microsurgery and as standalone sources of visualization to neurosurgeons. In our opinion, neuroendoscopy offers clear benefits in the treatment of intraventricular obstructive hydrocephalus by third ventriculostomy and in identifying neurovascular conflicts in trigeminal neuralgia and hemifacial spasm. Definitive objective proof of the value of endoscopy to many other applications is lacking, but it is the authors' belief that these techniques offer incremental improvements on well-established techniques and a minimally invasive emphasis. (Reprinted with permission from Barrow Neurological Institute.)

References

1. Hopf NJ, Perneczky A. Endoscopic neurosurgery and endoscope-assisted microneurosurgery for the treatment of intracranial cysts. Neurosurgery 1998;43(6):1330–1336, discussion 1336–1337
2. Teo C, Nakaji P, Mobbs RJ. Endoscope-assisted microvascular decompression for trigeminal neuralgia: technical case report. Neurosurgery 2006;59(4, Suppl 2):E489–E490, discussion E490
3. Valtonen HJ, Poe DS, Heilman CB, Tarlov EC. Endoscopically assisted prevention of cerebrospinal fluid leak in suboccipital acoustic neuroma surgery. Am J Otol 1997;18(3):381–385
4. Pillai P, Sammet S, Ammirati M. Image-guided, endoscopic-assisted drilling and exposure of the whole length of the internal auditory canal and its fundus with preservation of the integrity of the labyrinth using a retrosigmoid approach: a laboratory investigation. Neurosurgery 2009;65(6, Suppl):53–59, discussion 59
5. Wackym PA, King WA, Poe DS, et al. Adjunctive use of endoscopy during acoustic neuroma surgery. Laryngoscope 1999;109(8):1193–1201
6. Kadrian D, van Gelder J, Florida D, et al. Long-term reliability of endoscopic third ventriculostomy. Neurosurgery 2008;62(Suppl 2):614–621
7. Tamburrini G, Pettorini BL, Massimi L, Caldarelli M, Di Rocco C. Endoscopic third ventriculostomy: the best option in the treatment of persistent hydrocephalus after posterior cranial fossa tumour removal? Childs Nerv Syst 2008;24(12):1405–1412
8. Yamini B, Refai D, Rubin CM, Frim DM. Initial endoscopic management of pineal region tumors and associated hydrocephalus: clinical series and literature review. J Neurosurg 2004;100(5, Suppl Pediatrics):437–441
9. Di X. Endoscopic suboccipital decompression on pediatric Chiari type I. Minim Invasive Neurosurg 2009;52(3):119–125
10. Mobbs R, Teo C. Endoscopic assisted posterior fossa decompression. J Clin Neurosci 2001;8(4):343–344
11. Gawish I, Reisch R, Perneczky A. Endoscopic aqueductoplasty through a tailored craniocervical approach. J Neurosurg 2005;103(5):778–782

12. Sansone JM, Iskandar BJ. Endoscopic cerebral aqueductoplasty: a trans-fourth ventricle approach. J Neurosurg 2005;103(5, Suppl): 388–392
13. Little AS, Zabramski JM, Nakaji P. Endoscopic placement of aqueductal stent for isolated fourth ventricle in a patient with neurococcidiomycosis. Neurosurgery 2010;66: In press
14. Longatti P, Fiorindi A, Perin A, Martinuzzi A. Endoscopic anatomy of the cerebral aqueduct. Neurosurgery 2007;61(3, Suppl):1–5, discussion 5–6
15. Jannetta PJ, Levy EI. Trigeminal neuralgia: microvascular decompression of the trigeminal nerve for tic douloureux. In: Winn HR, ed. Youmans Neurological Surgery, 5th ed. Philadelphia, PA: W.B. Saunders; 2004:3005–3015
16. Jarrahy R, Berci G, Shahinian HK. Endoscope-assisted microvascular decompression of the trigeminal nerve. Otolaryngol Head Neck Surg 2000;123(3):218–223
17. Kabil MS, Eby JB, Shahinian HK. Endoscopic vascular decompression versus microvascular decompression of the trigeminal nerve. Minim Invasive Neurosurg 2005;48(4):207–212
18. Badr-El-Dine M, El-Garem HF, Talaat AM, Magnan J. Endoscopically assisted minimally invasive microvascular decompression of hemifacial spasm. Otol Neurotol 2002;23(2):122–128

26 Extended Endonasal Approaches to the Craniovertebral Junction

Yaron A. Moshel, Vijay K. Anand, Roger Härtl, and Theodore H. Schwartz

The endoscopic endonasal approach to the ventral craniovertebral junction (CVJ) offers an alternative to the traditional transoral, retropharyngeal upper cervical, and lateral skull base approaches to the CVJ. The endoscopic endonasal approach can be utilized to address pathology along the entire rostrocaudal extent of the clivus and ventral foramen magnum and upper cervical spine (**Fig. 26.1**).[1–7] Pathologies such as degenerative basilar invagination, odontoid fractures, rheumatoid arthritis with pannus or craniocervical settling, metastatic lesions, chordomas, and chondrosarcomas can be addressed with an endonasal endoscopic approach.[8,9] The dura can also be opened to address intradural lesions, such as foramen magnum and clival meningiomas, epidermoid tumors, and neurenteric cysts. The endoscopic endonasal approach has several benefits compared with the traditional transoral approach, including improved exposure of the upper clivus without the need for a hard or soft palate incision.[3,10–13] Incisions of the soft palate increase the risk of postoperative velopharyngeal insufficiency and can require a tracheostomy. The nasopharyngeal incision, as opposed to the oropharyngeal mucosal incision, permits earlier extubation and is less likely to become contaminated by food, saliva, and oral flora, enabling earlier feeding of the patient after surgery with little risk of infection and postoperative swallowing dysfunction.[5,8,9,14–18]

The endonasal endoscopic approach to the CVJ has several limitations. The most caudal exposure possible is limited by the extent to which the nasal bones and cartilaginous soft tissue around the nose can be elevated to increase the downward angled view. Another significant limitation is difficulty with obtaining lateral exposure. The lateral exposure with an endonasal approach is limited by the position of the medial pterygoid plate and the eustachian tube (**Fig. 26.2**). In contrast, with an open transoral approach, the parapharyngeal carotid artery can be easily controlled, and the wide exposure provides improved access to lateral tumor extensions.

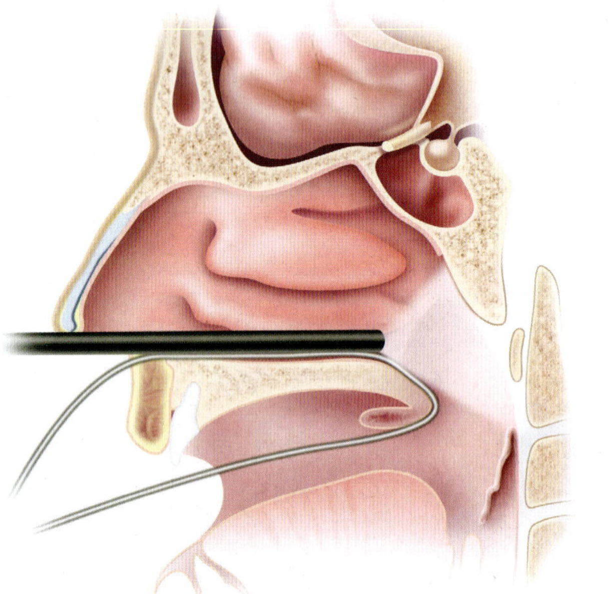

Fig. 26.1 Diagrammatic representation of the exposure afforded by the endoscopic approach to the craniovertebral junction. Using a flat angle, limited by the position of the nasal cartilage and the hard palate, exposure of the clivus, foramen magnum, C1, C2, and medial occipital condyle can be achieved. The use of angled endoscopes and inferior retraction of the soft palate can also improve the exposure of the C2 vertebral body.

■ Patient Selection

When evaluating a patient for an endonasal approach to a lesion in the CVJ, it is important to determine whether a suitable operative corridor is possible considering the individual patient's anatomy (**Tables 26.1** and **26.2**). For lesions in the clivus, such as chordomas or clival meningiomas, the most important limitation is the relationship between the carotid arteries and the tumor.[19] Midline and paramedian tumor extension can be addressed utilizing an endonasal, transmaxillary transpterygoid approach directed superiorly to the pterygopalatine fossa, petrous apex, and Meckel's cave.[20] Inferiorly, the transmaxillary approach can provide access to the infratemporal fossa, hypoglossal canal, and medial occipital condyle.[2,20–22] Although these paramedian endonasal approaches enable surgical access lateral to the carotid arteries through an endonasal approach, the risks of this maneuver must be identified before surgery and should be considered with other lateral skull base approaches, depending on the lateral extent of the lesion.[21] Large lesions in particular (>4 cm diameter) that are both medial and lateral to the lower cranial nerves may be best addressed in a staged fashion, removing the midline tumor endonasally and the lateral tumor transcranially.[9,17]

The need for exposure along the rostrocaudal axis must also be evaluated. Rostral lesions of the clivus may require extradural elevation of the sellar dura and a sphenoidotomy, and further rostral exposure may require pituitary transposition with extracapsular mobilization of the pituitary gland to access tumor extension in the retrosellar space, interpeduncular cistern, and along the posterior clinoids

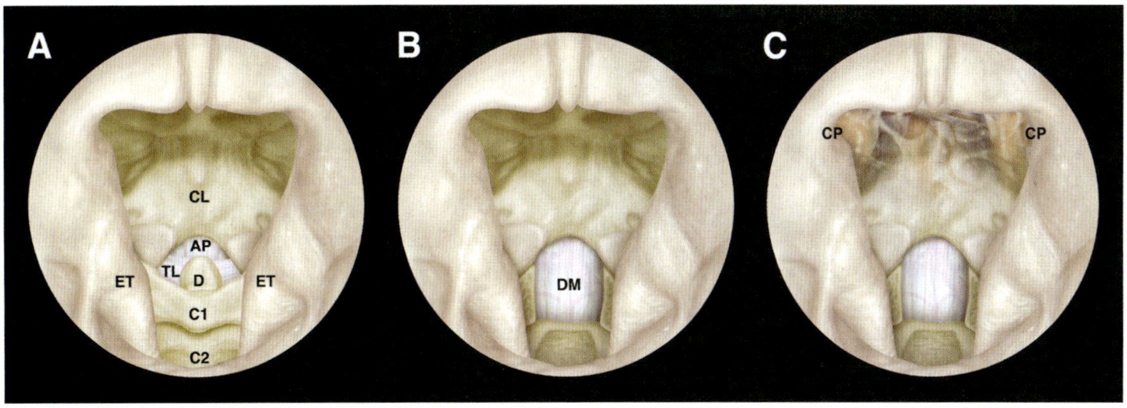

Fig. 26.2 Diagrammatic views of the endoscopic endonasal approach to the craniovertebral junction. **(A)** After inferior reflection of the pharyngeal mucosa, the clivus (*CL*), foramen magnum, anterior arch of C1, and odontoid process (*D*) can be visualized with the transverse (*TL*) and apical (*AP*) ligaments. The lateral limits of the exposure are the eustachian tubes (*ET*) and the associated carotid arteries, unless a transpterygoid approach is performed. **(B)** After removal of C1 and C2, the ventral dura matter (*DM*) of the craniovertebral junction and the underlying rostral spinal cord and pontomedullary junction are visible. **(C)** The position of the paraclival carotid protuberance (*CP*) adjacent to the eustachian tubes can be verified with intraoperative neuronavigation and a Doppler probe.

Table 26.1 Summary of Clinical Reports Utilizing an Endoscopic Endonasal Approach to Clival Chordomas

Authors	No. of Patients	No. of Patients Receiving GTR %	No. of Patients with CSF Leak %	Complications
Jho and Ha[7]	3	3 (100%)	1 (33%)	CN VI palsy
Solares et al.[41]	3	2 (67%)	0	–
Frank et al.[42]	9	3 (33%)	1 (11%)	ICA injury
Hwang and Ho[43]	3	0	0	Hydrocephalus
Dehdashti et al.[8]	12	7 (58%)	4 (33%)	Hematoma, hemiparesis, hydrocephalus
Hong Jiang et a.l[44]	9	6 (67%)	0	–
Zhang et al.[45]	7	6 (67%)	Not available	Subarachnoid hemorrhage
Stippler et al.[17]	20	9 (45%)	5 (25%)	ICA injury, brainstem hemorrhage, CN palsy
Fraser et al.[9]	7	5 (71%)	0	Pulmonary embolism

Abbreviations: CN, cranial nerve; CSF, cerebrospinal fluid; GTR, gross total resection; ICA, internal carotid artery; No., number.

Table 26.2 Summary of Clinical Reports Utilizing an Endoscopic Endonasal Odontoidectomy

Authors	No. of Patients	Pathology (No. of Patients)	Fusion (No.)	Extubation / Tracheostomy	CSF Leak %
Kassam et al.[28]	1	RA	Yes	Day 1 / no	0
Nayak et al.[16]	9	RA	Yes (8)	NA / 4 patients*	0
Laufer et al.[15]	1	RA	Yes	Day 1 / no	0
Magrini et al.[40]	1	Down syndrome, AA instability	Yes	Day 3 / no	0
Wu et al.[46]	3	RA (2), trauma (1)	Yes	Day 1 / no	0
Leng et al.[47]	1	AA instability	Yes	Day 1 / no	0
de Almeida et al.[26]	17	RA (14), metastatic (1), meningioma (1), chondrosarcoma (1)	Yes (16)	NA / no	

Abbreviations: AA, atlantoaxial; CSF, cerebrospinal fluid; NA, not available; No., number; RA, rheumatoid arthritis.
*Of the four patients who required a tracheostomy, two had documented preoperative pharyngeal dysfunction.

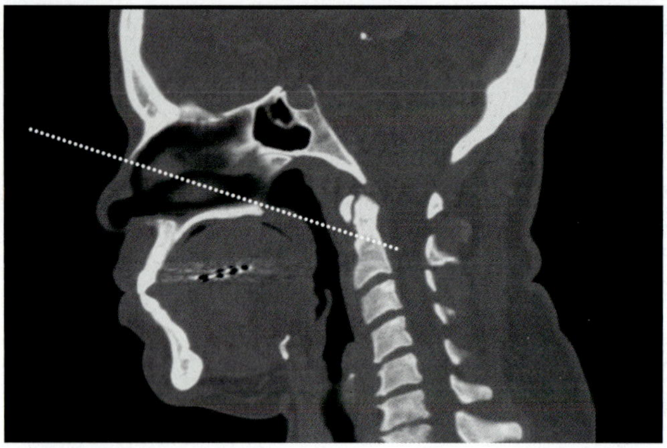

Fig. 26.3 Midsagittal contrast-enhanced computed tomography scan demonstrating the sphenoid sinus, clivus, craniovertebral junction, and their relationship to the nasal bones and hard palate. The *dotted line* represents the maximal angle of exposure that can be achieved with the use of a 0-degree endoscope. Compared with the dotted line, the actual intraoperative exposure is slightly more limited by the soft tissues of the nose; however, these limitations can be overcome with angled endoscopes.

and dorsum sella.[4,21,23–25] Preoperative imaging must also be scrutinized to identify the presence of intradural tumor extension so that harvesting of appropriate grafts for successful closure, such as fat, fascia lata, or a vascularized nasoseptal flap, are performed during the procedure.

In addressing lesions along the caudal aspect of the CVJ, such as upper cervical spine tumors or rheumatoid arthritis with pannus surrounding the odontoid process, endonasal exposure is limited superiorly by the nasal bones and cartilaginous soft tissues of the nose and, inferiorly, the exposure is limited by the hard palate and soft palate.[26] The line created by connecting the inferior edge of the nasal bone to the posterior edge of the hard palate on a midsagittal computed tomography (CT) scan represents the most caudal dissection possible with straight endoscopic instruments (**Fig. 26.3**). The most inferior limit of dissection is generally 0.9 cm above the base of the C2 vertebral body and even lower in patients with basilar invagination.[26] Patients with a high-positioned odontoid and platybasia often require removal of the anterior margin of the foramen magnum and lower clivus to expose the upper part of the odontoid, which can often be performed endonasally without disruption of the anterior rim of the atlas or alar and transverse ligaments because the superior to inferior angle is advantageous.[5,16] In contrast, with a transoral exposure, the body of C2 and anterior ring of C1 are exposed first, and it can be difficult to remove the odontoid without disruption of the C1 anterior arch.

Surgical Technique

A surgical team approach that includes an otolaryngologist and a neurosurgeon is used for all extended endoscopic skull base cases. Procedures are routinely performed under general anesthesia; antibiotics, glucocorticoids, and antihistamines are administered. Prior to the operation, a lumbar puncture is performed, and 0.2 mL of 10% fluorescein is injected in 10 mL of cerebrospinal fluid (CSF) to help visualize CSF leaks. A lumbar drain is placed prior to surgery in cases where a large skull base dural defect is anticipated. Topical 4% cocaine is used over the nasal mucosa for vasoconstriction, and then a mixture of lidocaine 1% and epinephrine (1:100,000) is injected. The patient's head is placed in three-point fixation, slightly elevated and slightly turned to the right, and intraoperative neuronavigation with magnetic resonance imaging (MRI) and/or CT angiography is used for all procedures. The patient's head is fixed in a slightly flexed position to improve the view to the clivus and the axial cervical spine. The lateral thigh is prepared for autologous fat and fascia lata grafts.

Under 0-degree endoscopic view (Karl Storz, Tuttlingen, Germany), the inferior, middle, and superior turbinates as well as the sphenoid ostia are identified bilaterally. The middle and superior turbinates are most often retracted laterally; however, in some patients the right middle turbinate is removed to optimize the exposure and allow easy passage of instruments and the endoscope.

Since 2008, we have used a nasoseptal flap as part of a multilayered closure of the skull base. The use of a pedicled nasoseptal vascular flap of the nasal septum mucoperiosteum based on the nasoseptal artery has become an important adjunct in the multilayered endoscopic reconstruction of large skull base defects.[27] The nasoseptal flap is generally harvested at the beginning of the operation—before tumor removal and before the posterior septectomy is performed. The vascular supply of the nasoseptal flap is derived from the posterior septal artery, a terminal branch of the internal maxillary artery.[27,28] The flap is raised by placing two parallel incisions in the septal mucosa, one along the nasal floor and the other just inferior to the most superior aspect of the septum. These incisions are joined anteriorly to create the flap and, posteriorly, these incisions are extended over the rostrum of the sphenoid superiorly and to the choana inferiorly. The flap is elevated anterior to posterior and lateral with a dissector and held out of the surgeon's way during the operation. For CVJ approaches, the flap can be stored in the sphenoid sinus or maxillary sinus so as not to interfere with the surgical corridor.

The endonasal approach to lesions of the clivus can require a sphenoidotomy, depending on the rostral-caudal extent of the pathology.[19] For lesions of the upper third of the clivus located behind the posterior wall of the sphenoid sinus, a bilateral transsphenoidal opening and removal of the posterior third of the septum is performed. The ostium of the sphenoid sinus is first enlarged to expose the sphenoid sinus, and the posterior third of the nasal septum adjacent to the vomer and maxillary crest is resected with a tissue shaver. At this point, a panoramic view is achieved and bimanual surgery with four separate instruments is possible. A graft of vomer or cartilage can be harvested to reconstruct the floor of the sella at the end of the operation. The anterior wall of the sphenoid sinus is drilled flush with the floor of the sinus. It is important to remove the entire anterior wall of the sphenoid sinus to provide enough room for the endoscope and instruments to sit in the sphenoid during the procedure. All sphenoid septae are removed with a drill, and the mucosa of the sphenoid sinus is completely removed so that a mucocele does not form under the nasoseptal flap. The carotid protuberance, optic protuberance, and medial and lateral opticocarotid recesses are identified. The lateral extent of the sphenoidotomy is verified using intraoperative neuronavigation, ensuring that optimal exposure is obtained in all dimensions before proceeding with progressively deeper exposure.

The lateral margins of the floor of the sphenoid sinus are marked by the course of the vidian nerve, which runs posteriorly along the floor into the vertical segment of the carotid artery. The sella can also be opened to mobilize the pituitary gland laterally or rostrally to allow drilling of the posterior wall of the sella, which forms the upper extent of the clivus and extends up behind the pituitary gland. With this maneuver, the posterior clinoid processes and the dorsum sella can be thinned with a microdrill and removed with a Kerrison rongeur.

The bone of the upper clivus can be opened from carotid to carotid artery with a microdrill, and the venous plexus can be controlled with hemostatic agents. The amount of drilling required will depend on the aeration of the sinus, and the location of the carotid arteries is verified using a Doppler ultrasound probe. The inferior intercavernous sinus is cauterized and transected. The dura is then opened in the midline to expose the basilar tip, superior cerebellar and posterior cerebral arteries, and cranial nerve III. The cranial nerve VI runs at the lateral edge of the exposure as it enters Dorello's canal.

The approach to the inferior two-thirds of the clivus is also combined with a transsphenoidal exposure to facilitate instrument placement. The basipharyngeal fascia and prevertebral musculature are dissected free from the clivus, cauterized, and cut laterally to create a U-shaped flap that is reflected inferiorly (**Fig. 26.4**). The lateral margins of the nasopharyngeal flap are the vidian nerves superiorly and eustachian tubes, which mark the location of the carotid arteries, laterally. The clivus is drilled back until flush with the dura. Extensive venous bleeding from the basilar plexus can be controlled with careful cautery, hemostatic agents, and gentle pressure. The use of cautery along the dural incision should only be performed after the position of the abducens nerves is determined. Opening the dura, when necessary, will expose the basilar trunk, anteroinferior cerebellar and vertebral arteries, and ventral pons. The dura is opened with an I-shaped incision to avoid damaging the near midline abducens nerve. The average distance between the abducens nerves at the dural emergence is 19.8 mm.[29]

The transodontoid approach is a continuation of the inferior extent of the transclival approach. Often, it is not necessary to perform a sphenoidotomy at this level unless there is a significant degree of basilar invagination, requiring removal of the inferior aspects of the clivus. However, bimanual dissection is achieved by removing the inferior part of the vomer. The approach courses parallel to the hard palate, and an angled scope can be helpful to gain an inferiorly directed view. The mucosal flap is reflected starting at the

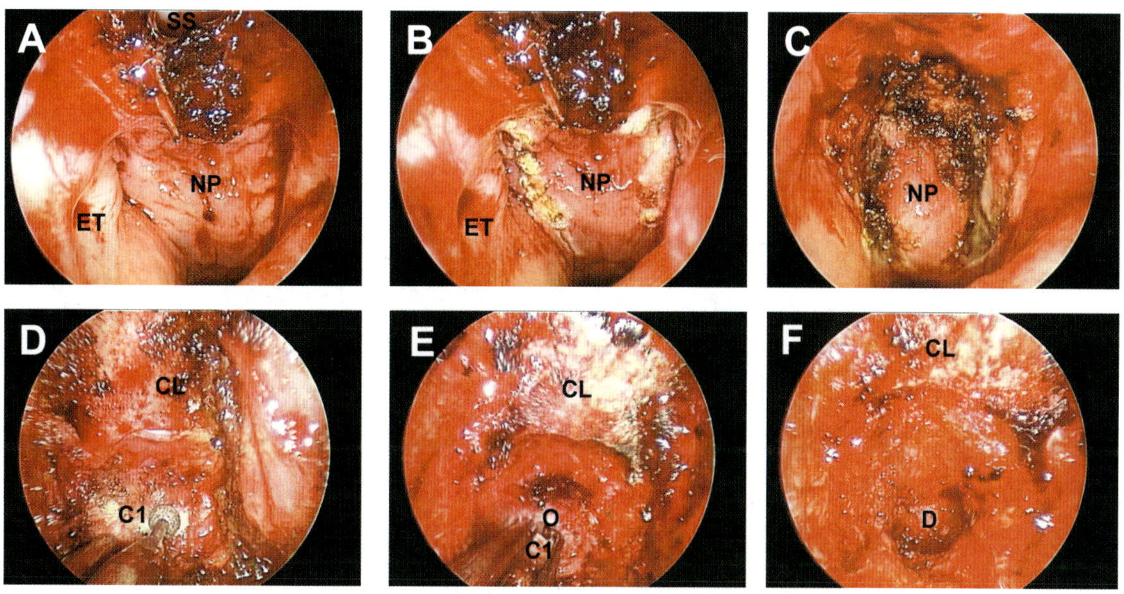

Fig. 26.4 Intraoperative endoscopic views of the approach to the craniovertebral junction. **(A)** Endoscopic view after exposure of the sphenoid sinus (*SS*) and identification of the eustachian tubes (*ET*) and the nasopharyngeal mucosa (*NP*). **(B)** With lateral limits demarcated by the opening of the eustachian tubes (*ET*), **(C)** the nasopharyngeal mucosa is incised in a U-shaped flap. **(D)** After inferior reflection of the mucosal flap, the clivus (*CL*) and anterior arch of C1 are identified. **(E)** After removing the anterior arch, C1 and the surrounding ligamentous attachments at the top of the odontoid process (*O*) are identified. **(F)** Further drilling of the arch of C1 reveals the body of the dens (*D*) at the bottom of the exposure.

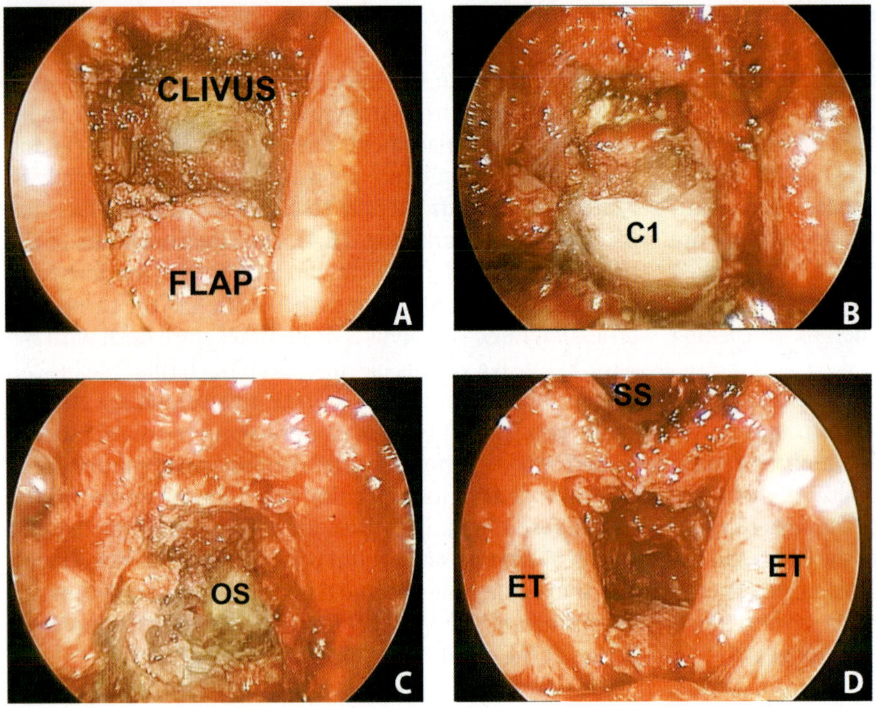

Fig. 26.5 **(A)** Intraoperative endoscopic views of the craniovertebral junction demonstrating the clivus and the inferiorly reflected nasopharyngeal mucosal flap. **(B)** Further dissection inferior to the clivus reveals the anterior arch of C1. **(C)** After removal of the anterior arch of C1, an os odontoideum (*OS*) can be visualized. **(D)** A demagnified view demonstrates the sphenoid sinus (*SS*), the lateral limits of the exposure determined by the eustachian tubes (*ET*), and the epidural space after removal of C1 and the odontoid process.

base of the sphenoid sinus and limited laterally by the eustachian tubes, exposing the lower third of the clivus. The bone at the base of the clivus is removed from medial occipital condyle to medial occipital condyle. Below this, the atlanto-occipital membrane, longus capitis, and longus colli muscles as well as the anterior aspects of C1 and C2 are exposed. If necessary, the anterior arch of C1 can be removed to expose the odontoid, which is then removed with a microdrill (**Fig. 26.5**). Once the central portion of the dens has been removed, the lateral aspects can be mobilized medially with a small curette. The use of intraoperative tomography is useful to ensure complete removal of the dens.[15] Retrodental inflammatory pannus can be resected with an ultrasonic aspirator until the dura is visualized. Stereotactic navigation is extremely useful for these maneuvers (**Fig. 26.6**).

Tumors that have a significant component extending lateral to the paraclival carotid artery and are to be exposed through an endonasal as opposed to a lateral skull base corridor require a transpterygoid approach to identify the vidian nerve and the paraclival carotid at the level of foramen lacerum. This approach requires maxillary antrostomy and posterior maxillary wall resection to gain access to the pterygopalatine fossa. The transmaxillary transpterygoid approach can be used to reach a variety of targets in the paramedian skull base, including the pterygopalatine fossa, infratemporal fossa, petrous apex, and Meckel's cave.[22] The approach

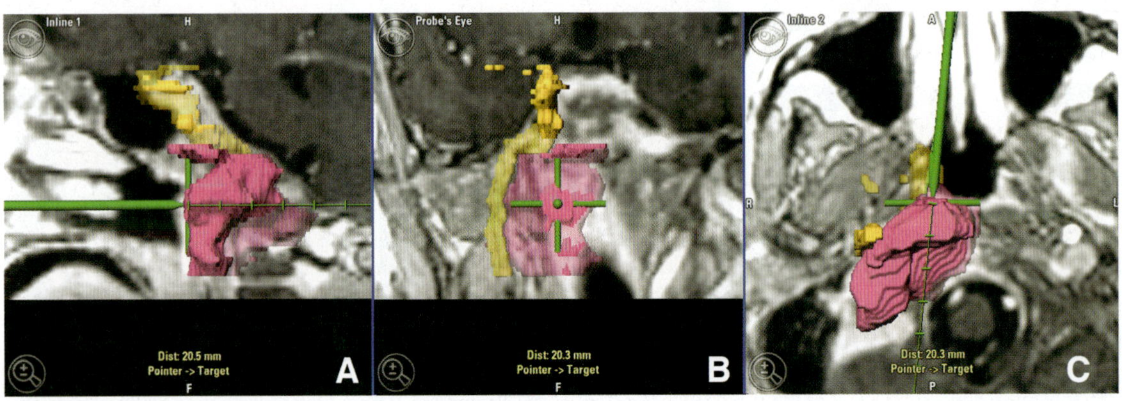

Fig. 26.6 Stereotactic neuronavigation is beneficial in planning endoscopic endonasal approaches to the craniovertebral junction. Representative **(A)** sagittal, **(B)** coronal, and **(C)** axial images are shown from the navigation screen during removal of a metastatic tumor (*pink volume*) involving the occipital condyle and displacing the carotid artery (*yellow volume*) laterally.

begins with an uncinectomy and opening of the maxillary ostium followed by elevation of the posterior maxillary sinus mucosa off the orbital process of the palatine bone and posterior wall of the maxillary sinus. The sphenopalatine artery is identified and ligated at the crista ethmoidalis, and the orbital process of the palatine bone and posteromedial wall of the maxillary sinus are removed to expose the pterygopalatine fossa. The anterior genu between the petrous carotid and the paraclival carotid at the foramen lacerum is then identified by following the vidian nerve in the pterygoid canal and drilling the medial pterygoid plate and sphenoid floor.

The exposure lateral to the carotid artery in the middle third of the clivus can then be extended superiorly to the petrous apex and Meckel's cave or inferiorly to the parapharyngeal carotid and occipital condyle, jugular foramen, and hypoglossal canal. The eustachian tube is the anatomical landmark to gain control of the parapharyngeal carotid artery during exposure of the occipital condyle, jugular foramen, and hypoglossal canal. Entry into Meckel's cave requires removal of the pterygoid process along the vidian nerve and identification of the infraorbital nerve up to the foramen rotundum. The so-called "quadrangular space," which is bounded medially by the vertical carotid artery and laterally by the maxillary nerve, can be drilled open to expose Meckel's cave.

Large chordomas or meningiomas should be internally decompressed using either two suctions or suction and microscissor. If the tumor is firm, a cavitational ultrasonic surgical aspirator (Valleylab, Boulder, CO), Elliquence monopolar ball or ring cautery (Elliquence, Oceanside, NY), or NICO Myriad tissue resection device (NICO, Indianapolis, IN) can be used to debulk the tumor. Visualization is enhanced with a 30-degree, 30-cm rigid 4-mm endoscope (Karl Storz). In a subset of cases, we have used a three-dimensional (3D) endoscope (Visionsense, Orangeburg, NY) for dissection to increase stereoscopic vision.[30,31] Once decompressed, the tumor capsule can be mobilized and sharply dissected. Care must be taken to preserve all perforator vessels to the midbrain and pons. Avoidance of coagulation and "pulling" are critical to the preservation of vital neurovascular structures while the remaining capsule is removed. The resection bed is examined with a 45-degree, 18-cm rigid 4-mm endoscope to ensure the absence of any residual tumor. Curved suctions, angled micropituitary rongeurs, and dissectors can be used to reach residual pieces of tumor. Once the tumor and cyst wall are completely removed, the resection bed is examined with a 45-degree, 18-cm rigid 4-mm endoscope to ensure the absence of residual tumor (**Fig. 26.7**).

Multilayered Closure

The use of intrathecal fluorescein helps to ensure adequate closure at two stages—identifying small CSF leaks and ensuring a watertight closure at the end of the case.[32] First, any dead space left behind after the tumor resection is filled with an autologous fat graft. Then a "gasket-seal" closure is performed, consisting of a fascia lata onlay placed over a rigid buttress of either vomer or Medpor (Porex Corporation, Newnan, GA) that is cut to the exact size of the defect and countersunk into the skull base defect.[33] Small areas of defect between the vomeric bone or the Medpor plate are filled in with an autologous fat graft. Finally, a vascularized nasoseptal flap is placed directly over the gasket seal construct followed by a final layer of DuraSeal (Covidien, Norwalk, CT) to hold everything in place and ensure a watertight closure.[27,28] No DuraSeal is placed between the flap and the gasket seal construct because it would prevent fibrosis and vascularization of the skull base. It is critical to assure that the nasoseptal flap is positioned over the entire defect, that it is not doubled over on itself, and that the mucosal surface is facing the nasal cavity. If fascia lata is used, it is critical that the nasoseptal flap lies beyond the edges of the fascia lata so that the flap is in contact with the sphenoid bone to fully cover the defect. For odontoid resection, merely replacing the fascial flap is adequate.

The nasal cavity is then filled with FloSeal (Baxter, Deerfield, IL) for hemostasis. A small piece of Telfa dressing (Covidien) is placed in each nostril overnight to absorb drainage and is removed in 1 to 2 days. If a lumbar drain is placed, it is typically drained at ~5 mL/hour for 1 to 2 days and then clamped and removed in the evening. The patient lies flat after its removal and sleeps to decrease the risk of spinal headache. Patients are placed on low doses of heparin to prevent deep venous thrombosis.

Fusion Considerations

Although it is possible to remove the very top of the odontoid and some of the retro-odontoid tissue without removing the anterior ring of C1 and its ligaments and without destabilizing the spine, in reality, the majority of cases will require occipitocervical fusion.[34,35] Furthermore, no consistent diagnostic criteria are available to predict whether an odontoidectomy will cause instability in patients with CVJ malformations. We recommend performing a fusion before the endonasal approach to avoid the risk of spinal cord injury when the patient is rotated into the prone position (**Figs. 26.8** and **26.9**).[3,36–38] We have, on one occasion, performed the endonasal odontoid resection with a nonfused patient in a halo vest. The fusion was then performed in a separate surgical procedure.[15] More commonly, patients will undergo both procedures in one operative setting. In this situation, we perform the occipitocervical fusion first followed by the endonasal procedure immediately afterward, with a brief wake-up test to ensure that there is no neurological deterioration.[14] Electrophysiologic monitoring is also utilized during the operation and is especially important during the repositioning of the patient between procedures.

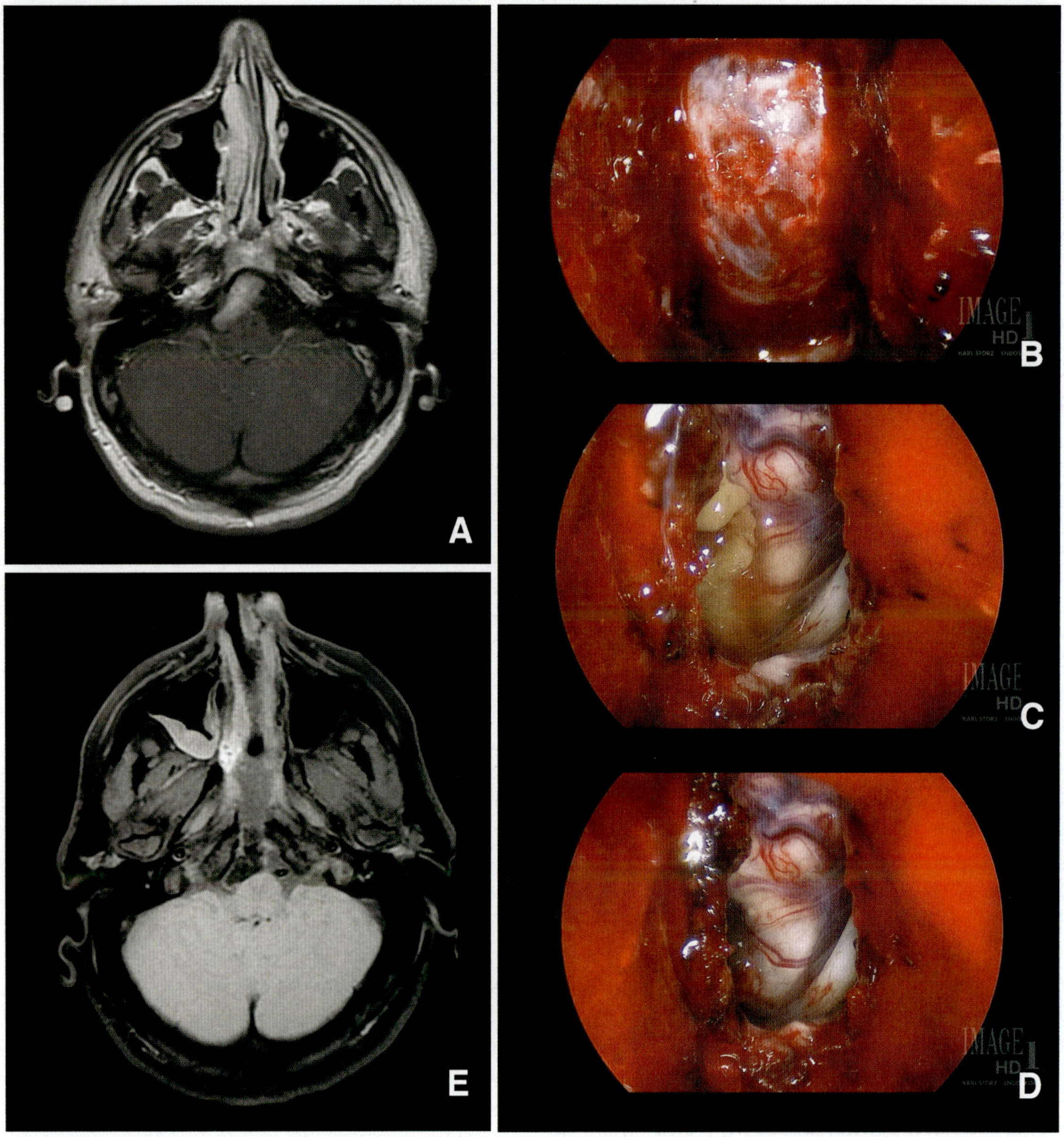

Fig. 26.7 **(A)** Preoperative, contrast-enhanced, magnetic resonance image (MRI) and **(B–D)** intraoperative endoscopic images in a patient with an epidermoid tumor located anterior and lateral to the ventral aspect of the medulla. **(B)** After the basipharyngeal fascia was reflected inferiorly, the clivus was removed to expose the dura, preserving some bone over the carotid arteries at the lateral limits of the exposure. **(C)** After opening the dura, the tumor was debulked and removed, **(D)** exposing the ventral brainstem. **(E)** Postoperative MRI demonstrates the tumor removal and the trajectory between the carotid arteries.

Conclusion

The endoscopic endonasal transclival approach uses a minimal access corridor but can provide the surgeon with excellent visualization of the entire rostrocaudal extent of the clivus, the foramen magnum, and the upper cervical spine. At our institution, the approach represents a joint effort between otolaryngology and neurosurgery. We have found that with the endonasal endoscopic approach to the CVJ, most lesions can be treated with a single endoscopic operation or, if necessary, combined in a staged fashion with lateral skull base approaches or posterior decompression and fusion. The endoscopic approach avoids many of the complications associated with the transoral approach, especially in relation to swallowing dysfunction, lengthy intubation, and early patient mobilization.[16,36,39,40]

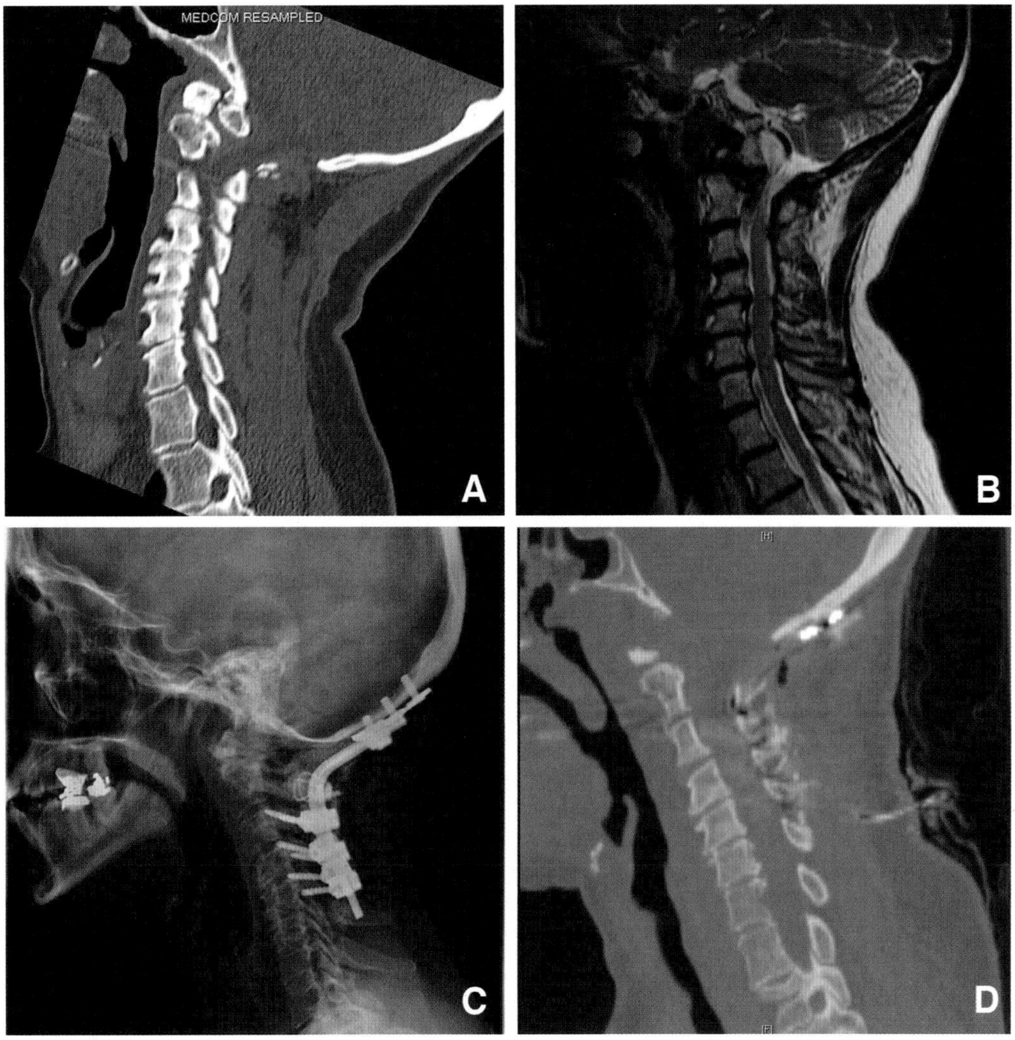

Fig. 26.8 Representative preoperative and postoperative sagittal **(A)** computed tomography and **(B)** magnetic resonance images of a patient with compression of the upper spinal cord secondary to an odontoideum and atlantoaxial instability. **(C)** The patient underwent occipitocervical fusion followed by **(D)** endonasal endoscopic removal of the odontoid and anterior arch of C1.

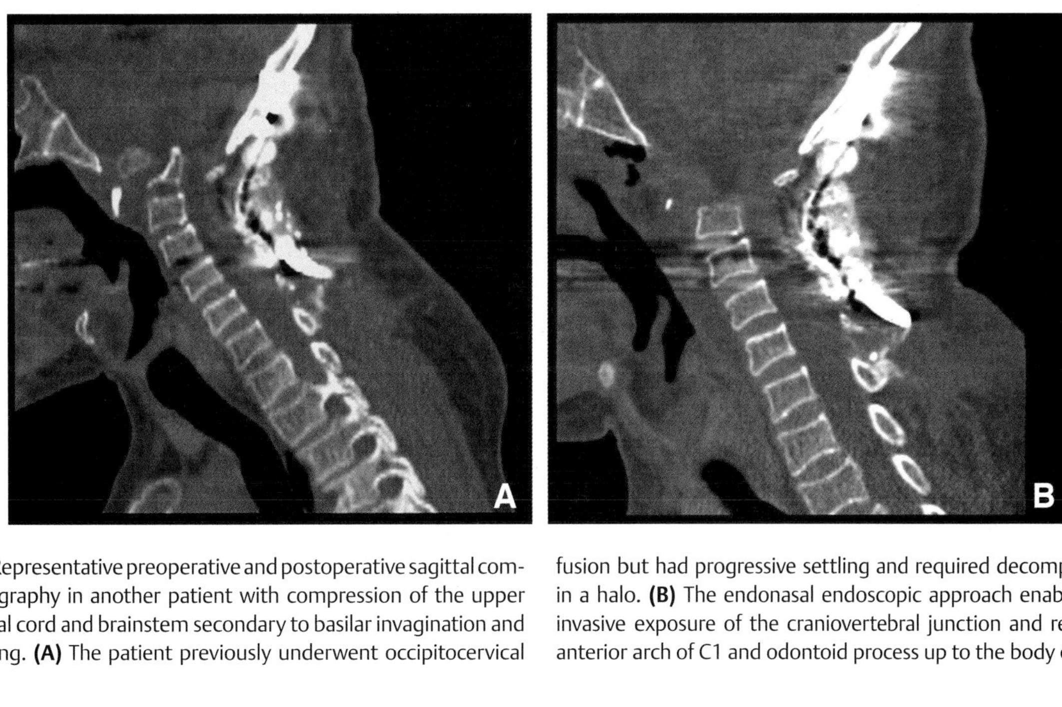

Fig. 26.9 Representative preoperative and postoperative sagittal computed tomography in another patient with compression of the upper cervical spinal cord and brainstem secondary to basilar invagination and cranial settling. **(A)** The patient previously underwent occipitocervical fusion but had progressive settling and required decompression while in a halo. **(B)** The endonasal endoscopic approach enabled minimally invasive exposure of the craniovertebral junction and removal of the anterior arch of C1 and odontoid process up to the body of C2.

References

1. Alfieri A, Jho HD, Tschabitscher M. Endoscopic endonasal approach to the ventral cranio-cervical junction: anatomical study. Acta Neurochir (Wien) 2002;144(3):219–225, discussion 225
2. Schwartz TH, Fraser JF, Brown S, Tabaee A, Kacker A, Anand VK. Endoscopic cranial base surgery: classification of operative approaches. Neurosurgery 2008;62(5):991–1002, discussion 1002–1005
3. Crockard HA, Sen CN. The transoral approach for the management of intradural lesions at the craniovertebral junction: review of 7 cases. Neurosurgery 1991;28(1):88–97, discussion 97–98
4. de Divitiis O, Conti A, Angileri FF, Cardali S, La Torre D, Tschabitscher M. Endoscopic transoral-transclival approach to the brainstem and surrounding cisternal space: anatomic study. Neurosurgery 2004;54(1):125–130, discussion 130
5. Kassam AB, Snyderman C, Gardner P, Carrau R, Spiro R. The expanded endonasal approach: a fully endoscopic transnasal approach and resection of the odontoid process: technical case report. Neurosurgery 2005;57(1, Suppl):E213, discussion E213
6. Jho HD, Carrau RL, McLaughlin MR, Somaza SC. Endoscopic transsphenoidal resection of a large chordoma in the posterior fossa. Acta Neurochir (Wien) 1997;139(4):343–347, discussion 347–348
7. Jho HD, Ha HG. Endoscopic endonasal skull base surgery: part 3—the clivus and posterior fossa. Minim Invasive Neurosurg 2004;47(1):16–23
8. Dehdashti AR, Karabatsou K, Ganna A, Witterick I, Gentili F. Expanded endoscopic endonasal approach for treatment of clival chordomas: early results in 12 patients. Neurosurgery 2008;63(2):299–307, discussion 307–309
9. Fraser JF, Nyquist GG, Moore N, Anand VK, Schwartz TH. Endoscopic endonasal transclival resection of chordomas: operative technique, clinical outcome, and review of the literature. J Neurosurg 2010;112(5):1061–1069
10. Apuzzo ML, Weiss MH, Heiden JS. Transoral exposure of the atlantoaxial region. Neurosurgery 1978;3(2):201–207
11. Blazier CJ, Hadley MN, Spetzler RF. The transoral surgical approach to craniovertebral pathology. J Neurosci Nurs 1986;18(2):57–62
12. Husain M, Rastogi M, Ojha BK, Chandra A, Jha DK. Endoscopic transoral surgery for craniovertebral junction anomalies. Technical note. J Neurosurg Spine 2006;5(4):367–373
13. Crockard HA, Pozo JL, Ransford AO, Stevens JM, Kendall BE, Essigman WK. Transoral decompression and posterior fusion for rheumatoid atlanto-axial subluxation. J Bone Joint Surg Br 1986;68(3):350–356
14. Leng LZ, Anand VK, Hartl R, Schwartz TH. Endonasal endoscopic resection of an os odontoideum to decompress the cervicomedullary junction: a minimal access surgical technique. Spine 2009;34(4):E139–E143
15. Laufer I, Greenfield JP, Anand VK, Härtl R, Schwartz TH. Endonasal endoscopic resection of the odontoid process in a nonachondroplastic dwarf with juvenile rheumatoid arthritis: feasibility of the approach and utility of the intraoperative Iso-C three-dimensional navigation. Case report. J Neurosurg Spine 2008;8(4):376–380
16. Nayak JV, Gardner PA, Vescan AD, Carrau RL, Kassam AB, Snyderman CH. Experience with the expanded endonasal approach for resection of the odontoid process in rheumatoid disease. Am J Rhinol 2007;21(5):601–606
17. Stippler M, Gardner PA, Snyderman CH, Carrau RL, Prevedello DM, Kassam AB. Endoscopic endonasal approach for clival chordomas. Neurosurgery 2009;64(2):268–277, discussion 277–278
18. Welch WC, Kassam A. Endoscopically assisted transoral-transpharyngeal approach to the craniovertebral junction. Neurosurgery 2003;52(6):1511–1512
19. Fraser JF, Nyquist GG, Moore N, Anand VK, Schwartz TH. Endoscopic endonasal minimal access approach to the clivus: case series and technical nuances. Neurosurgery 2010;67(3, Suppl Operative):ons150–ons158, discussion ons158
20. Kassam AB, Vescan AD, Carrau RL, et al. Expanded endonasal approach: vidian canal as a landmark to the petrous internal carotid artery. J Neurosurg 2008;108(1):177–183
21. Vescan AD, Snyderman CH, Carrau RL, et al. Vidian canal: analysis and relationship to the internal carotid artery. Laryngoscope 2007;117(8):1338–1342
22. Hofstetter CP, Singh A, Anand VK, Kacker A, Schwartz TH. The endoscopic, endonasal, transmaxillary transpterygoid approach to the pterygopalatine fossa, infratemporal fossa, petrous apex, and the Meckel cave. J Neurosurg 2010;113(5):967–974
23. Kassam AB, Prevedello DM, Thomas A, et al. Endoscopic endonasal pituitary transposition for a transdorsum sellae approach to the interpeduncular cistern. Neurosurgery 2008;62(3, Suppl 1):57–72, discussion 72–74
24. Cappabianca P, Cavallo LM, Colao A, et al. Endoscopic endonasal transsphenoidal approach: outcome analysis of 100 consecutive procedures. Minim Invasive Neurosurg 2002;45(4):193–200
25. Cavallo LM, Cappabianca P, Messina A, et al. The extended endoscopic endonasal approach to the clivus and cranio-vertebral junction: anatomical study. Childs Nerv Syst 2007;23(6):665–671
26. de Almeida JR, Zanation AM, Snyderman CH, et al. Defining the nasopalatine line: the limit for endonasal surgery of the spine. Laryngoscope 2009;119(2):239–244
27. Hadad G, Bassagasteguy L, Carrau RL, et al. A novel reconstructive technique after endoscopic expanded endonasal approaches: vascular pedicle nasoseptal flap. Laryngoscope 2006;116(10):1882–1886
28. Kassam A, Carrau RL, Snyderman CH, Gardner P, Mintz A. Evolution of reconstructive techniques following endoscopic expanded endonasal approaches. Neurosurg Focus 2005;19(1):E8
29. Puxeddu R, Lui MW, Chandrasekar K, Nicolai P, Sekhar LN. Endoscopic-assisted transcolumellar approach to the clivus: an anatomical study. Laryngoscope 2002;112(6):1072–1078
30. Roth J, Singh A, Nyquist G, et al. Three-dimensional and 2-dimensional endoscopic exposure of midline cranial base targets using expanded endonasal and transcranial approaches. Neurosurgery 2009;65(6):1116–1128, discussion 1128–1130
31. Tabaee A, Anand VK, Fraser JF, Brown SM, Singh A, Schwartz TH. Three-dimensional endoscopic pituitary surgery. Neurosurgery 2009;64(5, Suppl 2):288–293, discussion 294–295
32. Placantonakis DG, Tabaee A, Anand VK, Hiltzik D, Schwartz TH. Safety of low-dose intrathecal fluorescein in endoscopic cranial base surgery. Neurosurgery 2007;61(3, Suppl):161–165, discussion 165–166
33. Leng LZ, Brown S, Anand VK, Schwartz TH. "Gasket-seal" watertight closure in minimal-access endoscopic cranial base surgery. Neurosurgery 2008;62(5, Suppl 2):E342–E343, discussion E343
34. Dickman CA, Crawford NR, Brantley AG, Sonntag VK. Biomechanical effects of transoral odontoidectomy. Neurosurgery 1995;36(6):1146–1152, discussion 1152–1153
35. Dickman CA, Locantro J, Fessler RG. The influence of transoral odontoid resection on stability of the craniovertebral junction. J Neurosurg 1992;77(4):525–530
36. Menezes AH. Complications of surgery at the craniovertebral junction—avoidance and management. Pediatr Neurosurg 1991–1992–1992;17(5):254–266
37. Di Lorenzo N. Craniocervical junction malformation treated by transoral approach. A survey of 25 cases with emphasis on postoperative instability and outcome. Acta Neurochir (Wien) 1992;118(3–4):112–116

38. Naderi S, Crawford NR, Melton MS, Sonntag VK, Dickman CA. Biomechanical analysis of cranial settling after transoral odontoidectomy. Neurosurg Focus 1999;6(6):e7
39. Menezes AH, VanGilder JC. Transoral-transpharyngeal approach to the anterior craniocervical junction. Ten-year experience with 72 patients. J Neurosurg 1988;69(6):895–903
40. Magrini S, Pasquini E, Mazzatenta D, Mascari C, Galassi E, Frank G. Endoscopic endonasal odontoidectomy in a patient affected by Down syndrome: technical case report. Neurosurgery 2008;63(2):E373–E374, discussion E374
41. Solares CA, Fakhri S, Batra PS, Lee J, Lanza DC. Transnasal endoscopic resection of lesions of the clivus: a preliminary report. Laryngoscope 2005;115(11):1917–1922
42. Frank G, Sciarretta V, Calbucci F, Farneti G, Mazzatenta D, Pasquini E. The endoscopic transnasal transsphenoidal approach for the treatment of cranial base chordomas and chondrosarcomas. Neurosurgery 2006;59(1, Suppl 1):ONS50–ONS57, discussion ONS50–ONS57
43. Hwang PY, Ho CL. Neuronavigation using an image-guided endoscopic transnasal-sphenoethmoidal approach to clival chordomas. Neurosurgery 2007;61(5, Suppl 2):212–217, discussion 217–218
44. Hong Jiang W, Ping Zhao S, Hai Xie Z, Zhang H, Zhang J, Yun Xiao J. Endoscopic resection of chordomas in different clival regions. Acta Otolaryngol 2009;129(1):71–83
45. Zhang Q, Kong F, Yan B, Ni Z, Liu H. Endoscopic endonasal surgery for clival chordoma and chondrosarcoma. ORL J Otorhinolaryngol Relat Spec 2008;70(2):124–129
46. Wu JC, Huang WC, Cheng H, et al. Endoscopic transnasal transclival odontoidectomy: a new approach to decompression: technical case report. Neurosurgery 2008;63(1, Suppl 1):ONSE92–4, discussion E94
47. Leng LZ, Anand VK, Hartl R, Schwartz TH. Endonasal endoscopic resection of an os odontoideum to decompress the cervicomedullary junction: a minimal access surgical technique. Spine 2009;34(4):E139–E143

27 The Far-Lateral Approach and Its Variations

Nicholas C. Bambakidis, Cliff A. Megerian, and Robert F. Spetzler

A wide variety of surgical approaches has been described for lesions of the clivus, foramen magnum, and the inferior pontomedullary surface of the brainstem. Surgeons must balance the need to visualize the lesion and its surrounding eloquent structures adequately to ensure safe resection against the potential complications each approach entails. Exposure of the skull base in the posterior fossa is generally classified as a posterior or lateral approach (**Fig. 27.1A**). When viewed in the sagittal plane, the options include supratentorial and infratentorial directions (**Fig. 27.1B**). In terms of accessing the anterolateral craniovertebral junction (CVJ), the far-lateral approach[1,2] is the workhorse. Variations such as extreme lateral approaches[3] or the addition of other approaches can then be utilized to increase visualization as needed.

Both the far-lateral transcondylar approach, as described by Heros[4] and modified by Spetzler,[1,2] and the extreme lateral transcondylar approach, as described by Sen and

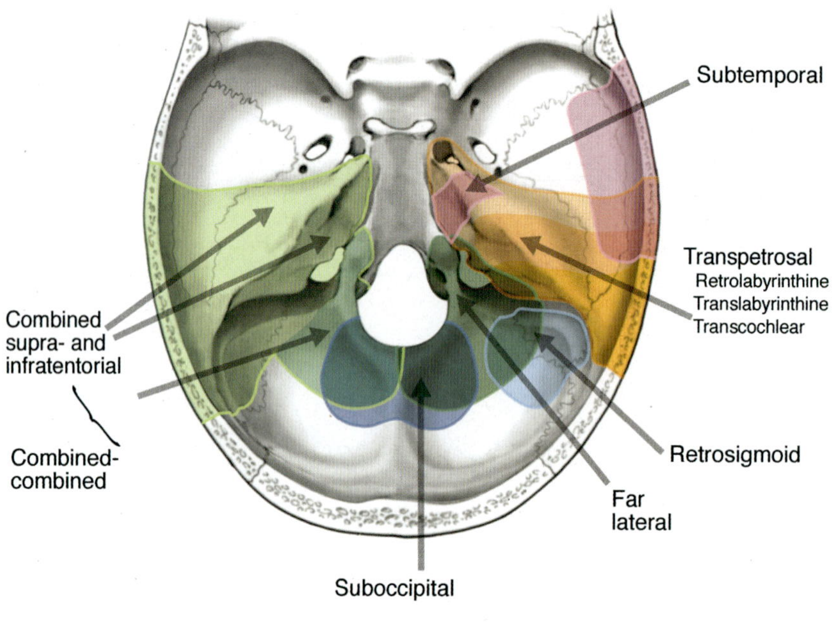

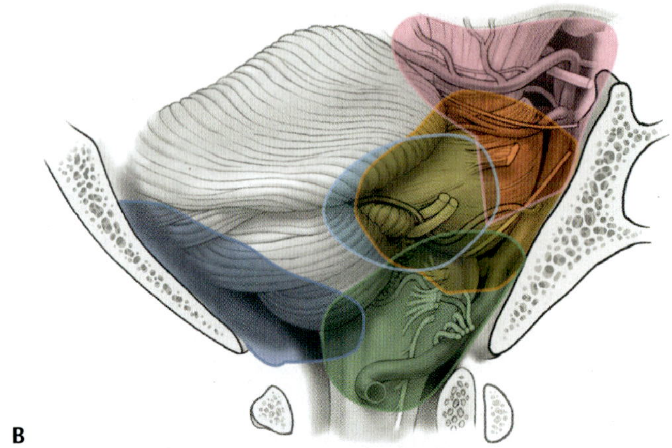

Fig. 27.1 Schematic representation of the surgical approaches to the skull base in the **(A)** axial and **(B)** sagittal planes. These can be broadly classified as posterior or lateral and supra- or infratentorial. (Reprinted with permission from Barrow Neurological Institute.)

Sekhar,[3] provide excellent surgical access to the lower third of the clivus, the pontomedullary junction, and the anterolateral foramen magnum. However, the far-lateral approach has several advantages over the extreme lateral approach. Although both approaches afford a wide lateral approach to the brainstem, the far-lateral approach requires significantly less bone dissection and mobilization of the vertebral artery. Therefore, it requires less time and entails a somewhat lower risk of vascular injury. Although both approaches require expertise with skull base techniques, the far-lateral approach is significantly faster to perform. In our experience, the far-lateral approach also carries a lower risk of cerebrospinal fluid (CSF) leak. Both techniques may be combined with additional cervical or cranial exposure to augment exposure of the petroclival and CVJ regions.[2,5] Because it entails significantly less bone and muscle dissection, the far-lateral approach is also less likely to create instability at the CVJ. Hence, unlike the extreme lateral approach, the far-lateral approach rarely requires subsequent craniovertebral fusion.

The most common indications for the far-lateral approach to the inferior clivus and anterolateral brainstem are neoplastic and vascular lesions. These include aneurysms of the posterior inferior cerebellar artery (PICA) and the confluence of the vertebral artery, cavernous vascular malformations of the brainstem, and tumors anterior to the lower pons and medulla. Meningiomas of the anterior foramen magnum, schwannomas of the lower cranial nerves, and occasionally intramedullary tumors at the CVJ are typical indications.

The far-lateral approach is an extremely versatile skull base technique that may be combined with subtemporal, petrous, and cervical approaches for enhanced exposure of the CVJ.[2] To maximize the exposure and minimize brain retraction, these approaches can be added individually or in combination, depending on the location and size of the lesion.

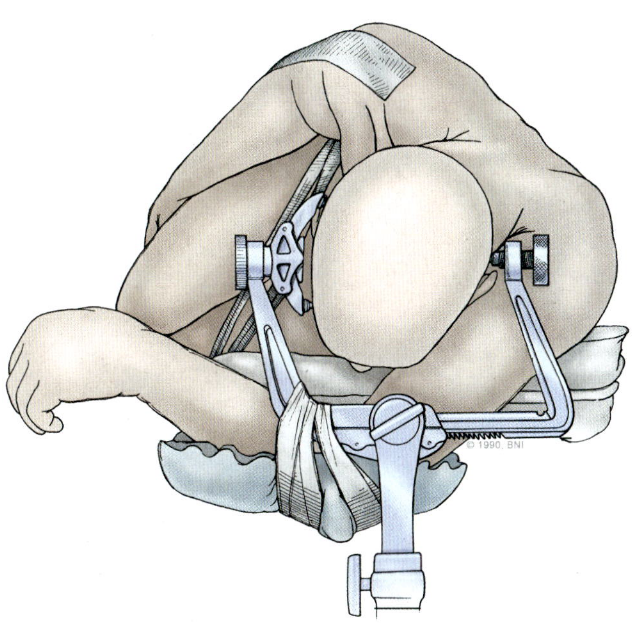

Fig. 27.2 Patient position for the right far-lateral approach. The patient is in a modified park bench position. The head has been secured in a Mayfield head holder after (1) cervical spine flexion in the anteroposterior plane; (2) head rotation 45 degrees to the contralateral side, leaving the mastoid process as the highest point in the operative field; and (3) lateral cervical flexion of 30 degrees toward the opposite shoulder, resulting in the cranial vertex pointing below the horizontal plane. The dependent arm is cradled from the Mayfield head holder and padded with a foam roll. (Reprinted with permission from Barrow Neurological Institute.)

■ Operative Technique

Patient Positioning

Perhaps to an even greater degree than in most cranial base exposures, positioning is critical to the success of the far-lateral approach. Difficulties with angle of approach, venous congestion, and inadequate exposure can be avoided with careful attention to positioning. After intubation and induction of anesthesia, the patient is placed in a modified park bench position. The head is secured with a Mayfield head holder, following three cardinal movements for optimal cranial positioning. First, the cervical spine is flexed in the anteroposterior plane, allowing at least two fingerbreadths between the patient's chin and sternum. Next, the head is rotated 45 degrees to the contralateral side, leaving the mastoid process as the highest point in the operative field. Finally, the cervical spine is flexed laterally 30 degrees toward the opposite shoulder, resulting in the cranial vertex pointing somewhat below the horizontal plane (**Fig. 27.2**). The head in this position places the craniotomy sufficiently inferior to provide generous exposure of the foramen magnum and provides an operating angle of approach that allows a surgical line of sight anterior to the brainstem and directly "up the clivus," which in this position stands almost vertical and inverted, perpendicular to the horizontal plane.[1] If the operative indication requires a combined subtemporal or petrosal exposure, the head may be positioned somewhat more parallel to the floor with the zygomatic arch elevated. The dependent arm should be positioned carefully and padded below the level of the body. The arm hangs independently from the end of the table, which is extended several inches with a ¾-inch plastic sheet. The arm is cradled underneath the edge of the table and attached to the Mayfield head holder with adhesive tape and copious foam padding. Care should be taken to ensure that the arm is not abducted severely. A foam roll is placed beneath the dependent axilla and between the patient's knees. The ipsilateral shoulder is pulled toward the feet and secured, like the entire body, with adhesive tape to allow full rotation of the table (**Fig. 27.3**). The trapezius muscle should be palpated to test its tension so that undue traction that could cause "positioning neural apraxia" can be avoided.

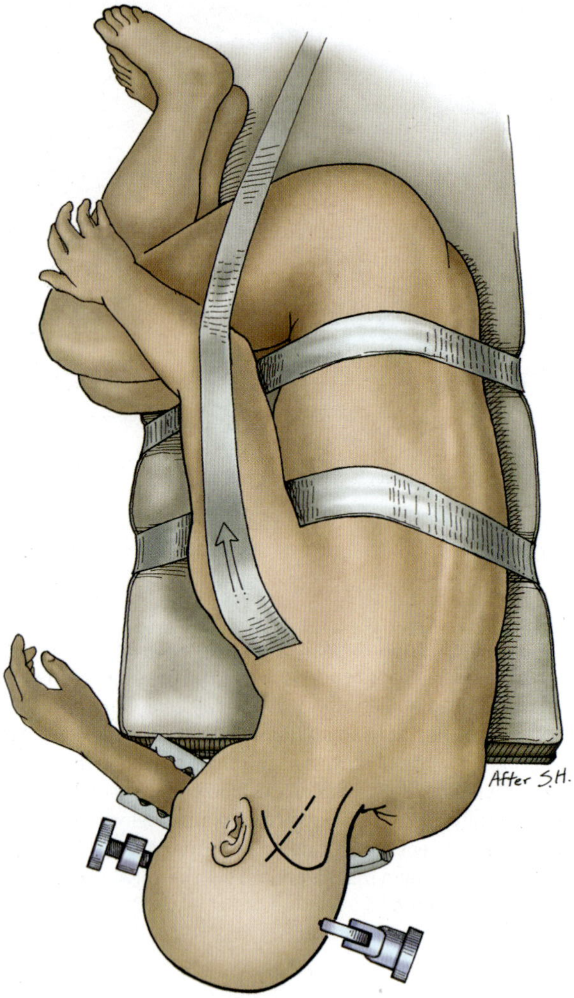

Fig. 27.3 Schematic of a patient positioned for the right lateral approach viewed from above. The right arm is pulled downward and secured with 3-inch tape. This maneuver opens up the cranial cervical angle. The patient is taped securely to the operating room table to permit axial rotation during microscopic dissection. (Modified figure from Baldwin HZ, Miller CG, van Loveren HR, Keller JT, Daspit CP, Spetzler RF. The far lateral/combined supra- and infratentorial approach. J Neurosurg 1994;81:60–68.)

Incision and Initial Soft Tissue Dissection

The opening of the far-lateral approach starts with an inverted hockey stick incision that begins just medial to the tip of the mastoid process and extends up to the superior nuchal line. The incision continues medially along the nuchal line to the midline, where it turns inferiorly down to the level of the C3 to C4 vertebrae (**Fig. 27.4**). A myocutaneous flap is elevated and reflected laterally. A 1-cm cuff of cervicalis fascia and splenius capitis is left attached to the superior nuchal line. Preservation of the osteoligamentous and nuchal attachments permits anatomical muscle reapproximation and helps to reestablish a watertight closure at the end of the procedure. A subperiosteal dissection is performed below the nuchal ligament down to the level of the foramen magnum and over the ipsilateral laminae of the C1 and C2 vertebrae. Identification of the C2 ganglion as it exits above its lamina allows preservation of cervical sensation and upper paraspinous musculature tone. The myocutaneous flap is retracted laterally and downward with the aid of fishhooks on a Leyla bar (Aesculap, San Francisco, CA).

If a subtemporal craniotomy is required, the incision should be modified to begin at the root of the zygoma. It extends superiorly and posteriorly in circumlinear fashion over the pinna and reaches posteromedially to the inion. The myocutaneous flap is dissected in a subperiosteal plane down to the level of the zygoma and the spine of Henle and then is retracted laterally by fishhooks to a Leyla bar.[6] The additional exposure permits petrosal dissection, if necessary.

Vertebral Artery Dissection

As the myocutaneous flap is turned laterally, surgical manipulation should remain in the subperiosteal plane. The vertebral artery, shrouded in its paravertebral venous

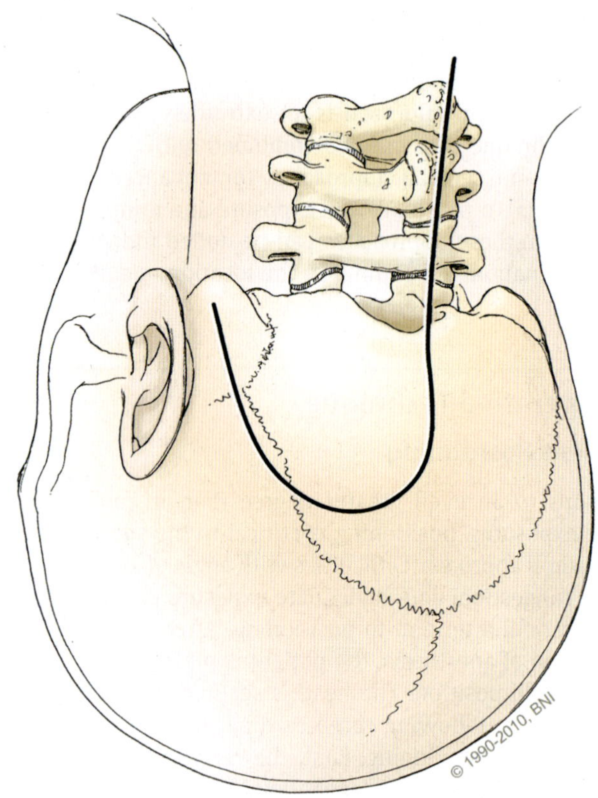

Fig. 27.4 Close-up view of the skin incision for the right far-lateral approach. Incision begins just medial to the tip of the mastoid process, extends up to the superior nuchal line, medial to the inion, and inferiorly to the C3 or C4 spinous process. (Reprinted with permission from Barrow Neurological Institute.)

plexus, is dissected in a subperiosteal plane from the superior lamina of C1 using a Key or an Adson periosteal elevator. The dissection begins at the sulcus arteriosus of the atlas and continues laterally to the foramen transversarium of the lateral mass. Once proximal control of the vertebral artery has been established, the dissection is carried medially to the entry point of the vertebral artery into the dura. It is unnecessary to skeletonize the paravertebral venous plexus off the vertebral artery. Blunt dissection usually provides adequate exposure of the vertebral artery over the atlas. The foramen magnum, the dorsal and ventral surfaces of the atlas, and the ipsilateral atlanto-occipital joint are dissected clean of soft tissue to prepare for the bony resection. The atlanto-occipital membrane may be resected if further dural exposure is desired, such as with a combined approach.

Care should be taken to avoid undue cauterization of the venous plexus around the second portion of the vertebral artery. Venous bleeding should be remedied easily by gentle tamponade with Surgicel strips (Ethicon, Somerville, NJ). Venous hypertension may cause excessive venous bleeding, so care must be taken during positioning to avoid exaggerated neck flexion and rotation. Repetitive use of bipolar cauterization and excessive packing with oxidized cellulose over the paravertebral venous plexus increase the risk of vertebral artery occlusion and usually can be avoided by attention to signs of venous congestion during the initial setup and positioning of the patient.

Craniotomy and Bony Exposure

Using a high-speed drill with a footplate, a hemilaminectomy of C1 is performed from the midline to just lateral to the sulcus arteriosus. The lamina may be replaced at the conclusion of the procedure. Any remaining atlantal bone is removed with the aid of a high-speed drill and a small bone rongeur. The foramen transversarium can then be opened over its dorsal aspect to allow mobilization of the vertebral artery, if necessary. Again, care is taken not to cause undue venous bleeding that would require packing with surgical gauze.

Attention is now turned to the retrosigmoid suboccipital craniotomy. With the same high-speed drill and footplate, the lip of the foramen magnum is used as the initial seating point for the drill bit to perform the craniotomy. With a Penfield no. 1 or Adson periosteal dissector, the condylar vein is carefully dissected away from the foramen magnum before the bone flap is turned. Alternatively, a single burr hole may be placed at the asterion, just lateral and inferior to the junction of the sigmoid and transverse sinuses. Ideally, the craniotomy begins from the foramen magnum lateral to the midline, continues medially up to the sigmoid sinus and jugular tubercle, and terminates at the contralateral aspect of the foramen magnum. If more lateral exposure is required, it can be achieved by use of rongeurs or high-speed drill. If irrigation is constant, the lateral foramen magnum, the posterior half of the occipital condyle, and the superolateral mass and facet of C1 can be removed.

The extracranial cervical vertebral artery (V2) is identified in its surrounding venous plexus and is carefully protected with a small dissector when bone is drilled in this region. Further lateral and ventral exposure may be obtained by drilling the lateral aspect of the foramen magnum to the jugular tubercle (**Fig. 27.5**). Cranial nerve XII lies in the anterior third of the occipital condyle; therefore, the posterior

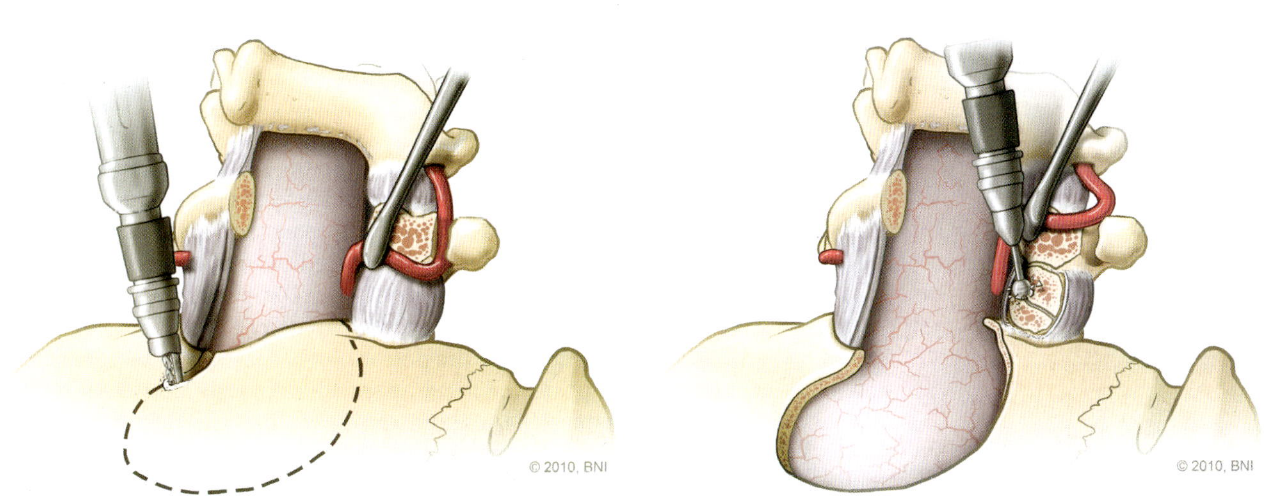

A B

Fig. 27.5 Intraoperative view after soft tissue dissection. The craniotomy is performed initially and incorporates the foramen magnum and removal of the arch of C1 **(A)**. The occipital condyle is then partially removed while the vertebral artery is carefully protected **(B)**. Approximately one-third of the condyle can be safely resected. Landmarks during resection include the condylar vein and hypoglossal canal. (Reprinted with permission from Barrow Neurological Institute.)

two-thirds of the occipital condyle and a medial portion of the superior lateral mass and facet of C1 may be removed with impunity.[7]

As the occipital condyle is removed, brisk venous bleeding heralds entry into the occipital condyle emissary vein. This bleeding can be controlled with judicious application of bone wax and Surgicel surgical gauze. If still greater bony exposure is required for a presigmoid approach, the mastoid process may be removed and the bony drilling carried to the occipital atlantal facet joint. If this joint is entered, however, bony fusion may be required to maintain postoperative stability of the CVJ. Nonetheless, it is this extreme lateral removal of bone from the occipital condyle, jugular tubercle, and the lateral mass of C1 that minimizes brain retraction and maximizes exposure of the anterolateral and inferior brainstem.

Intradural Dissection

The opening of the dura mater begins in the midline of the posterior fossa and extends down to the level of C1. The incision is extended laterally, at a right angle from the midline, toward and below the exposed vertebral artery (**Fig. 27.6**). The superior aspect of the dural incision is extended over the exposed cerebellar hemisphere laterally toward the sigmoid sinus. This exposure permits traction laterally to the level of the sigmoid sinus as well as retraction and mobilization of the proximal intradural vertebral artery. The entire dural flap is retracted inferolaterally and tacked to the surrounding soft tissues (**Fig. 27.6**). The operating microscope should be brought into play for opening the dura to allow early detection of a tethered vertebral artery or an aneurysm adherent to dura. Careful arachnoid dissection and division of the superior dentate ligament allow an inferolateral approach through the veil of cranial nerves VII to XII. This exposure affords an unobstructed view of the inferior clivus, anterolateral medulla, and the cervicomedullary junction. Gentle elevation of the ipsilateral cerebellar tonsil with minimal retraction permits visualization as far rostrally as the pontomedullary junction and vertebrobasilar confluence.[1]

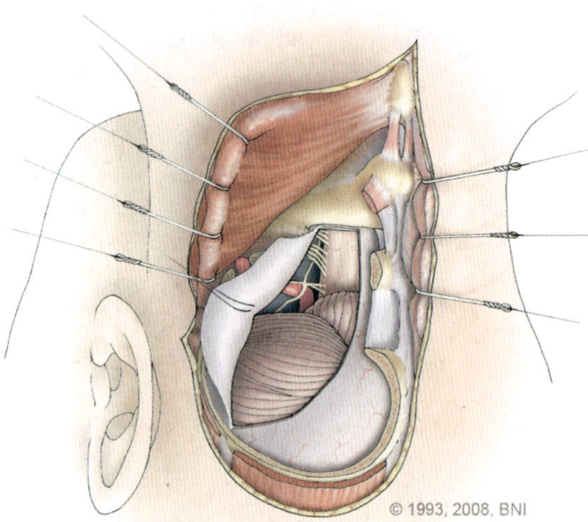

Fig. 27.6 Schematic of intraoperative view of the far-lateral approach after dural opening. The far-lateral suboccipital bone removal permits further lateral retraction of the reflected dura, and exposure of the inferolateral cerebellar hemisphere, inferior clivus, anterolateral medulla, and cervicomedullary junction, with minimal retraction of the vertebral artery or cerebellum. (Reprinted with permission from Barrow Neurological Institute.)

Cranial nerves IX through XII lie dorsal to the vertebral artery, and the ipsilateral origin and J-loop of the posterior inferior cerebellar artery are most often readily visible. Division of the dentate ligament permits gentle rotation of the upper cervical cord and brainstem and improves the anterolateral exposure for surgical manipulation.

The far-lateral approach has several advantages as an approach to the CVJ. First, the extremely flat approach to the clivus provided by removal of the posterior two-thirds of the occipital condyle allows a wide angle view along the cranial base. Second, it provides both proximal and distal control of the vertebral artery and its branches. Third, it offers excellent exposure of the inferior cranial nerves, the C1 and C2 spinal roots, and their relationship to the vertebral artery. Most importantly, this far-lateral approach into the cerebellopontine angle requires minimal, if any, retraction of brain and no retraction of neurovascular structures.

Combined Approaches

The exposure afforded by the far-lateral approach may be augmented with additional skull base approaches (**Fig. 27.7**). This may be done through the traditional curvilinear incision or through a linear paramedian incision. This linear incision can be advantageous as closure is easier to perform and more likely to be cosmetic; additionally, it may be associated with a lower incidence of postoperative pain and neuralgia than the larger hockey stick incision. Because the paramedian incision is located away from localizing midline structures, its use must be accompanied by careful palpation during opening to avoid injury to the vertebral artery.

Removal of the petrous bone through either a mid-fossa or posterior fossa approach offers greater versatility for lesions that extend above the CVJ. The retrolabyrinthine, translabyrinthine, transcochlear,[8–10] and anterior transpetrosal (Kawase)[11] approaches all offer various advantages and disadvantages, which may be tailored to the requirements of the exposure needed and the patient's preexisting neurological deficit. Specifically, the retrolabyrinthine approach[8,12] preserves both the cochlea and

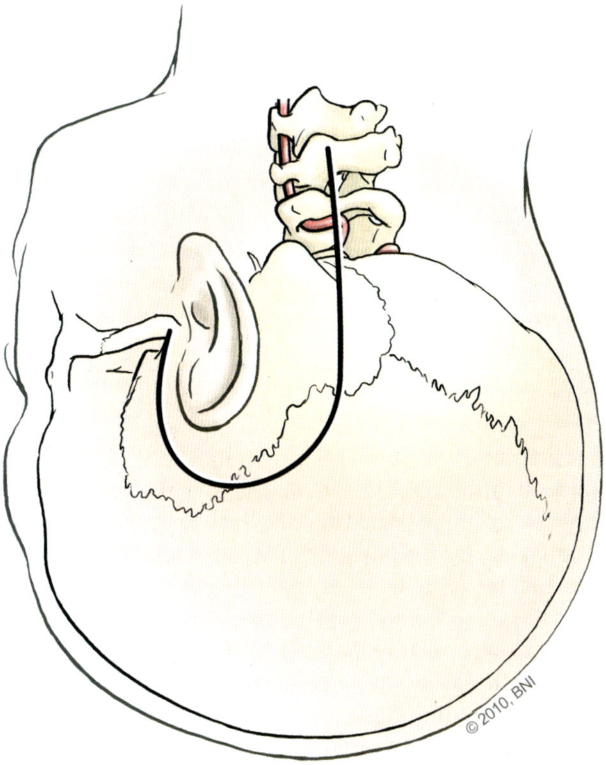

A

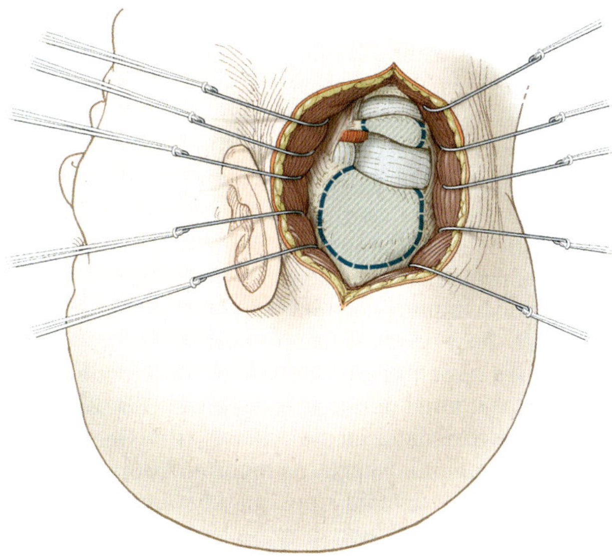

B

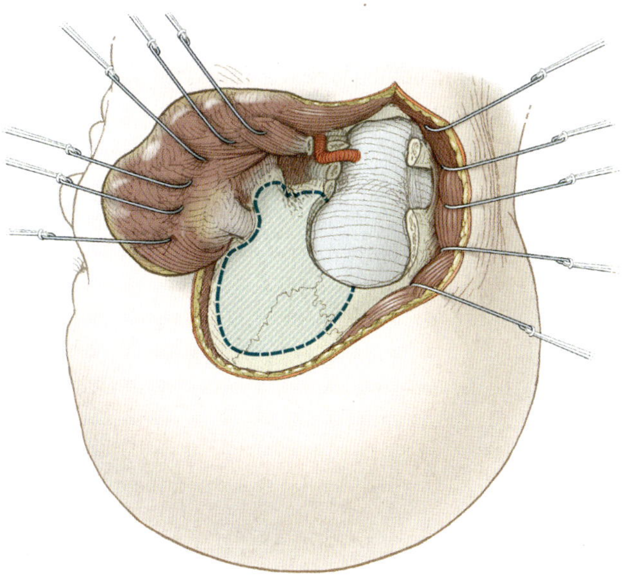

C

Fig. 27.7 Schematic drawing of the craniotomy performed during the far-lateral approach in a combined subtemporal-petrosal procedure. **(A)** In this variation, a linear incision is utilized and may extend below the foramen magnum. The incision can then be extended superiorly in a curvilinear fashion over the pinna to the root of the zygoma, allowing incorporation of a subtemporal craniotomy. **(B)** Using the paramedian muscle-splitting approach allows for exposure of the posterior fossa bone and subsequent bony removal (*dashed line*). The correct surgical orientation is important to maintain during soft tissue dissection to avoid inadvertent injury to the vertebral artery. **(C)** A subtemporal craniotomy (*dashed line*) can be combined with this approach or can be performed in isolation. Preservation of the transverse sinus during bony removal must be maintained. (Reprinted with permission from Barrow Neurological Institute.)

the labyrinth while the mastoidectomy portion of the petrosal resection is performed. This approach allows still greater lateral and superior exposure than the far-lateral approach alone.

The translabyrinthine approach[9] sacrifices hearing but provides an increased lateral, presigmoid approach to the upper brainstem and clivus. When combined with both the translabyrinthine and the Kawase extended middle fossa (transtentorial and anterior transpetrosal) approach,[11] the far-lateral approach affords excellent visualization of the entire lateral brainstem. Addition of the transcochlear approach with mobilization of the facial nerve permits even greater working space with a line of sight anterior to the brainstem and parallel to the clivus.[10]

When the far-lateral approach is combined with the transpetrosal approaches, the dura must be incised over the temporal lobe in the anterior region of the craniotomy. The dural incision is then extended posteriorly and inferiorly to the point where the superior petrosal sinus enters the sigmoid sinus. Care must be taken to avoid injury to the vein of Labbé, which may be either low-lying or attached to the temporal dura or tentorium. The dural opening should include an anterior opening from the jugular bulb to the sinodural angle and along the floor of the middle cranial fossa. The superior petrosal sinus should be cauterized, ligated, and divided so that the dural incision can be extended along the tentorium to the tentorial incisura. Care must be taken to avoid damage to the fourth cranial nerve as it passes along the tentorial edge as it may easily be injured during this maneuver (**Fig. 27.8**). An additional retrosigmoid incision allows still wider access to the cerebellopontine angle. As reported by Spetzler and colleagues,[2,13] the sigmoid sinus may be divided if temporary occlusion does not increase proximal intrasinus pressure by more than 10 mmHg (**Fig. 27.9**). The divided tentorium, posterior temporal lobe, and intact ipsilateral vein of Labbé may then be retracted and elevated superiorly as a single unit. Nevertheless, the venous structures can often be left intact.

Removal of portions of the temporal bone increases exposure to contents of the posterior and middle cranial fossae. Increasing amounts of bony removal translate into progressive increases in visualization but are also accompanied by increasing rates of procedure-related morbidity. They do offer the advantages of minimizing cerebellar retraction and allow for early visualization of the facial and lower cranial nerves. In general, the transtemporal approaches provide direct and superior access to lesions medial to the petrous bone along the length of the clivus. In all variations, the initial step of bony exposure is a mastoidectomy. Meticulous closure with dural patch materials, synthetic sealants, and autologous fat grafts along with postoperative lumbar drainage should be generously utilized to minimize complications.

The translabyrinthine exposure[9] is easily combined with the far-lateral approach to improve exposure of the lateral pontomedullary junction. This approach shortens the working distance in the brainstem while providing adequate exposure of the anterolateral pontomedullary junction without brain retraction. Hearing is inevitably lost with this approach, although, if desired, a less aggressive degree of bony resection sparing the labyrinth may be performed. If the translabyrinthine procedure is used in conjunction with the far-lateral approach, the patient is positioned as for the far-lateral approach but with the head in a less flexed position, almost parallel to the floor. A curved incision is made extending to the root of the zygoma. The ears are reflected anteriorly, and the temporal squama and mastoid processes are cleared of overlying pericranium and muscle. The section continues down to the spine of Henle to avoid entering the external auditory canal. After a complete mastoidectomy has been performed, the bone overlying the sigmoid sinus and adjacent retrosigmoid region is removed with a high-speed drill. Using the operating microscope, the

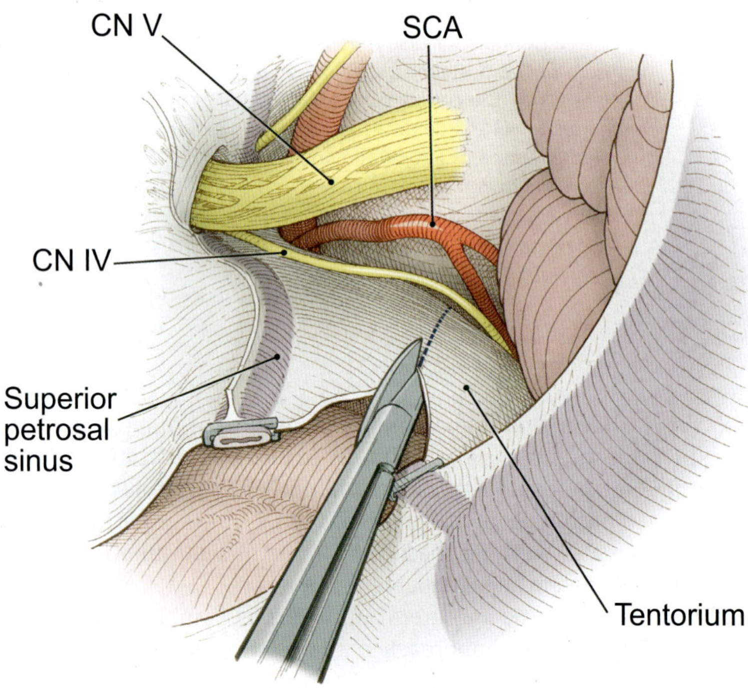

Fig. 27.8 Following ligation of the superior petrosal sinus, further exposure is obtained by dividing the tentorium. This must be done under direct vision while carefully avoiding damage to the trochlear nerve (*CN IV*), which travels just medial to the tentorial border. *CN V*, trigeminal nerve; *SCA*, superior cerebellar artery. (Reprinted with permission from Barrow Neurological Institute.)

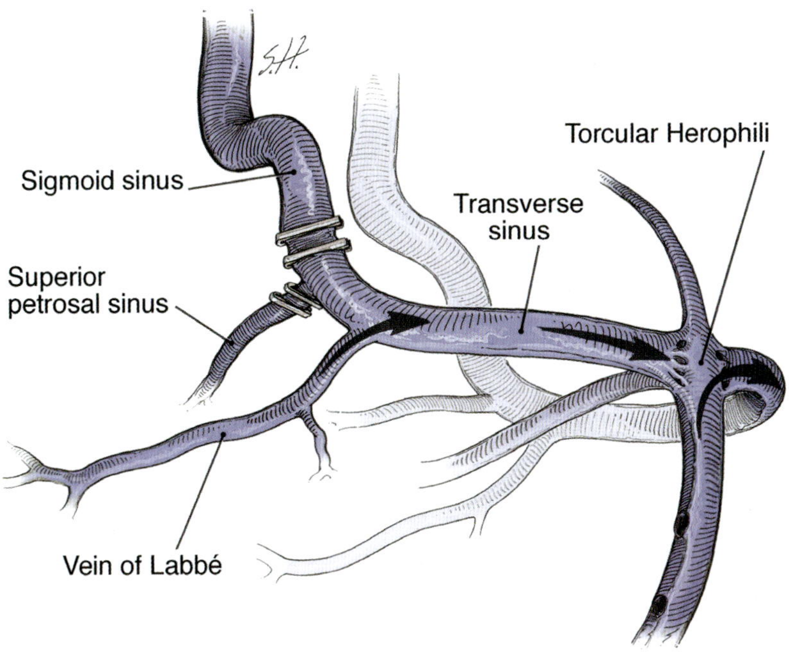

Fig. 27.9 Depiction of the venous sinuses. If ligation of the sigmoid sinus is considered, confirmation of patency of the contralateral jugular venous system must be made. With division of the superior sigmoid sinus and superior petrosal sinus, the vein of Labbé is able to drain through the medial transverse sinus across the torcula and down the transverse sigmoid to the opposite jugular vein. (Reprinted with permission from Barrow Neurological Institute.)

remaining air cells of the mastoid process are removed to the level of the lateral semicircular canal. This critical landmark delineates the location of the facial nerve, which is immediately inferior to the canal and parallel to its anterior border.[9] The mastoid portion of the facial nerve is identified, and a thin layer of bone is left over the nerve for its protection. After a labyrinthectomy has been performed (**Fig. 27.10**) the dura may be opened, providing a view of the facial nerve in its intracanalicular and subarachnoid segments.

Transcochlear Approach

Further expansion of the translabyrinthine approach may be performed through removal of the external auditory canal and middle ear along with further exposure of the extended facial recess.[9] This approach provides the widest avenue to the clivus and anterior brainstem. To accomplish the transcochlear or transotic approach, the normal dissection that occurs with the translabyrinthine bony extirpation is completed. Once this is accomplished, the facial nerve is skeletonized to the level of the stylomastoid foramen. Next, the external auditory canal skin and tympanic membrane are removed and the ear canal is oversewn. The ossicular chain is inspected, and the malleus and incus are removed as the posterior canal wall is lowered to the level of the facial nerve with diamond burrs. At this point, the thin bone over the fallopian canal is removed with a small diamond drill to the level of the geniculate ganglion. To accomplish the transcochlear approach, the nerve is mobilized from the fallopian canal and extratemporally via a parotid gland dissection and rotated anteriorly. The skeletonized facial nerve is transposed after the chordae tympani and the greater superficial petrosal nerves have been divided, affording unencumbered access to the entire cochlea, which is drilled away and gives exposure and access to the carotid artery, jugular bulb, and petrous apex for lesions such as large glomus tumors. The base of the cochlea is then drilled away, removing the stapes. This step allows identification of the internal carotid artery anteriorly and the jugular bulb inferiorly and exposes a triangular window of dura mater adjacent to the internal auditory canal and to the anterior petrous tip and clivus. Removal of the additional bone exposes the most anterior extent of the cerebellopontine angle. The disadvantage of this approach is postoperative facial paresis, which is often permanent.[10]

To avoid mobilization of the facial nerve and the potential facial nerve weakness that accompanies the mobilization maneuver, the transotic approach can be used where the nerve is left in situ. The cochlea can still be removed but needs to be approached anteriorly and posteriorly to the nerve as it remains in the fallopian canal. Completing the transcochlear exposure allows for the widest possible view of the posterior fossa contents (**Fig. 27.11**).

The far-lateral approach is best applied to lesions ventral and lateral to the medulla and lower half of the pons. Larger lesions that extend from the region of the upper clivus and mesencephalon down to the CVJ require the combined far-lateral and supra- and infratentorial approach. One must remember that, in performing such complex skull base approaches, there are several opportunities to

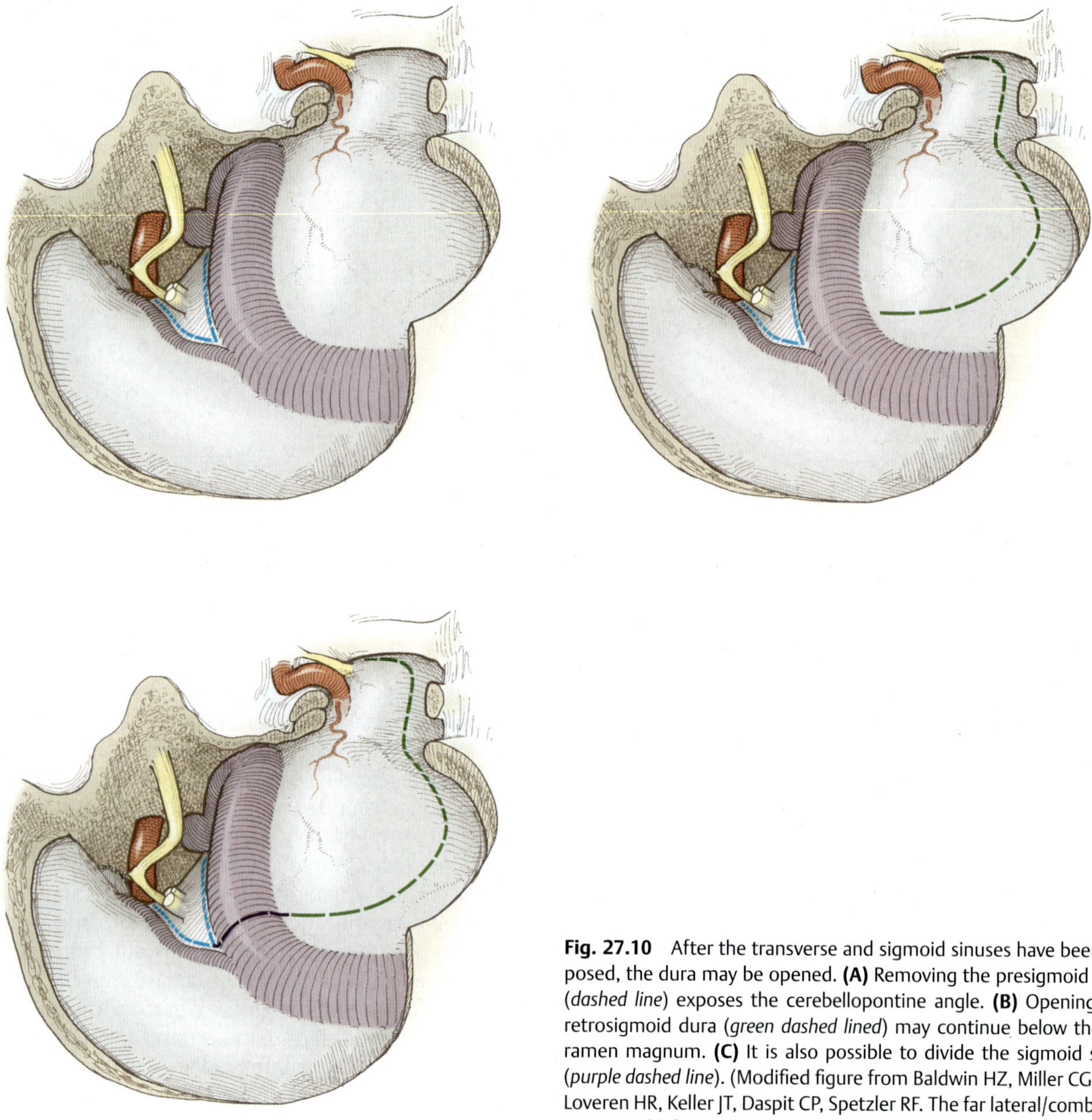

A

B

C

Fig. 27.10 After the transverse and sigmoid sinuses have been exposed, the dura may be opened. **(A)** Removing the presigmoid dura (*dashed line*) exposes the cerebellopontine angle. **(B)** Opening the retrosigmoid dura (*green dashed lined*) may continue below the foramen magnum. **(C)** It is also possible to divide the sigmoid sinus (*purple dashed line*). (Modified figure from Baldwin HZ, Miller CG, van Loveren HR, Keller JT, Daspit CP, Spetzler RF. The far lateral/combined supra- and infratentorial approach. J Neurosurg 1994;81:60–68.)

avoid complications (**Table 27.1**). Each approach has advantages in terms of extent of exposure as well as risks of injury to hearing and cranial nerve function and other complications, such as CSF leak (**Table 27.2**).[14–17] Positioning the patient is crucial and helps to provide a flat approach to the clivus and anterolateral brainstem. However, overzealous lateral and anterior flexion of the neck may cause venous hypertension, which may exacerbate bleeding from the paravertebral venous plexus. Hence, the head must be flexed laterally only 30 degrees and rotated no more than 45 degrees toward the contralateral shoulder. Care must also be taken to ensure that the incision over the medial tip of the mastoid bone is sufficiently lateral to expose the petrous bone adequately for drilling. Also critical for the success of this exposure is meticulous handling of the arterial dissection. The vertebral artery must not be compressed unduly during venous bleeding. Similarly, excessive use of bipolar cauterization, which may permanently injure the vertebral artery, should be avoided. During bony exposure, the anterior third of the occipital

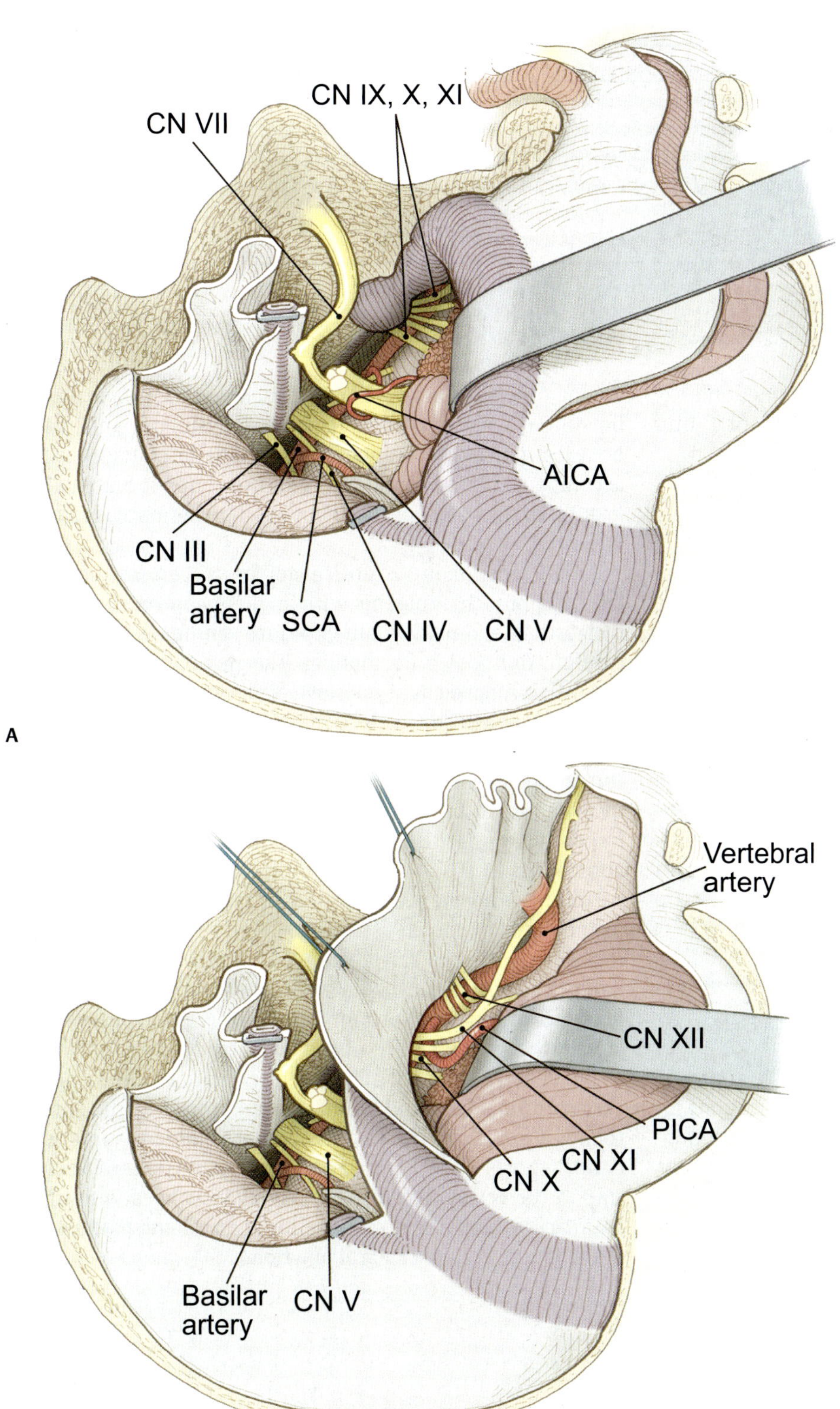

Fig. 27.11 Exposure of the posterior fossa contents following combined skull base approaches. Although ligation of the venous sinuses may be safely performed, sequential movement of the operating microscope and judicious retraction of the sigmoid sinus **(A)** posteriorly or **(B)** anteriorly often provides excellent visualization. This strategy minimizes the risk of venous injury and infarction. *AICA*, anterior inferior cerebellar artery; *CN*, cranial nerve; *PICA*, posterior inferior cerebellar artery; *SCA*, superior cerebellar artery. (Reprinted with permission from Barrow Neurological Institute.)

Table 27.1 Strategies to Avoid Complications with the Far-Lateral Approach

	Comment
Positioning	Provides flat approach and avoids venous hypertension
Vertebral artery section	Meticulous handling, avoidance of excessive venous bleeding tamponade, and avoidance of excessive bipolar coagulation of the perivertebral plexus prevent vascular injury.
Bony exposure	Remain in the posterior two-thirds of the occipital condyle to avoid cranial nerve XII and to avoid destabilization of the occipitoatlantal joint.
Closure	Aided by fat graft, lumbar drain, and multiple-layer myocutaneous flap closure

condyle, the otic structures of the petrous bone, and excessive destabilizing removal of the occipitoatlantal joint must be avoided.

Closure

Abdominal fat grafts are harvested to fill anatomical dead space in the region of the petrous bone resection. The dura is closed with dural graft or fascia lata, cadaveric dura, or temporalis fascia. Fibrin glue may be used as an additional CSF sealant. Bone plates from the subtemporal and suboccipital craniotomy are secured in their original location as is the arch of C1. The wound is closed in multiple layers, and the nuchal and temporalis muscles are reapproximated and secured to their respective ligamentous cuffs. Postoperative lumbar drainage is routinely utilized following combined skull base approaches in cases where the mastoid air cells and middle ear contents are encountered.

Conclusion

The far-lateral approach is often the most suitable approach for lesions of the anterolateral CVJ. Common indications for this approach to the inferior clivus and anterolateral brainstem include aneurysms of PICA and the vertebral artery, cavernous malformations of the brainstem, and tumors anterior to the lower pons and medulla (e.g., foramen magnum meningiomas and lower cranial nerve schwannomas), among others. Typically, a large curvilinear incision is used, but often a linear paramedian incision suffices and may be a less morbid technique. The extreme lateral approach accompanied by vertebral artery transposition is one modification to the basic approach but in our experience is rarely indicated.

Patient positioning is critical to the success of the far-lateral approach. Problems with angle of approach, venous congestion, and inadequate exposure can be avoided with careful attention to positioning. The risk of postoperative CSF leak is reduced by subperiosteal elevation and closure of a myocutaneous flap, watertight dural closure, and replacement of the bone flap. Exposure is enhanced most simply by retraction of the myocutaneous flap laterally and downward by fishhooks to a Leyla bar, but it is augmented, if necessary, by combination with the middle fossa and/or transtemporal approaches.

Drilling from the lateral aspect of the foramen magnum to the jugular tubercle is a critical step to assure maximal exposure with the far-lateral craniotomy. The posterior half of the occipital condyle is removed with a high-speed diamond drill under constant irrigation, as cranial nerve XII lays in the anterior third of the occipital condyle. Division of the dentate ligament allows gentle rotation of the upper cervical spinal cord and brainstem and improves the anterolateral exposure. The vertebrobasilar confluence, inferior cranial nerves, and C1 and C2 spinal roots and their relationship to the vertebral artery are readily visualized with this approach, which is a workhorse for approaching pathology in the lateral craniovertebral junction.

Table 27.2 Features of Posterior Petrosectomy Approaches

Approach	Hearing Preservation	Risk to Facial Nerve	Risk of CSF Leak	Extent of Exposure
Retrolabyrinthine	Possible	Minimal	Low	Least
Translabyrinthine	No	Minimal	Moderate	Mid
Transcochlear	No	High	Moderate	Most

Source: Bambakidis NC, Gonzalez LF, Amin-Hanjani S, et al. Combined skull base approaches to the posterior fossa. Technical note. Neurosurg Focus 2005;19(2):E8. Reprinted with permission.
Abbreviations: CSF, cerebrospinal fluid.

References

1. Spetzler RF, Grahm TW. The far lateral approach to the inferior clivus and the upper cervical region. Technical note. BNI Q 1990;6(4):35–38
2. Spetzler RF, Daspit CP, Pappas CTE. The combined supra- and infratentorial approach for lesions of the petrous and clival regions: experience with 46 cases. J Neurosurg 1992;76(4):588–599
3. Sen CN, Sekhar LN. An extreme lateral approach to intradural lesions of the cervical spine and foramen magnum. Neurosurgery 1990;27(2):197–204
4. Heros RC. Lateral suboccipital approach for vertebral and vertebrobasilar artery lesions. J Neurosurg 1986;64(4):559–562
5. Sen CN, Sekhar LN. Surgical management of anteriorly placed lesions at the craniocervical junction—an alternative approach. Acta Neurochir (Wien) 1991;108(1–2):70–77
6. Spetzler RF. Two technical notes for microsurgery. BNI Q 1988;4(2):38–39
7. de Oliveira E, Rhoton AL Jr, Peace D. Microsurgical anatomy of the region of the foramen magnum. Surg Neurol 1985;24(3):293–352
8. Hitselberger WE, House WF. A combined approach to the cerebellopontine angle. A suboccipital-petrosal approach. Arch Otolaryngol 1966;84(3):267–285
9. House WF. Translabyrinthine approach. In House WF, Luetje CM, eds. Acoustic Tumors. Baltimore, MD: University Park Press; 1979:43–87
10. House WF, Hitselberger WE. The transcochlear approach to the skull base. Arch Otolaryngol 1976;102(6):334–342
11. Kawase T, Toya S, Shiobara R, Mine T. Transpetrosal approach for aneurysms of the lower basilar artery. J Neurosurg 1985;63(6):857–861
12. Giannotta SL, Maceri DR. Retrolabyrinthine transsigmoid approach to basilar trunk and vertebrobasilar artery junction aneurysms. Technical note. J Neurosurg 1988;69(3):461–466
13. Wascher TM, Spetzler RF. Surgical approaches to lesions involving the brain stem. BNI Q 1992;8(4):19–28
14. Bambakidis NC, Kakarla UK, Kim LJ, et al. Evolution of surgical approaches in the treatment of petroclival meningiomas: a retrospective review. Neurosurgery 2007;61(5, Suppl 2):202–209, discussion 209–211
15. Gonzalez LF, Amin-Hanjani S, Bambakidis NC, Spetzler RF. Skull base approaches to the basilar artery. Neurosurg Focus 2005;19(2):E3
16. Bambakidis NC, Gonzalez LF, Amin-Hanjani S, et al. Combined skull base approaches to the posterior fossa. Technical note. Neurosurg Focus 2005;19(2):E8
17. Bambakidis NC, Safavi-Abbasi S, Spetzler RF. Combined surgical approaches. In: Bambakidis NC, Megerian CA, Spetzler RF, eds. Surgery of the Cerebellopontine Angle. Shelton, CT: BC Decker Inc/PMPH; 2009

28 The Transpetrosal Approaches

C. Phillip Daspit and Peter A. Weisskopf

The addition of neurotologic surgical techniques in the care of skull base diseases existing at the craniovertebral junction (CVJ) has significantly improved rates of morbidity and mortality in patients undergoing surgical treatment.

The CVJ is a small, restricted area encased in dense bone, making access challenging. The subarachnoid space is limited and filled with cranial nerve and vascular structures that can also limit access. Surgical treatment of CVJ lesions emphasizes maximizing surgical exposure of the pathology while minimizing brain retraction. Various surgical approaches are available to deal with lesions in different locations (**Table 28.1**) and include the transpetrosal,[1–3] combined supra- and infratentorial,[4,5] and far-lateral[6,7] approaches. These approaches often require the combined talents of a neurosurgeon well trained in vascular techniques, a neurotologic surgeon well versed in all transpetrosal approaches, and sometimes a craniofacial surgeon well versed in skull disassembly/reassembly techniques.

This chapter details the transpetrosal approach as performed at the Barrow Neurological Institute and explains how to combine these approaches with a supra-infratentorial craniotomy or far-lateral suboccipital approach to gain even more exposure. These procedures are performed by a team and require rapid removal of the temporal bone structures so that the neurosurgical aspects of the procedure can be completed in a reasonable time. The neurotologic surgeons should maintain technical expertise either by performing these operations frequently or by dissecting anatomical temporal bone specimens frequently.

■ Transpetrosal Approaches

The anterior brainstem, clivus, and CVJ can be accessed through the temporal bone. The entire exposure can be obtained by removing bone without retracting the brain or brainstem. More than one approach can be used, depending on the type of lesion and the amount of space needed to work safely. At times, the sacrifice of hearing is necessary to provide adequate exposure. Very large lesions can require transposition of the facial nerve, with a corresponding temporary facial paralysis. The potential for these complications demands a detailed discussion of the risks and benefits with the patient and family members.

There are three basic types of temporal (petrous) bone dissections. The most limited dissection is the extended retrolabyrinthine technique, which removes a large portion of the temporal bone but preserves the otic capsule (**Fig. 28.1**). This approach does not sacrifice hearing and offers limited exposure due to the overhanging semicircular canals. In comparison, the translabyrinthine technique removes more temporal bone and sacrifices hearing (**Fig. 28.2**). The most extensive modification is the transcochlear technique, which involves maximal removal of the temporal bone, sacrifices hearing (**Fig. 28.3**), and transposes the facial nerve. Moving through these three variations of surgical exposure gradually increases the amount of temporal (petrous) bone resection and, concomitantly, the exposure of the brainstem, clivus, and CVJ. These approaches can be combined with a supra-infratentorial craniotomy (i.e., combined approach) (**Fig. 28.4**) as well as a far-lateral approach (**Fig. 28.5**) if necessary to provide additional exposure of the skull base. The translabyrinthine and transcochlear approaches have the advantage of wide exposure of the cerebellopontine angle without extensive cerebellar retraction as well as access to the facial nerve in an area uninvolved with tumor.

Patient Positioning

Typically, the patient is positioned supine. The head is parallel to the floor, inclined slightly downward and flexed onto the opposite shoulder, and fixed to the operating table with a Mayfield three-pin head holder. A soft roll may be placed under the ipsilateral shoulder to provide support if necessary. In this position, the temporal bone can be dissected quickly and easily. Of note, the extreme rotation of the neck, which is advantageous for retrosigmoid approaches, is not necessary. Occasionally, however, the patient must be placed in the park bench position for the far-lateral position.[8] The neurotologist must become facile with far-lateral positioning because the usual relationships among bony landmarks and soft tissue are altered.

Table 28.1 Transpetrous and Modified Transpetrous Exposures

Transpetrosal Approaches	Combined Supra- and Infratentorial Approaches	Far-Lateral Combined Supra- and Infratentorial Approaches
Retrolabyrinthine	Retrolabyrinthine	Retrolabyrinthine
Translabyrinthine	Translabyrinthine	Translabyrinthine
Transcochlear	Transcochlear	Transcochlear

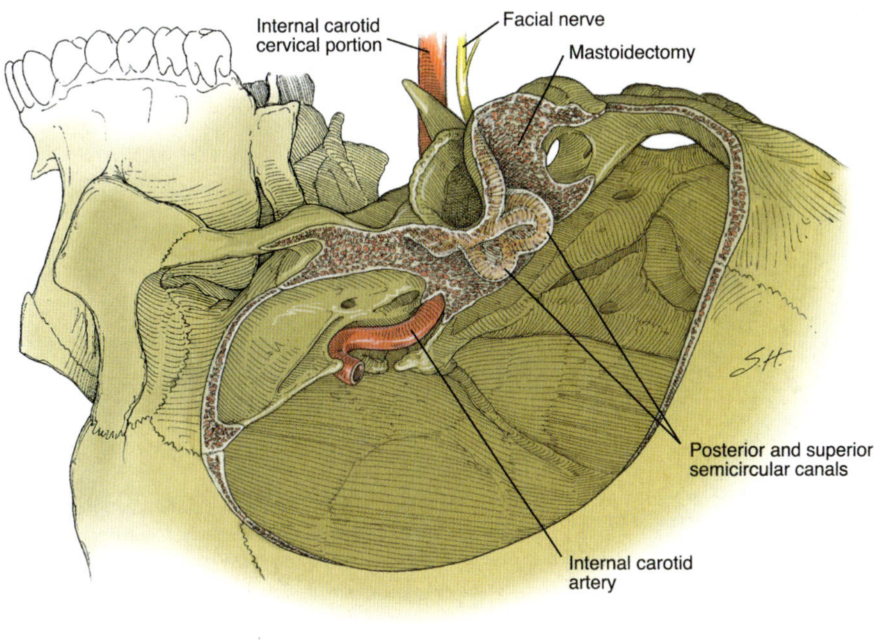

Fig. 28.1 The extended retrolabyrinthine approach consists of mastoidectomy and skeletonization of the semicircular canals. (Reprinted with permission from Barrow Neurological Institute.)

Skin Incision and Temporal Bone Drilling

The skin incision begins just in front of the auricle and continues in a gentle curving fashion around the auricle and into the upper neck behind the mastoid tip. Once the temporal and occipital bones are exposed, fish hooks attached to Leyla bars on both sides of the operating table allow generous room in which to work. The temporal squama, external auditory meatus, mastoid region, and bone overlying the foramen magnum are exposed. The temporal bone dissection is performed using the operating microscope, continuous suction irrigation, and a high-speed drill of the surgeon's choice.

Extended Retrolabyrinthine Approach

This technique is useful for small tumors or vestibular nerve sections for intractable vertigo, allowing access to the cerebellopontine angle while preserving hearing. Initially, bone is removed rapidly, exposing the sigmoid sinus, sinodural angle, and the tegmen plate. Bone must be removed at least 2 cm behind the sigmoid sinus. All dural surfaces as well as

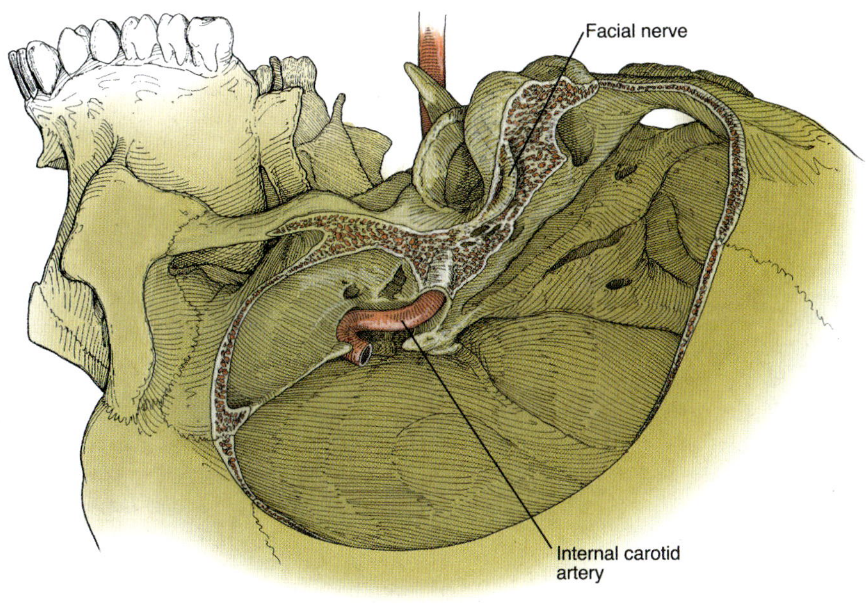

Fig. 28.2 The translabyrinthine approach removes the semicircular canals and skeletonizes the descending segment of the facial nerve and internal auditory canal. (Reprinted with permission from Barrow Neurological Institute.)

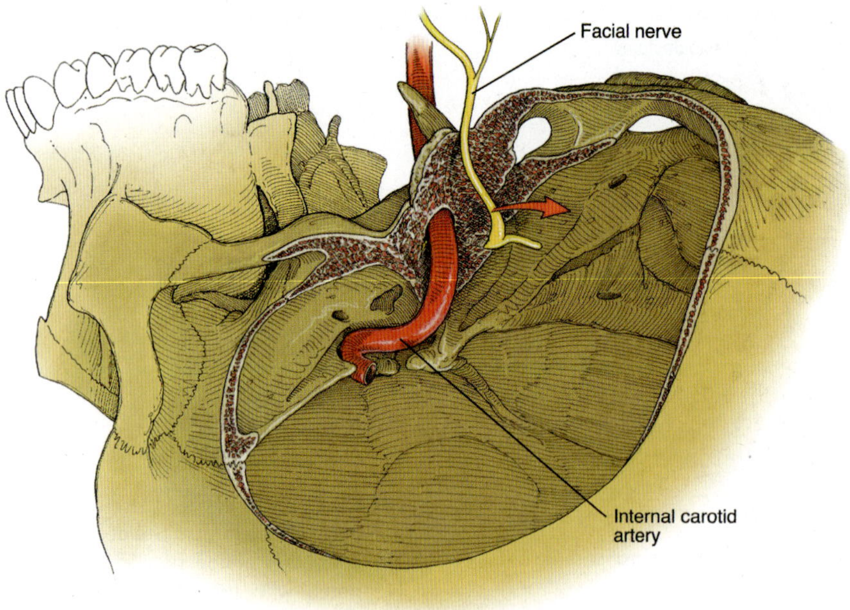

Fig. 28.3 The transcochlear approach requires transposition of the facial nerve posteriorly and removal of the cochlea. (Reprinted with permission from Barrow Neurological Institute.)

the sigmoid and superior petrosal sinuses are exposed using cutting and diamond burrs. A word of caution: Do not drill on the sinus wall with rough-cut or super-cut diamond burrs because they will perforate the sinus. The endolymphatic sac and duct, which lie in the dura in front of the lower portion of the sigmoid sinus, are identified. The posterior, superior, and horizontal semicircular canals are dissected by removing as much bone as possible without penetrating the canals (**Fig. 28.1**). It is important to remove bone underneath the crus commune (the junction of the posterior and superior canals). Bone along the tegmen is removed up to the heads of the malleus and incus but not beyond to prevent the brain from collapsing onto the ossicles. Otherwise, a conductive hearing loss could occur. In this manner, the dura can be exposed maximally without sacrificing hearing. This exposure is rarely used with CVJ lesions.

Translabyrinthine Approach

This approach permits greater exposure but at the expense of hearing. The initial approach is performed as described for the retrolabyrinthine approach, but all three semicircular (balance) canals are removed completely as is all bone from the posterior 270 degrees of the internal auditory canal

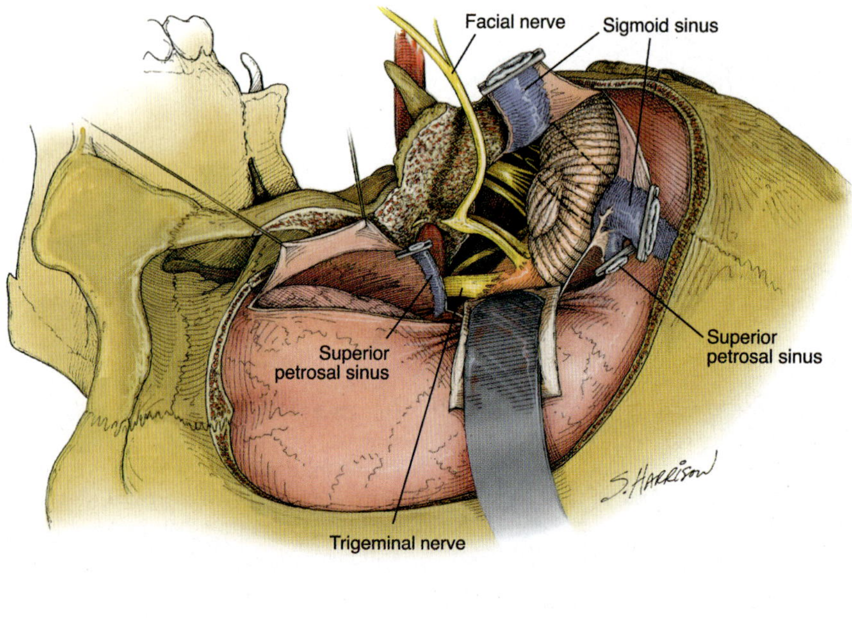

Fig. 28.4 The dural incision for the combined supra- and infratentorial approach crosses the superior petrosal sinus below where it enters the sigmoid sinus and then crosses the sigmoid sinus. The sigmoid sinus can be preserved by extending the dural incision inferiorly in front of the sinus. Incising the tentorium medially to the tentorial incisura exposes the cranial nerves, brainstem, vasculature, and clivus. Note that the sigmoid sinus has been divided. (Reprinted with permission from Barrow Neurological Institute.)

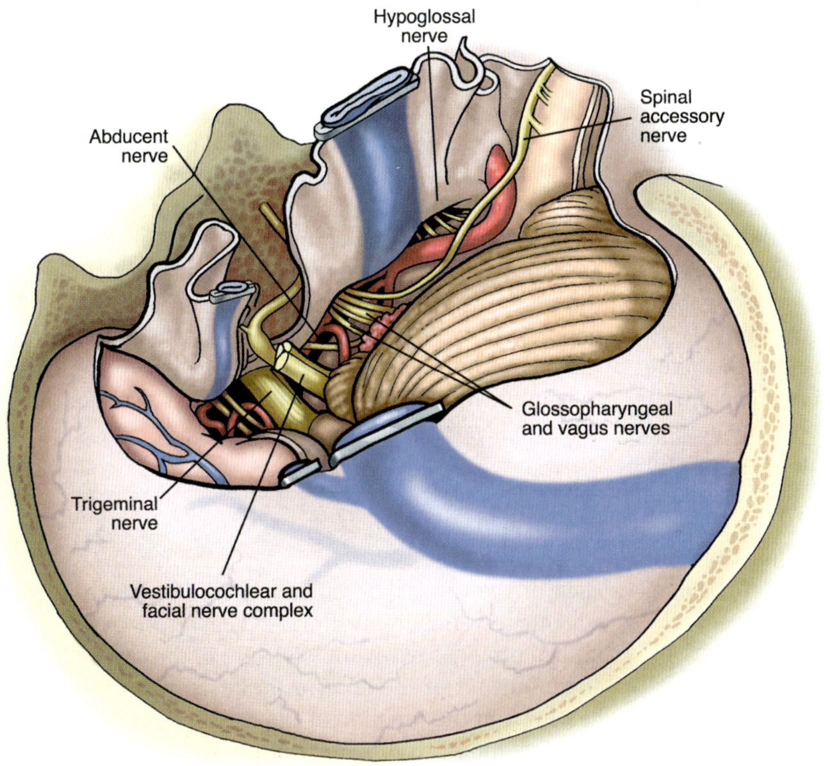

Fig. 28.5 The dural opening for the far-lateral, combined supra- and infratentorial ("combined-combined") approach. Alternatively, the dura can be opened in two flaps in front of and behind the sigmoid sinus to preserve this structure. Note that a transcochlear drilling was used with this approach. (From Baldwin HZ, Miller CG, van Loveren HR, et al. The far lateral/combined supra- and infratentorial approach. A human cadaveric prosection model for routes of access to the petroclival region and ventral brain stem. J Neurosurg 1994;81:60–68. Reprinted with permission from *Journal of Neurosurgery*.)

from the vestibule laterally to the porus acusticus medially (**Fig. 28.2**). The dissection removes the bone overlying the jugular bulb inferiorly, all bone overlying the posterior fossa as far anteriorly as the cochlear aqueduct, and bone anterosuperiorly over the internal auditory canal. This approach provides excellent exposure of the cerebellopontine angle once the dura is opened. Removal of bone overlying the mastoid segment of the facial nerve from the second genu to the stylomastoid foramen helps create space in which to work in the depths of the opening. The superior vestibular nerve in the lateral end of the internal auditory canal is identified as well as the vertical crest that separates the facial nerve anteriorly from the superior vestibular nerve posteriorly. The facial nerve in the labyrinthine segment is exposed using diamond bits under saline irrigation with continuous intraoperative facial electromyography (EMG).

Compared with the retrolabyrinthine approach, the translabyrinthine approach provides a more direct anterolateral approach to the cerebellopontine angle and provides greater exposure of the anterolateral brainstem, clivus, and CVJ. However, this exposure is obtained at the expense of hearing and an increased risk of cerebrospinal fluid (CSF) leakage. The degree of exposure needed must be balanced against the potential for these complications. The patient and family must understand that the extra exposure is frequently required to treat difficult lesions and that the unilateral loss of hearing is a reasonable compromise when lesions are large or hearing is already compromised. The ability to identify the facial nerve intact and uninvolved with tumor can make preservation of facial function much more likely. The hearing loss can easily be compensated by fitting the patient with a contralateral routing of signal hearing aid system, bone anchored hearing aid or Ponto (a surgically implanted bone conduction hearing device; Oticon Medical, Askim, Sweden), or other type of bone conduction hearing aid.

Transcochlear Approach

For maximum exposure via the temporal bone, the facial nerve must be transposed posteriorly and all bone of the petrous apex removed (**Fig. 28.3**). The external auditory canal is transected and oversewn in two layers. Although this appears to be a simple procedure, it can be quite time consuming to do correctly, and CSF leakage from the ear canal can be a devastating complication that is difficult to correct. The initial bone removal is identical to the translabyrinthine approach. The tympanic segment of the temporal bone is drilled away, allowing skeletonization of the facial nerve in the tympanic and mastoid segments. The anterior limit of the dissection is the periosteum of the temporal mandibular joint laterally and the horizontal segment of the carotid artery medially. Continuous EMG monitoring of the facial nerve during decompression minimizes trauma to the nerve. Once all bone has been removed from the nerve, transection of the greater superficial petrosal nerve permits the facial nerve to be elevated from its bony canal. The dura of the internal auditory canal is dissected free and used to protect the facial nerve during its mobilization posteriorly. Once the nerve is out of the way, it is protected with a piece of metal foil from a suture pack. The remaining temporal bone, including the cochlea down to the clivus, is removed rapidly, which can be relatively bloody because of the frequent venous channels. Intermittent packing with bone wax and the use of diamond burrs can improve visualization and decrease blood loss. The dura of the middle and posterior fossae is expanded, and the entire sinus is visualized. The jugular bulb is exposed completely, but injury to the lower cranial nerves in the jugular foramen must be avoided.

The transcochlear approach provides the greatest amount of exposure, furnishing a very flat angle of approach to the clivus and CVJ with excellent exposure of both the anterior and anterolateral aspects of the brainstem. However, this vast exposure is created at the expense of hearing and an increased risk of facial nerve paresis or paralysis. In addition, the risk of CSF leakage is high. Again, however, this additional exposure can be an essential aspect of the management of difficult lesions in the skull base.

Intradural Exposure

The dura mater is incised just inferior and parallel to the superior petrosal sinus and just superior to the jugular bulb. These two dural incisions meet at the sinodural angle and the porus acusticus. This exposure allows easy entry into the cerebellopontine angle.

Closure

Closure is accomplished in anatomical layers, with the dura reapproximated with 4–0 braided nylon sutures. A watertight closure is attempted but is rarely possible to achieve. Abdominal adipose tissue, temporalis muscle, and NuKnit (Ethicon, Somerville, NJ) are used to obliterate the eustachian tube (translabyrinthine, transcochlear approaches) and the void created by the temporal bone dissection. The fat is packed carefully in any residual dural clefts to prevent CSF leakage. Titanium mesh cranioplasty will help to maintain pressure on the packing to promote leak-free healing. When placing the cranioplasty, use only the minimal amount necessary to cover the defect. Overhanging edges can erode into the ear canal or hinder later placement of bone anchored hearing appliance abutments. In addition, temporary lumbar spinal drainage is used for several days to help prevent CSF leakage. A standard closure of the facial and skin layers is performed.

Conclusion

Each of the three different temporal bone techniques has advantages and disadvantages. The retrolabyrinthine approach provides excellent exposure of the cerebellopontine angle but not of the anterior brainstem. It preserves both hearing and the function of the facial nerve. The translabyrinthine approach provides additional exposure of the cerebellopontine angle and significantly improves exposure of the anterolateral and anterior brainstem. Additionally, it gives an excellent view of the facial nerve at its labyrinthine segment, prior to involvement with tumor. However, the exposure is accomplished at the expense of hearing and an increased risk of CSF leakage. The transcochlear approach furnishes the maximal exposure possible with an extremely flat angle of approach to the clivus and CVJ. This approach is associated with some disadvantages of the translabyrinthine approach, and facial nerve paresis or paralysis can be expected.

References

1. Al-Mefty O, Fox JL, Smith RR. Petrosal approach for petroclival meningiomas. Neurosurgery 1988;22(3):510–517
2. House WF. Translabyrinthine approach. In: House WF, Leutje CM, eds. Acoustic Tumors, Volume 2: Management. Baltimore, MD: University Park Press; 1979:43–87
3. House WF, Hitselberger WE. The transcochlear approach to the skull base. Arch Otolaryngol 1976;102(6):334–342
4. Spetzler RF, Daspit CP, Pappas CTE. The combined supra- and infratentorial approach for lesions of the petrous and clival regions: experience with 46 cases. J Neurosurg 1992;76(4):588–599
5. Daspit CP, Spetzler RF. The petrosal approach. In: Brackmann DE, Shelton C, Arriaga M, eds. Otologic Surgery. Philadelphia, PA: WB Saunders; 1994:667–689
6. Heros RC. Lateral suboccipital approach for vertebral and vertebrobasilar artery lesions. J Neurosurg 1986;64(4):559–562
7. Sen CN, Sekhar LN. An extreme lateral approach to intradural lesions of the cervical spine and foramen magnum. Neurosurgery 1990; 27(2):197–204
8. Spetzler RF, Grahm TW. The far-lateral approach to the inferior clivus and upper clinical region. Technical note. BNI Q 1990;6:35–38

29 Posterolateral Approach to the Upper Cervical Spine

Chandranath Sen

A variety of tumors occurs in the cervical spine and craniovertebral junction (CVJ). These tumors may arise from the bone, nerve root, or meninges; they may be intradural extramedullary, intradural intramedullary, primary, or metastatic. Several surgical approaches are available for accessing these tumors, and many factors are considered in selecting the most appropriate approach. With respect to intradural extramedullary spinal tumors and extradural bony tumors, the most important of these considerations is the location of the tumor in relation to the spinal cord.

Most intradural tumors are removed through a purely posterior approach, whereas tumors that involve the vertebral bodies and the anterior bony elements are removed through an anterior approach. The anterior approaches offer a direct route to such tumors. However, the exposure is usually limited (unless the tumor is strictly in the midline) and can be inadequate.[1–3] The posterior exposures are more extensive than the anterior approaches. However, the tumor is ventral to the spinal cord and the entire exposure cannot be utilized. Consequently, there is an attendant risk of excessively manipulating the already compromised cord. Furthermore, extradural tumors (chordomas or metastases) may involve the vertebral artery when they are located anteriorly or anterolaterally. The standard anterior and posterior approaches are inadequate for managing any significant degree of arterial involvement.[4]

The posterolateral approach is advantageous in overcoming these shortcomings.[5] The principle of the approach described here is that the muscles and soft tissues are reflected in a layer-by-layer fashion, clearing a wide area on the lateral aspect of the spine and providing the surgeon a substantially improved view of the area to ensure safe and complete removal of the tumor.

■ Operative Technique

Positioning and Initial Dissection

The patient is placed in a lateral decubitus position with the head fixed by a three-point pin head holder in a neutral position. Intraoperatively, somatosensory and motor evoked potentials are monitored. Specific anesthetic techniques are needed to allow real-time neurophysiological monitoring throughout the operation. The soft tissue and bony extent of the tumor are carefully noted on the preoperative evaluation of the patient's diagnostic imaging studies, which include thin-section magnetic resonance imaging (MRI) and computed tomography (CT). Any significant extension of the tumor into the foramen magnum and posterior fossa can be accessed through the lateral transcondylar approach, although the entire tumor may not need to be exposed.

Two alternative incisions can be used. The choice is based on whether the approach needs to be extended cephalad to the foramen magnum or the cervical spine. If the tumor extends above the foramen magnum, a wide C-shaped incision is centered on the ear and extended inferiorly, posterior and parallel to the sternomastoid muscle. To access a purely cervical tumor, an inverted L-shaped incision is used. The horizontal limb of the incision is made at the nuchal line, and the vertical limb starts from the mastoid tip and proceeds vertically along the lateral aspect of the neck (**Fig. 29.1**). If a posterior cervical fusion is needed, a separate midline incision can be made posteriorly, independent of the lateral cervical incision.

The dissection proceeds down along the muscle layers to the lateral masses of the vertebrae. The subcutaneous dissection along the inferior aspect of the incision must be performed carefully, with the surgeon looking for the accessory nerve as it exits the sternocleidomastoid muscle to enter the trapezius. This nerve can sometimes be mistaken for the cervical plexus of nerves formed by the branches of the upper cervical roots. The sternocleidomastoid muscle is detached from the mastoid and suboccipital region and reflected anteriorly (**Fig. 29.2A**). The splenius capitis and the longissimus capitis are detached from the mastoid region. The transverse process of C1 acts as a constant landmark that can be palpated easily just caudal to the mastoid process. The deepest muscle layer is formed by the uppermost slip of the levator scapulae and the superior and inferior oblique muscles and the rectus capitis lateralis, all of which attach to the transverse process of C1 (**Fig. 29.2B**). These attachments at the C1 transverse process are dissected and reflected inferiorly. The small segmental muscles deep to this layer are incised in a linear manner to access the lateral aspect of the spine.

Identification of the Vertebral Artery

Typically, the vertebral artery is identified, isolated, and mobilized mostly when extradural tumors are being treated. The lateral dissection through the muscles of the posterior triangle can produce troublesome bleeding from the rich plexus of veins. The vertebral artery is surrounded by a periosteal sheath, which encloses a venous plexus that communicates with the epidural plexus. The artery is identified

Fig. 29.1 (A,B) The lateral decubitus position and inverted L-shaped incision on the left side of the neck. **(C)** Intraoperative view after tumor resection. The vertebral artery (*VA*) is fully exposed from C4 to C1; the dura has been decompressed, and the internal carotid artery (*Carotid A.*) is seen anteriorly. The resection cavity is deep, with the pharynx as its anterior border and the dura as its posterior border.

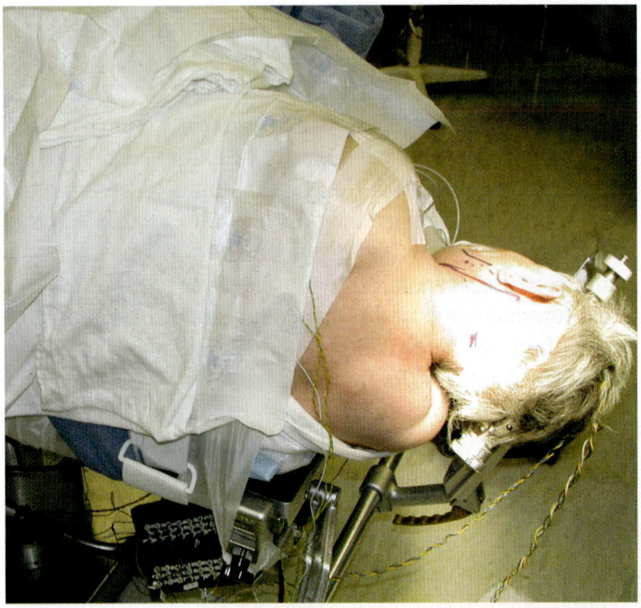

A

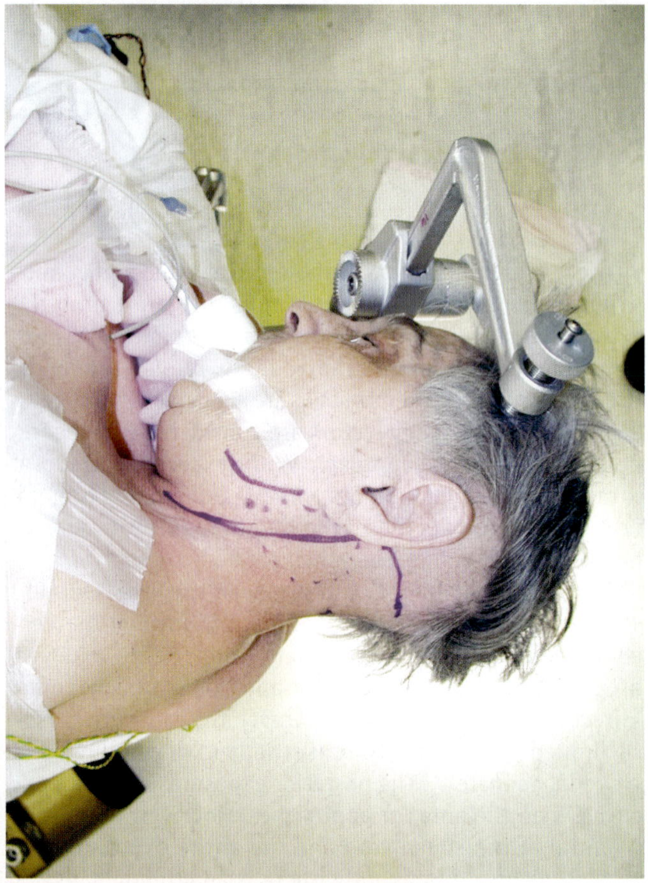

B

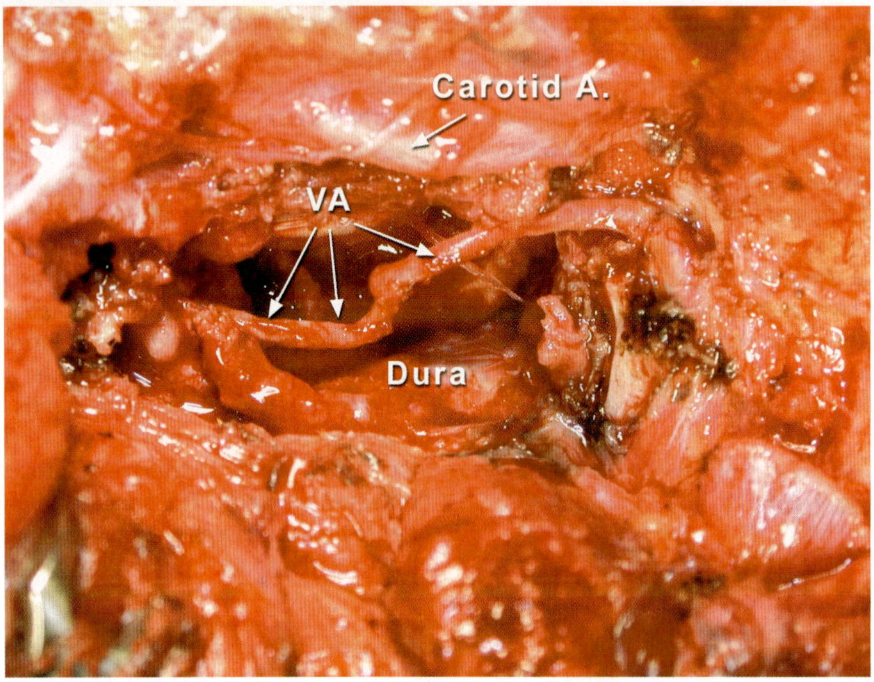

C

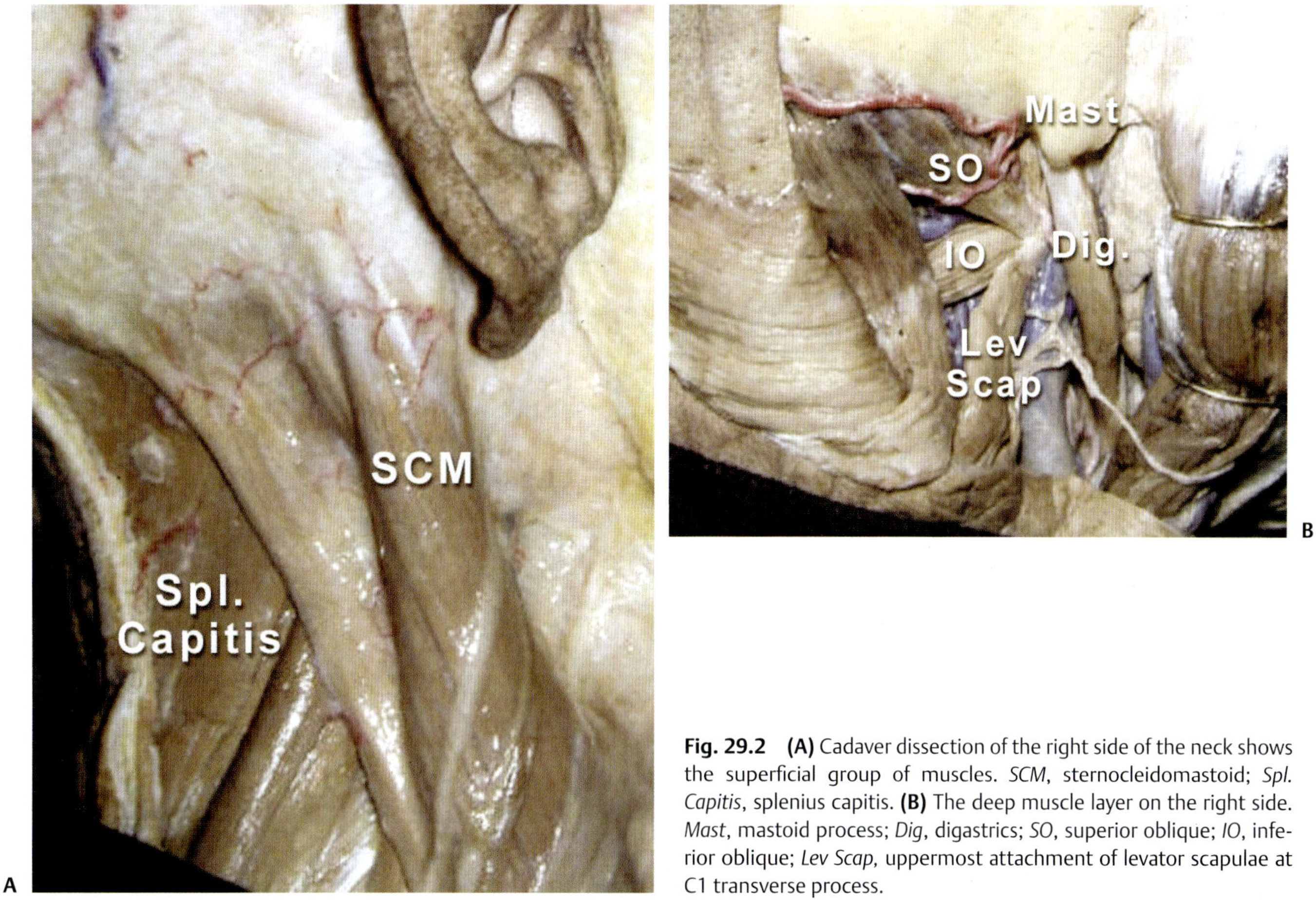

Fig. 29.2 **(A)** Cadaver dissection of the right side of the neck shows the superficial group of muscles. *SCM*, sternocleidomastoid; *Spl. Capitis*, splenius capitis. **(B)** The deep muscle layer on the right side. *Mast*, mastoid process; *Dig*, digastrics; *SO*, superior oblique; *IO*, inferior oblique; *Lev Scap*, uppermost attachment of levator scapulae at C1 transverse process.

by bony and muscular landmarks instead of by its pulsation, which may be imperceptible (**Fig. 29.3**). Between C2 and C1, the artery can be located caudal to the inferior border of the inferior oblique muscles. In the coronal plane, the artery exits at the superior portion of the foramen transversarium of C2, posterior to the plane at which it enters the foramen from below. Between C2 and C1, the ventral ramus of the C2 root crosses the lateral surface of the artery. After emerging on the superior surface of the C1 foramen, the artery turns posteriorly along the upper surface of the C1 posterior arch where it lies deep to the superior oblique muscle. The venous plexus about the vessel closely adheres to the joint capsule of the atlanto-occipital articulation as it winds around the joint to enter the dura. The artery can be variably redundant above C1 and between C2 and C1 to accommodate the motion at these spinal segments. Keeping the head and neck neutral minimizes distortion of the course of the vertebral artery and facilitates the dissection.

The arterial wall is exposed by opening the surrounding periosteal sheath and venous plexus. The venous plexus is coagulated and incised longitudinally and then opened circumferentially to expose the full circumference of the artery. The foramen transversarium is opened with rongeurs, and the artery is displaced from C1, if needed, to access the ventral C1-C2 region for extradural pathology (**Fig. 29.4**). Similarly, the foramen transversaria of C2-C3 can be opened, isolating the entire length of the artery as needed. Mobilizing the artery allows access to the entire lateral aspect of the spinal column (articular facets, lamina, transverse process, and side of the vertebral body).

Intradural Tumor

In purely intradural tumors, exposure of the vertebral artery may not be necessary. The bony opening consists of the ipsilateral hemilaminae and partial or total facetectomy of the levels involved with the lesion. This exposure may seem to be the same as that obtained through a standard posterior approach (**Fig. 29.5**). However, the lateral perspective that the surgeon gains by making the skin incision and muscle dissection from the side enables complete visualization of the area ventral to the spinal cord without retracting it (**Fig. 29.6**). The dura is opened in a linear fashion on the lateral aspect of the thecal sac immediately posterior to the C2 or other nerve roots. It is carried cephalad and caudal as needed, depending on the longitudinal extent of the tumor. For the treatment of tumors above the foramen magnum, it may be necessary to mobilize the vertebral artery. Epidural venous bleeding, which can be copious, is controlled with surgical packing and elevation of the head. The dural edges are held back with stay sutures, and the dentate ligaments in the exposure are divided.

A B

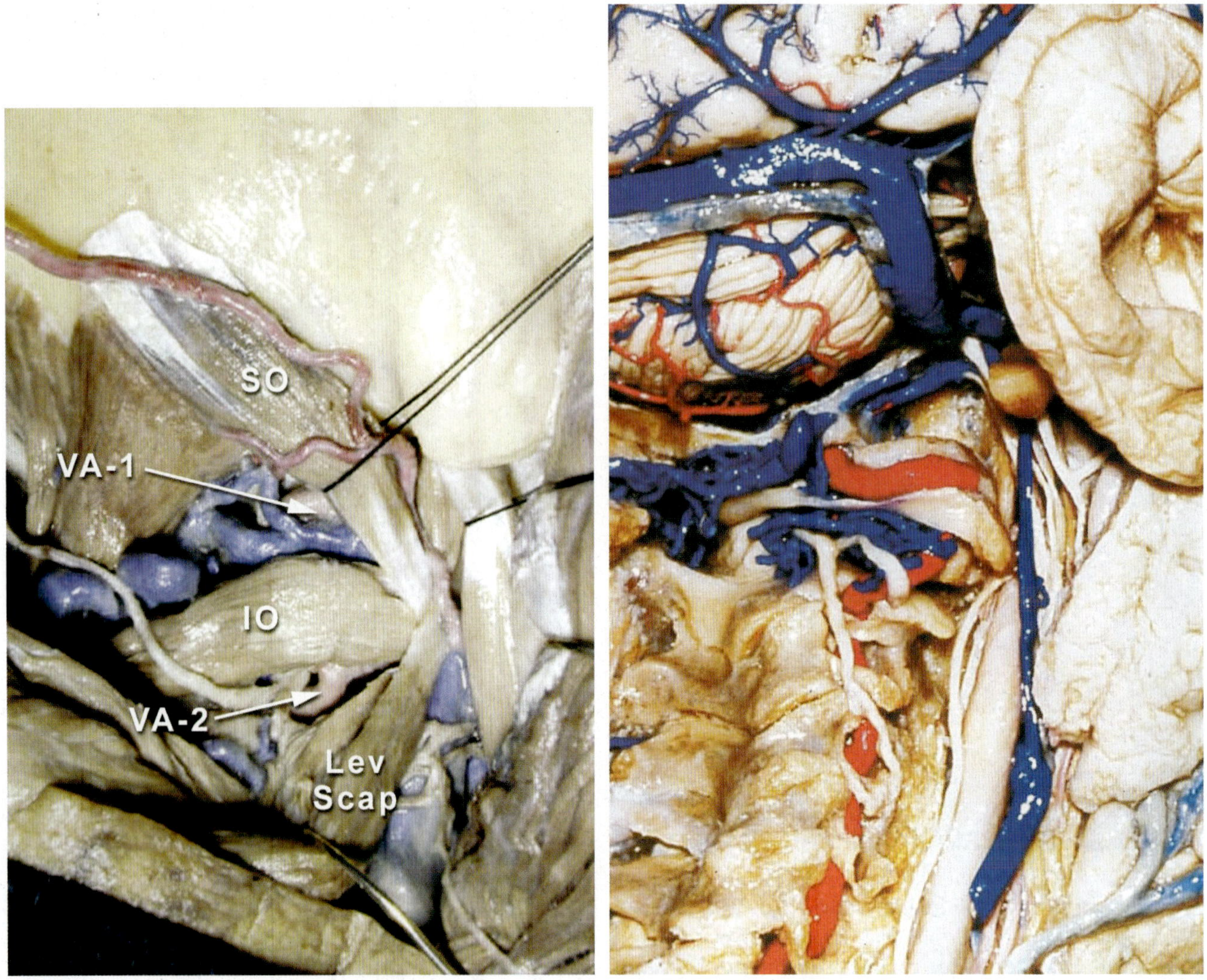

Fig. 29.3 **(A)** Cadaver dissection of the right side of the neck (nose is to the reader's right and vertex is at the top). *SO*, superior oblique; *IO*, inferior oblique; *Lev Scap*, uppermost attachment of levator scapulae at C1 transverse process. The vertebral artery above C1 (*VA-1*) is seen deep to the SO muscle while the artery between C2 and C1 (*VA-2*) is below the IO muscle. **(B)** Cadaver dissection of the right side after removal of muscles. The vertebral artery is coursing through the transverse processes of the vertebrae. Note the relation to the facet joints.

There are several ways to debulk the tumor, such as with the bipolar device and microscissor, ultrasonic aspirator, or laser. The crucial point is that the interface between the spinal cord should not be developed until substantial debulking has been achieved. This strategy allows the surgeon to separate the tumor capsule from the spinal cord with minimal manipulation of the cord itself. After the capsule has been removed, the ventral dural attachment can be excised. Dural closure usually requires a fascial patch graft, which is sutured under the microscope.

In the case of a dumbbell schwannoma, the intervertebral foramen is already widened. Therefore, the remnants of the adjacent facet joints are drilled away, permitting the intra- and extracanalicular portions of the tumor to be visualized simultaneously (**Fig. 29.7**). The entire tumor is easily removed through this exposure while the normal rootlets are preserved.

Extradural Tumors

Most extradural tumors involve the vertebral bodies and are eccentric to some degree, extending into the facet joints and vertebral artery more on one side than on the other. Such eccentric tumors are unsuitable for a direct anterior transoral approach or a mandibulotomy approach because their lateral access is inadequate. Furthermore, the contaminated field through the pharynx is an unnecessary hazard for manipulation of vascular structures. A more laterally oriented extrapharyngeal approach is preferred for such tumors in the upper cervical area. The posterolateral approach provides exposure of the vertebral body up to the opposite pedicle as well as excellent control and access to the artery for dissection from the tumor or reconstruction, as needed (**Fig. 29.4B,C**). Anterior stabilization cannot be performed via this route.

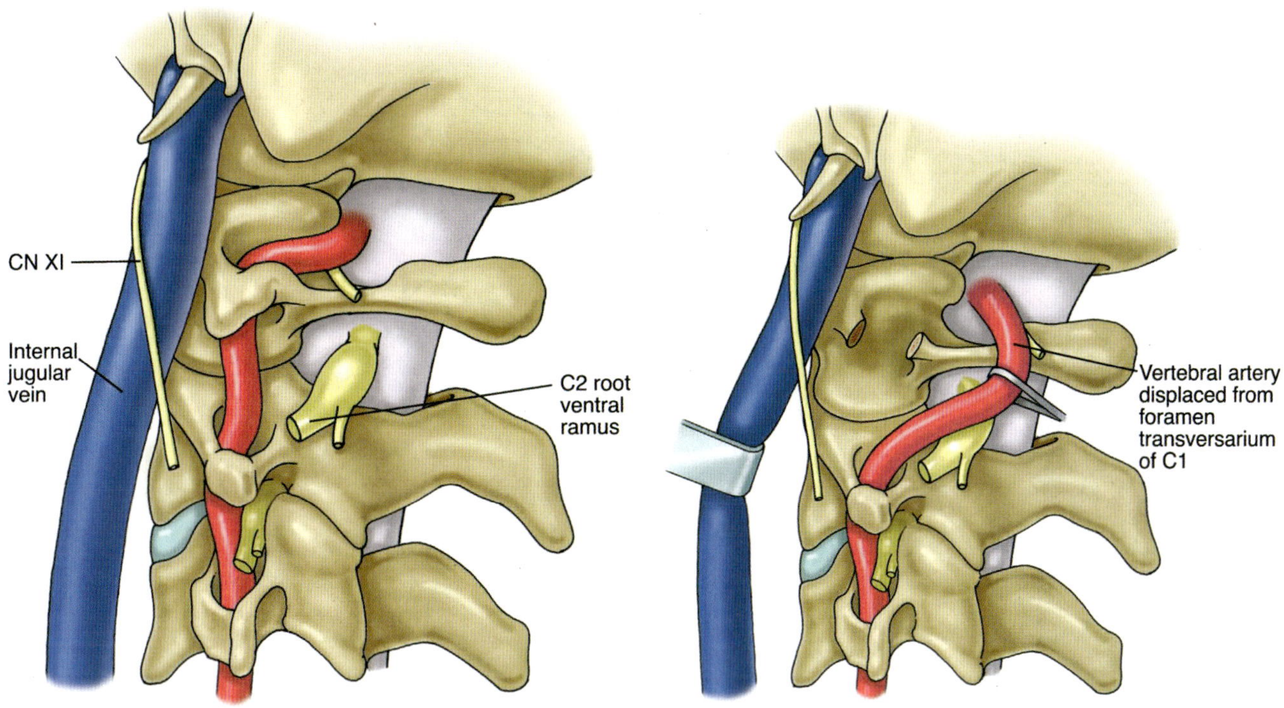

A

B

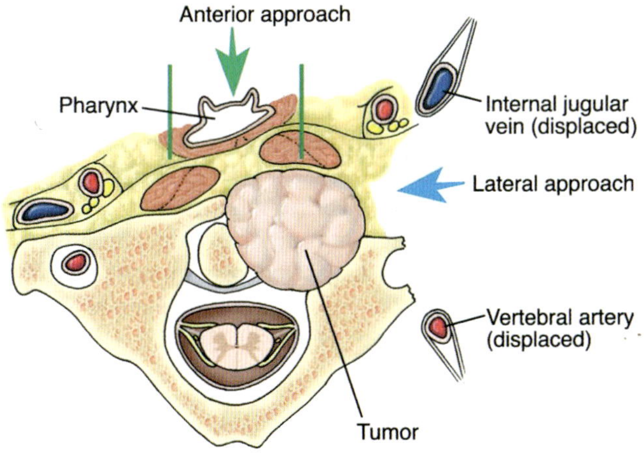

C

Fig. 29.4 **(A)** Diagram illustrating the left lateral aspect of the occiput C1-C2: the vertebral artery changes its course in the transverse foramen of C2, marking the beginning of the third portion of the artery. The relation of the C2 ventral ramus, the internal jugular vein, and cranial nerve XI (*CN XI*) to the artery is shown. **(B)** The artery is removed from the foramen transversarium of C1 and displaced posteriorly, providing access to the anterior portion of C1 and C2. **(C)** Axial view showing access to a ventrolateral tumor at C1-C2 through a lateral approach between the posteriorly displaced vertebral artery and the anteriorly retracted internal jugular vein. Note that a direct approach through the pharynx would not be adequate to reach the lateral portion of the tumor. (Reprinted with permission from Jon Coulter.)

Once the vertebral artery is controlled, the tumor can be removed relatively freely unless the dura, neighboring cranial nerves, or other vessels are involved. The surrounding bony margin can be drilled away aggressively until healthy bone is visible. If the tumor extends to the opposite side, a separate approach may be needed. Resection of the entire facet joints, pedicles, and part of the vertebral bodies would necessitate some form of stabilization. Depending on the extent of bone removal, a posterior stabilization operation may need to be performed at the same sitting.

Discussion

A lateral or posterolateral approach to the anterior aspect of the cervicomedullary junction is useful for accessing both intra- and extradural tumors anterior to the spinal cord. Using a lateral avenue of visualization, the surgeon has unimpeded access to the entire side of the spinal elements, including the ipsilateral half of the vertebral body, lateral mass, vertebral artery, and ipsilateral lamina, without contamination from the pharynx. The placement of the incision on the lateral aspect of the neck and dissection of the muscles in layers is an important aspect of the approach and helps to create a wide and shallow exposure that cannot be achieved when the muscles are divided in one line. The principle can be applied not only to the CVJ but also to the cervical spine to C7. Intradural tumors such as meningiomas and dumbbell schwannomas do not require a stabilization operation after such an approach. However, bony tumors always require a posterior stabilization because of the extensive bone removal that is involved in treating such tumors. Although anterolateral approaches have been described,[3,6,7] lateral and posterolateral approaches are best suited for

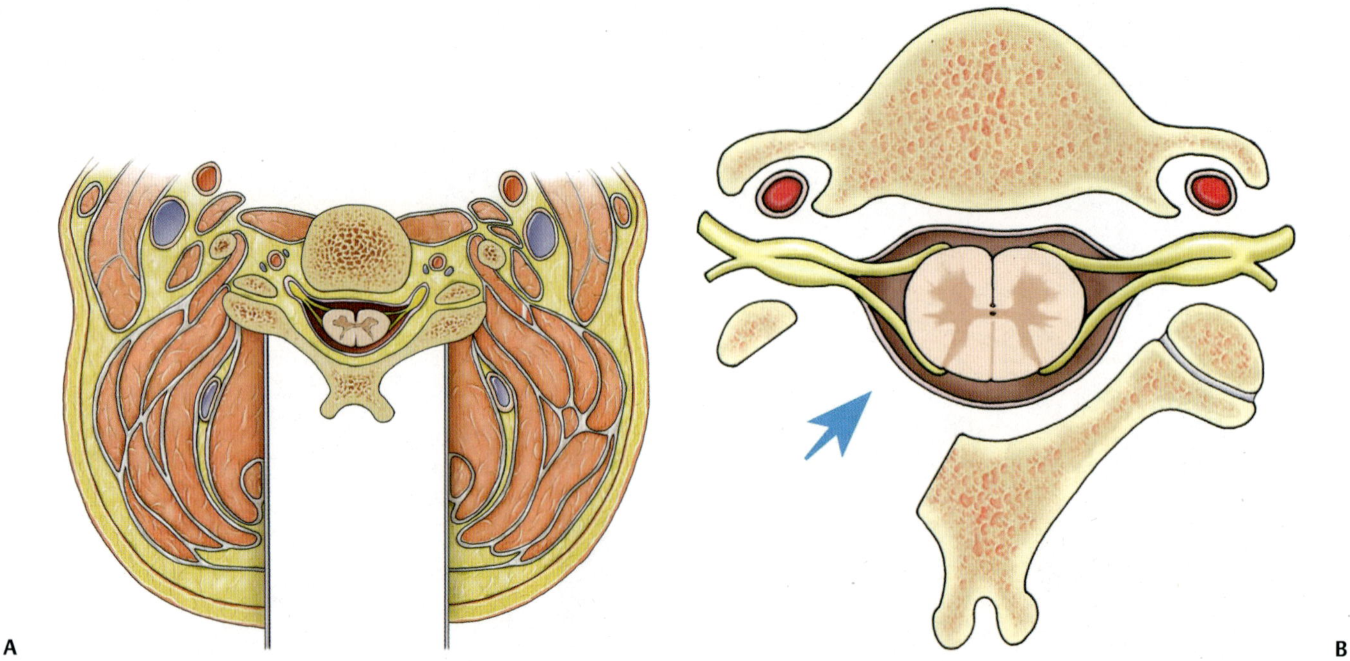

Fig. 29.5 (A,B) Axial sections diagrammatically illustrating the exposure and angle of visualization obtained through a posterior incision. The area ventral to the cord is difficult to visualize without retracting the spinal cord. (Reprinted with permission from Jon Coulter.)

the upper cervical spine[4,5,8,9] because the entry and exit of the carotid artery, internal jugular vein, and lower cranial nerves at the skull base limit their anterior displacement, thus restricting the anterior and anterolateral approaches. With intradural tumors, the surgeon's line of sight is along the interface between the tumor and the spinal cord. Consequently, the dissection can be performed under direct vision with minimum manipulation of the spinal cord.

Extradural tumors encountered in this region include chordomas and chondrosarcomas and may involve the vertebral body, lateral masses, vertebral artery, and epidural tissues (**Fig. 29.8**). For tumors situated strictly in the midline, a purely anterior approach is ideal because it is a direct approach to the disease process. In most cases, however, the tumor is more extensive and the lateral approach provides excellent access (**Figs. 29.1** and **29.9**). The lateral

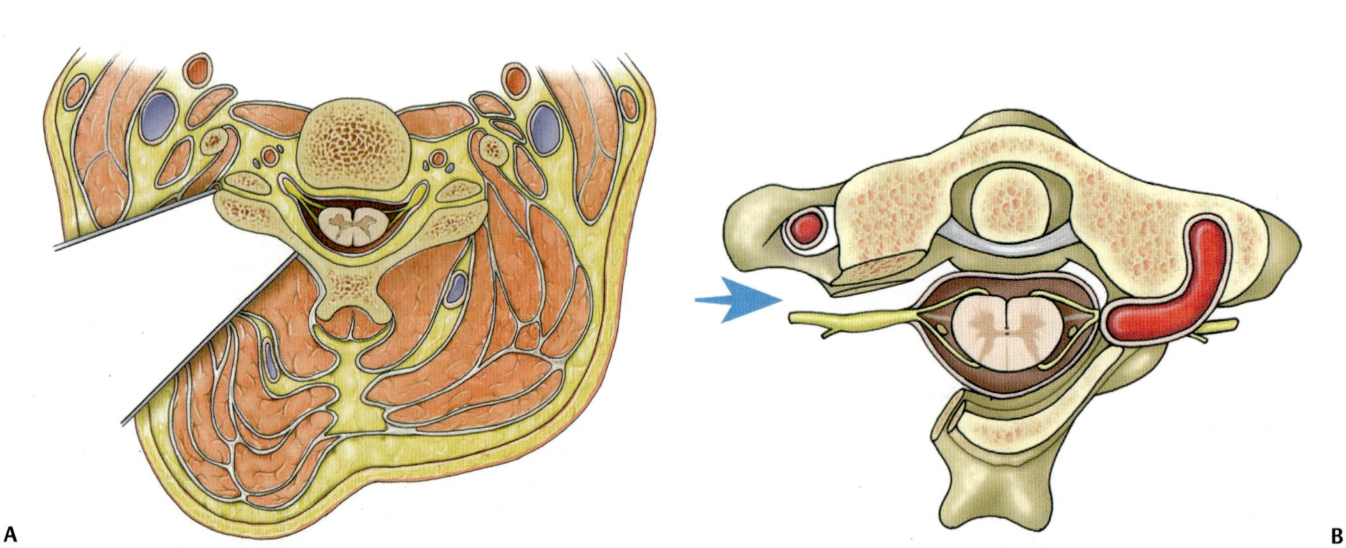

Fig. 29.6 (A,B) Axial sections diagrammatically illustrating the exposure and angle of visualization obtained through the laterally placed incision. The exposure of the area ventral to the spinal cord is much greater compared with Fig. 29.5A,B. (Reprinted with permission from Jon Coulter.)

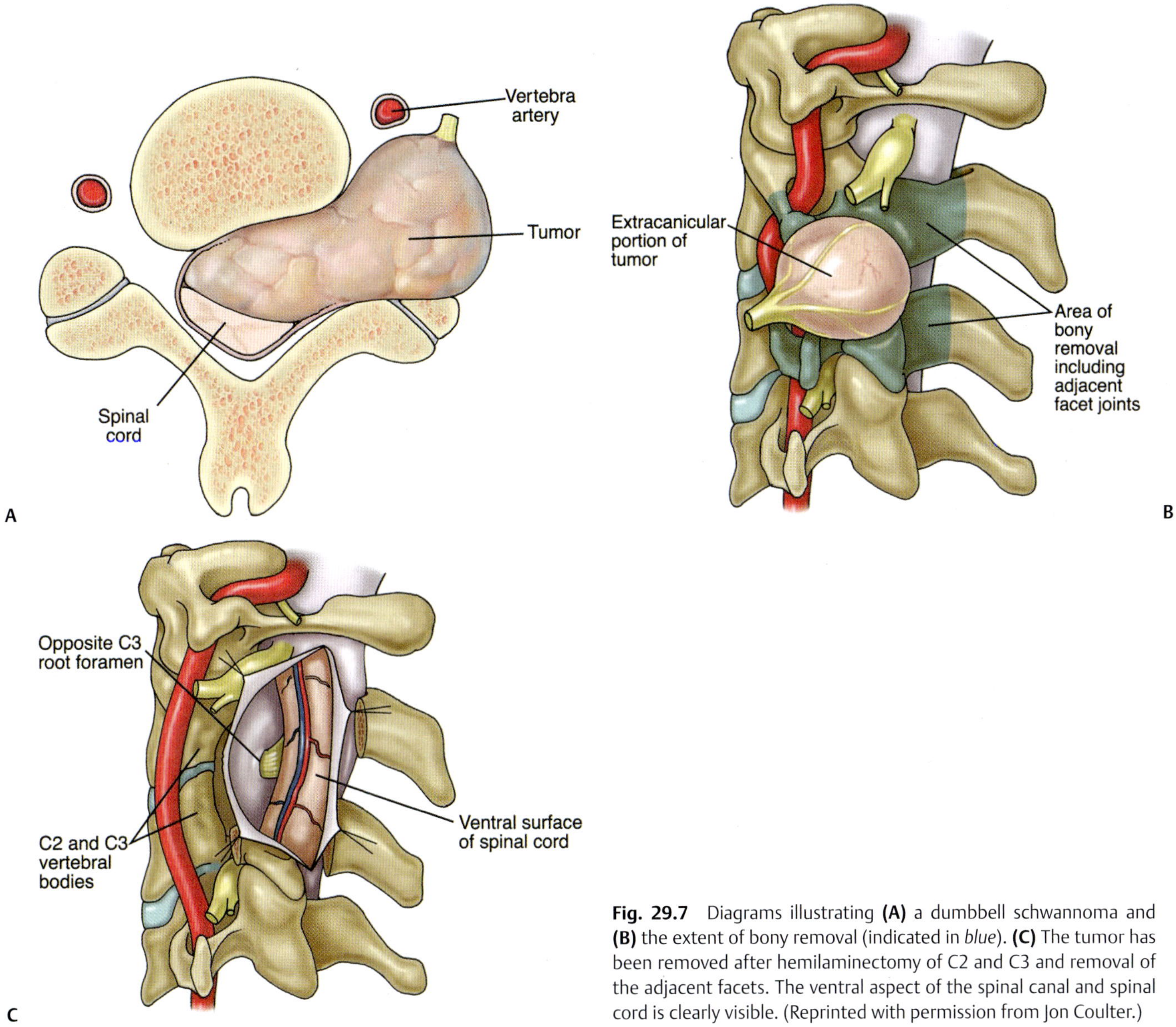

Fig. 29.7 Diagrams illustrating **(A)** a dumbbell schwannoma and **(B)** the extent of bony removal (indicated in *blue*). **(C)** The tumor has been removed after hemilaminectomy of C2 and C3 and removal of the adjacent facets. The ventral aspect of the spinal canal and spinal cord is clearly visible. (Reprinted with permission from Jon Coulter.)

approach is limited in the degree of access to the vertebral bodies across the midline; therefore, it may have to be combined with an anterior or lateral approach from the opposite side.

Among the intradural tumors, meningiomas can be located on any aspect of the spinal cord. Tumors located anteriorly and anterolaterally are best approached through the posterolateral approach as described. **Figure 29.10** shows an MRI of a young man with a meningioma that recurred after two previous operations performed through a midline laminectomy. The tumor was situated completely anterior to the spinal cord at C1-C2 and was approached from a posterolateral approach by making a new incision on the lateral aspect of the neck. The blood supply to the tumor from the vertebral artery was interrupted early from the posterolateral approach (**Fig. 29.11**). Schwannomas are often dumbbell shaped and have intraspinal and extraspinal components that need to be addressed simultaneously. The posterolateral approach is ideally suited for these tumors. **Figure 29.12** shows a young girl with neurofibromatosis who had a nerve sheath tumor (among others) at C1-C2 that was mostly intradural, although some of it extended out of the C1-C2 neural foramen. At surgery, the adjacent facets were drilled away with the hemilaminae, exposing the entire tumor (**Fig. 29.12C**). No stabilization was necessary because only the facet joints at one level were disrupted on one side.

The lateral perspective to the cervical spine, especially to the upper two vertebrae, adds greatly to the surgeon's ability to remove tumors that may be incompletely accessed via conventional anterior and posterior approaches. The technique, in itself, adds little to surgical morbidity.

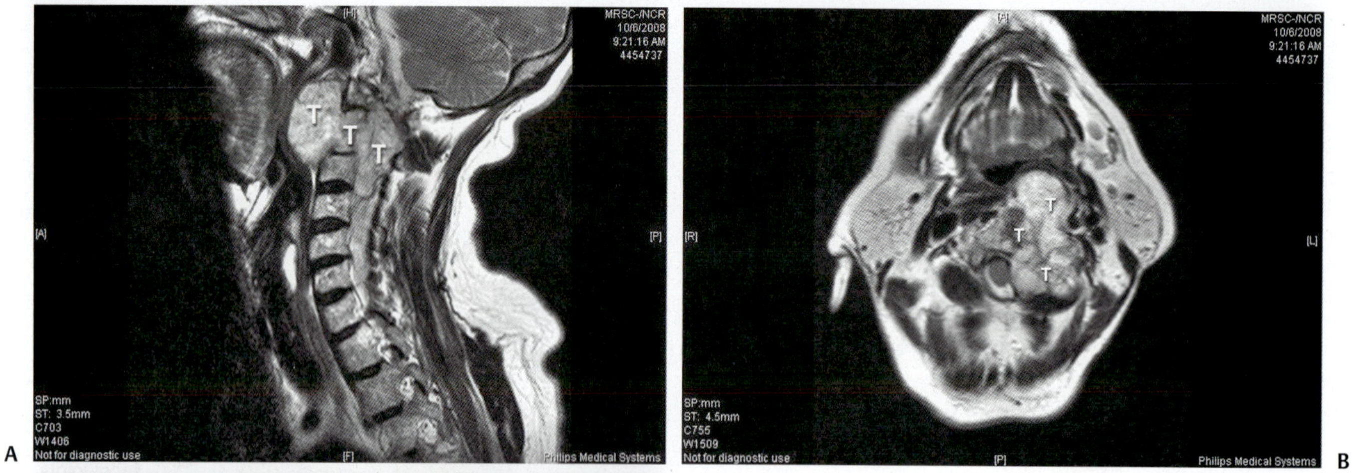

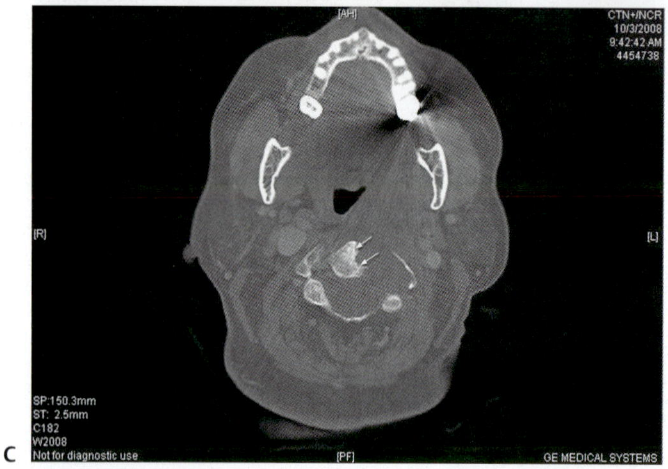

Fig. 29.8 **(A)** Sagittal and **(B)** axial magnetic resonance images show the large chordoma. *T*, tumor. **(C)** The axial computed tomography scan shows the bone destruction (*arrows*).

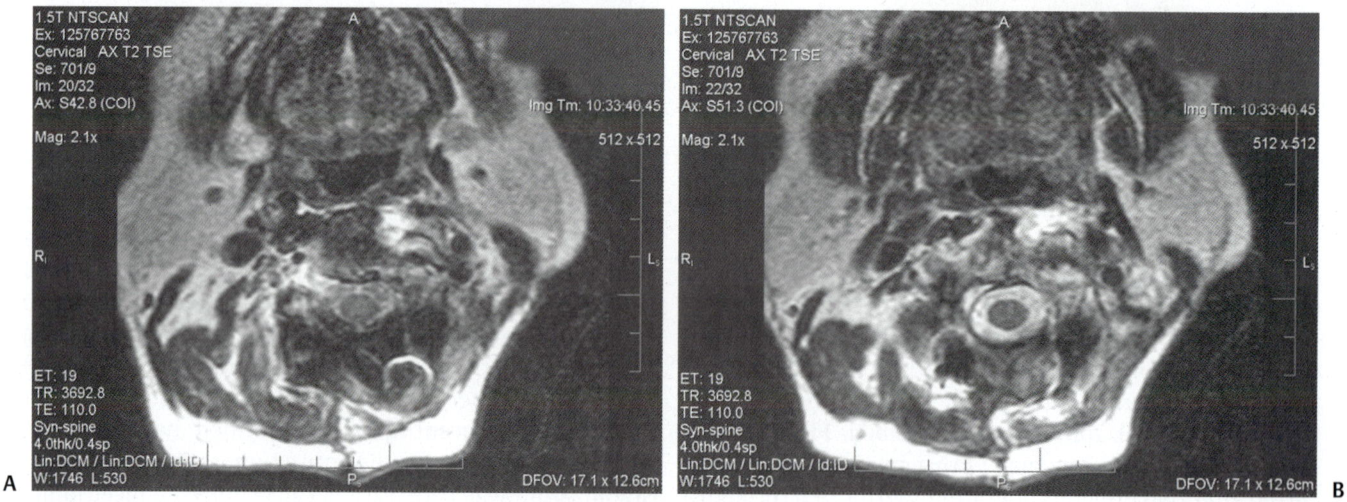

Fig. 29.9 **(A,B)** Axial slices after surgery showing the degree of tumor resection. Posterior instrumentation and fusion have been performed.

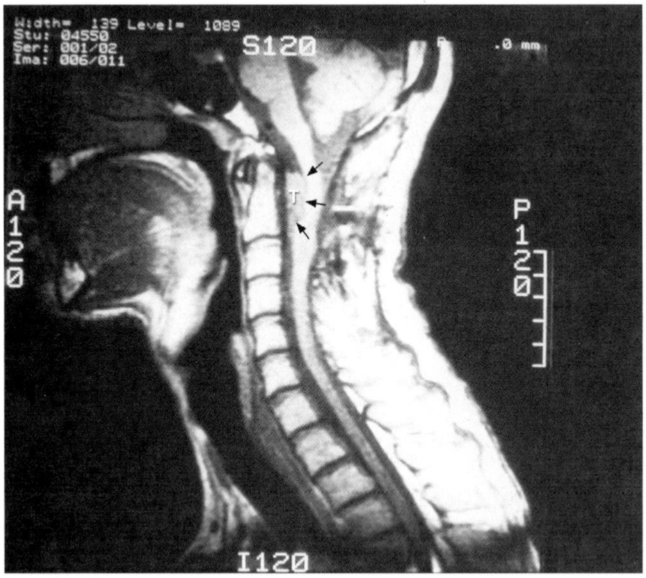
A

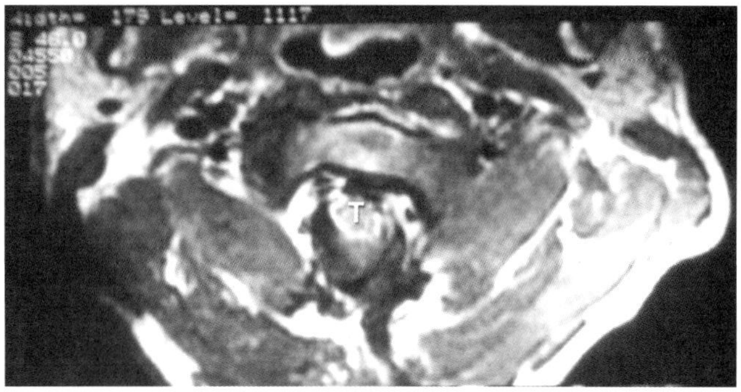
B

Fig. 29.10 **(A)** Sagittal magnetic resonance image (MRI) of a recurrent meningioma at C1-C2 (*arrows*) that had been previously resected through a laminectomy. **(B)** Axial MRI shows that the tumor (*T*) is entirely ventral to the spinal cord behind the vertebral body.

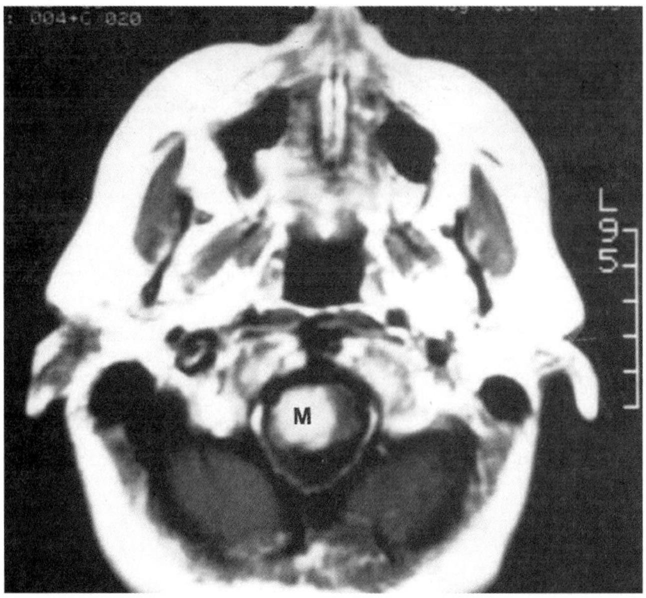
A

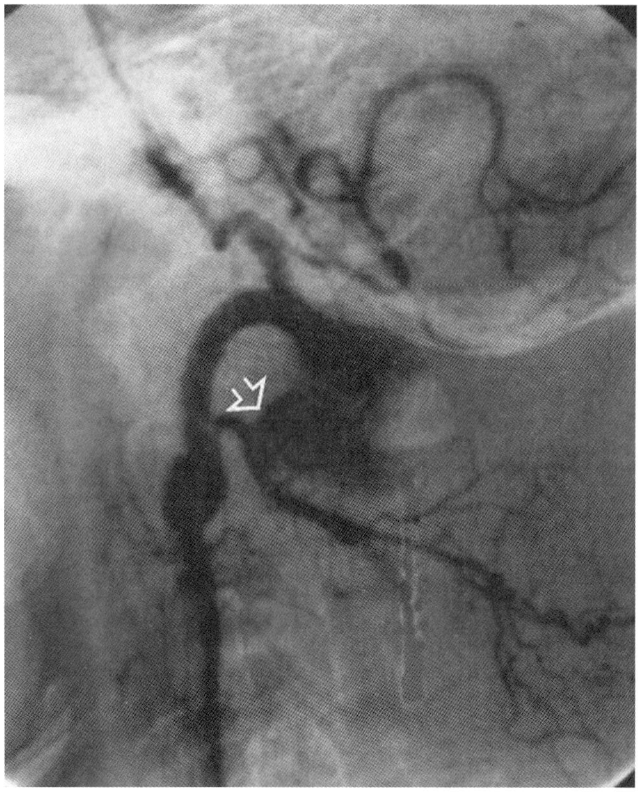
B

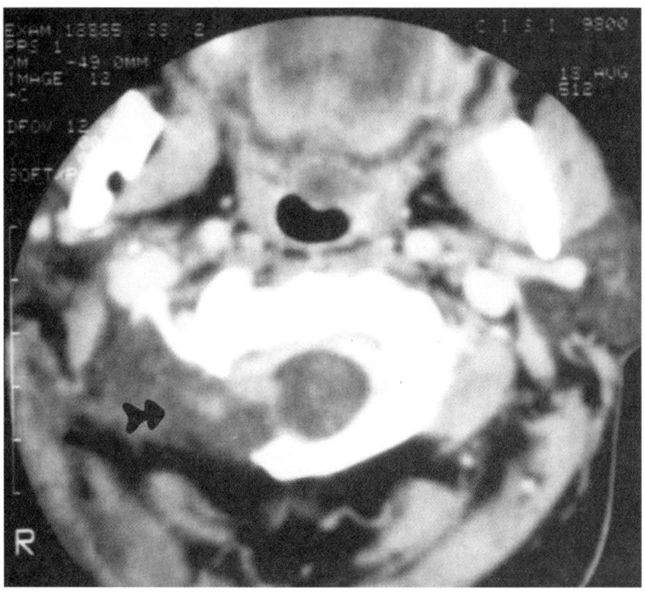
C

Fig. 29.11 **(A)** Axial magnetic resonance image obtained after administration of gadolinium shows a meningioma (*M*) arising from the right anterolateral aspect of the spinal canal. **(B)** The tumor received its blood supply from a branch of the vertebral artery arising between C1 and C2 (*arrow*). **(C)** Postoperative computed tomography scan showing the limited bony opening through the right posterolateral approach (*arrow*), which allowed interruption of the blood supply and resection of the tumor.

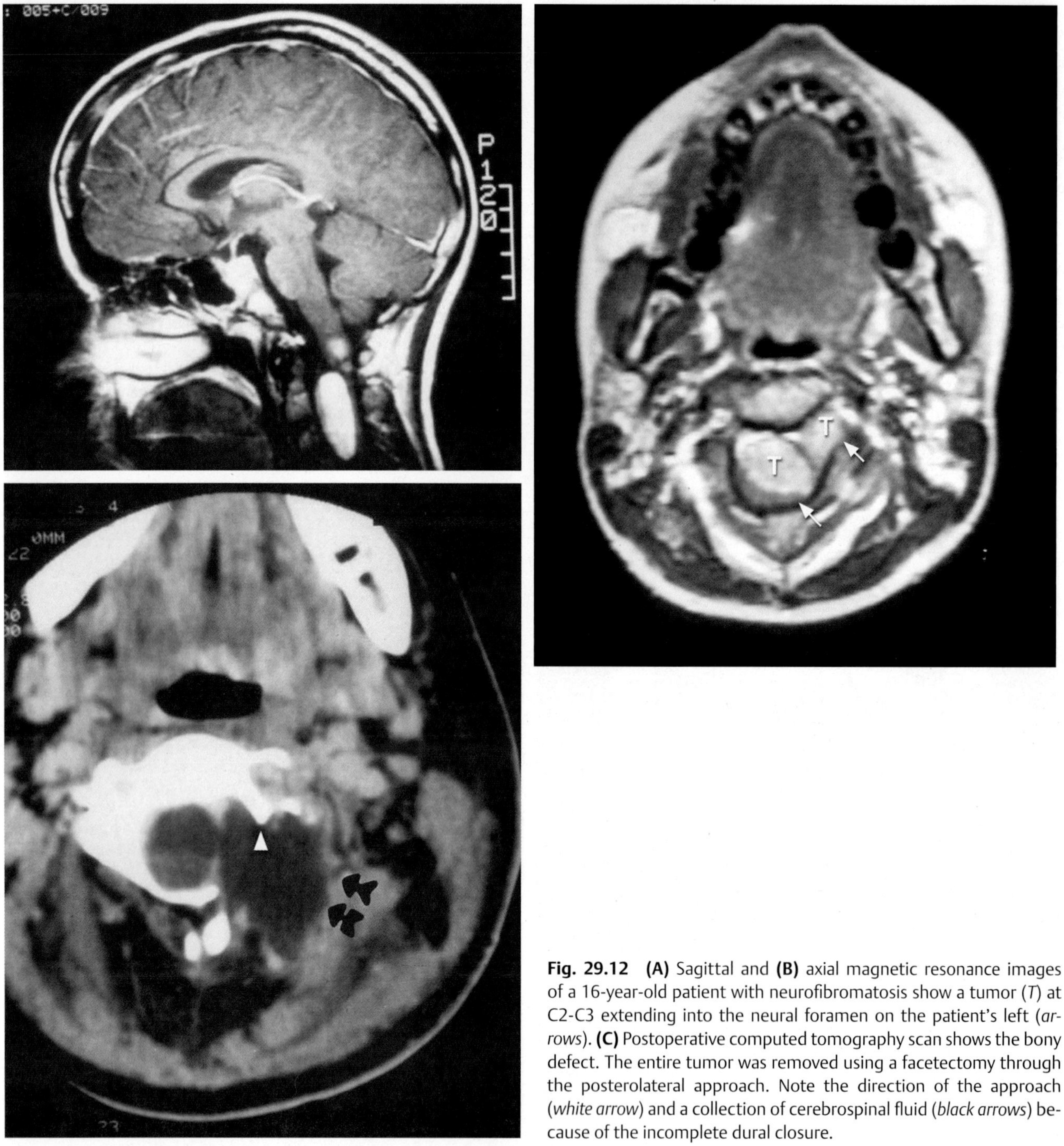

A

B

C

Fig. 29.12 **(A)** Sagittal and **(B)** axial magnetic resonance images of a 16-year-old patient with neurofibromatosis show a tumor (*T*) at C2-C3 extending into the neural foramen on the patient's left (*arrows*). **(C)** Postoperative computed tomography scan shows the bony defect. The entire tumor was removed using a facetectomy through the posterolateral approach. Note the direction of the approach (*white arrow*) and a collection of cerebrospinal fluid (*black arrows*) because of the incomplete dural closure.

References

1. Crockard HA, Sen CN. The transoral approach for the management of intradural lesions at the craniovertebral junction: review of 7 cases. Neurosurgery 1991;28(1):88–97, discussion 97–98
2. Menezes AH, VanGilder JC. Transoral-transpharyngeal approach to the anterior craniocervical junction. Ten-year experience with 72 patients. J Neurosurg 1988;69(6):895–903
3. George B, Zerah M, Lot G, Hurth M. Oblique transcorporeal approach to anteriorly located lesions in the cervical spinal canal. Acta Neurochir (Wien) 1993;121(3–4):187–190
4. Sen C, Eisenberg M, Casden AM, Sundaresan N, Catalano PJ. Management of the vertebral artery in excision of extradural tumors of the cervical spine. Neurosurgery 1995;36(1):106–115, discussion 115–116
5. Sen CN, Sekhar LN. An extreme lateral approach to intradural lesions of the cervical spine and foramen magnum. Neurosurgery 1990;27(2):197–204
6. Hakuba A, Komiyama M, Tsujimoto T, et al. Transuncodiscal approach to dumbbell tumors of the cervical spinal canal. J Neurosurg 1984; 61(6):1100–1106
7. Verbiest H. A lateral approach to the cervical spine: technique and indications. J Neurosurg 1968;28(3):191–203
8. George B, Laurian C. Surgical approach to the whole length of the vertebral artery with special reference to the third portion. Acta Neurochir (Wien) 1980;51(3–4):259–272
9. Shucart WA, Klériga E. Lateral approach to the upper cervical spine. Neurosurgery 1980;6(3):278–281

30 Endovascular Management of Posterior Fossa Atherosclerotic Disease

Ashish Nanda and Kristine A. Blackham

Intracranial atherosclerotic disease (ICAD) is the primary cause of ischemic stroke in a significant number of patients. Annually in the United States, there are roughly 795,000 new or recurrent strokes—of which 87% are ischemic.[1] ICAD accounts for 8 to 10% of ischemic strokes, with a disproportionate number of African American, Hispanic, and Asian individuals affected.[2] Increased incidence is noted among those with insulin-dependent diabetes mellitus, hypertension, hyperlipidemia, and a history of smoking.[3] The Warfarin versus Aspirin for Symptomatic Intracranial Disease (WASID) trial published in 2005 provided key information regarding the outcome of the medical treatment of ICAD and identified subsets of high-risk patients. Data accumulated from studies on the management of ICAD risk factors as well as the proliferation of small studies has resulted in the use of new and better equipment and techniques for the endovascular treatment of ICAD. Direct and subset analyses of the natural history and medical and endovascular treatment of vertebrobasilar ICAD have also been performed, which this chapter specifically discusses with data from intracranial atherosclerotic disease in general. Techniques for intracranial angioplasty and stenting in the posterior fossa are also reviewed.

■ Natural History and Medical Management

Conducted between 1999 and 2003, the WASID trial aimed to better understand the natural history of ICAD and choice of medical therapy, enrolling 569 patients with recent transient ischemic attack (TIA) or minor stroke and angiographically proven 50 to 99% stenosis of a major intracranial artery, attributable to ICAD. In this prospective, randomized controlled trial, roughly 40% of the patients had vertebrobasilar ICAD. The WASID study was stopped early—within 1.8 years of follow-up—as warfarin showed significantly higher rates of adverse events and provided no benefit over aspirin. In the territory of the stenosis, the overall rate of ischemic stroke was 11% at 1 year and 14% at 2 years, despite the use of aspirin or warfarin.[4] In subset analysis, the risk of subsequent stroke in the WASID population was found to be greatest in symptomatic patients with 70 to 99% stenosis (20% in the first year), which was significantly higher than those patients with moderate stenosis.[5] Although an earlier retrospective report from the WASID study group in 1996 showed patients with vertebrobasilar ICAD to be at particularly high risk of stroke, the prospective WASID trial determined that the location of the stenosis (i.e., vertebrobasilar disease versus carotid middle cerebral artery disease) was not significantly associated with an increased risk of stroke in the territory of the stenotic vessel.[6] Multiple other variables were examined, such as age, length of stenosis, and prior use of antithrombotic medications. No variables were found to be significantly associated with an increased risk of stroke in the territory of the stenotic artery.[5] Additional subgroup analysis of the posterior circulation showed that warfarin provided no definite benefit over aspirin.[7]

However, in 2009, it was reported that, in a population of 538 unselected patients, the prevalence of ≥50% vertebrobasilar stenosis was significantly greater than the prevalence of ≥50% carotid stenosis when comparing posterior versus anterior circulation TIA or minor stroke.[8] The same study also showed that ≥50% vertebrobasilar stenosis had a high 90-day risk of recurrent events, reaching 22% for stroke and 46% for stroke and TIA.[8] Looking at outcomes from a stroke-free survival perspective, a 2003 study determined stroke-free survival in 102 patients with symptomatic 50% or greater vertebrobasilar stenosis. The study found that 14% of patients experienced recurrent stroke over a mean follow-up period of 15 months. At 5 years, only half of the patients who had presented with ischemic symptoms were estimated to have survived without a second stroke. Death was attributable to initial and recurrent stroke (14 of 21 deaths), which the authors felt highlighted the high mortality associated with ischemic injury of the brainstem and its associated complications.[9]

Stroke prevention strategies for ICAD follow standard stroke prevention guidelines in addition to antiplatelet agents, including pharmacological treatments for blood sugar control for diabetics, statins for lipid disorders, and antihypertensive medications. Lifestyle management, including weight loss for overweight patients, moderate physical activity, and smoking cessation, are also part of the secondary stroke prevention strategies directed at atherosclerosis in general.[10] During WASID follow-up, poorly controlled blood pressure and low-density lipoprotein (LDL) levels were shown to be the most important risk factors for stroke, vascular death, or myocardial infarction.[11,12] Based on large studies of the link between serum cholesterol and ischemic stroke,[13,14] the lowering of cholesterol concentrations with atorvastatin has been shown in a randomized trial to reduce the risk of stroke in high-risk populations and in patients with noncardioembolic stroke or TIA.[15] The use of statins with intensive lipid-lowering effects is recommended in the updated American Heart Association guidelines for patients with atherosclerotic ischemic stroke or TIA without known coronary heart disease (**Fig. 30.1**).[16]

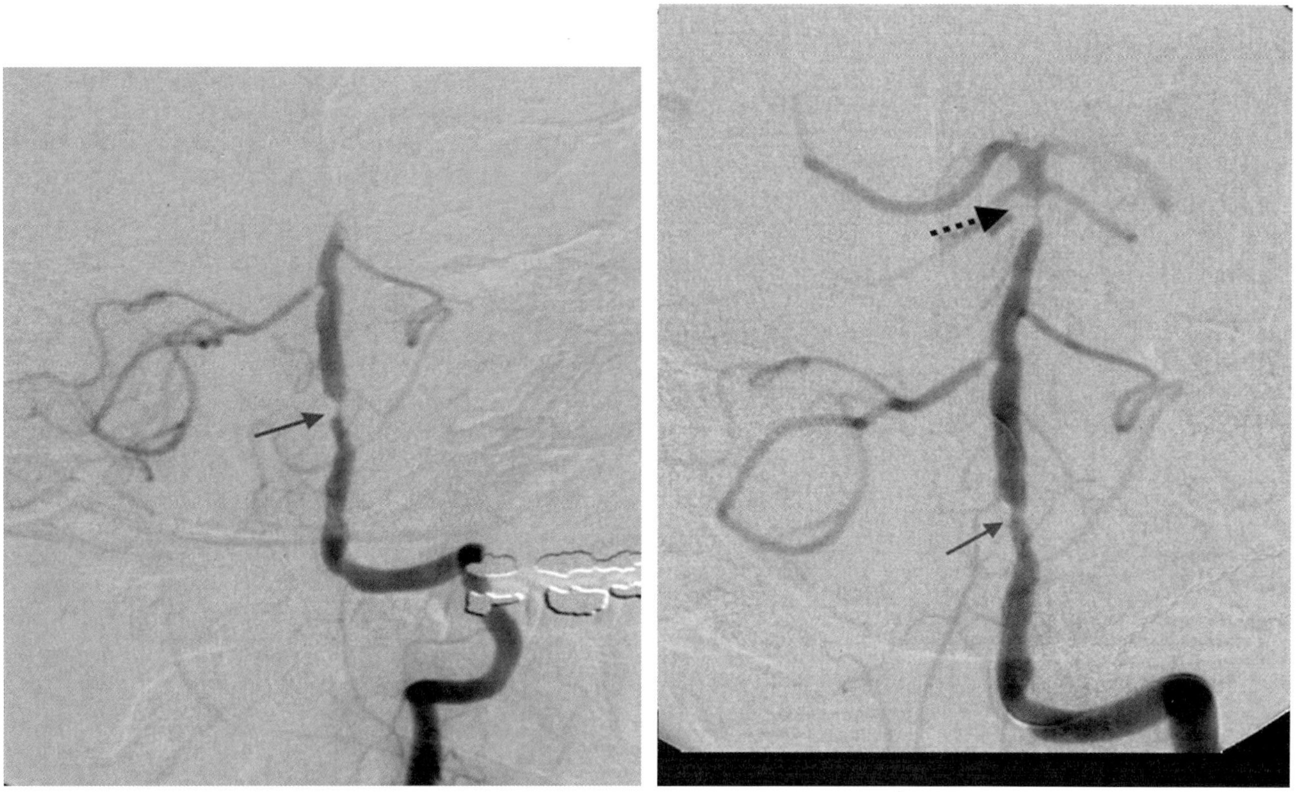

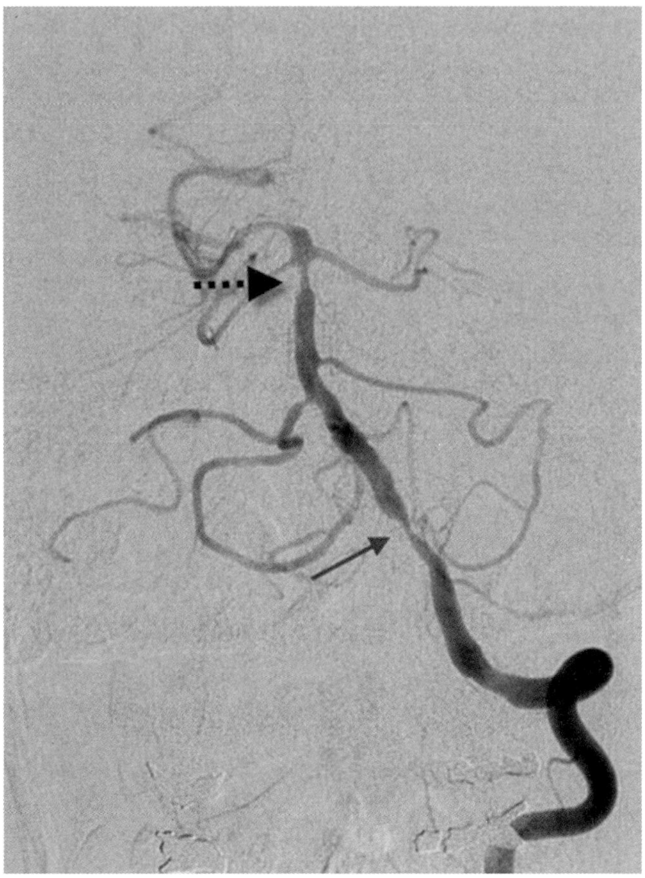

Fig. 30.1 A 50-year-old man presented with multiple transient ischemic attacks. The patient had multiple risk factors, including hypertension, diabetes, and morbid obesity. **(A)** Cerebral angiogram reveals distal left vertebral (*arrow*) and distal basilar stenosis, which were visualized from the anterior circulation injection with basilar apex opacification via a patent posterior communicating artery (not shown). **(B)** The distal vertebral stenosis was treated with angioplasty and a balloon-mounted coronary stent in 2004. Angioplasty was difficult and required high pressure to achieve the result shown (*solid arrow*). There was improved antegrade flow to the basilar apex with clear visualization of the distal stenosis (*dotted arrow*). The distal stenosis was left untreated. **(C)** At the 6-year follow-up, the patient had lost 100 pounds and had excellent control of his lipids, diabetes, and hypertension. Note the improved appearance of the untreated distal basilar stenosis (*dotted arrow*) and the recurrent stenosis within the stented distal vertebral lesion (*solid arrow*).

Endovascular Therapy

Due to the high rate of recurrent stroke and lack of successful medical therapy for intracranial stenosis secondary to ICAD, the investigation of endovascular intervention as an alternative treatment option has evolved since 1980, when Sundt and colleagues reported the first successful percutaneous intracranial transluminal angioplasty of the basilar artery,[17] on the premise that angioplasty alone or in conjunction with stenting may have a potential benefit for reducing recurrent stroke in these patients. Over the past 20 years, the development of microcatheters, balloons, and stents intended for cerebrovascular use has contributed to increased technical success by virtue of the increased compliance and navigability in the complex neurovascular anatomy.

Primary Angioplasty

Angioplasty is aimed at increasing perfusion of an arterial territory at risk, preventing vessel occlusion, and decreasing the risk of future embolic events. As flow is proportional to the fourth power of radius, any small improvement in vessel stenosis following angioplasty can lead to significant improvement in perfusion (**Fig. 30.2**). The risks of primary angioplasty of intracranial vessels include dissection, rebound stenosis, vessel rupture, thromboembolic events, and acute vessel closure. Thromboembolic complications in the posterior circulation can be significant and lead to death if brainstem perforators are involved. Early data regarding posterior circulation intracranial angioplasty without stent placement are retrospective and largely pertain to technical success and angiographic outcomes, with few reports of long-term follow-up.[18-21] These studies report less than 40% residual stenosis following angioplasty in a majority of patients and had complication rates ranging from 14 to 30%, with the periprocedural risk of stroke or death being 7 to 16%. When reported, the angiographic outcomes up to 1 year following angioplasty ranged from improvement or stability of stenosis to complete vessel occlusion.

After performing balloon angioplasty on 42 patients, 13 of whom had posterior circulation stenosis, Mori and colleagues described an angiographic classification of intracranial atherosclerotic lesions that indicated suitability for the

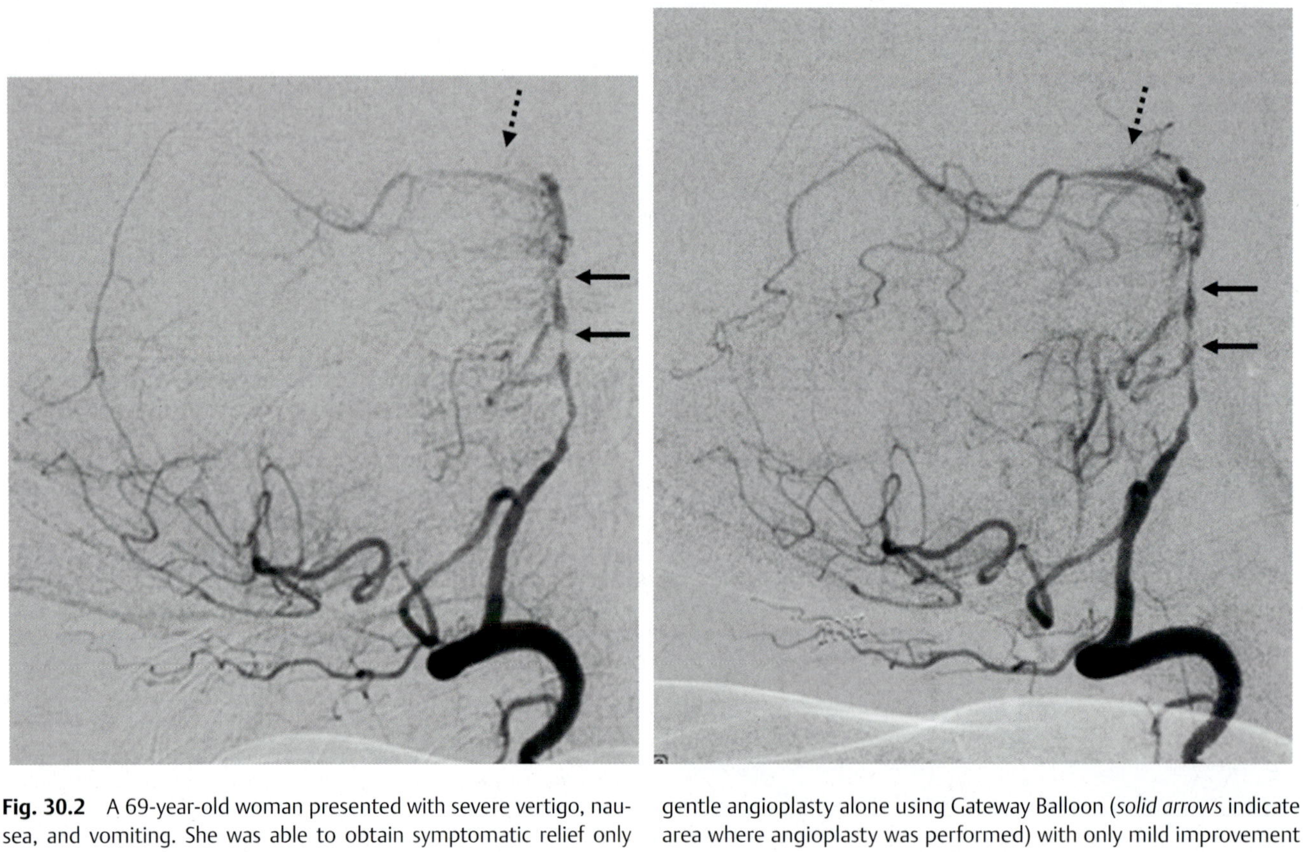
A B

Fig. 30.2 A 69-year-old woman presented with severe vertigo, nausea, and vomiting. She was able to obtain symptomatic relief only when lying down. **(A)** Cerebral angiogram reveals multifocal severe stenoses of the basilar artery (*solid arrows*) with diminutive filling of the posterior cerebral arteries (*dotted arrow*). **(B)** She underwent gentle angioplasty alone using Gateway Balloon (*solid arrows* indicate area where angioplasty was performed) with only mild improvement in degree of stenosis but significant improvement in posterior cerebral artery flow (*dotted arrow*). Her symptoms resolved following the procedure.

procedure. The three different lesions types described were as follows:

1. Type A: short (<5 mm), concentric or moderately eccentric, without vessel occlusion
2. Type B: 5 to 10 mm long, tubular configuration, eccentric, moderately angulated or totally occluded lesions but less than 3 months old
3. Type C: >10 mm long, tortuous configuration, angulated more than 90 degrees or totally occluded lesions and 3 or more months old

In this retrospective study, immediate clinical success rates of angioplasty in 80 hemodynamically significant extracranial and intracranial lesions for types A, B, and C were 92%, 86%, and 33%, with a 1-year restenosis rate of 0%, 33%, and 100%, respectively.[22]

In 1999, Connors and colleagues reported on their technique as it evolved over their retrospective 9-year experience with balloon angioplasty, with 35% of the 70 patients having posterior circulation intracranial stenosis. Their technique evolved from approximating the size of the balloon to the vessel caliber with rapid inflation to undersizing the balloon compared with the treated vessel with extremely slow inflation. Their technique of a very slow balloon inflation rate (1 atm/min) with an undersized angioplasty balloon resulted in lower periprocedural complication rates. Additionally, undersizing the balloon may have resulted in a suboptimal angiographic image but provided safer clinical results with reduced intimal damage, vessel dissection, and platelet aggregation.[23] In 2006, Marks and colleagues published long-term follow-up data on 120 patients (50% in the posterior circulation) with a mean posttreatment stenosis of 36%, a periprocedural stroke and death rate of 5.8%, and a 4.4% annual stroke rate for all strokes over a mean follow-up of 42 months.[24] Of note, this study contained patients with combined moderate and severe stenosis. A similarly large retrospective study by Wojak and colleagues on 84 lesions, all of which had greater than 70% initial stenosis and included 45% intracranial posterior circulation lesions, showed a low periprocedural stroke and death rate of 4.8% and a remarkably low annualized stroke and death rate of 3%, with a mean follow-up of 45 months.[25] Stents were used in 26% of the procedures, either primarily or secondarily, because of an inadequate response to angioplasty. Ten procedures had radiographic evidence of dissection that did not require treatment with a stent.

A 2008 retrospective comparison by Siddiq and colleagues confirms that angioplasty alone tends to have higher residual stenosis compared with stenting in 95 angioplasties and 98 stenting procedures.[26] However, this particular study found no statistically significant difference in the rates of periprocedural stroke, angiographic restenosis, or stroke-free and/or death-free survival between the two groups. The 2006 Wojak study states that only five were symptomatic, although 23% of their lesions developed restenosis. The degree of angiographic reduction to achieve clinical benefit has thus been controversial (i.e., whether less than 30 or 50% residual stenosis constitutes a technical success). Although stenting achieves an immediate greater reduction in degree of stenosis, this reduction may not translate into clinical benefit and is offset by greater technical difficulties. Several studies have suggested that stenting is technically more challenging than angioplasty,[27] though this challenge may become less of an issue with the widespread use of self-expanding stents, as discussed in the next section.

Stenting and Angioplasty

In a manner similar to the evolution of angioplasty balloons and techniques, endovascular treatment of ICAD with stents has evolved considerably in the past decade and was first explored in single-center studies with small numbers of patients. Furthermore, like primary angioplasty, prospective data on intracranial stenting for ICAD are limited and compounded by differing patient populations in terms of severity of stenosis and timing of treatment in regard to symptomatic qualifying events. Studies before 2005 utilized balloon-expandable stents borrowed from cardiology practice or balloon-expandable stents designed for intracranial circulation. These early, small, retrospective studies report periprocedural neurological complication rates of 8 to 30% using balloon-mounted coronary stents (BMCS), including those specifically involving the posterior circulation.[28–31]

In 2004, the results of the Stenting of Symptomatic Atherosclerotic Lesions in the Vertebral or Intracranial Arteries (SSLYVIA) study were published. A multicenter, nonrandomized, prospective, feasibility study, SSYLVIA evaluated the Neurolink stent system (Guidant Corporation, Indianapolis, IN) for treatment of vertebral and intracranial arteries. The Neurolink stent featured bare metal and was balloon-expandable. A total of 61 patients, including 43 intracranial and 18 extracranial with ≥50% atherosclerotic stenosis, were included. About two-thirds of the lesions were located in the posterior circulation, including 17 basilar, 5 intracranial, and 18 extracranial vertebral lesions (6 of which were ostial). The technical success rate of stent placement was 95%, with a 6.6% periprocedural stroke risk. The overall stroke rate at 1 year was 13.2% for all lesions and 14% for intracranial treated lesions. The stroke rate in the territory of the stented artery was 7.2% at 30 days and 10.9% at 1 year, which is comparable to WASID study results. At 6 months, high recurrent stenosis (≥50%) was noted in stented extracranial vertebral arteries (42.9%) in comparison to intracranial arteries (32.4%). Higher restenosis rates were noted for treated vertebral ostial lesions (67%). Factors that were significantly associated with restenosis were diabetes, postprocedure diameter stenosis >30%, and small vessel diameter.[32]

In 2007, Jiang and colleagues reported a 94% stent success rate specifically in the vertebrobasilar circulation with a balloon-mounted stent, with higher complication rates in the basilar artery compared with the vertebral artery.[33] A 2007 publication of a 7-year experience from Fiorella and colleagues also reported a 96% success rate with BMCS for symptomatic vertebrobasilar intracranial atheromatous disease. However, this group observed a 26% periprocedural complication rate.[34] A study by Kurre and colleagues of 21 patients with >70% intracranial stenosis, including more than 50% of patients with posterior circulation lesions, showed technical feasibility in achieving recanalization with the balloon-expandable Pharos stent (OBEX, Auckland, New Zealand) with stent failure in only one case.[35] Nevertheless, all groups noted difficulty with navigation distally and through marked tortuosity, necessitating aggressive distal parent-guide catheter access, stiff exchange-length microwires, which expose small vessels to risk of dissection and perforation, and aggressive angioplasty to free the stent from the balloon as detailed by Fiorella and colleagues.

In 2005, a self-expanding nitinol stent system newly designed specifically for intracranial arteries was approved by the U.S. Food and Drug Administration (FDA) for use under the Humanitarian Device Exemption. The Gateway Balloon Wingspan Stent System (Boston Scientific, Natick, MA) is designed to be more flexible and trackable, resulting in improved maneuverability through intracranial vasculature (**Figs. 30.3**

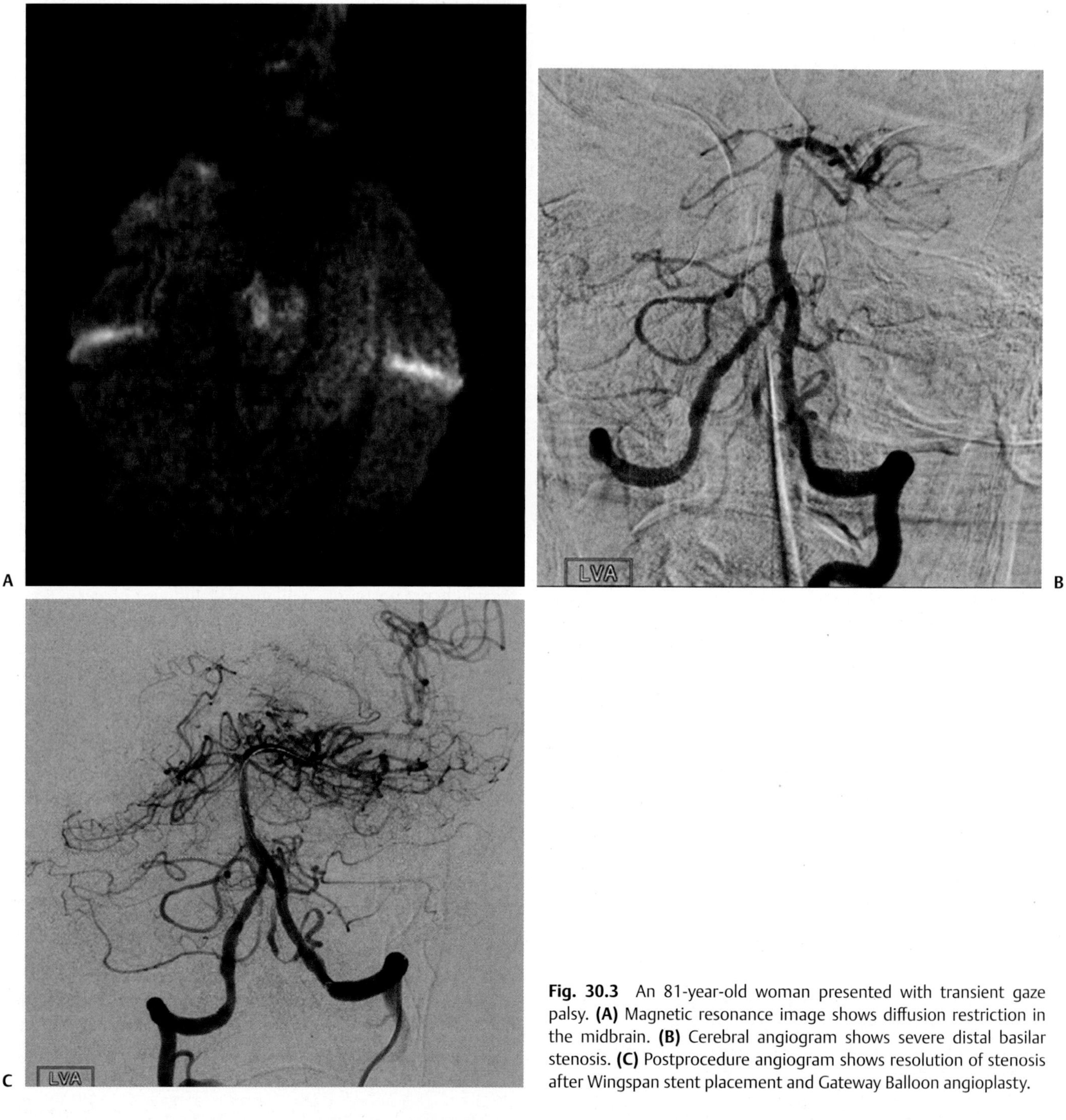

Fig. 30.3 An 81-year-old woman presented with transient gaze palsy. **(A)** Magnetic resonance image shows diffusion restriction in the midbrain. **(B)** Cerebral angiogram shows severe distal basilar stenosis. **(C)** Postprocedure angiogram shows resolution of stenosis after Wingspan stent placement and Gateway Balloon angioplasty.

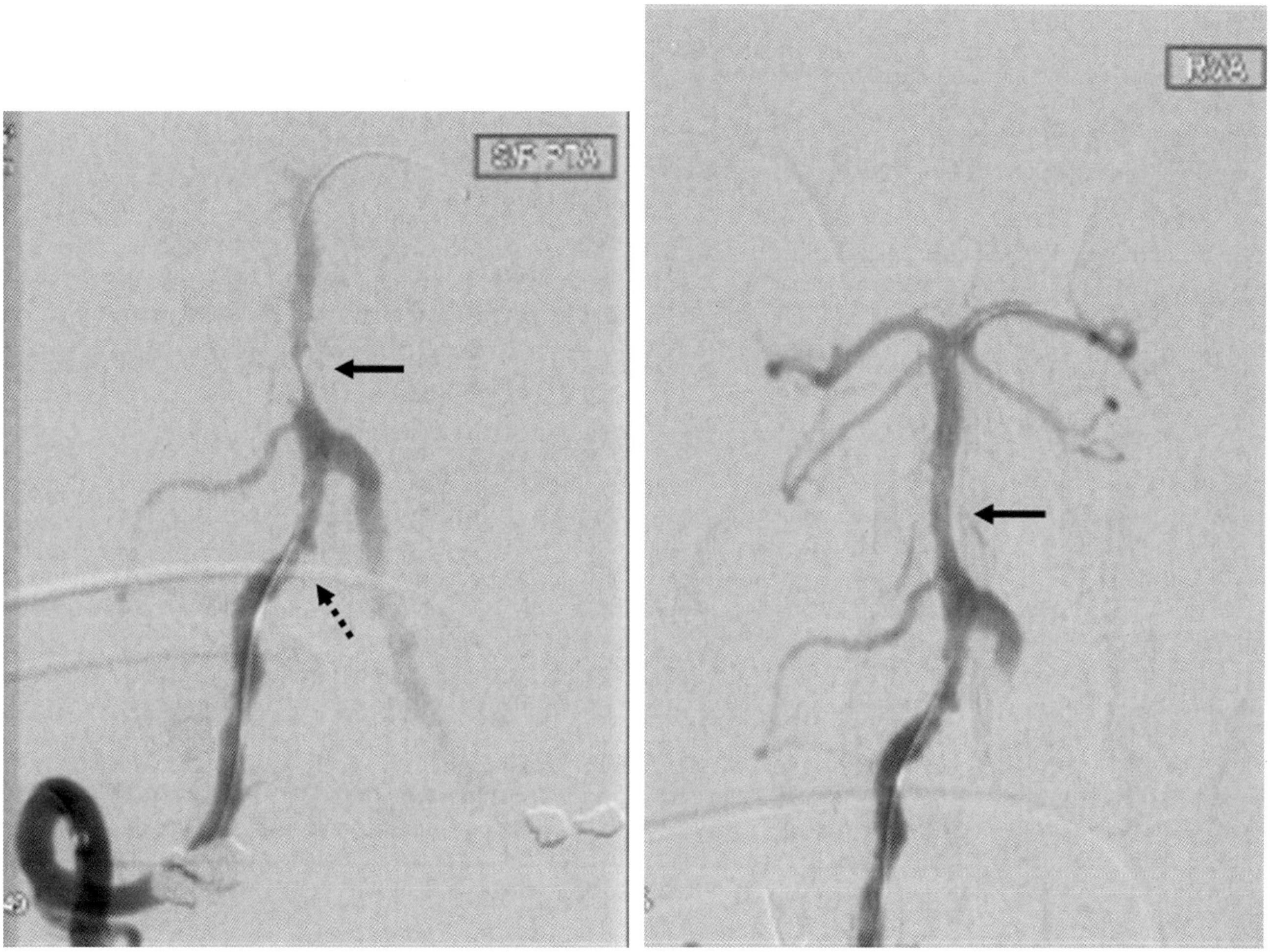

A B

Fig. 30.4 A 55-year-old right-handed man presented with three transient episodes of double vision and multiple episodes of dizziness. **(A)** Initial angiogram reveals a basilar stenosis of 75% (*arrow*). Note the diffuse atherosclerotic irregularity of the vertebral artery, necessitating careful catheterization (*dotted arrow*). Prestent angioplasty was performed with a 2.0 mm × 9.0 mm Gateway angioplasty balloon. A Wingspan 3 mm × 15 mm stent was then placed. **(B)** A final angioplasty was performed using a 3 mm × 15 mm Gateway angioplasty balloon leaving a residual 37% stenosis (*arrow*).

and **30.4**). The study that led to the approval evaluated the results of a prospective, single-arm, international multicenter investigation of the use of the Wingspan in 45 medically refractory patients with ≥50% stenosis in intracranial vessels with diameters of 2.5 to 4.5 mm. Almost half of the patients had posterior circulation stenosis. A high technical success rate (44 of 45 patients successfully treated), with an ipsilateral stroke/death rate of 4.5% at 30 days and 7% at 6 months, showed the Wingspan to be safe and effective.[36] Additional data reported in the multicenter Wingspan study of 78 patients in the United States showed a high technical success rate and low periprocedural rate of 6.1% within 30 days, and two-thirds of these patients had lesions with greater than 70% stenosis.[37] The overall rate of in-stent restenosis with the Wingspan was 31.2%, with a 9.7% symptomatic restenosis rate. The in-stent restenosis risk was high in younger patients with anterior circulation stenosis. In this study, the highest rates of both symptomatic and asymptomatic in-stent restenosis rates were observed in supraclinoid ICA stenosis.[38]

From the WASID study, it was evident that patients with 70 to 99% intracranial stenosis were at highest risk for recurrent strokes on medical therapy and were considered a subgroup that might benefit from endovascular therapy.[4] In 2008, Zaidat and colleagues published the results of the National Institutes of Health (NIH) Wingspan registry of 129 patients with 70 to 99% intracranial stenosis, with 40% of the lesions involving intracranial posterior circulation. A technical success rate of 97%, periprocedural risk rate of 6%, and 30-day stroke/death rate of 9.6% were reported. The rate of stroke, death, or intracerebral hemorrhage at 6 months was 14%, which was similar to the WASID endpoint in patients with 70 to 99% stenosis. The restenosis rate defined as ≥50% was noted in 25% of lesions.[39]

A 2009 review article examined 31 studies of angioplasty and stent placement in high-grade symptomatic stenosis and showed high technical success rates of 96%, with periprocedural stroke rates ranging widely from 0 to 50% (median 7.7%). Significantly higher periprocedural complication rates of 12.1% were noted in the posterior circulation as compared with 6.6% in the anterior circulation. No significant differences in the periprocedural complications rates were noted between balloon-mounted and self-expandable stents. Rates of restenosis of >50% were observed more frequently with self-expandable stents (17.4%) than with balloon-mounted stents (13.8%).[40]

Future Directions

The WASID study has helped to identify those patients who are at high risk of recurrent stroke despite medical therapy, suggesting the need for alternative therapies, such as extension of management of vascular risk factors and intracranial stenting. However, endovascular therapy of ICAD is not yet proven to be superior to medical therapy, especially given the new aggressive approaches to risk factor management. To discover whether endovascular therapy (i.e., angioplasty or stenting) of ICAD is superior to medical therapy, a randomized trial called Stenting and Aggressive Medical Management for Preventing Recurrent Strokes in Intracranial Stenosis (SAMMPRIS)[41] is underway. Funded by the NIH National Institute of Neurological Disorders and Stroke, this multicenter, prospective trial compares the best available medical therapy with endovascular angioplasty and stent placement (using the Gateway Balloon-Wingspan stent system) in symptomatic patients with 70 to 99% intracranial stenosis (**Fig. 30.5**). The primary endpoint is to determine whether there is a reduction of stroke or death within 30 days or ischemic stroke in the territory of symptomatic artery after 30 days during a 2-year follow-up from the start of the treatment regimen. Intensive medical therapy includes aspirin and clopidogrel, with aggressive management of blood pressure (target systolic blood pressure <140 mmHg), lipids (target LDL <70 mg/dL), and participation in a lifestyle modification program.

Patient Preparation and Techniques for Performing Intracranial Angioplasty and Stent Placement

Intracranial angioplasty and stenting should preferably be performed under general anesthesia to ensure adequate control over patient movement. The patient should be pretreated with antithrombotic medication prior to the performance of angioplasty or stenting procedures. The most commonly used choice of antithrombotic therapy is a combination of aspirin and clopidogrel. For elective cases, patients should receive both oral aspirin (325 mg) and clopidogrel (75 mg) daily for at least 5 days prior to the procedure. For emergency cases, a loading dose of clopidogrel (300 to 600 mg) with aspirin (325 mg) can be given orally 6 hours prior to the procedure or through a nasogastric tube at the time of the procedure, if necessary. Ticlopidine (250 mg) twice a day can replace clopidogrel in patients who cannot tolerate clopidogrel or who are allergic to it. Abciximab and eptifibatide are intravenous antiplatelet agents that can be used for emergencies.

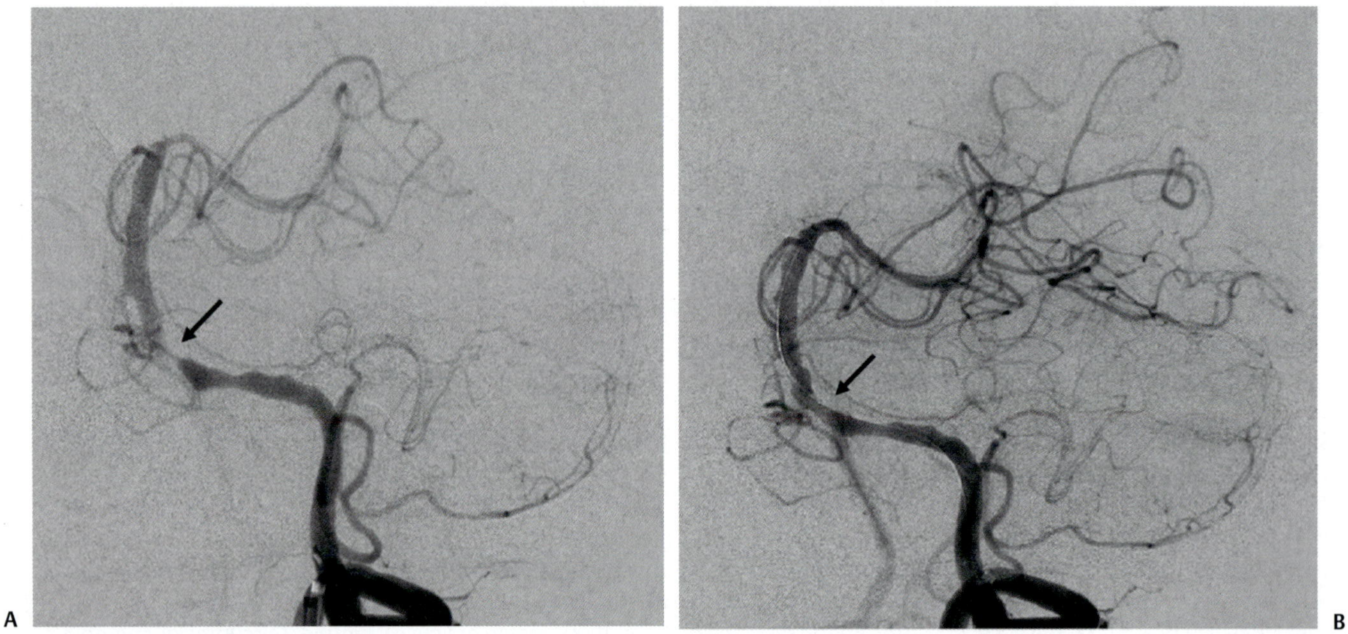

Fig. 30.5 A 54-year-old man presented with episodic double vision and dysarthria. **(A)** Cerebral angiogram reveals severe (>70%) stenosis of the proximal basilar artery (*arrow*). The patient underwent Wingspan stent placement. **(B)** There is a significant improvement in the degree of stenosis after stent placement (*arrow*) with improved opacification of the posterior cerebral arteries.

A firm, stable guide catheter of size 6-French or larger should be placed in the cervical vasculature for adequate base support. Baseline angiography should be obtained for initial evaluation of the intracranial vasculature to measure the degree of stenosis, length of stenosis, and parent vessel diameter and to obtain the best working views for the procedure. Patients should be systemically anticoagulated with heparin to keep baseline activated clotting time at least twice that of baseline value.

The choice of device will depend on the type of procedure to be performed, whether it is angioplasty alone or angioplasty with stent placement. Various balloons in smaller sizes are available for intracranial angioplasty. Balloon catheters commonly used for treatment of intracranial atherosclerotic lesions are Gateway (Boston Scientific) and Maverick (Boston Scientific). The balloon should be sized according to the vessel of interest and not exceed the normal vessel diameter but should be long enough to cover the entire segment of stenosis. Prior to insertion, the balloon catheter should be prepared according to manufacturer guidelines to eliminate air in the system. The balloon catheter can be navigated directly, preferably over an exchange length microguidewire measuring 0.014 inch and 300 cm, and the area of stenosis should be crossed gently. In more tortuous vessels, a microcatheter can be used to support the microguidewire to access the area of interest, which then can be exchanged for a balloon catheter over an exchange length microguidewire. All balloon catheters have fluoroscopic markers to help align the balloon catheter across the stenosis. After appropriate placement, the balloon should be slowly inflated to no more than 80% of normal vessel diameter followed by slow deflation. After performing angioplasty, the balloon catheter can be removed while leaving the exchange length microguidewire in place, thus maintaining distal access to the lesion. An angiographic run should be obtained to assess complications, including vessel dissection, vessel rupture, platelet aggregation, and distal embolization. The degree of stenosis and distal flow should be reassessed for possible stent placement, if needed.

Several stents are available, depending on their configuration, and include both balloon-mounted and self-expanding stents. The most commonly used stents are Driver (Medtronic, Minneapolis, MN), Cypher (Cordis, Bridgewater, NJ), Apollo (MicroPort, Shanghai, China), and Wingspan with Gateway Balloon (Boston Scientific). The stent should be sized according to the vessel of interest. Prestent angioplasty over an exchange microguidewire may be necessary if the degree of stenosis is too severe to allow primary stent placement. The diameter of the stent should be slightly larger or, at minimum, equal to the diameter of the normal vessel. The length of stent should be measured to cover the entire length of stenosis and 3 mm of normal vessel both proximal and distal to the stenosis. The stent catheter should be prepared according to manufacturer guidelines. The stent catheter should then be navigated over the exchange length microguidewire and positioned across the stenosis using stent position markers. Stent deployment should be done in a smooth fashion, neither too fast nor to slow, according to the manufacturer deployment technique, which may vary with the manufacturer and type of stent used.

After the stent is fully deployed, the delivery catheter can be removed, leaving the exchange length microguidewire in place, to maintain distal access. Again, an angiographic run should be obtained to assess possible complications, stent position, and degree of residual stenosis. These results should be compared with preprocedure images to assess improvement in the degree of stenosis and flow distal to the stenosis. If the degree of residual stenosis warrants angioplasty, the appropriate balloon-size catheter should be selected. The balloon catheter should be navigated over the exchange length wire and placed carefully within the stent lumen across the stenosis.

At this time, the Gateway Balloon and Wingspan stent system are the only FDA-approved endovascular devices for performing intracranial angioplasty and stenting of atherosclerotic lesions. Vital signs, particularly blood pressure and pulse, should be constantly monitored during the procedure. Any sudden rise in blood pressure with decline in pulse rate can indicate intracranial hemorrhage, which will require discontinuation of heparin drip and prompt reversal of heparin with protamine.

Postprocedure, the patient should be placed in an intensive care unit and closely monitored for changes in neurological status for 12 to 24 hours. Dual antiplatelet therapy, including aspirin and clopidogrel, should be continued for at least 30 days in patients who underwent angioplasty alone and for 6 to 8 weeks in patients who had angioplasty with stent placement. Aspirin should be continued afterward for an indefinite period.

Conclusion

ICAD of the posterior fossa is associated with a high risk of ischemic strokes. The WASID trial provides insight into the natural history of the disease and choice of medical therapy. Even with medical therapy, patients with severe intracranial stenosis are at high risk of recurrent stroke. Recent advances in stent and angioplasty techniques and availability of favorable intracranial catheters have made endovascular procedures an option for treatment of ICAD. Several prospective case series, single-arm studies, and retrospective studies have suggested a benefit of stenting and angioplasty in patients with >70% intracranial stenosis, with unanswered questions regarding the risk/benefit ratio of angioplasty alone versus stenting as well as the clinical implication of not insignificant restenosis rates. Randomized clinical trials like SAMMPRIS are underway to assess the benefit of endovascular therapy in this selected group of patients, bringing us a step closer toward evidence-based patient management of this serious disease.

References

1. Lloyd-Jones D, Adams RJ, Brown TM, et al; Writing Group Members; American Heart Association Statistics Committee and Stroke Statistics Subcommittee. Heart disease and stroke statistics—2010 update: a report from the American Heart Association. Circulation 2010;121(7):e46–e215
2. Waddy SP, Cotsonis G, Lynn MJ, et al. Racial differences in vascular risk factors and outcomes of patients with intracranial atherosclerotic arterial stenosis. Stroke 2009;40(3):719–725
3. Wityk RJ, Lehman D, Klag M, Coresh J, Ahn H, Litt B. Race and sex differences in the distribution of cerebral atherosclerosis. Stroke 1996;27(11):1974–1980
4. Chimowitz MI, Lynn MJ, Howlett-Smith H, et al; Warfarin-Aspirin Symptomatic Intracranial Disease Trial Investigators. Comparison of warfarin and aspirin for symptomatic intracranial arterial stenosis. N Engl J Med 2005;352(13):1305–1316
5. Kasner SE, Chimowitz MI, Lynn MJ, et al; Warfarin Aspirin Symptomatic Intracranial Disease Trial Investigators. Predictors of ischemic stroke in the territory of a symptomatic intracranial arterial stenosis. Circulation 2006;113(4):555–563
6. The Warfarin-Aspirin Symptomatic Intracranial Disease (WASID) Study Group. Prognosis of patients with symptomatic vertebral or basilar artery stenosis. Stroke 1998;29(7):1389–1392
7. Kasner SE, Lynn MJ, Chimowitz MI, et al; Warfarin Aspirin Symptomatic Intracranial Disease (WASID) Trial Investigators. Warfarin vs aspirin for symptomatic intracranial stenosis: subgroup analyses from WASID. Neurology 2006;67(7):1275–1278
8. Marquardt L, Kuker W, Chandratheva A, Geraghty O, Rothwell PM. Incidence and prognosis of > or = 50% symptomatic vertebral or basilar artery stenosis: prospective population-based study. Brain 2009;132(Pt 4):982–988
9. Qureshi AI, Ziai WC, Yahia AM, et al. Stroke-free survival and its determinants in patients with symptomatic vertebrobasilar stenosis: a multicenter study. Neurosurgery 2003;52(5):1033–1039, discussion 1039–1040
10. Taylor RA, Qureshi AI. Intracranial atherosclerotic disease. Curr Treat Options Neurol 2009;11(6):444–451
11. Derdeyn CP, Chimowitz MI. Angioplasty and stenting for atherosclerotic intracranial stenosis: rationale for a randomized clinical trial. Neuroimaging Clin N Am 2007;17(3):355–363, viii–ix viii–ix
12. Chaturvedi S, Turan TN, Lynn MJ, et al; WASID Study Group. Risk factor status and vascular events in patients with symptomatic intracranial stenosis. Neurology 2007;69(22):2063–2068
13. LaRosa JC, Grundy SM, Waters DD, et al; Treating to New Targets (TNT) Investigators. Intensive lipid lowering with atorvastatin in patients with stable coronary disease. N Engl J Med 2005;352(14):1425–1435
14. Lindenstrøm E, Boysen G, Nyboe J. Influence of total cholesterol, high density lipoprotein cholesterol, and triglycerides on risk of cerebrovascular disease: the Copenhagen City Heart Study. BMJ 1994;309(6946):11–15
15. Amarenco P, Labreuche J. Lipid management in the prevention of stroke: review and updated meta-analysis of statins for stroke prevention. Lancet Neurol 2009;8(5):453–463
16. Adams RJ, Albers G, Alberts MJ, et al; American Heart Association; American Stroke Association. Update to the AHA/ASA recommendations for the prevention of stroke in patients with stroke and transient ischemic attack. Stroke 2008;39(5):1647–1652
17. Sundt TM Jr, Smith HC, Campbell JK, Vlietstra RE, Cucchiara RF, Stanson AW. Transluminal angioplasty for basilar artery stenosis. Mayo Clin Proc 1980;55(11):673–680
18. Gress DR, Smith WS, Dowd CF, Van Halbach V, Finley RJ, Higashida RT. Angioplasty for intracranial symptomatic vertebrobasilar ischemia. Neurosurgery 2002;51(1):23–27, discussion 27–29
19. Higashida RT, Tsai FY, Halbach VV, et al. Transluminal angioplasty for atherosclerotic disease of the vertebral and basilar arteries. J Neurosurg 1993;78(2):192–198
20. Nahser HC, Henkes H, Weber W, Berg-Dammer E, Yousry TA, Kühne D. Intracranial vertebrobasilar stenosis: angioplasty and follow-up. AJNR Am J Neuroradiol 2000;21(7):1293–1301
21. Terada T, Higashida RT, Halbach VV, et al. Transluminal angioplasty for arteriosclerotic disease of the distal vertebral and basilar arteries. J Neurol Neurosurg Psychiatry 1996;60(4): 377–381
22. Mori T, Fukuoka M, Kazita K, Mori K. Follow-up study after intracranial percutaneous transluminal cerebral balloon angioplasty. AJNR Am J Neuroradiol 1998;19(8):1525–1533
23. Connors JJ III, Wojak JC. Percutaneous transluminal angioplasty for intracranial atherosclerotic lesions: evolution of technique and short-term results. J Neurosurg 1999;91(3):415–423
24. Marks MP, Wojak JC, Al-Ali F, et al. Angioplasty for symptomatic intracranial stenosis: clinical outcome. Stroke 2006;37(4): 1016–1020
25. Wojak JC, Dunlap DC, Hargrave KR, DeAlvare LA, Culbertson HS, Connors JJ III. Intracranial angioplasty and stenting: long-term results from a single center. AJNR Am J Neuroradiol 2006;27(9): 1882–1892
26. Siddiq F, Vazquez G, Memon MZ, et al. Comparison of primary angioplasty with stent placement for treating symptomatic intracranial atherosclerotic diseases: a multicenter study. Stroke 2008;39(9):2505–2510
27. Qureshi AI, Hussein HM, El-Gengaihy A, Abdelmoula M, K Suri MF. Concurrent comparison of outcomes of primary angioplasty and of stent placement in high-risk patients with symptomatic intracranial stenosis. Neurosurgery 2008;62(5):1053–1060, discussion 1060–1062
28. Gomez CR, Misra VK, Liu MW, et al. Elective stenting of symptomatic basilar artery stenosis. Stroke 2000;31(1):95–99
29. Kim DJ, Lee BH, Kim DI, Shim WH, Jeon P, Lee TH. Stent-assisted angioplasty of symptomatic intracranial vertebrobasilar artery stenosis: feasibility and follow-up results. AJNR Am J Neuroradiol 2005;26(6):1381–1388
30. Chow MM, Masaryk TJ, Woo HH, Mayberg MR, Rasmussen PA. Stent-assisted angioplasty of intracranial vertebrobasilar atherosclerosis: midterm analysis of clinical and radiologic predictors of neurological morbidity and mortality. AJNR Am J Neuroradiol 2005;26(4):869–874
31. Mori T, Kazita K, Chokyu K, Mima T, Mori K. Short-term arteriographic and clinical outcome after cerebral angioplasty and stenting for intracranial vertebrobasilar and carotid atherosclerotic occlusive disease. AJNR Am J Neuroradiol 2000;21(2): 249–254
32. SSYLVIA Study Investigators. Stenting of Symptomatic Atherosclerotic Lesions in the Vertebral or Intracranial Arteries (SSYLVIA): study results. Stroke 2004;35(6):1388–1392
33. Jiang WJ, Xu XT, Du B, et al. Long-term outcome of elective stenting for symptomatic intracranial vertebrobasilar stenosis. Neurology 2007;68(11):856–858
34. Fiorella D, Chow MM, Anderson M, Woo H, Rasmussen PA, Masaryk TJ. A 7-year experience with balloon-mounted coronary stents for the treatment of symptomatic vertebrobasilar intracranial atheromatous disease. Neurosurgery 2007;61(2):236–242, discussion 242–243
35. Kurre W, Berkefeld J, Sitzer M, Neumann-Haefelin T, du Mesnil de Rochemont R. Treatment of symptomatic high-grade intracranial stenoses with the balloon-expandable Pharos stent: initial experience. Neuroradiology 2008;50(8):701–708

36. Bose A, Hartmann M, Henkes H, et al. A novel, self-expanding, nitinol stent in medically refractory intracranial atherosclerotic stenoses: the Wingspan study. Stroke 2007;38(5):1531–1537
37. Fiorella D, Levy EI, Turk AS, et al. US multicenter experience with the wingspan stent system for the treatment of intracranial atheromatous disease: periprocedural results. Stroke 2007;38(3): 881–887
38. Turk AS, Levy EI, Albuquerque FC, et al. Influence of patient age and stenosis location on wingspan in-stent restenosis. AJNR Am J Neuroradiol 2008;29(1):23–27
39. Zaidat OO, Klucznik R, Alexander MJ, et al; NIH Multi-center Wingspan Intracranial Stent Registry Study Group. The NIH registry on use of the Wingspan stent for symptomatic 70–99% intracranial arterial stenosis. Neurology 2008;70(17):1518–1524
40. Gröschel K, Schnaudigel S, Pilgram SM, Wasser K, Kastrup A. A systematic review on outcome after stenting for intracranial atherosclerosis. Stroke 2009;40(5):e340–e347
41. SAMMPRIS Clinical Trials.gov Identifier: NCT00576693. http://www.clinicaltrials.gov/ct2/show/NCT00576693. Retrieved January 20, 2012

31 Bypass Options for the Posterior Fossa

Sepideh Amin-Hanjani and Fady T. Charbel

Various extracranial and intracranial bypass options are available for revascularization of the posterior fossa. Although advances in endovascular treatment have reduced the need for surgical approaches to neurovascular diseases that affect posterior circulation, these approaches remain important tools in patient management. This chapter focuses on surgical techniques for posterior fossa revascularization.

Indications

Indications for revascularization of the posterior fossa fall into two broad categories:

1. Flow augmentation for treatment of posterior circulation cerebral ischemia
2. Flow replacement to preserve distal blood flow for vessel sacrifice related to aneurysm or tumor treatment

Flow Augmentation

Patients presenting with refractory vertebrobasilar insufficiency (VBI) despite maximal medical therapy are potential candidates for posterior circulation revascularization. Bypass for revascularization for posterior fossa ischemia has been less studied than anterior circulation ischemia due to the relative prevalence of the conditions, the availability and evolution of endovascular techniques for treatment of vertebrobasilar stenosis, and the relatively high morbidity and technical complexity of posterior circulation bypass. However, various extracranial-intracranial (EC-IC) bypass options to the posterior circulation are feasible, including occipital artery (OA) to posterior inferior cerebellar artery (PICA), and superficial temporal artery (STA) to superior cerebellar artery (SCA) or posterior cerebral artery (PCA) bypasses.[1,2] A variety of surgical options for revascularization of the extracranial vertebral artery (VA) are also available.[3,4]

As with other stroke syndromes, standard evaluation for patients presenting with VBI includes cerebrovascular and parenchymal brain imaging, typically with a combination of magnetic resonance imaging (MRI) and magnetic resonance angiography (MRA). If vertebrobasilar occlusive disease is evident, imaging and clinical presentation can ascertain the etiology as atherosclerotic (versus dissection or extrinsic) compression. Compromised flow in the vertebrobasilar system and distal arterial tree is difficult to evaluate with traditional modalities but can be assessed with quantitative MRA (QMRA) using phase-contrast magnetic resonance technique to directly measure posterior circulation vessel flow.[5] The utility of hemodynamic assessment in identifying high-risk patients who may benefit from revascularization is currently under investigation.[6]

Presently, however, the indications for surgical revascularization are limited because no prospective or randomized studies have been performed to assess the efficacy of surgical intervention, and the procedures carry the risk of morbidity. Overall, surgical revascularization of the posterior circulation carries a higher risk and lower patency rates than anterior circulation bypass. Patency rates for OA–PICA bypass range from 88 to 100%, with mortality rates averaging 4%.[7] For STA–PCA and STA–SCA bypass, a review of 86 bypasses compiled from several series revealed patency rates in the 78 to 90% range, with mortality averaging 12%[7,8] and serious morbidity averaging 20%. Although these series reported improvement in symptoms in a subset of patients, the morbidity and mortality associated with such revascularization procedures have introduced caution when entertaining surgical bypass options, particularly for patients with a poor neurological condition or medical comorbidities. Nonetheless, recent advances in microsurgical and neuroanesthetic technique, as well as improvements in perioperative neurointensive care management, allow posterior circulation revascularization to be successfully undertaken in select patients without other options for management.

The approach to treatment is to first optimize all medical therapeutic options, including maximizing antithrombotic regimens, controlling blood pressure judiciously, lowering lipids aggressively with statins, controlling glycemic levels, and encouraging smoking cessation. Anticoagulation with warfarin has shown an increased risk of complications and no benefit over antiplatelet therapy in patients with intracranial atherosclerotic intracranial disease.[9] If the patient has recurrent ischemia despite these measures and the disease is not amenable to endovascular therapy, then bypass options will be considered but only if comorbid cardiac or medical conditions do not prohibit general anesthesia and surgery. Particular caution should be used in considering bypass distal to a high-grade vessel stenosis (e.g., distal bypass for severe basilar stenosis). Distal bypass can create a competing flow at the location of disease that has the potential to promote thrombosis at the site of stenosis[10] and cause local infarction with devastating consequence.

Flow Replacement

Preserving posterior circulation flow through revascularization may be necessary with large skull base tumors or with planned vessel sacrifice to treat complex aneurysms in the posterior fossa. Giant, fusiform, dolichoectatic, or partially thrombosed aneurysms of the vertebrobasilar system are not amenable to direct clipping and can be equally challenging for endovascular treatment. Proximal vessel occlusion and flow reversal, or trapping, is a treatment option.[11,12] Occlusion can be performed without the need for revascularization if collaterals are adequate, and it appears to be well tolerated for basilar trunk and apex aneurysms if both posterior communicating arteries (PCOAs) are greater than 1 mm in diameter.[11] However, the risk of complications increases to 26% if one PCOA is smaller; the risk increases to 45% if both are less than 1 mm. Tolerance to vessel occlusion can be evaluated by clinical testing and evoked potential monitoring over 20 to 30 minutes during endovascular balloon test occlusion, with neurological or electrophysiological failure indicating the need for bypass. Typically, revascularization in these cases will require a graft to the PCA or SCA to provide collateral flow prior to proximal occlusion.

Occasionally, fusiform or dissecting aneurysms can be well addressed with trapping but, if major branches are involved, revascularization of the branch distal territory is necessary. This situation is most commonly encountered with vertebral aneurysms that involve the PICA segment, in which case OA–PICA or PICA–PICA bypass can be performed[12,13]; alternatively, the PICA can be reimplanted into a more proximal intradural segment of the VA. For distal aneurysms of the major cerebellar branches, occlusion of the vessel without bypass can be tolerated if occlusion is performed distal to the proximal brainstem segments of the vessel and other cerebellar arteries are present and large, thus averting a major cerebellar stroke. Alternatively, fusiform distal aneurysms can be considered for bypass or direct excision and reanastomosis.[14]

Therefore, revascularization in the posterior fossa is necessary when aneurysm treatment requires proximal major arterial occlusion and the native collateral flow is inadequate, or when an individual arterial branch vessel is incorporated into an aneurysm.

General Considerations

Preoperative Assessment

Patients who are considered for posterior circulation bypass should undergo angiography to delineate the intracranial vasculature and selective external carotid injections to evaluate the caliber and course of donor branches, such as the STA or OA. If there is concern regarding the adequacy of the in situ donors, alternative bypass strategies using interposition grafts (saphenous vein or radial artery) can be entertained. In patients with VBI, where atherosclerosis is the primary etiology for the vertebrobasilar disease encountered in such patients, systemic atherosclerotic disease is often present. Therefore, preoperative cardiac and medical clearance for cardiac risk stratification, including echocardiography and stress testing, is an important element of preoperative assessment.

If interposition grafts are anticipated, a saphenous vein can be harvested from the calf or thigh following preoperative ultrasound mapping to determine the suitability (size and length) of the vein. For a radial artery, the vessel is generally harvested from the nondominant arm after ensuring adequate ulnar artery collaterals to the hand with the Allen test. Endoscopic harvesting is feasible for both,[15,16] although recent date from the cardiac literature would suggest worse long-term results with endoscopically harvested grafts.[17]

Perioperative and Anesthetic Considerations

Patients should be placed on full dose (325 mg) aspirin, ideally beginning a week prior to surgery but at least the morning of surgery. Other antiplatelet agents, such as clopidogrel, are generally avoided due to bleeding risk, particularly in cases involving intracranial surgery. For patients requiring dual antiplatelets due to high thrombotic risk, the second agent can be discontinued a week prior to surgery and replaced with enoxaparin or equivalent until the day prior to surgery. If patients have been on warfarin anticoagulation, they are converted to intravenous heparin, which is withheld 6 hours prior to surgery as antiplatelets are administered.

Arterial line and central venous access is routinely obtained for surgery. Antibiotic prophylaxis is administered prior to skin incision and maintained for 48 hours postoperatively. Throughout the surgery, normovolemia, normocapnia, and normotension (based on a patient's baseline blood pressure) are maintained. For tenuous patients with VBI who are blood pressure–dependent, even extreme hypertension is maintained until the bypass has been completed. Monitoring somatosensory evoked potential (SSEP) and motor evoked potential (MEP) during surgery can be useful in alerting the operative team to inadequate blood pressure maintenance during the case. Scalp electrodes for electroencephalographic monitoring are placed outside the surgical field to monitor induction of metabolic burst suppression during temporary vessel occlusion for bypass. Inhalational agents are used preferentially for burst suppression because they increase cerebral blood flow in comparison to barbiturates. Intravenous anesthetics for burst suppression may be required if SSEP and MEP are monitored; otherwise, evoked potentials may be suppressed.

For intracranial bypass operations, lumbar drain for cerebrospinal fluid (CSF) drainage is preferred for brain relaxation to avoid the need for intravenous diuretics (furosemide), hyperosmolar agents (mannitol), or hyperventilation. Prior to cross-clamping of major vessels, intravenous heparin is administered. For entirely extracranial operations, full dosing with weight-appropriate heparin (routine dose 5000 units) is performed 5 minutes prior to initial vessel occlusion; an additional 1000 to 2000 units are administered as needed for a second anastomosis. For intracranial operations, smaller doses (generally 2000 units) are administered prior to temporary vessel occlusion. Heparin is allowed to wear off on its own.

Postoperative Management

Patients are continued immediately on 325 mg of aspirin daily. If aspirin cannot be administered orally, it can be given rectally. Patients are observed in the intensive care unit postoperatively and are kept well hydrated, with avoidance of hypotension. Pressure from glasses or a nasal oxygen cannula over the location of the bypass graft is avoided to prevent direct mechanical occlusion. In patients with bypass for ischemia, it is especially important to avoid hypertension given the potential risk for hyperperfusion hemorrhage, although this event occurs less commonly in the posterior circulation and with STA or OA grafts compared with larger and higher flow interposition grafts. Potential postoperative complications include epidural hematoma, wound infection, and postoperative graft occlusion. Patients are discharged on daily aspirin.

Flow Measurement

Both intraoperatively and postoperatively, measurement of flow is an invaluable adjunct to successful posterior fossa bypass.[18,19] During surgery, blood flow in the recipient, donor, and graft can be readily measured quantitatively with devices such as a microvascular ultrasonic flow probe (Charbel Micro-Flowprobe; Transonics Systems Inc., Ithaca, NY).[20] During flow replacement surgery for aneurysms, measurement of flow in the recipient vessel provides a direct indication of the flow that the bypass must provide. When in situ donors, such as STA or OA, are being considered, the "cut flow" of the donor vessel is determined by measuring the free flow through the cut end of the vessel. The cut flow represents the maximal flow-carrying capacity of the donor and helps to determine whether the flow is adequate for flow replacement or whether a larger interposition graft is needed. After completion of the bypass, measurement of the flow through the graft provides direct confirmation of the adequacy and patency of the bypass.[19] When using STA or OA as donor vessels in a bypass for ischemia, the cut-flow index (ratio of bypass flow to the initial cut flow) provides an excellent indication of bypass success and is a sensitive predictor of bypass function.[20] Intraoperative conventional angiography is generally unnecessary if direct flow measurements and video indocyanine green (ICG) angiography are performed for physiologic and anatomic graft confirmation.

Postoperative assessment of bypass success and patency has traditionally relied on conventional angiography, although computed tomographic angiography (CTA) or MRA can be used. Alternatively or additionally, use of QMRA to measure flow in the graft and recipient vessels provides confirmation not only of patency but of graft function. QMRA provides a noninvasive option for serial monitoring over time.[21]

Extracranial Bypass Options

Extracranial revascularization procedures focus on diseases of the VA. The pathologies involved are primarily occlusive diseases, such as atherosclerotic stenosis, occlusion of the VA, or direct external compression. The most commonly utilized surgical options for treatment are vertebral–carotid transposition, carotid–vertebral bypass, and osteophyte foraminal decompression.

Vertebral–Carotid Transposition

Vertebral–carotid transposition (VCT) is performed for treatment of stenosis originating at the VA (**Fig. 31.1**). Performing a direct vertebral-origin endarterectomy[4] through a subclavian approach is also an option but is seldom used because VCT offers a simpler and more effective method of revascularization. The potential limitation of VCT is that it requires simultaneous occlusion of both carotid and vertebral arteries; however, given the proximal location of temporary occlusion on the common carotid and proximal vertebral arteries, cervical and muscular collaterals invariably prevent cerebral ischemia. If the carotid artery is stenotic or otherwise compromised, transposition to another location of the subclavian artery can be used. Similarly, if transposition is not feasible because of inadequate length of the proximal VA, an interposition vein or prosthetic graft bypass can be performed from the subclavian with end-to-end anastomosis to the VA.[22,23] Although this procedure does not interrupt carotid blood flow, it requires two anastomoses and is time consuming.

The proximal VA can be transposed from the subclavian artery to the thyrocervical trunk.[3,23] Occasionally, obstruction at the vertebral origin is extrinsic, caused by compression due to bands from the tendon of the anterior scalene or the longus colli muscle.[4,24] These ligaments, muscles, and bands overlying the artery can be excised. In some cases, the sympathetic ganglia or nerve fibers constrict the artery. If the ganglia are divided, a mild Horner syndrome will develop. Segmental resection and end-to-end anastomosis can be used when obstruction is caused by entrapment, but the VA must be long and its diameter adequate.

Positioning and Exposure

The patient's head is placed in extension on a donut head rest, in preparation for a supraclavicular approach (**Fig. 31.2A**). Downward traction of the arm and shoulder provides better exposure. The head is kept midline. A supraclavicular

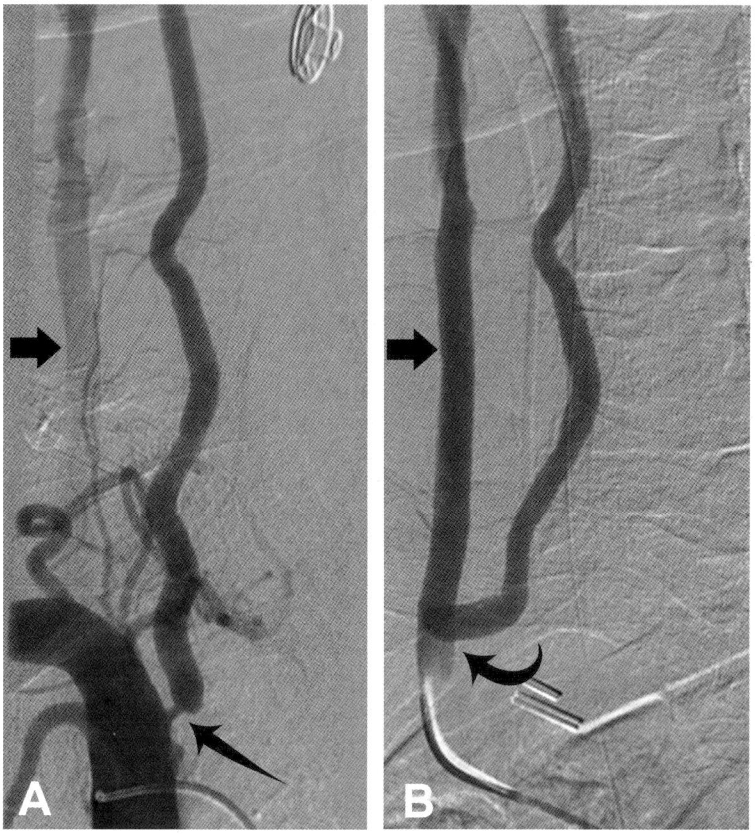

Fig. 31.1 Vertebral–carotid transposition (VCT). **(A)** An angiogram demonstrates severe right vertebral origin stenosis (*thin arrow*) and the common carotid artery (*thick arrow*). **(B)** Following VCT, carotid injection demonstrates transposition of the vertebral artery (*curved arrow*) with filling from the common carotid artery (*thick arrow*). (Reprinted with permission from the Department of Neurosurgery at University of Illinois at Chicago.)

incision is made ~2 cm above and parallel to the clavicle and extends from the suprasternal notch to 7 to 8 cm laterally. The skin is retracted superiorly and inferiorly, leaving the platysma, which is divided horizontally. The sternocleidomastoid muscle has two origins: the clavicular head from the superior surface of the medial third of the clavicle, and the sternal head from the anterior surface of the manubrium of the sternum. The clavicular head is divided, leaving a cuff on the clavicle, and the muscle is retracted superiorly and laterally. The underlying fat pad is mobilized superiorly by detaching it inferiorly. The omohyoid muscle can be divided if needed. The dissection is kept medial to expose the carotid sheath. The anterior scalene muscle lies laterally, with the phrenic nerve lying on top of it. This muscle is usually far-lateral to the exposure and rarely requires division. The carotid sheath is separated from the overlying fascia and opened. Within the sheath, the common carotid artery, the internal jugular vein, and the vagus nerve can be found. The jugular vein and vagus nerve are retracted laterally, and the carotid is retracted medially. From this point, dissection proceeds below the deep fascia layer caudally.

Specific concerns are related to the side of exposure. If the right side is exposed, it is important to recognize that lymphatic drainage on the right side of the neck differs from that on the left. Delicate lymphatic trunks empty into the right subclavian and jugular veins, which are usually smaller than the lymphatic ducts on the left. Because they do not coagulate completely, ligation is preferred if these structures are encountered. The right recurrent laryngeal nerve exits the vagus nerve and loops below the right subclavian artery as it approaches the trachea and larynx. Consequently, medial retraction of the trachea can cause ipsilateral paresis of the vocal cord. If the left side is exposed, the thoracic duct is encountered as it arches from the side of the esophagus laterally to the angle between the internal jugular and subclavian veins. The proximal portion of this duct should be ligated twice, and smaller branches are also ligated. The left recurrent laryngeal nerve can be retracted with greater ease than the right because it loops around the aortic arches and approaches the trachea much lower.

Working in the deep fascial layer, the VA can be identified as the first branch of the subclavian artery exiting from its posterosuperior surface (**Fig. 31.2B**). This feature distinguishes it from the thyrocervical trunk, which has multiple branches and exits from the anterosuperior surface. Alternatively, and more easily, the VA can be first located superiorly as it exits the transverse foramen of C6. The transverse process of C6 can be palpated adjacent to its foramen. The artery arises from the apex of the anterior scalene and longus colli muscles as they attach to the carotid tubercle. The vertebral vein, which overlies the artery, can be carefully coagulated and divided or retracted. The vertebral vein is formed at the lower end of the canal of the transverse foramina from a venous plexus within the canal around the VA. The vein is anterior to the artery and often adherent to it. It is important to identify and preserve the sympathetic

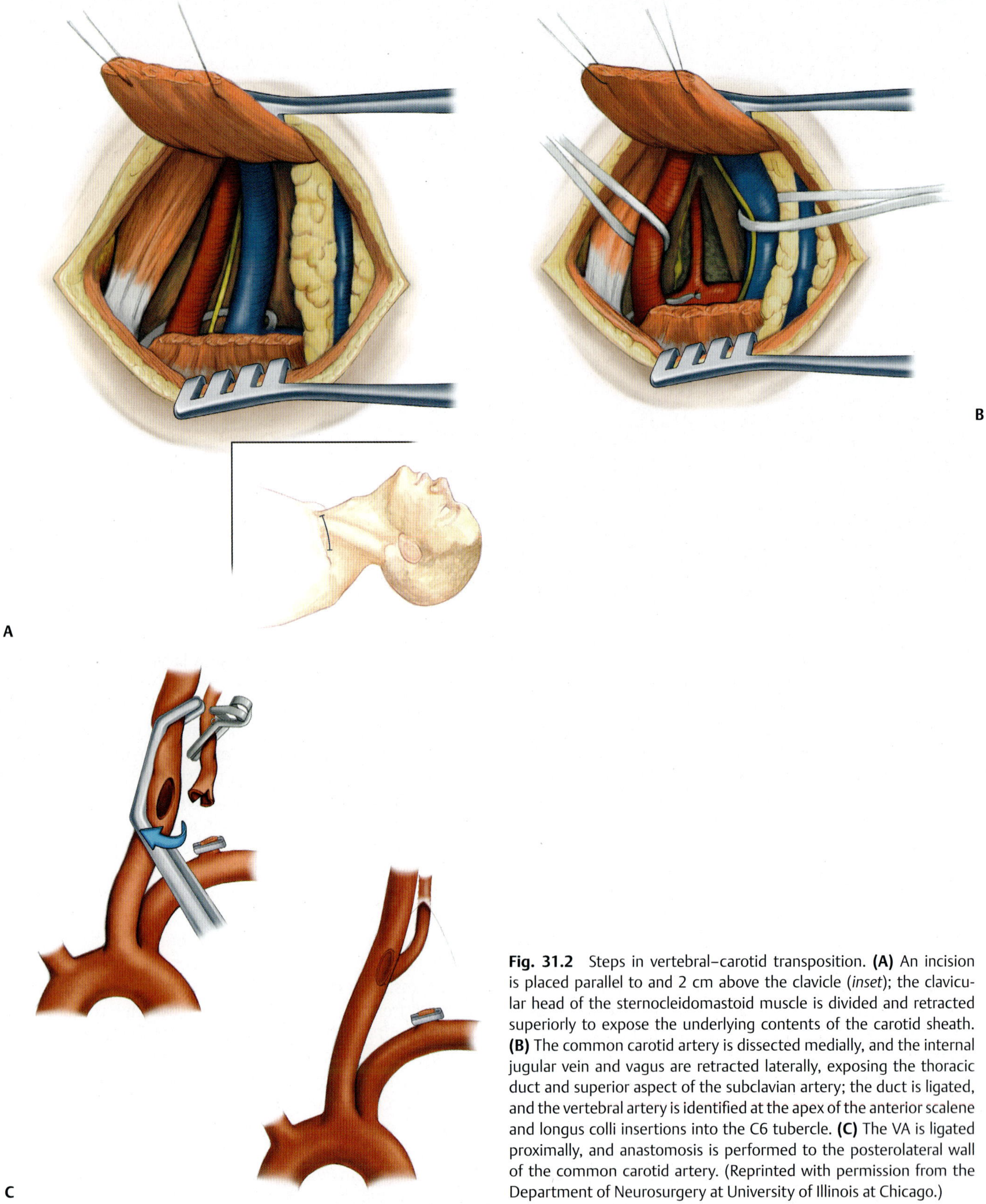

Fig. 31.2 Steps in vertebral–carotid transposition. **(A)** An incision is placed parallel to and 2 cm above the clavicle (*inset*); the clavicular head of the sternocleidomastoid muscle is divided and retracted superiorly to expose the underlying contents of the carotid sheath. **(B)** The common carotid artery is dissected medially, and the internal jugular vein and vagus are retracted laterally, exposing the thoracic duct and superior aspect of the subclavian artery; the duct is ligated, and the vertebral artery is identified at the apex of the anterior scalene and longus colli insertions into the C6 tubercle. **(C)** The VA is ligated proximally, and anastomosis is performed to the posterolateral wall of the common carotid artery. (Reprinted with permission from the Department of Neurosurgery at University of Illinois at Chicago.)

chain. The VA is dissected from C6 to the subclavian artery with care to avoid destroying the sympathetic trunks and stellate or intermediate ganglia that lie on it.

Transposition

The common carotid is prepared by clearing the adventitia. After heparin bolus, the VA is clamped at the level of C6 with a temporary clip. The proximal VA just above the stenosis is occluded with a hemo clip and transected. The artery is freed from the surrounding sympathetic trunk and moved medially toward the carotid. If the VA is not lax enough, it may be necessary to remove it from the C6 transverse process. A double-ended fish-mouth opening is made in the proximal end of the VA. An occluding clamp, such as a Satinsky clamp, is placed on the carotid artery at the selected level and used to rotate the vessel laterally (**Fig. 31.2C**). This maneuver allows the anastomosis to be performed on the posterolateral wall of the carotid in optimal orientation with the natural trajectory of the VA. The carotid is incised with a no. 15 or no. 11 blade, allowing the insertion of an appropriately sized aortic punch device for creation of the arteriotomy. With 7–0 monofilament nylon suture, the superior and inferior ends of the fish-mouth opening are sutured to the corresponding ends of the hole in the carotid artery. One suture is used to form a running anastomosis on the back wall and is tied to the opposite end on completion. The front wall is then sutured. Before the last suture is tied, the lumina of both arteries are flushed with heparinized saline. The VA and then the carotid are back-flushed. The final suture is tied, and all clamps are removed. If the suture line leaks, gentle pressure is placed over the anastomosis with Gelfoam (Baxter, Deerfield, IL). An additional interrupted suture can be placed for more significant leakage. After copious irrigation and hemostasis, the sternocleidomastoid muscle is reapproximated. A suction drain is placed in the neck for 24 hours, and the neck opening is closed in multiple layers.

Extracranial Carotid–Vertebral Bypass

Vein grafts can be used to bypass disease at a more proximal aspect of the VA by connecting the distal VA to the carotid artery.[25] The V2 segment of the VA is partially encased in a bony channel as it travels through the transverse foramina of the C1 through C6 cervical segments. Anatomically, however, the vertebral has more redundancy and is more easily accessible at the distal V2 segment (between C1 and C2) where anastomosis is favorable.[26] The graft can be attached to the external carotid artery, or the external carotid artery can be transposed onto the VA.[25] The advantage of the external carotid artery as the donor supply is that the proximal anastomosis does not interfere with the cerebral circulation. Although vein grafts to the mid-V2 segment can be performed successfully[27] with an anterior approach to expose the VA and the carotid artery, the C1-C2 VA segment accessed via the anterolateral approach is particularly amenable to bypass. In the C1-C2 interspace, a 2-cm segment of vessel can be exposed without the need for bony removal and unroofing of the vertebral canal that is necessary in the mid-V2 segment.

Positioning and Exposure

The exposure is made via an anterolateral approach, high in the anterior triangle (**Fig. 31.3A**). The patient's head is placed midline in rigid Mayfield fixation without turning the head so that the sternocleidomastoid does not obscure the exposure. Subluxation of the jaw to the contralateral side is a useful maneuver to provide additional exposure. The incision is made on the medial edge of the sternocleidomastoid muscle and extends in a curvilinear fashion over the mastoid bone. The auricular nerve may be encountered posterosuperiorly and may need to be transected. The incision is brought down to the platysma muscle and along the medial border of the sternocleidomastoid muscle. The carotid sheath is encountered, and the internal jugular vein is identified. The parotid gland is freed from the sternocleidomastoid muscle and reflected anteriorly. The internal jugular vein is then retracted medially and the sternocleidomastoid muscle laterally. Below and along the sternocleidomastoid muscle, the accessory nerve is visible. This nerve is protected by mobilizing the nerve, placing a loop around it, and retracting it, generally medially. The belly of the digastric muscle is retracted superiorly, or it can be divided. Below the digastric muscle, the C1 tubercle is palpated, and the location can be confirmed by obtaining a lateral cervical radiograph. The remainder of the dissection is best performed under microscopic magnification. The fascia is cleared, and the fibers of the levator scapulae and splenius cervicis become visible. The C2 tubercle is also palpated, and the levator scapulae is cut. Unlike the lower cervical nerves, the anterior ramus of the C2 nerve root lays anterior to the VA in its position between C1 and C2. Cutting the nerve root exposes the VA; the nerve should be cut posteriorly and retracted anteriorly and medially to avoid traction on the proximal root and spinal cord (**Fig. 31.3B**). Further dissection of the overlying tissue reveals a venous plexus surrounding the VA. Careful coagulation or the use of Gelfoam prevents injury to the artery. Approximately 2 cm of VA can be exposed in the C1-C2 intertransverse process interspace. Further exposure can be obtained by removing the lateral wall of the transverse foramen of C1.

Bypass

The preferred donor site is the external carotid artery or common carotid artery. The vein or radial artery graft is harvested in usual fashion and its end cut at a bevel. The patient is given heparin (5000 units). After 5 minutes, the VA is gently pulled up and temporary clips are used to isolate the segment. An incision is made, and an arteriotomy is created and sized to the cut end of the graft. With vein grafts, particular attention to graft orientation is necessary to ensure

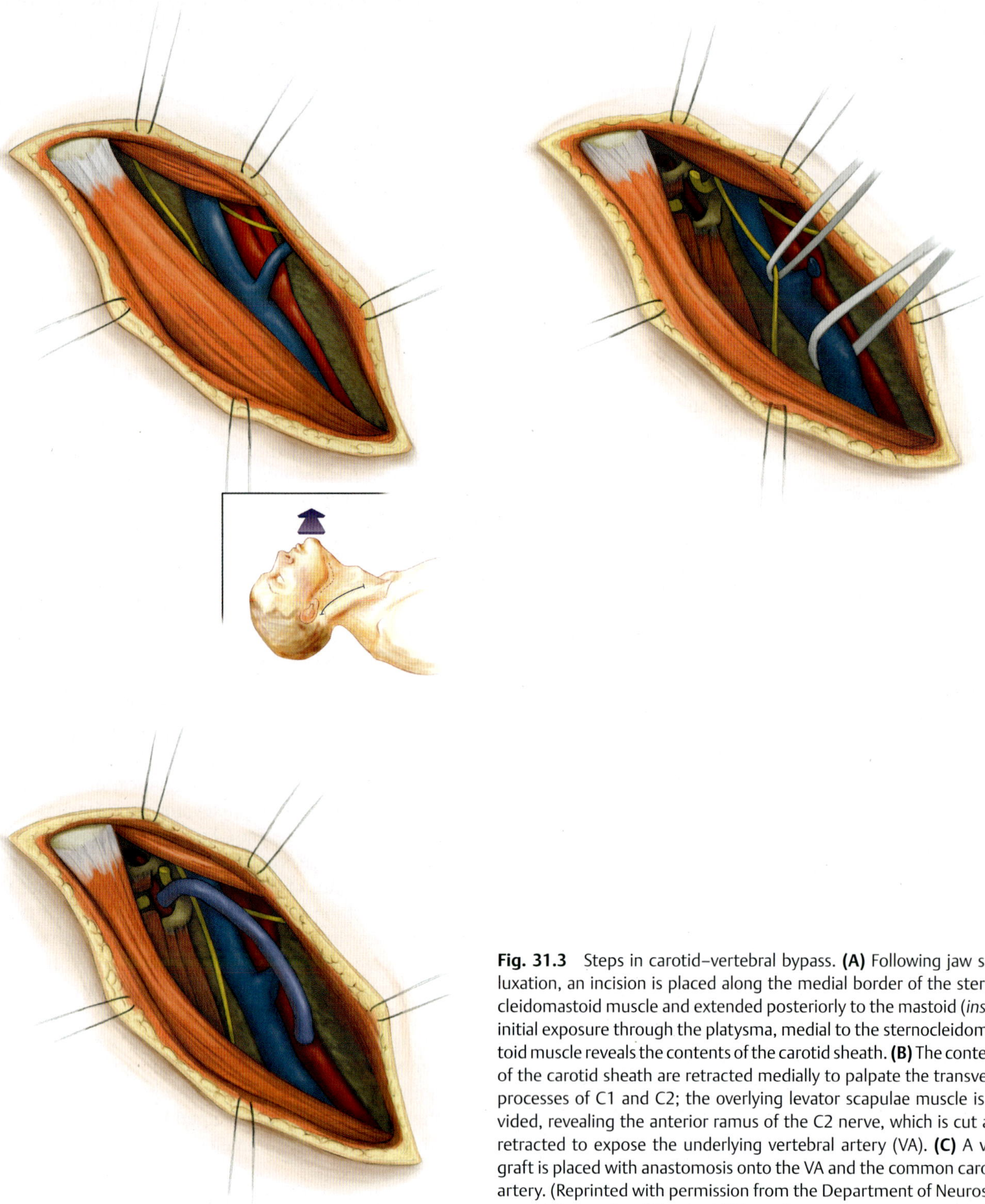

A B C

Fig. 31.3 Steps in carotid–vertebral bypass. **(A)** Following jaw subluxation, an incision is placed along the medial border of the sternocleidomastoid muscle and extended posteriorly to the mastoid (*inset*); initial exposure through the platysma, medial to the sternocleidomastoid muscle reveals the contents of the carotid sheath. **(B)** The contents of the carotid sheath are retracted medially to palpate the transverse processes of C1 and C2; the overlying levator scapulae muscle is divided, revealing the anterior ramus of the C2 nerve, which is cut and retracted to expose the underlying vertebral artery (VA). **(C)** A vein graft is placed with anastomosis onto the VA and the common carotid artery. (Reprinted with permission from the Department of Neurosurgery at University of Illinois at Chicago.)

flow is in the appropriate direction relative to the valves. The vein is connected to the VA with an end-to-side anastomosis using 8–0 Prolene (Ethicon, Somerville, NJ). Temporary clips are removed. If backflow through the graft is good, a temporary clip is used to occlude the graft just above the anastomosis. The donor portion of the carotid is cleared of surrounding tissue, and a cross-clamp is applied to its proximal and distal portions. Using an aortic punch, a 4-mm or 5-mm elliptical arteriotomy is made in the wall of the carotid. With 6–0 polypropylene, the vein graft is anastomosed in an end-to-side fashion. Backflow is allowed from the graft and distal carotid before the final suture is placed and tied. The clamps on the carotid and graft are then removed to establish flow in the bypass (**Fig. 31.3.C**). If the external carotid is used (**Fig. 31.4**), the graft can be anastomosed end-to-end to the proximal portion of the artery, and the distal portion of the artery can be tied off.

Osteophyte Decompression

Endovascular treatment is typically the first choice of treatment for intrinsic stenotic lesions affecting the posterior circulation, but extrinsic compression with osteoarthritic spurs in the cervical region is associated with good results from surgical decompression.[28–30]

Positioning and Exposure

Osteophytes generally affect the mid-V2 segment (C2-C5) where it is partially encased in the bony channel created by the cervical transverse foramina. In this region, the VA can be accessed most readily from an anterior approach.[28] The patient's head is placed in extension on a donut head rest. A horizontal skin incision in a skin crease or longitudinal incision along the anterior border of the sternocleidomastoid muscle can be made (**Fig. 31.5**) depending on whether the pathology involves one or multiple levels. A cervical radiograph is used to define the level of interest and should be repeated intraoperatively for verification of the level before the transverse process is drilled. After opening the skin, an incision is made longitudinally through the platysma along the anterior border of the sternocleidomastoid muscle. By blunt dissection, a plane is developed between the strap muscles and the carotid sheath, which contains the carotid, internal jugular vein, and vagus nerve. The carotid sheath along with the trachea and esophagus are bluntly dissected from the prevertebral fascia below, and its contents are gently retracted medially while the sternocleidomastoid muscle is retracted laterally. The prevertebral fascia is opened to expose the anterior longitudinal ligament and the longus colli muscles. The ligament is incised upon its lateral border to allow periosteal dissection of the prevertebral musculature (the longus colli and longus capitis) from the vertebral body and transverse processes laterally up to the anterior tubercle (**Fig. 31.5**). The bony canal of the VA lies deep and medial to the anterior tubercle. Further, dissection posterolaterally beyond the anterior tubercle must be avoided as it may lead to injury of the cervical nerve roots. The sympathetic ganglia should not be allowed to lie on the lateral aspect of the longus colli. A more lateral approach to this region can be performed by creating an incision lateral to the sternocleidomastoid and pulling this muscle medially while retracting the scalene muscles posteriorly; however, this extensive exposure has a high risk of Horner syndrome and other nerve palsies.

Decompression

Once the muscles have been reflected laterally, the anterior tubercle of the transverse process can be confirmed with an anteroposterior cervical radiograph. The anterior tubercle and associated osteophytes are removed using a high-speed drill, rongeur, or curet (**Fig. 31.5**) to unroof the bony canal and expose the VA. The periosteum must be removed; otherwise, adhesions to the artery can persist. Immediately below the transverse process, anterior to the VA, is the venous plexus, which is coagulated with care to avoid injury to the underlying artery. The artery is dissected

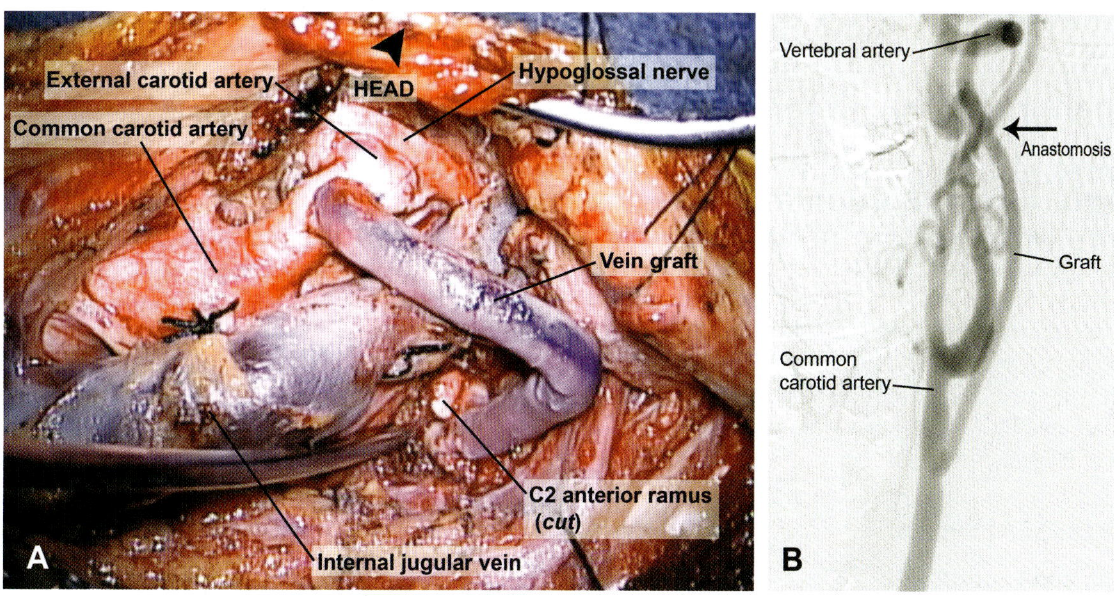

Fig. 31.4 Carotid–vertebral bypass. **(A)** An intraoperative photograph shows an external carotid artery to vertebral artery bypass using an interposition vein graft. **(B)** An angiogram (anteroposterior view) demonstrates a carotid–vertebral bypass with vein graft. (Reprinted with permission from the Department of Neurosurgery at University of Illinois at Chicago.)

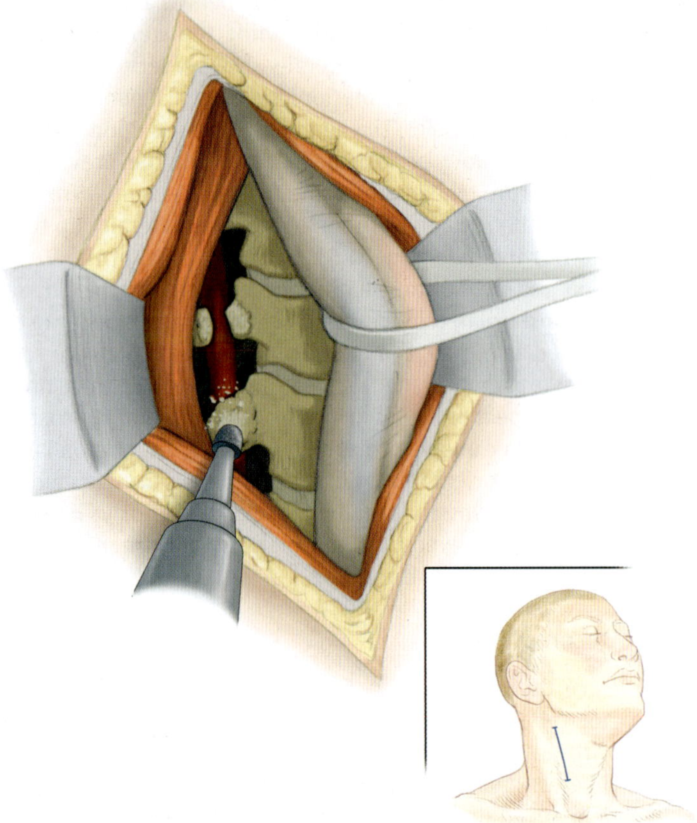

Fig. 31.5 Osteophyte decompression. An incision is placed along the medial border of the sternocleidomastoid muscle (*inset*); the carotid sheath and its contents are displaced medially, and the longus colli muscle is dissected laterally to expose the anterior tubercle of the transverse process; the bone can be removed with drills or rongeurs to remove osteophytes and relieve compression on the underlying vertebral artery. (Reprinted with permission from the Department of Neurosurgery at University of Illinois at Chicago.)

circumferentially and displaced laterally. During dissection, care must be taken to preserve radiculomedullary arteries that exit from the VA between C1 and C5 and supply the spinal cord. At the end of the procedure, the artery should be free of all restrictions.

Intracranial Bypass Options

The primary EC–IC bypass options for the posterior fossa include the STA to PCA or SCA bypass (**Fig. 31.6**) and the OA to PICA (**Fig. 31.7**) or anterior inferior cerebellar artery (AICA) bypass.[1,2] Other variants include the use of vein interposition graft to the SCA or PCA.[31–33] The general principles of position and approach for these variants are similar to the standard STA–PCA and OA–PICA bypasses that are described in the following text. Direct reimplantation, excision, end-to-end repair, and PICA–PICA bypass are further options for treatment of PICA aneurysms.

STA–PCA (or SCA) Bypass

Positioning and Exposure

A subtemporal approach to gain access to the PCA or SCA is used. The patient is placed in a lateral decubitus position, with axillary pad and other appropriate padding, or supine with the head turned and a shoulder roll to prevent the neck from rotating excessively. A lumbar drain is placed for CSF drainage and brain relaxation. The head is fixed in a lateral position with a rigid head holder (**Fig. 31.8**). The bypass is performed preferably on the right side so that manipulation of the temporal lobe is on the nondominant side. After shaving, a Doppler is utilized to map the trunk of the STA starting at the level of the zygoma as well as both anterior and posterior branches of the vessel (**Fig. 31.8**). A skin incision overlies the STA trunk just anterior to the tragus in the region of the zygoma and extends along the posterior branch in a linear fashion. If the posterior branch is inadequate as a donor vessel, the incision can be curved forward to elevate a skin flap and expose the anterior branch from the undersurface of the flap for harvesting. The initial incision through the epidermis and dermis is made along the midpoint of the projected course of the STA branch. Once the vessel is visualized, it is dissected proximally in the loose areolar plane above the vessel until the main trunk of the STA is reached. The same procedure is performed distally, although the tissue is more adherent to the vessel distally and dissection must proceed with caution. These steps are performed under loupe or microscopic magnification. The goal is to dissect at least 8–10 cm of STA to have enough length to reach subtemporally to the PCA or SCA. Once exposed, the STA and a cuff of surrounding tissue are skeletonized and wrapped in a papaverine-soaked Cottonoid

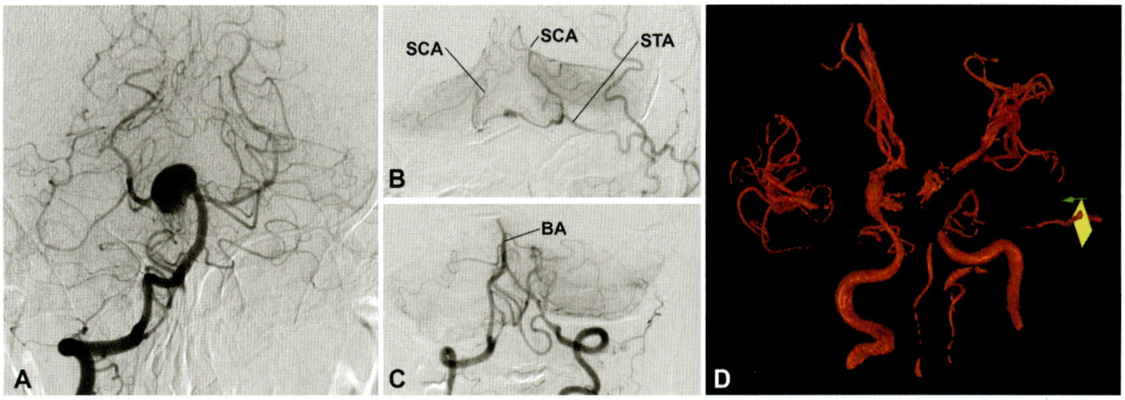

Fig. 31.6 Superficial temporal artery (*STA*) to superior cerebellar artery (*SCA*) bypass. **(A)** An angiogram (anteroposterior view) of a right vertebral injection demonstrates a partially fusiform basilar tip aneurysm incorporating the P1 origins not amenable to endovascular therapy or direct clipping. The patient was treated with staged aneurysm trapping (occluding the basilar and bilateral P1s) and STA–SCA bypass. **(B)** An angiogram (anteroposterior view) of left external carotid injection demonstrates the STA–SCA graft and filling of bilateral SCAs with near complete obliteration of the aneurysm through flow thrombosis and remodeling. **(C)** An angiogram (anteroposterior view) of a left vertebral injection demonstrates clip occlusion of the basilar artery (*BA*) above segments of the anterior inferior cerebellar artery. **(D)** A three-dimensional time-of-flight image from quantitative magnetic resonance angiography measures flow in the STA graft (*green arrow*) of 33 mL/min. (Reprinted with permission from the Department of Neurosurgery at University of Illinois at Chicago.)

(DuPuy, Raynham, MA) to alleviate vessel spasm induced by the mechanical manipulation of the vessel.

The temporalis muscle is cut along the line of the scalp incision and retracted anteriorly and posteriorly. Extending the linear incision to a T-shape or cruciate incision superiorly can facilitate retraction. The STA can be truncated at its most distal point and reflected inferiorly during the craniotomy to avoid injury to the vessel. It is important to flush the vessel with heparinized saline after truncation, placing a temporary clip proximally to avoid blood stagnating in the vessel. If the anterior branch is sacrificed, leaving a stump with a temporary clip will facilitate its use as a venting branch after anastomosis. A subtemporal craniotomy is performed (**Fig. 31.8**). The zygomatic arch and prominent elevations of the middle fossa floor are drilled to create a flat plane of approach. The dura is opened as a semicircular flap, which is retracted inferiorly.

Bypass

The microscope is utilized for all intradural aspects of the procedure. Using lumbar drainage for relaxation, the temporal lobe is elevated, with coagulation of small anterior bridging

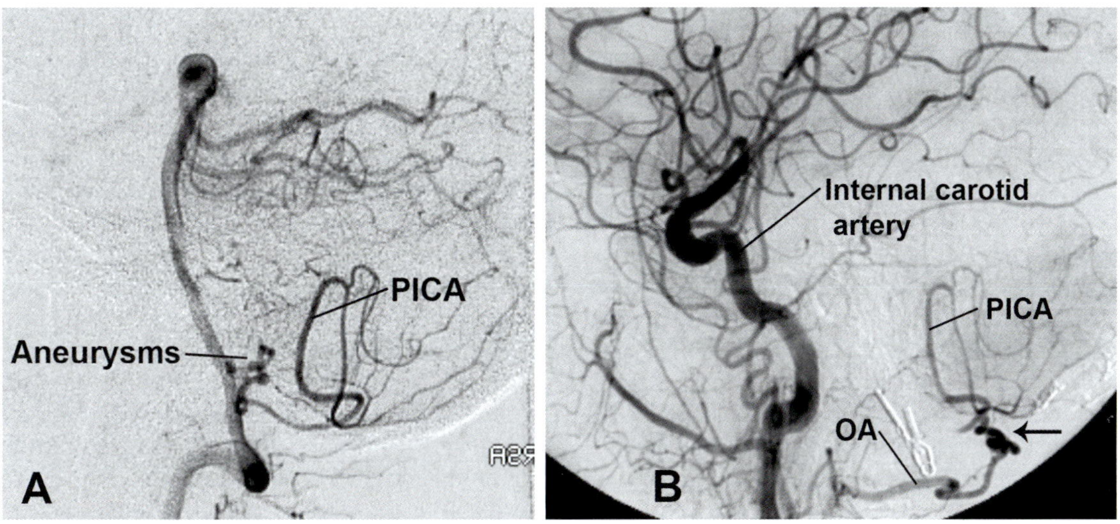

Fig. 31.7 Occipital artery (*OA*) to posterior inferior cerebellar artery (*PICA*) bypass. **(A)** An angiogram (lateral view) of a vertebral injection demonstrates fusiform proximal PICA pseudoaneurysms in a patient presenting with subarachnoid hemorrhage. The patient underwent OA–PICA bypass and trapping of aneurysmal segment. **(B)** A postoperative angiogram (lateral view) of carotid injection demonstrates OA filling of the distal PICA; the *arrow* indicates the site of anastomosis; later images show reflux filling of the PICA proximally to the clip location. (Reprinted with permission from the Department of Neurosurgery at University of Illinois at Chicago.)

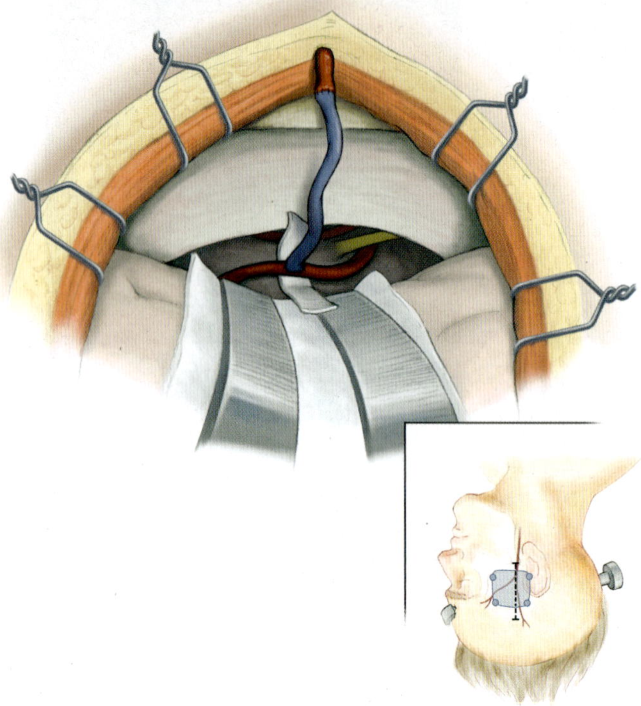

Fig. 31.8 Steps in a superficial temporal artery (STA) to posterior cerebral artery (PCA) bypass with interposition vein graft. An incision is placed overlying the STA, and a subtemporal approach exposes the PCA for anastomosis. (Reprinted with permission from the Department of Neurosurgery at University of Illinois at Chicago.)

veins as needed. Once the tentorial edge is reached, the third nerve anteriorly is apparent and the arachnoid is dissected. Typically, the SCA will come into view first, although it is often necessary to cut the tentorium to better view the lateral course of the vessel. The tentorium should be divided posteriorly behind the insertion of the cranial nerve IV and can be stitched laterally. Further elevation of the temporal lobe will bring the P2 segment of the PCA into view. The PCA provides a substantially larger recipient vessel than the SCA that can accommodate a higher flow bypass; in cases when the STA is inadequate and a radial artery or saphenous vein interposition graft is necessary, donor–recipient size mismatch precludes use of the SCA. When using the PCA, however, greater temporal lobe retraction is needed, and it can be more difficult to identify a perforator-free zone along the P2 segment than along the lateral SCA. Perforators in this region must be preserved and, if absolutely necessary, should be occluded with temporary clips during anastomosis rather than sacrificed. The chosen vessel is prepared by placing a rubber dam beneath it, and a papaverine-soaked cotton ball can be applied to the vessel surface to alleviate spasm prior to anastomosis. Next, the required length of STA to reach the anastomotic site without tension is gauged and marked on the vessel with a marking pen. The vessel is then dissected from its cuff of tissue to a point 1 inch proximal to the planned anastomosis length. Care must be taken to identify and coagulate side branches of the STA during dissection. Once the STA has been prepared, it is useful to check the cut flow of the vessel to determine its flow capacity and adequacy for bypass.

The STA–PCA or SCA anastomosis is performed in an end-to-side fashion. The STA is cut at a slight bevel and can be fish-mouthed to enlarge the opening. If an interposition vein or artery graft is used, it should be cut at a right angle; otherwise, the opening will be too long. It is important to examine the lumen of the STA carefully for intimal disease or dissection that would lead to an unsuccessful bypass. Temporary mini clips are placed proximally and distally on the recipient vessel, which is then incised with a sharp ophthalmic blade and opened to the required length with microscissor. The opened vessel lumen is flushed with heparinized saline, and 10–0 nylon suture is used to place anchoring sutures at the apices of the incision for the SCA and 8–0 or 9–0 nylon for the PCA. Due to the depth of the anastomosis, a continuous suture technique on each side of the anastomosis is more efficient and practical than interrupted sutures. The technique for running the suture involves leaving short loops of suture along the entire length of the vessel. The loops are tightened sequentially just prior to tying to achieve an even tension along the suture line. Placement of a small silastic stent into the recipient vessel during suturing can help to avoid inadvertent opposite-wall suturing; the stent is removed prior to tightening of the final suture line. Once the anastomosis is complete, the temporary clips on the recipient vessel are released. If a venting branch is available on the STA, it is used for back-bleeding prior to releasing the STA proximal clip. Gentle pressure is applied with cotton balls if the suture line is oozing. With careful attention to suture technique, additional sutures to control anastomotic leak are rarely necessary. If needed, a single 10–0 nylon suture can be placed at the bleeding site, generally without the necessity of reclipping the vessels unless there is profuse leakage. If an interposition artery or vein graft is utilized, a temporary clip is placed on the graft above the anastomosis after back-bleeding and the graft irrigated with heparinized saline prior to proximal anastomosis. The stump of the STA, if available, provides a convenient donor site for a short interposition graft. If necessary, tunneling the graft to the cervical region for anastomosis to the external or common carotid is feasible but requires a lengthy graft; in such a scenario, the radial artery is generally insufficient in length, and a saphenous vein would need to be utilized.

After completion of the bypass, blood flow measurement provides confirmation of the patency and function of the bypass. The dura is loosely tacked with a slit created for passage of the STA, and the dural opening is covered with a piece of Gelfoam. The bone is replaced, but the inferior opening is enlarged to accommodate the graft and avoid kinking or pressure on the vessel. The muscle is reapproximated loosely and left open inferiorly to avoid pressure on the graft. The skin is closed with care.

OA–PICA (or AICA) Bypass

Positioning and Exposure

The OA–PICA bypass is traditionally performed through a lateral suboccipital approach. The patient is placed in a prone or three-quarter prone position with the head rigidly fixed and flexed to optimize access to the posterior fossa. The scalp is shaved, and a Doppler can be utilized to map the distal OA, although the vessel is often difficult to localize prior to incision. The skin incision is planned as a hockey stick flap based over the midline and toward the side of interest, ending over the region of the mastoid process (**Fig. 31.9**). The occipital artery should be identified in the midpoint of the horizontal portion of the incision, where it can be transected, flushed with heparin solution, and occluded with a temporary clip on the proximal end. The suboccipital muscles are then dissected in the midline avascular plane. The skin and muscle flap are retracted laterally and inferiorly.

The OA is dissected from the undersurface of the flap to its exit point from the mastoid region and then wrapped in papaverine-soaked Cottonoids to relieve spasm. The OA is generally tortuous in its course and adherent to the surrounding tissue; therefore, dissection can be tedious but must be meticulous to avoid injury to the vessel. The suboccipital muscle is dissected laterally to the mastoid on the ipsilateral side and across the midline in preparation for the craniotomy. A standard lateral suboccipital craniotomy is performed, extending to the edge of the sigmoid sinus laterally to prevent kinking of the OA against the bony edge after muscle closure. The craniotomy also extends across the midline and foramen magnum to create a broader and flatter working space, reducing the depth and difficulty of the subsequent anastomosis. The dura is opened in a hockey

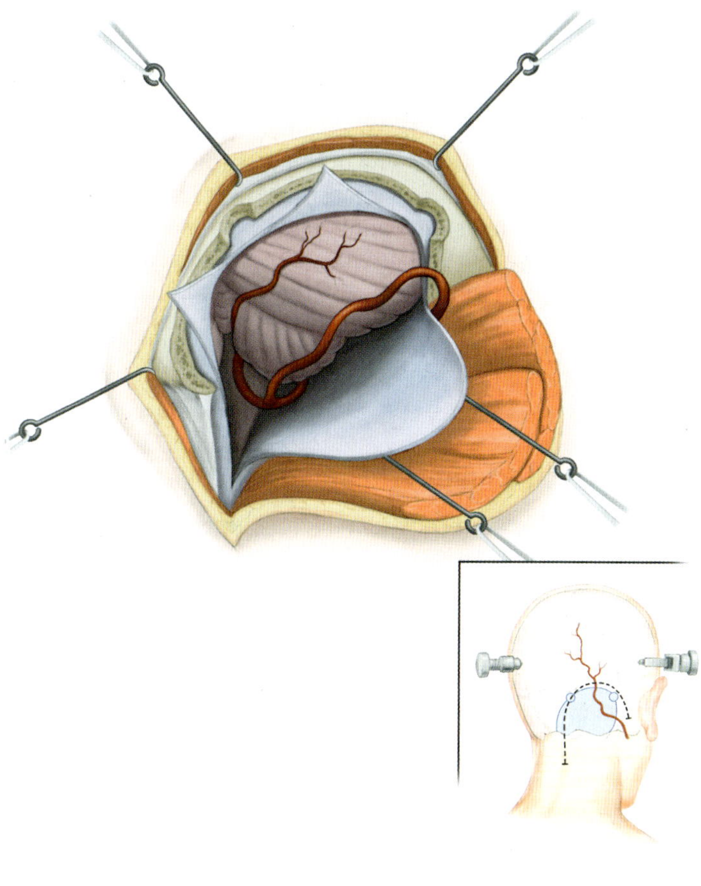

Fig. 31.9 Occipital artery (OA) to posterior inferior cerebellar artery (PICA) bypass. A hockey stick incision is placed extending from the mastoid to the midline (*inset*); the OA is dissected, and an anastomosis is performed at the tonsillomedullary loop of the PICA. (Reprinted with permission from the Department of Neurosurgery at University of Illinois at Chicago.)

stick fashion near the midline, with an additional limb crossing the midline to the contralateral side.

Bypass

A microscope is utilized for all intradural aspects of the procedure. Using lumbar drainage and opening the cisterna magna for relaxation, the ipsilateral cerebellar tonsil is elevated bringing the tonsillomedullary segment of the PICA into view. This location is preferred for anastomoses because a lengthy perforator-free portion can be readily obtained and the loop of vessel can be mobilized and elevated with cotton balls or Gelfoam to reduce the depth of the anastomosis (**Fig. 31.9**). If revascularization more distal to the PICA is needed, the AICA can be used as a recipient. The cerebellum is retracted to identify the region of the cranial nerves VI and VIII, allowing the AICA to be identified as it extends from the region of the foramen of Luschka to the anterior surface of the cerebellum. The vessel divides into a rostral and caudal branch at this point, and the branch with a segment free of brainstem perforators is identified for performing the anastomosis. Once the PICA or AICA recipient has been prepared, the required length of OA to reach the anastomotic site without tension is marked, and the OA is dissected free of adherent tissue 1 inch proximal to this location. The cut flow of the vessel can be checked to evaluate its flow capacity, and the vessel is flushed again with heparinized saline.

An end-to-side anastomosis of the OA–PICA or AICA is performed. The OA is beveled and fish-mouthed. Temporary clips are placed proximally and distally on the recipient. The vessel is then incised, opened to the required length, and flushed with heparinized saline. Typically, due to the large caliber of the vessels and thickness of the OA vessel wall, 9–0 nylon suture rather than 10–0 nylon suture is used for the anastomosis. The larger caliber of the vessels allows for a running suture technique. Temporary clips on the recipient and then the OA are removed following completion of the anastomosis, and the flow in the OA graft is measured. The dura is tacked loosely, and the dural opening is covered with a piece of Gelfoam. The superior portion of the bone should be replaced with care to avoid pressure on the graft. The lateral suboccipital musculature may need to be trimmed to prevent pressure on the exit point of the OA, and the midline muscle closure is performed with care to avoid kinking of the graft.

PICA–PICA Bypass

Positioning and Exposure

The PICA–PICA bypass is a useful option for cases requiring revascularization of the PICA territory as with proximal fusiform aneurysms.[13,14] It can be performed if the tonsillar loops of the PICA branches are of adequate length and proximity, which can be determined preoperatively on CTA or conventional angiography. Compared with the OA–PICA bypass, the PICA–PICA option avoids the more extensive dissection required for OA harvesting and can be performed quickly with little additional exposure if the need for bypass arises unexpectedly. However, it carries the relative downside of exposing both PICA branches to temporary clipping and the potential for bilateral PICA infarcts should the anastomosis fail. The patient is generally placed prone on rolls or three-quarter prone with the head held flexed in rigid fixation. A midline straight incision with dissection of the suboccipital muscles in the midline avascular plane is performed, and a standard suboccipital craniotomy is created, including removal of the foramen magnum (**Fig. 31.10**). A C1 laminectomy can be performed as needed to enlarge the working area. The dura is opened in a V-shaped fashion and the dural edges retracted to expose both cerebellar tonsils.

Bypass

Under the operative microscope, the cerebellar tonsils are separated and the tonsillar loop of both PICAs are released from their arachnoid attachments and mobilized so that they oppose each other without tension in preparation for side-to-side anastomosis. Both vessels are marked along the medial side and, following proximal and distal temporary clipping, an arteriotomy is created superficially to the medial equator of the vessel using a sharp blade and microscissor (**Fig. 31.10**). 10–0 or 9–0 nylon is used to place the first apical stitch, which is then passed through the vessel wall into the internal lumen so that the back wall of the anastomosis can be closed from the inside. Once back-wall suturing is complete, the needle is passed again through the vessel to the outside and tied to a newly placed apical stitch at the opposite corner of the anastomosis. Utilizing running sutures on the inside back wall of the anastomosis is more easily accomplished with only one apical stitch in place. The front wall of the anastomosis can be closed with running or interrupted suture and the temporary clips removed sequentially from both PICA branches. Patency of the anastomosis can be confirmed with flow measurements and video ICG angiography. The dura is closed in a watertight fashion, and the bone can be replaced prior to closure of the myocutaneous layers.

Direct Techniques

Direct vessel reconstruction or reimplantation is an option in the posterior fossa, most readily applicable to PICA pathology due to the relative redundancy of this vessel. If there is adequate laxity in the vessel, without compromising perforators, the PICA can be reimplanted into the proximal intradural portion of the VA.[12] This procedure can be useful in situations where trapping of the PICA segment of the VA is necessary for a dissecting aneurysm or for unclippable PICA-origin aneurysms. The approach is most readily performed through a lateral suboccipital exposure as described previously. Given that the lower cranial nerves traverse

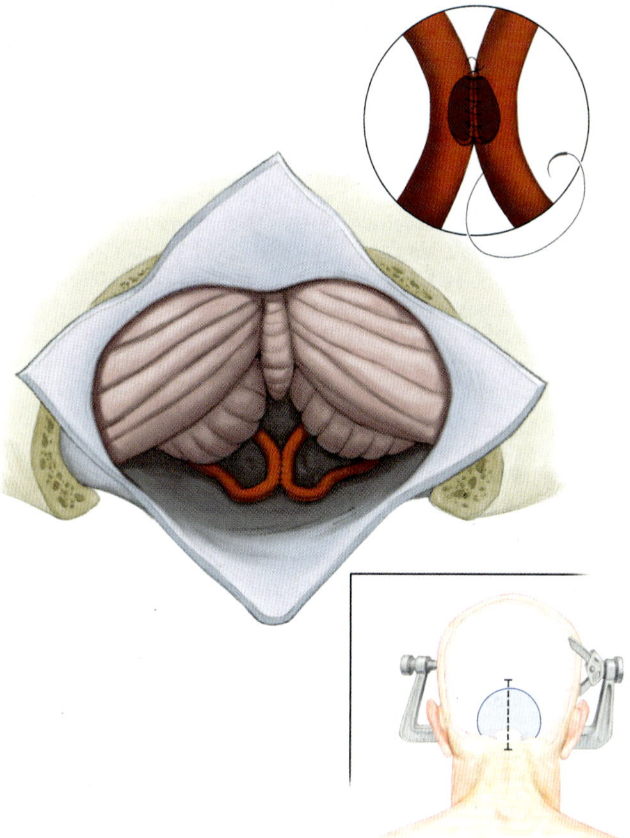

Fig. 31.10 Posterior inferior cerebellar artery (PICA) to PICA bypass. A suboccipital craniotomy is performed through a midline incision (*lower inset*) to expose the tonsillar loops of both PICAs; a side-to-side anastomosis is performed, sewing the back wall (*upper inset*) and then the front wall to complete the in situ bypass. (Reprinted with permission from the Department of Neurosurgery at University of Illinois at Chicago.)

posteriorly to the VA along its proximal intradural portion, care must be taken to avoid injury to these nerves during dissection, temporary clipping, and anastomosis. Reimplantation is performed in end-to-side fashion and requires at least an 8–0 suture due to the thickness of the VA.

Occasionally, transection with end-to-end anastomosis is a useful option.[12,14] This technique generally applies to the PICA for treatment of fusiform or dissecting aneurysms of a focal segment beyond the lateral medullary portion that carries brainstem perforators. For end-to-end reconstruction, the proximal and distal ends must be mobilized sufficiently to ensure a lack of tension on the anastomosis. Cutting the ends at an angle to create opposing beveled edges rather than cutting straight across creates a wider anastomosis that is easier to close with running suture along each side.

Conclusion

Surgical revascularization of posterior circulation can be performed through a variety of extracranial and intracranial bypass options, based on disease location and indication. Flow augmentation for ischemia and flow replacement for aneurysms that require vessel sacrifice can be achieved with existing surgical strategies. Success in these procedures depends on careful patient selection and meticulous technique.

References

1. Ausman JI, Diaz FG, Dujovny M. Posterior circulation revascularization. Clin Neurosurg 1986;33:331–343
2. Hopkins LN, Martin NA, Hadley MN, Spetzler RF, Budny J, Carter LP. Vertebrobasilar insufficiency. Part 2. Microsurgical treatment of intracranial vertebrobasilar disease. J Neurosurg 1987;66(5):662–674
3. Berguer R, Flynn LM, Kline RA, Caplan L. Surgical reconstruction of the extracranial vertebral artery: management and outcome. J Vasc Surg 2000;31(1 Pt 1):9–18
4. Spetzler RF, Hadley MN, Martin NA, Hopkins LN, Carter LP, Budny J. Vertebrobasilar insufficiency. Part 1: Microsurgical treatment of extracranial vertebrobasilar disease. J Neurosurg 1987;66(5):648–661
5. Amin-Hanjani S, Du X, Zhao M, Walsh K, Malisch TW, Charbel FT. Use of quantitative magnetic resonance angiography to stratify stroke risk in symptomatic vertebrobasilar disease. Stroke 2005; 36(6):1140–1145
6. Vertebrobasilar Flow Evaluation and Risk of Transient Ischemic Attach and Stroke (VERiTAS). Available at: http://veritas.neur.uic.edu. Accessed May 13, 2010.
7. Hopkins LN, Budny JL. Complications of intracranial bypass for vertebrobasilar insufficiency. J Neurosurg 1989;70(2):207–211
8. Ausman JI, Diaz FG, Vacca DF, Sadasivan B. Superficial temporal and occipital artery bypass pedicles to superior, anterior inferior,

and posterior inferior cerebellar arteries for vertebrobasilar insufficiency. J Neurosurg 1990;72(4):554–558
9. Chimowitz MI, Lynn MJ, Howlett-Smith H, et al; Warfarin-Aspirin Symptomatic Intracranial Disease Trial Investigators. Comparison of warfarin and aspirin for symptomatic intracranial arterial stenosis. N Engl J Med 2005;352(13):1305–1316
10. Massimo C, Orazio A, Felice F. Bypass surgery in patients with intracranial stenotic lesions. Postoperative morbidity and angiographic findings. J Neurosurg 1985;62(4):532–538
11. Steinberg GK, Drake CG, Peerless SJ. Deliberate basilar or vertebral artery occlusion in the treatment of intracranial aneurysms. Immediate results and long-term outcome in 201 patients. J Neurosurg 1993;79(2):161–173
12. Evans JJ, Sekhar LN, Rak R, Stimac D. Bypass grafting and revascularization in the management of posterior circulation aneurysms. Neurosurgery 2004;55(5):1036–1049
13. Lemole GM Jr, Henn J, Javedan S, Deshmukh V, Spetzler RF. Cerebral revascularization performed using posterior inferior cerebellar artery-posterior inferior cerebellar artery bypass. Report of four cases and literature review. J Neurosurg 2002;97(1):219–223
14. Nussbaum ES, Mendez A, Camarata P, Sebring L. Surgical management of fusiform aneurysms of the peripheral posteroinferior cerebellar artery. Neurosurgery 2003;53(4):831–834, discussion 834–835
15. Alexander MJ, Perna J. Endoscopic saphenous vein graft harvest for extracranial-intracranial bypass procedures. Surg Neurol 2005; 63(6):565–568, discussion 568
16. Ferroli P, Bisleri G, Nakaji P, et al. Endoscopic radial artery harvesting for U-clip EC-IC bypass in the treatment of a giant petrous internal carotid artery aneurysm: technical case report. Minim Invasive Neurosurg 2009;52(4):186–189
17. Lopes RD, Hafley GE, Allen KB, et al. Endoscopic versus open vein-graft harvesting in coronary-artery bypass surgery. N Engl J Med 2009;361(3):235–244
18. Ashley WW, Amin-Hanjani S, Alaraj A, Shin JH, Charbel FT. Flow-assisted surgical cerebral revascularization. Neurosurg Focus 2008;24(2):E20
19. Amin-Hanjani S, Charbel FT. Flow-assisted surgical technique in cerebrovascular surgery. Surg Neurol 2007;68(Suppl 1):S4–S11
20. Amin-Hanjani S, Du X, Mlinarevich N, Meglio G, Zhao M, Charbel FT. The cut flow index: an intraoperative predictor of the success of extracranial-intracranial bypass for occlusive cerebrovascular disease. Neurosurgery 2005;56(1, Suppl):75–85, discussion 75–85
21. Amin-Hanjani S, Shin J, Du X, et al. Evaluation of EC-IC bypass grafts using quantitative magnetic resonance angiography. J Neurosurg 2005;102:A791
22. Berguer R, Feldman AJ. Surgical reconstruction of the vertebral artery. Surgery 1983;93(5):670–675
23. Diaz FG, Ausman JI, de los Reyes RA, et al. Surgical reconstruction of the proximal vertebral artery. J Neurosurg 1984;61(5):874–881
24. Carney AL. VA surgery: pathology, hemodynamics, and technique. In: Robicsek F, ed. Extracranial Cerebrovascular Disease: Diagnosis and Management. New York: Macmillan; 1986:395–424
25. Berguer R, Morasch MD, Kline RA. A review of 100 consecutive reconstructions of the distal vertebral artery for embolic and hemodynamic disease. J Vasc Surg 1998;27(5):852–859
26. Carney AL, Anderson EM. Carotid distal vertebral bypass for carotid occlusion: case report and technique. Clin Electroencephalogr 1978;9:105–109
27. Kakino S, Ogasawara K, Kubo Y, Kobayashi M, Kashimura H, Ogawa A. Symptomatic occlusion at the origin of the vertebral artery treated using external carotid artery-cervical vertebral artery bypass with interposed saphenous vein graft. Surg Neurol 2008;69(2):164–168, discussion 168
28. Brink B. Approach to the second segment of the vertebral arteries. In: Berguer R, Bauer RB, eds. Vertebrobasilar Arterial Occlusive Disease: Medical and Surgical Management. New York: Raven; 1984:257–264
29. Diaz FG, Ausman JI, Shrontz C, et al. Surgical correction of lesions affecting the second portion of the vertebral artery. Neurosurgery 1986;19(1):93–100
30. Hardin CA, Williamson WP, Steegmann AT. Vertebral artery insufficiency produced by cervical osteoarthritic spurs. Neurology 1960;10:855–858
31. Russell SM, Post N, Jafar JJ. Revascularizing the upper basilar circulation with saphenous vein grafts: operative technique and lessons learned. Surg Neurol 2006;66(3):285–297
32. Sundt TM Jr, Piepgras DG, Houser OW, Campbell JK. Interposition saphenous vein grafts for advanced occlusive disease and large aneurysms in the posterior circulation. J Neurosurg 1982;56(2):205–215
33. Hopkins LN, Budny JL, Spetzler RF. Revascularization of the rostral brain stem. Neurosurgery 1982;10(3):364–369

32 Approaches to the Jugular Foramen

Madjid Samii, Marcos Tatagiba, and Venelin M. Gerganov

The complex bony and neurovascular anatomy of the jugular foramen has created the reputation for this region as one of the most difficult areas to access surgically. Developments in neuroradiology, microsurgical skull base approaches, and postoperative intensive care have transformed surgery of lesions in the jugular foramen area into a routine procedure with predictable postoperative results.

Among skull base pathologies, tumors arising in the region of the jugular foramen are relatively common. A variety of tumors can originate from the structures in or next to the jugular foramen. The differential diagnosis of primary jugular foramen tumors principally includes schwannomas and glomus jugular tumors. Several other skull base tumors may secondarily involve the jugular foramen, such as meningiomas, chordomas, chondrosarcomas, and carcinoma of the tympanic cavity. Surgery is the primary treatment option for most of these tumors. The objective of this chapter is to describe the current surgical management of jugular foramen tumors, based on the senior author's experience during the past four decades with more than 200 jugular foramen tumors among 5000 skull base lesions.

Surgical Anatomy of the Jugular Foramen

The jugular foramen is located between the lateral part of the occipital bone and the petrous part of the temporal bone. It usually has a triangular form, with the apex of the triangle situated anteriorly and medially.[1,2] From an intracranial-to-extracranial projection, the jugular foramen is described as a canal coursing anteriorly, inferiorly, and laterally. In earlier descriptions, the foramen was divided into two compartments: the anteromedial compartment, called the "pars nervosa," and the posterolateral compartment, called the "pars venosa" or "pars vascularis." The pars nervosa contained the inferior petrosal sinus, vena canaliculi cochleae, and glossopharyngeal nerve. The pars venosa contained the vagus and accessory nerves and the proximal part of the jugular bulb.

It is now recognized that the classic compartments of the jugular foramen are not always present. The cranial nerves IX to XI follow different patterns while traversing the foramen. The nerves are separated from the jugular bulb by bone, thick fibrous tissue, or thin connective tissue.[3,4]

The walls of the jugular bulb are very thin compared with the thick walls of the sigmoid sinus.[5] The inferior petrosal sinus commonly drains into the jugular bulb by one or more openings and usually passes between cranial nerve IX and cranial nerves X and XI.

A posterior meningeal branch of the ascending pharyngeal artery typically runs through the sheath of connective tissue in the jugular foramen to supply the bone and the dura mater. This meningeal artery is responsible for the vascular supply of most tumors in this area.

Diagnostic Evaluation

Patients with primary jugular foramen tumors usually present with a unilateral palsy of one or more of the lower cranial nerves (IX, X, or XI).[5,6] Patients can also present with hearing loss, raising the suspicion of a cerebellopontine angle (CPA) tumor. Patients with large tumors may present with involvement of cranial nerves VII and XII, increased intracranial pressure, papilledema, cerebellar symptoms, or brainstem signs.[7,8] Glomus jugulare tumors may produce sensorineural, conductive, or mixed hearing loss.[9] Pulsating tinnitus is present in several patients and may differentiate these tumors from schwannomas. The tumor may present as a neck mass, as a mass involving the lateral pharyngeal wall, or with a jugular foramen syndrome.

A variety of lesions other than schwannomas or glomus tumors may arise from the structures within or adjacent to the jugular foramen. Meningiomas, chordomas, chondromas, chondrosarcomas, metastases, and others lesions can often be differentiated on the basis of their radiological and imaging characteristics.[6,10]

Radiological Evaluation

The delineation of the tumor and its relationship with the bone, vessels, and neural tissues is essential for diagnosis and preoperative planning. The preoperative neuroradiological studies should include high-resolution computed tomography (CT), magnetic resonance imaging (MRI), and cerebral angiography.[10,11]

High-resolution CT is performed before and after intravenous administration of contrast material. Thin slice axial and coronal images (1.5-mm slice thickness) are preferred with bone windows to demonstrate the extent of bone involvement by the tumor. Enlargement or erosion of the foramen has a significant impact on the differential diagnosis of the lesion.

MRI studies are performed with intravenous administration of paramagnetic contrast medium. Sagittal, coronal, and axial projections allow for a three-dimensional delineation of tumor extension (**Fig. 32.1**). The tumor size and

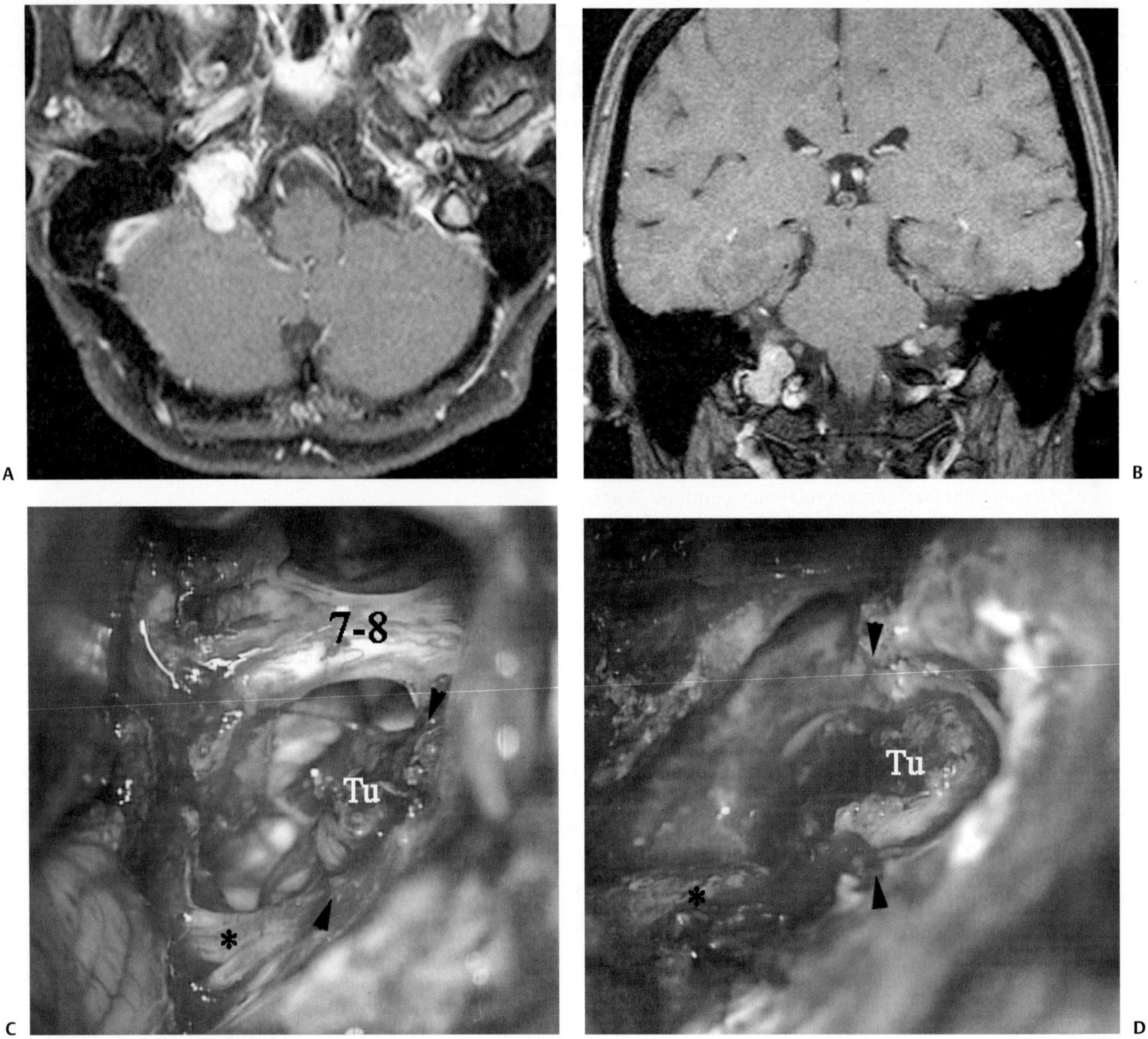

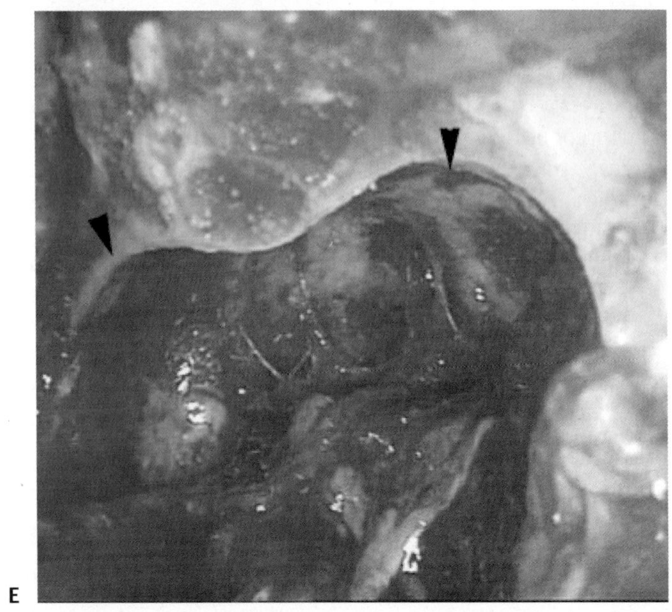

Fig. 32.1 **(A)** Axial and **(B)** coronal T1-weighted magnetic resonance images of a type B jugular foramen schwannoma. **(C)** The tumor (*Tu*) part in the cerebellopontine angle has been removed. The intraforaminal part is seen. 7–8, cranial nerves VII and VIII; *, lower cranial nerves. **(D)** The dorsal wall of the jugular foramen has been drilled off (*arrowheads*), and the intraforaminal tumor part is well exposed. **(E)** Endoscopic view of the jugular foramen demonstrating complete tumor removal (*arrowheads*).

its relationship to surrounding tissues can be defined. Magnetic resonance angiography (MRA) can demonstrate the vascular involvement by the lesion, including displacement or occlusion of the venous sinuses and arteries. In selected cases, MRA has replaced the use of cerebral angiography.

Cerebral angiography can be performed to evaluate the tumor vascularization, the type and number of feeding vessels, the displacement of major cerebral vessels, and the venous drainage (**Fig. 32.2**). Angiography might be essential for decision making in tumor management.[12,13] The most important role of cerebral angiography is for the preoperative embolization of highly vascularized tumors, such as glomus jugulare tumors.

■ Surgical Technique

The most frequent primary tumors of the jugular foramen are schwannomas of cranial nerves IX, X, and XI, followed by glomus jugulare tumors.[7–9,14] Schwannomas may be localized mainly to the CPA with little extension into the jugular foramen (type A), may be located primarily in the jugular foramen with small intracranial extension (type B), may be primarily extracranial with extension into the jugular foramen (type C), or may become extensive dumbbell-shaped tumors extending from the CPA through the jugular foramen down into the cervical region (type D).[14] Type A and some

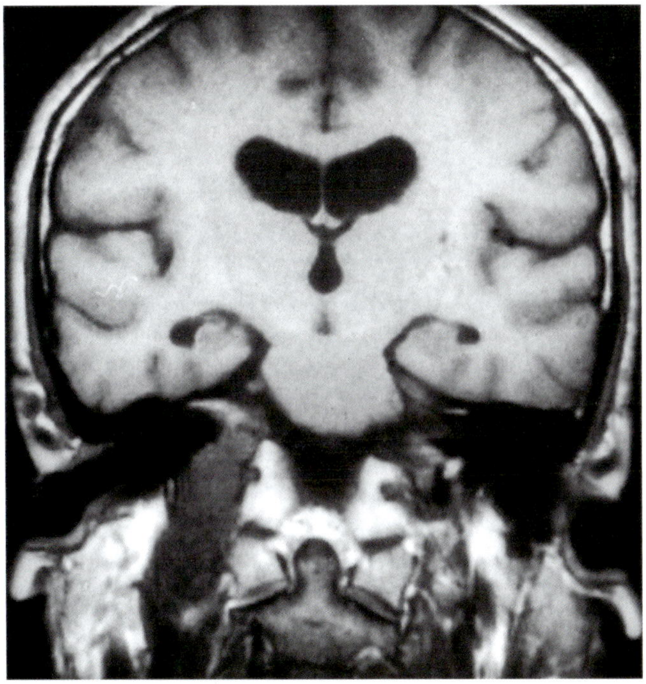
A

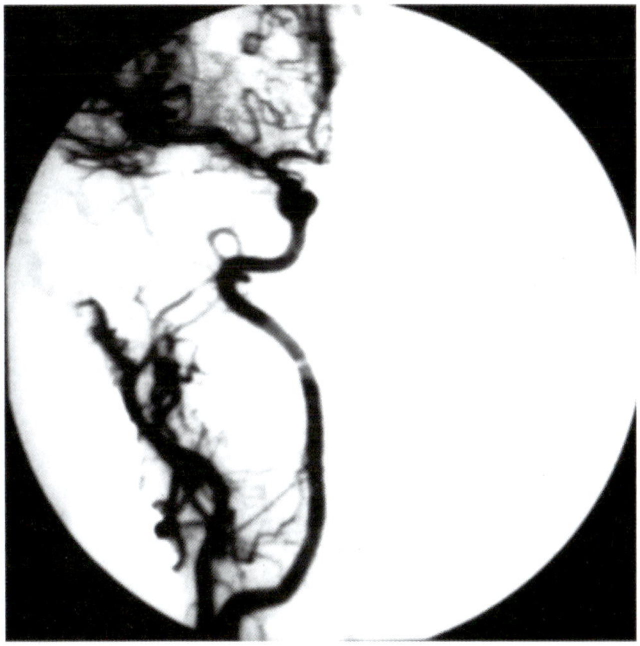
B

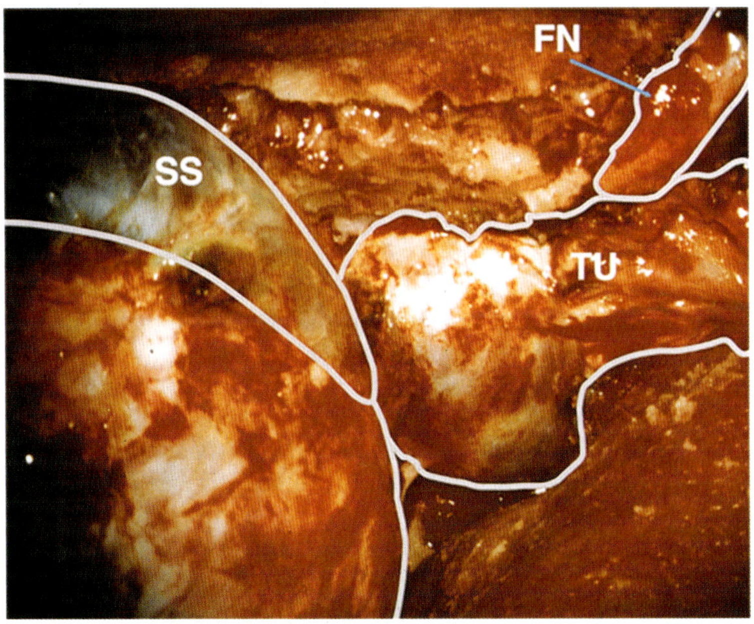

C

Fig. 32.2 **(A)** Nonenhanced coronal magnetic resonance image of a 43-year-old man with a 2-year history of progressive tongue atrophy, hoarseness, swallowing problems, and hearing dysfunction. The tumor is well delineated in the neck region, extending anteriorly to the lateral retropharyngeal space. The tumor extension into the cerebellopontine angle (*CPA*) was thought to be the cause of the hearing loss. **(B)** The angiography reveals a poorly vascularized tumor that displaces and stretches the internal carotid artery. **(C)** Intraoperative photograph after performing a retrosigmoid craniectomy and partial mastoidectomy with opening the jugular foramen. The dura of the posterior fossa is seen with the sigmoid sinus (*SS*). The facial nerve (*FN*) is exposed below the partially resected mastoid. The extracranial part of the tumor (*TU*) is demonstrated. *(continued)*

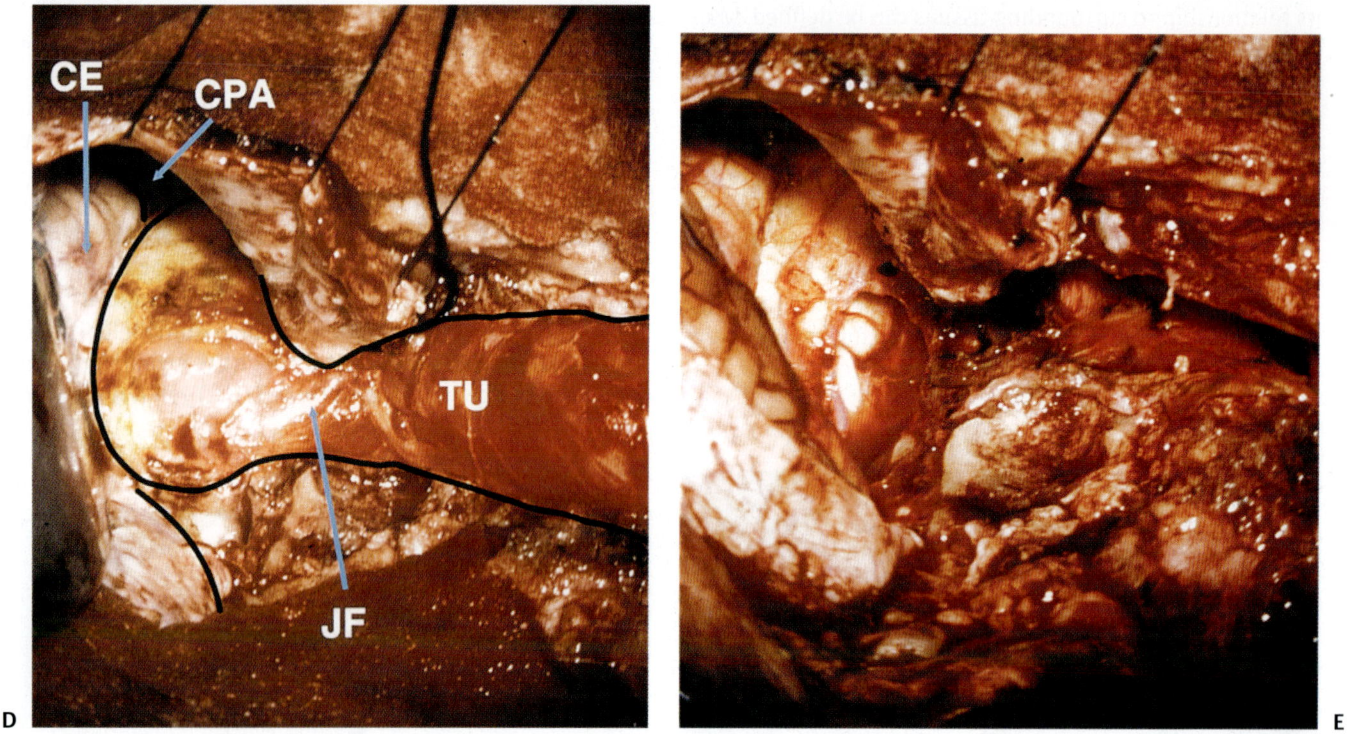

Fig. 32.2 *(continued)* **(D)** The dura is opened behind the sigmoid sinus. The dural incision extends to the jugular foramen (*JF*), which is completely exposed. The cerebellum (*CE*) is retracted, and the tumor is seen in its entire extension from the CPA to the neck region. **(E)** Complete intracranial and extracranial tumor resection. Histological examination revealed a schwannoma.

type B schwannomas are resected by a lateral suboccipital route. Schwannomas with a cervical extension or large foraminal part are resected by a combined cervical and lateral extradural transmastoid infralabyrinthine approach.[12]

Glomus jugulare tumors are benign, highly vascularized tumors that arise extracranially, but they may be complicated by intracranial extension and internal carotid artery involvement.[9,15,16] The tumor is usually unilateral, but bilateral tumors may occur. Complete surgical tumor resection is the preferred treatment in the majority of cases. Preoperative embolization of major feeding vessels reduces intraoperative bleeding, facilitates obtaining a complete surgical resection, and shortens the time required for surgery. Preoperative medical treatment is required for catecholamine-secreting tumors. Radiation therapy is reserved for rare aggressive tumors or when surgery is contraindicated.

Surgical Approaches

The choice of surgical approach is determined by the location, extension pattern, and type of lesion.[12–14,17] The tumor may be located primarily in the jugular foramen and grow outside it, or the tumor may arise from structures surrounding the jugular foramen and involve it secondarily.[18] Depending on these factors, two major approaches to the jugular foramen can be considered: a primary intradural approach through the CPA and a primary extradural approach through a mastoidectomy. The approaches can be used separately or together to permit a multidirectional view.

Primary Intradural Approach to the Jugular Foramen

Prophylactic antibiotics are administered. Dexamethasone is initiated to reduce the risk of postoperative edema. The patient is usually intubated nasally. Monitoring for air embolism includes intraoperative electrocardiography, arterial oximetry, capnometry, precordial Doppler ultrasonography, catheterization of the right atrium, and central venous catheterization.

The patient is placed in the semi-sitting position, with the head flexed and rotated ~30 degrees toward the side of the tumor.[14,19] The legs are elevated to the level of the right cardiac atrium, and the head is fixed in place with a Mayfield head holder. All body parts subject to pressure are supported with cushions. The legs are slightly flexed to avoid stretching the peroneal nerves. Sensory evoked potentials for the median nerve are monitored throughout surgery. Cochlear nerve function is monitored by measurement of brainstem auditory evoked potentials. Subdermal needle electrodes are implanted in the orbicularis oris and orbicularis oculi muscles for continuous electromyographic monitoring of the facial nerve. The glossopharyngeal, accessory, and hypoglossal nerves are monitored by placing the electrodes in the soft palate, trapezius muscle, and tongue, respectively.

Part of the occipital and suboccipital area of the scalp is shaved; the skin is prepared, and the drapes are stapled into position. A slightly curved incision is made behind the ear. The neck muscles are divided vertically and retracted. A burr hole is created and enlarged with rongeurs to form a craniectomy that exposes the transverse sinus superiorly and the sigmoid sinus laterally (**Fig. 32.3**). The bone opening should extend to the floor of the posterior fossa.

The dura mater is then opened in a curvilinear manner 1.5 to 2 mm medial to the sigmoid and inferior to the transverse sinus. The cerebellum is not retracted primarily. First, cerebrospinal fluid (CSF) is released from the cerebellomedullary cistern, and then a retractor is inserted to gently support but not compress the cerebellar hemisphere (**Fig. 32.4**).

The intracranial aspect of the tumor is exposed at the CPA. After identification of the main anatomical landmarks and cranial nerves, the tumor is debulked with ultrasonic aspiration, suction, or platelet knife. Dissection of cranial nerves is performed only when sufficient internal decompression has been achieved. A two-handed technique is used and performed always in the arachnoidal planes. Usually, the intraforaminal part of the tumor can be pulled out of the foramen, into the CPA, and removed. The access to this tumor part, if required, can be extended by opening the dorsal part of the jugular foramen in a technique similar to the opening of the internal auditory canal in a case of vestibular schwannoma (**Fig. 32.1**). The dura overlying the dorsal part of the foramen is stripped off, and its bony wall is removed using high-speed diamond drills. The intraforaminal tumor part is initially debulked, and then its capsule is dissected from the cranial nerves. An angled endoscope is routinely used to "look around the corner" and inspect the entire jugular foramen (**Fig. 32.1**). Tumor remnants can be readily viewed and removed under direct endoscopic or microscopic control.

After tumor removal, the dura is closed in a watertight fashion, and the mastoid air cells are sealed with fat and fibrin glue. If the jugular foramen has been opened, it should be sealed

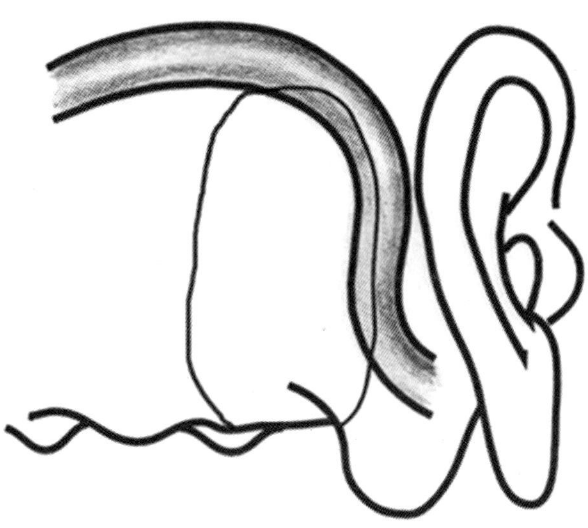

Fig. 32.3 The position of the craniotomy for the retrosigmoid intradural approach to the cerebellopontine angle and the jugular foramen.

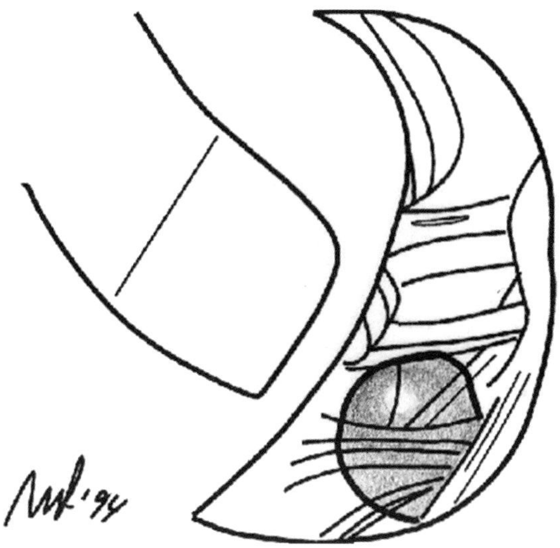

Fig. 32.4 The dura is opened, cerebrospinal fluid is released after opening the cerebellomedullary cistern, and the cerebellum is held with a retractor. The anatomy of the cerebellopontine angle (CPA) and the jugular foramen are shown. This jugular foramen tumor grows into the CPA.

with several small pieces of fat and fixed with fibrin glue. The craniectomy is reconstructed with methyl methacrylate.

Combined Intradural-Extradural Approach

Prophylactic antibiotics and dexamethasone are administered. General anesthesia is initiated with appropriate monitoring techniques. For large tumors with brainstem compression, endoscopic nasotracheal intubation is used to avoid hyperextending the head. The auditory, facial, glossopharyngeal, accessory, and hypoglossal nerves are monitored, if necessary.

The patient is placed in a supine position. The head is turned 60 degrees to the contralateral side and slightly extended. The head is fixed in position with a Mayfield head holder. The scalp is shaved for a suboccipital approach. After the skin is prepared, a slightly curved line is marked from the retro-auricular region above the mastoid tip to the anterior border of the sternocleidomastoid muscle (**Fig. 32.5**). Drapes are stapled into position to allow for exposure of the occiput and neck.

Surgery consists of the following steps: (1) exposure of the cervical region, vessels, and nerves; (2) craniectomy and mastoidectomy; (3) intradural exposure; (4) tumor removal; and (5) reconstruction of the dura and skull base.[12,13]

A retro-auricular skin incision is made. A dissection plane is created between the parotid gland and the anterior border of the sternocleidomastoid muscle. The greater auricular nerve is identified and preserved. The mastoid is exposed after mobilizing the sternocleidomastoid muscle and the posterior belly of the digastric muscle. The facial nerve is identified anterior to the mastoid process at the stylomastoid foramen (**Fig. 32.6A**). The caudal cranial nerves are exposed in the neck, along with the internal jugular vein, and followed cranially to the skull base (**Fig. 32.6B**).

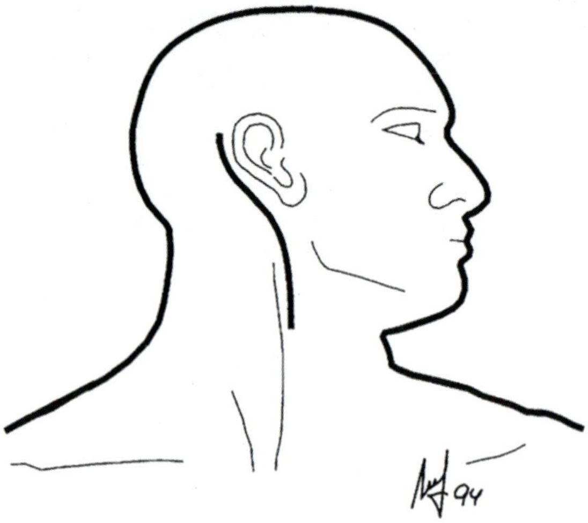

Fig. 32.5 Drawing of the skin incision for large jugular foramen tumors. The incision extends from behind the ear over the mastoid to the anterior border of the sternocleidomastoid muscle in the neck.

A retromastoid craniectomy is performed, exposing the transverse and sigmoid sinuses. The sigmoid sinus is mobilized caudally from its bony groove to the jugular foramen. The mastoid tip is removed. To extend the exposure, the posterior part of the occipital condyle may be removed, thus opening the jugular foramen dorsolaterally. Through this approach, the sigmoid sinus, the jugular bulb, and the internal jugular vein are exposed (**Fig. 32.6C**).

The petrous bone is further drilled away anteromedial to the fallopian canal, up to the styloid process, inferior to the labyrinth. Gradual bone removal exposes the antrum, the lateral semicircular canal, and the vertical portion of the facial nerve (**Fig. 32.6D**). Rerouting the facial nerve is necessary only if the tumor extends to the middle ear cavity or to the carotid canal, which occurs in cases of extensive glomus jugulare tumors. When the facial nerve is rerouted, care is taken to keep the vascularized fascia and soft tissue attached to the nerve at the stylomastoid foramen to avoid severe postoperative facial nerve palsy.

The dura may be opened posterior to the sigmoid sinus, extending the incision to the jugular foramen, or it may be opened anterior to the sigmoid sinus. The transverse sinus is kept intact. The dura, transverse and sigmoid sinuses, and the jugular bulb are retracted anteriorly. The cerebellopontine cistern is opened to release the CSF; then the cerebellum is gently retracted posteriorly. The intracranial portion of the tumor is exposed.

The extracranial portion of the tumor is usually resected first using microsurgical technique. The caudal cranial nerves are identified, and piecemeal complete tumor resection is performed. Schwannomas may displace the internal carotid artery anteriorly, whereas glomus jugulare tumors may surround or infiltrate the walls of the internal carotid arteries. In such cases, subtotal tumor resection is preferred to carotid resection and reconstruction.

The intracranial portion of the tumor is removed through the widened jugular foramen and the suboccipital craniectomy. The cranial nerves are identified and separated from the tumor. Schwannomas of the jugular foramen usually displace the nerves ventrally and the jugular bulb dorsally. Glomus jugulare tumors arise from the dome of the jugular bulb and can extend intraluminally in the sigmoid sinus and internal jugular vein. In such cases, radical tumor removal requires ligation of the sigmoid sinus and the internal jugular vein. In contrast, the sigmoid sinus should be left intact in cases of schwannomas.

A

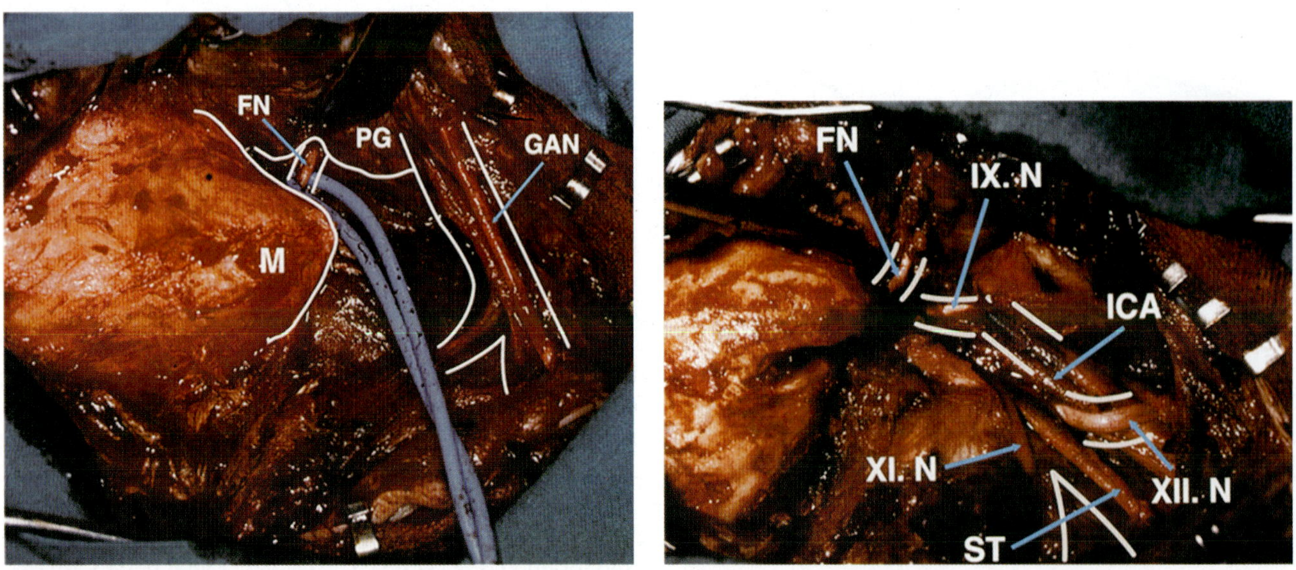

B

Fig. 32.6 **(A)** Intraoperative photograph after exposing the mastoid (*M*), the facial nerve (*FN*) at the stylomastoid foramen, the parotid gland (*PG*), and the greater auricular nerve bundle (*GAN*). **(B)** The neurovascular anatomy of the neck region is exposed: the facial nerve, the glossopharyngeal nerve (*IX. N*), the internal carotid artery (*ICA*), the hypoglossal nerve (*XII. N*), the accessory nerve (*XI. N*), and the sympathetic trunk (*ST*). *(continued)*

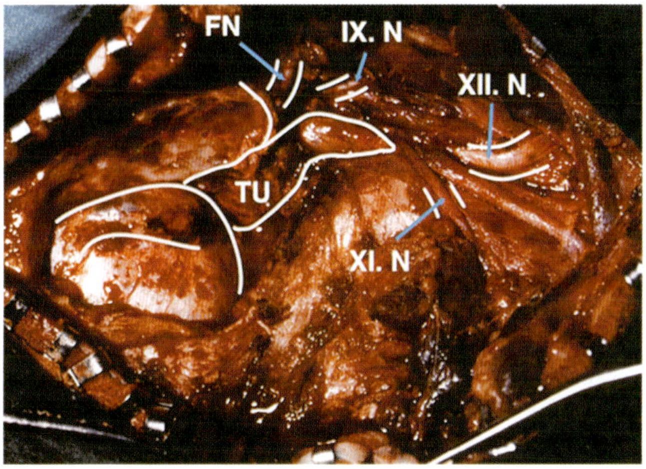

C

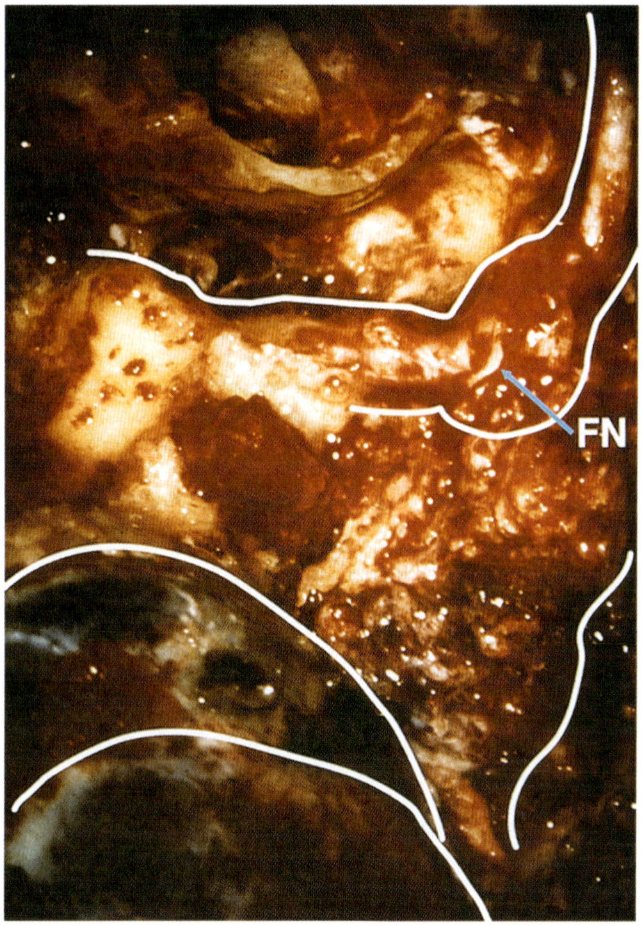

D

Fig. 32.6 *(continued)* **(C)** A craniectomy with a partial mastoidectomy is performed to expose the sigmoid sinus and part of the tumor (*TU*) in the opened jugular foramen. **(D)** An intraoperative microphotograph of the mastoidectomy shows the facial nerve after opening the fallopian canal and the stylomastoid foramen. Note the preservation of vascularized tissue at the facial nerve near the opened stylomastoid foramen (*arrow*) to help reduce ischemic facial palsy postoperatively.

A combined intradural and extradural resection of a jugular foramen schwannoma is illustrated in **Fig. 32.2**.

After the tumor has been resected, the dura is closed in a watertight fashion. Fat and fibrin glue are used to close the jugular foramen, which is reinforced with the posterior belly of the digastric muscle. The sternocleidomastoid muscle is sutured back at its insertion on the occipital bone. With this reconstruction technique, CSF leaks are exceptionally rare.

Complications

Major complications of jugular foramen surgery include CSF leakage, meningitis, and cranial nerve deficits.[5,7,8,14] CSF leaks can be largely avoided by performing watertight dural closure and using fat and fibrin glue, as described previously. If a CSF leak develops, lumbar drainage is inserted and kept for at least 7 days. A persisting CSF leak necessitates surgical revision but is rarely required. Resection of jugular foramen tumors may worsen deficits of the lower cranial nerves, resulting in breathing difficulty, dysphagia, and hoarseness. The significance of the neurological deficits depends on the type and number of cranial nerves involved. Deficit of a single nerve usually does not produce a major disability. However, the presence of two or more lesions, particularly in combination with the vagus nerve, increases tremendously the risk of aspiration pneumonia.

We have observed that, if a deficit of the caudal cranial nerves has developed over months or years, the altered mechanism of swallowing is usually compensated, yet deficits of acute onset in patients having normal function preoperatively are not tolerated. Intensive patient observation and care are essential in the immediate postoperative period. The moment of extubation is a critical instant; it should be performed only when the patient is completely awake. The nasogastric tube is kept in place to allow gastric fluids to drain.

If a slow recovery of swallowing dysfunction is expected, or if cranial nerves are injured at surgery, temporary tracheostomy with a cuffed tube is performed. We maintain the tracheostomy until the patient is able to swallow. As swallowing begins to recover, a special uncuffed tube that allows the patient to speak may be used temporarily during meals. For intractable aspiration, or if a prolonged recovery is anticipated, a gastrostomy is performed.

Acknowledgments

Special thanks are given to Mr. S. Brinkmann for his photographic assistance.

References

1. Rhoton AL Jr. Jugular foramen. Neurosurgery 2000;47(3, Suppl): S267–S285
2. Roche PH, Mercier P, Sameshima T, Fournier HD. Surgical anatomy of the jugular foramen. Adv Tech Stand Neurosurg 2008;33:233–263
3. Saleh E, Naguib M, Aristegui M, Cokkeser Y, Sanna M. Lower skull base: anatomic study with surgical implications. Ann Otol Rhinol Laryngol 1995;104(1):57–61
4. Lang J. Clinical Anatomy of the Posterior Fossa and Its Foramina. New York, NY: Thieme; 1991
5. Ramina R, Maniglia JJ, Fernandes YB, Paschoal JR, Pfeilsticker LN, Coelho Neto M. Tumors of the jugular foramen: diagnosis and management. Neurosurgery 2005;57(1, Suppl):59–68, discussion 59–68
6. Bakar B. Jugular foramen meningiomas: review of the major surgical series. Neurol Med Chir (Tokyo) 2010;50(2):89–96, 96–97
7. Fayad JN, Keles B, Brackmann DE. Jugular foramen tumors: clinical characteristics and treatment outcomes. Otol Neurotol 2010;31 (2):299–305
8. Bulsara KR, Sameshima T, Friedman AH, Fukushima T. Microsurgical management of 53 jugular foramen schwannomas: lessons learned incorporated into a modified grading system. J Neurosurg 2008;109(5):794–803
9. Borba LA, Araújo JC, de Oliveira JG, et al. Surgical management of glomus jugulare tumors: a proposal for approach selection based on tumor relationships with the facial nerve. J Neurosurg 2010;112(1):88–98
10. Löwenheim H, Koerbel A, Ebner FH, Kumagami H, Ernemann U, Tatagiba M. Differentiating imaging findings in primary and secondary tumors of the jugular foramen. Neurosurg Rev 2006;29(1):1–11, discussion 12–13
11. Ong CK, Fook-Hin Chong V. Imaging of jugular foramen. Neuroimaging Clin N Am 2009;19(3):469–482
12. Samii M, Bini W. Surgical strategy for jugular foramen tumors. In: Sekhar LN, Janecka IP, eds. Surgery of Cranial Base Tumors. New York, NY: Raven Press 1993:379–87
13. Samii M, Draf W. Surgery of the Skull Base. Heidelberg: Springer; 1989
14. Samii M, Babu RP, Tatagiba M, Sepehrnia A. Surgical treatment of jugular foramen schwannomas. J Neurosurg 1995;82(6):924–932
15. Al-Mefty O, Teixeira A. Complex tumors of the glomus jugulare: criteria, treatment, and outcome. J Neurosurg 2002;97(6):1356–1366
16. Jackson CG. Glomus tympanicum and glomus jugulare tumors. Otolaryngol Clin North Am 2001;34(5):941–970, vii
17. Carvalho GA, Tatagiba M, Samii M. Cystic schwannomas of the jugular foramen: clinical and surgical remarks. Neurosurgery 2000;46 (3):560–566
18. Bruneau M, George B. The juxtacondylar approach to the jugular foramen. Neurosurgery 2008;62(3, Suppl 1):75–78, discussion 80–81
19. Samii M, Gerganov VM. Surgery of extra-axial tumors of the cerebral base. Neurosurgery 2008;62(6, Suppl 3):1153–1166, discussion 1166–1168

33 Suboccipital and Retrosigmoid Approaches

Albert L. Rhoton, Jr. and Guilherme L. Ribas

The suboccipital approaches are directed through the portion of the occipital bone located between the inion and transverse sinuses above, the sigmoid sinuses laterally, and the foramen magnum inferiorly. The suboccipital approaches can be divided into three variants: midline, paramedian, and lateral. The retrosigmoid approach is a variant of the lateral suboccipital approach in which the cranial opening extends up to or over the back edge of the sigmoid sinus.[1,2]

The midline suboccipital approach is commonly selected for the removal of tumors involving the fourth ventricle, cerebellar tonsils, and medial part of the cerebellar hemispheres. The midline exposure is combined with an upper cervical laminectomy for tumors of the posterior and posterolateral part of the foramen magnum, for intra- and extramedullary lesions involving the cervicomedullary junction, and for decompression of Chiari malformations. The midline approach may be extended upward to provide a route between the tentorium and superior surface of the cerebellum to reach lesions in the quadrigeminal cistern and pineal region. It can also be combined with an occipital craniotomy for the management of selected lesions of the tentorium and quadrigeminal cistern.

The lateral suboccipital approach was once combined with extensive retraction or resection of the lateral part of the cerebellar hemisphere to reach tumors in the cerebellopontine angle. However, the development of microsurgical techniques allows lesions in the cerebellopontine angle to be exposed by the lateral suboccipital approach with minimal brain retraction and without resecting any cerebellum, if the bony opening extends to or over the posterior edge of the sigmoid sinus. The strict adherence of the lateral suboccipital approach to the posterior margin of the sigmoid sinus has led to it being referred to as the retrosigmoid approach.

A combined midline and lateral suboccipital exposure can be obtained using a hockey stick incision, which extends upward in the midline from the upper cervical region to the inion and laterally and downward near the superior nuchal line to the mastoid tip. This combined approach would be selected for lesions that involve both the cervicomedullary junction and the cerebellopontine angle. Lesions that involve both the region of the fourth ventricle and the lateral recess can also be approached by this combined route.

The retrosigmoid variant of the suboccipital approach also can be combined with a temporo-occipital craniotomy to give a combined supra- and infratentorial approach to lesions involving the posterior and middle fossae or with a presigmoid approach directed through the mastoid and labyrinth to reach lesions involving the petrous apex, clivus, and cavernous sinus. The lateral suboccipital variant can be extended downward to expose the transverse processes of the upper cervical vertebrae and the condyles forming the atlanto-occipital joint to give a variant referred to as the extreme lateral approach, which is commonly selected for meningiomas and other lesions located anterolateral or anterior to the medulla or cervicomedullary junction.

The paramedian suboccipital approach exposes the area over the cerebellar hemisphere intermediate between the regions exposed in the midline and lateral suboccipital approaches. It is commonly selected for lesions in the central part of one cerebellar hemisphere.

Osseous and Muscular Relationships, Transverse and Sigmoid Sinuses, and External Surgical Landmarks

When dealing with suboccipital and retrosigmoid approaches, surgeons initially confront the occipital and temporal bones and their related structures. Careful exposure, particularly of the bony sutures and other osseous prominences and depressions, enables these sites to be used as important landmarks for surgical orientation and for more restricted and appropriate approaches.

The occipital bone surrounds the foramen magnum and is divided into a squamosal part above and behind the foramen magnum, a basal portion in front of the foramen magnum, and paired condylar portions lateral to the foramen magnum.[3] The squamous portion is an internally concave plate, and its upper margins articulate with the parietal bones at the lambdoid sutures. Its lower margins articulate with the mastoid portion of the temporal bones at the occipitomastoid sutures. The convex external surface has several prominences on which the muscles of the neck attach. The largest prominence, the external occipital protuberance, or inion, is situated at the central portion of the external surface and over the inferior margin of the confluence of the sagittal and transverse sinuses. Two parallel ridges radiate laterally from the protuberance. The highest nuchal line is the upper and thinner ridge; the superior nuchal line is lower and more prominent. The rough and irregular area below the nuchal lines serves as the site of attachment of numerous muscles. A vertical ridge, the external occipital crest, descends from the external occipital protuberance to the midpoint of the posterior margin of the foramen magnum. The inferior nuchal lines run laterally from the midpoint of the crest (**Fig. 33.1**).

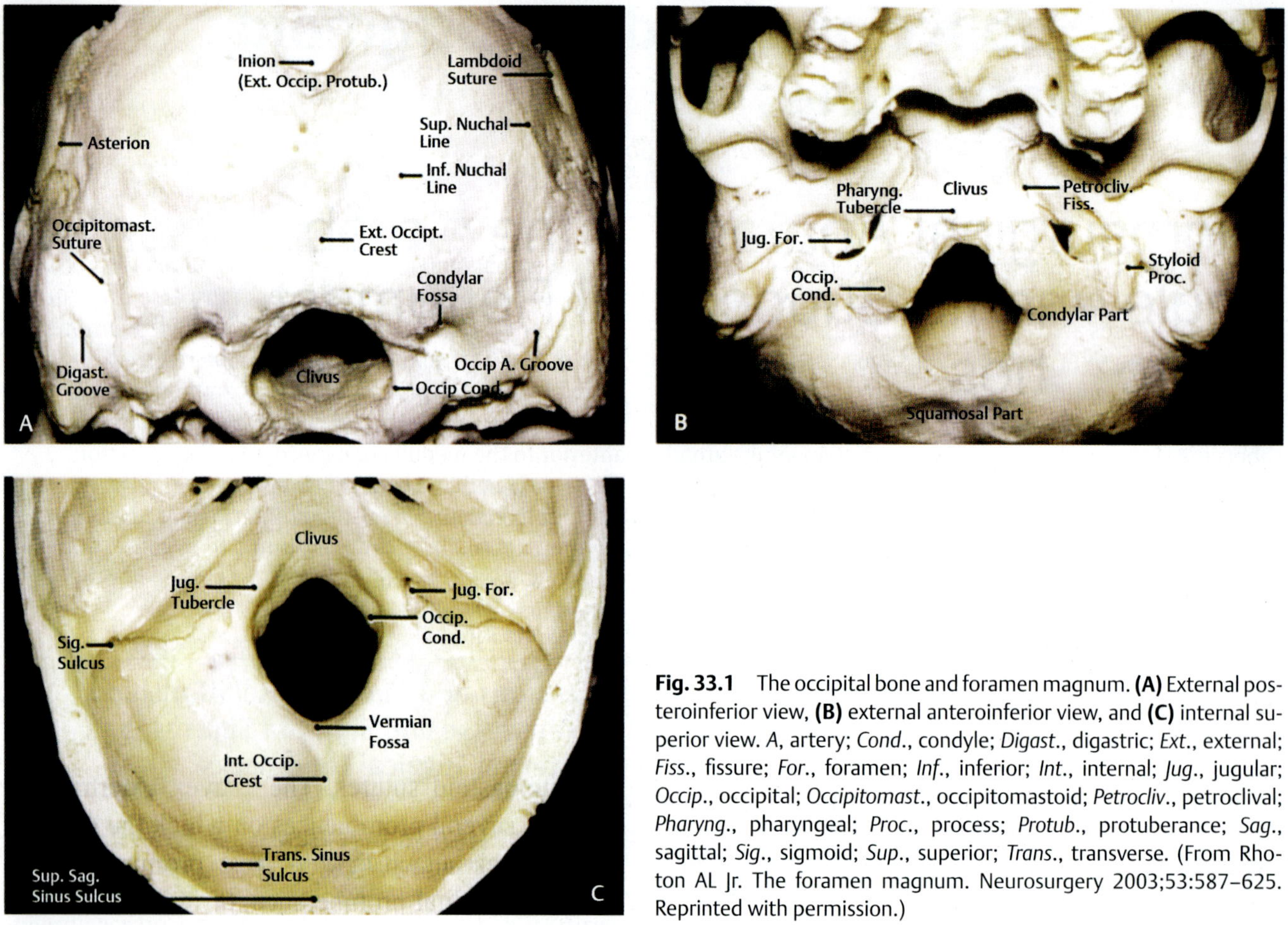

Fig. 33.1 The occipital bone and foramen magnum. **(A)** External posteroinferior view, **(B)** external anteroinferior view, and **(C)** internal superior view. *A*, artery; *Cond.*, condyle; *Digast.*, digastric; *Ext.*, external; *Fiss.*, fissure; *For.*, foramen; *Inf.*, inferior; *Int.*, internal; *Jug.*, jugular; *Occip.*, occipital; *Occipitomast.*, occipitomastoid; *Petrocliv.*, petroclival; *Pharyng.*, pharyngeal; *Proc.*, process; *Protub.*, protuberance; *Sag.*, sagittal; *Sig.*, sigmoid; *Sup.*, superior; *Trans.*, transverse. (From Rhoton AL Jr. The foramen magnum. Neurosurgery 2003;53:587–625. Reprinted with permission.)

The basilar portion of the occipital bone, also referred to as the clivus, is a thick quadrangular plate of bone that extends anteriorly and superiorly at about a 45-degree angle from the foramen magnum. It joins the sphenoid bone at the spheno-occipital synchondrosis just below the dorsum sellae.[4] The superior surface of the clivus is concave from side to side and is separated on each side from the petrous portion of the temporal bone by the petroclival fissure. This fissure has the inferior petrosal sinus on its upper surface and ends posteriorly at the jugular foramen. On the inferior surface of the basilar part in front of the foramen magnum, a small elevation called the pharyngeal tubercle attaches to the fibrous raphe of the pharynx.

The paired lateral or condylar portions are situated at the sides of the foramen magnum. The occipital condyles, which articulate with the atlas, protrude from the external surface of this part. These condyles are located lateral to the anterior half of the foramen magnum. They are oval, convex downward, and face downward and laterally. Their long axes are directed anteriorly and medially. A tubercle that attaches to the alar ligament of the odontoid process is situated on the medial side of each condyle. The hypoglossal canal, which transmits the hypoglossal nerve, is situated above the condyle and is directed anteriorly and laterally from the posterior cranial fossa. The canal may be partially or completely divided by a bony septum.

The superior nuchal lines, which extend laterally and horizontally from the external occipital protuberance, are the boundary between the scalp and neck. These lines are often sharp.[5] Each is located at the level of an imaginary line formed by the inion and external acoustic meatus.[6] Along this imaginary line, the trapezius inserts medially. The sternocleidomastoid muscle, which covers the semispinalis and splenius capitis muscles, inserts laterally. The highest nuchal lines, which are more arched than the superior nuchal lines, are eventually identified. Medially, the galea aponeurotica inserts, and laterally the occipitofrontalis muscle inserts. The slightly arched inferior nuchal lines are located below the external occipital protuberance. The semispinalis capitis and the superior oblique muscles are inserted medially and laterally between the inferior and superior nuchal lines. The rectus capitis posterior minor and major muscles are inserted medially and laterally, respectively, below each inferior nuchal line (**Fig. 33.2**).

The suboccipital triangle is a region bound superiorly and medially by the rectus capitis posterior major muscle, superiorly and laterally by the superior oblique muscle, and inferiorly and laterally by the inferior oblique muscle. It is covered by the semispinalis capitis muscle medially and by the splenius capitis muscle laterally. The floor of the triangle is formed by the posterior atlanto-occipital membrane and the posterior arch of the atlas. The structures in the triangle

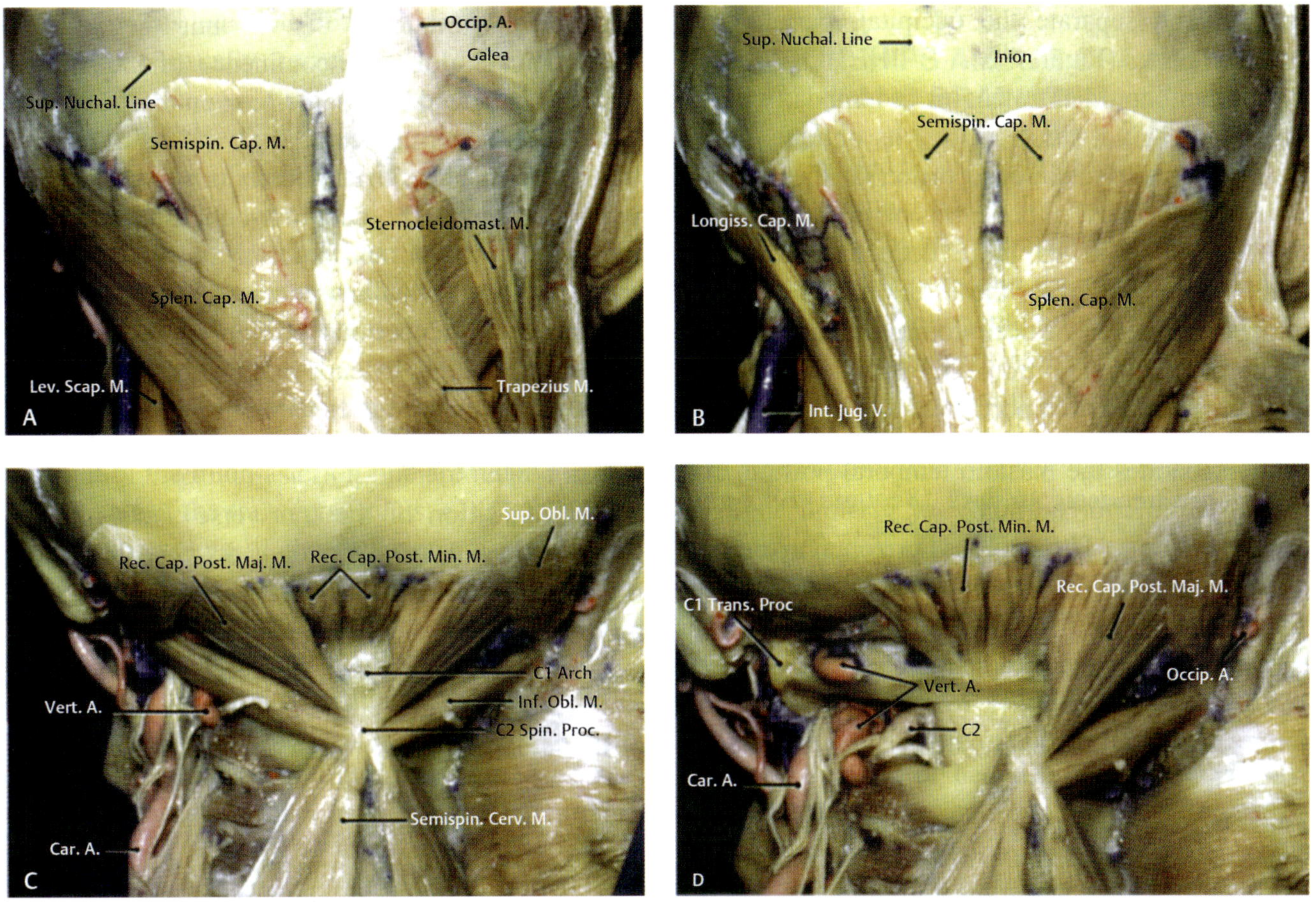

Fig. 33.2 The suboccipital muscles. **(A)** The right trapezius and sternocleidomastoid muscles have been preserved. The left trapezius and sternocleidomastoid muscles have been reflected with the galea aponeurotica to expose the underlying semispinalis capitis, splenius capitis, and levator scapulae muscles. **(B)** The right sternocleidomastoid and trapezius muscles have been reflected to expose the splenius capitis muscles. The left splenius capitis has been removed to expose the underlying semispinalis and longissimus capitis muscles. **(C)** Both semispinalis capitis muscles have been reflected laterally to expose the suboccipital triangles bilaterally. **(D)** The muscles forming the left suboccipital triangle have been removed. The vertebral artery ascends slightly lateral from the transverse process of C2 to reach the transverse process of C1. Behind the superior facet of C1, the artery turns medially to reach the upper surface of the posterior arch of C1. The C2 ganglion is located between the posterior arch of C1 and the lamina of C2. The dorsal ramus of C2 produces a medial branch that forms most of the greater occipital nerve. *A.*, artery; *Cap.*, capitis; *Car.*, carotid; *Inf.*, inferior; *Int.*, internal; *Jug.*, jugular; *Lev.*, levator; *Longiss.*, longissimus; *M.*, muscle; *Maj.*, major; *Min.*, minor; *Obl.*, oblique; *Occip.*, occipital; *Post.*, posterior; *Proc.*, process; *Rec.*, rectus; *Scap.*, scapulae; *Semispin.*, semispinalis; *Spin.*, spinalis; *Splen.*, splenius; *Sternocleidomast.*, sternocleidomastoid; *Sup.*, superior; *Trans.*, transverse; *V.*, vein; *Vert.*, vertebral. (From Rhoton AL Jr. The foramen magnum. Neurosurgery 2003;53:587–625. Reprinted with permission.)

are the terminal extradural segment of the vertebral artery and the first cervical nerve.[3]

The external occipital crest descends from the external occipital protuberance, with the nuchal ligamentum attached. The lambdoid, occipitomastoid, and parietomastoid sutures[3,7–11] are united at the asterion and separate the occipital, parietal, and temporal bones.

The lambdoid suture begins at the lambda, where it meets the sagittal suture. Along its oblique course, it separates the squamous part of the occipital bone from the parietal bone. It is particularly evident superiorly due to its deeper and prominent serrations.[11] Inferior to the asterion, the lambdoid suture continues as the occipitomastoid suture, which separates the lower portion of the occipital squamous from the petromastoid portion of the temporal bone, ending at the jugular foramen. The parietomastoid suture separates the mastoid temporal portion from the posteroinferior portion,[11] or mastoid angle, of the parietal bone. The suture is horizontal to the skull base. Occasionally, sutural bones are present, usually along the lambdoid suture. An isolated bone at the lambda is named the Inca bone.

Laterally and parallel to the occipitomastoid suture, along and medial to the mastoid process, the deep groove of the mastoid notch is where the posterior belly of the digastric muscle inserts. Parallel and between this notch and the occipitomastoid suture, the occipital artery lies in a shallow occipital groove.[11] The sulcus of the transverse sinus extends laterally from the protuberance on each cranial side; the tentorium cerebelli attaches to its margins.[12] Frequently, the larger sulcus, usually the right one, is continuous with

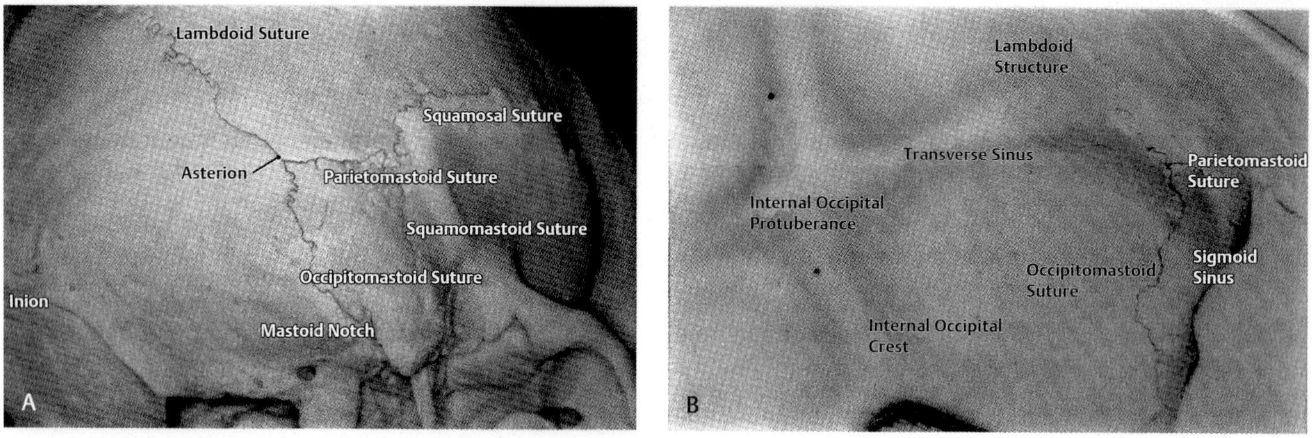

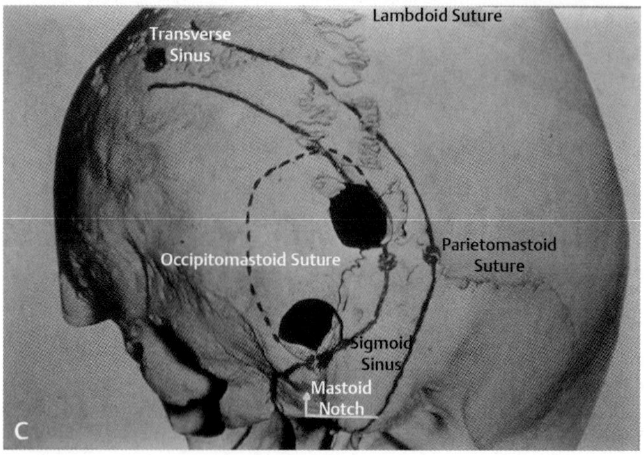

Fig. 33.3 **(A)** External cranial surface with the cranial sutures, **(B)** internal cranial surface with cranial sutures and sinus groove, and **(C)** initial burr hole sites for suboccipital/retromastoid approaches (*1*) at the asterion and (*2*) over the occipitomastoid suture just behind the superior aspect of the mastoid notch. (From Ribas GC, Rhoton AL Jr, Cruz OR, et al. Suboccipital burr holes and craniectomies. Neurosurg Focus 2005;19(2):E1. Reprinted with permission.)

the sulcus of the superior sagittal sinus. The smaller sulcus is usually better related with the straight sinus (**Fig. 33.3**).[11,13]

The transverse sinuses are sites of frequent anatomical variations,[11,14–21] but they usually communicate along the confluence of the sinuses, which is indicated by a depression on one side of the internal occipital protuberance.[11] Each transverse sinus is situated posteriorly over the squamous portion of the occipital bone and anteriorly over the posterior and inferior portion of each parietal bone. This sinus ends at the posterolateral extremity of the petrous portion of the temporal bone from where it extends inferiorly as the sigmoid sinus. Along their course, the transverse sinuses can receive occipital, temporal, cerebellar, and tentorial veins.[12,13,22–26]

The transition of the transverse sinus into the sigmoid sinus occurs at the point where the former receives the superior petrosal sinus, at the level of the so-called sinodural angle of Citelli. The sigmoid sulcus lies over a deep, curved groove on the inner surface of the mastoid portion of the temporal bone, which is anteriorly separated from the mastoid air cells by a thin lamina of bone. It ends at the jugular fossa, where the sinus enters the jugular foramen.[4,27,28]

The relationships between the cranial sutures and venous sinuses can be used in surgical planning.[29,30] The asterion corresponds to the meeting point of the lambdoid, occipitomastoid, and parietomastoid sutures. This important anthropological point is usually located over the lower aspect of the transverse sinus at its distal margin. The midpoint of the inion-asterion line is particularly related to the bottom of the transverse sinus. This relationship has led to the observation that the inion-asterion line usually corresponds to the inferior aspect of the transverse sinus.[29,30]

The occipitomastoid suture always crosses the posterior margin of the sigmoid sinus at the level of the superior aspect of the mastoid notch. This crossing point coincides with the intersection of the occipitomastoid suture and an imaginary line between the inion and mastoid tip. The relationships among these external landmarks can be specified relative to the transverse and sigmoid sinuses. In particular, (1) the asterion and the midpoint of the inion-asterion line are related to the inferior half of the transverse sinus; (2) the superior and inferior points of the transverse and sigmoid sinus junction, respectively, are situated above and below the posterior portion of the parietomastoid suture; (3) the intersection of the parietomastoid and squamous sutures is located at the level of the posterior aspect of the superior surface of the petrous bone; and (4) the occipitomastoid suture and the posterior margin of the sigmoid sinus crossing point is situated at the level of the superior and posterior aspect of the mastoid notch. This point corresponds to the intersection of the occipitomastoid suture with the inion-mastoid tip line.[29,30]

These relationships can be used intraoperatively to plan the placement of burr holes during suboccipital and retromastoid exposures. An initial burr hole placed just anterior to the asterion can expose the transition between the transverse and sigmoid sinuses. A second burr hole placed over the occipitomastoid suture posterior to the mastoid process at the most posterior level of the mastoid notch demarcates the posterior margin of the sigmoid sinus.

■ Retrosigmoid Approach

The retrosigmoid approach is most commonly selected for approaching the structures in the cerebellopontine angle (**Figs. 33.4** and **33.5**). A detailed understanding of the complex microsurgical anatomy of this area is essential to optimize operative results.[3,25,31–33] The retrosigmoid exposure is performed with the patient in the three-quarter prone position with the midsagittal plane roughly parallel to the floor, with the top of the head tilted slightly downward to the floor to reduce the possibility that the shoulder will obstruct access to the operative field (**Fig. 33.5**). The table is tilted so that the head is slightly above the chest and abdomen. The vertical lateral suboccipital scalp incision for the retrosigmoid approach is situated in the lateral half of the middle third of the distance between the midline and the mastoid process so that it crosses the asterion at the junction of the parietomastoid, occipitomastoid, and lambdoid sutures. The surgeon is seated above the head of the patient for operations in the upper part of the cerebellopontine angle and behind the head for operations in the middle and lower part of the cerebellopontine angle.

The muscle opening is carried inferiorly to just lateral to the foramen magnum, with care taken to avoid injury to the vertebral artery as it courses behind the atlanto-occipital joint and posterior arch of the atlas. A bone flap medial to

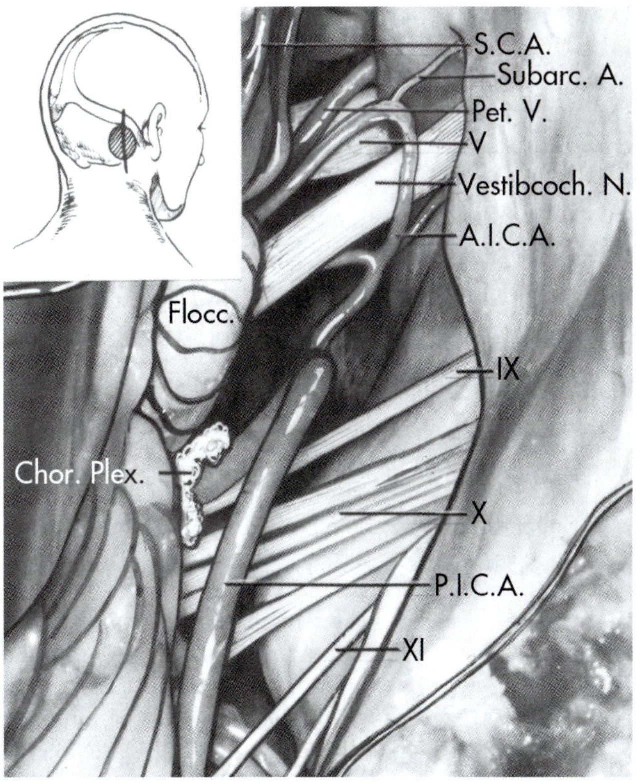

A

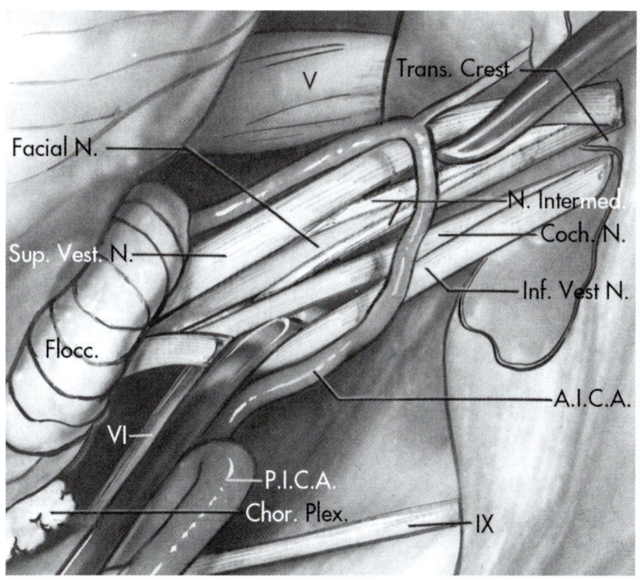

B

Fig. 33.4 Microsurgical anatomy of the retrosigmoid approach. A to D are matched black and white and color photographs of a stepwise cadaveric dissection. **(A)** The *inset* shows the site of the scalp incision (*solid line*) and bone opening (*oblique lines*). The cerebellum has been elevated to expose the trigeminal nerve (*V*), vestibulocochlear nerve (*Vestibcoch. N.*), glossopharyngeal nerve (*IX*), vagus nerve (*X*), accessory nerves (*XI*), the superior cerebellar artery (*S.C.A.*), anterior inferior cerebellar artery (*A.I.C.A.*), posterior inferior cerebellar artery (*P.I.C.A.*), and petrosal vein (*Pet. V.*). Choroid plexus (*Chor. Plex.*) protrudes from the foramen of Luschka behind the glossopharyngeal nerve. The flocculus (*Flocc.*) is located behind the vestibulocochlear nerve. The subarcuate artery (*Subarc. A.*) arises from the anterior inferior cerebellar artery and penetrates the dura behind the internal acoustic meatus. **(B)** The posterior wall of the internal auditory canal has been removed, and the cleavage planes between the superior vestibular nerve (*Sup. Vest. N.*), inferior vestibular nerve (*Inf. Vest. N.*), and cochlear nerve (*Coch. N.*) has been extended medially to the brainstem. The superior vestibular nerve has been elevated and the inferior vestibular nerve depressed to expose the facial nerve (*Facial N.*), cochlear nerve, and two small bundles of the nervus intermedius (*N. Intermed.*). The transverse crest (*Trans. Crest*) separates the facial and superior vestibular nerve above from the cochlear and inferior vestibular nerves below. *(continued)*

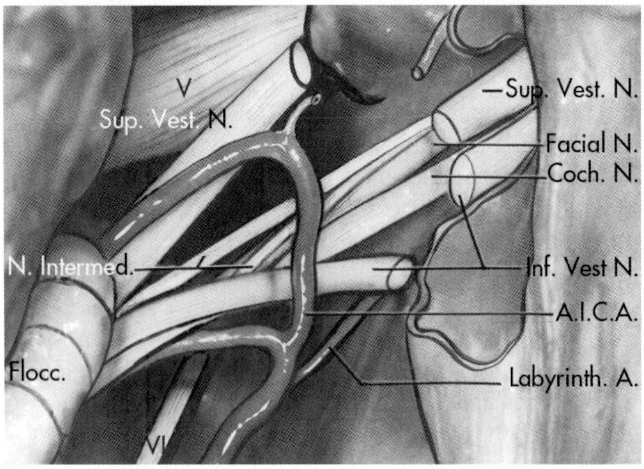

C

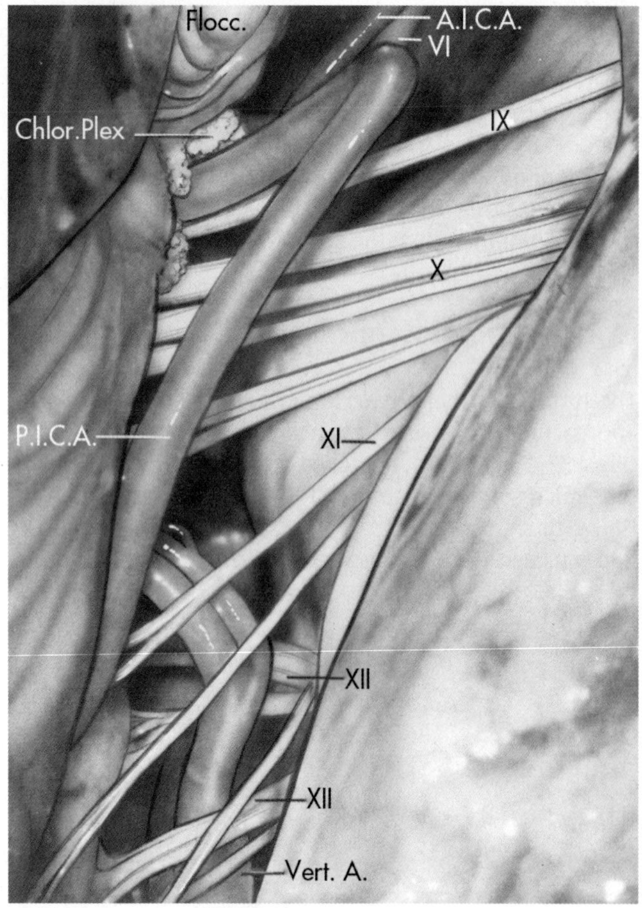

D

Fig. 33.4 *(continued)* **(C)** The superior and inferior vestibular nerves have been divided to show the facial nerve and nervus intermedius in front of the superior vestibular nerve and the cochlear nerve in front of the inferior vestibular nerve. A labyrinthine artery (*Labyrinth. A.*) passes into the internal acoustic meatus. The abducens nerve (*VI*) ascends in front of the pons. **(D)** Enlarged view of the nerves entering the jugular foramen. There is a dural septum between the glossopharyngeal and vagus nerves where they enter the jugular foramen. The hypoglossal nerve (*XII*) passes behind the vertebral artery (*Vert. A.*). (From Tedeschi H, Rhoton AL Jr. Lateral approaches to the petroclival region. Surg Neurol 1994;41:180–216. Reprinted with permission.)

the sigmoid sinus is elevated, and the opening is enlarged to the lower margin of the transverse sinus and the posterior margin of the sigmoid sinus (**Fig. 33.5**). The osteotome cut around the margin of the bone flap is made after placing a burr hole medial to the sigmoid sinus and stripping the dura from the inner table. The foramen magnum does not routinely need to be opened to remove a tumor in the cerebellopontine angle. The mastoid air cells entered in the lateral part of the craniectomy are closed with bone wax. The dura is opened with the pedicle medially. The dural cuff bordering the transverse and sigmoid sinuses is tacked up to the muscles and fascia bordering the craniectomy margin with sutures to minimize the need for cerebellar retraction. The cerebellum, which commonly bulges outward upon opening the dura, usually relaxes after opening the arachnoid membrane over the cisterna magna or the superolateral margin of the cerebellum and allowing cerebrospinal fluid (CSF) to escape. Cerebellar resection is infrequently needed, even when removing large tumors.

All of the intradural part of the procedure is conducted with the operating microscope. The surface of the cerebellum facing the posterior surface of the temporal bone is elevated to expose a tumor in the cerebellopontine angle (**Fig. 33.6**). Self-retaining retraction rather than handheld retraction is used. A wide retractor blade that will cover most of the lateral margin of the cerebellum and does not need to be moved as the operation progresses causes less damage than smaller blades that must be shifted repeatedly. A tapered blade 15 to 25 mm wide at its base and 10 to 15 mm at its tip is commonly used.

The operation for a cerebellopontine angle tumor should be planned so that the tumor surface is allowed to settle away from the neural tissue rather than the neural structures being retracted away from the tumor. No attempt is made to see the whole tumor on initially elevating the cerebellum when removing meningiomas. The surface of the tumor is then opened and biopsied, and the intracapsular contents are removed. As the intracapsular contents are evacuated, the tumor shifts laterally, making it possible to remove more of it through the small exposure. Carefully applied, fine bipolar coagulation is preferred for controlling bleeding and shrinking small deposits of tumor. In the final step, the last thin sheet of tumor capsule is removed from the neural and vascular structures using fine dissecting instruments. The most common reason for the tumor appearing to be tightly adherent to neural structures is not adhesions between the capsule and surrounding tissue; rather, it is residual tumor in the capsule wedging the tumor into position. Only rarely are tumors so densely adherent that they defy easy removal after their intracapsular

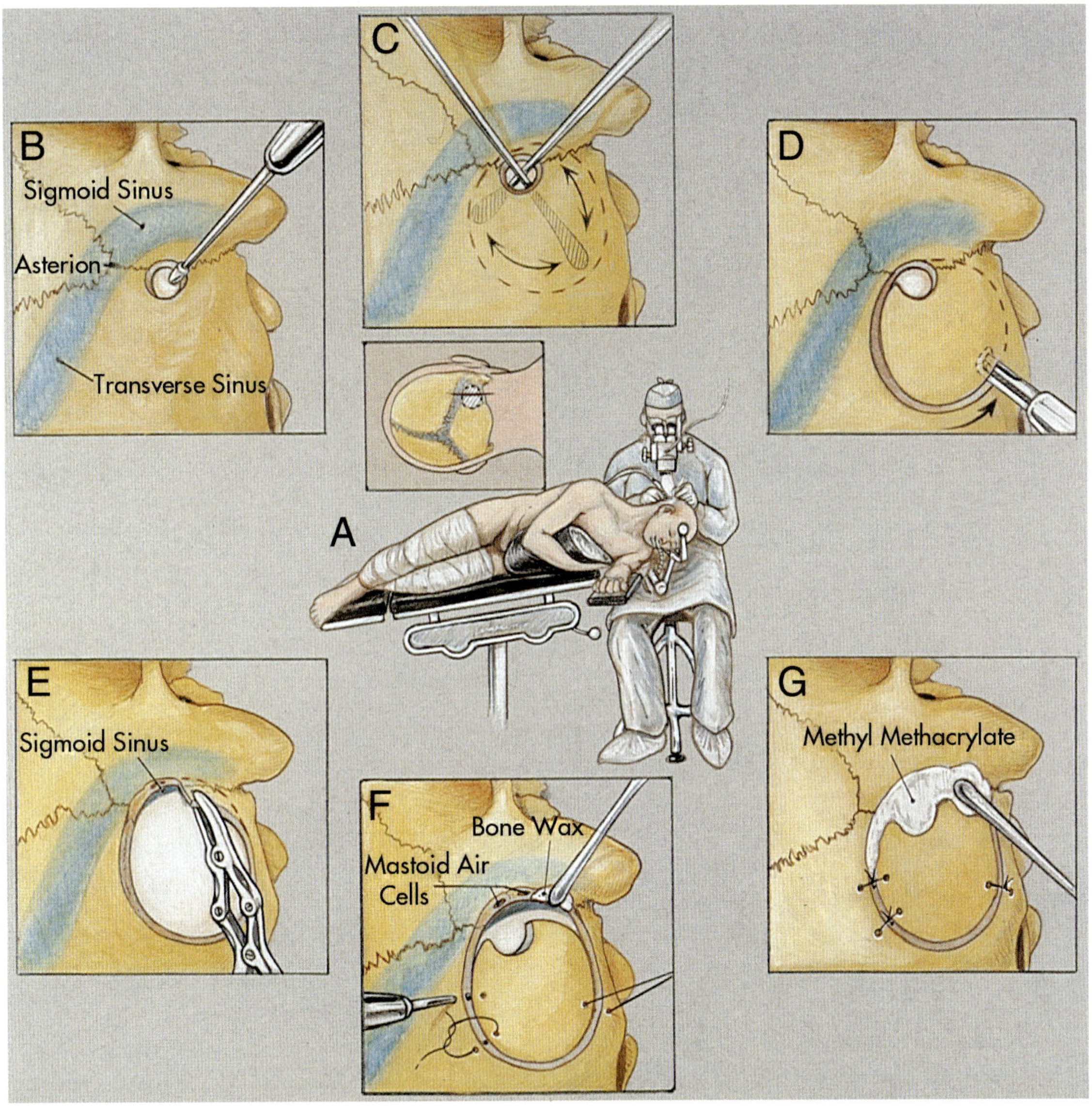

Fig. 33.5 Steps in elevation of suboccipital craniotomy flap. **(A)** The patient is placed in the park bench position. The *inset* shows the site of the bone flap (*oblique lines*) and the vertical paramedian scalp incision (*solid line*) that crosses the asterion. **(B)** A burr hole is placed medial to the sigmoid sinus. **(C)** A Penfield dissector strips the dura from the lower margin of the flap in the area below the transverse sinus and medial to the sigmoid sinus. **(D)** A craniotome opens the margin of the bone flap. **(E)** A rongeur removes bone to extend the opening to the margin of the sigmoid and transverse sinuses. **(F)** The bone flap is replaced and fixed in position with several 0-silk sutures after completing the intradural part of the operation. Bone wax is pressed into the openings in the mastoid air cells. **(G)** Methylmethacrylate is molded around the margins of the flap to give a solid and cosmetically satisfactory closure.

contents are removed. A remnant of tumor capsule may be left if it is so firmly adherent to vital neural or vascular structures that removing it would damage these structures.

If the pia-arachnoid is adherent to the tumor capsule or a mass of tumor in the capsule prevents collapse of the capsule away from the pia-arachnoid, there is a tendency to apply traction to both the capsule and pia-arachnoid and to tear vessels running on the neural structures. Gentle irrigation directed into the plane between the tumor capsule and brain will often open the appropriate cleavage plane. Under magnification, individual adhesions between vital structures and tumor can be divided with microinstruments. Prior to separating the pia-arachnoid from the capsule, it is important that the entire tumor be removed so that the capsule is so thin that it is almost transparent. If one is uncertain about the margin between the capsule and the pia-arachnoid, several sweeps of a fine dissector through the area while gently irrigating the area will help clarify the appropriate plane for dissection.

Any vessel that stands above or is stretched around the tumor capsule should be dealt with initially as if it were a vessel that runs over the tumor surface to supply the

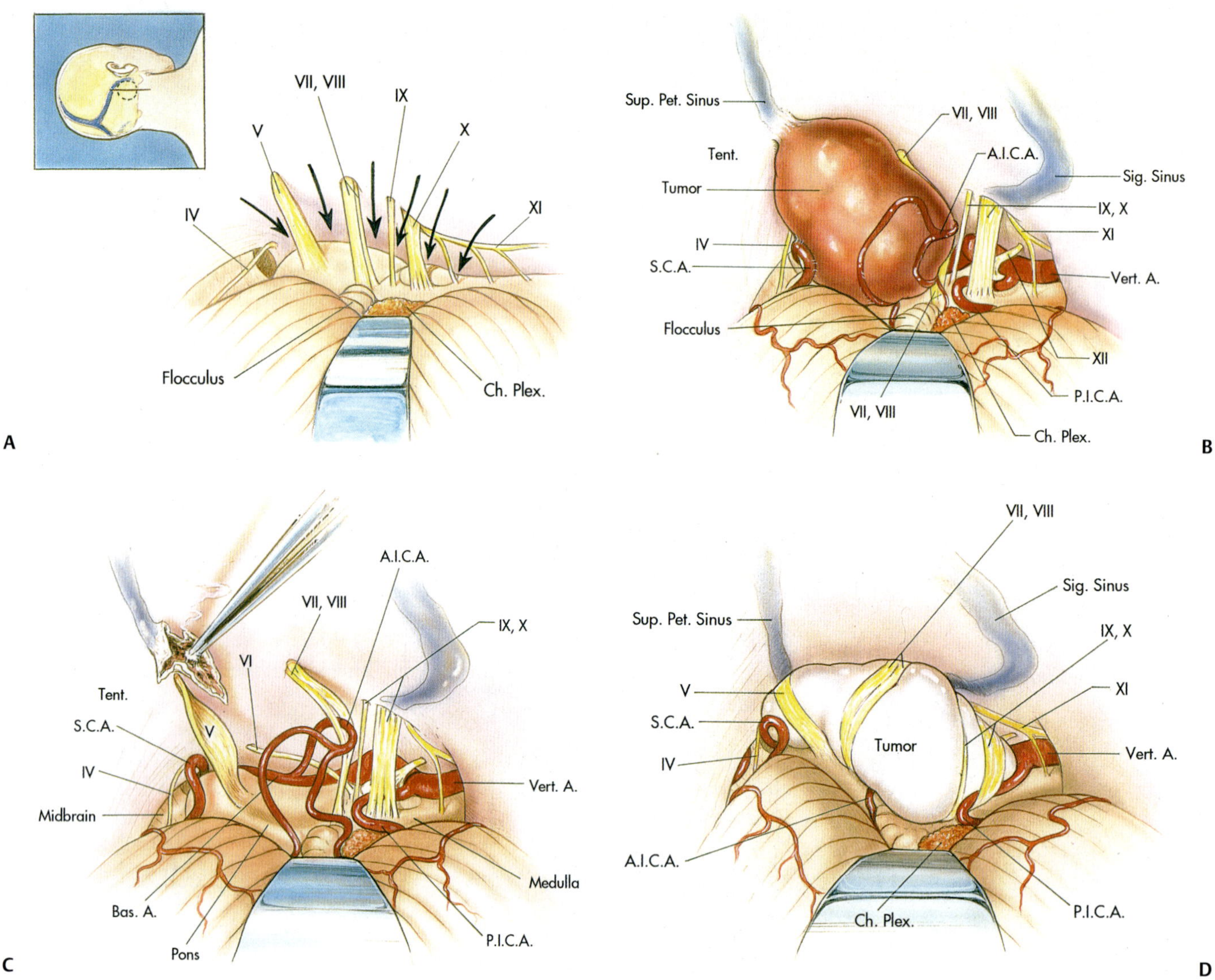

Fig. 33.6 Approach to meningiomas of the cerebellopontine angle. **(A)** Routes that can be taken between the cranial nerves to expose and remove a tumor situated medial to and involving multiple cranial nerves. The patient is positioned in the three-quarter prone position. The *inset* (upper left) shows the site of the vertical scalp incision and craniectomy. The approach to pathology located medial to the nerves can be directed (*arrows*) between the trochlear nerve (*IV*) above and the trigeminal nerve (*V*) below; between the trigeminal nerve above and the facial (*VII*) and vestibulocochlear nerves (*VIII*) below; between the facial and vestibulocochlear nerves above and the glossopharyngeal nerve (*IX*) below; between the glossopharyngeal and vagus nerves (*X*); between the vagus nerve and accessory rootlets (*XI*); and between the widely separated rootlets of the accessory nerve. A tumor located medial to the nerves will often widen the intervals between the nerves, depending on the site of origin of the tumor. Choroid plexus (*Ch. Plex.*) protrudes from the foramen of Luschka. **(B)** Meningioma attached lateral to the trigeminal nerve in the region of the superior petrosal sinus (*Sup. Pet. Sinus*). The trochlear nerve is elevated, the trigeminal nerve is pushed medially, and the facial and vestibulocochlear nerves are stretched below the tumor. Other structures exposed include the vertebral artery (*Vert. A.*), superior cerebellar artery (*S.C.A.*), anterior inferior cerebellar artery (*A.I.C.A.*), posterior inferior cerebellar artery (*P.I.C.A.*), sigmoid sinus (*Sig. Sinus*), and hypoglossal nerve (*XII*). **(C)** The tumor has been removed. The thin distorted nerves have been preserved, and the remaining dural attachment is removed or cauterized with bipolar coagulation. The basilar artery (*Bas. A.*) and abducens nerve (*VI*) are exposed. **(D)** Large meningioma arising from the clivus in the region of the inferior petrosal sinus with involvement of the cranial nerves IV to XI. The nerves are displaced laterally around the tumor. The tumor is removed by working through the intervals between the nerves. *(continued)*

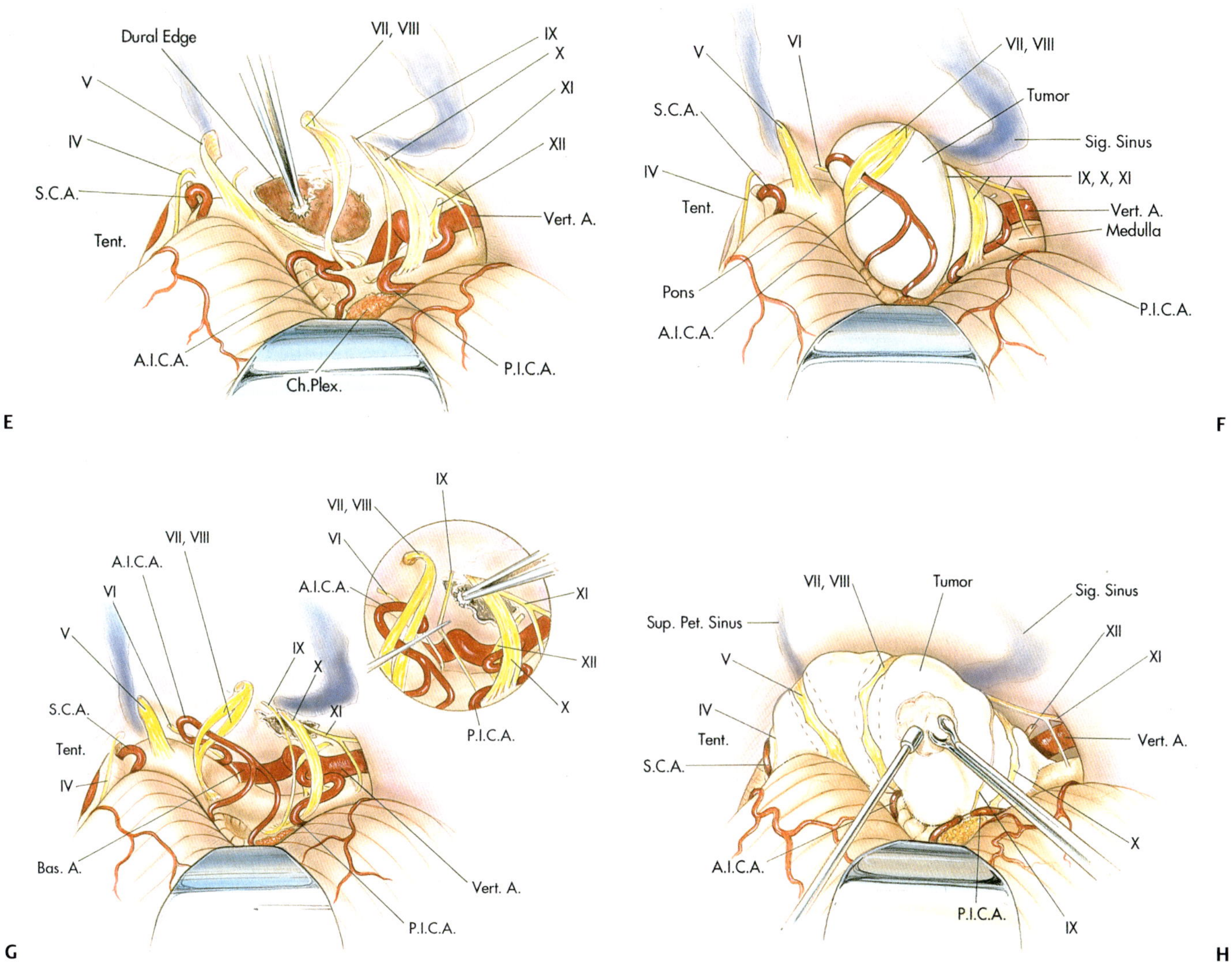

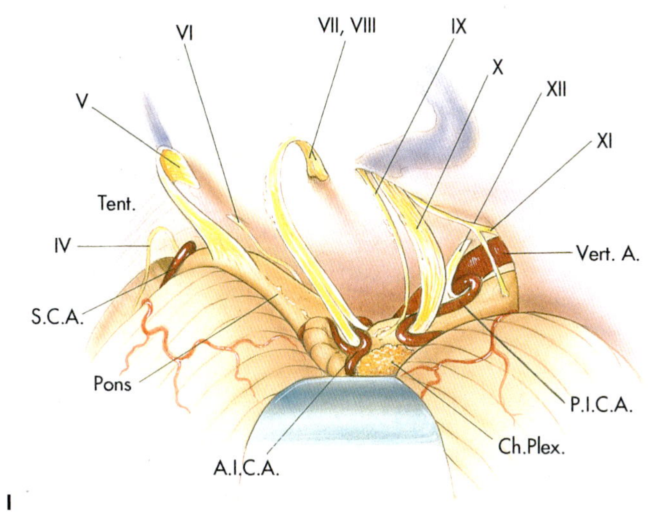

Fig. 33.6 *(continued)* **(E)** The meningioma has been removed. The dural attachment has been partially removed, and the base is being cauterized. **(F)** Meningioma arising medial to the jugular bulb in the region of the jugular tubercle. The tumor involves the lower cranial nerves. **(G)** The tumor was removed by operating through the intervals between the facial and vestibulocochlear nerves above and the glossopharyngeal nerve below and between the glossopharyngeal and vagus nerves (*round inset*). **(H)** Large epidermoid tumor being removed by working through the intervals between the nerves. **(I)** Distorted nerves after the removal of the epidermoid tumor. (From Rhoton AL Jr. Microsurgical anatomy of posterior fossa cranial nerves. In: Barrow DL, ed. Surgery of the Cranial Nerves of the Posterior Fossa: Neurosurgical Topics. Chicago, IL: American Association of Neurological Surgeons; 1993:1–103. Reprinted with permission.)

brain. An attempt should be made to displace the vessel off the tumor capsule using a small dissector after the tumor has been removed from within the capsule. When dissected free of the capsule, vessels that initially appear to be adherent to the capsule often prove to be neural vessels. Occlusion of a cerebellar artery is one of the most common causes of morbidity and mortality in removing cerebellopontine angle tumors.[32] One of the most dangerous aspects of surgery in the cerebellopontine angle is removing a tumor from an encased vertebral artery. The site of encasement is commonly near the site of passage of the artery through the dura. The cutting loop should be avoided. A remnant of tumor may be left on an artery if removing it might lead to major hemorrhage or occlusion of the artery.

The number of veins sacrificed should be kept to a minimum because of the undesirable consequences of their loss.[25] Obliteration of the petrosal veins, which pass from the surface of the cerebellum and brainstem to the superior petrosal sinus, is inescapable in reaching and removing some cerebellopontine angle tumors. Occlusion of these veins, which drain much of the cerebellum and brainstem, may infrequently cause hemorrhagic edema of the cerebellum and brainstem. Some of these veins will need to be sacrificed if the tumor extends into the area above the internal acoustic meatus; however, small tumors located in the middle or lower part of the cerebellopontine angle may be removed without sacrificing a petrosal vein.

Preserving the arachnoidal walls of the cisterns bordering the cerebellopontine angle aids in protecting adjacent neural and vascular structures during the removal of some tumors. Meningiomas commonly arise outside the outer arachnoidal membrane and compress the cisterns without extending directly into them. Some cerebellopontine angle meningiomas can be removed without opening the outer arachnoid membrane because the membrane is displaced around the inner surface of the tumor.

In removing meningiomas, the initial intradural approach is directed toward obliterating the blood supply of the tumor at the point that it comes through the dura (**Fig. 33.6**).[34] In the initial approach, avoid entering the dome of the tumor opposite its vascular supply because this will allow bleeding throughout the operation. Meningiomas in the upper part of the cerebellopontine angle receive their predominate blood supply from the meningohypophysial branch of the intracavernous segment of the internal carotid artery, and those in the lower part of the posterior fossa receive their predominate supply from the branches of the external carotid artery that pass through the hypoglossal canal and jugular foramen. Only the dural base of the tumor is exposed initially, and the bipolar forceps are used to coagulate the base of the tumor and separate it from its blood supply and site of attachment. As the dissection crosses the dural base of a meningioma, the outer circumference is composed of soft tumor that separates easily from the dura. As the dissection and coagulation of the base are carried deeper, the hyperostosis and fibrous attachment are encountered. Finally, on the opposite side of the base, soft tumor is encountered again. It may not be possible to completely cross the base of the tumor until some tumor has been removed from within the capsule near the base.

Meningiomas and other tumors that arise lateral to the nerves in the cerebellopontine angle and displace them medially are easier to remove than those that arise medial to the cranial nerves and displace them laterally (**Figs. 33.6** and **33.7**). In exposing and removing medially placed tumors in the upper part of the cerebellopontine angle, the approach can be directed through the interval between the lower margin of the tentorium and the trigeminal nerve. Care is needed to protect the trochlear nerve and superior cerebellar artery in this area. Further inferiorly, the medially placed tumor is approached through the interval between the trigeminal nerve above and the facial and vestibulocochlear nerves below. If the tumor has an even lower attachment near the jugular foramen, it can be approached through the interval between the facial and vestibulocochlear nerves above and the glossopharyngeal nerve below or through the interval between the lower rootlets of the vagus nerve and the upper part of the spinal accessory nerve, or between the widely separated accessory rootlets. The intervals between the glossopharyngeal nerve above and vagus nerve below and between the individual vagal rootlets are too small to work through unless they have been widened by the tumor.

Meningiomas may infrequently extend into the internal acoustic meatus, in which case it may be necessary to remove the posterior wall of the internal auditory canal.

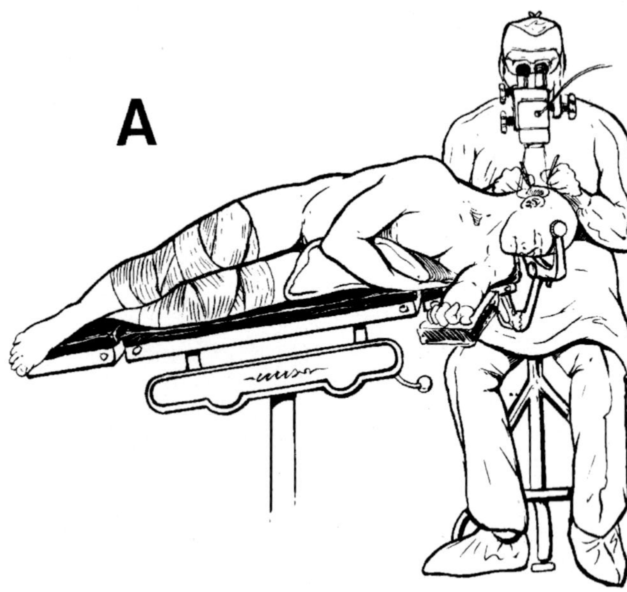

Fig. 33.7 Retrosigmoid approach for the removal of acoustic neuromas. **(A)** Right side: The patient is positioned in the three-quarter prone position with the surgeon behind the head. *(continued)*

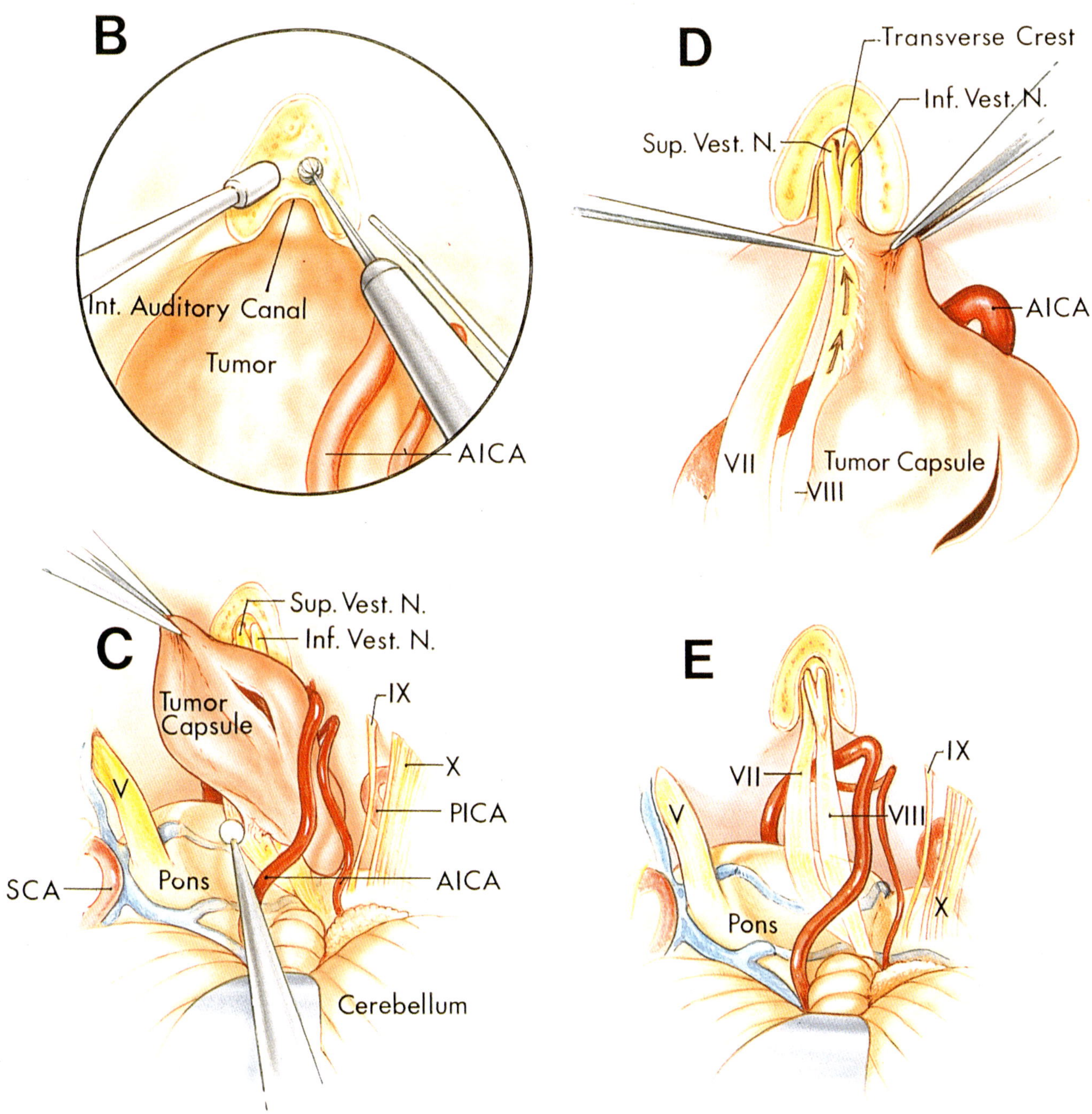

Fig. 33.7 *(continued)* **(B)** The posterior wall of the internal (*Int.*) auditory canal is removed. The anterior inferior cerebellar artery (*AICA*) courses around the lower margin of the tumor. **(C)** The intracapsular contents of the tumor have been removed. The capsule of the tumor is separated from the pons and the posterior surface of the superior vestibular nerve (*Sup. Vest. N.*) and inferior vestibular nerve (*Inf. Vest. N.*). The trigeminal nerve (*V*) and superior cerebellar artery (*SCA*) are above the tumor, and the glossopharyngeal nerve (*IX*), vagus nerve (*X*), and posterior inferior cerebellar artery (*PICA*) are below the tumor. **(D)** The dissection along the vestibulocochlear nerve (*VIII*) is done in a medial to lateral direction (*arrows*) to avoid tearing the tiny filaments of the cochlear nerve in the lateral end of the canal where they pass through the lamina cribrosa. The transverse crest separates the superior and inferior vestibular nerves in the lateral end of the canal. The facial nerve (*VII*) is anterior to the superior vestibular nerve. **(E)** Cerebellopontine angle and internal auditory canal after tumor removal, with the facial and cochlear nerves preserved. (From Rhoton AL Jr, Tedeschi H. Microsurgical anatomy of acoustic neuroma. Otolaryngol Clin North Am 1992;25:257–294. Reprinted with permission.)

Greater care is required in opening the meatus with a meningioma than with an acoustic neuroma because the facial nerve is more commonly displaced posteriorly on the back side of the tumor than with an acoustic neuroma, which commonly displaces the nerve around the anterior half of the tumor.

During the craniectomy and removal of the posterior meatal lip or a hyperostosis, the mastoid air cells may be opened and must then be sealed to prevent CSF leakage and meningitis. The air cells that are opened in removing the posterior meatal lip are carefully closed with bone wax. A patch of fat taken from a small transverse incision on the lower abdomen will settle into the depression created by the drilling and is then laid over the drilled meatal margin. The patient's own dura is carefully closed. If some openings are left in the dura along the suture line, a small patch of suboccipital muscle or fat can be sutured over the opening.

The operation for removal of an acoustic neuroma differs from that for a meningioma because the acoustic neuroma has its firmest attachment to the area around the internal acoustic meatus rather than to the dura on the posterior surface of the petrous bone (**Fig. 33.7**). After opening the dura to expose an acoustic neuroma, the lateral margin of the tumor is exposed using gentle self-retaining retraction, and the posterior wall of the internal auditory canal is removed using an irrigating drill. No attempt is made to see the whole tumor on initial retraction of the cerebellum. The posterior wall of the internal canal is removed as an initial step if the tumor is small. The intracapsular contents of the tumor are removed before opening the meatus if the tumor is large and deforms the brainstem. Care is required to avoid injury to the anterior inferior cerebellar artery if it is adherent to the dura covering the posterior wall of the internal auditory meatus. After removing the posterior wall of the meatus, the dura that lines the meatus is opened to expose its contents. The facial nerve is identified near the origin of the facial canal at the anterior superior quadrant of the meatus rather than in a more medial location where the direction of displacement is variable. The tumor within the meatus is separated from the posterior surface of the facial and vestibulocochlear nerves. There are several landmarks that are helpful in identifying the facial and vestibulocochlear nerves at the brainstem on the medial side of the tumor. These nerves, although distorted by the tumor, can usually be identified on the brainstem side of the tumor at the lateral end of the pontomedullary sulcus, just rostral to the glossopharyngeal nerve and just anterosuperior to the foramen of Luschka, flocculus, and choroid plexus protruding from the foramen of Luschka. After the facial and vestibulocochlear nerves are identified on the medial and lateral sides of the tumor, the final remnant of the tumor is separated from the intervening segment of the nerves.

Epidermoid tumors in the cerebellopontine angle are easily recognized on computed tomography and magnetic resonance images by their characteristic appearance. They occasionally may be confused with arachnoid cysts or cystic acoustic neuromas. Epidermoid tumors are removed by completing an intracapsular removal and then by excising the portions of the capsule that are not firmly adherent to the brainstem, cranial nerves, and vascular structures. The intracapsular contents are usually soft and easily removed with gentle suction; however, portions of the capsule, although thin, may need to be left in place because they are firmly adherent to the cranial nerves or brainstem. The surface of the adherent capsule should be carefully cleaned of squamous debris, which may cause aseptic meningeal reaction if it mixes with the CSF. Epidermoid tumors are often situated medial to the nerves in the cerebellopontine angle and must be removed by working between the nerves. Subarachnoid cysts in the cerebellopontine angle are treated by removing enough of their wall that they communicate freely with the adjacent subarachnoid cisterns.

Gliomas may grow into the cerebellopontine angle and mimic other tumors there. The senior author has operated on several exophytic gliomas that displaced but did not infiltrate the nerves in the cerebellopontine angle. After completing the intracapsular removal of the exophytic portion of the tumor, it became obvious that the medial part of these tumors infiltrated the side of the pons near the facial and vestibulocochlear nerves. With the use of gentle traction on the remaining tumor and microdissection, these tumors were delivered from the side of the pons, thus achieving gross total removal. Ependymomas may extend into the cerebellopontine angle from their origin along the lateral recess or from the area surrounding the foramen of Luschka. The tumor protrudes into the area behind the glossopharyngeal and vagus nerves and below the facial and vestibulocochlear nerves.

At the time of the craniectomy and the removal of the posterior meatal lip or a hyperostosis, the mastoid air cells may be opened and must then be sealed to prevent CSF leakage and meningitis. The air cells that are opened in removing the posterior meatal lip are closed with bone wax, after which a pledget of fat taken from a small incision on the abdomen is laid over the drill site and onto the dura surrounding the opening. The craniotomy margin is closed by bone wax that is carefully and heavily applied (**Fig. 33.5**). In most cases, a watertight dural closure is obtained using the patient's own dura. A dural graft, commonly from cadaveric dura or fascia lata, is infrequently needed. The patient's pericranium or fascia lata may also be used. Small openings in the dura may be closed with pledgets of muscle or fat taken from the wound margin.

There are several other variants of the retrosigmoid approach in addition to those used for tumor removal (**Figs. 33.8** and **33.9**).[1,35] The superior variant, in which a small cranial opening is centered adjacent to the upper part of the sigmoid sinus, is commonly selected for vascular decompression operations for trigeminal neuralgia. The surgeon is positioned at the head of the patient for this type

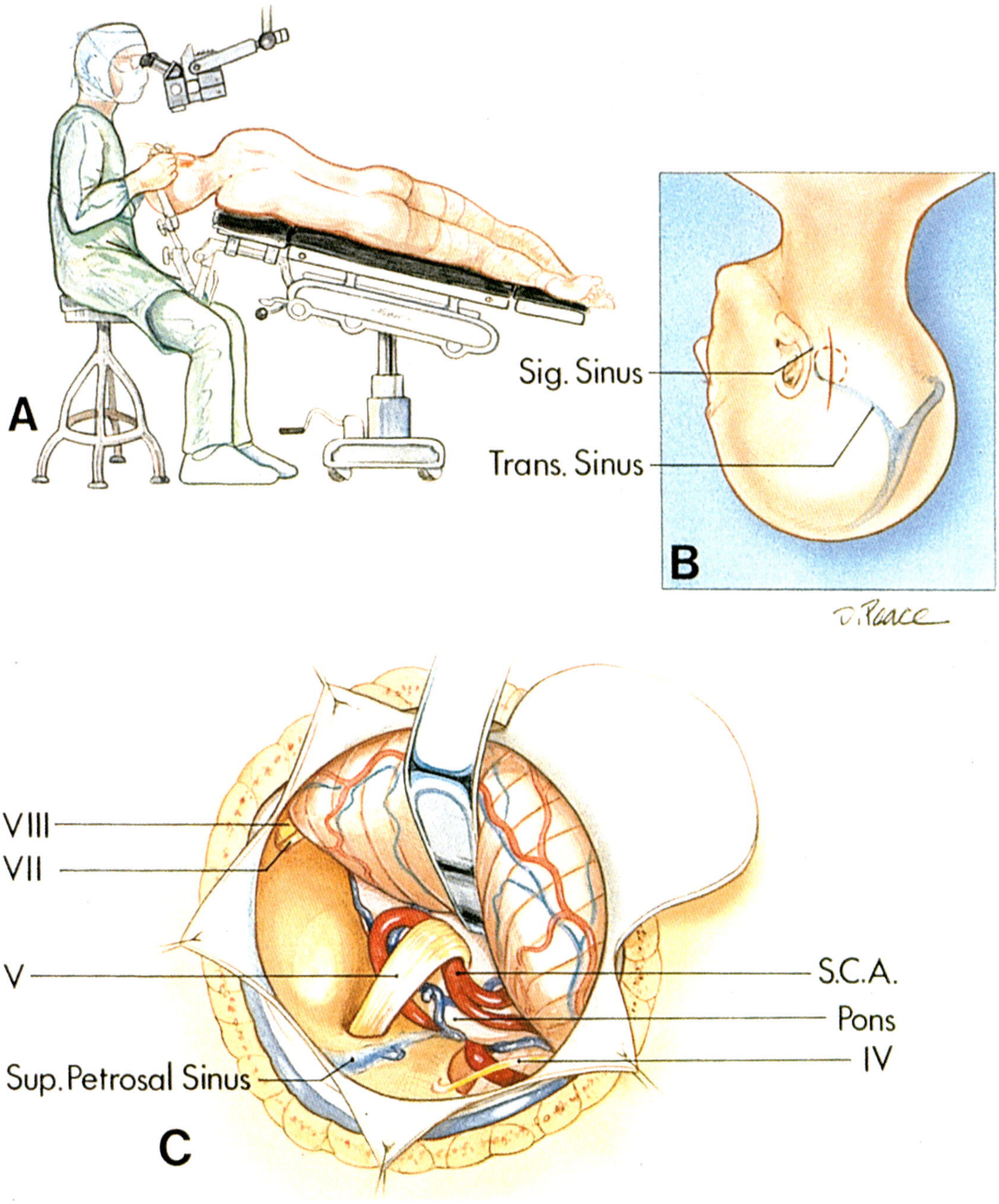

Fig. 33.8 Retrosigmoid approach to the trigeminal nerve for a decompression operation. **(A)** The patient is positioned in the three-quarter prone position. The surgeon is seated at the head of the table. The table is tilted so that the feet are lower than the heart. **(B)** The vertical paramedian incision crosses the asterion. The superolateral margin of the craniectomy is positioned at the junction of the transverse sinus (*Trans. Sinus*) and sigmoid sinus (*Sig. Sinus*). **(C)** The superolateral margin of the cerebellum is gently elevated using a brain spatula tapered from 10 mm at the base to 3 or 5 mm at the tip to expose the site at which the trigeminal nerve (*V*) enters the pons. The brain spatula is advanced and aligned parallel to the superior petrosal sinus (*Sup. Petrosal Sinus*). The trochlear nerve (*IV*) is at the superior margin of the exposure, and the facial (*VII*) and vestibulocochlear nerves (*VIII*) are at the lower margin. The dura is tacked up to the adjacent muscles to maximize the exposure along the superolateral margin of the cerebellum. The main trunk of the superior cerebellar artery (*S.C.A.*) loops down into the axilla of the trigeminal nerve. (From Rhoton AL Jr. Microsurgical anatomy of decompression operations on the trigeminal nerve. In: Rovit RL, Murali R, Jannetta PJ, eds. Trigeminal Neuralgia. Baltimore, MD: Williams & Wilkins; 1990:165–200. Reprinted with permission.)

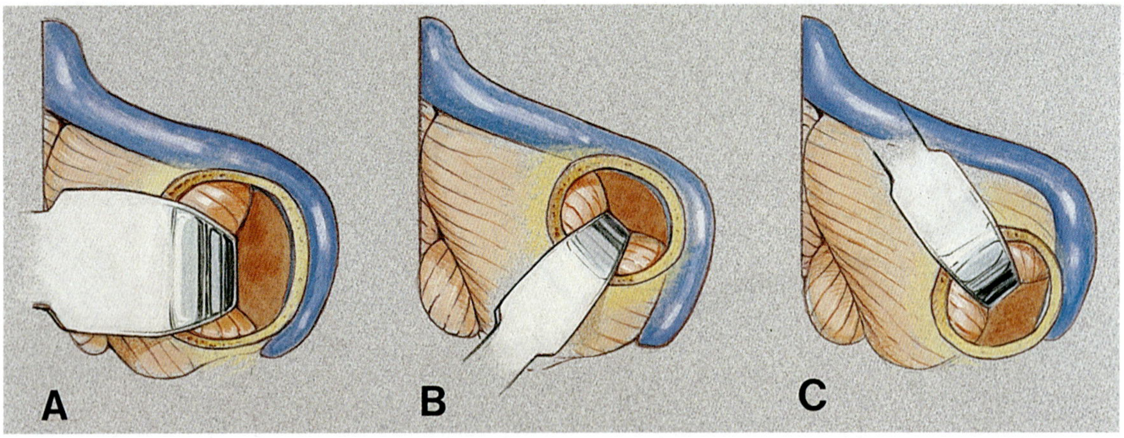

Fig. 33.9 Direction of application of brain spatulas for surgery in the various compartments of the cerebellopontine angle. **(A)** Lateral exposure for a lesion in the midportion of the cerebellopontine angle, such as an acoustic neuroma. The site of the craniectomy below the transverse sinus and medial to the sigmoid sinus is shown for removing an acoustic neuroma or other lesions involving multiple neurovascular complexes. The spatula protects the lateral surface of the cerebellum. A brain spatula tapered from 20 or 25 mm at the base to 15 or 20 mm at the tip is commonly used during acoustic neuroma removal. **(B)** Spatula application for exposing the upper neurovascular complex for a decompression operation for trigeminal neuralgia. A spatula tapered from 10 mm at the base to 3 or 5 mm at the tip is commonly selected. The spatula is placed parallel to the superior petrosal sinus. **(C)** Retractor application for exposure of the lower neurovascular complex. This approach is also used in hemifacial spasm because the nerve root exit zone of the facial nerve is located only a few millimeters above the glossopharyngeal nerve and the posterior inferior cerebellar artery is commonly the compressing vessel. A brain spatula tapered from 10 mm at the base to 3 or 5 mm at the tip is commonly used for operations for hemifacial spasm. (From Rhoton AL Jr. Instrumentation. In: Apuzzo MLJ, ed. Brain Surgery: Complication Avoidance and Management, vol 2. New York, NY: Churchill-Livingstone; 1993:1647–1670. Reprinted with permission.)

of retrosigmoid approach (**Fig. 33.8**). Another variant, in which a small opening is centered behind the lower part of the sigmoid sinus, is used to approach lesions in the lower part of the cerebellopontine angle or for a decompression operation for hemifacial spasm. For operations in the mid and lower part of the cerebellopontine angle, the surgeon is seated behind the head of the patient (**Fig. 33.7**).

Midline Suboccipital Approach

The midline approach is commonly used for meningiomas in the upper spinal canal and posterior or posterolaterally at the foramen magnum (**Fig. 33.10**). The midline exposure also can be used for tumors of the fourth ventricle, cerebellar vermis, medial part of the cerebellar hemisphere, and one or both cerebellar tonsils. Elevation, gentle lateral displacement, or resection of a cerebellar tonsil may provide access to tumors arising in the fourth ventricle or those that extend laterally from the foramen of Luschka into the region behind the nerves in the cerebellopontine angle.

The three-quarter prone position is routinely used, with the side of greatest expansion of the tumor uppermost (**Fig. 33.10**). Turning the head to the side of the lesion facilitates access to the front of the cervicomedullary junction. The vertical midline skin incision is of sufficient length to complete a craniectomy above the foramen magnum and a laminectomy of the axis and atlas. The subcutaneous tissues are separated from the underlying fascia near the inion to gain room for a Y-shaped fascial incision. The upper limbs of the "Y" begin at the level of the superior nuchal line, lateral to the external occipital protuberance, and join several centimeters below the inion, leaving a musculofascial flap along the superior nuchal line for closure. The inferior limb of the "Y" incision extends downward in the midline. Care is taken to avoid injury to the vertebral artery as it courses along the lateral part of the posterior arch of the atlas. This artery is not encountered if the incision is strictly midline, but it is frequently apparent in the floor of the suboccipital triangle if the muscle incision deviates laterally, or when the muscles are stripped from the lateral part of C1. The emissary veins and vertebral venous plexus should be quickly obliterated if they are opened.

The dura is opened with a Y-shaped incision, and dural tack-up sutures are placed. The marginal and occipital sinuses encountered in opening the dura are controlled with gentle bipolar coagulation to minimize dural shrinkage. Posterior or posterolateral lesions may separate easily from the surface of the brainstem and spinal cord.

Anterolaterally situated tumors displace the spinal cord dorsally and rotate it away from the side on which the main tumor mass is located. The ventral rootlets are often pushed dorsally by such lesions. They must be identified and separated from the dorsal rootlets and dentate ligaments. Spinal rootlets of cranial nerve XI are frequently draped over the tumor. Rarely should it be necessary to sacrifice the rootlets of the upper cervical levels. It is usually possible to separate them sufficiently to afford piecemeal resection of the tumor between them. Care should be taken to avoid injury to

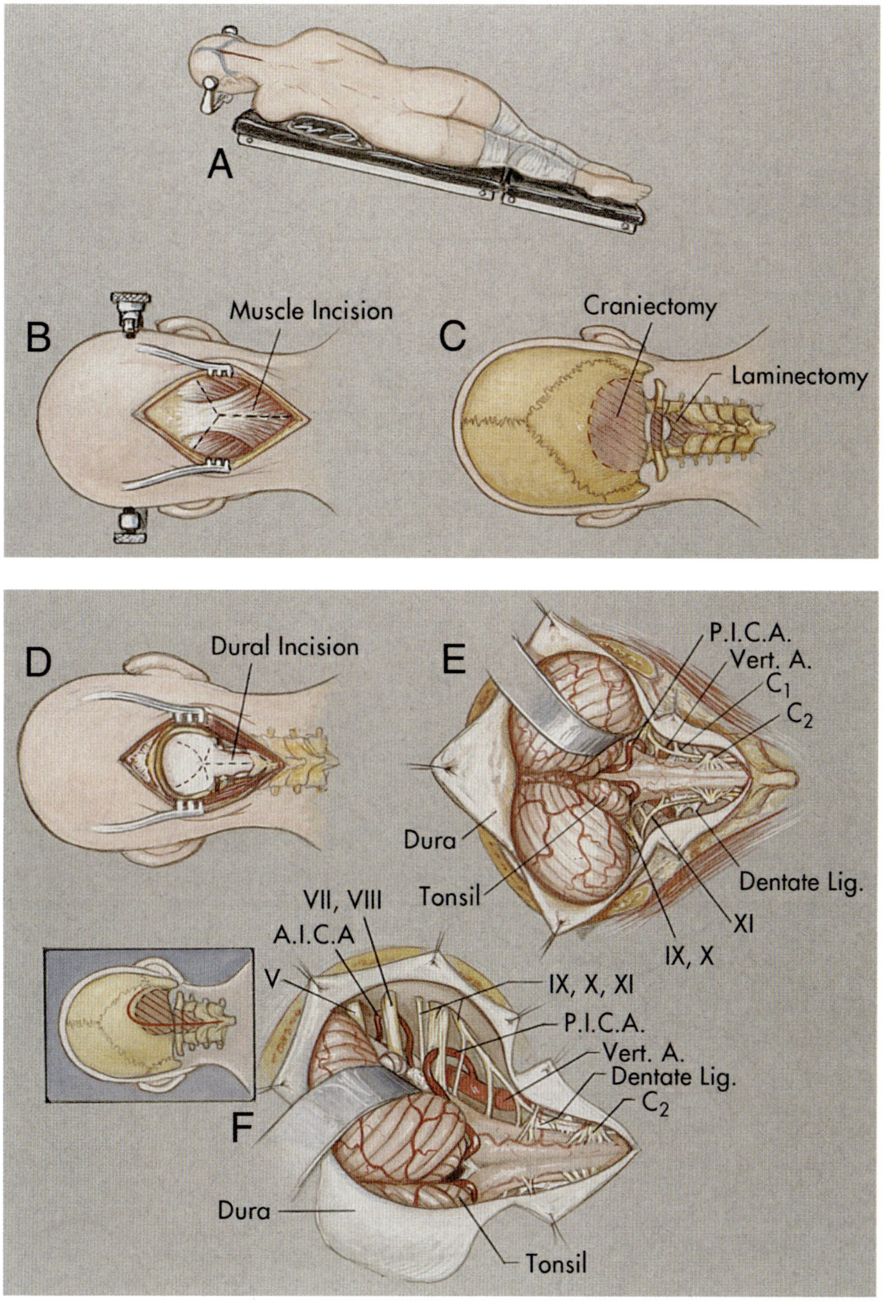

Fig. 33.10 Midline suboccipital approaches for a foramen magnum tumor. The lesion is exposed through a suboccipital craniectomy and upper cervical laminectomy. **(A)** The patient is placed in the three-quarter prone position. The vertical midline incision is selected for lesions posterior or posterolateral in the area of the foramen magnum, or those involving the cerebellar vermis and tonsil and fourth ventricle, or the medial part of the cerebellar hemispheres. **(B)** The subcutaneous tissues are separated from the underlying fascia near the inion to gain room for a Y-shaped incision in the muscles. The upper limbs of the Y begin at the level of the superior nuchal line lateral to the external occipital protuberance and join several centimeters below the inion, permitting a musculofascial flap to be reflected upward from the superior nuchal line. The inferior limb of the Y extends downward in the midline. **(C)** The incision is of sufficient length to complete a suboccipital craniectomy and a laminectomy of the axis and atlas (*oblique lines*). **(D)** Dural incision (*interrupted lines*). **(E)** Intradural exposure. The major extracranial hazard is injury to the vertebral artery (*Vert. A.*) as it courses along the lateral part of the posterior arch of the atlas. The vertebral arteries give rise to the posterior inferior cerebellar arteries (*P.I.C.A.*). The glossopharyngeal (*IX*), vagus (*X*), and accessory nerves (*XI*) pass toward the jugular foramen. The upper attachment of the dentate ligament (*Dentate Lig.*) is at the level of the foramen magnum behind the vertebral artery. **(F)** Hockey stick incision combining the midline and lateral exposure. Skin incision (*solid line*) and bone removal (*inset*). The hockey stick incision extends from the mastoid process along the superior nuchal line and downward in the midline. This incision is selected if a lesion arising in the craniovertebral junction extends anterolateral or anterior to the brainstem into the cerebellopontine angle. This exposure permits the removal of the posterior rim of the foramen magnum and the posterior elements of the atlas and axis; additionally, it allows completion of a unilateral suboccipital craniectomy of sufficient size to expose the anterolateral surface of the brainstem and the trigeminal (*V*), facial (*VII*), and vestibulocochlear nerves (*VIII*), and the anterior inferior cerebellar artery (*A.I.C.A.*) in the cerebellopontine angle.

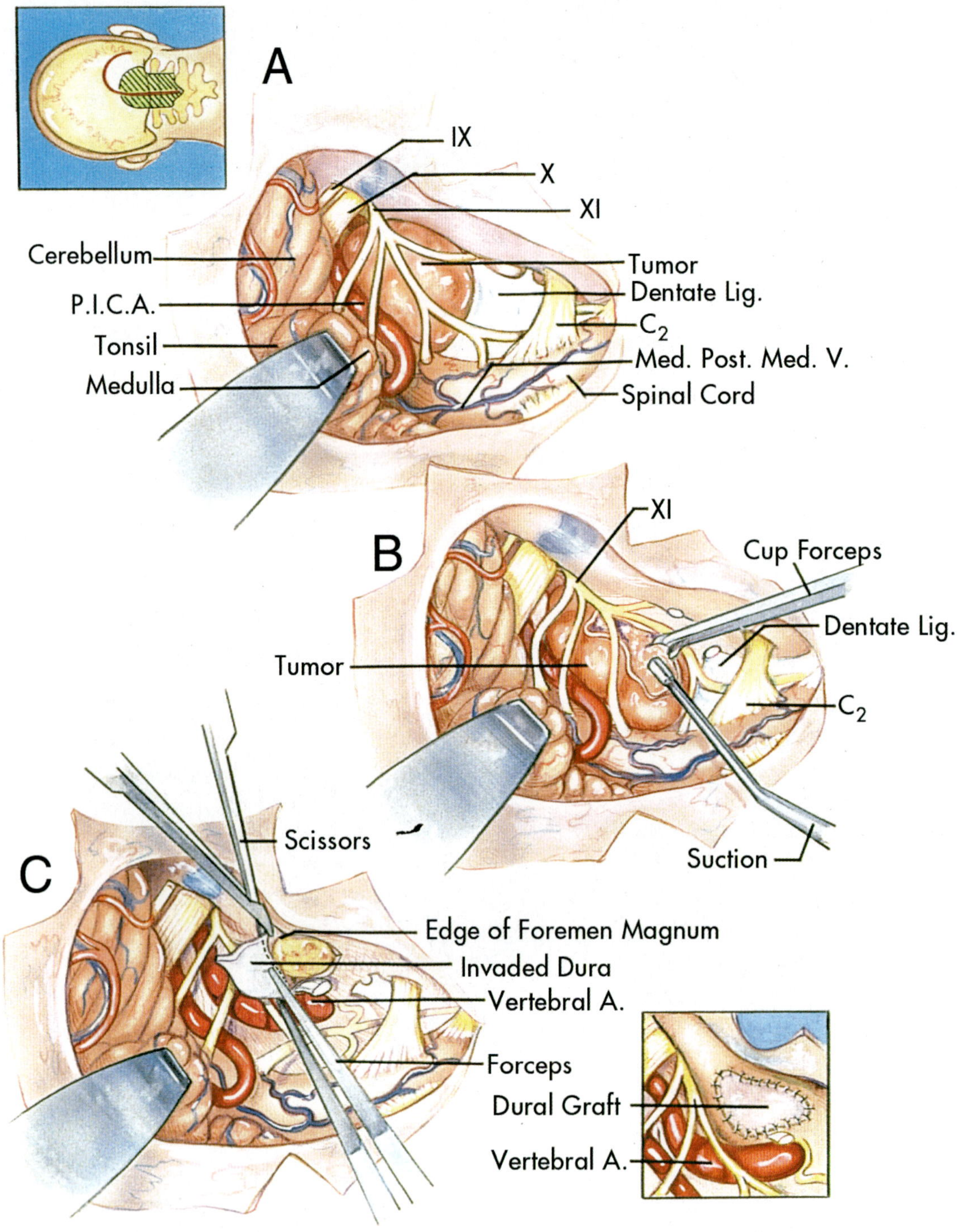

Fig. 33.11 **(A)** Removal of encapsulated foramen magnum meningioma in an anterolateral location displacing the cervicomedullary junction. The patient is positioned in the park bench or prone position. The inset (*upper left*) shows the hockey stick incision (*solid line*) and area of the suboccipital craniectomy and C1 to C2 laminectomy (*diagonal lines*). The right cerebellar tonsil is gently elevated to expose the tumor. The posterior inferior cerebellar artery (*P.I.C.A.*), spinal accessory nerve (*XI*), and rootlets of C2 are draped over the tumor. The glossopharyngeal (*IX*) and vagus (*X*) nerves are uninvolved. The vertebral artery is hidden anterior to the tumor. The dentate ligament (*Dentate Lig.*) has been sectioned to facilitate the exposure. **(B)** A fine suction with a blunt tip and 3-mm cup forceps debulk the intracapsular portion of the tumor. **(C)** Despite the large bulk of some of these tumors, they usually arise from a small vascular pedicle off the anterolateral dura. The involved dura is resected with microscissor. (*Inset lower right*) A dura graft may be necessary if closure of the patient's own dura constricts the neural structures. (From Rhoton AL Jr. Meningiomas of the cerebellopontine angle and foramen magnum. Neurosurg Clin North Am 1994;5:349–377. Reprinted with permission.)

radicular vessels running with the upper cervical roots, which may provide essential blood supply to the spinal cord.

A useful landmark is the most rostral dentate ligament, which lies at the level of the foramen magnum and indicates the point at which the vertebral artery pierces the dura.[3] The upper two or three attachments of the dentate ligament may be sectioned to reduce traction on the spinal cord during manipulation. The capsule is opened and the intracapsular contents are removed in a piecemeal fashion. Extreme care should be utilized when cutting into tumors situated anterolateral to the brainstem, as they may encase a segment of the vertebral or posterior inferior cerebellar arteries. Occasionally, a small tab of tumor is tightly adherent to the vertebral artery and will need to be left behind.

Although some authors claim that the dural attachment of spinal meningiomas should be radically removed to prevent recurrence, others have demonstrated no clear correlation between late recurrence and the extent of dural resection. When tumor resection is completed, an attempt should be made to excise the involved dura. Failing this, scraping the inner dural surface with a Penfield dissector or curette followed by vigorous bipolar coagulation is usually sufficient to complete the elimination of the tumor. A fascia lata, pericranial, or cadaver dural graft is used when closure of the patient's own dura might constrict the neural structures. Complications related to this approach have included injury to the vertebral artery, epidural hematoma, and destabilization of the craniocervical junction.

The hockey stick incision, which permits a combined midline and lateral approach, is selected if the lesion extends anterior or anterolateral to the brainstem toward the jugular foramen or the cerebellopontine angle (**Figs. 33.10** and **33.11**). The skin incision extends from the mastoid process along the superior nuchal line to the inion and downward in the midline. A muscular cuff is left attached along the superior nuchal line to facilitate the closure. This incision permits removal of the full posterior rim of the foramen magnum, the posterior elements of the atlas and axis, and a unilateral suboccipital craniectomy of sufficient size to expose the anterolateral surface of the brainstem and the nerves in the cerebellopontine angle. The amount of suboccipital craniectomy and cervical laminectomy varies depending on the rostrocaudal extent of the tumor and its size. Despite the large bulk of some of the more anteriorly located meningiomas, they usually arise from a small vascular pedicle off the anterolateral dura and are thus fully resectable via this approach. The laminectomy should be performed widely and may include the medial margin of the facet joints on the side of the tumor, although it is often not necessary to sacrifice the stability of the joints themselves.

The so-called extreme lateral approach is a modification of the suboccipital approach devised to facilitate removal of more anteriorly placed lesions and to minimize the need for retraction on the medulla, lower cranial nerves, and spinal cord.[2,36] The extreme lateral approach provides the access to the foramen magnum and cerebellopontine angle provided by the hockey stick incision. In addition, the lateral limb of the incision extends lower to provide access to the transverse foramen of C1, the occipital condyle, and the lateral mass of C1. The dural incision can be extended completely around the vertebral artery, leaving a cuff of dura encircling the artery. This dural incision, along with removal of a portion of the occipital condyle and lateral mass of C1, allows the vertebral artery to be mobilized and gives a more direct approach to the anterior rim of the foramen magnum and the structures ventral to the brainstem and upper cervical cord.

Paramedian Approach

This approach is commonly selected for lesions involving the central part of one cerebellar hemisphere in which it is not necessary to expose the midline or the cerebellopontine angle. A vertical incision situated in the midline third of the area between the inion and mastoid tip provides access for a bony opening, which exposes the posterior surface of one cerebellar hemisphere. The approach may be selected for tumors such as gliomas, hemangioblastomas, or metastases situated in the central part of one cerebellar hemisphere. The bony opening could be extended up to the transverse sinus for exposure of a tumor attached to the lower surface of the tentorium. The patient is placed in the three-quarter prone position, with the side of the lesion uppermost. A cortical incision is commonly used to reach the lesion. The bone flap is usually replaced at the end of the operation.

References

1. Rhoton AL Jr. Microsurgical anatomy of posterior fossa cranial nerves. In: Barrow DL, ed. Surgery of the Cranial Nerves of the Posterior Fossa: Neurosurgical Topics. Chicago, IL: American Association of Neurological Surgeons; 1993:1–103
2. Tedeschi H, Rhoton AL Jr. Lateral approaches to the petroclival region. Surg Neurol 1994;41(3):180–216
3. de Oliveira E, Rhoton AL Jr, Peace D. Microsurgical anatomy of the region of the foramen magnum. Surg Neurol 1985;24(3): 293–352
4. Dichiro G, Anderson WB. The clivus. Clin Radiol 1965;16:211–223
5. Watt JC, McKillop AN. Relation of arteries to roots of nerves in posterior cranial fossa in man. Arch Surg 1935;30:336–345
6. Bremond G, Garcin M, Magnan JI. Preservation of hearing in the removal of acoustic neuroma. ('minima' posterior approach by retrosigmoidal route). J Laryngol Otol 1980;94(10):1199–1204
7. Lang J. Inferior skull base anatomy: In: Sekhar LN, Schramm VL Jr, eds. Tumors of the Cranial Base: Diagnosis and Treatment. New York: Futura; 1987:461–529
8. McMinn RMH, Hutchings RT, Logan BM. Color Atlas of Head and Neck Anatomy. Chicago, IL: Year Book Medical Publishing; 1981
9. Pernkoff E. Atlas of Topographical and Applied Human Anatomy. Baltimore, MD: Urban & Schwarzenberg; 1980
10. Waddington M. Atlas of the Human Skull. Athens, GA: Rutland Academy Books; 1981

11. Williams PL, Warwik R, eds. Gray's Anatomy, 36th ed. Philadelphia: Saunders; 1980
12. Ono M, Ono M, Rhoton AL Jr, Barry M. Microsurgical anatomy of the region of the tentorial incisura. J Neurosurg 1984;60(2): 365–399
13. Oka K, Rhoton AL Jr, Barry M, Rodriguez R. Microsurgical anatomy of the superficial veins of the cerebrum. Neurosurgery 1985;17(5):711–748
14. Bisaria KK. Anatomic variations of venous sinuses in the region of the torcular Herophili. J Neurosurg 1985;62(1):90–95
15. Kaplan HA, Browder A, Browder J. Narrow and atretic transverse dural sinuses: clinical significance. Ann Otol Rhinol Laryngol 1973;82(3):351–354 PubMed
16. Kaplan HA, Browder J. Neurosurgical consideration of some features of the cerebral dural sinuses and their tributaries. Clin Neurosurg 1976;23:155–169
17. Kaplan HA, Browder J, Knightly JJ, Rush BF Jr, Browder A. Variations of the cerebral dural sinuses at the torcular herophili. Importance in radical neck dissection. Am J Surg 1972;124(4):456–461
18. Saxena RC, Beg MA, Das AC. Double straight sinus. Report of six cases. J Neurosurg 1973;39(4):540–542
19. Waltner JG. Anatomic variations of the lateral and sigmoid sinuses. Arch Otolaryngol 1944;39:307–312
20. Wolf-Heidgger G. Atlas de Anatomia Humana, 2nd ed. Rio de Janeiro: Guanabara Koogan; 1972
21. Woodhall B, Seeds AE. Cranial venous sinuses: correlations between skull markings and roentgenograms of the occipital bone. Arch Surg 1936;33:867–875
22. Browder J, Kaplan HA, Krieger AJ. Anatomical features of the straight sinus and its tributaries. J Neurosurg 1976;44(1):55–61
23. Duval JM, Latouche X, Mondine P, Robillard D. [Sinus of the cerebellar tentorium]. Bull Assoc Anat (Nancy) 1975;59(167):855–862 French.
24. Kaplan HA, Browder J, Krieger AJ. Venous channels within the intracranial dural partitions. Radiology 1975;115(3):641–645
25. Matsushima T, Rhoton AL Jr, de Oliveira E, Peace D. Microsurgical anatomy of the veins of the posterior fossa. J Neurosurg 1983; 59(1):63–105
26. Ono M, Rhoton AL Jr, Peace D, Rodriguez RJ. Microsurgical anatomy of the deep venous system of the brain. Neurosurgery 1984;15(5):621–657
27. Haas LL. The posterior condylar fossa, foramen and canal, and the jugular foramen. Radiology 1957;69(4):546–552
28. Rhoton AL Jr, Buza RC. Microsurgical anatomy of the jugular foramen. J Neurosurg 1975;42(5):541–550
29. Ribas GC, Rhoton AL Jr, Cruz OR, Peace D. Suboccipital burr holes and craniectomies. Neurosurg Focus 2005;19(2):E1
30. Ribas GC, Rhoton AL Jr, Cruz OR, et al. Temporo-parieto-occipital burrhole sites study and systematized approaches proposal. In: Samii M, ed. Skull Base Surgery, First International, Skull Base Congress, Hannover 1992. Basel: Karger; 1994:723–730
31. Lister JR, Rhoton AL Jr, Matsushima T, Peace DA. Microsurgical anatomy of the posterior inferior cerebellar artery. Neurosurgery 1982;10(2):170–199
32. Martin RG, Grant JL, Peace DA, Theiss C, Rhoton AL Jr. Microsurgical relationships of the anterior inferior cerebellar artery and the facial-vestibulocochlear nerve complex. Neurosurgery 1980;6(5):483–507
33. Rhoton AL Jr. Microsurgical anatomy of the brainstem surface facing an acoustic neuroma. Surg Neurol 1986;25(4):326–339
34. Rhoton AL Jr. Meningiomas of the cerebellopontine angle and foramen magnum. Neurosurg Clin N Am 1994;5(2):349–377
35. Rhoton AL Jr. Microsurgical anatomy of decompression operations on the trigeminal nerve. In: Rovit RL, Murali R, Jannetta PJ, eds. Trigeminal Neuralgia. Baltimore, MD: Williams & Wilkins; 1990:165–200
36. Sen CN, Sekhar LN. An extreme lateral approach to intradural lesions of the cervical spine and foramen magnum. Neurosurgery 1990;27(2):197–204
37. Rhoton AL Jr. The foramen magnum. Neurosurgery 2000;47 (3, Suppl):S155–S193

IV Fixation and Fusion Techniques

34 Biology of Spinal Fusion

David J. Hart and Curtis A. Dickman

This chapter reviews the anatomy, histology, and physiology of bone healing and the biology of spinal fusion. Bone is a dynamic biological tissue composed of metabolically active cells that are integrated into a rigid environment. The healing potential of bone is influenced by biomechanical, biochemical, cellular, hormonal, and pathological mechanisms. Normally, bone is in a constant state of flux because its deposition, resorption, and remodeling are continuous. The goals of spinal internal fixation procedures are to achieve anatomical alignment, to protect the neural elements, and to stabilize the spine mechanically while preserving the motion of normal spinal segments. These goals may be attained only by achieving arthrodesis. Ultimately, the success of a fusion depends on satisfactory bone healing. Instrumentation provides immediate but often temporary spinal fixation. Metal instrumentation is susceptible to fatigue, loosening, breakage, and failure even after a fusion has formed. Only a solid osseous union ensures long-term spinal stability. The surgical success for fusion depends on preparation of the fusion site, the ability of the graft material to induce bone healing, and the effect of systemic and local factors.

Bone Anatomy and Histology

There are three primary types of bone in humans: woven, cortical, and cancellous.[1,2] Typically, woven bone has randomly arranged collagen bundles and irregularly shaped vascular spaces lined with osteoblasts. The disordered arrangement of woven bone makes it relatively weak. Woven bone is found during rapid bone formation: at birth, during fracture healing (callus formation), and in some disease states (hyperparathyroidism and Paget disease).[2] Woven bone normally is remodeled and replaced with cortical or cancellous bone.

Cortical bone, also called compact or lamellar bone, forms the internal and external tables of flat bones and the external surfaces of long bones (**Fig. 34.1**).[1,2] Microscopically, cortical bone consists of densely packed regions called osteons bound on the endosteal and periosteal surface by inner and outer circumferential lamellae. Osteons, the fundamental structural units of bone, are lamellar cylinders of bone that surround longitudinally oriented vascular channels (haversian canals). Horizontally oriented canals (Volkmann's canals) connect adjacent osteons.

Cancellous bone is interposed between cortical bone surfaces and is referred to as spongy bone, trabecular bone, or marrow. Cancellous bone has honeycombed hematopoietic interstices and bony trabeculae. The trabeculae are predominantly oriented perpendicular to external forces to provide structural support.[3,4]

Cellular components of bone include osteoblasts, osteoclasts, osteocytes, osteogenic precursor cells, and hematopoietic elements of the bone marrow.[1,2] Mature bone cells differentiate from mesenchymal precursors.[2,5,6] Osteoblasts, osteoclasts, and osteocytes are present in all types of bone.

Osteoblasts are metabolically active bone-forming cells. They are plump, cuboidal cells that secrete osteoid. As bone-forming activity nears completion, some osteoblasts are trapped within the osteon and become osteocytes incorporated into the bone structure. Other osteoblasts remain on the periosteal or endosteal surfaces as lining cells.

Osteocytes are mature osteoblasts entrapped within the bone matrix. Their cell bodies are found in lacunae. Multiple cytoplasmic processes extend to blood vessels and other osteocytes via canaliculi, which are 1 to 2 lumens in diameter (**Fig. 34.2**).

Osteoclasts are multinucleated, bone-resorbing cells controlled by hormonal and cellular mechanisms. They resorb bone by releasing acid and proteolytic enzymes and reside in shallow pits called Howship's lacunae. Working in groups called cutting cones, osteoclasts can dissolve the inorganic and organic matrices of bone and calcified cartilage.

Bone Biochemistry

Bone is composed of organic and inorganic components. Water constitutes ~20% of the weight of bone tissue.[2] The weight of dry bone consists of inorganic calcium phosphate molecules (65 to 70%) and an organic matrix of fibrous protein and collagen (30 to 35%).[1,2,6,7]

Osteoid is the unmineralized organic matrix produced by osteoblasts and subsequently undergoes mineralization. In mature human lamellar bone, a 1-lumen layer of osteoid is produced each day. Osteoid is composed of 90% collagen and 10% ground substance, which consists primarily of noncollagenous proteins, glycosaminoglycans, and glycoproteins.[2,7] The strength and rigidity of bone reflect the presence of inorganic mineral salts embedded in the organic matrix.[3,4]

The inorganic mineral content of bone constitutes 50% of bone volume and 70% of bone weight.[2] The primary bone

Modified from Dickman CA, Maric Z: The biology of bone healing and techniques of spinal fusion. *BNI Quarterly* 1994; 10(1):2-12. (Modified with permission from Barrow Neurogolical Institute.)

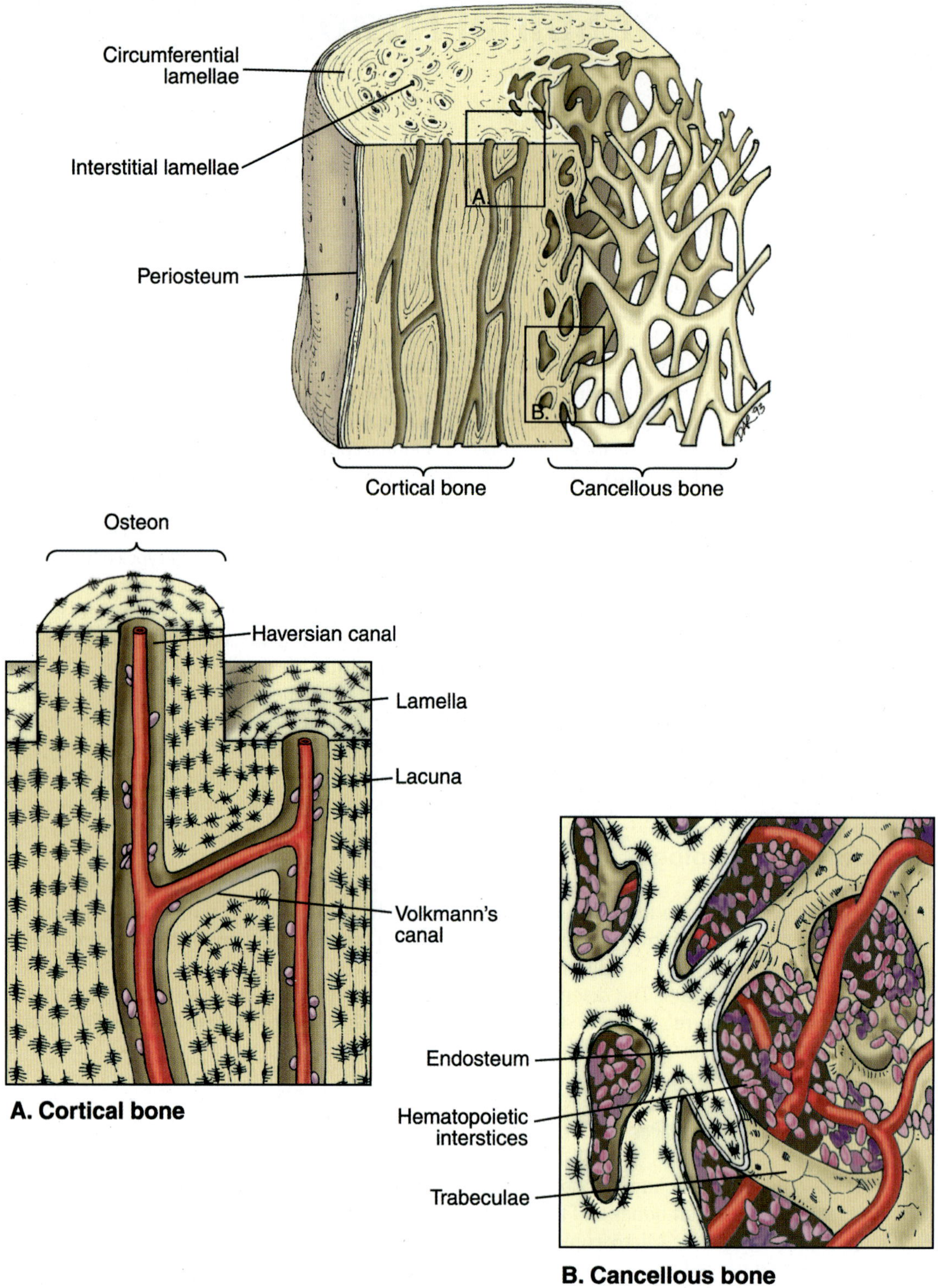

Fig. 34.1 Cross-section of bone showing its components. **(A)** Cortical bone is composed of compact, cylindrical osteons, which are the fundamental structural units of bone. **(B)** Cancellous bone is porous and contains hematopoietic elements, vascular interstices, and bone trabeculae. The trabeculae are oriented to resist the external loads placed on the bone. (Reprinted with permission from Barrow Neurological Institute.)

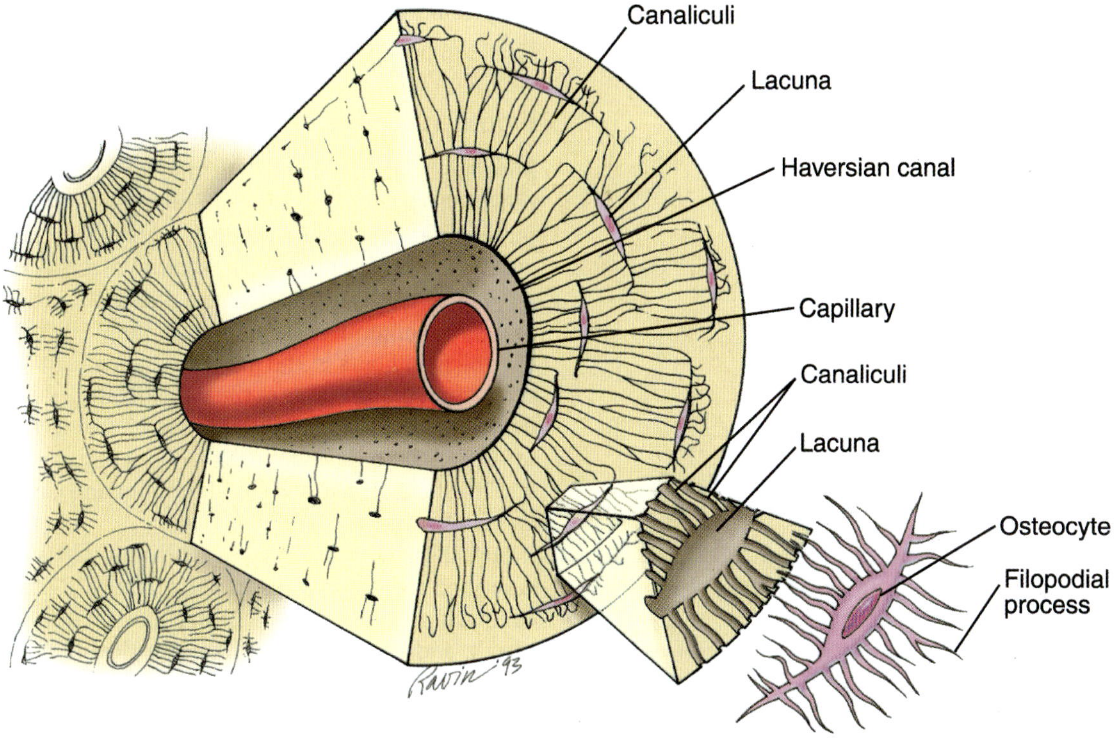

Fig. 34.2 An osteon or haversian system is composed of a haversian canal and the surrounding lamellar bone. Osteocytes live within the lacunae and have cytoplasmic processes that extend via canaliculi to the blood vessels and adjacent lacunae. (Reprinted with permission from Barrow Neurological Institute.)

minerals are calcium phosphate and calcium carbonate, with small quantities of magnesium, fluoride, and sodium. The mineral crystals form hydroxyapatite, $Ca_{10}(PO_4)_6(OH)_2$.

Hydroxyapatite precipitates in an orderly arrangement around the collagen fibers of the osteoid. These collagen fibers are type I collagen, found in skin, tendon, and fascia.[1,2] Type I collagen molecules have a helical structure with extensive cross-linking and are composed of two α_1 chains and one α_2 chain. Osteoid initially becomes calcified within a few days; however, calcification is completed only after several months.

Bone Growth Factors

The mineral and nonmineral components in both cancellous and cortical bone undergo constant remodeling. Coupling of bone absorption and formation is mediated through bone-cell-derived growth factors, local factors, and biomechanical stresses.[7–10]

Several proteins cause healing bone to vascularize, solidify, incorporate, and function mechanically. Bone healing also can be influenced directly by neurotransmitters, hormones, vitamins, and minerals (**Tables 34.1** and **34.2**).

Proteins that enhance bone healing include bone morphogenic proteins (BMPs), insulin-like growth factors, transforming growth factors (TGF-β), platelet-derived growth factor, and fibroblast growth factor, among others. A few of these proteins have been synthesized using recombinant DNA technology and have the potential to revolutionize our approach to spinal surgery.

The most well known of these proteins are BMPs, which are osteoinductive glycoproteins extracted from bone matrix. BMPs induce mesenchymal cells to differentiate into bone cells.[11–13] Several BMP subtypes have been defined: osteoinductive factor, osteogenic protein, osteogenin, and osteopontin. BMP has a molecular weight of 17,500 daltons.[11–13] It has a concentration of less than 1 mg/kg of bone and is most abundant in cortical bone.[11–13] BMP may be extracted from gelatinized bone matrix prepared from demineralized bone, or it may be prepared from recombinant DNA techniques. Clinically, it has tremendous potential for

Table 34.1 Proteins That Promote Bone Healing

Protein	Abbreviation
Bone morphogenic protein	BMP
Epidermal growth factor	EGF
Cartilage-derived growth factor	CDGF
Insulin-like growth factor	IGF
Platelet-derived growth factor	PDGF
Fibroblast growth factor	FGF
Transforming growth factor	TGF
Bone-derived growth factor	BDGF
Osteoinductive factor	OIF

Table 34.2 Factors That Enhance Bone Healing

Anabolic steroids
Calcitonin
Cancellous bone exposure of fusion bed
Electrical stimulation
Estrogen
Growth hormone
Insulin
Large bone surface area of fusion bed
Local growth factors
Mechanical loading
Mechanical stability
Parathyroid hormone
Somatomedins
Testosterone
Thyroxine
Vitamins A and D

stimulating bone healing and for promoting spinal fusion (see Bone Morphogenic Protein section).

Several other proteins influence bone healing in different ways. TGF-β regulates angiogenesis, bone formation, and extracellular matrix syntheses and primarily controls cell-mediated activities. Osteonectin, fibronectin, osteoponectin, and osteocalcin function as osteoconductive elements to promote cell attachment, to encourage cell migration, and to activate cells.[2,7,14]

Bone Growth and Development

Bones are formed by intramembranous or endochondral ossification.[1,2] Intramembranous ossification occurs de novo from mesenchymal cells. Mesenchymal cells form a sheet of tissue with an abundant vascular supply and subsequently differentiate into osteoblasts. These cells then deposit collagen and osteoid, which ossifies. The collagen is arranged randomly and initially forms woven or primitive bone. The woven bone is remodeled into flat plates with an outer and inner cortical shell and intervening cancellous bone. Membranous bone forms directly without an intermediate process. Membranous bone is found in the skull, face, mandible, and clavicle.

Endochondral ossification occurs through an intermediary step in which cartilage is transformed to bone. Primitive hyaline cartilage forms from mesenchymal tissue. The cartilage is invaded by blood vessels and bone-forming cells. The cartilage becomes calcified and is reabsorbed by osteoclasts. Simultaneously, osteoblasts deposit new bone. The intermediary cartilaginous phase distinguishes endochondral from intramembranous bone formation. The skull base and the bones of the axial skeleton are formed by this process.

Throughout life there is a continuous, highly regulated process of bone reabsorption by osteoclasts and bone deposition by osteoblasts. All bone formed by remodeling is called secondary bone. In contrast, bone formed by endochondral ossification or by direct subperiosteal deposition is called primary bone.[1,2]

Biomechanics of Bone Grafts

Bone is a living tissue with hard and rigid characteristics that reflect the orderly deposition of minerals.[2,4,14,15] Bone resists force better in compression than in tension.[4] The composite arrangement of bone forms a material that is very strong for its weight and is much stronger than either the organic or inorganic components would be alone.[2,3] The orientation of the collagen fibers in the matrix, which affects the material properties, is analogous to the way that the grains of lumber determine the strongest orientation of wood.[2] The strength-to-weight ratio of bone is very high compared with other structural materials, such as aluminum and cast iron, and it is half as strong as steel.[2,3]

Cortical bone grafts are used primarily in areas that are subjected to compressive or shear stress.[3] Cortical bone is compact, provides immediate structural support, and resists tensile and compressive forces.[3] Cortical bone grafts have to be fixated properly to produce a satisfactory mechanical result. In comparison, cancellous bone is much weaker than cortical bone under compressive or tensile loads.[3,4] Because cancellous bone grafts are relatively weak, they should be used with rigid fixation in areas subjected to large mechanical stresses. Cancellous bone has several advantages: it is more cellular and porous, becomes rapidly vascularized, and promotes fusion better than cortical bone. Therefore, the ideal reconstruction graft contains a mixture of cortical and cancellous bone (i.e., corticocancellous iliac crest struts), which combines optimum mechanical strength and bone-healing properties.

Allograft bone can be weakened during sterilization, procurement, processing, or preparation.[7,15–17] Although freezing does not alter bone strength, freeze-drying significantly reduces the three-point bending, torsional stiffness, and compressive strength of allografts.[17,18] Irradiation of bone grafts can reduce their bending, compression, and torsional strength and reduce their osteoinductive properties.[7,17] High-dose irradiation and freeze-drying should be avoided whenever possible to preserve the biomechanical integrity of the graft. Freeze-dried allografts need to be reconstituted in saline for 30 minutes before shaping.

Mechanical and Structural Bone Adaptation

Bone remodeling and healing are dynamic phenomena that are strongly influenced by the local biomechanical environment. Functional adaptation of bone tissue is a widely recognized property. The geometry, thickness, trabecular orientation, and density of bone can change depending on the mechanical demands placed on it. Bone placed under compressive or tensile stress is remodeled. Bone is formed where stresses require its presence, and bone is absorbed where stresses do not require it. Bone can become hypertrophic or atrophic.

In 1892, J. Wolff[19] developed his ideas regarding the structural adaptation of bone. It is worthwhile to understand the English translation of Wolff's ideas: "Every change in the form and function of bones, or of their function alone, is followed by certain definite changes in their internal architecture and equally definite secondary alteration in their external conformation, in accordance with mathematical laws."[19] The modern version of Wolff's law is the following: "Loaded areas of bone have increased deposition of bone in an effort to increase the structural strength."[2]

Stress shielding is another important concept of functional adaptation that applies to spinal fixation.[10,20] Rigid fixation can shield the bones from physiological stresses and can cause osteopenia or osteoporosis. However, in clinical and experimental studies, rigid instrumentation significantly improves the fusion rates in spinal surgery.[20] The beneficial effects of rigid spinal instrumentation on fusion clearly outweigh the potential disadvantages of instrument-related osteoporosis. The "ideally rigid" spinal instrument system has not yet been developed. Theoretically, this device would provide temporary rigid fixation until a satisfactory fusion developed and would then eventually dissolve or loosen to allow the healed bone to be subjected to normal mechanical stresses.

■ Physiology of Bone Repair

A bone graft can possess several properties that can enhance healing: osteogenic, osteoconductive, and osteoinductive properties (**Table 34.3**).[6–8,15,21] Osteogenesis, the ability of the graft to make bone, requires live bone cells within the graft. Autogenous cortical bone and bone marrow are osteogenic.[6]

Table 34.3 Comparison of Graft Materials

Graft Material	Osteogenic	Osteoinductive	Osteoconductive
Cancellous autograft	+	+	+ +
Cortical autograft	+	+ +	+
Cancellous allograft	0	+	+ +
Cortical allograft	0	+ +	+
Demineralized bone matrix	0	+ +	+ +
Ceramics	0	0	+
Bone morphogenic protein	0	+ + +	0
Collagen	0	0	+

Abbreviations: + +, strong effect; +, weak effect; 0, no effect.
Source: Modified from Muschler GF, Lane JM, Dawson EG. The biology of spinal fusion. In: Cotler JM, Cotler HP, eds. Spinal Fusion Science and Technique. Berlin: Springer-Verlag; 1990:9–21.With permission from Springer-Verlag.

Osteoconduction is the ability of the graft to act as a scaffolding to facilitate bone healing over the entire volume of the graft. Osteoconductive materials include collagen, bone, demineralized bone matrix, hydroxyapatite, and calcium phosphate.[6] Osteoconductive activity is secondary to structural properties that influence cell attachment, cell migration, cell differentiation, and vascular ingrowth.[6] Osteoinduction refers to the ability to induce stem cells to differentiate into mature bone cells. BMP is the principal osteoinductive agent.[6]

Stages of Fracture Healing

Bone healing responses are strikingly similar in fractured bone and in bone grafts. Fracture healing restores the tissue to its original physical and mechanical properties and is influenced by local and systemic factors (**Tables 34.1, 34.2,** and **34.4**). The healing occurs in three distinct histological stages: inflammation, repair, and remodeling.[1,2,6,8,10,19,21]

A hematoma initially forms and an inflammatory response occurs at the fracture site during the first hours and weeks. Inflammatory cells (macrophages, monocytes, lymphocytes, and polymorphonuclear cells) and fibroblasts infiltrate the bone under the direction of chemical messengers. The initial inflammatory stage of bone healing is characterized by formation of granulation tissue, ingrowth of vascular tissue,

Table 34.4 Factors That Inhibit Bone Healing

Anemia
Antineoplastic drugs
Bone devascularization
Bone healing
Bone necrosis
Bone wax
Castration
Corticosteroids
Deficiency of vitamin D, calcium, or iron
Diabetes
Excessive mechanical motion
Fibrous dysplasia
Infection
Intoxication by vitamin A or D
Irradiation
Local marrow pathology (thalassemia, sickle cell disease)
Malnutrition
Nonsteroidal anti-inflammatory drugs
Obesity
Osteoporosis
Paget disease
Primary or metastatic tumors
Rheumatoid arthritis
Scar tissue
Syndrome of inappropriate secretion of antidiuretic hormone (SIADH)
Smoking

and migration of mesenchymal cells. If anti-inflammatory drugs or cytotoxic drugs are given during the first week of healing, they may modify the inflammatory response and inhibit bone healing.

A callus subsequently forms to bridge the bone defect and extends across the periosteal and endosteal surfaces, restoring the continuity of the bone. The proliferation of callus tissue is a critical step in spontaneous fracture repair. During the first 4 to 6 weeks of bone healing, callus tissue is very weak and requires adequate protection to avoid refracture and reinjury. The callus subsequently ossifies to form a bridge of woven bone between bone fragments. During this phase, adequate bone healing requires immobilization. Persistent fibrous tissue or fibrous transformation of callus tissue (fibrous union) may occur if the fixation is inadequate or the gaps between the fracture fragments are large.

Fracture healing is completed by remodeling of the bone to the original shape, structure, and mechanical strength. Remodeling occurs slowly and is facilitated by mechanical stress placed on the bone. Adequate strength of a spinal fusion is achieved only after 3 to 6 months of osseous healing. Maximum strength may develop months to years later, after the bone is remodeled and subjected to physiological stresses.

Primary (contact) fracture healing occurs by direct remodeling of areas of bone that are in apposition. Primary healing allows direct revascularization of the fracture fragments and reconstitution of the cortical bone structure; however, it also requires an exact reduction of the fractures, restoration of alignment, stable fixation, and a sufficient blood supply. Primary bone healing occurs at compressed surfaces and only with rigid internal fixation.[10]

Secondary (spontaneous) fracture healing occurs with formation of periosteal and endosteal callus. The callus forms an envelope that encases and bridges the fracture fragments to immobilize the injured site. The callus becomes ossified and is subsequently replaced by new bone.

The healing of a spinal fusion is more complicated than the healing of a long-bone fracture.[10] The grafts are usually nonvascularized and are replaced with a continuous bone mass.[10] Only superficial cells in the bone graft survive by diffusion of nutrients; the remaining graft cells die.[22] Bone grafts are incorporated by an integrated process in which old necrotic bone is reabsorbed and simultaneously replaced with new viable bone. This process of incorporation is called creeping substitution.[7,10]

The processes of inflammation and revascularization are critical to bone graft healing.[22,23] Incorporation and remodeling require that mesenchymal cells from the host bed have vascular access to the graft and differentiate into osteoclasts and osteoblasts.

Factors that can inhibit bone healing include malnutrition, obesity, cigarette smoking, diabetes, rheumatoid arthritis, medications, and variety of other factors (**Table 34.4**). The most critical period in determining the ultimate success or failure of a fusion attempt is during the first 3 to 7 days of healing. Exposure to steroids, cytotoxic drugs (e.g., methotrexate, doxorubicin), nicotine, nonsteroidal anti-inflammatory agents, and radiation is particularly harmful during the first postoperative week.

Radiation has acute and chronic effects that inhibit bone healing. If bone is irradiated within the first 2 weeks of surgery, the effect is pronounced—radiation inhibits cell proliferation and induces an acute vasculitis.[24] Delayed effects include osteonecrosis and scar tissue formation that create poor substrates for fusion.[24]

■ Bone Grafts

There are several different types of bone grafts, including autografts, allografts, syngrafts, and xenografts.[7] Autografts are transplanted from one part of the body to another part of the same individual. Allografts are transplanted from genetically nonidentical members of a species. Syngrafts are transfers of tissue between identical members of a species (as between twins), and xenografts are transplants between species.

Autogenous Bone Grafts

Autogenous cancellous bone has osteogenic, osteoconductive, and osteoinductive properties and is currently the most successful bone grafting material.[2,7,10,21] Cortical bone grafts are less ideal than cancellous grafts. Cortical bone has fewer osteoblasts and osteocytes, has less surface area per unit weight, and provides a barrier to vascular ingrowth and bony remodeling.[2,7,10,21] The only advantage of cortical bone is its mechanical strength.[2,4]

The healing of cortical and cancellous bone grafts differs in several ways, primarily in the rate of revascularization and the capacity for osteoinduction.[7–9,25,26] Cortical bone grafts are slowly revascularized and minimally osteoinductive.[25]

Cortical and cancellous autografts have different mechanical characteristics during remodeling.[17] Initially, the predominant response in cortical bone is osteoclastic (resorptive), whereas in cancellous bone it is osteoblastic. Cancellous bone becomes progressively strengthened because of early, rapid new bone formation.[7,8] In comparison, cortical autografts can become progressively weaker because of bone resorption and slow, incomplete remodeling.[7–9]

Autografts have several advantages: the graft is sterile, nonreactive, live, and genetically identical to the host.[7] Disadvantages include potential morbidity of the donor site and the potential for quality or quantity of the graft to be insufficient.[7]

Vascularized Bone Grafts

Vascularized bone autografts from the fibula, rib, or iliac crest have been used for spinal fusion. A vascular pedicle is transposed locally or is anastomosed using microsurgical techniques. Vascularized bone grafts have superior healing capabilities and mechanical properties compared with nonvascularized grafts.

An intact blood supply to the bone allows rapid incorporation and maintenance of structural integrity of the bone. Vascularized bone grafts perform better mechanically than nonvascularized grafts. Vascularized bone grafts can hypertrophy when subjected to mechanical stress.[14] In comparison, nonvascularized grafts can demonstrate early resorption and weakening.[4,14] Vascularized bone grafts may be particularly helpful when the recipient bed is devascularized, irradiated, or scarred.[4,24]

Disadvantages of vascularized bone grafts include difficulty with maintaining patency of the anastomosis, difficulty finding suitable donor sites, limited graft volume, and prolonged operating time.

Allograft Bone

Identical stages of bone healing (inflammation, repair, and remodeling) occur in allograft and autograft, but the rates differ. Vascular ingrowth is slower and less extensive in allografts; therefore new bone formation is subsequently delayed.[7,10,11]

Allografts avoid the complications of the donor site and are readily available in the desired configuration and quantity. Disadvantages of allograft include delayed vascular penetration, slow formation of bone, prominent resorption of bone, encapsulation of fibrous tissue, delayed or incomplete incorporation, and possible infection or graft rejection.[6,7,14,16,27–31] Allografts elicit an immunological reaction similar to other transplanted tissue.[9,28,30,31] Proteins are identified as nonself in the graft, evoking an immunological response.[27–29]

Allografts have been used extensively for spinal surgery. Allograft struts can be useful if a multilevel cervical corpectomy has been performed or if a very long bone graft is needed. Typically, allograft bone is reserved for fusions when the patient's bone stock is inadequate or diseased. When allograft fibula struts are used for reconstruction of the vertebral body, the bone healing process can be augmented by filling the hollow center of the fibula strut graft with autogenous cancellous bone.

Clinical and experimental reports using allograft for spinal fusions have had mixed results.[16,18,32–42] Some reports find allograft significantly inferior to autograft; other reports find little or no difference between them. However, when histological fusion is examined, autogenous bone appears to be superior. Allograft bone has a higher incidence of nonunion or delayed union.[8,9,14,18,27,34,39,40,42,43]

Several clinical reports compare allograft and autograft for anterior cervical fusions. Allograft and autograft have similar fusion rates for single-level anterior cervical fusions.[33,35,36,38] Allografts tend to have more delayed unions and instances of graft collapse.[18] However, autograft is clearly superior for multiple level anterior cervical fusions.[18,32,34,41] Allografts for multilevel cervical fusions can have a 60 to 70% pseudarthrosis rate.[18,34] For posterior cervical spinal fusions, autograft produces a higher fusion rate compared with allograft.[26,27,35,40,44]

Allograft Banking

Bone banks procure allografts and should be certified by the American Association of Tissue Banks. There are established standards for tissue harvesting and processing of the graft.[7,10] Bone grafts are harvested in a sterile fashion, processed, and freeze-dried or stored fresh-frozen. Allograft bone is prepared to reduce the immunogenicity, to provide sterility, and to preserve mechanical integrity.[7,28,29,31,45] Serological testing, autopsy evaluation, and careful donor screening are performed to minimize the risk of contamination by the human immunodeficiency virus (HIV).[46,47] The risk of transplanting HIV-infected bone has been estimated at less than 1 in 1 million when stringent screening criteria are used.[46] The risk can escalate to 1 in 161 if only HIV antibodies are screened. HIV has been cultured from bone after freezing and freeze-drying; these methods offer no protection from infection.[35,46,47]

Immunogenicity of bone is reduced by ethylene oxide, freezing to $-20°C$, or freeze-drying.[7,10,16,48,49] Freeze-drying reduces the immunogenicity but significantly decreases the mechanical strength of the graft.[17,50] Heating, autoclaving, or irradiating bone disrupts the matrix proteins in bone and should be avoided.[7,35] Ethylene oxide reduces immunogenicity, provides sterilization, preserves osteoinductive character, and preserves the mechanical integrity of bone grafts. It can be combined with freeze-drying for ease of storage.[7,16,17,35,49]

Demineralized Bone Matrix

Demineralized bone is a type of allograft bone prepared to reduce antigenicity and to uncover BMP and other bioactive proteins in the bone matrix to augment healing.[6,7,11–13] Demineralized bone is osteoinductive and osteoconductive. Although demineralized bone can act as a stimulant to grafts, it has no mechanical function. No clinical trials have yet demonstrated the efficacy of demineralized bone for spinal fusions.

Ceramic

Ceramics are osteoconductive, but they are not osteogenic or osteoinductive.[14,44] Osteoblasts form bone directly on the ceramic surface. Tricalcium phosphates, hydroxyapatite, and other materials have been used; however, the efficacy of ceramics as a graft material has not been established clinically. Ceramics are biocompatible, but they are brittle and much weaker than bone. Improvements in ceramic strength, porosity, reabsorbability, and the addition of osteoinductive factors (i.e., BMP) may eventually make these materials clinically useful.[44,46,51,52]

Bone Morphogenic Protein

The characteristics and biological activity of BMPs are discussed previously. Currently, there are two clinically available recombinant human BMP (rhBMP) preparations that are approved by the U.S. Food and Drug Administration (FDA) for spinal fusion purposes. Infuse (Medtronic, Minneapolis, MN), which is a preparation of rhBMP-2 on a collagen sponge carrier, is approved only for anterior lumbar interbody fusion in conjunction with a specific threaded interbody cage device (LT cages) in the lower lumbar spine. A preparation of rhBMP-7 known as OP-1 putty (Stryker Biotech, Hopkinton, MA) has been approved under a humanitarian device exemption for posterolateral lumbar spinal fusion. Despite the limited regulatory approval, use of rhBMP in spinal fusion surgery has exploded over the last decade. Just within a 6-month period at the end of 2009, Medtronic reported $439 million in biologics sales, the majority of which comes from sales of Infuse. Their total spine revenue in the same 6-month period was $1.777 billion, making biologics 25% of their total spine sales.[53]

Biologics is commonly used for fusion via anterior and posterior approaches in all regions of the spine, either as a stand-alone graft substitute or combined with various amounts of autograft, allograft, and/or other synthetic bone graft extenders, such as ceramics or hydroxyapatite-based materials. Clinical results have been impressive, although not quite as universally successful as early animal studies suggested it would be. As an example, a 2002 study reported 6-month fusion rates in a sheep anterior lumbar interbody fusion model comparing rhBMP-2 with autologous iliac crest bone.[54] They found a 100% fusion rate with the BMP versus 37% for autograft. Other animal studies were performed in goats, rabbits, dogs, and various primates, leading to the first human trial with rhBMP-2. This small pilot study was performed in 1996 and reported in 2000.[55] Only 14 patients were studied, with 11 of 11 BMP patients judged fused and 2 of 3 autograft patients judged fused. Clinical outcomes based on ODI were judged superior in the BMP group. This led to a larger pivotal trial, also a randomized controlled multicenter trial, but this time enrolling 280 patients, all undergoing anterior lumbar interbody fusion with threaded titanium cages.[56] They found a 100% versus 96% fusion rate for BMP versus autograft, with a slightly higher overall clinical success rate in the BMP group. They also reported a greater than 30% rate of donor site pain in the autograft group at 2-year follow-up. This trial was reported in 2002 and led to the FDA approval of BMP for this application. A similar study with similar results but using either BMP or autograft packed in the center of an allograft ring was reported the same year.[57] This BMP preparation has also been studied in lumbar posterolateral fusions with good results compared with autograft.[58] Lessons learned from animal studies led to recognition that the dose and carrier needed to be modified for posterolateral lumbar fusions. Using this paradigm has led to good results. A recent study randomized patients to iliac crest autograft versus rhBMP-2 combined with a ceramic-granule bulking agent for single-level instrumented posterior lumbar arthrodesis.[59] Fusion rate at 24 months was 95% for BMP and 70% for autograft, with overall clinical success rates of 81% versus 55%.

The earliest human trial for rhBMP-2 in the cervical spine was published in 2003 and demonstrated high fusion rate in a small patient population.[60] By March 2006, however, concerns developed over soft tissue complications related to this usage, leading to extensive edema, hematoma, and/or seroma with high doses of BMP.[61] Several other studies confirmed this subsequently. Due to the severity of the reaction in some patients, on July 1, 2008, the FDA issued a warning letter against the use of BMP products in anterior cervical fusion surgery. Nevertheless, many authors have continued to explore the use of this product, and several reports over the last few years suggest that these complications are directly linked to use of relatively high doses of BMP. Most of the early complication reports were in patients given doses of BMP similar to what is used in the lumbar spine. Many surgeons continue to use BMP in anterior cervical fusions but in much lower doses and have reported acceptably low complication rates and excellent fusion rates in abstracts at recent meetings. Similar concerns with soft tissue swelling leading to a higher rate of wound complications have also been raised in the posterior cervical spine.[62]

Many authors have pointed out concerns about the widespread use of these products, with much of the attention focused on Infuse. First, it is an extremely expensive product. A standard small kit of Infuse, which might often be used for a single-level lumbar interbody fusion, costs several thousand dollars, depending on the local market. Most other graft materials would cost less than half as much. Second, its potency is indiscriminate and, therefore, careful handling and surgical technique is necessary. Spread of BMP at the time of surgery can lead to bone formation, where such is undesirable. Extension of BMP-mediated bone growth through annular defects has led to ossification in the neuroforamen or spinal canal after transforaminal lumbar interbody fusion (TLIF)[63] or posterior lumbar interbody fusion procedures and has caused vascular impingement after anterior lumbar interbody fusion procedures through the same mechanism. This is particularly likely if portions of the BMP material are placed outside the interbody cage. Third, it is now believed that if an excessive dose of BMP is applied, there is a risk of osteolysis[64] with fairly extensive endplate erosion leading to graft collapse, hardware failure, and eventual pseudoarthrosis. Fourth, as discussed previously, some patients appear susceptible to an intense inflammatory reaction to the BMP that can cause massive local tissue edema. Shortly after BMPs were adopted for use in anterior cervical discectomy and fusion procedures, reports surfaced regarding patients developing severe prevertebral edema, dysphagia, and airway compromise. Many of these early patients were taken emergently back to surgery for exploration for presumed hematoma, but intraoperative findings revealed only extensive edema in some and seromas in others. Lateral radiographs often revealed massive soft tissue thickening and tracheal displacement. It is now recognized that this condition responds well to treatment with corticosteroids, if the clinical presentation is appropriate.

Stem Cells and Bone Marrow

As awareness of the importance of osteogenesis grew in the latter 20th century, the contribution of mesenchymal stem cells, osteoblastic precursor cells, and other constituents of bone marrow toward the fusion process became more evident. Interest in the use of autologous bone marrow—with allograft, synthetic graft materials, and/or BMP—dates back several decades. One of the first studies used allogenic demineralized bone matrix and autologous bone marrow to attain posterior fusion in rabbits and was published in 1987.[65] Over the next 20 years, a majority of studies used rabbit (or occasionally other animal) models to evaluate various marrow aspirate-enhanced graft constructs, but human studies continued to be largely absent. In 2005, McLain and colleagues determined that aspirate from lumbar vertebral bodies contained as many or more osteogenic precursor cells as iliac crest marrow aspirate.[66] In 2006, a British group reported type I collagen/hydroxyapatite combined with iliac crest bone marrow aspirate to be equivalent to autograft for posterior lumbar fusion in a case-controlled series of 50 patients but found the same graft material to be ineffective for interbody fusions in this group.[67] However, a later study examining the same graft construct used for instrumented TLIF with posterolateral fusion found high fusion rates.[68]

In the first several years of the 21st century, many different preclinical and animal studies were reported using various methods of either selective retention of nucleated cells from whole bone marrow aspirate (BMA)[69] or ex vivo culture of autologous stem cells for eventual spinal fusion purposes.[70] More recent studies include a 2009 publication of 30 human patients with thoracolumbar spinal trauma, who were treated with posterolateral fusion and pedicle screw fixation. Fusion material consisted of autograft on one side and hydroxyapatite/β-tricalcium phosphate with bone marrow aspirate on the other side. All levels fused by 1 year, except one side treated with autologous bone graft in one patient.[71] Another study randomized patients undergoing single-level lumbar laminectomy and posterior fusion with pedicle screw fixation. Both groups had autologous iliac crest bone marrow on one side (control side). On the contralateral side, patients were randomized to local laminectomy bone plus BMA versus calcium sulfate pellets plus BMA. In the local bone plus BMA group, fusion rate was equivalent to autograft; in the calcium sulfate plus BMA group, the fusion rate was poor.[72] As of this writing, there is still significant debate as to the merits of bone marrow preparations in spinal fusions, with ongoing questions regarding the ideal matrix or substrate as well as techniques (e.g., addition of platelet-rich plasma) for improving the osteogenic potential of any marrow graft.

Gene Therapy

A very new approach to spinal fusion involves the use of gene therapy techniques. This research is in preliminary stages as of this writing, with no human trials currently reported. The first report of this technique was published in 1998 and described application of an adenoviral vector containing a human BMP-2 gene to bone marrow-derived mesenchymal stem cells in culture. The transfected cells were then implanted between the lumbar transverse processes of five donor rabbits. One rabbit developed bone formation.[73] Other reports of animal models with successful fusion followed, using various viral vectors to transfect genes for several different osteoinductive proteins.[74–77] Further topics of investigation have included means of modifying the immune response to the virus vectors.[78] This is a highly complex biological system, and much research remains to be done in to clarify the ideal transfection method (e.g., adenovirus versus lentivirus versus nonviral strategy), the ideal gene product, and the ideal scaffold or carrier matrix. Defining these solutions and transferring the information obtained from animal studies to humans will be a great challenge. To date, no studies have been published in higher order animals (rabbits and athymic nude rats have been the usual subjects). In addition, potential long-term consequences of gene therapy are poorly understood, and public fears about "genetic manipulation" will need to be overcome for this strategy to be brought into the mainstream.

Methylmethacrylate

Methylmethacrylate is not osteoconductive, osteoinductive, or osteogenic. Methylmethacrylate should be avoided whenever possible because it does not promote bone healing.[79] It acts as a spacer that resists compression but readily fails under tension, so it must be anchored to bone (with wires, screws, or Steinmann pins) because it can loosen. Methylmethacrylate becomes encapsulated and elicits a foreign body response. Gentamicin, tobramycin, or clindamycin powder can be mixed into the methylmethacrylate during preparation to reduce the risk of infection. Because methylmethacrylate does not generate an adequate bone fusion response, it should be reserved for patients with tumors and life expectancies of less than 6 months.

Electromagnetic Stimulation

Pulsed electromagnetic fields promote bone healing without evidence of hazardous side effects. Electromagnetic fields trigger rapid angiogenesis, which improves bone union. Collars, belts, or implantable stimulators may be used to deliver the fields. Electrical stimulation has been used successfully to treat nonunions of long bone fractures, failed arthrodesis, and congenital pseudarthrosis.[80]

Few clinical or basic science studies have evaluated electromagnetic stimulation for spinal fusion. In animals, lumbar facet fusion and dorsal lumbar fusion may be enhanced with electrical stimulation.[81,82] In clinical trials in humans, Kane[83] found electromagnetic fields useful for improving the fusion rates in 59 patients with a previous lumbar pseudarthrosis. An 81% fusion rate occurred in stimulated patients compared with a 54% fusion rate in nonstimulated patients. In a blind randomized study, Mooney[37] evaluated electromagnetic stimulation in 195 patients with posterior lumbar interbody fusion. He found a significant difference in the fusion rates between stimulated and nonstimulated patients (92 versus 65%). Other investigators found no advantage to direct current or pulsed magnetic fields for spinal fusion.[80,84] The efficacy of electrical stimulation is not yet established for spinal fusion. No clinical data are available on the effects of electromagnetic stimulation on cervical fusion.

Conclusion

The fundamental physiology of bone healing was reviewed to optimize the probability of attaining spinal fusion. A solid bone fusion is the foundation for permanent spinal stability because internal fixation devices can fatigue and break. The clinician can manipulate a variety of clinical, pharmacological, and surgical strategies to enhance bone healing. Newer developments such as the use of recombinant osteoinductive proteins, bone marrow, and gene therapy represent modern attempts to provide a suitable alternative grafting strategy to what is still the gold standard in spinal fusion: autologous bone graft.

References

1. Copenhaver WM, Kelly DE, Wood RL. The connective tissues: cartilage and bone. In: Copenhaver WM, Kelly DE, Wood RL, eds. Bailey's Textbook of Histology, 17th ed. Baltimore, MD: Williams & Wilkins; 1978:170–205
2. Recker RR. Embryology, anatomy, and microstructure of bone. In: Coe FL, Favus MJ, eds. Disorder of Bone and Mineral Metabolism. New York, NY: Raven Press; 1992:219–240
3. Hayes WC. Biomechanics of cortical and trabecular bone: implications for assessment of fracture risk. In: Mow VC, Hayes WC, eds. Basic Orthopaedic Biomechanics. New York, NY: Raven Press; 1991:93–142
4. White AA III, Panjabi MM. Clinical Biomechanics of the Spine. Philadelphia, PA: JB Lippincott; 1990
5. Chalmers J, Gray DH, Rush J. Observations on the induction of bone in soft tissues. J Bone Joint Surg Br 1975;57(1):36–45
6. Muschler GF, Lane JM, Dawson EG. The biology of spinal fusion. In: Cotler JM, Cotler HP, eds. Spinal Fusion Science and Technique. Berlin: Springer-Verlag; 1990:9–21
7. Prolo DJ. Biology of bone fusion. Clin Neurosurg 1990;36:135–146
8. Burchardt H. Biology of bone transplantation. Orthop Clin North Am 1987;18(2):187–196
9. Burchardt H, Enneking WF. Transplantation of bone. Surg Clin North Am 1978;58(2):403–427
10. Kaufman HH, Jones E. The principles of bony spinal fusion. Neurosurgery 1989;24(2):264–270
11. Urist MR. Bone transplants and implants. In: Urist MR, ed. Fundamentals and Clinical Bone Physiology. Philadelphia, PA: JB Lippincott; 1980:331–368
12. Urist MR, Dawson E. Intertransverse process fusion with the aid of chemosterilized autolyzed antigen-extracted allogeneic (AAA) bone. Clin Orthop Relat Res 1981;154(154):97–113
13. Urist MR, Mikulski A, Lietze A. Solubilized and insolubilized bone morphogenetic protein. Proc Natl Acad Sci U S A 1979;76(4):1828–1832
14. Habal MB. Different forms of bone grafts. In: Habal MB, Reddi AH, eds. Bone Grafts and Bone Substitutes. Philadelphia, PA: WB Saunders; 1992:6–8
15. Prolo DJ, Rodrigo JJ. Contemporary bone graft physiology and surgery. Clin Orthop Relat Res 1985;200(200):322–342
16. Herron LD, Newman MH. The failure of ethylene oxide gas-sterilized freeze-dried bone graft for thoracic and lumbar spinal fusion. Spine 1989;14(5):496–500
17. Pelker RR, Friedlaender GE. Biomechanical aspects of bone autografts and allografts. Orthop Clin North Am 1987;18(2):235–239
18. Zdeblick TA, Ducker TB. The use of freeze-dried allograft bone for anterior cervical fusions. Spine 1991;16(7):726–729
19. Wolff J. Das Gesetz der Transformation der Knochen. Berlin: Hirschwold; 1892
20. McAfee PC, Farey ID, Sutterlin CE, Gurr KR, Warden KE, Cunningham BW. 1989 Volvo Award in basic science. Device-related osteoporosis with spinal instrumentation. Spine 1989;14(9):919–926
21. Freidberg SR, Gumley GJ, Pfeifer BA, Hybels RL. Vascularized fibular graft to replace resected cervical vertebral bodies. Case report. J Neurosurg 1989;71(2):283–286
22. Deleu J, Trueta J. Vascularization of bone grafts in the anterior chamber of the eye. J Bone Joint Surg Br 1965;47:319–329
23. Kingma MJ, Hampe JF. The behavior of blood vessels after experimental transplantation of bone. J Bone Joint Surg Br 1964;46:141–150
24. Emery SE, Brazinski M, Bensusan J, et al. Effects of irradiation on the biologic and biomechanical properties of anterior spine fusion in a canine model. Washington, DC: Orthopaedic Research Society 38th Annual Meeting; 1992. Abstract
25. Enneking WF, Eady JL, Burchardt H. Autogenous cortical bone grafts in the reconstruction of segmental skeletal defects. J Bone Joint Surg Am 1980;62(7):1039–1058
26. Knapp DR Jr, Jones ET. Use of cortical cancellous allograft for posterior spinal fusion. Clin Orthop Relat Res 1988;229(229):99–106
27. Aurori BF, Weierman RJ, Lowell HA, Nadel CI, Parsons JR. Pseudarthrosis after spinal fusion for scoliosis. A comparison of autogeneic and allogeneic bone grafts. Clin Orthop Relat Res 1985;199(199):153–158
28. Bos GD, Goldberg VM, Powell AE, Heiple KG, Zika JM. The effect of histocompatibility matching on canine frozen bone allografts. J Bone Joint Surg Am 1983;65(1):89–96
29. Brooks DB, Heiple KG, Herndon CH, Powell AE. Immunological factors in homogenous bone transplantation. IV. The effect of various methods of preparation and irradiation on antigenicity. J Bone Joint Surg Am 1963;45:1617–1626

30. Burchardt H, Glowczewskie FP, Enneking WF. Short-term immunosuppression with fresh segmental fibular allografts in dogs. J Bone Joint Surg Am 1981;63(3):411–415
31. Friedlaender GE, Strong DM, Sell KW. Studies on the antigenicity of bone. II. Donor-specific anti-HLA antibodies in human recipients of freeze-dried allografts. J Bone Joint Surg Am 1984;66(1):107–112
32. Brown MD, Malinin TI, Davis PB. A roentgenographic evaluation of frozen allografts versus autografts in anterior cervical spine fusions. Clin Orthop Relat Res 1976;119(119):231–236
33. Cloward RB. Gas-sterilized cadaver bone grafts for spinal fusion operations. A simplified bone bank. Spine 1980;5(1):4–10
34. Fernyhough JC, White JI, LaRocca H. Fusion rates in multilevel cervical spondylosis comparing allograft fibula with autograft fibula in 126 patients. Spine 1991;16(10, Suppl):S561–S564
35. Hollowell JP. Surgery of the Cervical Spine. Park Ridge, IL: American Association of Neurological Surgeons Instructional Course Manual; 1992
36. Malinin TI, Rosomoff HL, Sutton CH. Human cadaver femoral head homografts for anterior cervical spine fusions. Surg Neurol 1977;7(4):249–251
37. Mooney V. A randomized double-blind prospective study of the efficacy of pulsed electromagnetic fields for interbody lumbar fusions. Spine 1990;15(7):708–712
38. Rish BL, McFadden JT, Penix JO. Anterior cervical fusion using homologous bone grafts: a comparative study. Surg Neurol 1976; 5(2):119–121
39. Sachs B, Brennan W. Comparison of freeze-dried allograft versus autograft in anterior cervical spine fusions. Palm Desert, CA: Cervical Spine Research Society; 1992:140–141. Abstract
40. Stabler CL, Eismont FJ, Brown MD, Green BA, Malinin TI. Failure of posterior cervical fusions using cadaveric bone graft in children. J Bone Joint Surg Am 1985;67(3):371–375
41. Sypert GW. Thoracolumbar fusion techniques. Clin Neurosurg 1990;36:186–216
42. Zdeblick TA, Cooke ME, Kunz DN, Wilson D. Anterior cervical discectomy, fusion, and plating. A comparative animal study. Palm Desert, CA: Cervical Spine Research Society; 1992:106–107. Abstract
43. Bucholz RW, Carlton A, Holmes RE. Hydroxyapatite and tricalcium phosphate bone graft substitutes. Orthop Clin North Am 1987; 18(2):323–334
44. Nasca RJ, Lemons JE, Deinlein DA. Synthetic biomaterials for spinal fusion. Orthopedics 1989;12(4):543–548
45. Goldberg VM, Bos GD, Heiple KG, Zika JM, Powell AE. Improved acceptance of frozen bone allografts in genetically mismatched dogs by immunosuppression. J Bone Joint Surg Am 1984;66(6): 937–950
46. Buck BE, Malinin TI, Brown MD. Bone transplantation and human immunodeficiency virus. An estimate of risk of acquired immunodeficiency syndrome (AIDS). Clin Orthop Relat Res 1989;240(240): 129–136
47. Buck BE, Resnick L, Shah SM, Malinin TI. Human immunodeficiency virus cultured from bone. Implications for transplantation. Clin Orthop Relat Res 1990;251(251):249–253
48. Friedlaender GE, Strong DM, Sell KW. Studies on the antigenicity of bone. I. Freeze-dried and deep-frozen bone allografts in rabbits. J Bone Joint Surg Am 1976;58(6):854–858
49. Prolo DJ, Pedrotti PW, White DH. Ethylene oxide sterilization of bone, dura mater, and fascia lata for human transplantation. Neurosurgery 1980;6(5):529–539
50. Wittenberg RH, Moeller J, Shea M, White AA III, Hayes WC. Compressive strength of autologous and allogenous bone grafts for thoracolumbar and cervical spine fusion. Spine 1990;15(10): 1073–1078
51. Holmes R, Mooney V, Bucholz R, Tencer A. A coralline hydroxyapatite bone graft substitute. Preliminary report. Clin Orthop Relat Res 1984;188(188):252–262
52. Ohgushi H, Goldberg VM, Caplan AI. Heterotopic osteogenesis in porous ceramics induced by marrow cells. J Orthop Res 1989; 7(4):568–578
53. United States Securities and Exchange Commission form 10-q quarterly report under section 13 or 15(d) of the Securities Exchange Act of 1934. For the quarterly period ended October 30, 2009. Commission File Number 1-7707. Available at: http://www.faqs.org/sec-filings/091209/MEDTRONIC-INC_10-Q/#A003#ixzz0keBBuXYo. Accessed April 13, 2010
54. Sandhu HS, Toth JM, Diwan AD, et al. Histologic evaluation of the efficacy of rhBMP-2 compared with autograft bone in sheep spinal anterior interbody fusion. Spine 2002;27(6):567–575
55. Boden SD, Zdeblick TA, Sandhu HS, Heim SE. The use of rhBMP-2 in interbody fusion cages. Definitive evidence of osteoinduction in humans: a preliminary report. Spine 2000;25(3):376–381
56. Burkus JK, Gornet MF, Dickman CA, Zdeblick TA. Anterior lumbar interbody fusion using rhBMP-2 with tapered interbody cages. J Spinal Disord Tech 2002;15(5):337–349
57. Burkus JK, Transfeldt EE, Kitchel SH, Watkins RG, Balderston RA. Clinical and radiographic outcomes of anterior lumbar interbody fusion using recombinant human bone morphogenetic protein-2. Spine 2002;27(21):2396–2408
58. Boden SD, Kang J, Sandhu H, Heller JG. Use of recombinant human bone morphogenetic protein-2 to achieve posterolateral lumbar spine fusion in humans: a prospective, randomized clinical pilot trial: 2002 Volvo Award in clinical studies. Spine 2002;27(23): 2662–2673
59. Dawson E, Bae HW, Burkus JK, Stambough JL, Glassman SD. Recombinant human bone morphogenetic protein-2 on an absorbable collagen sponge with an osteoconductive bulking agent in posterolateral arthrodesis with instrumentation. A prospective randomized trial. J Bone Joint Surg Am 2009;91(7):1604–1613
60. Baskin DS, Ryan P, Sonntag V, Westmark R, Widmayer MA. A prospective, randomized, controlled cervical fusion study using recombinant human bone morphogenetic protein-2 with the CORNERSTONE-SR allograft ring and the ATLANTIS anterior cervical plate. Spine 2003;28(12):1219–1224, discussion 1225
61. Shields LB, Raque GH, Glassman SD, et al. Adverse effects associated with high-dose recombinant human bone morphogenetic protein-2 use in anterior cervical spine fusion. Spine 2006;31(5):542–547
62. Crawford CH III, Carreon LY, McGinnis MD, Campbell MJ, Glassman SD. Perioperative complications of recombinant human bone morphogenetic protein-2 on an absorbable collagen sponge versus iliac crest bone graft for posterior cervical arthrodesis. Spine 2009;34(13):1390–1394
63. Chen NF, Smith ZA, Stiner E, Armin S, Sheikh H, Khoo LT. Symptomatic ectopic bone formation after off-label use of recombinant human bone morphogenetic protein-2 in transforaminal lumbar interbody fusion. J Neurosurg Spine 2010;12(1):40–46
64. Rihn JA, Patel R, Makda J, et al. Complications associated with single-level transforaminal lumbar interbody fusion. Spine J 2009; 9(8):623–629
65. Ragni P, Lindholm TS, Lindholm TC. Vertebral fusion dynamics in the thoracic and lumbar spine induced by allogenic demineralized bone matrix combined with autogenous bone marrow. An experimental study in rabbits. Ital J Orthop Traumatol 1987;13(2): 241–251
66. McLain RF, Fleming JE, Boehm CA, Muschler GF. Aspiration of osteoprogenitor cells for augmenting spinal fusion: comparison of progenitor cell concentrations from the vertebral body and iliac crest. J Bone Joint Surg Am 2005;87(12):2655–2661

67. Neen D, Noyes D, Shaw M, Gwilym S, Fairlie N, Birch N. Healos and bone marrow aspirate used for lumbar spine fusion: a case controlled study comparing healos with autograft. Spine 2006; 31(18):E636–E640
68. Carter JD, Swearingen AB, Chaput CD, Rahm MD. Clinical and radiographic assessment of transforaminal lumbar interbody fusion using HEALOS collagen-hydroxyapatite sponge with autologous bone marrow aspirate. Spine J 2009;9(6):434–438
69. Gupta MC, Theerajunyaporn T, Maitra S, et al. Efficacy of mesenchymal stem cell enriched grafts in an ovine posterolateral lumbar spine model. Spine 2007;32(7):720–726, discussion 727
70. Jiang H, Secretan C, Gao T, et al. The development of osteoblasts from stem cells to supplement fusion of the spine during surgery for AIS. Stud Health Technol Inform 2006;123:467–472
71. Bansal S, Chauhan V, Sharma S, Maheshwari R, Juyal A, Raghuvanshi S. Evaluation of hydroxyapatite and beta-tricalcium phosphate mixed with bone marrow aspirate as a bone graft substitute for posterolateral spinal fusion. Indian J Orthop 2009;43(3):234–239
72. Niu CC, Tsai TT, Fu TS, Lai PL, Chen LH, Chen WJ. A comparison of posterolateral lumbar fusion comparing autograft, autogenous laminectomy bone with bone marrow aspirate, and calcium sulphate with bone marrow aspirate: a prospective randomized study. Spine 2009;34(25):2715–2719
73. Riew KD, Wright NM, Cheng S, Avioli LV, Lou J. Induction of bone formation using a recombinant adenoviral vector carrying the human BMP-2 gene in a rabbit spinal fusion model. Calcif Tissue Int 1998;63(4):357–360
74. Boden SD, Titus L, Hair G, et al. Lumbar spine fusion by local gene therapy with a cDNA encoding a novel osteoinductive protein (LMP-1). Spine 1998;23(23):2486–2492
75. Alden TD, Pittman DD, Beres EJ, et al. Percutaneous spinal fusion using bone morphogenetic protein-2 gene therapy. J Neurosurg 1999;90(1, Suppl):109–114
76. Helm GA, Alden TD, Beres EJ, et al. Use of bone morphogenetic protein-9 gene therapy to induce spinal arthrodesis in the rodent. J Neurosurg 2000;92(2, Suppl):191–196
77. Viggeswarapu M, Boden SD, Liu Y, et al. Adenoviral delivery of LIM mineralization protein-1 induces new-bone formation in vitro and in vivo. J Bone Joint Surg Am 2001;83-A(3):364–376
78. Kim HS, Viggeswarapu M, Boden SD, et al. Overcoming the immune response to permit ex vivo gene therapy for spine fusion with human type 5 adenoviral delivery of the LIM mineralization protein-1 cDNA. Spine 2003;28(3):219–226
79. McAfee PC, Bohlman HH, Ducker T, Eismont FJ. Failure of stabilization of the spine with methylmethacrylate. A retrospective analysis of twenty-four cases. J Bone Joint Surg Am 1986;68(8):1145–1157
80. Lindsey RW, Grobman J, Leggon RE, Panjabi M, Friedlaender GE. Effects of bone graft and electrical stimulation on the strength of healing bony defects in dogs. Clin Orthop Relat Res 1987;222(222):275–280
81. Kahanovitz N, Arnoczky SP. The efficacy of direct current electrical stimulation to enhance canine spinal fusions. Clin Orthop Relat Res 1990;251(251):295–299
82. Nerubay J, Marganit B, Bubis JJ, Tadmor A, Katznelson A. Stimulation of bone formation by electrical current on spinal fusion. Spine 1986;11(2):167–169
83. Kane WJ. Direct current electrical bone growth stimulation for spinal fusion. Spine 1988;13(3):363–365
84. Kahanovitz N, Arnoczky SP, Hulse D, Shires PK. The effect of postoperative electromagnetic pulsing on canine posterior spinal fusions. Spine 1984;9(3):273–279

35 Techniques of Bone Graft Harvesting and Spinal Fusion

Curtis A. Dickman

In the preparation of bone grafts and surfaces for spinal fusion, meticulous surgical techniques are the best way to ensure proper bone healing. Careful preparation of the fusion site combined with rigid internal fixation optimizes surgical success. Internal fixation immobilizes the bone until fusion occurs; however, long-term stability can be guaranteed only if a fusion is achieved. This chapter emphasizes the surgical techniques for spinal fusion, bone graft harvesting, and bone graft preparation.

Surgical Techniques of Harvesting Autologous Bone Grafts

Iliac Crest Bone Grafts

Autologous bone grafts for spinal fusion are usually obtained from the anterior or posterior iliac crest.

Anterior Iliac Crest

The most anterior osteotomy for anterior iliac crest bone grafts should be made at least 2 to 3 cm behind the anterior superior iliac spine to avoid an avulsion fracture of the bone remaining anterior to the harvest site (**Fig. 35.1**).[1,2] The skin and fascia are incised parallel to the cortex of the iliac crest directly over the graft harvest site. Careful subperiosteal dissection should be performed to avoid injury to the ilioinguinal nerve, lateral femoral cutaneous nerve, blood vessels, or viscera.[2,3] The periosteum of the iliac bone is incised with monopolar cautery; the linear incision is made longitudinally along the top of the iliac crest (**Fig. 35.2**). A cuff of fascia and periosteum is elevated from the top and sides of the iliac crest with a Cobb periosteal elevator. This cuff of tissue is preserved to provide a secure fascial closure to reduce muscular pain when the patient ambulates postoperatively.

Bone grafts are harvested carefully with an oscillating saw or an osteotome after the medial and lateral surfaces of the graft harvest site have been exposed subperiosteally with a Cobb periosteal elevator. All bone cuts are made with sharp cutting tools while the surgeon visualizes the tips of the instruments directly to prevent complications. If bone grafts are used for mechanical reconstruction to bear loads (i.e., tricortical blocks), they should be harvested with an oscillating saw whenever possible. Osteotomes create microfractures, which can weaken the grafts. Hemostasis of the iliac crest donor bed is obtained with Gelfoam (Baxter, Deerfield, IL) or bone wax. A multilayer wound closure is performed. The fascial and periosteal tissues are reapproximated securely with interrupted sutures.

Posterior Iliac Crest

Posteriorly, bone grafts are obtained from the medial 6 to 8 cm of the posterior iliac crest. A more lateral exposure can

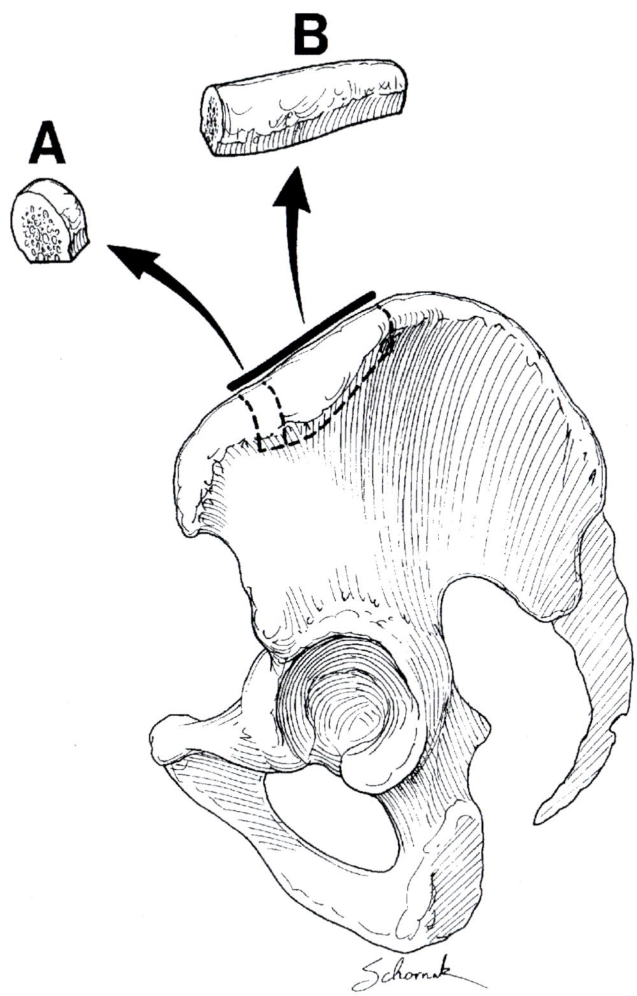

Fig. 35.1 Bone grafts harvested from the anterolateral ileum should remain 2 to 3 cm behind the anterior superior iliac spine to avoid an avulsion fracture. Tricortical bone grafts can be harvested for **(A)** single-level interbody fusions or for **(B)** multisegment vertebral body reconstruction. (Reprinted with permission from Barrow Neurological Institute.)

Portions of this chapter have been reprinted from Dickman CA, Maric Z. The biology of bone healing and techniques of spinal fusion. *BNI Quarterly* 1994;10(1):2–12. With permission from Barrow Neurological Institute.

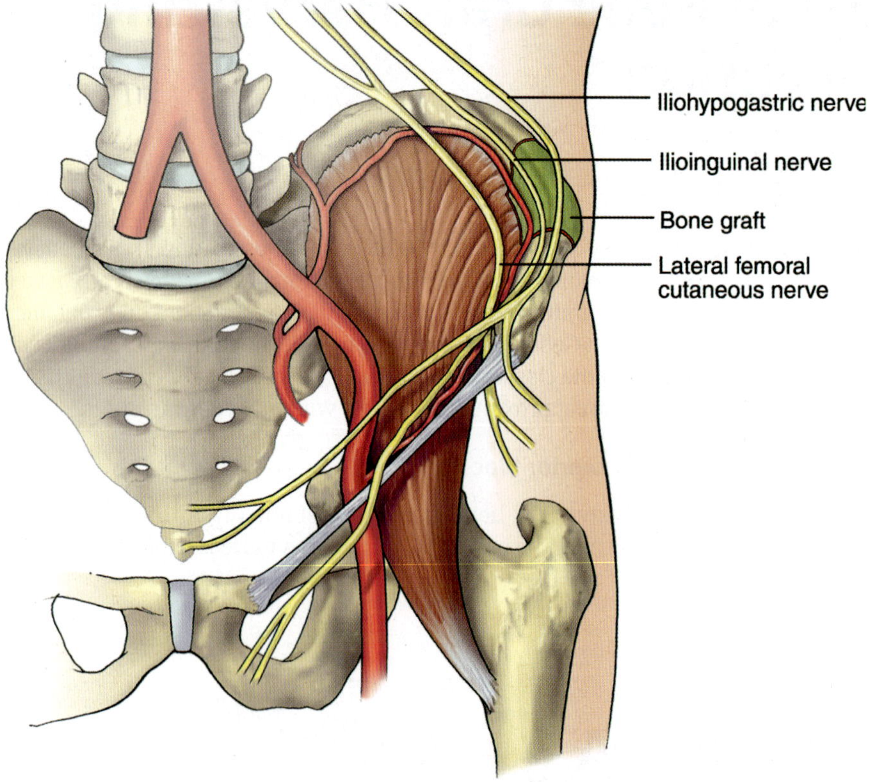

A

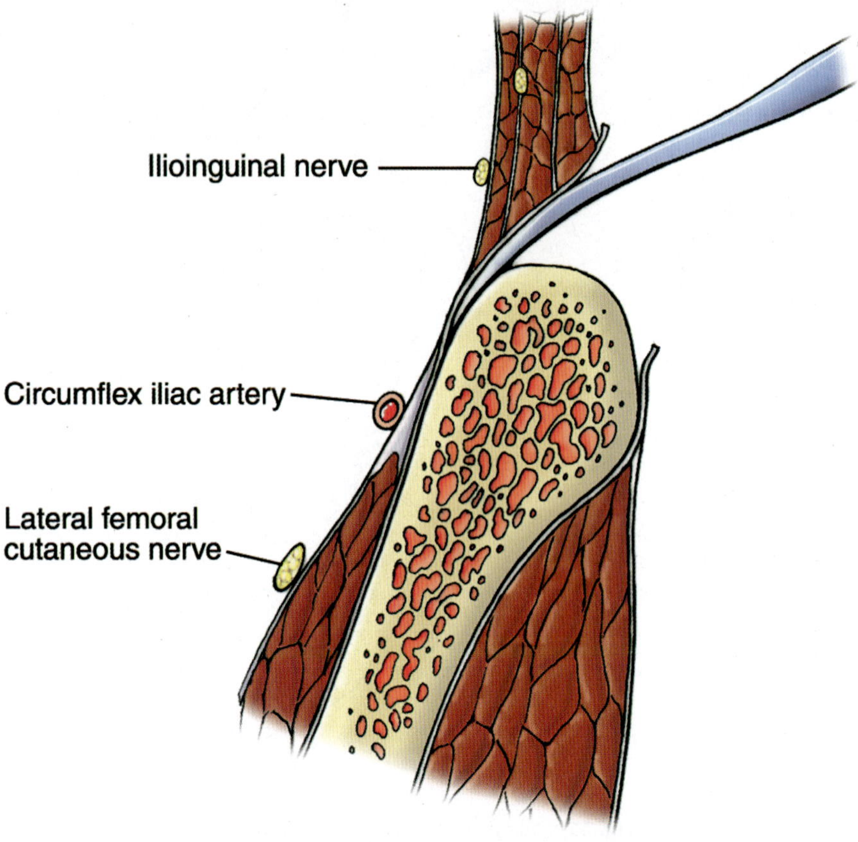

B

Fig. 35.2 **(A)** Fascial and periosteal incisions used for exposure of bone over the anterolateral iliac crest. **(B)** The dissection should remain in a subperiosteal plane, avoiding cautery along the medial surface of the ileum, to avoid injuring the ilioinguinal, iliohypogastric, and lateral femoral cutaneous nerves. (Reprinted with permission from Barrow Neurological Institute.)

cause buttock numbness or painful neuromas from injuring the superior cluneal nerves. Tricortical grafts, cortical matchstick grafts, a large corticocancellous plate, or cancellous bone strips can be harvested posteriorly (**Fig. 35.3**).

A curved skin incision is made over the medial iliac crest, beginning at the posterior iliac spine and continuing superolaterally. As with anterior osteotomies, careful anatomical tissue dissection must be performed under direct visualization to preserve the normal tissue planes whenever a bone graft is obtained. Tissue cuffs also are preserved during subperiosteal dissection of the bone surfaces to allow secure anatomical tissue closure.

All bone and soft tissue are dissected under direct visualization to prevent complications.[1,2,5,6] Monopolar cauterization and Cobb periosteal elevators are used to dissect the muscles from the iliac crest. Dissection of the bone surfaces should remain subperiosteal to avoid the branches of the gluteal arteries within the muscles. If the superior gluteal arteries are torn or cut, they can retract into the muscles and cause brisk, protracted bleeding. A Taylor (Aesculap, San Francisco, CA) retractor is useful for retracting soft tissues laterally from the ileum during graft harvest. The tissue dissection is restricted cephalad and lateral to the posterior iliac spine (**Fig. 35.4**) to avoid the sacroiliac joint (medially) and the sciatic notch (inferiorly). The sacroiliac ligaments should be preserved to maintain stability of the sacroiliac joint.[1,2,6] If a tricortical bone graft is needed, the anterior surface of the iliac crest should be dissected carefully with a curved Cobb periosteal elevator. The retroperitoneal fat pad is visualized, and within this fat pad, the ureter must be avoided. The muscles must be detached from the ventral, dorsal, and superior edges of the iliac crest to remove the tricortical graft.

Sharp instruments (e.g., osteotomes, oscillating saws, bone curettes, and bone gouges) are used to incise the bone to obtain grafts. These tools should be used with precision. After bone grafts have been harvested, meticulous hemostasis should be obtained with bone wax or Gelfoam. Bone wax provides an excellent method to obtain complete or almost complete hemostasis. However, bone wax inhibits bone healing and precludes accessing the same donor site if a new graft is needed in the future. Sheets of Gelfoam compressed onto the donor site provide reasonably good hemostasis and allow further grafts to be obtained from the same donor site if needed. Suction drains are placed if any blood

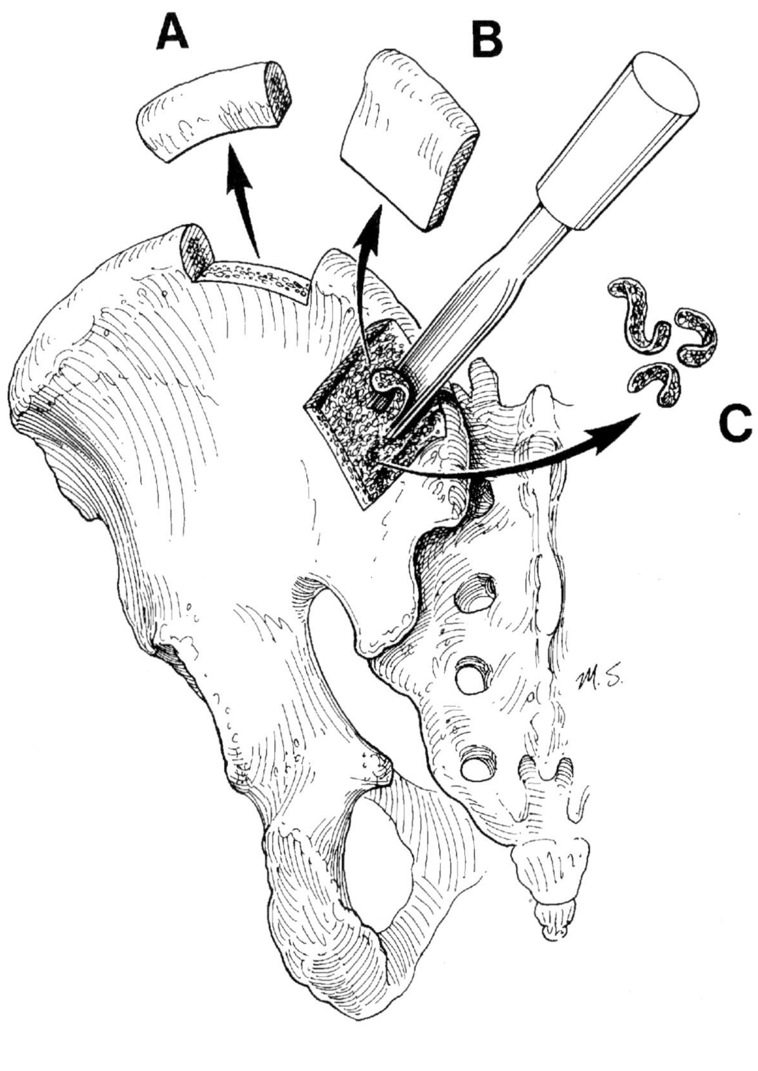

Fig. 35.3 A variety of bone grafts can be harvested from the posterior ileum: **(A)** tricortical strut graft, **(B)** corticocancellous plate, and **(C)** cancellous bone strips. (Reprinted with permission from Barrow Neurological Institute.)

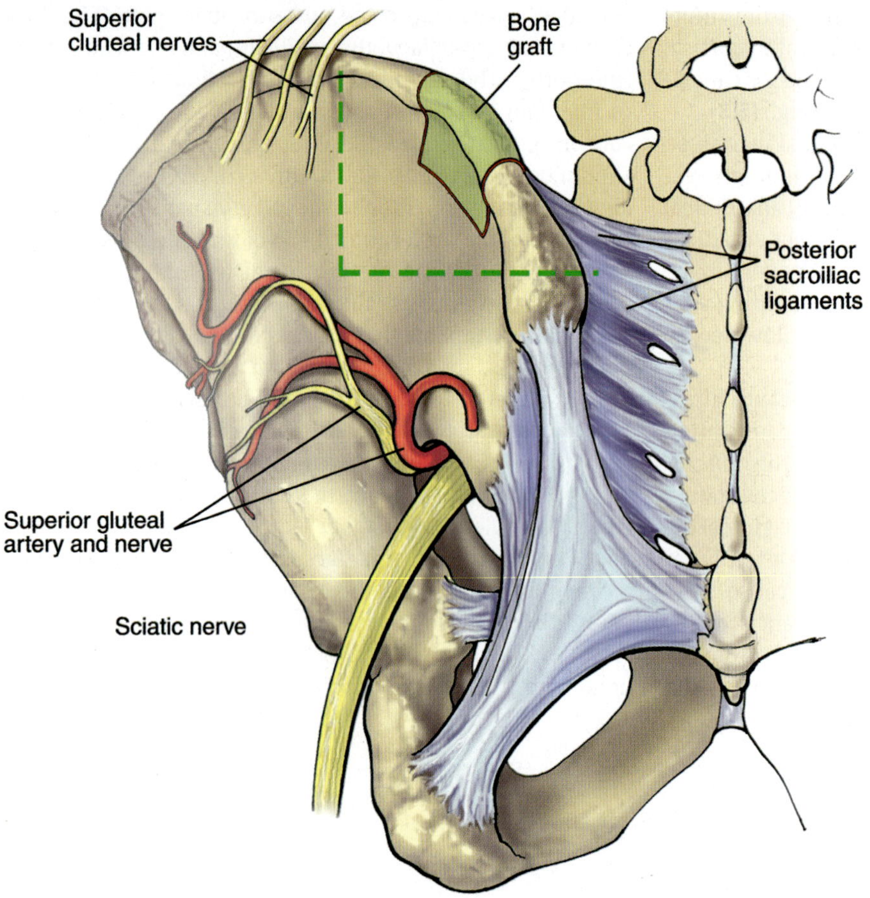

Fig. 35.4 The bone dissection at the posterior iliac crest is kept above a line intersecting the posterior superior iliac spine. The sacroiliac ligaments (medially), sciatic nerve (caudally), gluteal vessels (caudally and submuscularly), superior cluneal nerves (laterally), and ureter (anteriorly) should be avoided. (Reprinted with permission from Barrow Neurological Institute.)

persistently oozes from the graft donor site. All periosteal and fascial layers are closed to obliterate dead space, to reattach the muscles to their sites of origin or insertion, to prevent herniation of abdominal contents, and to reduce postoperative muscular pain.

Rib Grafts

Although not a favored source of bone grafts for cervical spinal fusion, ribs are a useful alternative if other autologous sites cannot be used.[7–9] Ribs have a relatively thin cortex, are weak mechanically in resisting compressive and tensile loads, and provide a relatively limited volume of bone graft. Rib grafts can be obtained for struts or as sources of cancellous bone (**Fig. 35.5**). Straight or curved rib segments can be obtained for spinal fusion. Rib grafts can be wired to the occiput and cervical spine for internal fixation (**Fig. 35.5D**). Ribs have a large area of cancellous bone with a thin cortical shell and do not tolerate strong compressive, shear, or torsional loads without breaking or splintering. Consequently, they should be avoided for reconstruction of any major spinal deformity unless supplemented with a rigid internal fixation device.

Rib grafts are obtained in the following manner. A skin incision is made parallel to and directly over the surface of the rib (**Fig. 35.5A**). The muscles and periosteum are incised over the outer surface of the rib. The neurovascular bundle is detached carefully from the inferior margin of the rib using a curved periosteal elevator. A Doyen rib dissector is used to detach the intercostal muscles from the superior and inferior margins of the rib (**Fig. 35.5B**). The parietal pleura is preserved carefully and detached with blunt dissection from the undersurface of the rib. The ends of the segment of rib are then transected sharply. A rib cutter or an oscillating saw can be used to cut the rib. Oscillating or reciprocating saws are preferred to cut the rib precisely. The rib cutter is sharp but tends to crush, splinter, and weaken the rib adjacent to the cut surfaces. Two cuts are created, one proximally and one distally, to detach the rib (**Fig. 35.5C**).

The rib harvest site is examined carefully. Bone spicules are removed and bone edges are waxed to prevent a pneumothorax. The pleura is examined to ensure that it was not violated. After hemostasis is completed, a multilayer wound closure is performed. A postoperative chest radiograph is obtained to monitor for a pneumothorax.

Fibula Grafts

Vascularized or nonvascularized fibula grafts are obtained from the middle third of the fibula shaft.[9–13] The proximal head of the fibula is avoided to preserve the function of the peroneal nerve. Its distal end is preserved to maintain ankle

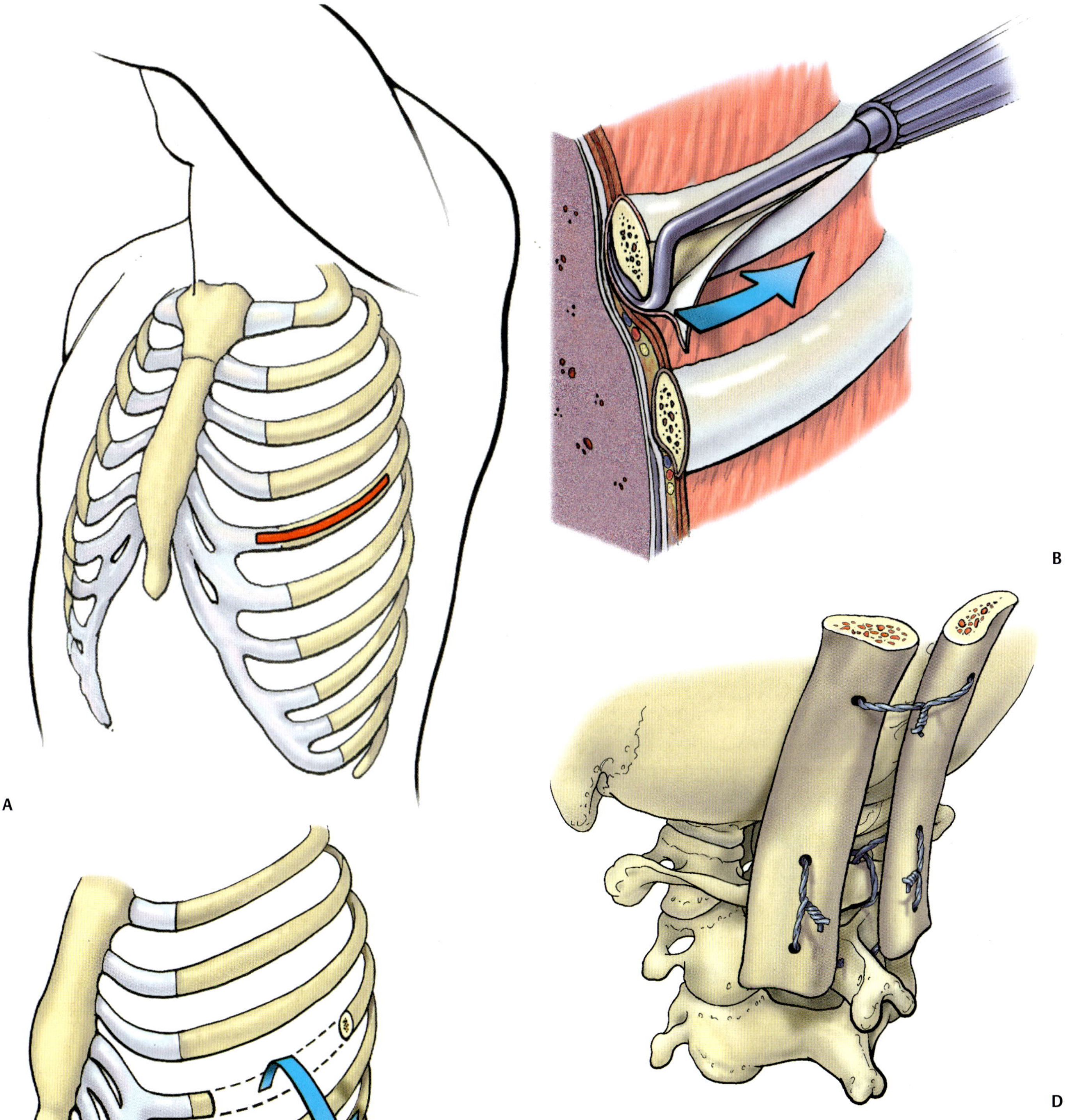

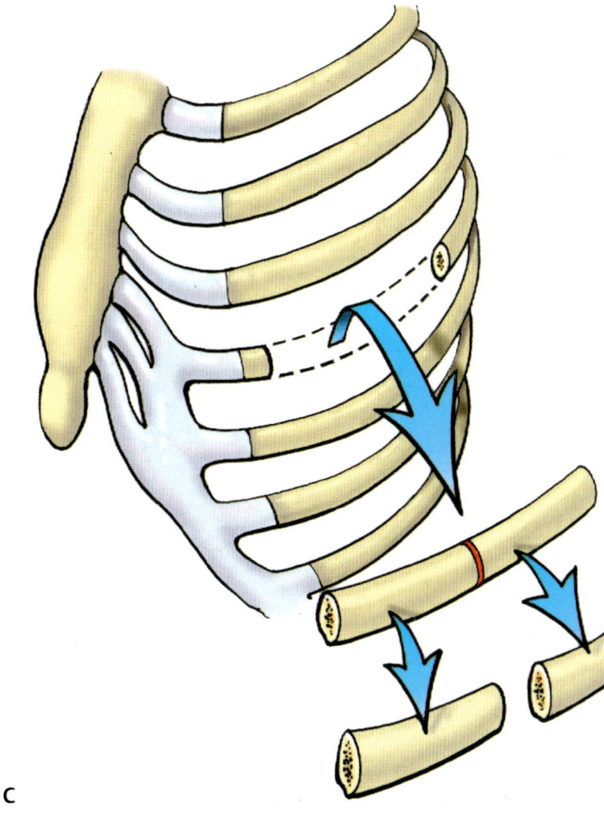

Fig. 35.5 **(A)** The incision over the ribs exposes two ribs along a curved segment. **(B)** A Doyen periosteal elevator is used to dissect the neurovascular bundle and muscle attachments from rib, remaining extrapleural. **(C)** Ribs are cut sharply with a cutting tool. **(D)** The ribs are wired to the occiput and the cervical laminae for occipitocervical fusion. (Reprinted with permission from Barrow Neurological Institute.)

function. The fibula can be removed with no functional consequences as long as the patient's tibia is normal.[9–13] The fibula provides a dense cortical strut graft with relatively little cancellous bone. It is used primarily for anterior reconstruction of long segment vertebral body defects.

An incision is made over the lateral surface at the middle of the leg, parallel to the fibula (**Fig. 35.6A**). Nonvascularized grafts are obtained after subperiosteal exposure of the desired segment circumferentially. For vascularized fibula grafts, a muscular cuff is preserved around the fibula graft along with the nutrient vessels. The muscles and fascia are dissected from the distal ends of the fibula surface. A vascular pedicle of the peroneal artery and vein, along with the nutrient vessels to the midshaft of the fibula, is preserved for the anastomosis (**Fig. 35.6B,C**).

The graft is measured to the desired length. Proximally and distally, the bone is transected sharply with a Gigli saw or an oscillating saw. The leg incision is closed with a routine multilayered wound closure. In the anterior cervical spine, the vessels of the fibula graft can be anastomosed with the superior thyroid artery and vein or other accessible large vessels. In the posterior cervical spine the graft can be anastomosed to the occipital artery. The fibula provides a strong graft with dense cortical bone, which can be used for reconstruction in areas with large loads or high stress. There is relatively little cancellous bone, and the dense cortical bone may be incorporated slowly and remodeled incompletely. However, vascularized grafts are usually incorporated rapidly as long as the graft is well fixated and the anastomoses remain patent.[9–13] Because of the time and

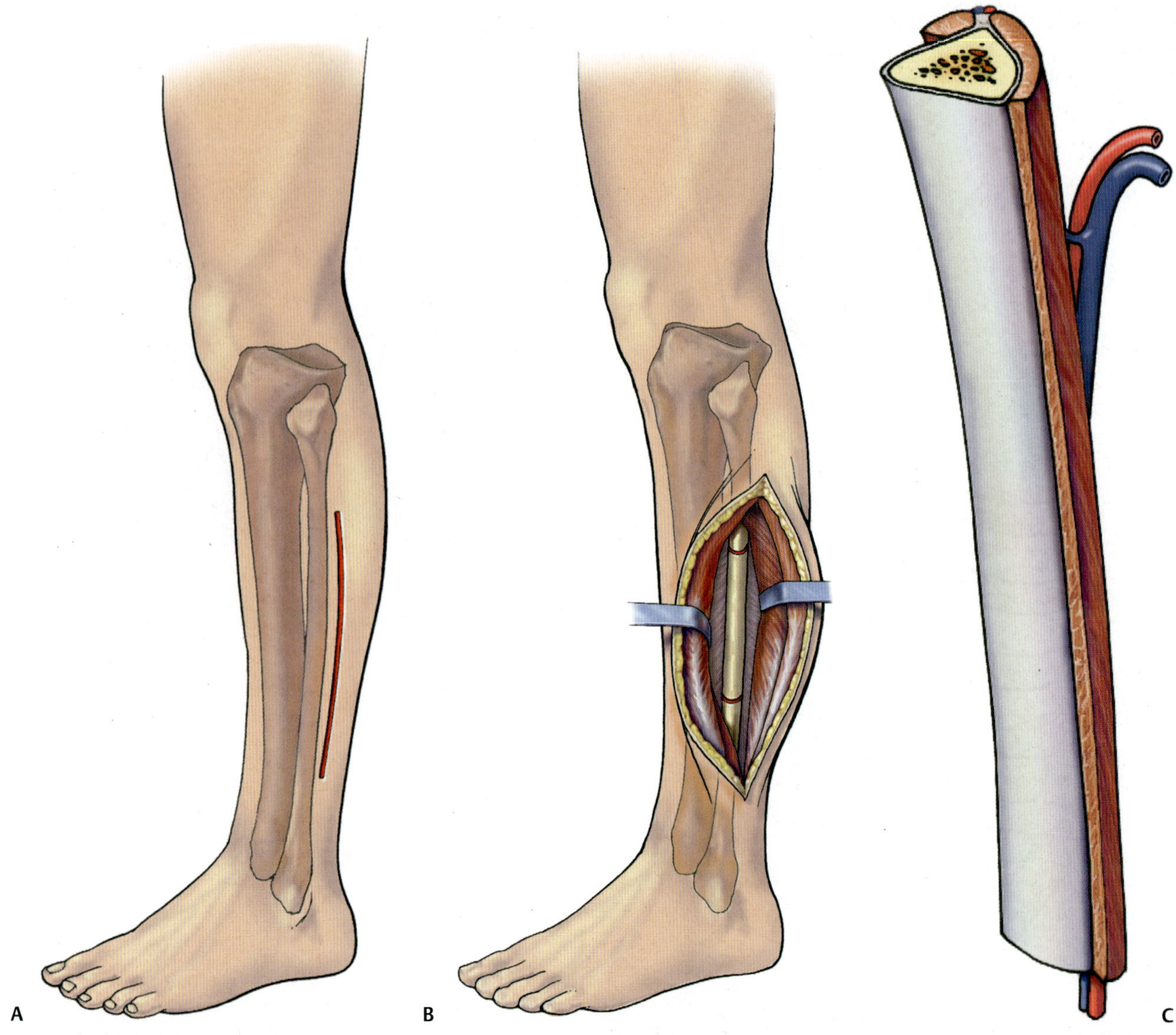

Fig. 35.6 Vascularized fibula graft. **(A)** An incision is made parallel to the fibula to expose its middle third segment. **(B)** Periosteal incisions are made proximally and distally along the fibula. The proximal and distal peroneal vessels are isolated, and the bone is harvested. A muscle cuff and a margin of periosteum are preserved around the graft. **(C)** The vascularized graft is harvested, preserving a muscle cuff and the peroneal vascular pedicle. The vascular pedicle is anastomosed to vessels within the host site. (Reprinted with permission from Barrow Neurological Institute.)

difficulty involved in maintaining patent graft anastomoses, vascularized grafts are reserved for special circumstances (i.e., irradiated, devascularized fusion beds).

Calvarial Grafts

Calvarial bone grafts are particularly useful for fusions in young children because the iliac crest and the fibula are primarily nonossified.[9,14–17] Full-thickness calvarial bone grafts can be obtained from the midline occipital bone (**Fig. 35.7A**); split-thickness grafts can be harvested from the parietal bones (**Fig. 35.7B**). Both of these calvarial sources provide dense cortical bone, with relatively little cancellous bone. The grafts are moderately rigid but are often thin.

Occipital bone grafts have been used for cervical fusion.[9,15–17] Full-thickness rectangular grafts are harvested from a cephalad extension of the patient's posterior midline neck incision (**Fig. 35.7A**). A burr hole is used to expose the dura beneath the occipital squamosa. The atlanto-occipital membrane is dissected sharply from the edge of the foramen magnum. A craniotome is used to cut the margins of the rectangular-shaped bone graft. The dura should be separated carefully from the bone before the craniectomy is removed. This technique is useful as a salvage technique. If, however, an occipital extension of the fusion is needed, the large defect in the occipital bone may preclude reliable fixation of the occiput.

The parietal bone can be used as a source of split-thickness bone grafts (**Fig. 35.7B**). A bicoronal or "C"-shaped scalp incision is made at the vertex. Full-thickness, paramedian craniotomy flaps are removed bilaterally, leaving the midline bone intact over the superior sagittal sinus. A reciprocating saw is used to split the diploic layer of the bone grafts longitudinally. The top half of each of the grafts is reattached to the skull with wires or miniplates. The scalp is closed routinely with galeal and skin sutures. The split-thickness parietal bone grafts are contoured to the desired shape and fixated to the spine.

Allografts

Allograft bone usually must be reconstituted by soaking the grafts in sterile saline solution before the bone is shaped or cut. An unreconstituted graft remains brittle and will

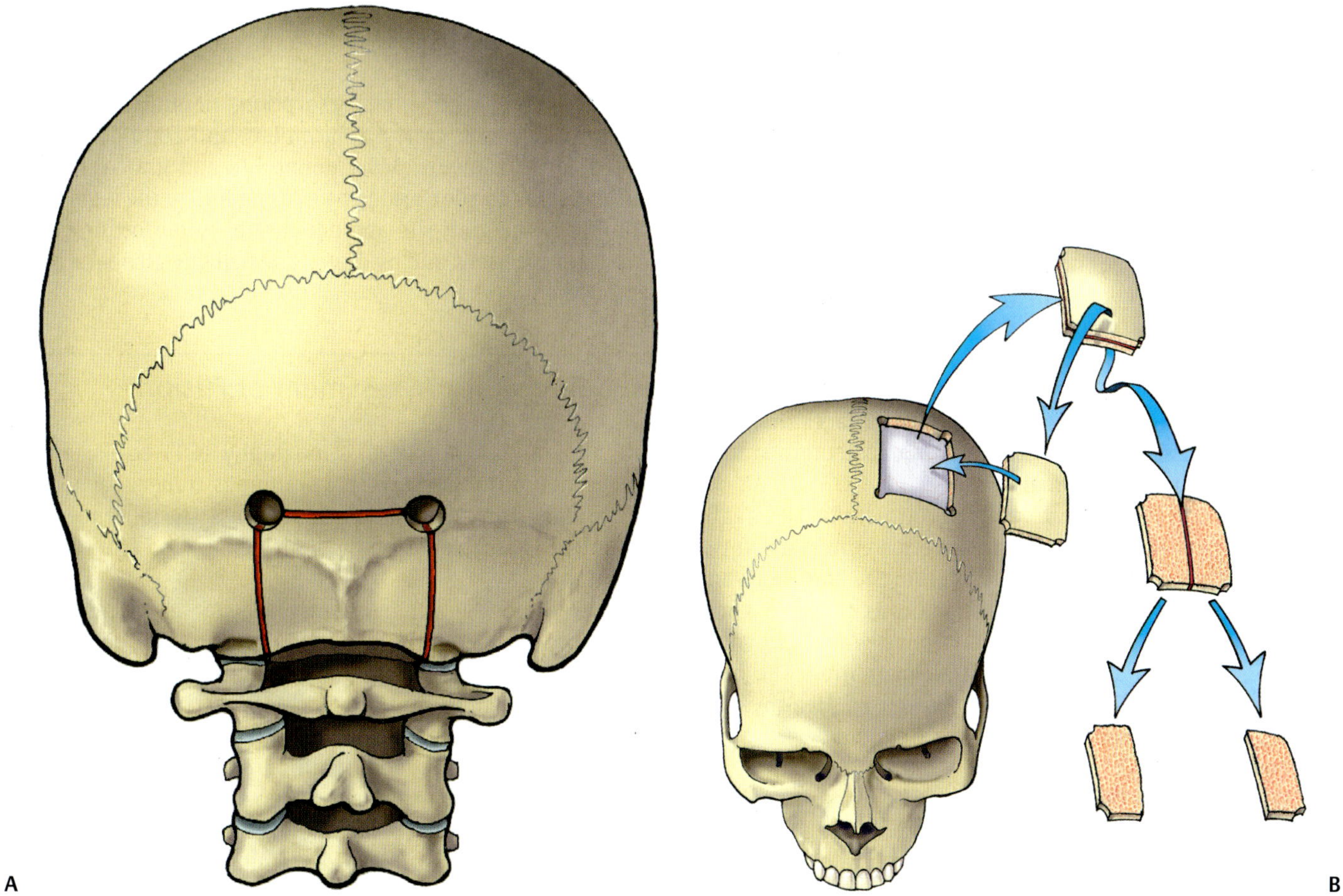

Fig. 35.7 Calvarial bone grafts. **(A)** An occipital, full-thickness, rectangular bone graft is harvested with a craniotome. **(B)** A split-thickness parietal calvarial graft. A full-thickness bone flap is removed with a craniotome. The grafts are divided with a microreciprocating saw. The upper layer of the calvarial flap is reattached with miniplates. The bone grafts are contoured and wired to the spine. (Reprinted with permission from Barrow Neurological Institute.)

splinter and fracture when it is cut or drilled. The grafts should be soaked for 30 minutes or more before they are used. The length of time for reconstitution depends on the size and thickness of the graft and on the method of preparation (i.e., freeze-dried bone must be reconstituted longer than fresh-frozen allograft). Typically, the length of time for reconstitution is specified by the tissue bank that provides the bone graft.

Allografts are perceived by the body as "foreign" even though they are processed to reduce their immunogenicity.[18–29] Therefore, we prefer to reserve allograft for patients who lack adequate autograft or when very long reconstructive grafts are needed for areas subjected to strong mechanical stresses. Allograft struts used for mechanical reconstruction of the vertebral bodies also can be augmented with autografts. To promote bone healing, the hollow center of an allograft fibula strut can be packed with autogenous bone obtained from removal of the vertebrae.

Surgical Preparation of Bone Grafts and Fusion Site

Surgical technique plays a critical role in determining the outcome of bone grafting. Bone healing requires living cells; however, few of the osteocytes and osteoblasts transplanted in an autogenous graft survive.[30–35] The tissue bed is the source of almost all of the active processes of the healing response.[30–38] The primary goal is to maximize the surface area of healthy vascularized bone in the fusion bed.

Diseased or poorly vascularized tissue should be debrided. Local tissue trauma should be minimized. Atraumatic dissection technique should be used. Devascularization and heating of bone should be avoided. Hemostasis should be obtained with bipolar coagulation when possible. Cauterization heats the bone and should be used judiciously. If high-speed drills are used, irrigation must be used to minimize thermal injury. Whenever possible, the bone surfaces should be decorticated with a Leksell rongeur or an osteotome rather than a drill to avoid thermal injury.

Preparation of bone grafts and the recipient bed is equally important for successful fusion. All periosteum and soft tissue must be removed meticulously from the bone graft and fusion bed. Soft tissue can provide a fibrous interface where a nonunion can form. Autogenous bone grafts should be harvested within 30 minutes of transplantation. The bone is stored in blood-soaked sponges until used. Healthy, vascularized, nondessicated muscle tissue should be preserved to cover the fusion.

When adjacent bone surfaces are to be fused, osteogenic cells are exposed by segmentally decorticating the bone to expose the bone marrow. Sufficient cancellous bone should be exposed; however, excessive decortication can weaken the bone and should be avoided. The articular cartilage should be removed from articular surfaces. Curettes, osteotomes, or drills can be used to decorticate the bone surfaces of the vertebral end plates or facet joints to promote arthrodesis across the articular surfaces.

Bone grafts should fit precisely into the fusion site to maximize the surface area for bone-to-bone contact. Meticulous carpentry of the graft and recipient sites is required to obtain an ideal fitting. Grafts should be compressed against the recipient bed, and dead space within the fusion bed should be obliterated. Cancellous bone can be used to fill residual gaps in the fusion bed; however, a margin is always preserved adjacent to the dura to prevent neural compression.

The local mechanical environment has a strong bearing on the outcome of bone healing.[7,9,20,27,32,35,36,39] Excessive movement promotes differentiation of fibrous tissue that can cause pseudarthrosis. By decreasing this excessive movement, fixation enhances the rate of union in the grafted segment. External orthoses, internal fixation, or both may be needed to control postoperative spinal motion adequately.

Complications of Bone Grafts

Donor site complications include acute pain from graft harvest, infection, hemorrhage, nerve injury, pelvic instability, cosmetic deformity, gait disturbance, pelvic fracture, chronic pain, and hernia formation, among others.[1–6,40] Complications at the fusion bed include neural compression, graft breakage, graft resorption, nonunion, infection, graft fracture, graft displacement, and complications related to instruments. Most donor site and graft-related complications can be avoided by understanding the regional anatomy of the graft site and donor site, by performing all dissection precisely, and by directly visualizing all operative maneuvers.

Radiographic Assessment of Fusion

On radiographs, computed tomography (CT) scans, and tomograms, fusion appears as continuous trabecular bone that bridges the adjacent bone surfaces. The absence of movement is assessed with dynamic flexion and extension radiographs.

Failure of bone grafts frequently appears as progressive resorption. Radiographically, failure appears as a decrease in the size and density of the graft. Nonunion (pseudarthrosis) or fibrous union can be recognized on radiographs as persistent lucencies between the graft and the host bone. Thin-section CT scans or tomograms are helpful because radiolucencies are often thin and may be difficult to identify on plain radiographs. Dynamic radiographs (flexion and extension views) are helpful for determining nonunion. Motion across a grafted motion segment confirms inadequate healing. Resorption of bone around internal fixation devices, with lucency around the screws, may indicate failure of the fixation devices.

There are several types of nonunions, among which are hypertrophic, oligotrophic, dystrophic, necrotic, deficit, and atrophic nonunions.[7,31–33,35,41] Hypertrophic nonunion derives from inadequate stabilization or premature weight bearing. Oligotrophic nonunion occurs when bones are separated too widely for callus to bridge the defect. In dystrophic nonunions only one side of a fracture unites. Necrotic nonunion occurs because of vascular insufficiency and the presence of nonviable tissue. A deficit nonunion occurs when the parts are too distant. Atrophic nonunion occurs when the bone graft becomes reabsorbed.

Conclusion

Meticulous preparation of the bone graft and fusion bed are equally important for achieving bone healing. Autogenous bone grafts are preferred to allografts whenever possible because they heal better, are incorporated more completely and remodeled rapidly, and evoke no immunological response. Donor site complications can be avoided by understanding the anatomy of the regions of the donor sites and by using careful dissection techniques.

References

1. Coventry MB, Tapper EM. Pelvic instability: a consequence of removing iliac bone for grafting. J Bone Joint Surg Am 1972;54(1): 83–101
2. Kurz LT, Garfin SR, Booth RE Jr. Harvesting autogenous iliac bone grafts. A review of complications and techniques. Spine 1989;14(12):1324–1331
3. Ghent WR. Further studies on meralgia paresthetica. Can Med Assoc J 1961;85:871–875
4. Dougherty PJ, Jones AAM, Sharkey N, et al. Iliac crest bone graft: osteotome versus saw. Cervical Spine Res Soc 1992;148. Abstract
5. Fernyhough JC, Schimandle JJ, Weigel MC, Edwards CC, Levine AM. Chronic donor site pain complicating bone graft harvesting from the posterior iliac crest for spinal fusion. Spine 1992; 17(12):1474–1480
6. Lichtblau S. Dislocation of the sacro-iliac joint. A complication of bone-grafting. J Bone Joint Surg Am 1962;44:193–198
7. Habal MB. Different forms of bone grafts. In: Habal MB, Reddi AH, eds. Bone Grafts and Bone Substitutes. Philadelphia, PA: WB Saunders; 1992:6–8
8. Prolo DJ, Rodrigo JJ. Contemporary bone graft physiology and surgery. Clin Orthop Relat Res 1985;200(200):322–342
9. Sullivan JA. Bone grafting. Sources and methods. In: Weinstein SL, ed. The Pediatric Spine: Principles and Practice. New York, NY: Raven Press; 1994:1299–1310
10. Freidberg SR, Gumley GJ, Pfeifer BA, Hybels RL. Vascularized fibular graft to replace resected cervical vertebral bodies. Case report. J Neurosurg 1989;71(2):283–286
11. Conley FK, Britt RH, Hanbery JW, Silverberg GD. Anterior fibular strut graft in neoplastic disease of the cervical spine. J Neurosurg 1979;51(5):677–684
12. Rossier AB, Hussey RW, Kenzora JE. Anterior fibular interbody fusion in the treatment of cervical spinal cord injuries. Surg Neurol 1977;7(2):55–60
13. Whitecloud TS, LaRocca H. Fibular strut graft in reconstructive surgery of the cervical spine. Spine 1976;1:33–43
14. Tanaka T, Ninchoji T, Uemura K, et al. Multilevel anterior cervical fusion using skull bone grafts. Case report. J Neurosurg 1992;76(2):298–302
15. Sagher O, Malik JM, Lee JH, et al. Fusion with occipital bone for atlantoaxial instability: technical note. Neurosurgery 1993;33(5): 926–928, discussion 928–929
16. Duong DH, Chadduck WM. Reconstruction of the hypoplastic posterior arch of the atlas with calvarial bone grafts for posterior atlantoaxial fusion: technical report. Neurosurgery 1994;35(6): 1168–1170
17. Chadduck WM, Boop FA. Use of full-thickness calvarial bone grafts for cervical spinal fusions in pediatric patients. Pediatr Neurosurg 1994;20(1):107–112
18. Brooks DB, Heiple KG, Herndon CH, Powell AE. Immunological factors in homogenous bone transplantation. IV. The effect of various methods of preparation and irradiation on antigenicity. J Bone Joint Surg Am 1963;45:1617–1626
19. Brown MD, Malinin TI, Davis PB. A roentgenographic evaluation of frozen allografts versus autografts in anterior cervical spine fusions. Clin Orthop Relat Res 1976;119(119):231–236
20. Burchardt H, Enneking WF. Transplantation of bone. Surg Clin North Am 1978;58(2):403–427
21. Burchardt H, Glowczewskie FP, Enneking WF. Short-term immunosuppression with fresh segmental fibular allografts in dogs. J Bone Joint Surg Am 1981;63(3):411–415
22. Emery SE, Brazinski M, Bensusan J, et al. Effects of irradiation on the biologic and biomechanical properties of anterior spine fusion in a canine model. Orthopaedic Research Society 38th Annual Meeting; 1992. Abstract
23. Fernyhough JC, White JI, LaRocca H. Fusion rates in multilevel cervical spondylosis comparing allograft fibula with autograft fibula in 126 patients. Spine 1991;16(10, Suppl):S561–S564
24. Friedlaender GE, Strong DM, Sell KW. Studies on the antigenicity of bone. II. Donor-specific anti-HLA antibodies in human recipients of freeze-dried allografts. J Bone Joint Surg Am 1984;66(1):107–112
25. Goldberg VM, Bos GD, Heiple KG, Zika JM, Powell AE. Improved acceptance of frozen bone allografts in genetically mismatched dogs by immunosuppression. J Bone Joint Surg Am 1984;66(6):937–950
26. Herron LD, Newman MH. The failure of ethylene oxide gas-sterilized freeze-dried bone graft for thoracic and lumbar spinal fusion. Spine 1989;14(5):496–500
27. Pelker RR, Friedlaender GE. Biomechanical aspects of bone autografts and allografts. Orthop Clin North Am 1987;18(2):235–239
28. Stabler CL, Eismont FJ, Brown MD, Green BA, Malinin TI. Failure of posterior cervical fusions using cadaveric bone graft in children. J Bone Joint Surg Am 1985;67(3):371–375
29. Wittenberg RH, Moeller J, Shea M, White AA III, Hayes WC. Compressive strength of autologous and allogenous bone grafts for thoracolumbar and cervical spine fusion. Spine 1990; 15(10):1073–1078
30. Chalmers J, Gray DH, Rush J. Observations on the induction of bone in soft tissues. J Bone Joint Surg Br 1975;57(1):36–45
31. Kaufman HH, Jones E. The principles of bony spinal fusion. Neurosurgery 1989;24(2):264–270
32. Muschler GF, Lane JM, Dawson EG. The biology of spinal fusion. In: Cotler JM, Cotler HP, eds. Spinal Fusion Science and Technique. Berlin: Springer-Verlag; 1990:9–21
33. Prolo DJ. Biology of bone fusion. Clin Neurosurg 1990;36:135–146
34. Recker RR. Embryology, anatomy, and microstructure of bone. In: Coe FL, Favus MJ, eds. Disorders of Bone and Mineral Metabolism. New York, NY: Raven Press, 1992:219–240

35. Urist MR. Bone transplants and implants. In Urist MR, ed. Fundamentals and Clinical Bone Physiology. Philadelphia, PA: JB Lippincott; 1980:331–368
36. Burchardt H. Biology of bone transplantation. Orthop Clin North Am 1987;18(2):187–196
37. Deleu J, Trueta J. Vascularization of bone grafts in the anterior chamber of the eye. J Bone Joint Surg Br 1965;47:319–329
38. Kingma MJ, Hampe JF. The behavior of blood vessels after experimental transplantation of bone. J Bone Joint Surg Br 1964;46:141–150
39. Wolff J. Das Gesetz der Transformation der Knochen. Berlin: Hirschwold; 1892
40. Weikel AM, Habal MB. Meralgia paresthetica: a complication of iliac bone procurement. Plast Reconstr Surg 1977;60(4): 572–574
41. Hayes WC. Biomechanics of cortical and trabecular bone: Implications for assessment of fracture risk. In: Mow VC, Hayes WC, eds. Basic Orthopaedic Biomechanics. New York, NY: Raven Press; 1991:93–142

36 General Principles of Spinal Wire and Cable Fixation

Curtis A. Dickman and Volker K. H. Sonntag

This chapter reviews the fundamental principles for successful fixation with wires and cables as they apply to cervical and occipitocervical stabilization. Wires have diverse uses, are simple to apply, and are familiar to most surgeons. They create a mechanical tension band for the posterior cervical spine. They can be used to attach adjacent vertebral surfaces together, or they can be used to bind bone grafts or metal implants to the surface of the occiput and posterior cervical spine. Wires also can be attached directly to several adjacent motion segments to achieve multiplanar control of segmental motion.

The spinous processes, the laminae, the facets, or the occiput can serve as points of bony attachments for wire. The goal of wiring is to fixate the spine until a solid bone fusion develops.

Techniques of Wire Application

There are several different types of wires available for surgical use. Monofilament wire, double-stranded, twisted wire, or braided wire cables are used for cervical or occipital fixation.

Traditionally, monofilament stainless steel has been the most common wire used for spinal fixation. Monofilament wire is available in a variety of diameters (**Table 36.1**). For the cervical spine, 20-gauge wire is the most convenient; it is easy to work with and relatively strong. In comparison, 18-gauge wire is stronger than 20-gauge wire, but it is stiff and therefore difficult to twist, contour, and manipulate. Twenty-two-gauge wire is more flexible than 20-gauge wire, but it is weaker and more likely to fatigue and break. Usually, 20-gauge monofilament wire is used to fixate the occiput, spinous processes, or cervical laminae. Bone grafts or the cervical facets are fixated with either 20- or 22-gauge wire. These applications are modified depending on the individual circumstances.

Double-stranded twisted monofilament wire has mechanical advantages over single-stranded monofilament wire. Taitsman and colleagues demonstrated that double-stranded, 24-gauge twisted wire is much stronger than monofilament 24-gauge wire. The tensile strength increases up to 8 turns/inch (2.5 turns/cm) and decreases thereafter.[1] Double-stranded wires can be prepared easily using a hand drill or a "Robinson" wire twister. The end of a pair of wires is held by the wire twister or is inserted into the shaft of the twist drill. The free ends of the wires are held with a Kocher clamp. The wires are pulled taut and twisted uniformly by rotating the twist drill or the wire twister. A ruler is used to measure the number of twists in the wire.

The preferred method of fixating monofilament wire to the spine is by twisting the wire. A loop of wire is wrapped around a bone surface. The free ends of the wire are brought together; they are crossed and twisted to remove slack from the loop of wire around the bone surfaces. Twisting sets progressive tension in the wire. Wire can be twisted with a needle holder or with a Robinson wire twister (**Fig. 36.1**). The free ends of the wires are crossed, and one or two twists are placed in the wire. The intersection of the wires is grasped with a wire twister. The wires are pulled upward to

Table 36.1 Wire Size Comparisons*

Wire Gauge	Size (mm)	Diameter (in)	Suture Sizes
28	0.3	0.0126	2–0
26	0.4	0.0159	0
24	0.5	0.0201	#2
22	0.6	0.0254	#4
20	0.8	0.032	#5
18	1.0	0.04	#7
16	1.2	0.05	

*Wire gauge varies depending on the manufacturer.
Source: Stauffer ES. Wiring techniques of the posterior cervical spine for the treatment of trauma. Orthopedics 1988;11(11):1543–1548. Reprinted with permission.

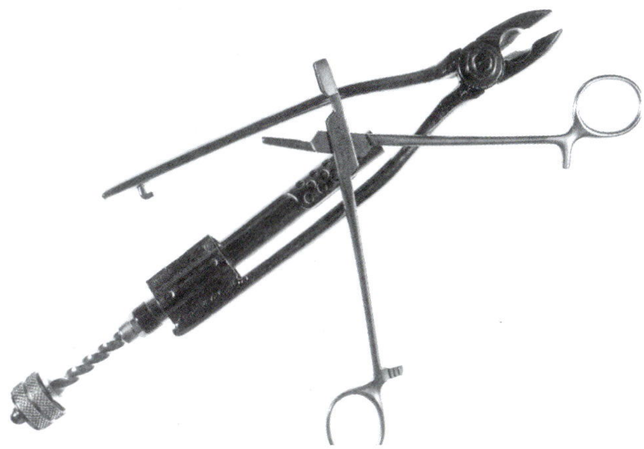

Fig. 36.1 Wire twisting devices. The Robinson wire twister is shaped like a pliers. The wire holding forceps are shaped like a needle holder. (Reprinted with permission from Barrow Neurological Institute.)

Modified from Dickman CA, Sonntag VKH. Wire fixation for the cervical spine: biomechanical principles and surgical techniques. *BNI Quarterly* 1993;9(4):2–16.

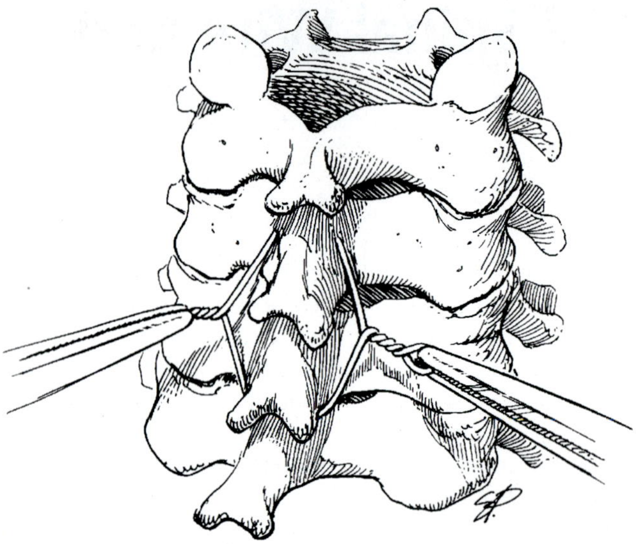

Fig. 36.2 Bilateral wire twisting evenly distributes tension in the wire. (Reprinted with permission from Barrow Neurological Institute.)

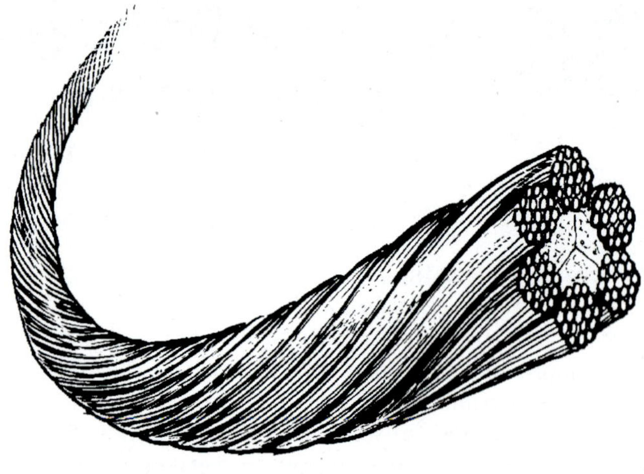

Fig. 36.3 Braided cables have a core surrounded by wire strands. Each strand is composed of several individual wires. Cross-sectional view. (Reprinted with permission from Barrow Neurological Institute.)

distribute tension uniformly in the wire and to remove slack from the wire while it is twisted. Although stiff, the monofilament wires are malleable and retain the twisted configuration permanently. Wires should not be over-twisted or they will weaken and break. Wire also should not be overtightened or it will pull through soft, osteoporotic bone.

Single-stranded or double-stranded monofilament wire usually is twisted at one site to remove slack from the wire. Alternatively, the wire can be twisted bilaterally to distribute the tension in the wire more evenly (**Fig. 36.2**).

The twists should be uniform. Excessive twisting will change the color of the wire and secondary turns will appear. Kinking of the wire must be avoided when wires are bent, passed, or tightened. Wire should not be kinked, notched, or bent in an acute angle. Acute angles or excessive twisting in the wire make it extremely susceptible to fatigue and breakage.

Braided Cables

"Wire rope" has been used extensively in mechanical engineering in the construction of bridges, elevators, and heavy machinery, among other things. Wire rope consists of several cable strands laid vertically about a metallic or nonmetallic core (**Fig. 36.3**). Such ropes are very flexible yet strong and resist crushing and distortion. Multistranded braided wire cables were developed as an adaptation of this concept for spine surgery.[2,3] Wire cables for spinal fixation were developed by a surgeon, Dr. Matthew Songer, and his father, Robert Songer, an engineer.[2] Cables are stronger, more flexible, and more fatigue-resistant than monofilament wire; however, they also cost considerably more. Within the past few years, wire cables have almost completely replaced monofilament wires for spinal fixation. Because the cables are flexible, the risk of neurological injury during wire placement or wire removal is reduced. Wire cables conform to the surface of the laminae. The flexibility allows an even distribution of tension in the cable. Several types of braided cables are marketed for use in spinal fixation. Two representative types of cables (**Table 36.2**) are discussed later.

Danek Cables

Danek cables (Sofamor, Memphis, TN) are braided wires that are attached to a stiff monofilament leader wire for sublaminar passage. There are 49 wire strands in each cable, arranged in a 7 × 7 array. The cables are composed of titanium or stainless steel.[2,3] Single cables or two cables are welded to each leader wire; the double cables are used for sublaminar wire passage. A crimping cylinder is welded to the distal end of the cables. The end of the cable is passed through the cylinder to create a loop. After slack is removed from the cable, the crimp is pinched to fixate the cable permanently.

The double cables have the same crimping mechanism as the single cables (**Fig. 36.4**). The leader wire is passed

Table 36.2 Comparison of Two Types of Braided Wire Cables

Features	Danek Cable	Sof'wire
Wire array	7 × 7	19 × 7
No. strands	7	19
No. wires per strand	7	7
Total no. wires	49	133
Diameter	0.041 in	0.034 in
Materials	Stainless steel or titanium	Stainless steel or titanium
Appearance of crimp device	Cylindrical crimp	Cylindrical crimp
Tensioning device	Tensioner, torque wrench	No torque measuring wrench
Comparable diameter of monofilament wire	18 g	20 g

Source: Reprinted permission from Barrow Neurological Institute.

through the cylindrical crimp welded on the end of the cable; tension is applied to engage the wire. The crimp is pinched to permanently fix the cable. The cables are permanently, irreversibly secured into position with a metal crimp shaped like a cylinder. The crimp is pinched with a tool that binds it to the cable. Two different tensioner devices are available (**Figs. 36.5** and **36.6**). The larger combined tensioner and crimper is easiest to use. The tensioner device is used to remove slack from the wire, and a torque wrench is used to adjust the desired wire tension. The desired tension is adjusted using a knob on the base of the torque wrench. The torque measurement is indicated by calibrations, which are marked on the shaft of the torque wrench in inch-pounds and Newton-meters. The torque applied with the wrench is directly proportional to the tension applied to the cable (**Table 36.3**). The cable is threaded through the crimp, which is held in the jaws of the crimping device. The cable is fed through a locking nut on the end of the crimper. The torque wrench is attached to a locking gear that winds the cable around a post. The torque wrench has a ratchet mechanism

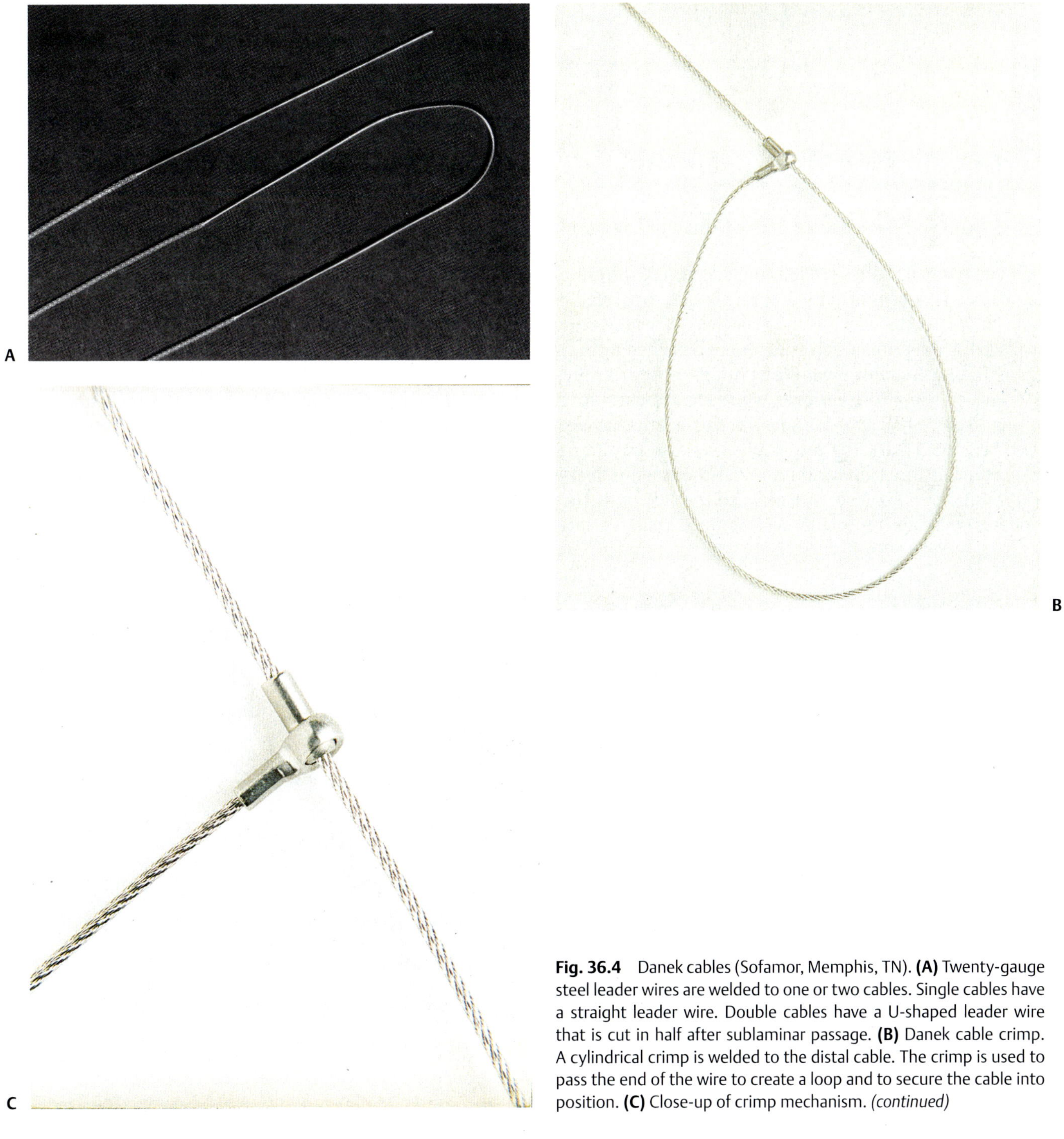

Fig. 36.4 Danek cables (Sofamor, Memphis, TN). **(A)** Twenty-gauge steel leader wires are welded to one or two cables. Single cables have a straight leader wire. Double cables have a U-shaped leader wire that is cut in half after sublaminar passage. **(B)** Danek cable crimp. A cylindrical crimp is welded to the distal cable. The crimp is used to pass the end of the wire to create a loop and to secure the cable into position. **(C)** Close-up of crimp mechanism. *(continued)*

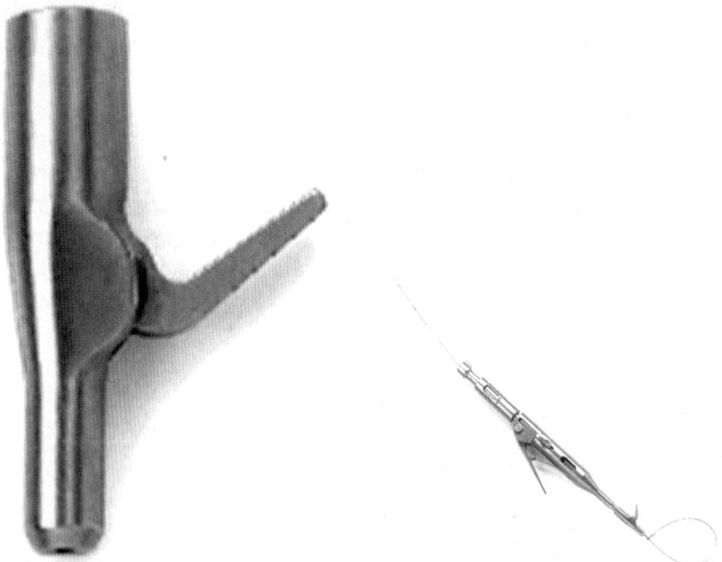

D E

Fig. 36.4 *(continued)* **(D,E)** Temporary crimp allows cable tension to be adjusted before the crimp is fixated permanently. (Reprinted with permission from Barrow Neurological Institute.)

that yields when the desired tension is achieved. The crimping device is squeezed until a spring-loaded bar releases, indicating that the crimp is fully pinched. After the crimp is placed, the tensioner and crimper are detached from the cable. The excess cable is cut flush with the crimp.

A smaller cylindrical tensioner, which has a ratchet-driven spring-loaded shaft that tensions the cable, also has been used (**Fig. 36.5 A,B**). The leader wire is threaded through the center of the cylindrical unit, and the cable is locked into position with a lever. A handle on the side of the tensioner is depressed repeatedly against the shaft and released to progressively set the wire tension. A scale on the side of the unit displays the cable tension (in pounds). The crimp is pinched and the cable is cut flush with the end of the crimp.

The ability to set the cable tension precisely is valuable because overtightened cables can pull through weak or osteoporotic bone. A torque of 8 to 12 in-lb is recommended for normal laminae,[2,3] and 6 to 8 in-lb are used for facets or weak osteoporotic bone. **Table 36.3** displays the relationship between torque and cable tension.[4]

Danek cables and other wire cables are flexible but should not be bent or kinked. An acute angle weakens the cable and

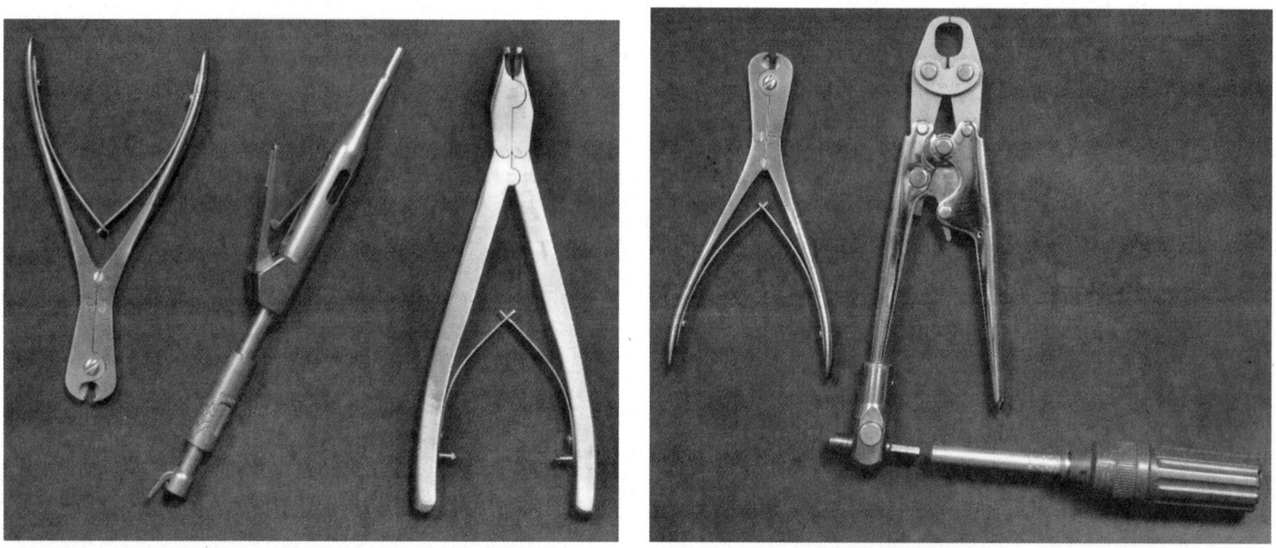

A B

Fig. 36.5 Tensioners for Danek cables (Sofamor, Memphis, TN). **(A)** Cable cutter, tensioner, and crimper (*left to right*). **(B)** Cable cutter and combined tensioner-crimper, and torque wrench (*left to right*). (Reprinted with permission from Barrow Neurological Institute.)

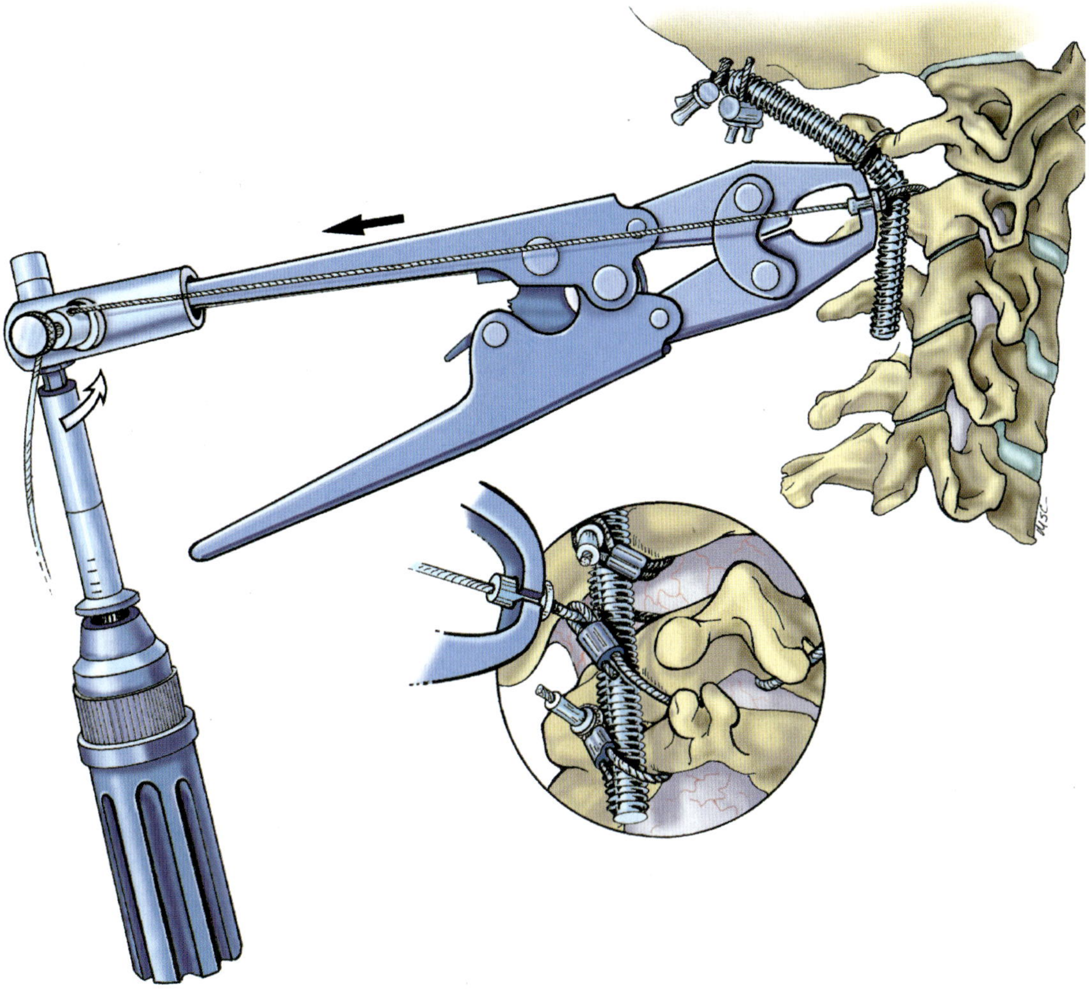

Fig. 36.6 Cables are applied with a combined torque wrench, tensioner, and crimper. The cables are used to secure a threaded Steinmann pin for occipitocervical fusion. (Reprinted with permission from Barrow Neurological Institute.)

creates a stress riser where the cable can break. The cables are strong under static and dynamic mechanical loading conditions.

Danek cables have a maximum yield strength 2.85 to 2.94 times greater than double 0.05-inch stainless steel wire loops. In fatigue tests, steel cables require 6 to 22 times more cycles to failure than stainless steel wires.[4]

Titanium cables have failure mechanisms different from steel cables.[2] Steel cables are stronger than titanium. Steel cables tend to break under relatively high loads. Titanium cables can fail under high loads because the crimp can slip or the cables can break. In general, we reserve titanium cables for tumor patients or when postoperative magnetic resonance imaging (MRI) is needed. A satisfactory myelogram and computed tomography (CT) scan can still be obtained with steel cables present.

Table 36.3 Cable Tension for Danek Cables*

Torque (in-lb)	Cable Tension (lbs × 1–2 lbs)
2	10
4	20
6	30
8	40
10	50

*Data supplied by Sofamor Danek, Inc.
Source: Sofamor Danek Medical, Inc., Memphis, TN. Reprinted with permission.

Sof'wire

Sof'wire is a braided cable (Codman, Raynham, MA) with 133 wires in an array of 19 strands with 7 wires per strand. Sof'wire has a narrower diameter than Danek cables (**Table 36.2**) and is more flexible than Danek cables.

The Sof'wire has a flexible tip rather than a stiff leader. The crimping mechanism differs from the Danek cable (**Fig. 36.7**). The crimp is a hollow cylinder through which the cable is fed. After the Sof'wire is passed or positioned, the ends of the cable are wrapped into the locking gear of a plastic tensioner device. The tensioner is twisted with a

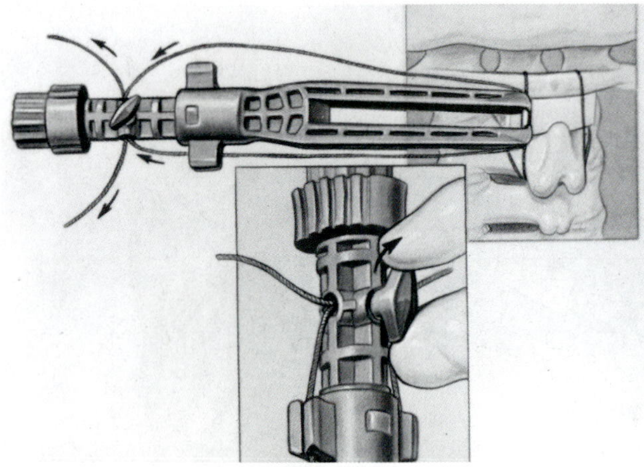

A

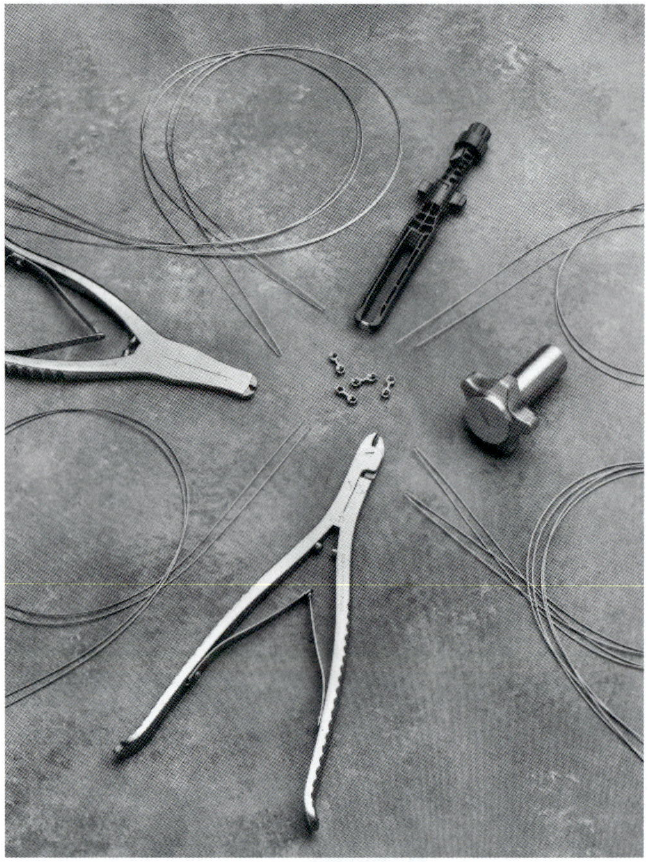

B

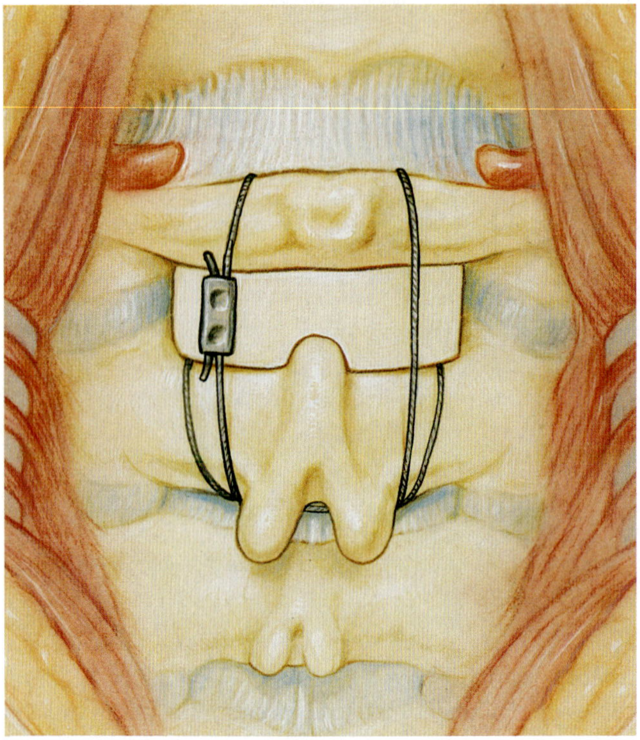

C

Fig. 36.7 Sof'wire (Codman, Raynham, MA). **(A)** Cables are passed through a cylindrical crimp and locked onto the plastic tensioner device with a screw mechanism. The cable is wrapped around the shaft of the tensioner using a steel hand wrench. **(B)** Tools for inserting Sof'wire cables. **(C)** The cable and crimp used for a C1-C2 interspinous fusion. (Reprinted with permission from Codman, Inc.)

hand wrench to remove slack from the cable to progressively set the tension. The crimp is squeezed with a separate crimping tool to pinch the metal crimp and to bind the cable strands. Excess cable is cut flush with the crimp. No torque wrench or tension measuring device is used to assess tension with this cable system. However, tension can be assessed clinically by palpating the cable.

Biomechanical testing has compared Sof'wire to monofilament wire. The flexibility, tensile strength, and fatigue characteristics of single loops of Codman Sof'wire cable (diameter, 0.034 in); 20-gauge (diameter, 0.032 in); 18-gauge (diameter, 0.040 in); and 16-gauge (diameter, 0.050 in) monofilament wire were determined. Stainless steel Sof'wire was 60 times more flexible than 20-gauge monofilament wire and had a higher tensile strength than 20- and 18-gauge wire. When these cables failed, they tended to break at the crimp. In comparison, the monofilament wires failed by unraveling and elongating. They failed at the beginning of the first twist of the wire.

Operative Techniques

Spinous Process Wiring

Spinous process wires can be used to fixate single or multiple cervical motion segments.[5–8] A hole is made in the center of the base of the spinous process with a bone awl or a drill. The hole is positioned at the junction of the spinous processes and laminae with a wide margin of bone preserved adjacent to the hole to resist wire pullout. The hole is completed with a towel clip or a Lewin clamp. The end of a cable or wire is passed through this hole. The wire is looped beneath the inferior adjacent spinous process or passed through a similar hole in the adjacent spinous process (**Fig. 36.8A–D**).

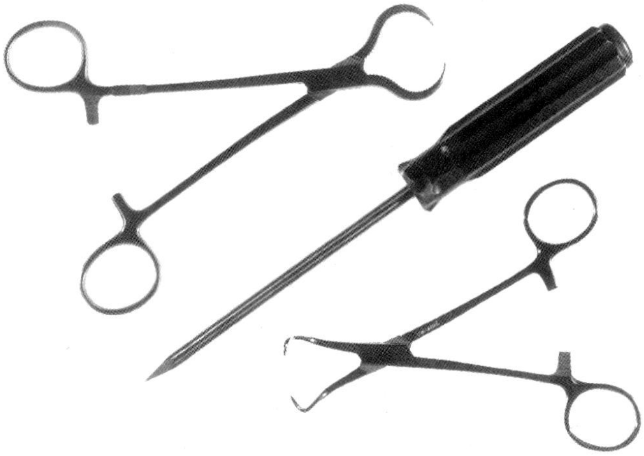
A

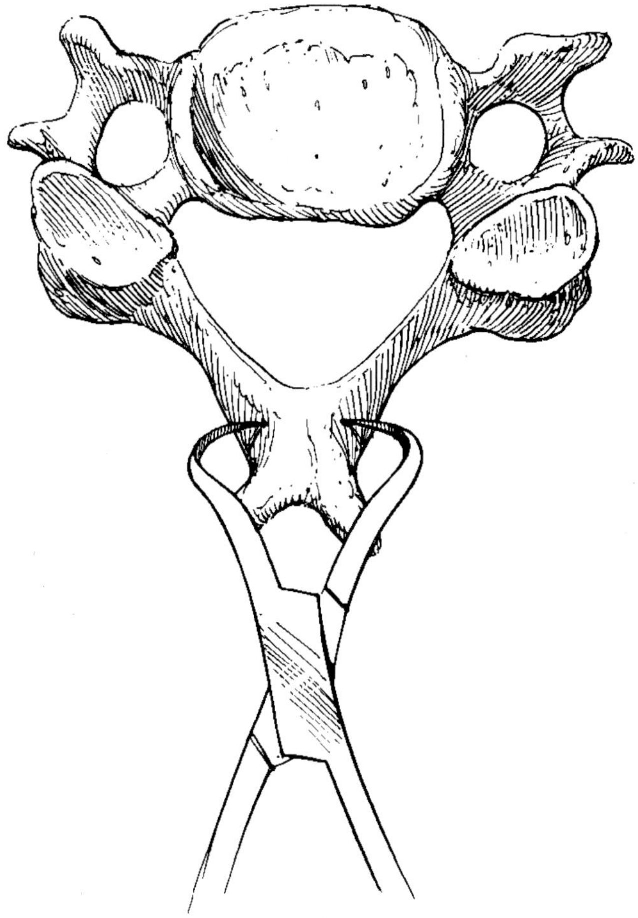
B

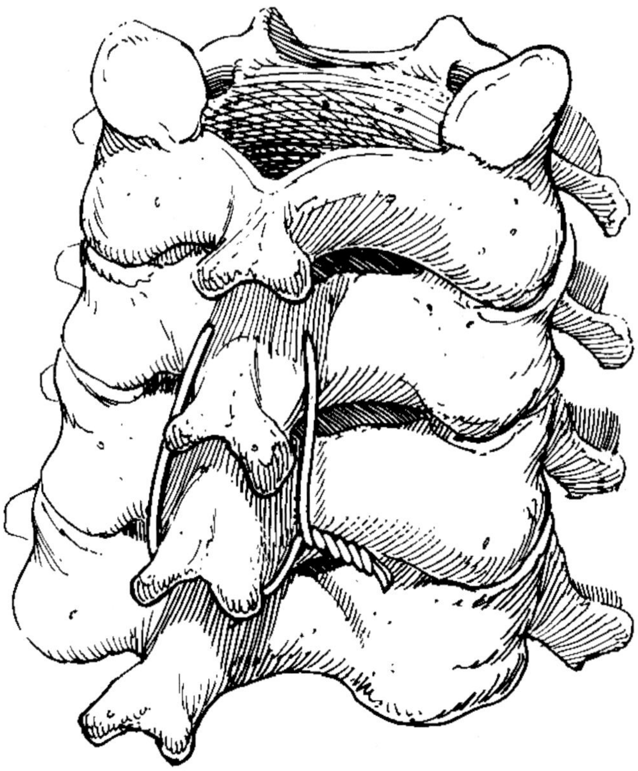
C

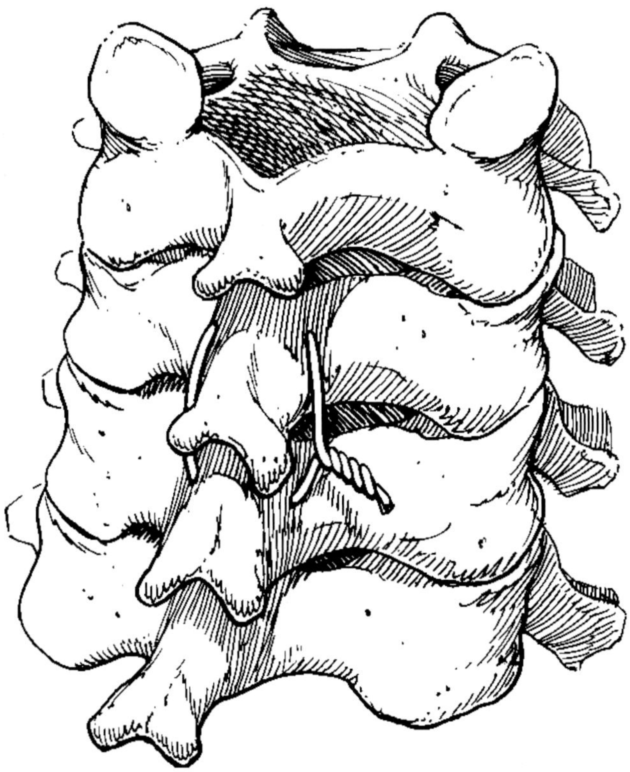
D

Fig. 36.8 Spinous process wiring techniques. **(A)** Tools to create holes in the spinous processes: Lewin clamp, bone awl, and a towel clip (*top to bottom*). **(B)** A hole is made in the spinous process with a towel clip or Lewin clamp. **(C)** The wire is looped beneath the inferior adjacent spinous process. **(D)** The wire also can fixate the inferior vertebrae through a hole in the adjacent spinous process. *(continued)*

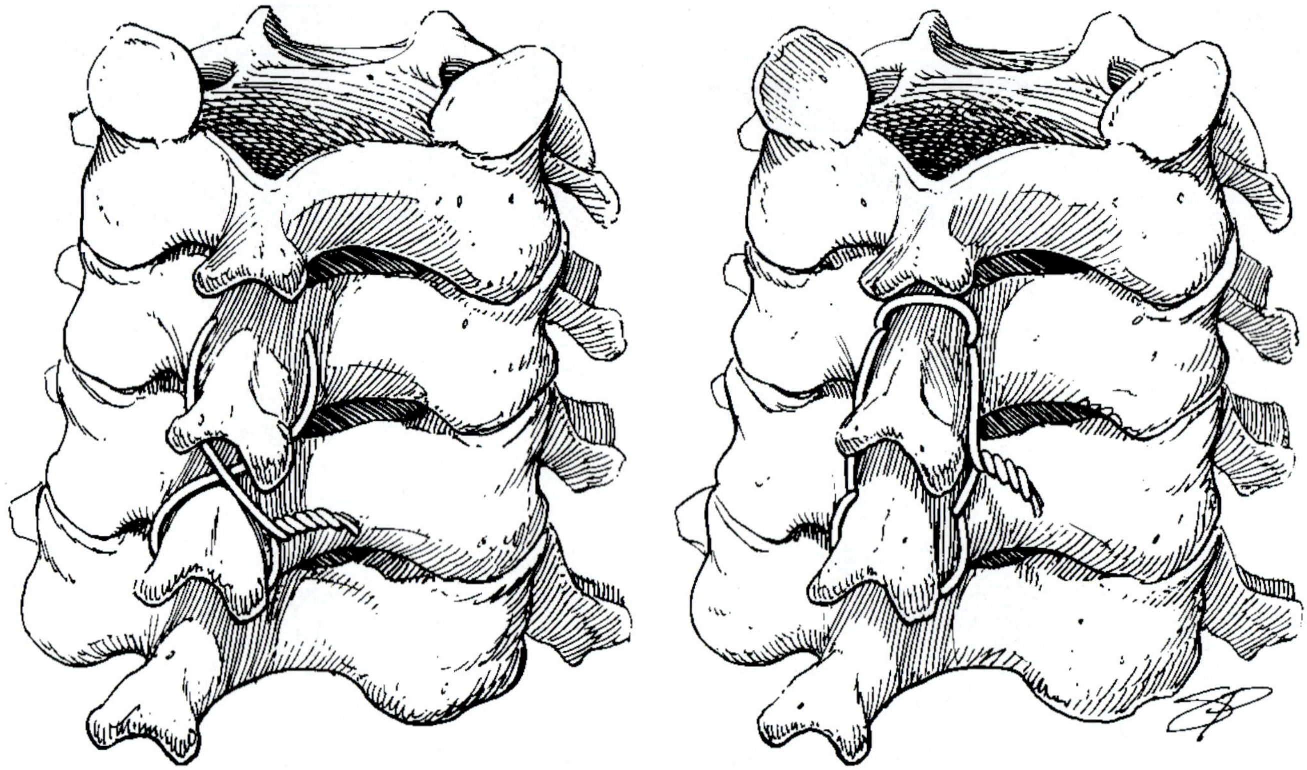

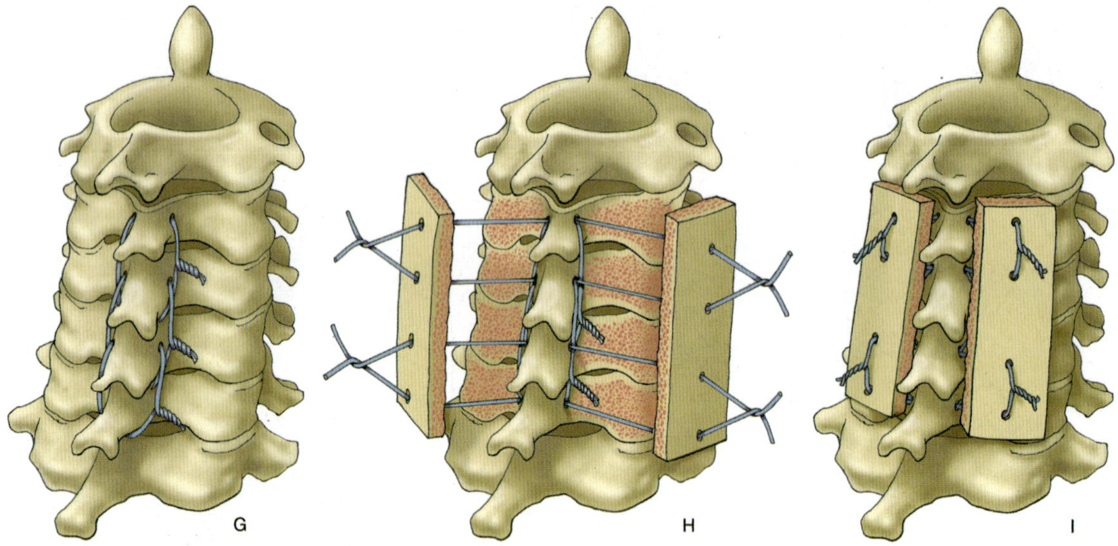

Fig. 36.8 *(continued)* **(E)** A figure-eight configuration can help resist axial rotation. **(F)** Looping the wire around the distal bone surfaces of the spinous processes can help resist wire pullout. **(G–I)** Bohlman triple wire technique. Segmentally wired bone struts are added to the spinous process wires to improve the mechanical fixation. (Reprinted with permission from Barrow Neurological Institute.)

A simple loop or "figure eight" of wire can be created to wire the segments together (**Fig. 36.8E**). The wire also can be wrapped around the distal cortical bone of the spinous process to prevent pullout and to increase the fixation strength (**Fig. 36.8F**). The interspinous and supraspinous ligaments are preserved at levels adjacent to the fused segments.

Spinous process wires offer a safe, easy method of providing a tension band. They avoid the risks associated with sublaminar instrumentation.[9] However they do not resist extension, weakly inhibit rotation and lateral bending, and cannot be used after a laminectomy.[5,10–13] The strength of spinous process wires can be augmented by attaching segmentally fixated bone struts with additional wires passed through the spinous processes (**Fig. 36.8G–I**).

Facet Wiring

Facet wires are placed into the inferior articular facets of the cervical lateral masses.[7,8,14–16] The facet joint surface is opened with a small curette and is held open with a Penfield dissector (**Fig. 36.9A**). A drill hole is placed through the inferior facet into the facet joint. Twenty- or 22-gauge wires are passed through the holes. The facet wires can be used to attach bone struts or metal implants to the vertebrae (**Fig. 36.9B**). Facet-to-spinous process wiring also can be performed (**Fig. 36.9C**).

As the facets are relatively thin, wires can pull the facets out if enough force is applied, if the wires are overtightened, or if the bone is soft or osteoporotic. Facet wires are an excellent alternative after a laminectomy has been performed. However, facet wires are weaker than sublaminar or spinous process wires.[10–12] If facet wires are used, a rigid orthosis may need to be considered to supplement the wiring until a fusion occurs.

Sublaminar Wiring

Sublaminar wires can be used to fixate adjacent motion segments or to wire struts or implants to the vertebrae (**Fig. 36.10**).[2,7,9,16–18] Sublaminar wires carry a risk of neurological injury especially at the middle and lower cervical levels. It is safest to pass wire beneath only one laminae. Spanning multiple laminae during sublaminar wire passage markedly increases the risk of neurological injury.[9] Precise technique and cautious maneuvers are required to avoid complications. Compressive pathology should be removed and the dura should be visualized directly before sublaminar wires are passed. The ligamentum flavum is removed from the upper and lower surfaces of the laminae (**Fig. 36.10A**). Small laminotomies in the medial edges of the laminae facilitate wire passage. However, the bone should not be weakened with an extensive laminotomy (**Fig. 36.10B**). When neural compression exists and sublaminar wires are needed for fixation, a decompression should be performed first! Passing sublaminar wires in a stenotic canal can cause neurological injury.[19]

A wire passer or heavy silk suture can help position and guide the wire beneath the undersurface of the lamina (**Fig. 36.10C**). The wire is bent to conform to the "C" shape of the laminae. Sublaminar wires should be passed with a two-handed process, simultaneously feeding and pulling the wire to avoid displacing the wire or manipulating the unstable vertebrae. The wire should hug the undersurface of the bone during sublaminar passage. After wires are positioned, the ends are positioned across the bone surface to avoid displacing a loop of wire against the spinal cord. This technique is mechanically strong and effective but has risks and should be used with caution and precise technique.

Occipital Wiring

The occiput can be fixated with wires or cables. The bone surfaces are anchored using burr holes or holes drilled tangentially into the midline occipital crest. The bone near the base of the occiput is wired after enlarging the rim of the foramen magnum and making burr holes 5- to 10-mm above the foramen magnum. The dura is separated from the inner table of bone before the occipital wires are passed. The complete details of occipital wiring are discussed in Chapter 47.

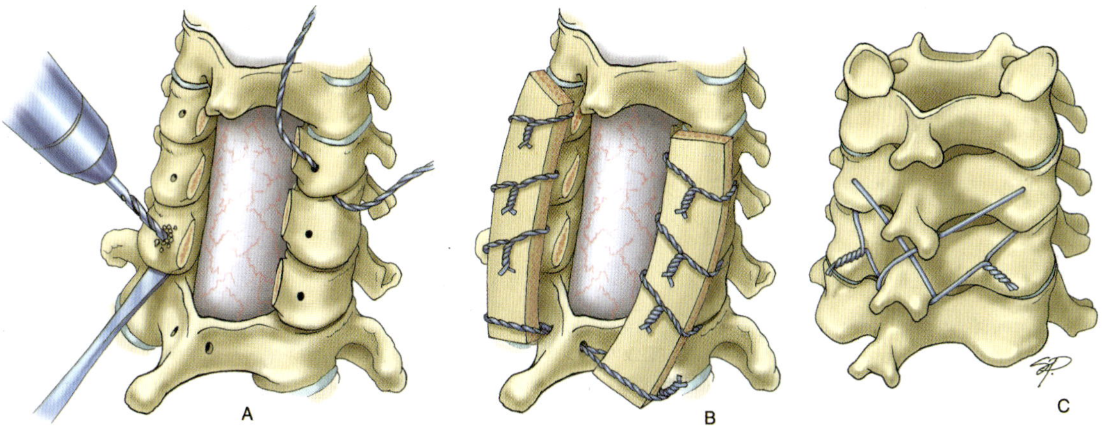

Fig. 36.9 Facet wiring techniques. **(A)** The facet joints are opened and holes are drilled into the facets. Wires are passed through the holes. **(B)** The wires are used to fixate bone grafts to the facet surfaces. **(C)** Facet-to-spinous process wiring can be used to immobilize a motion segment. (Reprinted with permission from Barrow Neurological Institute.)

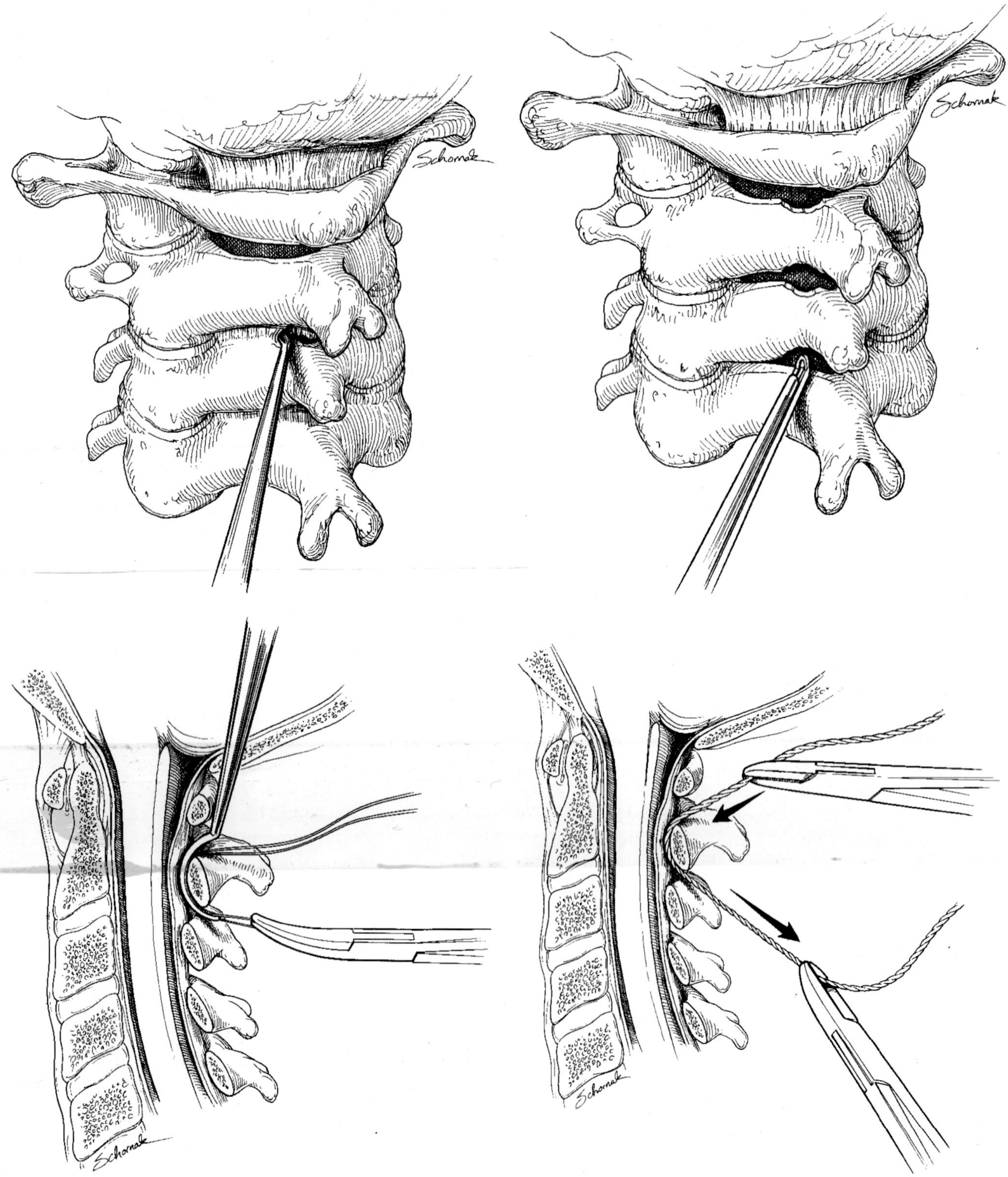

A B C D

Fig. 36.10 Sublaminar wiring techniques. **(A)** The ligamentum flavum is removed with curettes to visualize the dura. **(B)** Small laminectomies are made to make room for wire passage. **(C)** A heavy suture or a wire guide is used to feed the wire so it hugs the bone surface. **(D)** A two-handed process is used to feed and pull the wire simultaneously to control its movement precisely to avoid neurological injury. (Reprinted with permission from Barrow Neurological Institute.)

Conclusion

Wiring techniques have been used extensively for cervical spinal internal fixation and have the advantage of being familiar to most spinal surgeons. These techniques can be used relatively safely if details are given close attention. The biomechanical features of the injury and the biomechanics of the fixation technique need to be considered carefully. Wiring techniques are unsatisfactory for three-column spine injuries or when the bone is osteoporotic, weak, or extensively destroyed. These circumstances require a supplementary halo brace or an alternative fixation technique.

Wire affects a tension band for the posterior surface of the spine that is relatively strong in preventing flexion but that weakly resists other cervical motions (i.e., rotation, lateral bending, and extension). The mechanical fixation can be improved by using segmentally fixated bone struts, which add multiplanar control of motion. The merits, limitations, and mechanical effects of wires must be remembered to plan rational treatment strategies to fixate unstable cervical segments.

References

1. Taitsman JP, Saha S. Tensile strength of wire-reinforced bone cement and twisted stainless-steel wire. J Bone Joint Surg Am 1977; 59(3):419–425
2. Songer MN, Spencer DL, Meyer PR Jr, Jayaraman G. The use of sublaminar cables to replace Luque wires. Spine 1991;16(8, Suppl): S418–S421
3. Huhn SL, Wolf AL, Ecklund J. Posterior spinal osteosynthesis for cervical fracture/dislocation using a flexible multistrand cable system: technical note. Neurosurgery 1991;29(6):943–946
4. Danek Medical Inc. Songer cable system. Memphis, TN: Danek Medical, Inc.; 1990,
5. White AA III, Panjabi MM. Clinical Biomechanics of the Spine. Philadelphia, PA: JB Lippincott; 1978:191–271
6. Rogers WA. Fractures and dislocations of the cervical spine; an end-result study. J Bone Joint Surg Am 1957;39-A(2):341–376
7. Stauffer ES. Wiring techniques of the posterior cervical spine for the treatment of trauma. Orthopedics 1988;11(11):1543–1548
8. Robinson RA, Southwick WO. Surgical approaches to the cervical spine. In: American Academy of Orthopedic Surgeons, ed. Instructional Course Lectures. St. Louis, MO: CV Mosby; 1960:299–330
9. Geremia GK, Kim KS, Cerullo L, Calenoff L. Complications of sublaminar wiring. Surg Neurol 1985;23(6):629–635
10. Ulrich C, Woersdoerfer O, Kalff R, Claes L, Wilke HJ. Biomechanics of fixation systems to the cervical spine. Spine 1991;16(3, Suppl):S4–S9
11. Pelker RR, Duranceau JS, Panjabi MM. Cervical spine stabilization. A three-dimensional, biomechanical evaluation of rotational stability, strength, and failure mechanisms. Spine 1991;16(2): 117–122
12. Sutterlin CE III, McAfee PC, Warden KE, Rey RM Jr, Farey ID. A biomechanical evaluation of cervical spinal stabilization methods in a bovine model. Static and cyclical loading. Spine 1988;13(7): 795–802
13. Fielding JW, Hawkins RJ, Ratzan SA. Spine fusion for atlanto-axial instability. J Bone Joint Surg Am 1976;58(3):400–407
14. Callahan RA, Johnson RM, Margolis RN, Keggi KJ, Albright JA, Southwick WO. Cervical facet fusion for control of instability following laminectomy. J Bone Joint Surg Am 1977;59(8): 991–1002
15. Garfin SR, Moore MR, Marshall LF. A modified technique for cervical facet fusions. Clin Orthop Relat Res 1988;230(230):149–153
16. Abdu WA, Bohlman HH. Techniques of subaxial posterior cervical spine fusions: an overview. Orthopedics 1992;15(3):287–295
17. Brooks AL, Jenkins EB. Atlanto-axial arthrodesis by the wedge compression method. J Bone Joint Surg Am 1978;60(3):279–284
18. Griswold DM, Albright JA, Schiffman E, Johnson R, Southwick W. Atlanto-axial fusion for instability. J Bone Joint Surg Am 1978;60(3):285–292
19. Hamblen DL. Occipito-cervical fusion. Indications, technique and results. J Bone Joint Surg Br 1967;49(1):33–45

37 General Principles of Spinal Screw Fixation

Curtis A. Dickman and Volker K. H. Sonntag

Internal spinal fixation can be achieved with wire and bone grafts, cables, clamps, screws, plates, rods, or hooks.[1–10] The ideal system would provide immediate rigid fixation with few risks. It would be nonfatiguing, promote fusion, and preserve normal motion segments. Screw fixation provides diverse alternatives for fixating the cervical spine. Screws or screw plates are indicated for internal spinal fixation when wire cannot be used, when wire is inadequate to fixate the spine, or when a biomechanically rigid fixation is needed. The rate and strength of spinal fusions are improved quantitatively and qualitatively as the rigidity of implants increases,[11] and screws offer the advantage of providing immediate rigid fixation of spinal segments.[12–15]

In the cervical spine, screws have been used for odontoid fixation, atlantoaxial facet fixation, C2-pedicle fixation, anterior vertebral body screw-plate fixation, posterior lateral mass screw-plate fixation, and posterior occipitocervical screw-plate fixation. Screws are used either to fasten metal plates onto bone or as lag screws to hold together fragments of bone. Both techniques have merit in the cervical spine. This chapter reviews the fundamental principles of screw fixation for the cervical spine.

■ Types of Vertebral Screws

Surgical bone screws are usually constructed of stainless steel, pure titanium, or alloyed titanium. Screws should be nontoxic, biocompatible, strong, and noncorrosive. Steel consists of a mixture of iron, chromium, and nickel and has traditionally been used for bone implants and screws. Pure titanium, or an alloy of titanium, aluminum, and vanadium, is also popular for implants. Titanium and alloyed titanium are safe, strong, and malleable. Titanium is resistant to corrosion and is inert and biocompatible. Titanium has 90% of the strength of steel.[16] Titanium, however, is notch sensitive, cracks when bent, and may fatigue and break more readily than steel. Titanium has a significant advantage over steel—it produces minimal artifact with magnetic resonance imaging (MRI), thereby allowing postoperative assessment of the spinal cord. When using titanium implants, one should consider the mechanical stresses placed on the implants, as well as the possible need for postoperative radiographic evaluation.

Portions of this chapter are reprinted from Dickman CA, Sonntag VKH, Marcotte P. Techniques of screw fixation of the cervical spine. *BNI Quarterly* 1992;8(2):9–26; 1993;9(4):27–39.

Screw Components

Screws are composed of a head, a tip, a shaft, and a threaded portion. The major diameter refers to the widest diameter of the screw shaft (i.e., diameter of the threads). The minor screw diameter, also called the core or inner diameter, refers to the diameter of the shaft beneath the threads. Screws can be characterized as cortical or cancellous screws, lag screws, fragment screws, self-tapping or non–self-tapping screws, cannulated or noncannulated screws, solid or hollow screws, or locking screws.

Self-Tapping and Non–Self-Tapping Screws

Self-tapping and non–self-tapping screws are differentiated by the design of their threads and screw tips. They require different surgical techniques for insertion (**Fig. 37.1**). Both types of screws require drilling a pilot hole in the bone to create a tract for the screw. The diameter of the pilot hole should match the minor diameter of the screw. Self-tapping screws have sharp threads and a sharp tip with a distal cutting channel. The sharp self-tapping screws cut their path into the bone as they are inserted. The threads of non–self-tapping screws are less sharp than those of self-tapping screws. The tip is blunt and has no cutting flute. Before non–self-tapping screws are inserted, the screw thread pattern is cut into the bone using a tap, which is inserted into the pilot hole. The width and pitch of the threads of the tap correspond to the thread characteristics of the screw.

Non–self-tapping screws (unlike self-tapping screws) can usually be removed and reinserted without a high risk of inadvertently creating a new tract. Theoretically, the purchase of self-tapping screws in the bone is slightly less secure than that of non–self-tapping screws. However, no proven biomechanical advantage supports tapping a screw site.[14,17–19]

Cortical and Cancellous Bone Screws

Cortical bone screws are usually non–self-tapping screws, have relatively narrow threads, and are usually threaded along their entire length (**Fig. 37.1**). They are available in a variety of diameters and lengths, and each size has its corresponding drill bit and tap. The diameter of the drill bit corresponds to the minor diameter of the screw; the diameter of the tap corresponds to the major diameter of the screw.

Cancellous bone screws can be non–self-tapping or self-tapping screws. Their minor diameter is small and their thread is wide and deep. These dimensions increase the holding power of the screw in trabecular bone. Cancellous

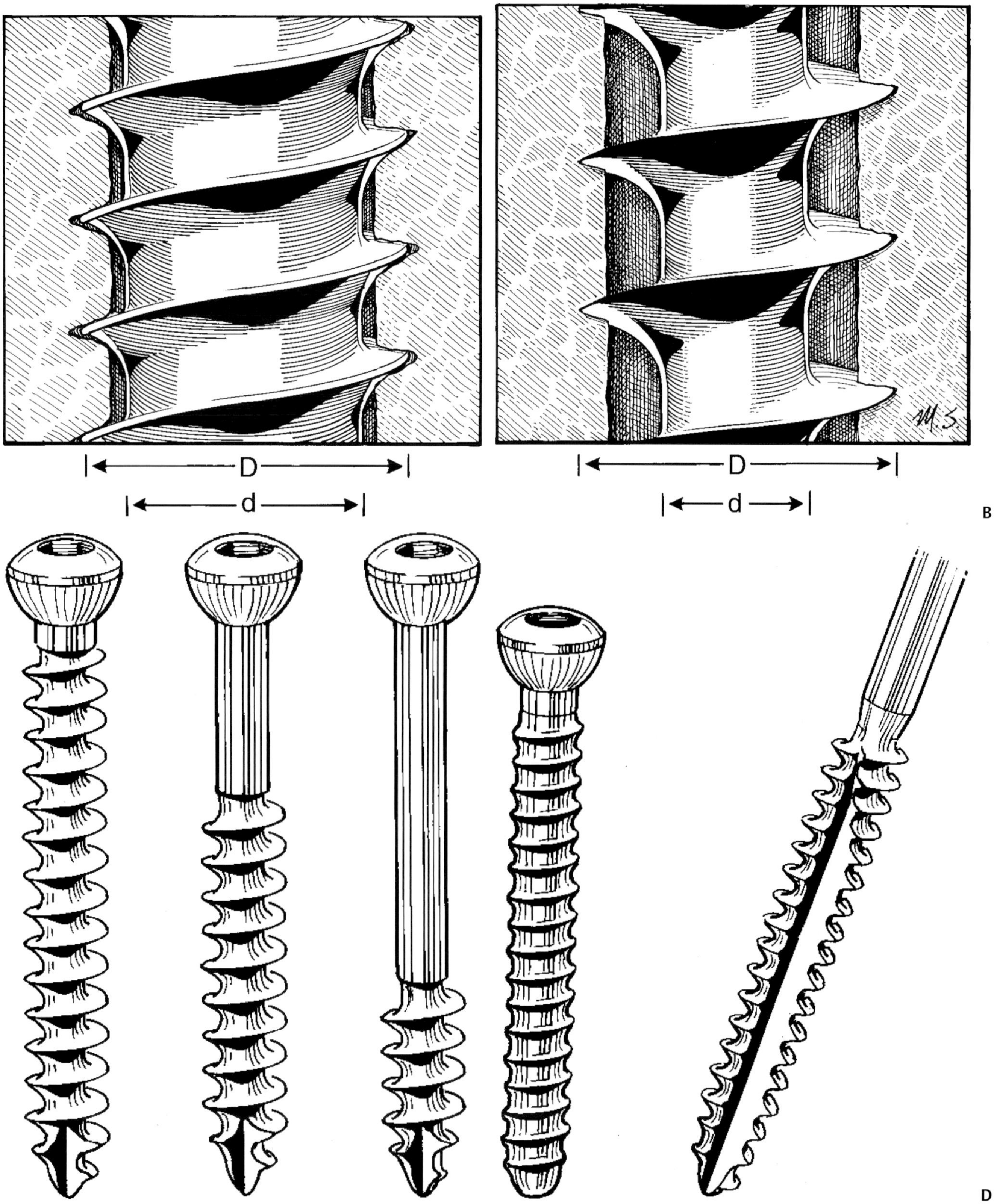

Fig. 37.1 **(A)** Screw thread profiles for cortical and **(B)** cancellous bone screws. Cortical and cancellous screws differ primarily in the design of the screw threads and tips and in the methods of insertion. **(C)** Self-tapping screws have a sharp tip with a distal cutting channel and sharp, wide threads. They can be inserted into a pilot hole without tapping the bone. Self-tapping screws are usually used in cancellous bone or in bone with thin cortices. **(D)** Non–self-tapping screws have a dull tip and narrower threads and are usually used for bone with thick, dense cortices. The pilot hole must be tapped to cut threads into the bone before the non–self-tapping screw is inserted. (Reprinted with permission from Barrow Neurological Institute.)

bone screws have either partially or fully threaded shafts. Fully threaded screws are used for attaching plates to bone or as lag screws; partially threaded screws are used as lag screws. Engaging the tip of the screw in a distal bone cortex increases the holding power of cancellous screws.[16,18]

Lag Screws

In the spine, lag screws are used to fixate odontoid fractures and the C1-C2 facets. Lag screws restore structural continuity. They place adjacent bone fragments under compression and thereby facilitate healing. The threads of a lag screw should engage the distal bone but not the proximal bone fragment. When the threads engage only the distal fragment, the bone fragments can be reduced and compressed. As the screw is tightened, the lag effect (i.e., compression) is generated as long as the functioning screw threads do not cross the fracture line (**Fig. 37.2**).

Screw purchase in the proximal bone is avoided by one of two mechanisms. Either the proximal screw shaft must have

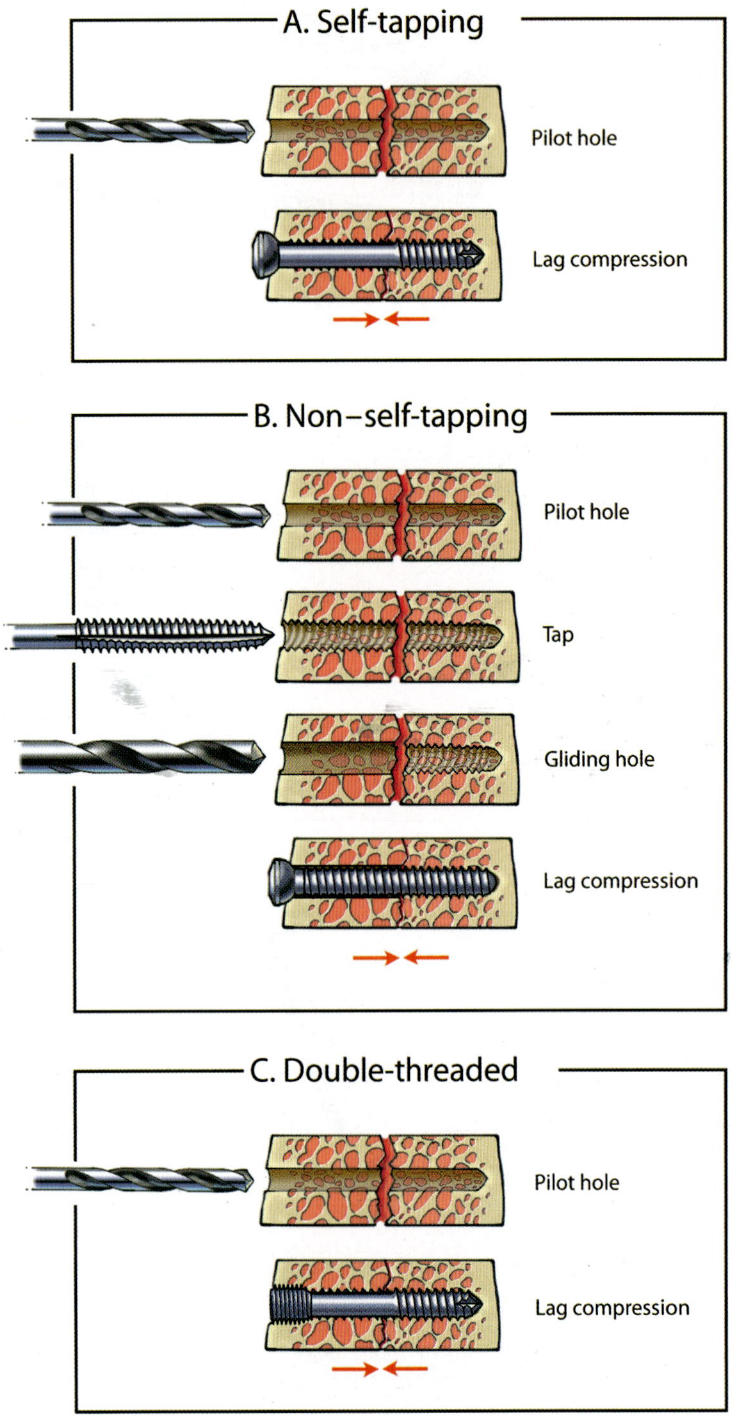

Fig. 37.2 Techniques for lag screw insertion. **(A)** Self-tapping screws are inserted directly into the pilot hole. **(B)** With fully threaded screws, a pilot hole is drilled and the hole is tapped. The proximal bone is overdrilled to create a gliding hole that is wider than the screw diameter. The screw threads purchase only the distal bone and reduce the fracture. **(C)** Double-threaded compression screws are inserted directly into a pilot hole. No threads cross the fracture line. The pitch of the threads on the proximal and distal ends of the screws differs so that when the screw is inserted, the fracture is reduced and a lag effect is created. (Reprinted with permission from Barrow Neurological Institute.)

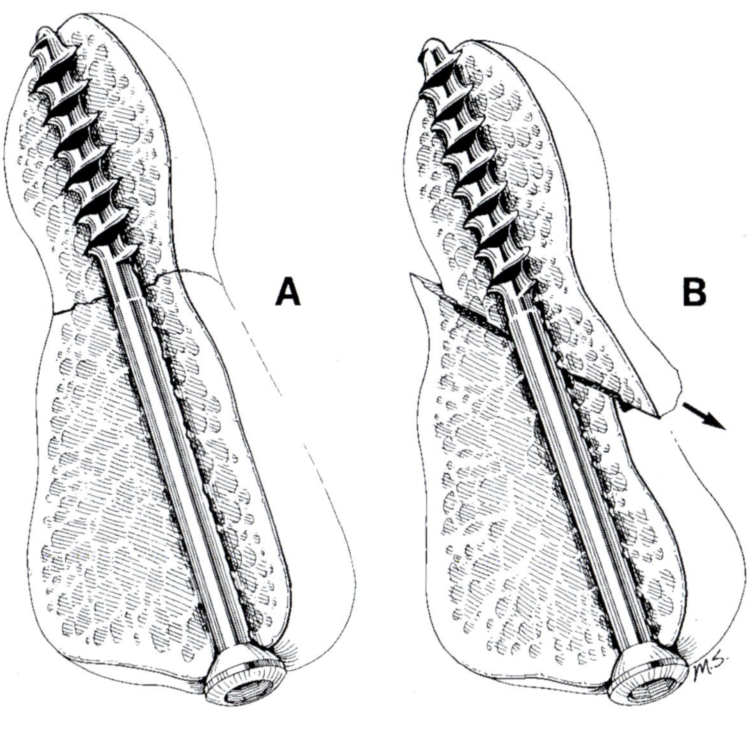

Fig. 37.3 **(A)** Lag screws are ideally inserted at right angles to the fracture line. This technique is best for transverse fractures across the base of the dens (i.e., odontoid type II fractures). **(B)** Lag screw reduction of an oblique odontoid fracture can theoretically cause malalignment because shearing forces are generated during reduction. If an oblique odontoid fracture is fixated, the fracture should be anatomically reduced with postural or open techniques prior to inserting a screw. (Reprinted with permission from Barrow Neurological Institute.)

no threads, or the hole in the proximal bone must be drilled wider than the major diameter of the screw. Such a wide proximal hole is called a gliding hole (**Fig. 37.2**). The gliding hole lag technique is used with fully threaded screws.

Partially threaded screws with threads confined to the distal portion of the screw provide another method for lag screw fixation. Lag screw fixation can also be achieved by using double-threaded compression screws.[20,21] The pitch of the proximal and distal screw threads differs, so that the distal fragments are compressed as the screws are tightened (**Fig. 37.2C**).

Lag screws should be inserted at a right angle to the fracture line. Otherwise, shearing forces can shift the bone fragments when the screw is tightened (**Fig. 37.3**). Oblique fractures of the odontoid are particularly susceptible to this problem. When possible, fractures should be reduced and alignment restored before a lag screw is placed.

Cannulated Screws

Cannulated screw systems consist of a long Kirschner wire (K-wire), a drill guide, a hollow drill, a hollow tap, a hollow screw driver, and hollow screws.[16,22] The thin, 1.2-mm diameter K-wires permit screws to be placed precisely within small bones with minimal injury. They are particularly useful for odontoid or C1-C2 facet fixation. The thin, end-threaded K-wires serve to guide the placement of the screws. The K-wires are inserted with a high-speed, reversible, pneumatic drill to the desired depth and trajectory in the vertebrae (**Fig. 37.4**). Cannulated non–self-tapping or self-tapping screws can be used. The hollow drills, instruments, and screws are threaded sequentially over the K-wire so that they maintain the intended trajectory into the bone. Power tools (such as drills) are usually not inserted over the K-wire because they can bind and advance the K-wire intradurally. Self-tapping cannulated screws can be inserted directly over the K-wire without drilling a pilot hole. After the screw is inserted, the K-wire is removed.

If the K-wire is misdirected, it can be repositioned easily without affecting the screw purchase site. In comparison, a wide screw hole that is malpositioned can destroy the purchase site if the bone adjacent to the screw site is weakened. The risk of potential inadvertent intradural advancement of the K-wire can be prevented using several appropriate techniques. The techniques for cannulated screw insertion are reviewed in detail in Chapter 39.

Biomechanical Principles of Screw Fixation

Although screw fixation techniques for the cervical spine typically provide more rigid and stronger fixation than wire,[12,15,23] these methods do have limitations. Their weakest component is the bone-screw thread interface. The holding power of a screw is a function of two variables: the design of the screw and the characteristics of the bone adjacent to the screw. Holding power depends on changes induced in the bone by the trauma of insertion, the reaction of the bone to the implant, and resorption and remodeling of bone as a result of healing.[18]

Pullout strength depends on the purchase of the screw within the bone. Fixation will be inadequate and likely to fail if the bone adjacent to a screw is diseased, fractured, softened, or weakened. Screws that purchase solid cortical bone will be more rigidly fixed than screws in cancellous trabecular bone. Besides bone quality, the pullout strength

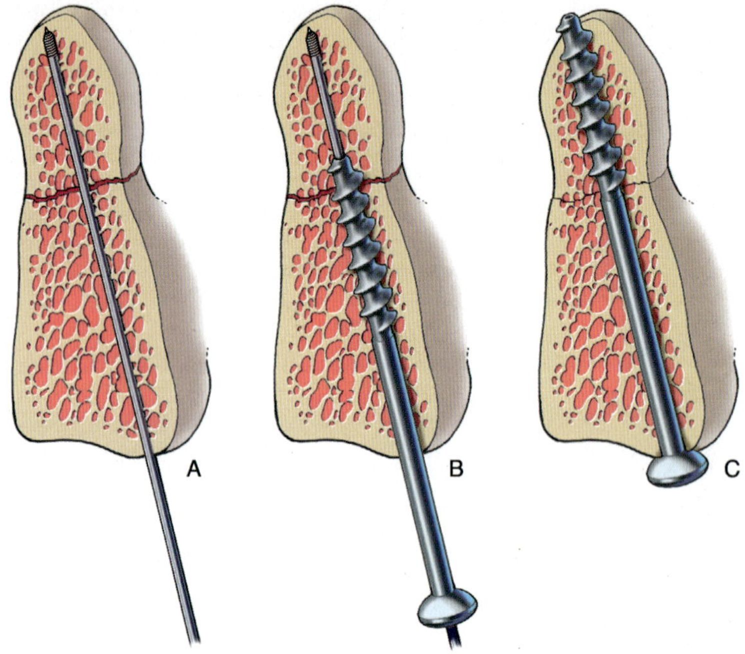

Fig. 37.4 Technique of cannulated screw insertion for fixation of an odontoid fracture. **(A)** A threaded K-wire is inserted into the dens. Hollow tools and screws are subsequently threaded over the K-wire into the bone. **(B)** A self-drilling, self-tapping, partially threaded lag screw is placed over the K-wire. The screw threads should engage only the distal bone fragment. **(C)** The tip of the screw should barely penetrate the tip of the dens. The K-wire is removed. (Reprinted with permission from Barrow Neurological Institute.)

of screws is determined by the depth of screw insertion and by the major screw diameter.[14,17–19,24,25] A direct linear relationship exists between screw length and pullout strength. Longer, wider screws resist pullout more than narrow, shallow screws.[14,17]

Thorough irrigation during drilling will cool the bone and minimize subsequent screw loosening. Excessive heating of the bone during drilling will damage the bone and can cause its resorption around the screw. Screws in the cervical spine should be "finger tight" (i.e., use two fingers for twisting when tightening the screwdriver). Overtightening the screw will strip the screw hole and result in an inadequate screw purchase. If a screw hole becomes stripped, the hole can be filled with cancellous bone or methylmethacrylate to recover a screw purchase. Screws with a wider diameter than regular screws (i.e., rescue screws) are also available to recover a stripped screw hole.

Chronic movements of the neck (i.e., repetitive subfailure cyclic loads) or large single loads may loosen, bend, or break screws. The strength of the metallic implants is particularly important, as metal is susceptible to fatigue and can break with repetitive stress. The bending strength of screws is directly proportional to the third power of the minor screw diameter.[14,17] A twofold increase in the minor diameter produces an eightfold increase in bending strength (**Fig. 37.5**).[13] When screws bend or break, they tend to fail at the site of the first screw thread (i.e., where the shaft and threaded portions join) or at the site of the greatest leverage or stress.[14]

Biomechanical testing of transarticular screw fixation of the C1-C2 facets has shown that this technique is more rigid than C1-C2 wiring techniques. Furthermore, atlantoaxial facet screws resist translation and rotation considerably more than wiring.[12,15,26] The biomechanical properties of cervical fixation devices are discussed fully in Chapter 3.

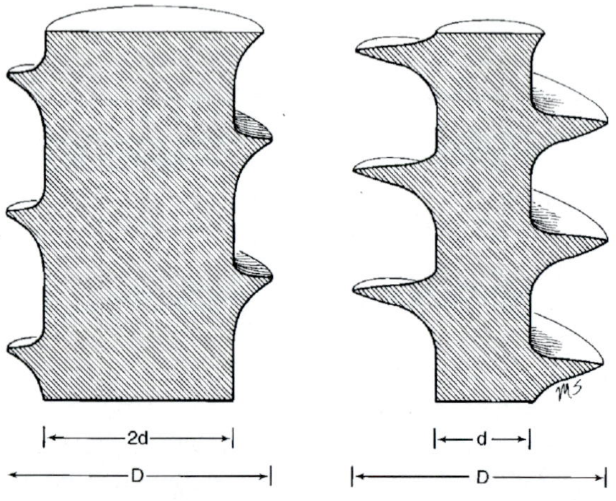

Pullout strength $(^D/_D)^2 = 1$
Bending strength $(^{2d}/_d)^3 = 8$

Fig. 37.5 The bending strength of a screw is directly proportional to the third power of the minor screw diameter (*d*). The pullout strength of a screw is determined by the major diameter (*D*) and by the volume and density of bone beneath the screw threads. A twofold increase in the minor screw diameter increases the bending strength by eightfold. (Reprinted with permission from Barrow Neurological Institute.)

Conclusion

Screw fixation for the upper cervical spine is useful for achieving rigid internal fixation to facilitate bone fusion. Knowledge of the different types of bone screws and basic principles for screw insertion provides a foundation for successful spinal screw application.

Metallic implants are only temporary measures for spinal fixation while an osseous union develops. Long-term stability can be guaranteed only by achieving a fusion. Meticulous preparation of the fusion site is necessary to ensure development of a fusion. Soft tissue must be removed from the fusion site, the fusion bed must be decorticated to expose cancellous bone, and articular surfaces must be obliterated with curettes or drills. Autologous bone grafts are preferred; they should fit precisely and be placed under compression. Although instrumentation must be precise, it is not a substitute for meticulous grafting and fusion methods.[3,4,27,28]

References

1. Aldrich EF, Crow WN, Weber PB, Spagnolia TN. Use of MR imaging-compatible Halifax interlaminar clamps for posterior cervical fusion. J Neurosurg 1991;74(2):185–189
2. Brooks AL, Jenkins EB. Atlanto-axial arthrodesis by the wedge compression method. J Bone Joint Surg Am 1978;60(3):279–284
3. Dickman CA, Douglas RA, Sonntag VKH. Occipitocervical fusion: posterior stabilization of the craniovertebral junction and upper cervical spine. BNI Q 1990;6(2):2–14
4. Dickman CA, Sonntag VKH, Papadopoulos SM, Hadley MN. The interspinous method of posterior atlantoaxial arthrodesis. J Neurosurg 1991;74(2):190–198
5. Holness RO, Huestis WS, Howes WJ, Langille RA. Posterior stabilization with an interlaminar clamp in cervical injuries: technical note and review of the long term experience with the method. Neurosurgery 1984;14(3):318–322
6. Huhn SL, Wolf AL, Ecklund J. Posterior spinal osteosynthesis for cervical fracture/dislocation using a flexible multistrand cable system: technical note. Neurosurgery 1991;29(6):943–946
7. Magerl F, Grob D, Seemann P. Stable dorsal fusion of the cervical spine (C2-Th1) using hook plates. In: Kehr P,Weidner A, eds. Cervical Spine I. New York, NY: Springer-Verlag; 1987:217
8. Ransford AO, Crockard HA, Pozo JL, Thomas NP, Nelson IW. Craniocervical instability treated by contoured loop fixation. J Bone Joint Surg Br 1986;68(2):173–177
9. Sonntag VKH, Dickman CA. High cervical and occipitocervical stabilization. In: American Association of Neurological Surgeons, ed. Operative Atlas of Neurosurgery. Chicago, IL: American Association of Neurological Surgeons; 1991:327–337
10. Sonntag VKH, Dickman CA. Operative management of occipitocervical and atlantoaxial instability. In: Holtzman RN, Farcy J, McCormick P, eds. Spinal Instability. Berlin: Springer-Verlag; 1993:255–294
11. McAfee PC, Farey ID, Sutterlin CE, Gurr KR, Warden KE, Cunningham BW. 1989 Volvo Award in basic science. Device-related osteoporosis with spinal instrumentation. Spine 1989;14(9):919–926
12. Hanson PB, Montesano PX, Sharkey NA, Rauschning W. Anatomic and biomechanical assessment of transarticular screw fixation for atlantoaxial instability. Spine 1991;16(10):1141–1145
13. Kostuik JP, Smith TJ. Pitfalls of biomechanical testing. Spine 1991;16(10):1233–1235
14. Krag MH. Biomechanics of thoracolumbar spinal fixation. A review. Spine 1991;16(3, Suppl):S84–S99
15. Montesano PX, Juach EC, Anderson PA, Benson DR, Hanson PB. Biomechanics of cervical spine internal fixation. Spine 1991;16(3, Suppl):S10–S16
16. Muller ME, Allgower M, Schneider R, et al. Manual of Internal Fixation. Techniques Recommended by the AO-ASIF Group. Berlin: Springer-Verlag; 1991
17. Krag MH, Fredrickson BE, Yuan HA. Spinal instrumentation. In: Weinstein JN, Wiesel SW, eds. The Lumbar Spine. Philadelphia, PA: WB Saunders; 1990:916–940
18. Schatzker J, Sanderson R, Murnaghan JP. The holding power of orthopedic screws in vivo. Clin Orthop Relat Res 1975; 108(108):115–126
19. Sell P, Collins M, Dove J. Pedicle screws: axial pull-out strength in the lumbar spine. Spine 1988;13(9):1075–1076
20. Knoringer P. Double-threaded compression screws for osteosynthesis of acute fractures of the odontoid process. In: Voth D, Glees P, eds. Diseases in the Cranio-Cervical Junction. Anatomical and Pathological Aspects and Detailed Clinical Accounts. Berlin: de Gruyter; 1987:127–136
21. Weidner A. Internal fixation with metal plates and screws. In: Cervical Spine Research Society, ed. The Cervical Spine, 2nd ed. Philadelphia, PA: JB Lippincott; 1989:404–421
22. Etter C, Coscia M, Jaberg H, Aebi M. Direct anterior fixation of dens fractures with a cannulated screw system. Spine 1991;16(3, Suppl):S25–S32
23. Sutterlin CE III, McAfee PC, Warden KE, Rey RM Jr, Farey ID. A biomechanical evaluation of cervical spinal stabilization methods in a bovine model. Static and cyclical loading. Spine 1988;13(7):795–802
24. Skinner R, Maybee J, Transfeldt E, Venter R, Chalmers W. Experimental pullout testing and comparison of variables in transpedicular screw fixation. A biomechanical study. Spine 1990;15(3):195–201
25. Smith TJ. In vitro spinal biomechanics. Experimental methods and apparatus. Spine 1991;16(10):1204–1210
26. Grob D, Crisco JJ III, Panjabi MM, Wang P, Dvorak J. Biomechanical evaluation of four different posterior atlantoaxial fixation techniques. Spine 1992;17(5):480–490
27. Fielding JW. The status of arthrodesis of the cervical spine. J Bone Joint Surg Am 1988;70(10):1571–1574
28. Kaufman HH, Jones E. The principles of bony spinal fusion. Neurosurgery 1989;24(2):264–270

38 CT-Based Image Guidance in Fixation of the Craniovertebral Junction

John H. Shin, Iain H. Kalfas, Edward C. Benzel, and Michael P. Steinmetz

Image guidance technology has had a dramatic effect on the practice of neurosurgery in the past two decades. Initially developed for intracranial surgery, advances in imaging have allowed for the application of stereotactic techniques in the placement of screws throughout the spine. In light of the proximity of vital structures in the region of the craniovertebral junction (CVJ), the use of image guidance has increased the precision and accuracy of placing screws at C1 and C2. Several fixation strategies have been developed over the past several decades to minimize vascular and neurological complications often associated with screws in this region. As such, surgeons have traditionally relied on intraoperative fluoroscopy for confirmation of screw trajectory during surgery. However, these techniques do not provide three-dimensional (3D) views of the anatomy and risk increased exposure to radiation.

Specific anatomic landmarks used for successful placement of screws at the CVJ may be difficult to identify on lateral radiographs during surgery and subject patients to additional risks of either neurological or vascular injury due to suboptimal visualization. Particularly in revision surgery or cases in which the normal bony landmarks have been disrupted due to congenital variances, tumor, infection, degeneration, or metabolic disease, image guidance can be a useful adjunct that requires little additional preparation or operative time.

Since its inception, several image guidance modalities specific to spinal navigation have been developed. These include systems based on images acquired preoperatively, such as computed tomography (CT) or magnetic resonance imaging (MRI) and images acquired intraoperatively. These intraoperative imaging systems include fluoroscopy-based navigation or "virtual" fluoroscopy, 3D C-arm fluoroscopy, and O-arm CT-fluoroscopy. Although each system has its strengths and limitations, a full discussion of each is beyond the scope of this chapter. Herein, we review the principles of image guidance and the application of preoperatively acquired CT-based guidance technology to fixation of the CVJ.

Principles of Image-Guided Spinal Navigation

Image-guided spinal navigation is a computer-based surgical technology that was developed to improve intraoperative orientation to unexposed anatomy during complex spinal procedures.[1,2] It evolved from the principles of stereotaxy that have been used by neurosurgeons for several decades to help localize intracranial lesions. Stereotaxy is defined as the localization of a specific point in space using 3D coordinates. The application of stereotaxy to intracranial surgery initially involved the use of an external frame attached to the patient's head. However, the evolution of computer-based technologies has eliminated the need for a frame and has allowed for the expansion of stereotactic technology into spinal surgery.

The management of complex spinal disorders has been greatly influenced by the increased acceptance and use of spinal instrumentation as well as the development of complex operative exposures. Many of these techniques require the surgeon to have a precise orientation to spinal anatomy that is not exposed and, therefore, not directly visualized in the surgical field. With the proper surgical exposure, direct visualization of the rostral, caudal, medial, and lateral aspects of the exposed bony anatomy is straightforward. However, it is the imprecise estimation of structures deep to the exposed anatomy that potentially confounds surgeons and leads to misplaced instrumentation and possible neurological or vascular injury. In particular, the various fixation techniques that require placing screws into the lateral masses of C1 and across the C1-C2 joint space require "see-through visualization" of the unexposed spinal anatomy.

Although conventional intraoperative imaging techniques such as fluoroscopy are helpful, they are limited in that they provide only two-dimensional imaging of a complex 3D structure. Consequently, the surgeon is required to extrapolate the third dimension based on an interpretation of the images as well as the surgeon's knowledge of spinal anatomy. This "dead reckoning" of anatomy can result in varying degrees of inaccuracy when placing screws into the unexposed spinal column.[3–6]

The main objective of computer-based image guidance is to establish a spatial relationship between image data of the surgical field and its corresponding intraoperative anatomy. The image data typically used for navigation purposes can be a preoperatively or intraoperatively acquired CT scan or an intraoperatively acquired fluoroscopic image. A spatial relationship can be created between the image data and the corresponding surgical anatomy because each represents a series of points, or coordinates, in a 3D space. Each point can be defined by a specific x, y, and z Cartesian coordinate. With defined mathematical algorithms, a specific point in the image dataset can be matched to its corresponding point in the surgical field. After several of these points are matched, or registered, it becomes possible to select random points in the surgical field and have the corresponding points in the image dataset displayed. These image data points can then be reformatted into multiplanar images of the surgical field, greatly enhancing the surgeon's intraoperative visualization of the pertinent surgical anatomy.

CT-based image-guided spinal navigation was developed to provide real-time axial imaging of selected screw trajectories. It allows for the intraoperative manipulation of multiplanar CT images that can be oriented to a selected point in the surgical field and helps minimize much of the guess work associated with complex spinal surgery. Although it is not an intraoperative imaging device, it provides the spinal surgeon with superior image data compared with conventional intraoperative fluoroscopy. It improves the speed, accuracy, and precision of complex spinal surgery while, in most cases, eliminating the need for an intraoperative fluoroscopy.

A variety of navigational systems have evolved over the past decade. Although each of these systems may differ slightly, the common components of these systems include an image-processing computer workstation interfaced with a two-camera optical localizer (**Fig. 38.1**). When positioned during surgery, the optical localizer emits infrared light toward the operative field. A handheld navigational probe mounted with a fixed array of passive reflective spheres serves as the link between the surgeon and the computer workstation (**Fig. 38.2**). Alternatively, passive reflectors may be attached to standard surgical instruments.

The spacing and positioning of the passive reflectors on each navigational probe or customized trackable surgical instrument are known by the computer workstation. The infrared light transmitted toward the operative field is reflected back to the optical localizer by the passive reflectors. The information is then relayed to the computer workstation, which can then calculate the precise location of the instrument tip in the surgical field as well as the location of the anatomic point on which the instrument tip is resting. Multiplanar images through the selected point are generated, providing the surgeon with optimal spatial information for performing the surgical plan.

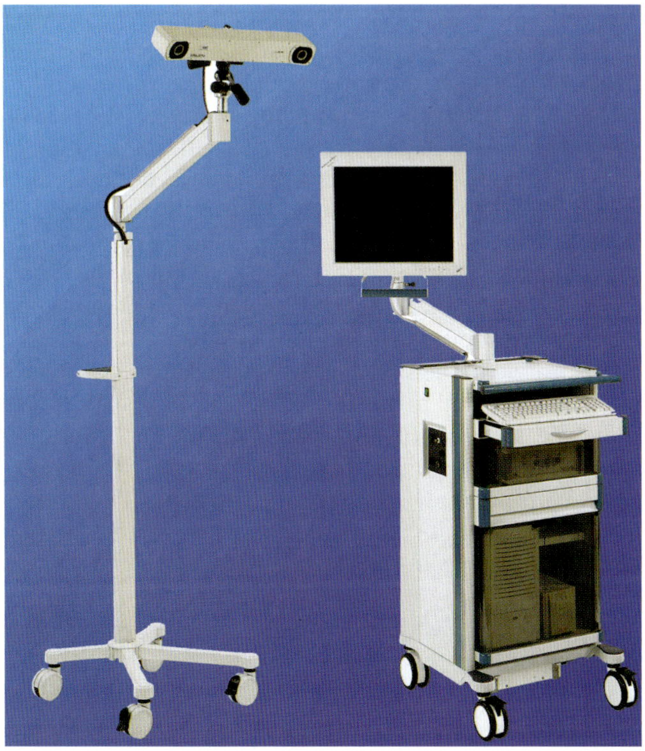

Fig. 38.1 Image-guided navigational workstation with infrared camera localizer system.

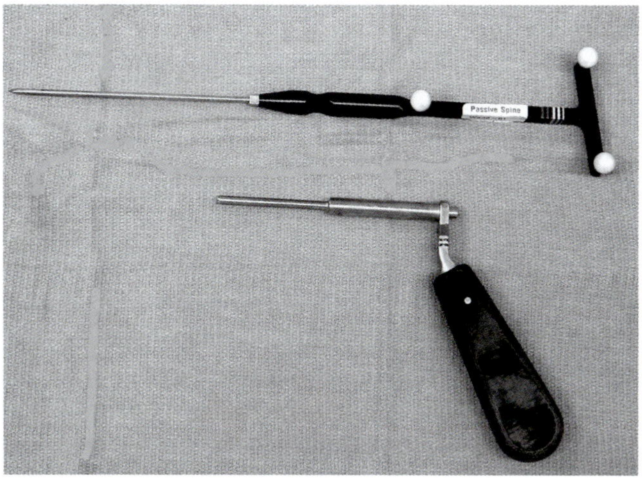

Fig. 38.2 Navigation probe and drill guide for spinal surgery.

Spinal anatomy itself can be used as a frame of reference to establish the spatial relationship between image data and surgical anatomy. Accordingly, neither a stereotactic frame nor surface-mounted fiducials are necessary because bone landmarks on the exposed surface of the spinal column provide the points of reference necessary for image-guided navigation. Specifically, any anatomic landmark that can be identified intraoperatively as well as in the preoperative image dataset can be used as a reference point. The tip of a spinous or transverse process, a facet joint, or a prominent osteophyte can serve as potential reference points (**Fig. 38.3**). Because each vertebra is a fixed and rigid body, the spatial relationship of the selected registration points to the vertebral anatomy at a single spinal level is not affected by changes in body position.

The initial step of spinal navigation is the creation of a spatial relationship between the image data and the corresponding surgical anatomy. This step is called registration. Three different registration techniques can be used for spinal navigation: paired point registration, surface matching, and automated registration. Paired point registration involves selecting a series of points in a CT dataset and matching them to their corresponding points in the exposed spinal anatomy. The registration process is performed immediately after surgical exposure and prior to any planned decompressive procedure, allowing for the use of the spinous processes as registration points.

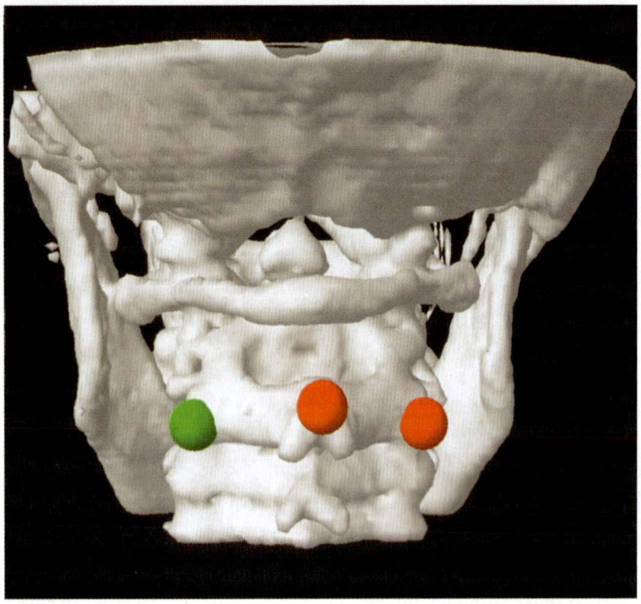

Fig. 38.3 Navigational workstation screen demonstrating a paired point registration plan for the insertion of C2 pedicle screws. Three discreet bony landmarks are selected at the C2 level. In this case, the lateral margins of the two C2-C3 facets (*green dot* and *right red dot*) and the spinous process tip of C2 (*center red dot*) have been selected.

A specific registration point in the CT image dataset is selected by highlighting it with the computer cursor. The tip of the probe is then placed on the corresponding point in the surgical field, and the reflective spheres on the probe handle are aimed toward the camera. Infrared light from the camera is reflected back, allowing the spatial position of the probe's tip to be identified. This initial step of the registration process effectively matches the point selected in the image data with the point selected in the surgical field. When a minimum of three such points are registered, the probe can be placed on any other point in the surgical field and the corresponding point in the image dataset will be identified on the computer workstation. Additionally, multiple planar images centered on the selected point will be displayed.

Alternatively, a second registration technique called surface matching can be used. This technique involves the selection of multiple, nondiscreet points on the exposed and debrided surface of the spine in the surgical field. This technique does not require a prior selection of points in the image set though several discreet points in both the image dataset and surgical field are frequently required to improve the accuracy of surface mapping. The positional information of these points is transferred to the workstation, and a topographic map of the selected anatomy is created and matched to the patient's image set.

A third registration technique is termed automated registration. This technique is used with navigation, employing intraoperatively acquired fluoroscopic or CT images. During image acquisition, a reference grid internal to the imaging device is interposed between the image source and the spinal anatomy. Registration is then performed by the imaging system itself without a need for input from the surgeon. Up to five spinal levels can be registered with this technique without compromising accuracy.

The purpose of the registration process is to establish a precise spatial relationship between the image space of the data with the physical space of the patient's corresponding surgical anatomy. If the patient is moved after registration, this spatial relationship is distorted, making the navigational information inaccurate. This problem can be minimized by the optional use of a spinal tracking device that consists of a separate set of passive reflectors mounted on an instrument that can be attached to the exposed spinal anatomy. The position of the reference frame can be tracked by the camera system. Movement of the frame alerts the navigational system to inadvertent movement of the spine. The system can then make correctional steps to keep the registration process accurate and eliminate the need to repeat the registration process.

When CT-based navigation is used, registration is performed and the navigational probe is placed on a surface point on the registered vertebrae. When activated, the system will immediately display three separate reformatted CT images centered on the corresponding point in the image dataset. Each reformatted image is referenced to the long axis of the probe. If the probe is placed on the spinal anatomy directly perpendicular to its long axis, the three images will be in the sagittal, coronal, and axial planes.

A trajectory line representing the orientation of the long axis of the probe will overlay the sagittal and axial planes. A cursor representing a cross-section through the selected trajectory will overlay the coronal plane. The insertional depth of the trajectory can be adjusted to correspond to selected screw lengths. As the depth is adjusted, the specific coronal plane will adjust accordingly with the position of the cursor demonstrating the final position of the tip of a screw placed at that depth along the selected trajectory.

As the probe is moved to another point in the surgical field, the reformatted images as well as the position of the cursor and trajectory line will change. The planar orientation of the three reformatted images will also change as the probe's angle relative to the spinal axis changes. When the probe's orientation is not perpendicular to the long axis of the spine, the images displayed will be in oblique or orthogonal planes. Regardless of the probe's orientation, the navigational workstation will provide the surgeon with a greater degree of anatomic information than can be provided by any intraoperative imaging technique.

Surgical Technique

CT-based image-guided navigation requires the acquisition of a preoperative CT scan through the appropriate spinal segments to be instrumented. Image data are then transferred to the computer workstation through optical disk or a high-speed data link. If paired point registration is to be used, three to five reference points for each spinal segment to be instrumented are selected and stored in the image dataset. For most cervical procedures, the camera can be positioned at the head of the table with the navigation workstation positioned across from the surgeon. If fluoroscopy is used, it can be positioned next to the workstation (**Fig. 38.4**).

For fixation of the CVJ, the patient is typically positioned prone with the head secured to the operating table with a halo or Mayfield device. Following a standard surgical exposure, either the paired point or surface matching registration technique is performed. When the registration process has been completed, the navigational workstation will calculate a registration error (expressed in millimeters) that is directly dependent on the surgeon's registration technique.

The error presented does not represent a linear error but rather a volumetric calculation comparing the spacing of registration points in the surgical field to the spacing of the corresponding points in the image dataset. This figure is, at best, a relative indicator of accuracy and is a feature of CT-based navigation systems. Systems based on intraoperative imaging, such as the O-arm, do not require registration of anatomic structures by the surgeon and thus do not provide an indicator of accuracy.

A more practical method of assuring registration accuracy is the verification step. This step is typically performed immediately after completing either registration process. The surgeon places the navigational probe on a discreet landmark in the surgical field. With the navigational system now tracking the movement and position of the probe, the trajectory line and cursor on the workstation screen will move to the corresponding point in the image dataset (**Fig. 38.5A**). If registration accuracy has not been achieved, the cursor and trajectory line may rest on something other than the point selected in the surgical field (**Fig. 38.5B**). If this occurs to a significant degree, the registration process needs to be repeated. This step is an absolute indicator of registration accuracy and a necessary step to perform prior to proceeding with navigation.

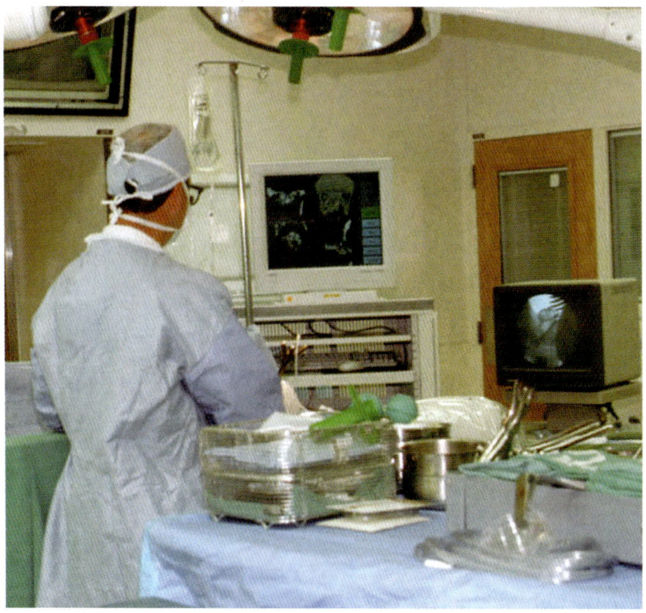

Fig. 38.4 Positioning of image-guided system for a C1-C2 transarticular screw fixation procedure. The camera is positioned at the head of the table in a vertical orientation, minimizing a potential visual obstruction between the camera and the surgical field. The workstation is positioned across the table from the surgeon. The fluoroscopic monitor sits next to the navigational workstation.

C1-C2 Transarticular Screw Fixation

C1-C2 transarticular screw fixation as described by Magerl gained widespread popularity for its superior immobilization of C1-C2 and improved fusion rates compared with wiring techniques.[7] However, transarticular screw fixation is technically demanding with a potential risk for vertebral artery injury, particularly as the artery courses through the transverse foramen of C2.[8] The risk of vertebral artery injury is reported to range from 0 to 8.2%, with a higher susceptibility in patients with a large tortuous high-riding vertebral artery, enlarged transverse foramen, or hypoplastic C2 pars interarticularis.[9,10] It is estimated that as many as 23% of patients are unable to undergo C1-C2 transarticular screw placement due to these aforementioned anatomical variations.[11–13]

Successful placement of this screw involves insertion of a screw through the pars interarticularis of C2, across the facet joint, and into the lateral mass of C1. The insertion of a screw on either side may be contraindicated if the pars interarticularis of C2 is too narrow. The procedure is typically performed bilaterally using fluoroscopic guidance. Due to the complications associated with placement of this particular screw and the poor visualization of key anatomic structures using fluoroscopy, many surgeons have abandoned this technique and have adopted alternative strategies for fixation across the C1-C2 joint. These will be discussed in subsequent sections.

The selection of the appropriate screw entry site and trajectory requires a thorough understanding of atlantoaxial anatomy. It should be emphasized that the use of image guidance does not replace a surgeon's understanding of the local neural and vascular anatomy. Instead, it helps visualize the intended trajectory of the screw. Although fluoroscopy provides real-time imaging of the relevant spinal anatomy, the views generated represent only two-dimensional images of a complex 3D anatomic region. Visualization of key anatomic landmarks is often difficult, and the cumulative exposure to radiation is not trivial.

A preoperative CT that extends from, at least, the lower occipital region to C3 is used for surgical planning and navigation. Image data are transferred to the computer workstation, and a preoperative trajectory is planned. The image dataset can then be manipulated in multiple planes

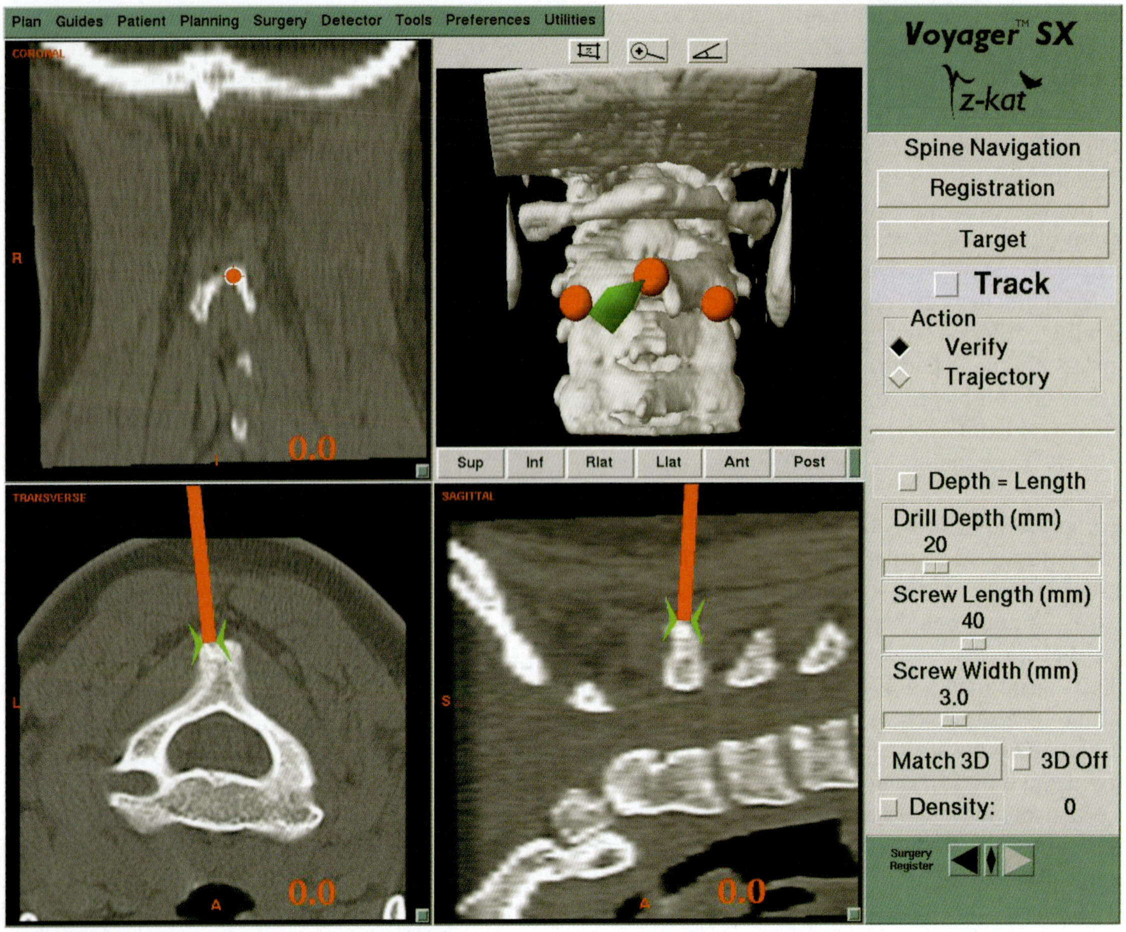

A

Fig. 38.5 **(A)** Navigational workstation screen demonstrating satisfactory verification of registration accuracy. While the navigational probe is positioned on the C2 spinous process in the surgical field, the workstation screen should show the cursor and trajectory line in a correlative position in the computed tomography image set. *(continued)*

to demonstrate the position of a screw placed along the selected trajectory. In addition to a sagittal image that demonstrates the same information provided by lateral fluoroscopy, two other images are presented. One of the images lies perpendicular to the sagittal image along the selected trajectory. It represents an orthogonal view that lies approximately midway between the coronal and axial planes through the spine.

A third view demonstrates an image oriented perpendicular to the long axis of the probe and, therefore, the selected trajectory. A cursor superimposed on this image can show the position of the screw tip along the selected trajectory at millimetric increments. By scrolling through this image, the surgeon can assess the proposed position of the screw along the selected trajectory along its entire path. Although this planning technique does not assure safe screw placement intraoperatively, it can preoperatively alert the surgeon to avoid screw placement in patients with insufficient anatomy and to select an alternate approach.

Intraoperatively, the patient is positioned prone and the dorsal C1-C2 complex is exposed. If a reference frame is used, it can be attached to the spinous process of C2. Three to five registration points are then selected at the C1 and C2 level. Although the spatial relationship of C1 and C2 may change between the preoperative scanned position and the intraoperative position, the ability of image-guided navigation to facilitate accurate screw placement is not significantly affected. The lateral mass of C1 is a relatively large target. It can be easily accessed by an inserted screw, provided there is satisfactory atlantoaxial alignment.

The technical difficulty of this procedure is the accurate passage of the screw through the narrow pars interarticularis of C2. Although the relative position of C1 and C2 in both the preoperative image set and surgical field is important, it is not critical enough to interfere with the process of image-guided navigation.

Two separate stab incisions are made on either side of the midline at the C7-T1 level. A drill guide is placed through one of the stab incisions and passed through the paravertebral muscles into the operative field. A small divot is drilled at the proposed entry site to provide a secure dock for the drill guide. The registration process is performed at

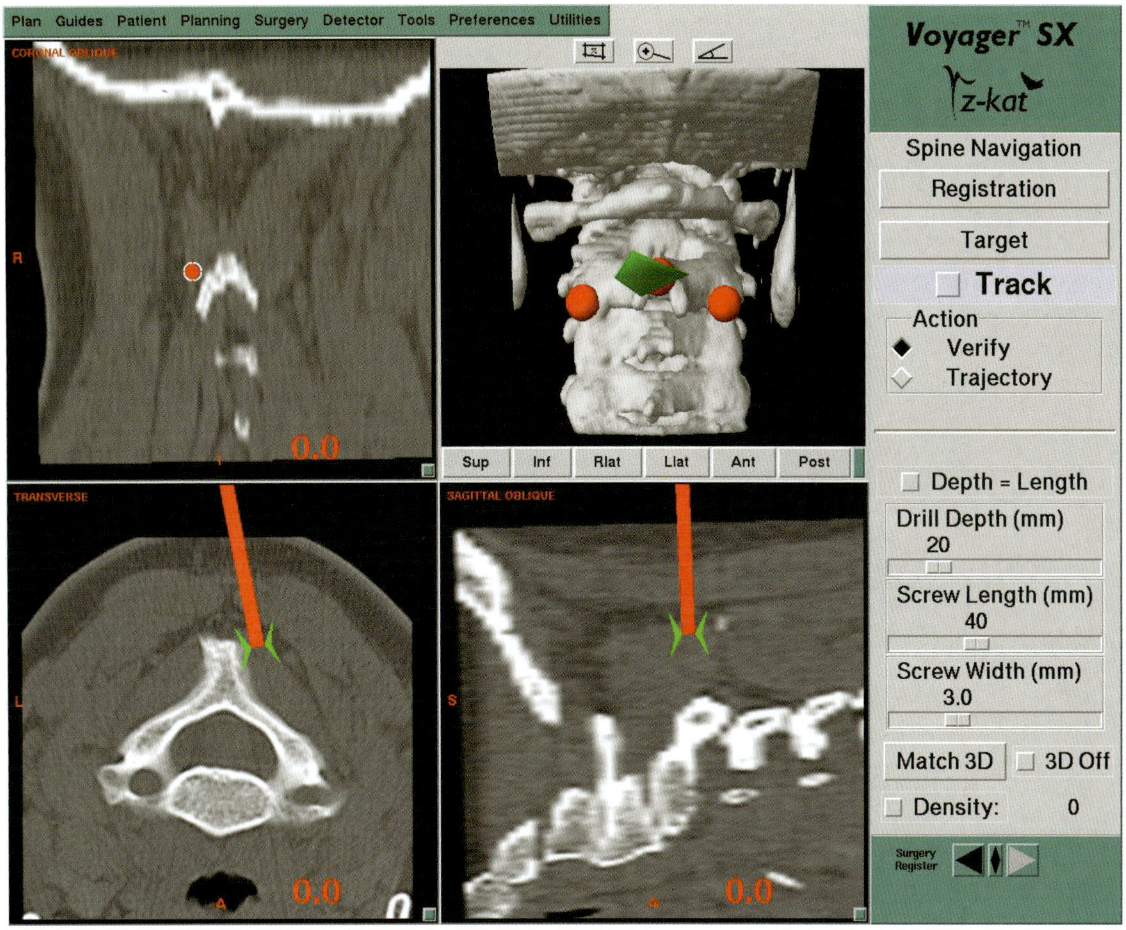

B

Fig. 38.5 *(continued)* **(B)** Navigational workstation screen demonstrating an unsatisfactory verification of registration accuracy. If the navigational probe is positioned on the C2 spinous process in the surgical field but the workstation screen shows the cursor and the trajectory line is a noncorrelative position (i.e., not on the C2 spinous process), accurate registration has not been achieved and the registration process needs to be repeated before proceeding with navigation.

the C2 level and its accuracy confirmed using the verification step. The probe is passed through the drill guide and, as its position is adjusted in the surgical field, the images on the workstation screen adjust accordingly to show the corresponding trajectory in two separate planes and the projected location of the screw tip in the third plane. Orientation to the correct screw position can be assessed rapidly and accurately (**Fig. 38.6**). Errors in trajectory or entry point selection can be determined and corrected by adjusting the position of the probe and the drill guide through which it passes. When the correct screw insertion parameters have been selected, the probe is removed from the drill guide and a drill is inserted. A hole is drilled along the selected trajectory and tapped, and the appropriate length of screw is inserted. The process is repeated on the opposite side.

The purpose of the drill guide is to preserve the physical trajectory and entry point information just acquired through the navigation of that pedicle. If a drill guide is not used, it may be difficult to precisely position a drill or pedicle probe on the same point and with the same trajectory previously conveyed by the navigational probe after probe removal.

C1 Lateral Mass Screws

As an alternative to transarticular screw fixation, segmental fixation of C1-C2 can be used for managing atlantoaxial instability.[14–16] This fixation involves placing a screw into each of the two lateral masses of C1 and two screws through either the pedicles, pars, or lamina of C2. The polyaxial screw heads on each side are then connected with rods. Although this approach potentially reduces the risk of injury to the vertebral artery during screw insertion, it does not completely eliminate this risk. As with the transarticular technique, precise anatomic orientation is required to avoid arterial or neural injury. Image guidance can supplement intraoperative fluoroscopy and provide an added degree of orientation for accurate screw insertion.

As with the transarticular screw fixation technique, a preoperative CT is obtained. Registration is first performed

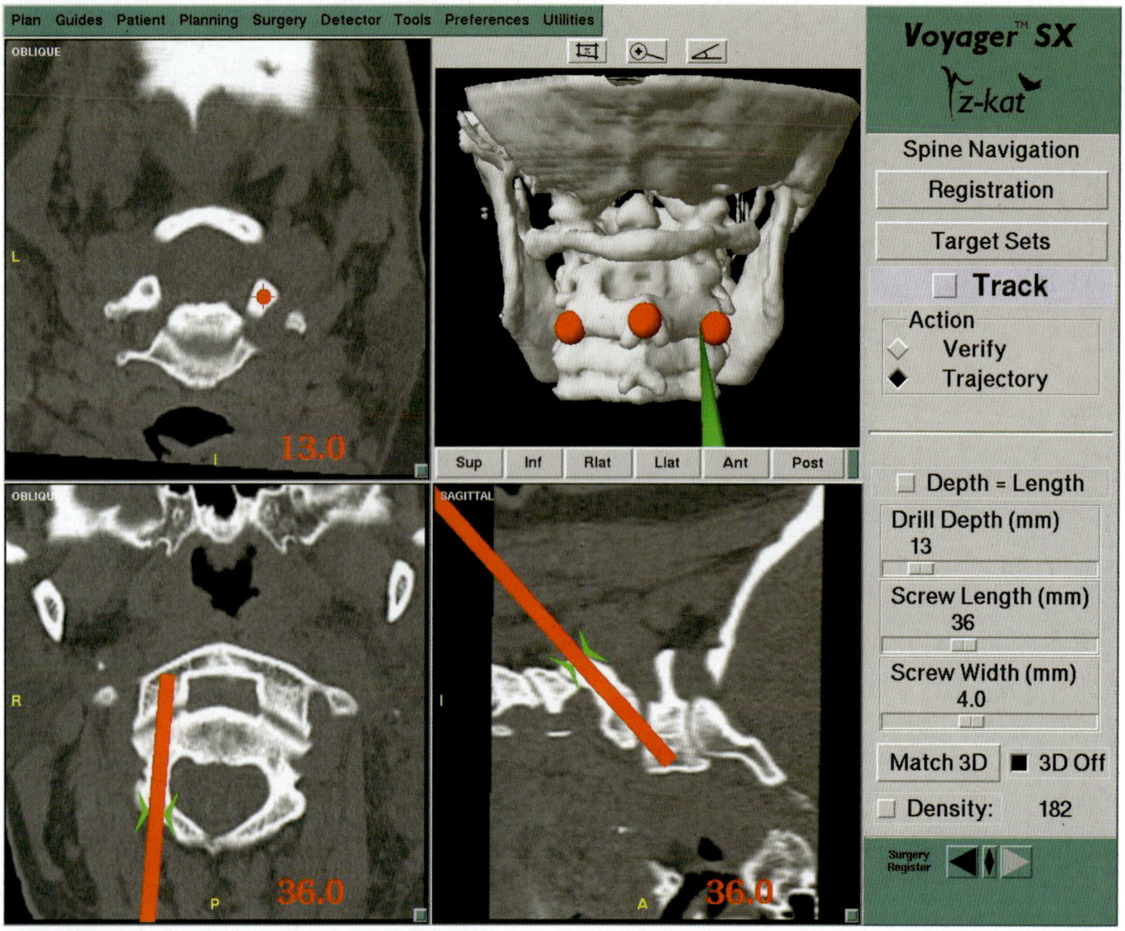

Fig. 38.6 Workstation screen demonstrating a trajectory for insertion of a C1-C2 transarticular screw. The lower right screen shows the trajectory in the sagittal plane. The lower left screen represents an orthogonal plane lying between the axial and coronal planes. It conveys the medial-lateral trajectory. The upper left screen represents a plane that is perpendicular to the two other images. It demonstrates the location of the screw tip (*arrow*) inserted along the selected trajectory (*arrow*) at the indicated depth. The screw trajectory and tip location are highlighted by *arrows*.

at C1 for placement of the C1 lateral mass screws. The three registration points typically used at C1 include the midline posterior tubercle and the bilateral points marked by the junction of the small pedicle of C1 with its lateral mass (immediately above the two exiting C2 nerve roots). Once registered, the correct trajectory into the lateral masses can be displayed on the workstation screen and the screws inserted using the technique described previously (**Fig. 38.7**).

C2 Pedicle Screws

To utilize image guidance for inserting C2 pedicle screws, the surgeon will use the same registration points at C2 as those used for transarticular fixation (the C2 spinous process and the two lateral margins of the C2-C3 facet). The entry point for the screw is more lateral and the trajectory more medially oriented than for a transarticular screw. The navigation probe is placed through a drill guide onto this entry point, and the selected trajectory is displayed on the workstation screen. When the correct entry point and trajectory have been selected, the probe is removed, a drill is inserted, and the pilot hole is drilled (**Fig. 38.8**). The process is then repeated for the other side. The heads of the screws are then connected with two short rods.

C2 Pars Interarticularis Screws

Another strategy for fixation at C2 is placement of pars interarticularis screws. Determining whether it is safe to place a screw in this structure requires careful review of the preoperative CT imaging. The course of the vertebral artery varies in this region and, in some cases, precludes safe placement of a pars screw. Sagittal reconstruction is usually most helpful in identifying the course of the vertebral artery in the vicinity of the pars. Unlike the C2 pedicle screw, however, the pars screw stops short of the pedicle and the transverse foramen, minimizing the risk of vertebral artery injury.

Similar in many ways to the insertional technique described for the transarticular screw, the starting point is essentially the same. However, due to the shorter length of

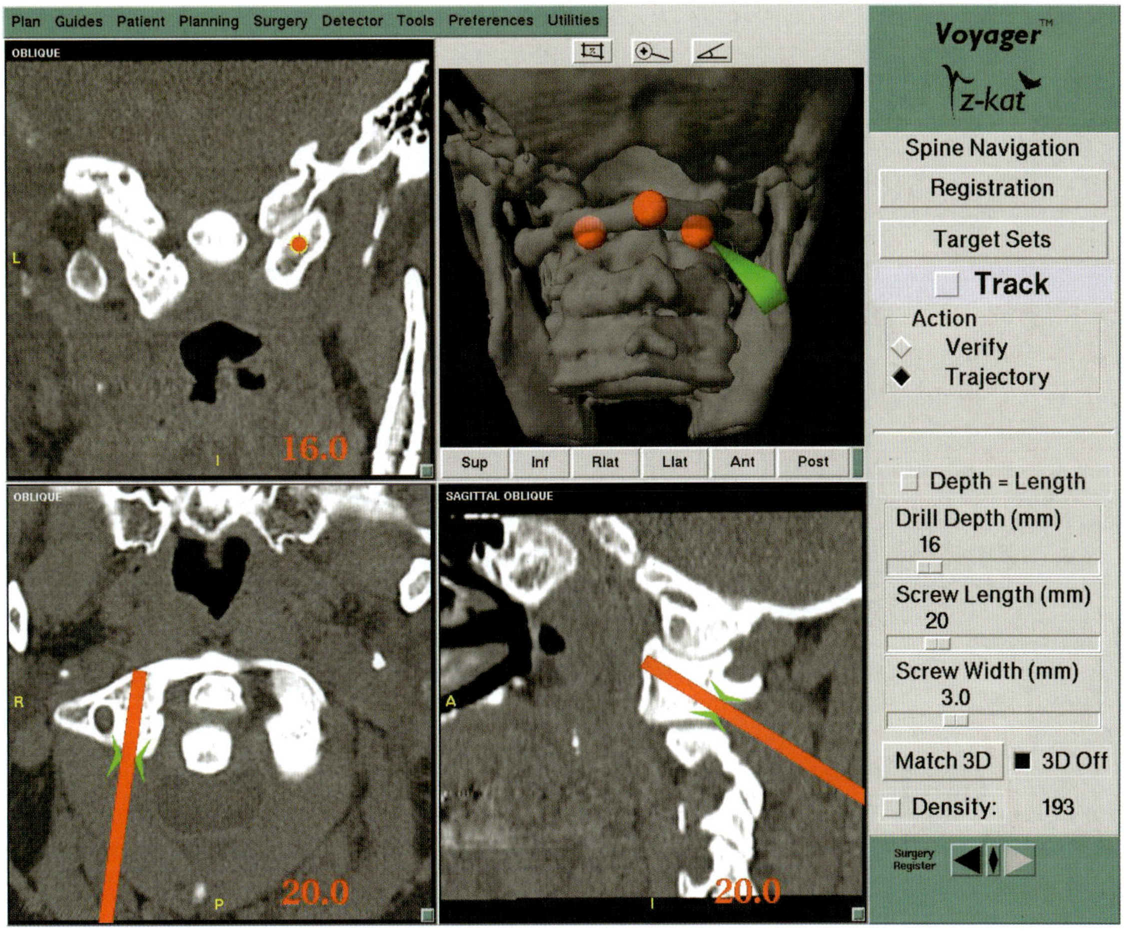

Fig. 38.7 Workstation screen demonstrating navigational information for placement of a screw into the lateral mass of C1.

the pars, the trajectory required is less steep than that of the transarticular screw. As such, a separate stab incision is not required and the drill guide can be placed directly over the starting point through the operative exposure. With the image guidance probe placed within the drill guide and docked on the starting point, the ideal trajectory can be visualized on the workstation screen in several planes. The navigation probe is then removed from the drill guide, the trajectory drilled, and the screw placed.

C2 Crossed Translaminar Screws

To minimize risk to the vertebral artery, the technique of crossed translaminar screws through the lamina of C2 to provide alternative fixation of the atlas was introduced.[17,18] This technique has been advocated as a biomechanically viable salvage strategy in failed C2 pars or pedicle fixation.[19–21] It is also a safe alternative in cases of high-riding anomalous vertebral arteries.[22] Biomechanical analysis in cadaveric specimens has demonstrated crossed translaminar fixation to be superior to pars screws in pullout strength and insertional torque.[20]

For proper registration, the spinous process, lamina, and lateral masses of C2 are exposed. Easily recognized bony landmarks, such as the spinous process and lateral aspect of the lateral masses, are used for registration. Once registered, the drill guide is placed at the estimated entry point at the junction of the spinous process and the lamina at the superior laminar margin. The navigation probe is inserted into the drill guide, and the trajectory of the intended screw is checked on the navigation workstation. Once verified, the navigation probe is removed and the lamina drilled. After placement of the screw, the inferior ledge of the lamina can be palpated with an instrument to verify integrity of the ventral wall of the lamina. The contralateral screw is inserted in a similar manner, with the entry point at the inferior margin of the C2 lamina and spinous process junction.

Potential complications with this technique, including cortical breach into the spinal canal with resultant cerebrospinal fluid leak and spinal cord injury, can be largely avoided with navigation. The 3D reconstructions provided on the computer workstation provide visualization of the intended screw path that would be impossible to see with fluoroscopy. Although placement of these screws is relatively safe considering that the anatomy through which instrumentation is being placed is entirely exposed, navigation provides the surgeon with greater confidence

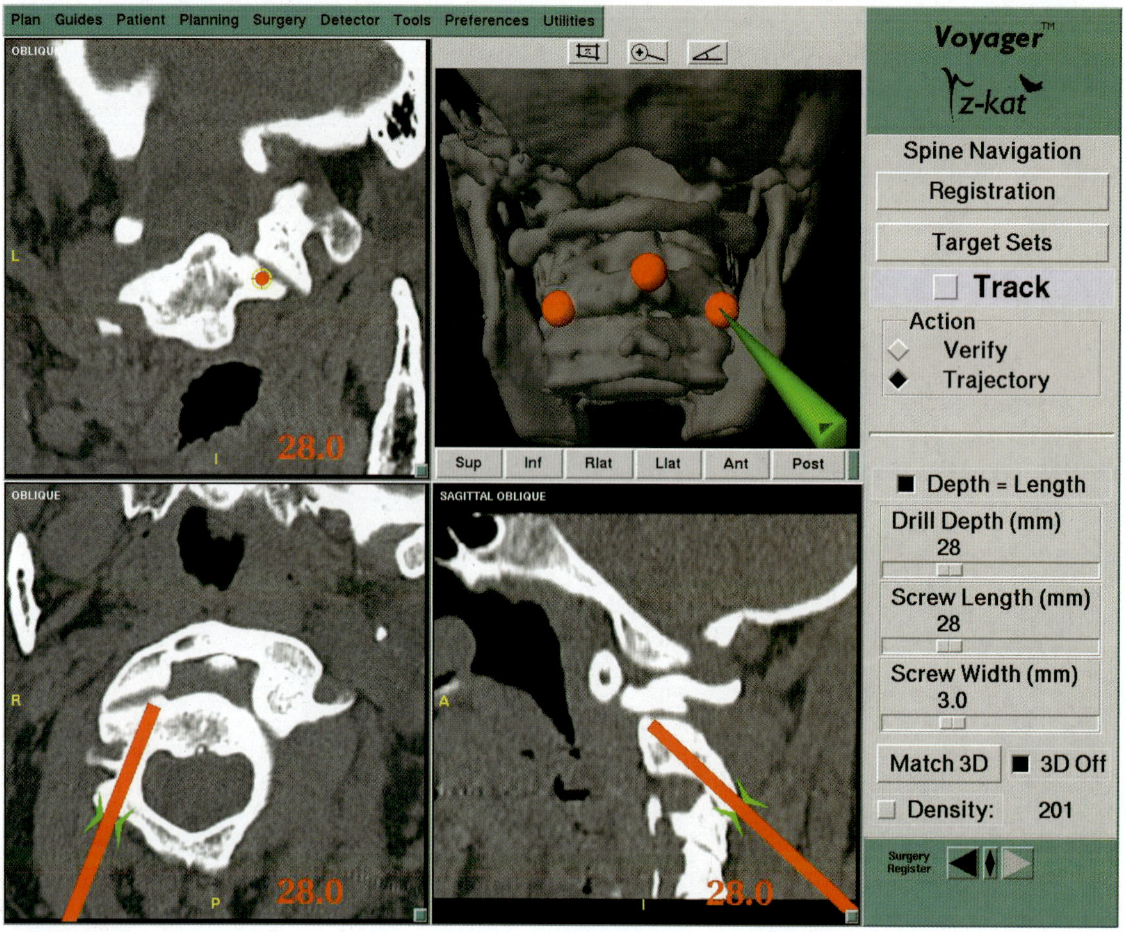

Fig. 38.8 Workstation screen demonstrating navigational information for placement of a screw into the pedicle of C2.

that the ventral cortical laminar surface is not violated during screw placement.

Transoral Surgery

Although instrumentation is not often applied directly through the transoral route, image-guided navigation facilitates the appropriate approach vector to the area of interest. Transoral decompression of the upper cervical spine typically requires intraoperative fluoroscopy to help maintain proper anatomic orientation during the procedure. Although orientation in the sagittal plane is easy to obtain with fluoroscopy, depth and medial–lateral orientation are more difficult to assess. Image-guided technology can be used to orient the surgeon in multiple planes during transoral surgery.[23]

Unlike other spinal applications of image guidance, discreet registration points are not readily available during transoral surgery. In this setting, surface-mounted markers (fiducials) are applied to the patient prior to obtaining the preoperative CT. Typically, two fiducials are applied to the mastoid processes and two are applied to the lateral orbital margins or to both malar eminences. The nasal septum can also be used as a registration point. Following surgical exposure, registration points in the surgical field, such as the ventral arch of C1 or the base of the odontoid, can be used.

The patient is positioned in a three-point head holder. The registration process is performed prior to draping the patient, using the surface-mounted fiducials. Because the registration points will not be accessible during the procedure, a reference frame is used for transoral navigation, allowing for changes in patient positioning during surgery without the need to reregister. The reference frame can be attached to the three-point head holder.

During the decompressive procedure, the probe can be intermittently placed in the surgical field. Reformatted sagittal, axial, and coronal CT images are immediately generated, providing the surgeon with a precise orientation to the pertinent surgical anatomy. In particular, orientation in the axial plane minimizes the risk of lateral deviation toward the vertebral artery during the decompression (**Fig. 38.9**). If dorsal fixation is performed following transoral decompression, the same CT image dataset can be used for C1-C2 screw placement.

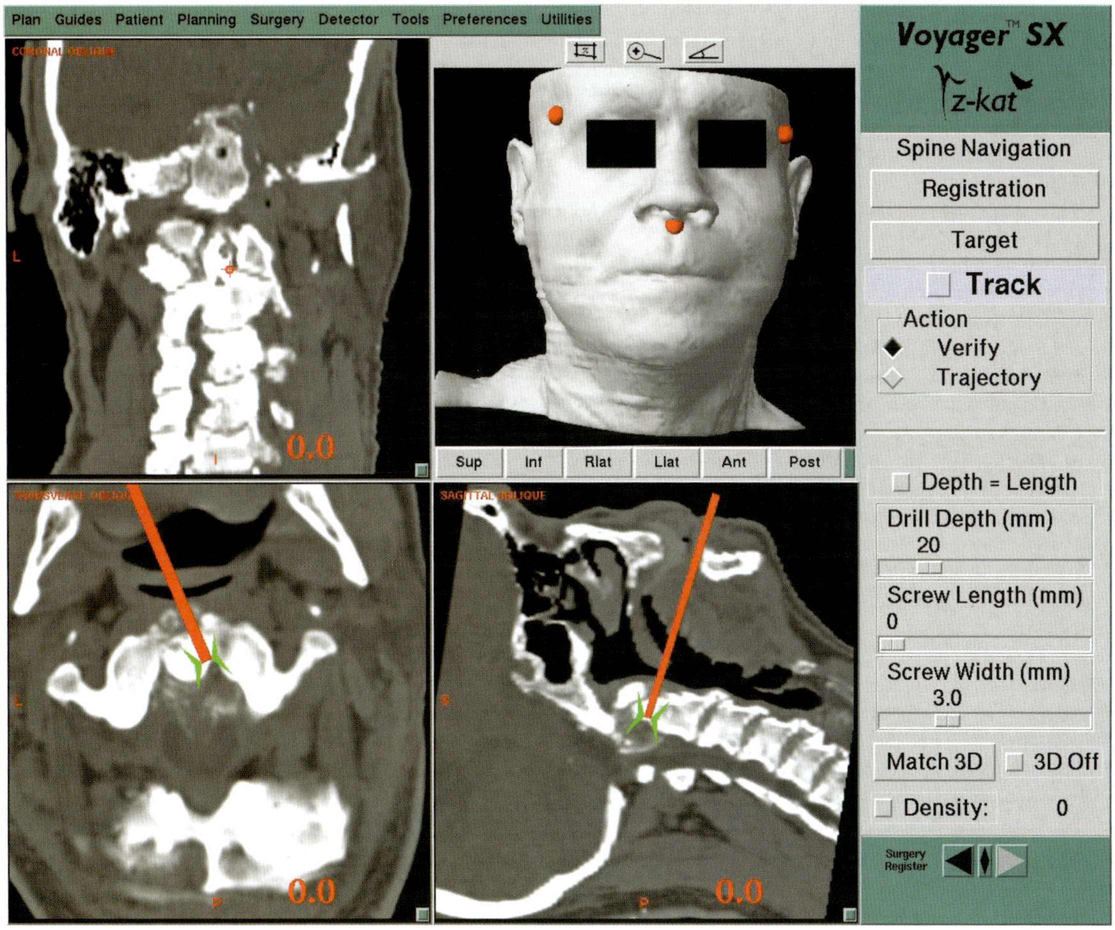

Fig. 38.9 Workstation screen demonstrating navigational information during transoral decompression. The probe tip location and trajectory are highlighted by *arrows*.

Conclusion

Like any other computer-based technology, image-guided navigation is highly dependent on the quality of the information imported into the system. While obtaining the properly formatted CT images and having them correctly transferred to the navigational workstation is important, the critical step of image guidance is the registration process. If registration is not performed properly, the images displayed during navigation may be inaccurate. Confirming registration accuracy prior to proceeding with navigation is imperative.

An important concept of image guidance is understanding that the navigational information presented during surgery must correlate with the surgeon's knowledge of surgical anatomy and the appropriate screw trajectories through that anatomy. Image-guided navigation is not a replacement for knowledge of the pertinent spinal anatomy and surgical technique. With the various options for fixation at the CVJ, image-guided navigation helps minimize potential injury to neurological and vascular structures.

As image-guided navigation continues to evolve, its ease of use and practicality will continue to improve, creating a greater acceptance of the technology, expanding its clinical applications, and helping reduce operative time and morbidity. Ultimately, with continued improvement, it can develop into a routine, cost-effective standard of care in spinal surgery.

References

1. Murphy MA, McKenzie RL, Kormos DW, Kalfas IH. Frameless stereotaxis for the insertion of lumbar pedicle screws. J Clin Neurosci 1994;1(4):257–260
2. Kalfas IH, Kormos DW, Murphy MA, et al. Application of frameless stereotaxy to pedicle screw fixation of the spine. J Neurosurg 1995;83(4):641–647
3. Holly LT, Foley KT. Image guidance in spine surgery. Orthop Clin North Am 2007;38(3):451–461, abstract viii
4. Mueller CA, Roesseler L, Podlogar M, Kovacs A, Kristof RA. Accuracy and complications of transpedicular C2 screw placement without the use of spinal navigation. Eur Spine J 2010;19(5):809–814

5. Weinstein JN, Spratt KF, Spengler D, Brick C, Reid S. Spinal pedicle fixation: reliability and validity of roentgenogram-based assessment and surgical factors on successful screw placement. Spine 1988;13(9):1012–1018
6. Steinmann JC, Herkowitz HN, el-Kommos H, Wesolowski DP. Spinal pedicle fixation. Confirmation of an image-based technique for screw placement. Spine 1993;18(13):1856–1861
7. Grob D, Magerl F. [Surgical stabilization of C1 and C2 fractures]. Orthopade 1987;16(1):46–54
8. Hoh DJ, Liu CY, Wang MY. A radiographic computed tomography-based study to determine the ideal entry point, trajectory, and length for safe fixation using C-2 pars interarticularis screws. J Neurosurg Spine 2010;12(6):602–612
9. Dickman CA, Sonntag VK. Posterior C1-C2 transarticular screw fixation for atlantoaxial arthrodesis. Neurosurgery 1998;43(2): 275–280, discussion 280–281
10. Gluf WM, Brockmeyer DL. Atlantoaxial transarticular screw fixation: a review of surgical indications, fusion rate, complications, and lessons learned in 67 pediatric patients. J Neurosurg Spine 2005;2(2):164–169
11. Kazan S, Yildirim F, Sindel M, Tuncer R. Anatomical evaluation of the groove for the vertebral artery in the axis vertebrae for atlanto-axial transarticular screw fixation technique. Clin Anat 2000;13(4):237–243
12. Abou Madawi A, Solanki G, Casey AT, Crockard HA. Variation of the groove in the axis vertebra for the vertebral artery. Implications for instrumentation. J Bone Joint Surg Br 1997;79(5):820–823
13. Mandel IM, Kambach BJ, Petersilge CA, Johnstone B, Yoo JU. Morphologic considerations of C2 isthmus dimensions for the placement of transarticular screws. Spine 2000;25(12): 1542–1547
14. Harms J, Melcher RP. Posterior C1-C2 fusion with polyaxial screw and rod fixation. Spine 2001;26(22):2467–2471
15. Goel A, Laheri V. Plate and screw fixation for atlanto-axial subluxation. Acta Neurochir (Wien) 1994;129(1–2):47–53
16. Mummaneni PV, Lu DC, Dhall SS, Mummaneni VP, Chou D. C1 lateral mass fixation: a comparison of constructs. Neurosurgery 2010;66(3, Suppl):153–160
17. Wright NM. Translaminar rigid screw fixation of the axis. Technical note. J Neurosurg Spine 2005;3(5):409–414
18. Wright NM. Posterior C2 fixation using bilateral, crossing C2 laminar screws: case series and technical note. J Spinal Disord Tech 2004;17(2):158–162
19. Cassinelli EH, Lee M, Skalak A, Ahn NU, Wright NM. Anatomic considerations for the placement of C2 laminar screws. Spine 2006;31(24):2767–2771
20. Lehman RA Jr, Dmitriev AE, Helgeson MD, Sasso RC, Kuklo TR, Riew KD. Salvage of C2 pedicle and pars screws using the intralaminar technique: a biomechanical analysis. Spine 2008;33(9): 960–965
21. Parker SL, McGirt MJ, Garcés-Ambrossi GL, et al. Translaminar versus pedicle screw fixation of C2: comparison of surgical morbidity and accuracy of 313 consecutive screws. Neurosurgery 2009;64(5, Suppl 2):343–348, discussion 348–349
22. Ma W, Feng L, Xu R, et al. Clinical application of C2 laminar screw technique. Eur Spine J 2010;19(8):1312–1317
23. Welch WC, Subach BR, Pollack IF, Jacobs GB. Frameless stereotactic guidance for surgery of the upper cervical spine. Neurosurgery 1997;40(5):958–963, discussion 963–964

39 Odontoid Screw Fixation

Curtis A. Dickman and Volker K. H. Sonntag

Anterior screw fixation of the odontoid process is clinically useful for the internal fixation of unstable type II odontoid fractures.[1–8] A variety of other methods has been used for the internal fixation of unstable dens fractures. These other atlantoaxial fixation techniques, however, sacrifice all C1-C2 motion. The major advantage of the odontoid screw technique is that it fixates the odontoid fracture directly yet completely preserves normal C1-C2 motion. This chapter reviews the clinical techniques for odontoid screw fixation.

Table 39.1 Indications for Odontoid Screw Fixation

Type II odontoid fractures
Acute, widely displaced (6 mm or more dens dislocation)
Subacute, unstable (alignment not maintained with orthoses)
Chronic nonunion
Inability to wear halo brace for a displaced fracture
Type III odontoid fractures*
Shallow fractures if nonunion develops or if unstable with an orthosis

*Acute type III fractures can usually be managed nonoperatively.

Indications

The Anderson and D'Alonzo[9] classification system divides odontoid fractures into three subtypes. The system is based on fracture morphology and healing capabilities, and both factors are used to guide treatment. Type I fractures involve the tip of the dens. Type II fractures involve the neck of the dens. Type III fractures extend from the base of the dens into the body of C2 (**Fig. 39.1**). Odontoid screw fixation is designed primarily for treating unstable type II dens fractures because of their morphology and their predisposition to nonunion. Most odontoid fractures (type I, nondisplaced type II, and type III) heal satisfactorily with a cervical orthosis. Widely displaced type II odontoid fractures (>6 mm), however, are predisposed to nonunion when treated nonoperatively.[6,9–14]

Odontoid screw fixation is reserved for patients with widely displaced type II fractures (6 mm or more), fracture nonunions, or patients who are unable to wear a halo brace (**Table 39.1**). The probability of a type II fracture uniting when treated with an orthosis primarily depends on the extent of bone displacement.[6,9–14] Nondisplaced fractures or fractures displaced less than 6 mm have a 90% chance of healing with an orthosis.[10,14] In comparison, type II fractures displaced 6 mm or more have 78% chance of nonunion when treated with an orthosis.[10] Type II fractures with extensive bone comminution at the base of the dens (type IIA fractures) also have a high risk for nonunion and should be considered for early surgical fixation (**Fig. 39.2**).[15]

If there are no medical contraindications to surgery, odontoid screw fixation can be considered for the initial treatment of fractures that are at a high risk for nonunion. Surgery also may be considered for patients with a displaced dens fracture who object to wearing a halo brace, those who cannot tolerate a halo brace (i.e., because of cosmetics, psychological concerns, or multiple skull fractures), or those who prefer to have surgery rather than to wear a halo brace.

Odontoid fractures that fail treatment with an orthosis require surgery. Orthotic failures include recurrent subluxations of the dens, an inability to restore satisfactory C1-C2 alignment, and nonunions. If the dens heals in a malaligned

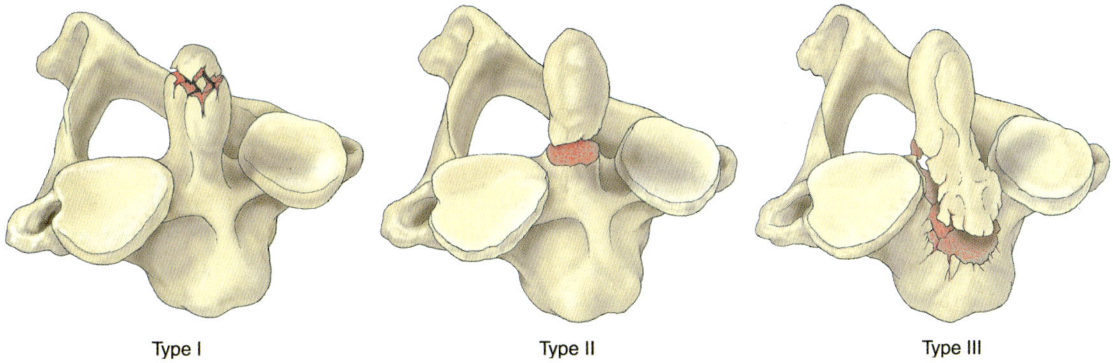

Fig. 39.1 Anderson and D'Alonzo[9] classification of odontoid fractures. Type I fractures are through the apex of the dens. Type II fractures extend across the neck of the dens. Type III fractures extend into the body of C2. (Reprinted with permission from Barrow Neurological Institute.)

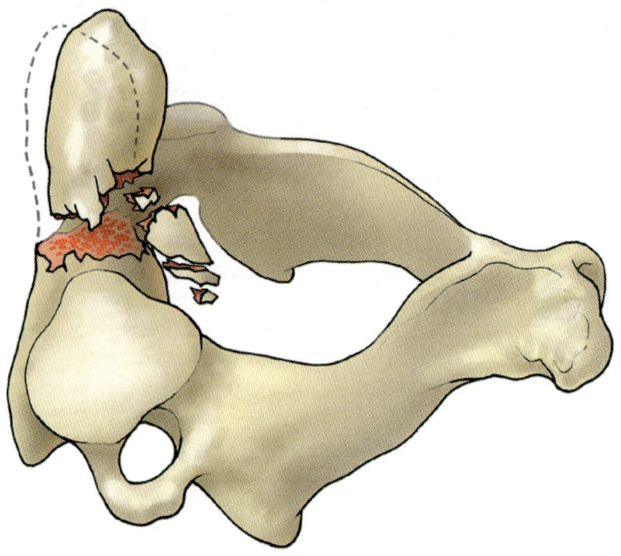

Fig. 39.2 Type IIA fractures have extensive comminution and are at high risk for nonunion when treated with an orthosis.[15] (From Hadley M, Browner C, Liu S, et al. New subtype of acute odontoid fractures (type IIA). Neurosurgery 1988;22(1):67–71. Reprinted with permission.)

position, chronic spinal cord compression and neurological deficits may develop. When the alignment of the dens cannot be maintained satisfactorily with a halo brace, surgical fixation should be considered. All patients treated with an orthosis require meticulous follow-up to detect nonunion and persistent atlantoaxial instability.

Contraindications

There are a variety of contraindications to odontoid screw fixation (**Table 39.2**): severe osteoporosis, fractures that extend deeply into the body of the dens (type III), or extensively comminuted bone fragments that have weakened the bone and will not hold a screw securely. If the transverse ligament is disrupted, an odontoid screw will not restore C1-C2 stability even if the dens is fixated solidly.[16] Odontoid screw fixation cannot be performed if C1-C2 alignment cannot be restored. Alignment is best restored preoperatively. Intraoperative realignment of the dens can be achieved with direct methods (i.e., manipulation of C1, C2, or both with instruments) or by altering the position of the head. All realignment maneuvers are monitored directly with fluoroscopy. Large chests, short necks, and fixed cervical flexion deformities prohibit the proper trajectory of the screws parallel to the anterior surface of the spine. Os odontoideum and chronic nonunions are associated with poor outcomes when treated with odontoid screws. Os odontoideum has sclerotic bone, which does not heal satisfactorily. Chronic nonunions have a higher nonunion rate than acute fractures because the fibrous tissue that forms between the fracture surfaces interferes with bone healing.

Table 39.2 Contraindications for Odontoid Screw Fixation

Severe osteoporosis
Extensive bone comminution
Disrupted transverse atlantal ligament
Os odontoideum
Type III odontoid fractures (with deep extension into C2 body)
Inability to restore C1-C2 alignment
Inability to achieve the appropriate trajectory for screw insertion
Short neck
Large barrel chest, large breasts
Fixed cervical flexion deformity
Inability to extend patient's head and neck
Chronic nonunions of type II odontoid fractures (relative contraindication)

Preoperative Radiographic Evaluation

Preoperative thin-section computed tomography (CT) is required to evaluate the bone architecture and to assess abnormalities that may preclude screw placement, (e.g., an aberrant course of the vertebral artery or extensive concurrent cervical fractures). Magnetic resonance imaging (MRI) of the cervical ligaments can be used to detect a disrupted transverse atlantal ligament preoperatively.[16,17] The relationship of an odontoid fracture associated with a disrupted transverse ligament has been reported in several cases.[16] Odontoid screw fixation is contraindicated when this disruption occurs because the screw will not restore atlantoaxial stability.

Surgical Procedure

Operating Room and Patient Positioning

Precise imaging using simultaneous anteroposterior (AP) open-mouth and lateral plane fluoroscopy is mandatory to visualize C2 intraoperatively so that the screw trajectory can be guided accurately. Fluoroscopy is an essential aspect of performing this operation and is achieved with two separate C-arms. The fracture must be reduced to anatomical alignment by positioning the head or by intraoperative manipulation before the screw is inserted. The screws compress the adjacent bone fragments together but will not restore alignment if the dens is malaligned horizontally. A malaligned fixation must be avoided because it can cause neural compression.

Odontoid screw fixation is performed using an anterior cervical operative exposure while the patient is supine. The patient's head and neck are extended to provide the proper screw trajectory into the tip of the dens (**Fig. 39.3**). Extension is performed carefully under fluoroscopic monitoring to avoid distraction or subluxation of the fracture. Extension is needed to position the drill and screw trajectory

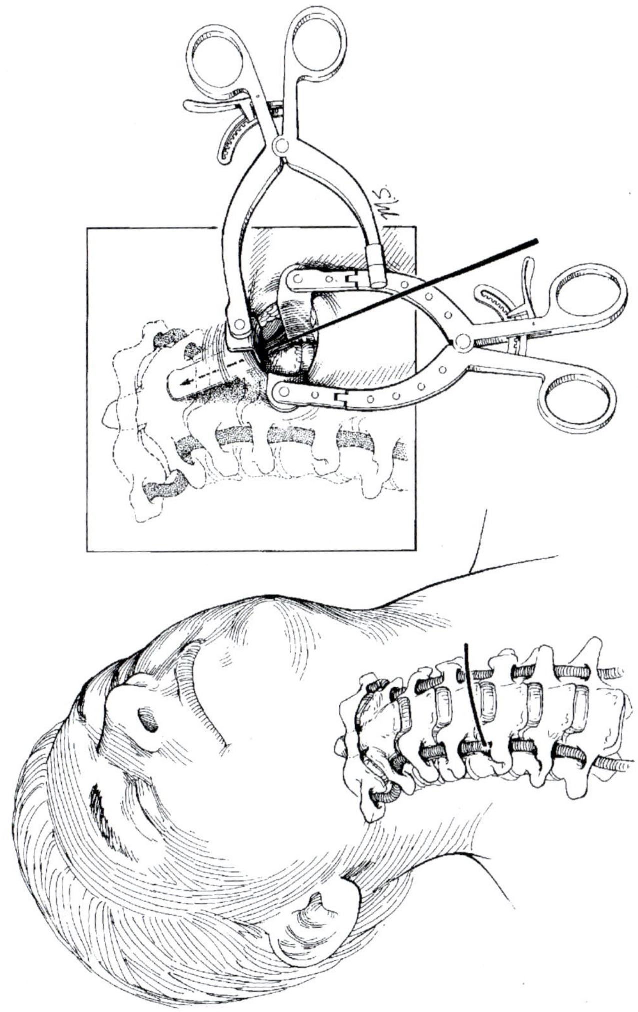

A

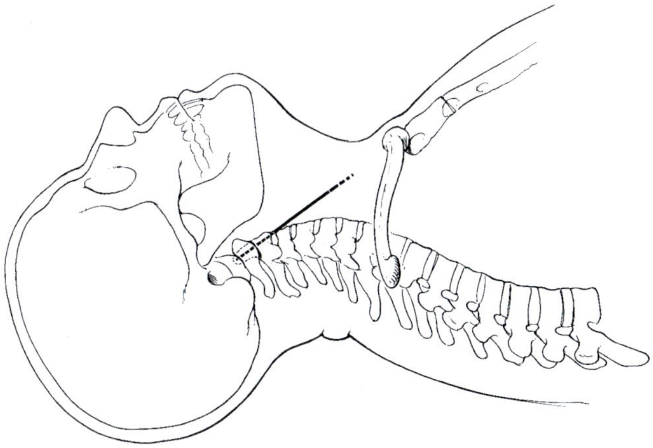

B

Fig. 39.3 **(A)** Patients are positioned supine with the head and neck extended to facilitate placing the screw into the tip of the dens. A transverse incision is made over the C4-C5 interspace to provide horizontal trajectory, parallel to the anterior surface of the spine. The Apfelbaum retraction system (Aesculap, San Francisco, CA) and the screw trajectory are depicted *(insert)*. **(B)** The proper screw trajectory cannot be achieved in patients with a short neck or a barrel chest.[20] (Reprinted with permission from Barrow Neurological Institute.)

parallel to the anterior surface of the cervical spine so that the screw can be aimed into the tip of the dens. The proper screw trajectory cannot be achieved in individuals with barrel-shaped large chests, short necks, or fixed cervical flexion deformities. Instead of odontoid screw fixation, such patients should undergo a posterior C1-C2 fixation.

Skull fixation with a Mayfield head holder interferes with positioning the C-arms and with obtaining the intraoperative radiographs. The head is best positioned on a radiolucent headrest, supported on a doughnut. Enough space must be maintained to position the two C-arms around the patient's head. Alternatively, the patient can be kept in a halo brace until screw fixation is achieved. To allow AP open-mouth fluoroscopy, the mouth is propped open widely with cloth, gauze, or other radiolucent materials.

Patient positioning and setup of the C-arms are critical for the success of this procedure (**Fig. 39.4**). These maneuvers often take longer than the surgical insertion of the screw. The AP C-arm is positioned above the head of the operating table. The lateral C-arm advances from the patient's left side. The anesthesia machines are positioned on the patient's left, near the thorax. The surgeon is on the patient's right side.

Ideally, the dens should be realigned preoperatively, and the alignment should be verified after the patient is positioned on the operating table. However, it is not always possible to restore C1-C2 alignment preoperatively. When the dens is displaced posteriorly, alignment may be restored intraoperatively by directly pushing the C2 body posteriorly with a curette. When the dens is displaced anteriorly, alignment can be restored by extending the patient's head and by positioning C1 and the dens more posteriorly.

Exposure

A transversely oriented cervical incision is made in the neck over the C4-C5 level. This lower neck incision facilitates a drill trajectory parallel to the anterior border of the cervical spine. The platysma muscle is undermined widely to allow adequate soft tissue retraction. The deep cervical fascia is dissected to separate the carotid sheath from the trachea and esophagus. The dissection is deepened to the level of the prevertebral fascia. The exposure is extended in a cephalad direction. The fascial planes are opened superiorly and a handheld retractor is inserted up to the level of the C2

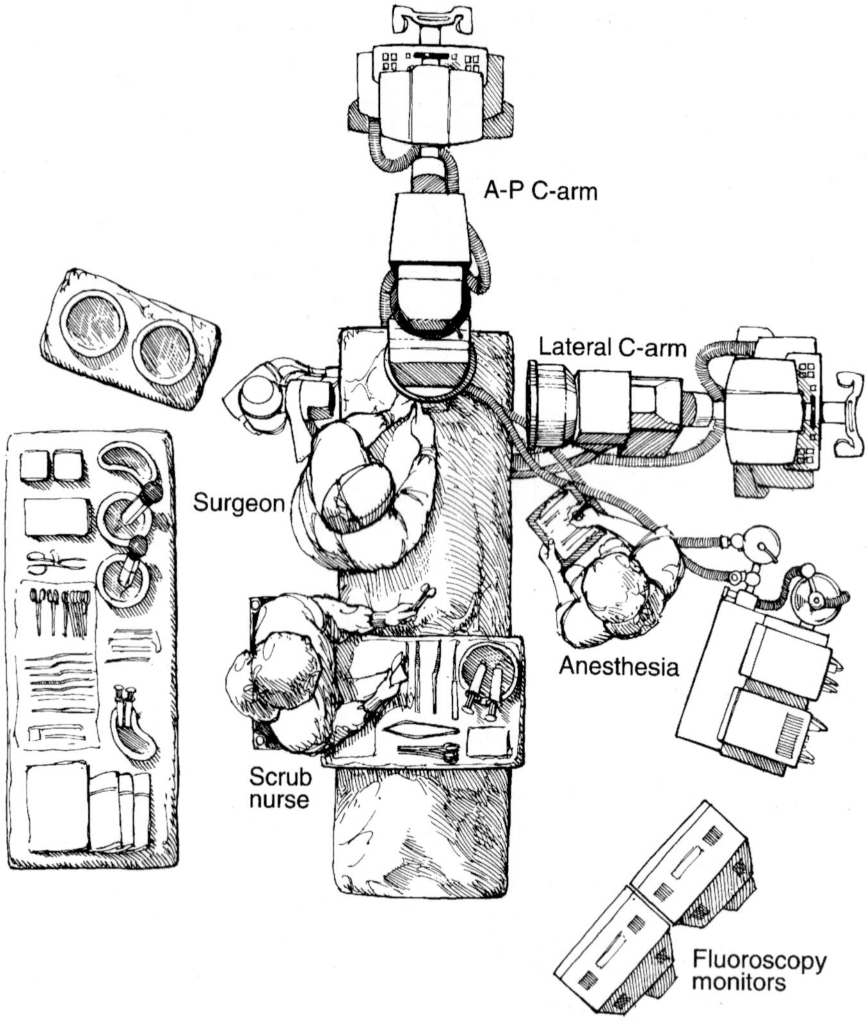

A

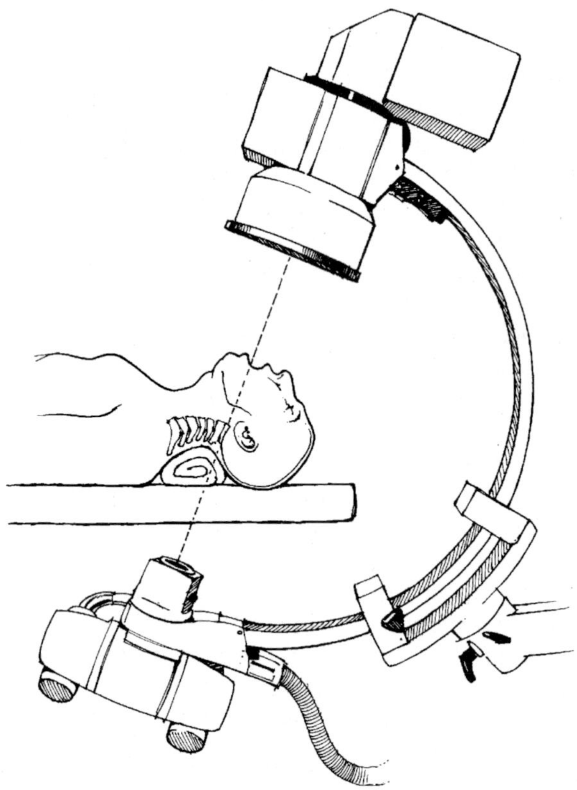

B

Fig. 39.4 **(A)** Organization of the surgical suite demonstrating the relative positions of the patient, personnel, and equipment. **(B)** The patient's neck is extended and the anteroposterior C-arm is positioned to provide an open-mouth view of the dens.[20] (Reprinted with permission from Barrow Neurological Institute.)

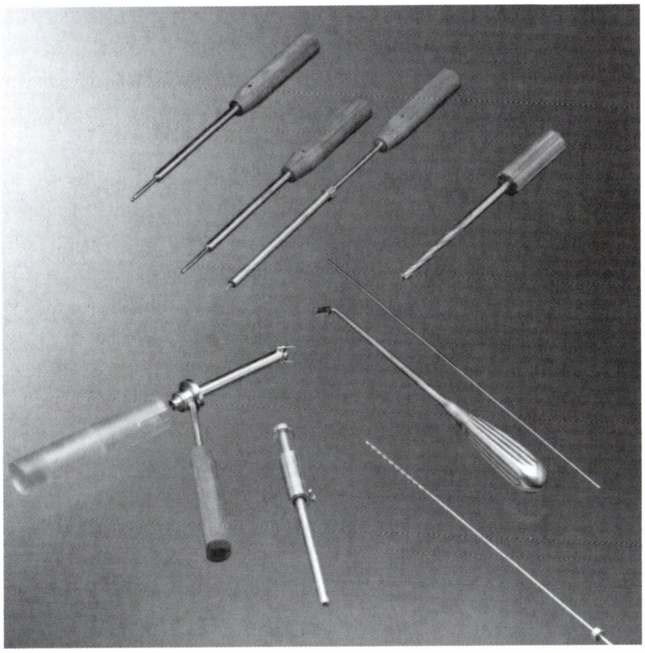

Fig. 39.5 The Apfelbaum instrumentation system (Aesculap, San Francisco, CA). Clockwise: screwdrivers, tap, hand drill, Kirschner wire, double-edged curette, drill bit, inner drill guide, outer drill guide.[8] (Provided courtesy of Aesculap, Inc., San Francisco, CA.)

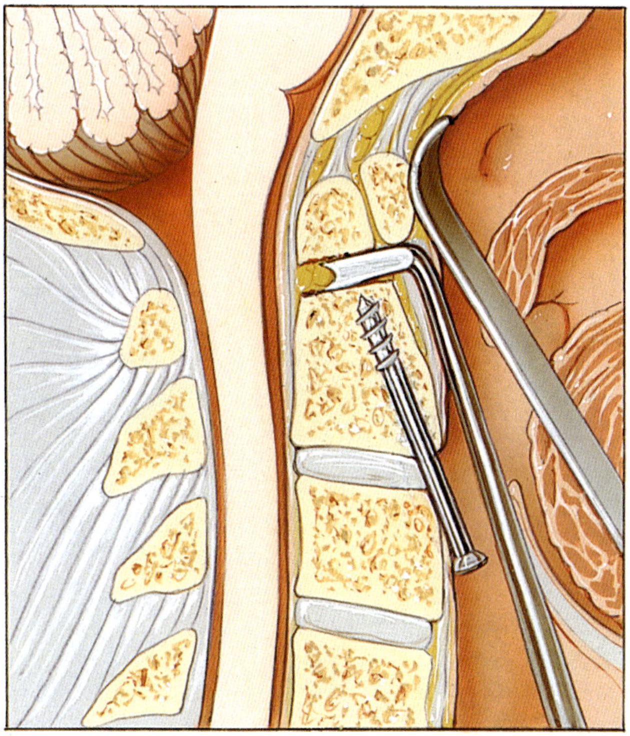

Fig. 39.6 Illustration showing use of an angled retractor blade and a double-edged curette.[8] (Provided courtesy of Aesculap, Inc., San Francisco, CA.) (Modified from Apfelbaum: Anterior screw fixation of odontoid fractures. In Rengachery SS, Wilkins RH (eds), Neurosurgical Operative Atlas, Vol. 2, Baltimore: Williams and Wilkins, 1992. Reprinted with permission from AANS.)

vertebral body. The exposure is achieved by dissecting directly over the anterior longitudinal ligament and requires no exposure or mobilization of the hypoglossal nerve, superior laryngeal nerve, or branches of the external carotid artery.

Kittner dissectors are used to dissect bluntly the prevertebral fascia up to the anterior C2-C3 level. The longus colli muscles adjacent to the C2-C3 disc space are coagulated at their medial borders and are elevated from the surface of the bone. A Hardy self-retaining retractor, used for transsphenoidal surgery, keeps the soft tissues away from the spine during the surgery. Handheld retractors, Apfelbaum retractors (Aesculap, San Francisco, CA), or Caspar retractors also can be used. Radiolucent retractors are recommended to facilitate inoperative radiographic imaging.

Specialized retractors and instrumentation (Apfelbaum odontoid instrument, Aesculap) have been developed to facilitate odontoid screw fixation (**Fig. 39.5**).[8] Self-retaining retractor blades maintain soft tissue retraction medially and laterally. An angled retractor blade retains the soft tissues superiorly in the midline to provide access for drilling and screwing. A double-edged curette can be used to remove soft tissue from bone surfaces in the event of a chronic nonunion (**Fig. 39.6**).

Screw Insertion Techniques

Typically, only one screw is needed to fixate the dens. There is no biomechanical advantage to inserting two screws; the second screw does not strengthen the fixation.[18,19] However, if the first screw does not reduce the fracture gap satisfactorily, a second screw may be needed. The entry points for drill and screw insertion are selected. When one screw is placed, a midline entry point is used. When two screws are placed, each enters 5 mm lateral to the midline and is directed 5 to 10 degrees medially into the tip of the dens (**Fig. 39.7**). If two screws are planned, the preoperative CT should be reviewed to determine whether the dens is wide enough to accommodate both screws.

A midline trough is cut into the anterosuperior edge of the C3 vertebral body and the C2-C3 annulus with a rongeur. The trough facilitates the flat screw trajectory into the tip of the dens (**Fig. 39.8**). The drill and screw should enter into the inferior C2 end plate, and the drill should not be inserted into the anterior body of C2. The cortical bone at the entry point for insertion of the drill is penetrated with a bone awl or high-speed drill to allow the drill bit to securely engage the bone as the pilot hole drilling is initiated.

The drill and screw are aimed into the center of the tip of the dens. The trajectory should be as horizontal as possible to capture the tip of the dens. If the trajectory is not horizontal enough, the drill and screw will penetrate through the posterior cortex of the dens into the spinal canal. When the drill and screw penetrate rostrally through the tip of the dens, they are adjacent to the alar and apical ligaments and

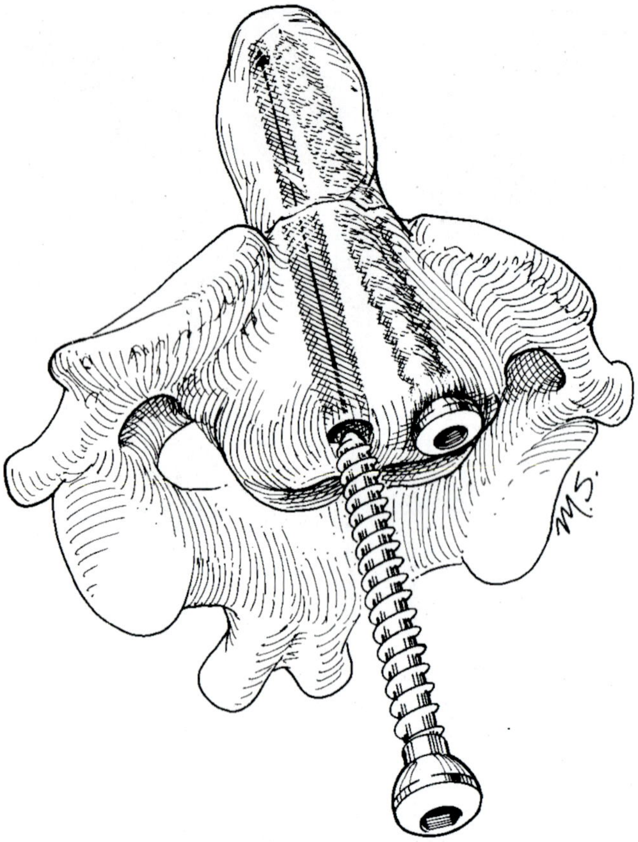

Fig. 39.7 When two screws are placed into the dens, the screws are angled 5 to 10 degrees medially.[20] (Reprinted with permission from Barrow Neurological Institute.)

do not endanger the spinal cord. The drill trajectory is carefully monitored with fluoroscopic guidance. The trajectory is adjusted as needed. Intradural penetration is avoided using precise maneuvers and careful radiographic monitoring throughout the procedure.

The screw length is measured with a depth gauge or by measuring the length of the drill within the bone (**Fig. 39.9**). The screw is inserted into the bone with a screwdriver. The screw tip barely penetrates the tip of the dens. If the odontoid fragment is distracted from the C2 body, a screw is selected that is shorter than the length of the pilot hole, because the gap will be obliterated as the bone fragment is reduced. The screw head should sit flush against the C2 body so that it does not protrude into the C2-C3 interspace. If the screw extends into the interspace, a lever effect can occur and cause the screw to loosen or to break.

■ Types of Screws for Odontoid Fixation

There are several methods to insert screws into the odontoid. Cannulated screws, noncannulated screws, self-tapping screws, or non–self-tapping screws can be used. The details of each type of screw system are reviewed in Chapter 37. Cannulated self-tapping screws provide the simplest method for odontoid screw fixation. This technique allows the screw fixation to be achieved in a few simple steps. The screw trajectory can be repositioned if needed, and the bones are fixated in continuity as the screws are inserted.

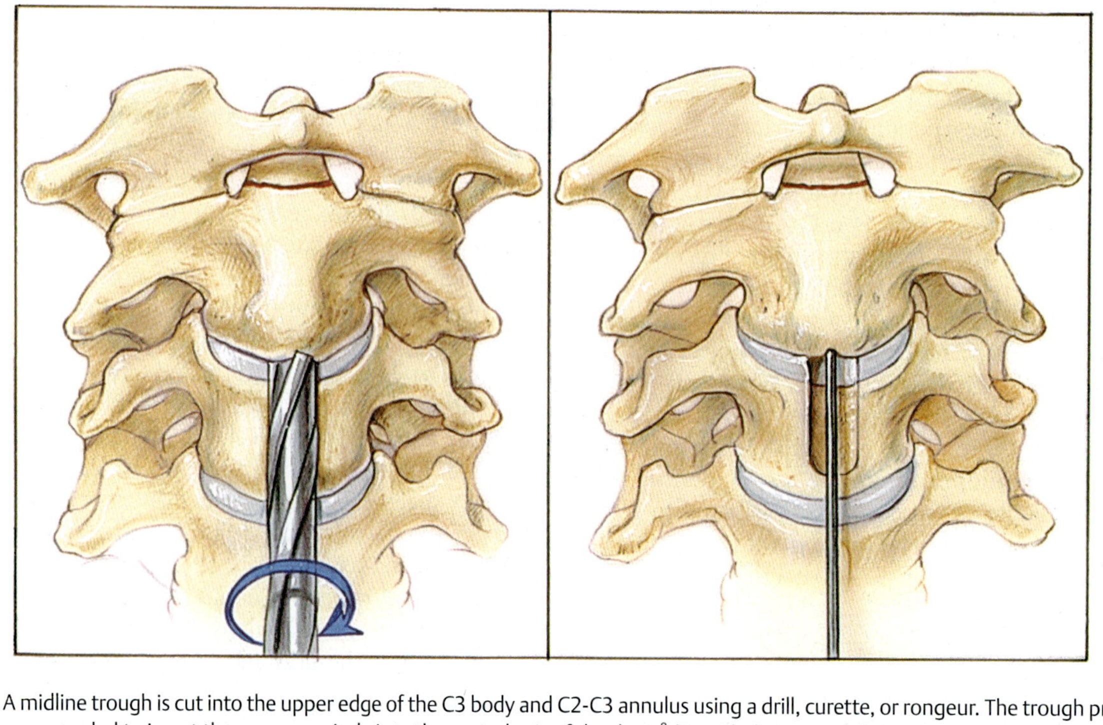

Fig. 39.8 A midline trough is cut into the upper edge of the C3 body and C2-C3 annulus using a drill, curette, or rongeur. The trough provides the additional space needed to insert the screw precisely into the central axis of the dens.[8] (Provided courtesy of Aesculap, Inc., San Francisco, CA.)

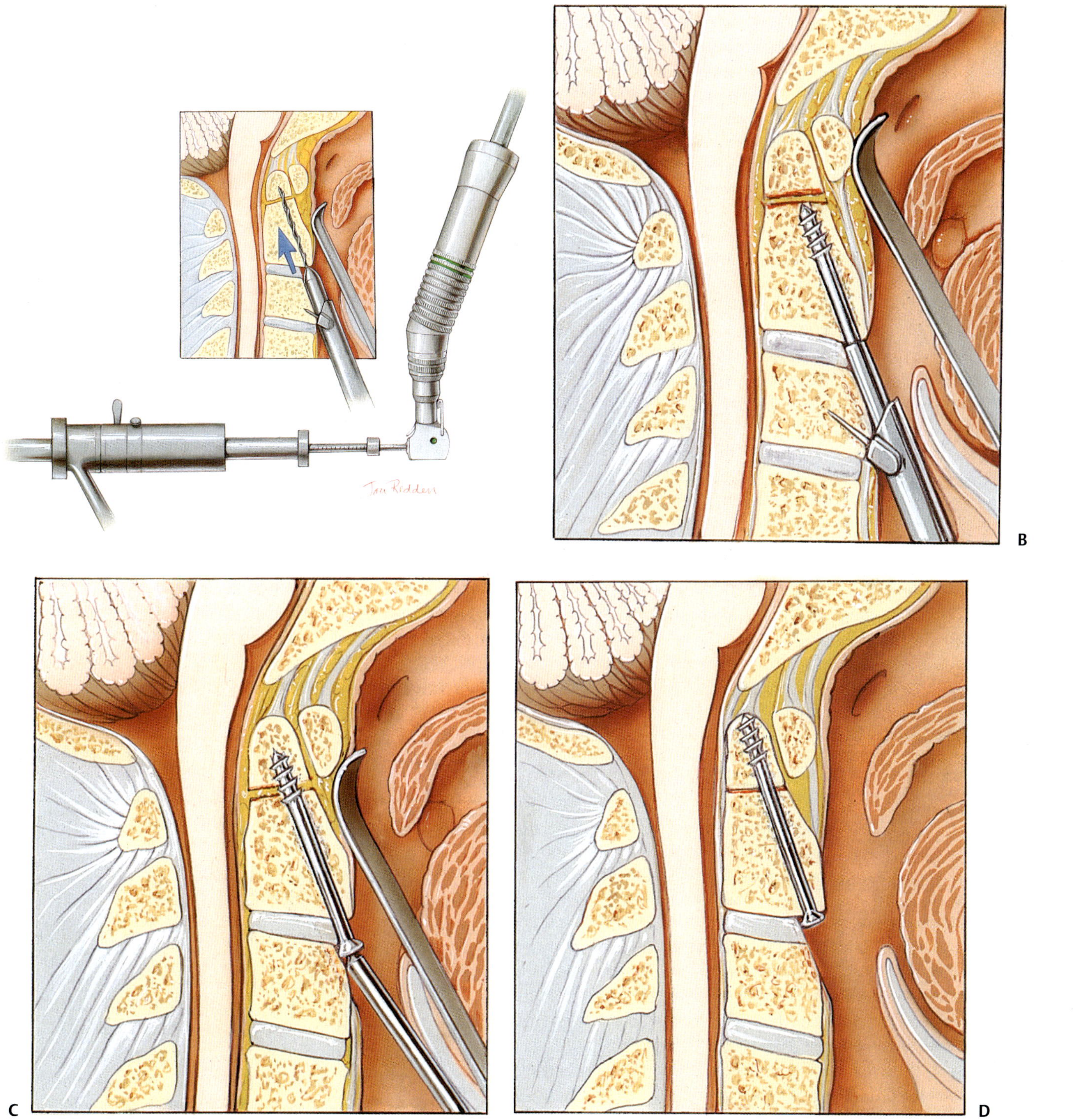

Fig. 39.9 **(A)** The Apfelbaum drill guide has sharp spikes that anchor it to the C3 vertebral body. An inner sheath is used to drill the pilot hole. The screw length is measured from calibrated markings on the proximal drill bit. **(B)** Subsequently, the pilot hole is tapped to cut the screw thread profile into the bone. **(C)** The screw is inserted into the bone using an Allen screwdriver. **(D)** In its final position, the head of the screw should sit flush against the body of C2 and should not protrude into the C2-C3 interspace.[8] *(continued)*

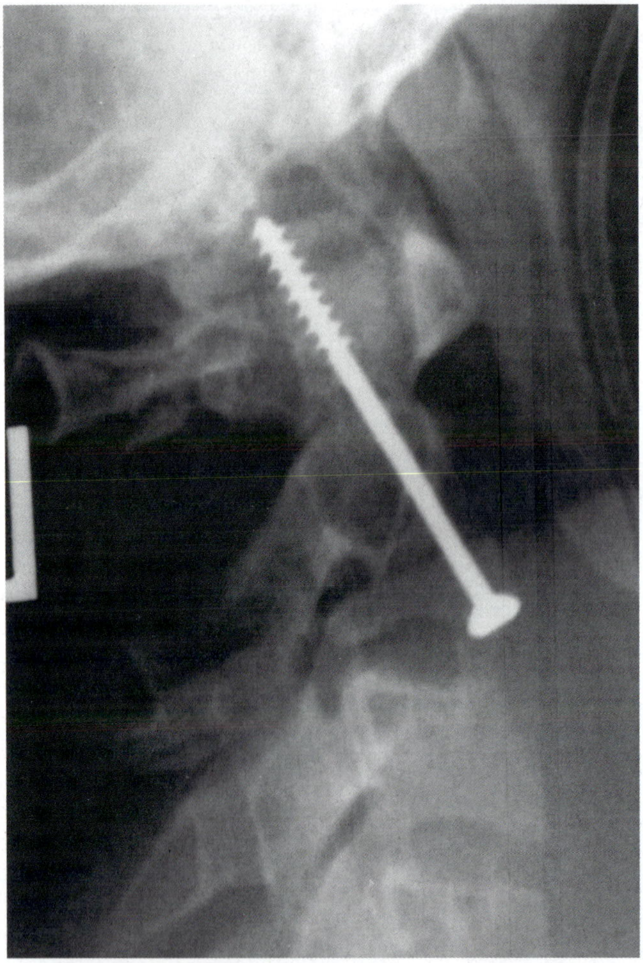

E

Fig. 39.9 *(continued)* **(E)** Postoperative lateral cervical radiograph of the final position of the odontoid screw. (Fig. 39.9A–D provided courtesy of Aesculap, Inc., San Francisco, CA.)

Cannulated Screw Systems

Cannulated screw systems use a thin (1.2-mm diameter) Kirschner wire (K-wire) to drill a precise trajectory into the bone (**Fig. 39.10**).[3,20] Hollow screws and hollow tools are threaded sequentially over the K-wire, which guides the intended trajectory into the bone. Cannulated screw systems have several advantages. First, if the K-wire trajectory was not ideal, the wire can be repositioned without destroying the bone. In comparison, if wide drill bits or wide screws are malpositioned, the screws often cannot be repositioned in the adjacent bone because a wide bone defect has been created. Second, the K-wire holds adjacent unstable bone fragments together during screw insertion, preventing loss of alignment of the pilot holes. Cannulated screws are associated with the disadvantage of potential intradural advancement of the K-wire during manipulation with tools. This problem is avoided by using long K-wires, grasping the end of the K-wire with a needle holder, and monitoring all maneuvers with fluoroscopy.

The details of cannulated screw insertion are provided fully in Chapter 40. Only a few simple steps are required. The K-wire is drilled into C2 until its tip engages the tip of the dens. The screw length is measured and a 3.5- or 4.0-mm diameter self-tapping screw is inserted directly over the K-wire. The K-wire is then removed.

Noncannulated Screws

Noncannulated bone screws can be used relatively easily for odontoid fixation.[1,2,4–8,18,19] A pilot hole is drilled with a drill bit that matches the core diameter (i.e., inner diameter, minor diameter) of the screw (i.e., a 2.5-mm bit for a 3.5-mm diameter screw). The pilot hole is relatively wide; therefore, a new pilot hole cannot be drilled if the initial drill trajectory was malpositioned. The drill and screw trajectory are monitored with fluoroscopy. Self-tapping or non–self-tapping screws can be inserted into the pilot hole. Self-tapping screws have sharp threads and a sharp tip with a cutting channel. They can be inserted directly into the bone without using a tap. In comparison, non–self-tapping screws have dull tips and dull threads. They require tapping to cut the thread profile into the pilot hole before the screw is inserted.

Lag Screw Fixation

A lag effect is required for odontoid fixation regardless of the type of screw used.[1,2,6,20] Lag screws compress bone fragments together to facilitate bone healing. The dens is compressed against C2 using this technique. A lag effect is achieved when the screw threads purchase only the distal and not the proximal bone fragment. This effect is provided by an end-threaded screw or by using a fully threaded screw after a wide gliding hole has been drilled in the proximal bone (**Fig. 39.11**).[20]

Postoperative Care

A Philadelphia collar or semirigid cervical orthosis is worn postoperatively until the bone unites satisfactorily. The immediate fixation strength of an odontoid screw is only half the strength of the normal odontoid.[18,19] Therefore, excessive loads placed on the screw before the bone heals can cause the screw to bend or to lever out of the anterior C2 vertebral body. An orthosis of some type is needed until the bone heals satisfactorily, usually within 10 to 12 weeks after surgery. Meticulous follow-up with flexion-extension radiographs is needed to monitor for osseous union and screw integrity.

Biomechanics of Odontoid Screw Fixation

Oblique type II dens fractures are not well suited for placing a screw. If a displaced oblique dens fracture is fixed with a screw, shearing forces are generated as the screw is tightened. These forces can cause the bone fragments to shift and therefore to fixate in a malaligned position (**Fig. 39.12**).

Odontoid screws do not restore normal strength to the dens immediately. Until the fracture heals, they restore

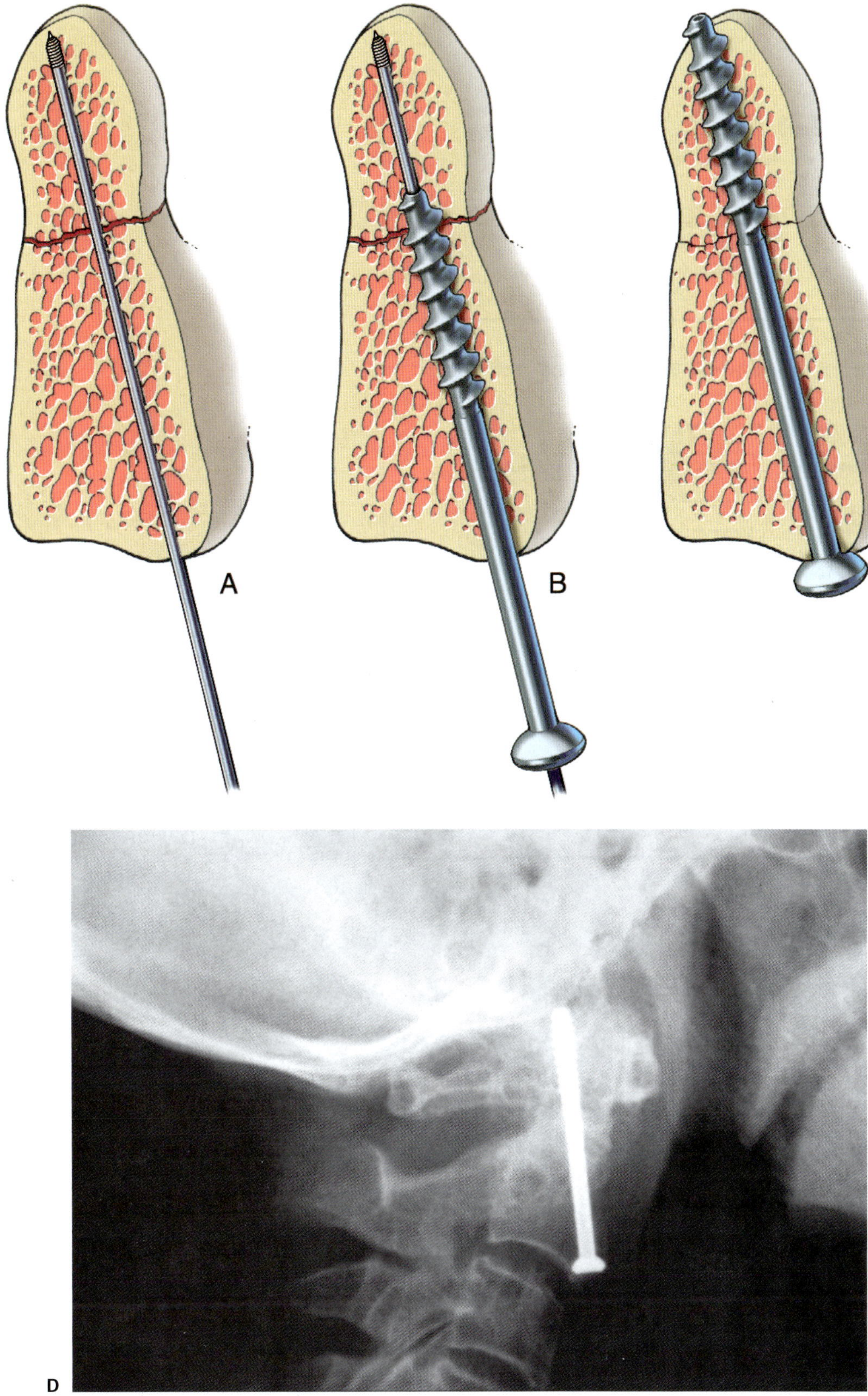

Fig. 39.10 Cannulated screws use a Kirschner wire (K-wire) to direct the insertion of hollow tools and hollow screws into the bone. **(A)** The K-wire is drilled into the dens to fixate the fracture and to provide a guide for the screw. **(B)** A self-tapping screw is inserted directly over the K-wire. **(C)** The K-wire is removed. **(D)** Radiograph of a cannulated screw 3 months after surgery. A solid fusion has formed.[20] (Reprinted with permission from Barrow Neurological Institute.)

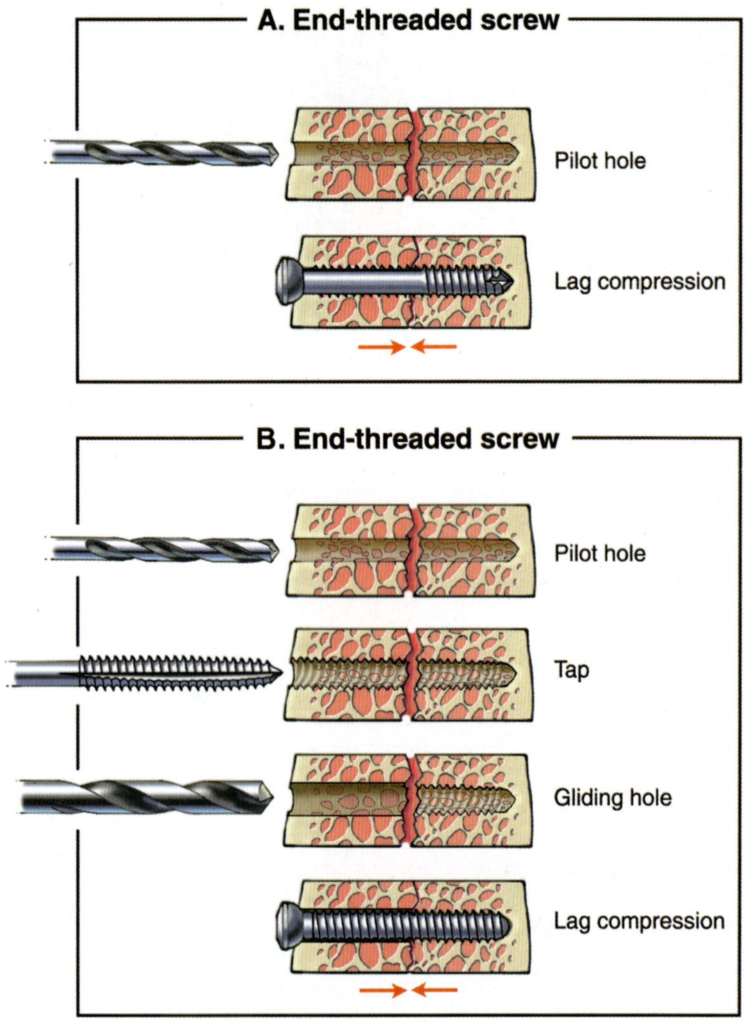

Fig. 39.11 Lag screws compress adjacent bone fragments together. A lag effect is achieved by several methods. **(A)** An end-threaded screw engages only the distal fragment of bone. If the threads purchase the proximal bone, a lag effect (i.e., compression) will not be generated. **(B)** A lag effect can be achieved with a fully threaded screw by drilling a wide gliding hole in the proximal bone so that the proximal threads of the screw do not engage the bone.[20] (Reprinted with permission from Barrow Neurological Institute.)

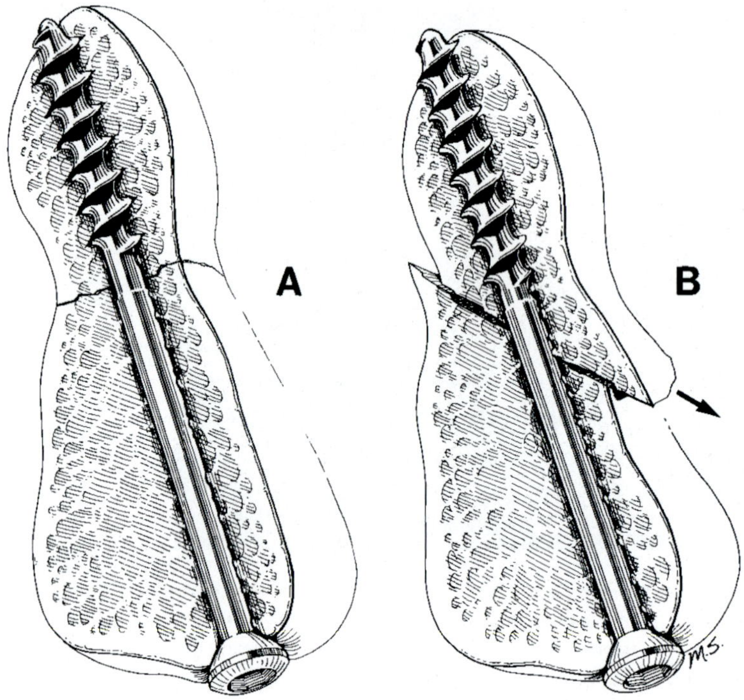

Fig. 39.12 Lag screws used to reduce an oblique dens fracture may generate shearing forces that can cause the bone fragments to shift as the bones are compressed together. **(A)** A transverse type II fracture is ideal for an odontoid screw. **(B)** An oblique, malaligned type II fracture may shift during reduction.[20] (Reprinted with permission from Barrow Neurological Institute.)

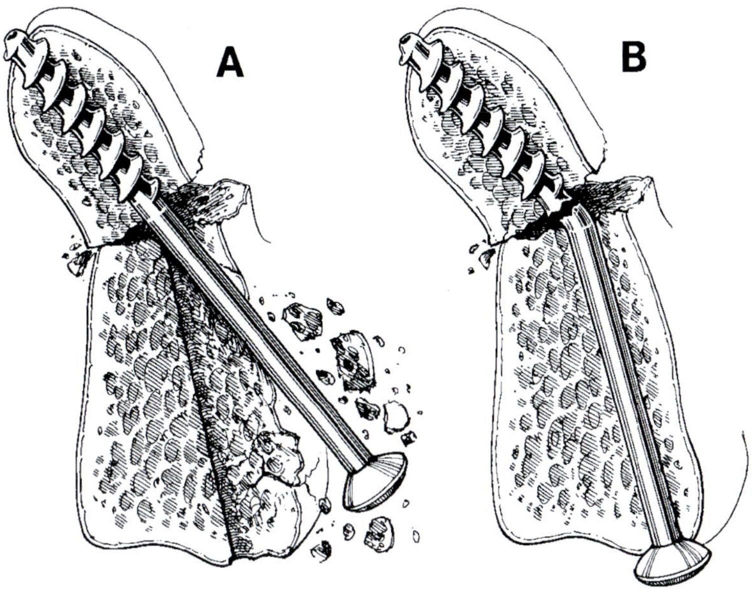

Fig. 39.13 Mechanisms of odontoid screw failure. **(A)** The proximal shaft of the screw can lever through the anterior vertebral body of C2 if the bone is thin or weakened. **(B)** The screws can bend or break across the fracture if excessive torque is applied to the spine.[20] (Reprinted with permission from Barrow Neurological Institute.)

only half of the original mechanical strength to the dens.[18,19] When odontoid screws are excessively loaded and fail, a lever effect occurs. Either the screw bends or breaks across the fracture site or the proximal screw shaft can fracture through the anterior C2 vertebral body (**Fig. 39.13**). Therefore, screws should not be relied on as the only source of mechanical fixation needed during the immediate postoperative phase. An orthosis also should be used.

There is no mechanical difference in the immediate fixation strength, whether one or two screws are used.[19] Theoretically, two screws provide some rotational control of the dens; however, the risk of inserting a second screw must be weighed against its potential benefit.

Conclusion

Odontoid screw fixation is unique compared with other methods of spinal stabilization because it stabilizes the fracture directly and completely preserves all normal cervical motion. Normal motion at C1-C2 is particularly important because of the prominent axial rotation at this level. More than half of all cervical axial rotation occurs at C1-C2.

Acute displaced type II dens fractures are best suited for an odontoid screw. Chronic nonunions have scar tissue that can be difficult to remove in an attempt to promote fusion. Os odontoideum should not be treated with odontoid screws because the bone surfaces cannot be prepared properly to ensure fusion.

Odontoid screws are contraindicated when the bone will not hold a screw securely (e.g., if the bone is soft or fractured excessively), when the transverse ligament is disrupted, or when the screws cannot be inserted properly (irreducible fractures or an unsuitable body habitus). In these patients a different method of C1-C2 fixation should be performed.

Odontoid screws are reasonably strong, but they do not immediately restore normal strength to the dens. An orthosis is suggested as a postoperative load-sharing device that can minimize stress on the fixation until the bone heals.

References

1. Barbour JR. Screw fixation in fracture of the odontoid process. South Aust Clin 1971;5:20–24
2. Borne GM, Bedou GL, Pinaudeau M, Cristino G, Hussein A. Odontoid process fracture osteosynthesis with a direct screw fixation technique in nine consecutive cases. J Neurosurg 1988;68(2):223–226
3. Etter C, Coscia M, Jaberg H, Aebi M. Direct anterior fixation of dens fractures with a cannulated screw system. Spine 1991;16 (3, Suppl):S25–S32
4. Geisler FH, Cheng C, Poka A, Brumback RJ. Anterior screw fixation of posteriorly displaced type II odontoid fractures. Neurosurgery 1989;25(1):30–37, discussion 37–38
5. Knoringer P. Double-threaded compression screws for osteosynthesis of acute fractures of the odontoid process. In: Voth D, Glees P, eds. Diseases in the Cranio-Cervical Junction. Anatomical and Pathological Aspects and Detailed Clinical Accounts. Berlin: de Gruyter; 1987;127–136
6. Böhler J. Anterior stabilization for acute fractures and non-unions of the dens. J Bone Joint Surg Am 1982;64(1):18–27
7. Donovan MM. Efficacy of rigid fixation of fractures of the odontoid process. Retrospective analysis of fifty-four cases. Orthop Trans 1979;3:309
8. Apfelbaum R. Anterior screw fixation of odontoid fractures. In: Rengachary SS, Wilkins RH, eds. Neurosurgical Operative Atlas, 2nd ed. Baltimore, MD: Williams & Wilkins; 1992:189–199
9. Anderson LD, D'Alonzo RT. Fractures of the odontoid process of the axis. J Bone Joint Surg Am 1974;56(8):1663–1674

10. Hadley MN, Dickman CA, Browner CM, Sonntag VK. Acute axis fractures: a review of 229 cases. J Neurosurg 1989;71(5 Pt 1):642–647
11. Apuzzo MLJ, Heiden JS, Weiss MH, Ackerson TT, Harvey JP, Kurze T. Acute fractures of the odontoid process. An analysis of 45 cases. J Neurosurg 1978;48(1):85–91
12. Clark CR, White AAI III. Fractures of the dens. A multicenter study. J Bone Joint Surg Am 1985;67(9):1340–1348
13. Dunn ME, Seljeskog EL. Experience in the management of odontoid process injuries: an analysis of 128 cases. Neurosurgery 1986; 18(3):306–310
14. Ekong CEU, Schwartz ML, Tator CH, Rowed DW, Edmonds VE. Odontoid fracture: management with early mobilization using the halo device. Neurosurgery 1981;9(6):631–637
15. Hadley MN, Browner CM, Liu SS, Sonntag VK. New subtype of acute odontoid fractures (type IIA). Neurosurgery 1988;22(1 Pt 1):67–71
16. Greene KA, Dickman CA, Marciano FF, Drabier J, Drayer BP, Sonntag VK. Transverse atlantal ligament disruption associated with odontoid fractures. Spine 1994;19(20):2307–2314
17. Dickman CA, Mamourian A, Sonntag VKH, Drayer BP. Magnetic resonance imaging of the transverse atlantal ligament for the evaluation of atlantoaxial instability. J Neurosurg 1991;75(2): 221–227
18. Doherty BJ, Heggeness MH, Esses SI. A biomechanical study of odontoid fractures and fracture fixation. Spine 1993;18(2): 178–184
19. Sasso RC, Doherty BJ, Crawford MJ, Heggeness MH. Biomechanics of odontoid fracture fixation. Comparison of the one- and two-screw technique. Spine 1993;18(14):1950–1953
20. Dickman CA, Sonntag VKH, Marcotte PJ. Techniques of screw fixation of the cervical spine. BNI Q 1992;8(2):9–26

40 Posterior Atlantoaxial Screw Fixation

Nicholas C. Bambakidis, David J. Hart, and Curtis A. Dickman

Traditionally, atlantoaxial instability has been treated surgically using posterior C1-C2 wiring and bone grafts. However, bone grafts and wires do not provide rigid internal fixation of C1-C2, and they have high nonunion rates unless supplemented with a halo brace.[1-4] There are several techniques to fixate C1 and C2 with screws. Magerl[5] initially developed posterior atlantoaxial facet screw fixation as a way to achieve rigid internal fixation of C1-C2 by eliminating motion, promoting arthrodesis, and treating instability. The technique is useful but has risks as well as advantages. Alternatively, the technique of C1-C2 fixation utilizing the lateral mass of C1 and pars interarticularis, lamina or pedicle of C2 with screw-rod fixation is an excellent method of achieving solid fixation, as described by Harms[6] and modified by Goel.[7,8] This chapter describes the operative techniques for posterior atlantoaxial facet screw fixation, C1 lateral mass screw fixation, C2 pars and C2 lamina screw fixation, and strategies to minimize or avoid complications.

Indications

Atlantoaxial instability

Contraindications

1. Aberrant course of vertebral artery (as seen on computed tomography [CT] or magnetic resonance angiography)
2. Destruction of C2 pars interarticularis and C1 lateral mass
3. Severe osteoporosis

Preoperative Evaluation

1. Flexion and extension radiographs (evaluate reducibility and instability)
2. CT with sagittal reconstructions through the screw path (**Fig. 40.1**)

Patient Positioning and Preparation

1. Prone
2. Flexed position of the neck (**Fig. 40.2**)
3. Fluoroscopic monitoring during neck positioning (lateral C-arm)

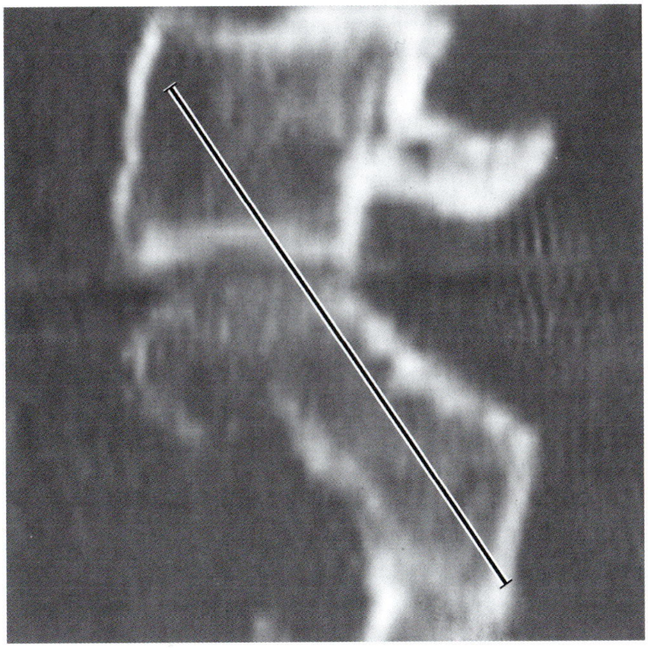

A

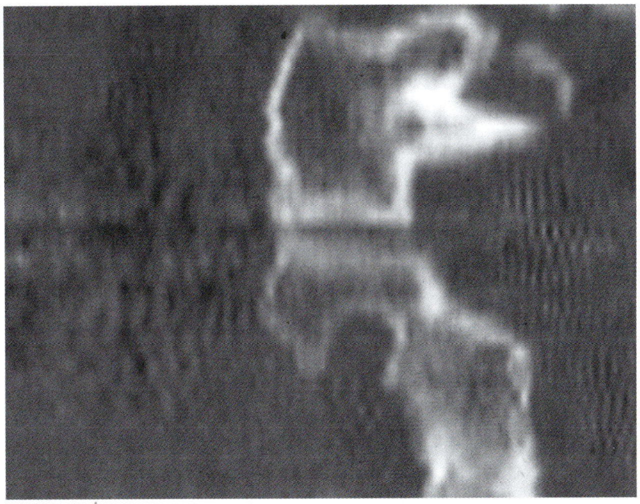

B

Fig. 40.1 Sagittal reformatted computed tomography images through the C2 pars interarticularis and the C1 lateral mass. **(A)** Normal bone structures permit insertion of a transarticular screw. **(B)** In this patient, an aberrant foramen transversarium precluded placing a screw on one side.

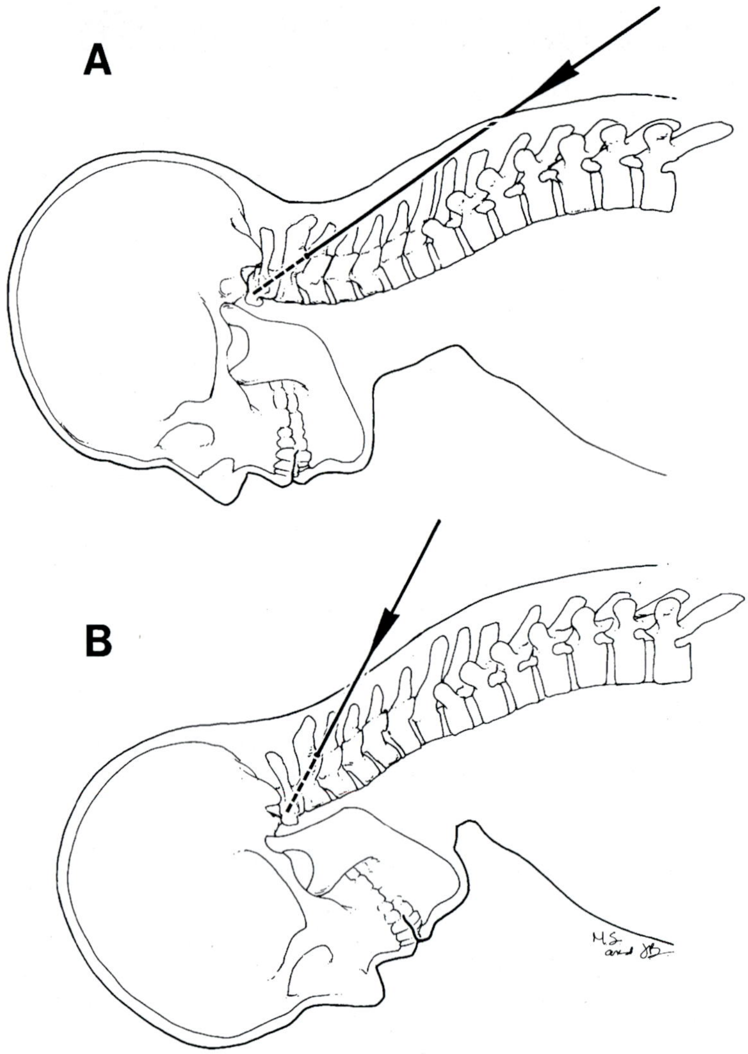

Fig. 40.2 Neck flexion helps to obtain the appropriate trajectory for drilling and screw insertion. **(A)** If the neck cannot be flexed, percutaneous drilling is performed. **(B)** When the neck can be flexed, drilling often can be performed directly through the incision used to expose C1 and C2. The patient is positioned while the cervical alignment is monitored with real-time fluoroscopy to avoid subluxation and neurological injury. (From Marcotte P, Dickman C, Sonntag VK, Karahalios DG, Drabier J. Posterior atlantoaxial facet screw fixation. J Neurosurg 1993;79:234–237. Reprinted with permission.)

4. Head fixation with Mayfield skull clamp and halo ring
5. Intraoperative somatosensory evoked potential monitoring

Operative Technique of Transarticular Screw Fixation

Neck flexion helps obtain the proper trajectory for the drills and screws, which should be almost parallel to the posterior surface of the spine (**Fig. 40.2**). Lateral fluoroscopic monitoring is used to assess spinal alignment during positioning, drilling, and screw insertion.

A posterior cervical incision is made to access the atlas and axis. The incision extends from the inion to the spinous process of C7 or to the spinous process of C3, if percutaneous drilling technique is planned. The skin over the upper thoracic level is prepared if percutaneous access is needed for drilling (**Fig. 40.2A**).

C1 and C2 are exposed using a subperiosteal dissection. The C2 pars interarticularis and the C1-C2 articular surfaces are exposed and visualized directly. The ligamentum flavum is removed adjacent to the C2 laminae and pars interarticularis. A thin Kirschner wire (K-wire) or a no. 4 Penfield dissector is placed directly along the upper surface of the C2 pars interarticularis into the atlantoaxial facet joint and retracted upward to displace the C2 nerve root and venous plexus superiorly. Removal of the ligament and retraction of the C2 nerve root enable direct visualization of the C2 pars interarticularis and C1-C2 facet joint during drilling (**Fig. 40.3**). Bleeding around the C2 root from the venous plexus is controlled by gentle packing with Surgicel (Ethicon, Somerville, NJ) and bipolar cauterization. Various commercially available products utilizing preparations of powdered Gelfoam (DuPuy, Raynham, MA) and thrombin (e.g., FloSeal [Baxter, Deerfield, IL], Surgifoam [Ferrosan, Soeborg, Denmark]) are extremely effective for this as well.

If needed, the atlas and axis are realigned by manual reduction. Anterior atlantoaxial subluxations are reduced by gently displacing C2 anteriorly and by pulling C1 posteriorly. Opposite forces are applied for posterior C1-C2 subluxations. A wire or braided cable is placed around the ring of

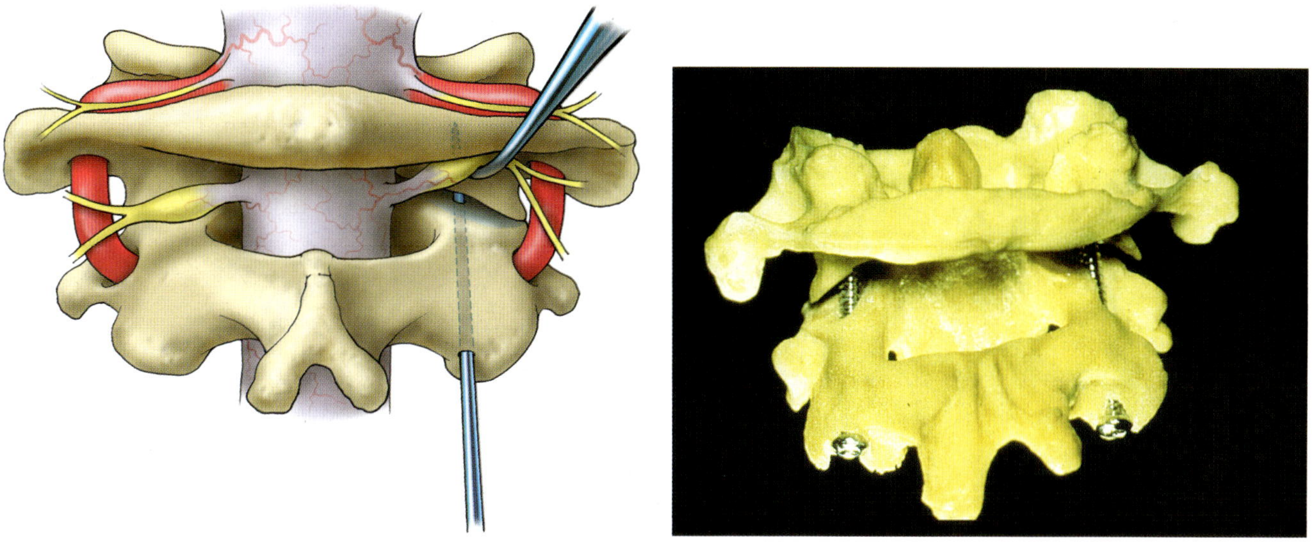

Fig. 40.3 Dorsal view of C1-C2. **(A)** The C2 nerve root and venous plexus are retracted superiorly, and the ligamentum flavum is removed to allow direct visualization of the C2 pars interarticularis and facet joint during drilling. The drill enters C2 just above the C2-C3 facet joint. **(B)** The screws positioned in a model of C1-C2. (Reprinted with permission from Barrow Neurological Institute.)

C1 for traction and for later fixation of an interspinous bone graft. Direct traction of C2 is applied with an Allis clamp attached to the C2 spinous process. The C2 spinous process is retracted gently toward the base of the occiput to obtain an ideal trajectory for drilling.

The drill enters the caudal aspect of the C2 inferior facet, 2 to 3 mm lateral to the medial edge of the C2-C3 facet (**Fig. 40.3**). Occasionally, the entry point is adjusted 1 to 2 mm to compensate for the altered anatomical relationships of the vertebrae. First, the posterior cortical bone of C2 is penetrated with a bone awl or high-speed drill. This step precisely directs the drill insertion for the pilot hole to prevent the bit from migrating as drilling begins.

Lateral fluoroscopic monitoring is used to adjust the drill trajectory toward the dorsal cortex of the anterior arch of C1 (**Fig. 40.4**). In the anteroposterior direction, the drill is placed through the central axis of the C2 pars interarticularis. A sagittal trajectory between 0 and 10 degrees medially is required (**Fig. 40.5**). Typically, the screw trajectory is straight in a sagittal orientation. The sagittal trajectory is oriented along the central axis of the C2 pars interarticularis, which is visualized directly by retracting the C2 root during the drilling.

Cannulated or noncannulated screws can be used for C1-C2 fixation. The tract for the screw is created with a drill while the path is monitored with lateral plane fluoroscopy and direct visualization. A K-wire is used for drilling when cannulated screws are used. For noncannulated screws, a wider cylindrical drill bit (2.5 mm diameter) is used to drill the pilot hole.

After the length of the screw has been measured, the screw is inserted into the bone with a screwdriver. On lateral fluoroscopic imaging, the tip of the screw should be positioned behind the dorsal cortical rim of the anterior arch of C1 (**Fig. 40.6**). Screws ventral to this cortical rim can penetrate through C1 anteriorly. Screws should not extend cephalad or they could cross the occipitoatlantal joint.

As the screws cross the joint space into Cl, the atlas and axis become rigidly coupled. The surgeon can feel the vertebrae lock together with characteristic stiffness as the screws

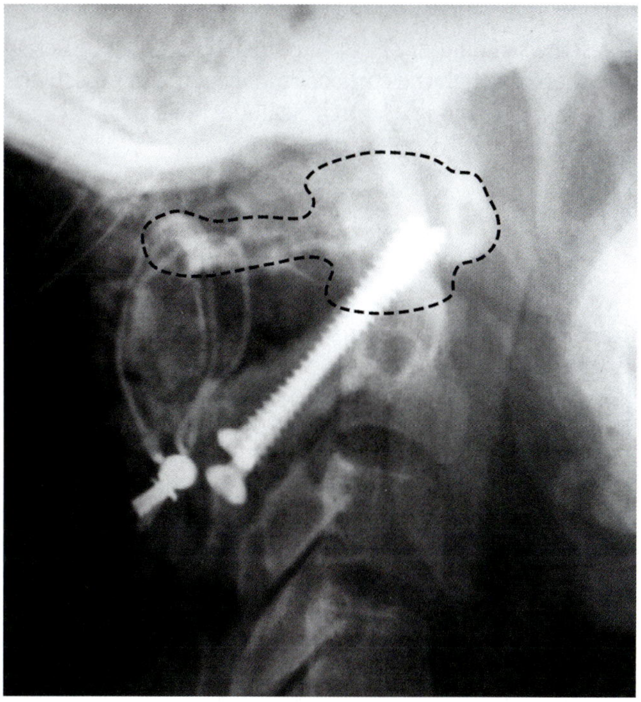

Fig. 40.4 A postoperative lateral cervical radiograph demonstrates the screw trajectory. Screws are directed through the center of the C2 pars interarticularis. Lateral fluoroscopy is used to adjust the screw path toward the anterior arch of Cl. The tips of the screws are positioned behind the posterior cortex of the anterior arch of C1.

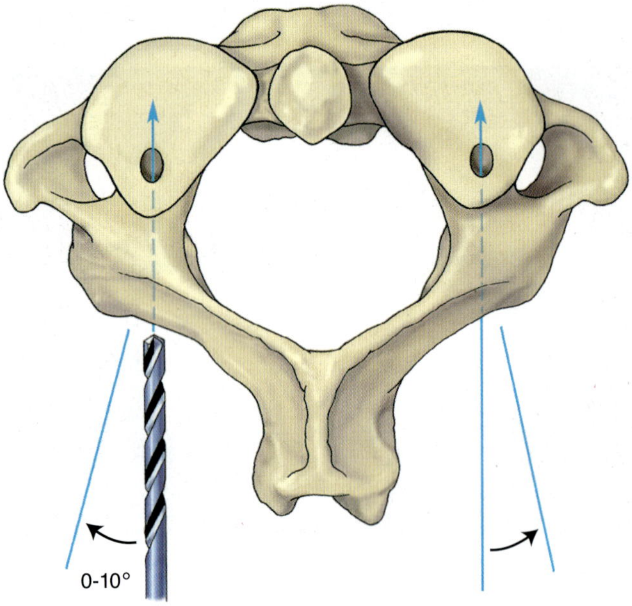

Fig. 40.5 The screws are positioned sagittally through the center of the C2 pars interarticularis. The angle varies between 0 and 10 degrees medially and depends on the position of the entry site of the screw relative to the pars interarticularis. (From Marcotte P, Dickman C, Sonntag VK, Karahalios DG, Drabier J. Posterior atlantoaxial facet screw fixation. J Neurosurg 1993;79:234–237. Reprinted with permission.)

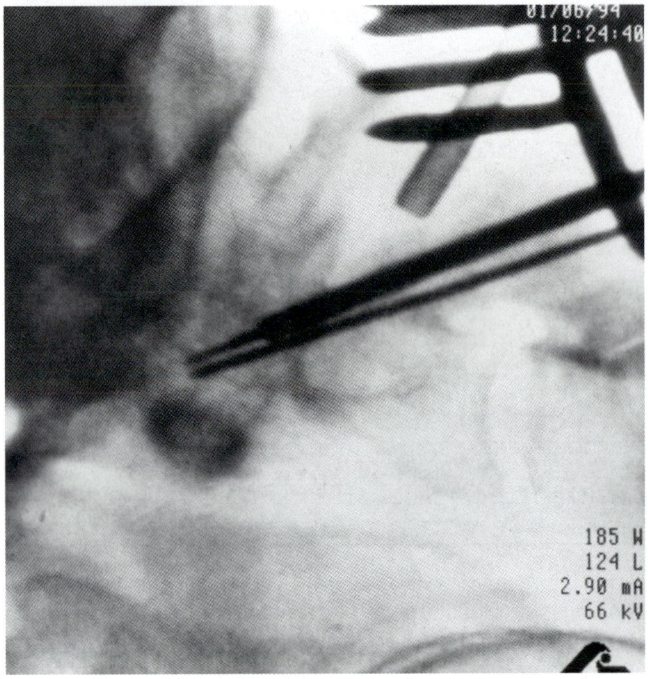

Fig. 40.6 Intraoperative lateral fluoroscopic image of percutaneous screw insertion using long cannulated tools. Pilot holes are drilled bilaterally using long guide pins or Kirschner wires. The screws are positioned with their tips behind the dorsal cortex of the anterior ring of C1.

are inserted. The screw heads are positioned flush against the bone surfaces or recessed slightly into the bone to prevent the screws from levering against the C2-C3 joint space. The screws should not be overtightened because the screw will shear through the cortex of the C2 pars interarticularis and facet, destroying its purchase in the bone.

After the screws have been inserted bilaterally, a bicortical interspinous strut graft is placed using autologous iliac crest bone.[1] The graft is fitted precisely and wired into position to compress it between C1 and C2 (**Fig. 40.7**). The graft provides the substrate for fusion. The wire provides three-point fixation (two screws plus the wire)

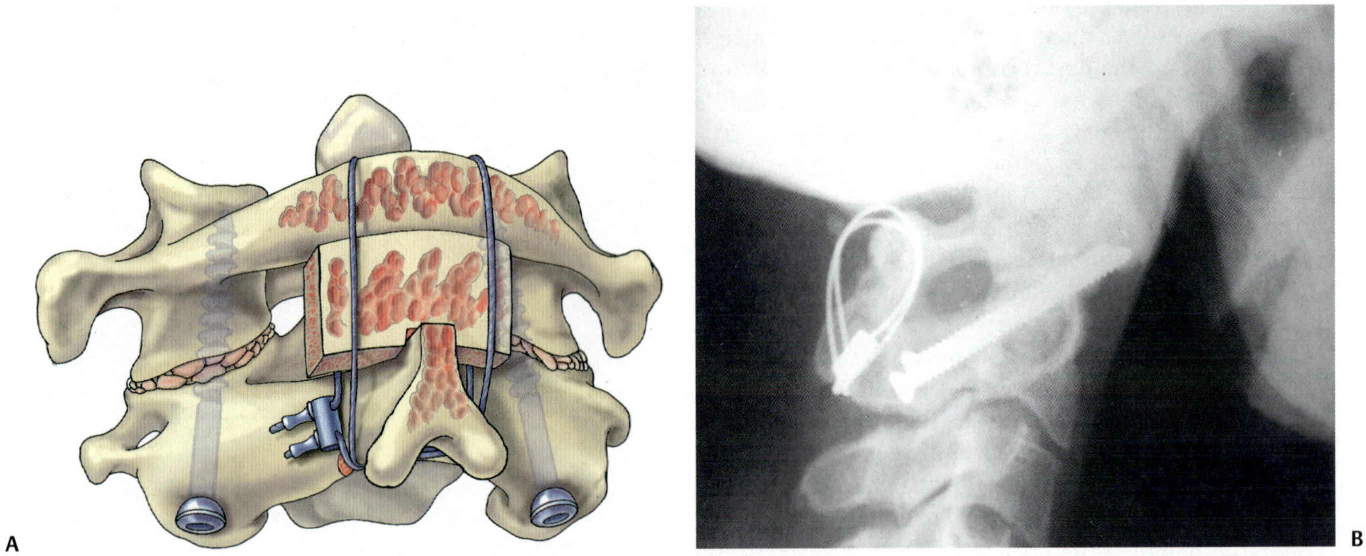

Fig. 40.7 Illustration of a three-point fixation construct. **(A)** A bicortical strut graft is wired so that it is compressed between C1 and C2. The wired graft facilitates fusion and provides additional mechanical stabilization. **(B)** Postoperative lateral cervical radiograph demonstrates the position of the screws, cables, and a well-developed osseous union. (From Marcotte P, Dickman C, Sonntag VK, Karahalios DG, Drabier J. Posterior atlantoaxial facet screw fixation. J Neurosurg 1993;79:234–237. Reprinted with permission.)

and compresses the graft between C1 and C2 to promote fusion.

Percutaneous Drilling and Screw Insertion

After C1 and C2 have been exposed subperiosteally through a neck incision, the surgeon must decide whether the proper screw trajectory can be achieved directly through the incision or whether a percutaneous method is needed. If the patient's neck can be flexed adequately, pilot holes are drilled directly through the neck incision used to expose C1 and C2 (**Fig. 40.2B**). Often, however, the patient's neck cannot be flexed sufficiently without dislocating C1-C2; therefore, percutaneous drilling is used to achieve the proper drill trajectory (**Fig. 40.2A**). Long tools, long drill bits, and a tissue sheath are required for percutaneous screw insertion (**Fig. 40.6**). Percutaneous drilling should not be used exclusively without the subperiosteal exposure of C1 and C2 to visualize the proper medial-lateral screw trajectory and to prepare the entry point for the drill on the C2 inferior facet. Also, the bone surfaces must be exposed to prepare them for fusion. The percutaneous drilling is performed only after C1 and C2 have been exposed directly through the neck incision. Many surgeons prefer the percutaneous technique for routine use, arguing that it results in less injury to the musculoligamentous structures between C3 and C7, leaves less dead space, and promotes more rapid recovery due to the incision being less than half as long and avoiding subperiosteal muscle dissection of the mid to lower cervical spine.

The position of the percutaneous tunnel is judged by holding a long instrument adjacent to the patient's neck and thorax and imaging the trajectory with fluoroscopy. Stab incisions are made in the skin lateral to the midline in the upper thoracic region. A tunneler inserted into a tissue sheath is inserted through the stab incisions to the soft tissues of the neck. The tip of the tissue sheath is positioned adjacent to the C2 inferior facet. A handle on the tissue sheath is used to manipulate the sheath to alter the trajectory of the drills and screws.

Cannulated Screws

A 50-cm long, 1.2-mm diameter K-wire is used to drill the initial screw trajectory into the bones. The tip and threads along the distal 1 cm of the K-wire sharply cut its path into the bone. The K-wire is inserted with a reversible pneumatic drill. A K-wire drill guide is inserted into the tissue sheath to stabilize the K-wire.

After the K-wire is positioned, its drill guide is removed and the screw length is measured. Under fluoroscopic monitoring, a self-tapping screw is inserted into the bone directly over the K-wire. The position of the K-wire is monitored to prevent it from advancing. After the screw is seated into the bone, the K-wire is removed with the reversible drill. The contralateral screw is then inserted in the same fashion.

Noncannulated Screws

Percutaneous drilling is achieved using the tissue sheath and tunneler. The drill bit used matches the minor diameter of the screw to be inserted (i.e., 2.5-mm diameter drill for a 3.5-mm or 4.0-mm screw). A 9-inch, calibrated, end-threaded guide pin (Zimmer Inc., Warsaw, IN) for hip fixation can be used to drill the pilot hole into the bone (**Fig. 40.6**).[9] This drill creates a wide pilot hole; therefore, the pilot hole must be positioned accurately on the first pass. Otherwise, the pilot hole will be too wide and will fail to anchor the screw properly.

The guide pins are drilled into the C1 lateral masses on each side. The first pin is left in place while the second pin is inserted on the contralateral side. The pins anchor C1 to prevent movement and to avoid loss of alignment of the pilot holes during manipulation with taps or screws. One guide pin is removed, the length of the pilot hole is measured, and a screw is inserted into the bone. After the first screw is inserted, the second guide pin is removed from the contralateral site and the second screw is inserted (**Fig. 40.8**).

If non–self-tapping screws are used, the profile of the screw's thread is cut into the bone with a tap before the screws are inserted. In contrast, self-tapping screws have a sharp tip with a cutting channel that cuts a path into the bone as they are inserted. Self-tapping screws avoid the extra maneuver of tapping the pilot hole; however, they cannot be reinserted easily because the wide channel that they cut in the bone can compromise fixation. All screw manipulations are observed with fluoroscopy to prevent complications.

Screw Selection

The widest possible diameter screw should be used because the screw's minor diameter is the primary determinant of its bending strength.[10,11] For C1-C2 facet screw fixation, 3.5-mm or 4.0-mm diameter screws usually are used. The length of a posterior C1-C2 transarticular screw averages 40 mm (range 35 to 50 mm). Steel or titanium screws can be used.

Operative Technique of C1-C2 Screw-Rod Fixation

In some cases, surgical or anatomical factors limit the ability to perform transarticular screw fixation. If there is a need for reduction, placement of screws in the lateral mass of C1 and into C2 allows for such manipulation after placement of the connecting rods. Such a technique also allows for more flexibility in cases of vertebral artery aberrancy or when bony abnormalities results in destruction of the C1-C2 articulation.

This technique requires careful exposure of the C1 lateral mass, which is obscured by the venous plexus adjacent to the vertebral artery. This venous plexus may be quite extensive and further engorged by the prone patient position required for the procedure, and careful microdissection is

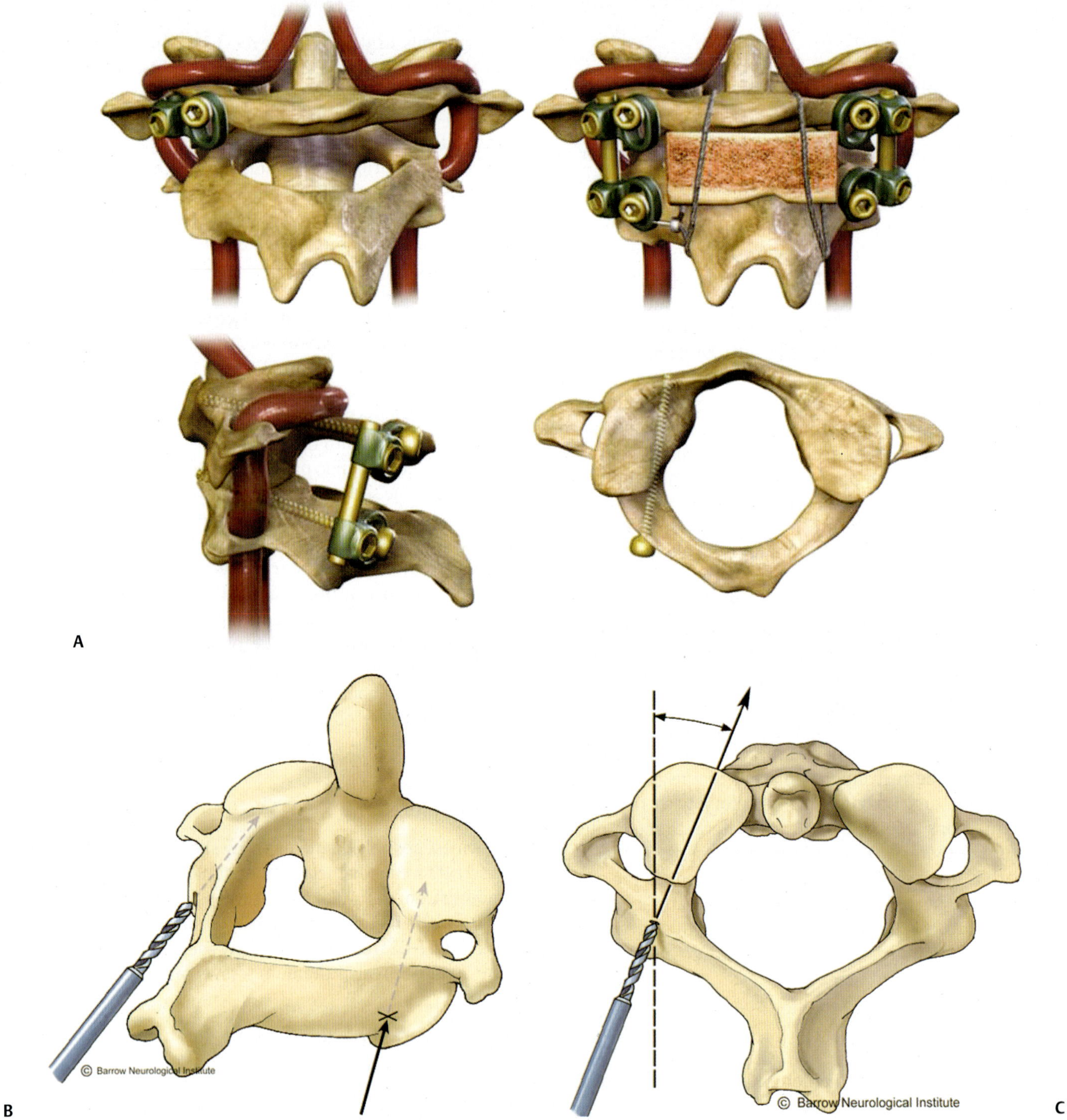

Fig. 40.8 **(A)** Illustration demonstrating the Harms construct with lateral mass screws in C1 and pedicle screws in C2. **(B)** Entry into C1 is at the midpoint on the lateral mass with a medial trajectory of 10 to 15 degrees pointed toward the anterior tubercle of C1. **(C)** Entry into C2 is at the same point as the entry of transarticular screws, with a medial trajectory of 30 degrees to avoid the vertebral artery, and a length of 35 to 40 mm. *(continued)*

D

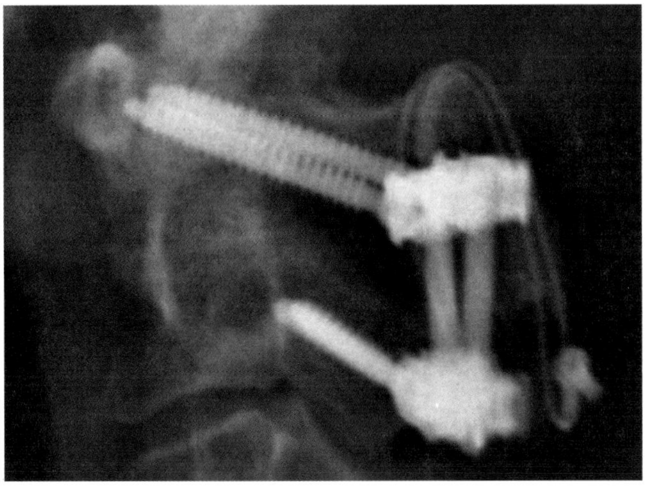

Fig. 40.8 *(continued)* **(D)** Alternately, short pars screws, which avoid the vertebral artery altogether but are only 10 to 12 mm in length, can be placed into C2. (Reprinted with permission from Barrow Neurological Institute.)

often required to dissect bone free and allow for adequate exposure of the lateral mass. The ideal entry point for the C1 lateral mass screw is directly into the posterior aspect of the inferior articular process of the C1 lateral mass, below the point at which the posterior arch attaches to the lateral mass (**Fig. 40.8**). Care must be taken when dissecting the arch, as it may often be quite thin with the vertebral artery laying on its superior surface. Depending on patient anatomy, when the posterior arch is very thick in the cranial-caudal axis, it may be impossible to fit the screw below the arch without penetrating the C1-C2 joint space. In these cases, *very* cautious drilling away from the caudal lip of the posterior arch can create enough room for the screw, but this should only be attempted if a preoperative CT angiogram has demonstrated the course of the vertebral artery clearly and a ponticulus posticus (deviation of the vertebral artery through the center of the posterior arch via an accessory foramen) has been ruled out. Some authors have actually proposed dissection of the vertebral artery out of its groove in C1 followed by direct screw placement through the posterior arch, but this has not gained widespread popularity.

In some cases, sacrifice of the C2 nerve root may be required to ensure adequate bony exposure and identification of the lateral and medial margins of the lateral mass. In the author's experience, this is a safe procedure that is well tolerated by patients without significant morbidity. If the nerve root is left intact, it should be retracted inferiorly while drilling commences in the midposition of the lateral mass parallel to the arch of C1. The drill should be angled medially ~10 to 15% to gain the greatest degree of bony purchase. Typically, the tip of the drill is aimed toward the C1 tubercle.

Careful preoperative evaluation of axial CT images should be performed to gauge the length of the lateral mass, as some C1 arches are fairly flat in shape anteriorly.[12] This may lead to inadvertent penetration of the anterior bony cortex, despite careful use of intraoperative fluoroscopy.[13] Intraoperative guidance may also be utilized in screw placement and has been advocated by some authors.[14] If a traditional posterior interpositional C1-C2 bone graft and cable construct is not planned or is not possible due to absent C1-C2 posterior elements, an intra-articular fusion of C1-C2 is possible by retracting the C2 nerve root superiorly, following the C2 pars interarticularis down to the C1-C2 joint space, and then using a curette and/or very small high-speed drill (the author prefers a curette) to decorticate the joint surfaces. Morcellized bone graft material can then be packed into the joint space. This step must be done prior to C1 lateral mass screw placement. Once the C1 screw is in place, access to the C1-C2 joint space becomes essentially impossible due to the caudal displacement of the C2 nerve root by the C1 screw. Even if the C2 nerve root is sacrificed, access to the joint space is still extremely difficult once the C1 screw is placed. Modern C1-C2 screw sets typically include "smooth-shank" or partially threaded polyaxial 3.5-mm and/or 4-mm screws for C1 lateral mass fixation. These have the advantage of a smooth bore at the proximal end of the screw, just below the polyaxial screw head. The theoretical advantage of this is decreased irritation of the C2 nerve root compared with a fully threaded screw (**Fig. 40.9**).

Once a contralateral screw is placed at C1, attention may be turned to fixation at C2. The entry point and trajectory for C2 pars screws are similar to that utilized for the placement of transarticular screws, except that the screw does not need to traverse the C1-C2 joint and typically has a length of 10 to 12 mm. If additional purchase is desired, then pedicle screws

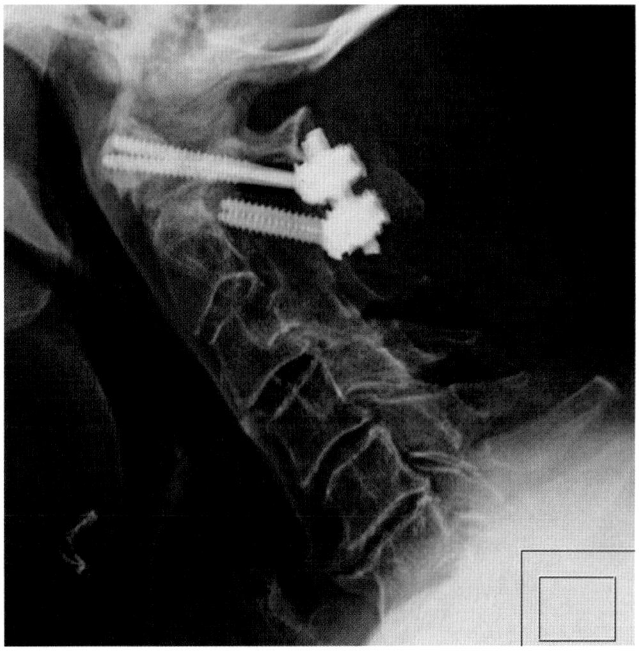

Fig. 40.9 Partially threaded screws are used in accessing the C1 lateral mass. These reduce irritation of the C2 nerve root.

may be placed. Such screws are longer (often 35 to 40 mm) and angle medially 30 degrees. The entry point for C2 pedicle screws is usually 3 mm above the C2-C3 joint but significantly farther lateral than the entry point for transarticular or C2 pars screws in many patients. Careful evaluation of preoperative axial CT scans is mandatory. A line is drawn along the bore of the pedicle and projected posterolaterally onto the dorsal surface of the C2 lateral mass to determine how lateral the entry point must be. In practice, there is little advantage to placement of a C2 pedicle screw over a pars screw and the risk of vertebral artery injury is higher.[15] Another alternative is the placement of crossing laminar screws in C2, assuming an intact C2 lamina is present (**Fig. 40.10**). Of all screw options, this one has as its main advantage the nearly complete lack of risk to the vertebral artery, and still the construct is biomechanically quite strong with typical

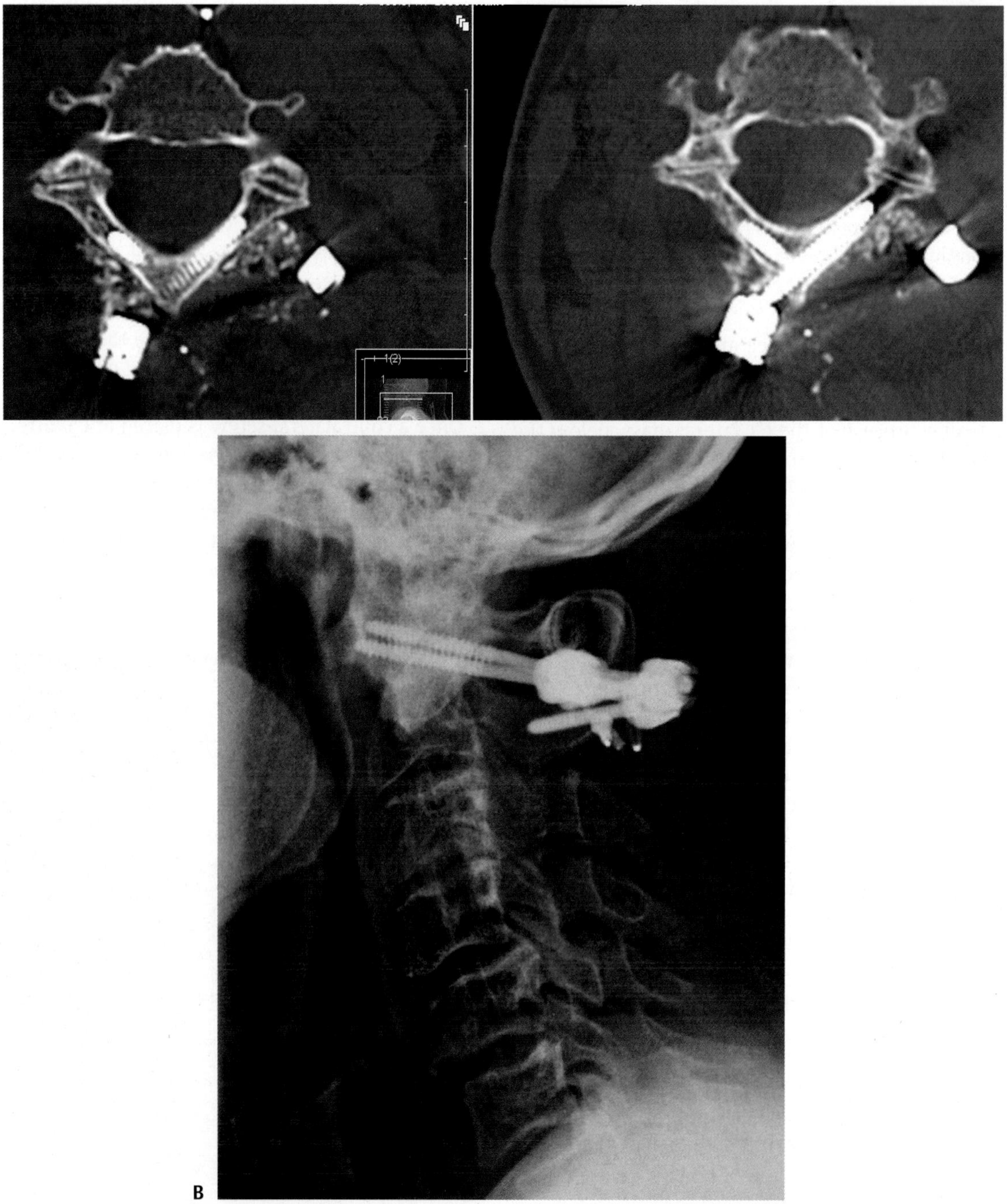

A

B

Fig. 40.10 (A) Laminar screws may be placed in C2 and provide another option for fixation, as shown in axial computed tomography slices. **(B)** These may then be included in lateral mass constructs and allow for increased surgical versatility in a variety of pathological conditions and anatomical variations.

screw lengths between 30 and 40 mm. Another potential advantage is that fluoroscopy is usually not necessary for this portion of the procedure. Main drawbacks to this option include the risk of dural injury if the screw is not directed parallel along the lamina as well as the fact that the screw heads are offset from the lateral mass line, making extension to longer constructs challenging without utilization of screw head spacers or offset connectors, which may predispose to a higher rate of pseudoarthrosis in such constructs.[16] A final option if screw placement into C2 is impossible for anatomic reasons is placement of a sublaminar wire bilaterally and extension of the construct to C3 lateral mass screws.[17]

Clinical Pearls

Meticulous preoperative planning and precise operative techniques are required to achieve success with this technique. Preoperatively, plain radiography and CT are necessary. Plain radiographs are used to assess the alignment of C1-C2 and to verify that the C1-C2 complex can be reduced adequately. The architecture of the C1 lateral masses and C2 facets can be assessed with sagittal CT reconstructions. Pathology of the lateral masses of C1 must be identified so that the screw trajectory can be altered accordingly. Comminuted fractures or tumors destroying the C1 lateral masses preclude screw placement. C1-C2 alignment must be restored to obtain the proper screw trajectory and to gain adequate bone purchase in C1. Although not universally accepted, the authors strongly recommend obtaining preoperative CT angiography in all patients without contraindications, such as intravenous contrast allergies. Although the position of the vertebral artery relative to the C2 pars interarticularis and its course along the C1 posterior arch can often be inferred from the size, shape, and position of bony notches, foramina, or grooves in the bone on a plain CT scan with reconstructions, CT angiography often reveals potentially disastrous deviations and anomalies of the vertebral artery that can radically affect surgical planning, such as the choice between C2 pars screws versus laminar screws.

Intraoperatively, the C2 pars interarticularis and the C1-C2 facet must be visualized directly to direct the screw trajectory precisely. Identification of these structures prevents inadvertent perforation through the C2 pars interarticularis and allows medial-lateral adjustment of the drill trajectory.

Several strategies help to obtain the proper screw trajectory. Flexion of the neck provides an unobstructed drill trajectory through the incision. Manual reduction and direct upward traction on C2 with an Allis clamp also can improve the screw trajectory into the C1-C2. When the patient's neck cannot be flexed and direct drilling cannot be performed, percutaneous drilling is performed. The tissue sheath, tunneler, long tools, K-wires, or guide pins provide an excellent method to insert the screws percutaneously.

Biomechanically, C1-C2 facet screw fixation is significantly more rigid than wiring techniques or Halifax clamps for fixating C1-C2.[2–4,9,18] Immediate, multidirectional, atlantoaxial stability is achieved after the screws have been placed properly. The construct resists translational and rotational forces.

The C1-C2 screw fixation is always supplemented with an autologous bone graft to guarantee fusion. Some authors have demonstrated successful C1-C2 fusions using allograft iliac crest bone wired or cabled in as a C1-C2 interpositional graft with rigid screw fixation, pointing out that the dogma against allograft in C1-C2 fusion stems from the time of nonrigid wire fixation and halo vest placement, which is biomechanically inferior. This practice is not universally accepted, however. Cable or wire fixation is used unless the posterior arches of C1 or C2 are fractured or incompetent, in which case, as described above, an intra-articular fusion can be performed. Three-point fixation of C1-C2 with two screws plus a cable provides greater mechanical stability than either technique used alone.[2,18]

Conclusion

These fixation techniques require considerable expertise and technical precision. If screws are misdirected, vertebral artery injury, neurological injury, or inadequate fixation may occur. Despite these limitations, several clinical series demonstrate that this technique can be used safely with acceptable risks and minimal complication rates.[5,9,14–16,19–21] Superior mechanical rigidity and excellent fusion rates are obtained compared with wiring techniques. The fusion rate associated with this method of fixation exceeds 90% and minimizes the need for a postoperative cervical orthosis. It is a particularly useful way to salvage C1-C2 pseudarthrosis and has been effective in reducing the need for long occipital to midcervical fusions to adequately stabilize limited C1-C2 pathology. Careful and detailed preoperative planning is mandatory for good outcomes. Surgeons experienced in all of these techniques are able to combine or "mix-and-match" techniques, creating hybrid constructs (e.g., a transarticular screw on one side with C1-C2 screw rod fixation contralaterally) to optimally suit each patient's anatomy and pathology and obtain optimal results.

References

1. Dickman CA, Sonntag VKH, Papadopoulos SM, Hadley MN. The interspinous method of posterior atlantoaxial arthrodesis. J Neurosurg 1991;74(2):190–198
2. Grob D, Crisco JJ III, Panjabi MM, Wang P, Dvorak J. Biomechanical evaluation of four different posterior atlantoaxial fixation techniques. Spine 1992;17(5):480–490
3. Montesano PX, Juach EC, Anderson PA, Benson DR, Hanson PB. Biomechanics of cervical spine internal fixation. Spine 1991;16(3, Suppl):S10–S16
4. Hanley EN Jr, Harvell JC Jr. Immediate postoperative stability of the atlantoaxial articulation: a biomechanical study comparing simple midline wiring, and the Gallie and Brooks procedures. J Spinal Disord 1992;5(3):306–310

5. Magerl F, Seemann PS. Stable posterior fusion of the atlas and axis by transarticular screw fixation. In: Kehr P, Weidner A, eds. Cervical Spine I. New York, NY: Springer-Verlag; 1987:322–327
6. Harms J, Melcher RP. Posterior C1-C2 fusion with polyaxial screw and rod fixation. Spine 2001;26(22):2467–2471
7. Goel A. C1-C2 pedicle screw fixation with rigid cantilever beam construct: case report and technical note. Neurosurgery 2002; 51(3):853–854, author reply 854
8. Goel A. Techniques of posterior C1-C2 stabilization. Neurosurgery 2008;62(6):E1384, author reply E1384
9. Marcotte P, Dickman CA, Sonntag VKH, Karahalios DG, Drabier J. Posterior atlantoaxial facet screw fixation. J Neurosurg 1993; 79(2):234–237
10. Dickman CA, Sonntag VKH, Marcotte PJ. Techniques of screw fixation of the cervical spine. BNI Q 1992;8(2):9–26
11. Krag MH, Fredrickson BE, Yuan HA. Spinal instrumentation. In: Weinstein JN, Wiesel SW, eds. The Lumbar Spine. Philadelphia, PA: WB Saunders; 1990:916–940
12. Rocha R, Safavi-Abbasi S, Reis C, et al. Working area, safety zones, and angles of approach for posterior C-1 lateral mass screw placement: a quantitative anatomical and morphometric evaluation. J Neurosurg Spine 2007;6(3):247–254
13. Wait SD, Ponce FA, Colle KO, Parry PV, Sonntag VK. Importance of the C1 anterior tubercle depth and lateral mass geometry when placing C1 lateral mass screws. Neurosurgery 2009;65(5):952–956, discussion 956–957
14. Acosta FL Jr, Quinones-Hinojosa A, Gadkary CA, et al. Frameless stereotactic image-guided C1-C2 transarticular screw fixation for atlantoaxial instability: review of 20 patients. J Spinal Disord Tech 2005;18(5):385–391
15. Mummaneni PV, Lu DC, Dhall SS, Mummaneni VP, Chou D. C1 lateral mass fixation: a comparison of constructs. Neurosurgery 2010;66(3, Suppl)153–160
16. Parker SL, McGirt MJ, Garcés-Ambrossi GL, et al. Translaminar versus pedicle screw fixation of C2: comparison of surgical morbidity and accuracy of 313 consecutive screws. Neurosurgery 2009; 64(5, Suppl 2)343–348, discussion 348–349
17. Horn EM, Hott JS, Porter RW, Theodore N, Papadopoulos SM, Sonntag VK. Atlantoaxial stabilization with the use of C1-3 lateral mass screw fixation. Technical note. J Neurosurg Spine 2006;5(2):172–177
18. Hanson PB, Montesano PX, Sharkey NA, Rauschning W. Anatomic and biomechanical assessment of transarticular screw fixation for atlantoaxial instability. Spine 1991;16(10):1141–1145
19. Grob D, Jeanneret B, Aebi M, Markwalder TM. Atlanto-axial fusion with transarticular screw fixation. J Bone Joint Surg Br 1991; 73(6):972–976
20. Stillerman CB, Wilson JA. Atlanto-axial stabilization with posterior transarticular screw fixation: technical description and report of 22 cases. Neurosurgery 1993;32(6):948–954, discussion 954–955
21. Jeanneret B, Magerl F. Primary posterior fusion C1/2 in odontoid fractures: indications, technique, and results of transarticular screw fixation. J Spinal Disord 1992;5(4):464–475

41 Occipitocervical Fixation

Nicholas C. Bambakidis, David J. Hart, and Curtis A. Dickman

A variety of surgical techniques has been described for the treatment of patients with occipitocervical instability. Originally, surgeons used onlay grafts with subsequent subperiosteal dissection of the bone to promote fusion but had a very high failure rate.[1–5] In response, they began using bone struts (ribs or iliac crest bone grafts) wired to the occiput and cervical vertebrae.[6–10] More recently, metal implants (e.g., rods, plates, or metallic loops) were wired into position. Such methods provided immediate internal fixation of unstable motion segments. Early attempts using rods and steel loops showed promising results but still resulted in failure rates between 5 and 30%.[2,11–19]

Newer techniques have evolved, with screws and plates or rods used for rigid internal fixation. Extensions of this technique include the use of occipitoatlantal transarticular screws alone.[20,21] These techniques are technically demanding, but the published clinical series on screw-rod or plate methods demonstrate that they are superior to previously developed methods of achieving stable occipitocervical fusion.[22–31] These techniques have the advantage of avoiding sublaminar instrumentation and are especially useful as an alternative if a cervical laminectomy has been performed.

Screws, plates, and rods are similar to other internal fixation techniques that use hardware and provide only temporary internal fixation. Bone grafts must be added, and the fusion bed must be prepared to achieve fusion and permanent spinal stability. The plates are anchored to the bone surfaces with screws placed in the midline occipital crest and in the spine with lateral mass screws, C2 pars/pedicle/translaminar screws, or C1-C2 posterior transarticular screws.

Indications

1. Occipitoatlantal instability
   A. Cranial settling, basilar invagination
   B. Occipitoatlantal dislocation
   C. Destruction of occipitoatlantal joints
2. Atlantoaxial instability with inability to fixate C1, C2, or both

Contraindications

1. Severe osteoporosis (relative contraindication)
2. Destruction of bone surfaces (occiput, C1, C2)

Preparation and Positioning

1. Prone position
2. Neck slightly flexed to neutral and head neutral. Head positioning is far more critical for occipitocervical fusions than other cervical surgeries because the patient's head position will be fixed for the rest of his or her life. If fixed into extension, patients will have great difficulty seeing the ground they walk on, leading to high risk for falls and great difficulty with activities of daily living, such as dressing oneself and toileting. If fixed into flexion, patients develop chronic axial neck and back pain from having to constantly hyperextend the neck and back to look straight ahead. They are unable to reach into high cupboards or shelves. In some cases, fixed flexion can lead to dysphagia.
3. Somatosensory evoked potential monitoring (consider baseline prior to positioning)
4. Lateral fluoroscope monitoring (C-arm)
5. Rigid head fixation (halo brace or Mayfield skull clamp)
6. Traction to reduce cranial settling
7. Preoperative computed tomography (CT) with angiographic reconstruction to assess the thickness of the occipital crest and the integrity of the cervical bone and to exclude an anomalous vertebral artery

Operative Exposure

Access to the posterior occipitocervical region is achieved using a standard midline cervical exposure. A linear skin incision extends from the inion to the spinous process of the cervical vertebra one level below the lowest planned instrumented vertebra (e.g., for an occiput to C4 fusion, the incision extends to the C5 spinous process). The nuchal fascia and posterior cervical muscles are divided in the midline sagittal plane, which affords a relatively avascular dissection. Subperiosteal dissection is used to expose the occiput and dorsal arches of the upper cervical vertebra. The suboccipital and cervical paraspinous muscles are swept laterally using lightweight, broad-surfaced periosteal elevators. Careful operative technique prevents dislocation of unstable vertebral segments. The laterally situated vertebral arteries should be avoided during the operative exposure.

Curettes, periosteal elevators, and bone rongeurs are used to remove the soft tissue, interspinous ligaments, and ligamentum flavum from the vertebrae to be fused. The posterior occipitoatlantal membrane is detached from the rim of the foramen magnum and C1. Curettes and/or a high-speed drill are used to decorticate the cervical facet joints to facilitate fusion.

Screw-Plate Constructs

Following surgical exposure, the fixation plates of choice are contoured until they fit the patient's individual anatomy precisely. The plates are removed, and the pilot holes are drilled for the screws. After the pilot holes are prepared, the plates are repositioned. Bone grafts are positioned between the plate and the fusion surfaces to compress the grafts onto the bone (**Fig. 41.1**). Screws are inserted through holes in the plates into the occiput and the cervical vertebrae.

Surgeons have adapted a variety of devices from other applications to use for occipitocervical fixation. Occipitocervical screw plate fixation has been described using single plates, paired plates, titanium plates, steel plates, Y-shaped ankle reconstruction plates, curved pelvic reconstruction plates, and modified bone fixation plates.[22–25,32–34] Several anatomical and technical issues need to be considered in the insertion of occipitocervical plates. Acute angles (90 to 120 degrees) occur between the surface of the occiput and dorsal surface of the cervical spine. Implants must be fabricated to approximate these angles or must tolerate adjustments in curvatures without weakening. Titanium weakens significantly when bent extensively; therefore, if titanium plates are used, bending should be minimized.

Screw-Rod Constructs

Despite the development of a wide variety of plating techniques, surgeons had remained frustrated with the limitations of plating systems. Plates cannot be bent in multiple planes simultaneously (e.g., sagittal and coronal), and precisely aligning the holes or slots of plates with the ideal entry points for cervical screw fixation can be tedious or impossible. Consequently, once posterior cervical screw-rod constructs became widely available, they rapidly replaced screw-plate instrumentation in most practices. As these

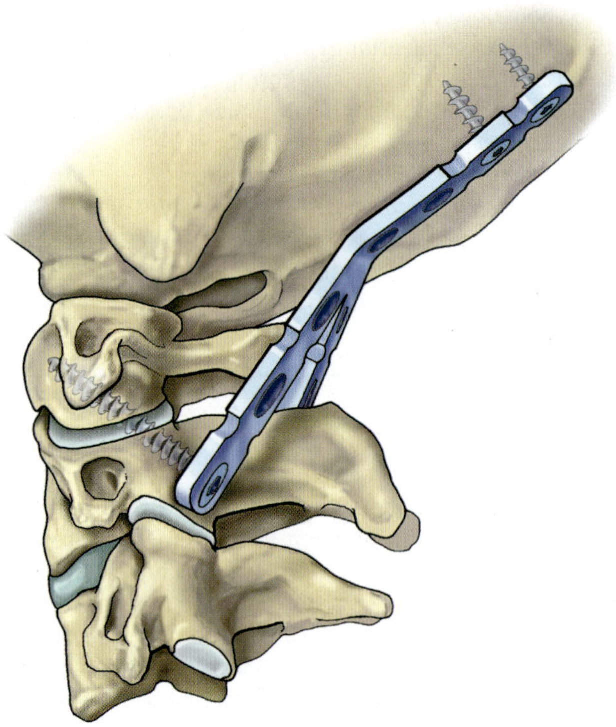
A

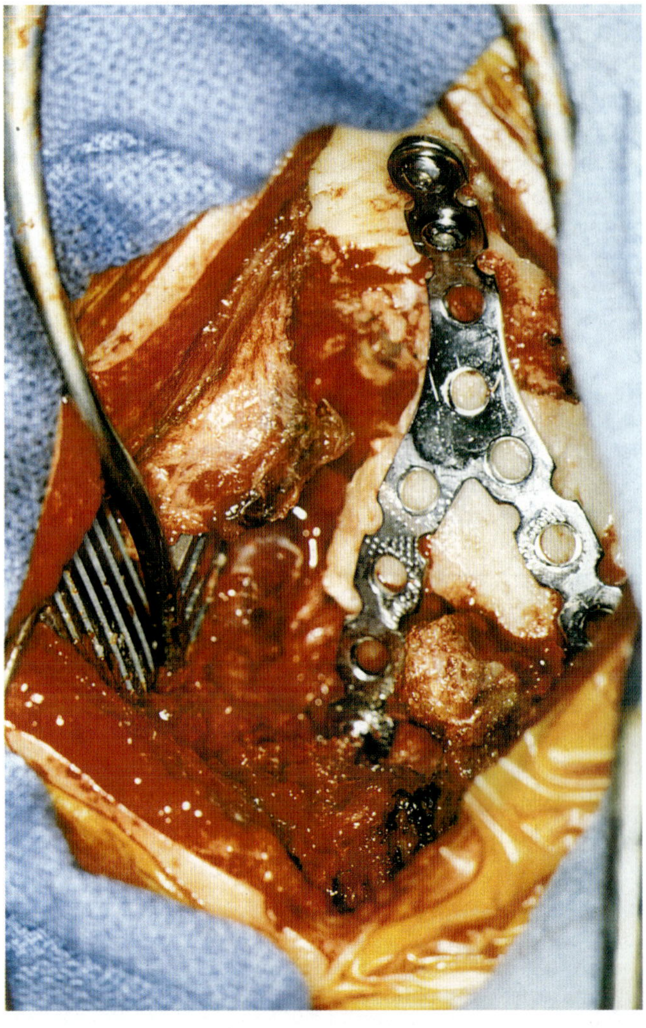
B

Fig. 41.1 **(A)** Illustration and **(B)** intraoperative photograph of the Y-plate. The plate was anchored to the occiput with two midline screws and to the cervical spine with two transarticular screws. A plate of corticocancellous iliac crest autograft was interposed between the plate, the occiput, C1, and C2. *(continued)*

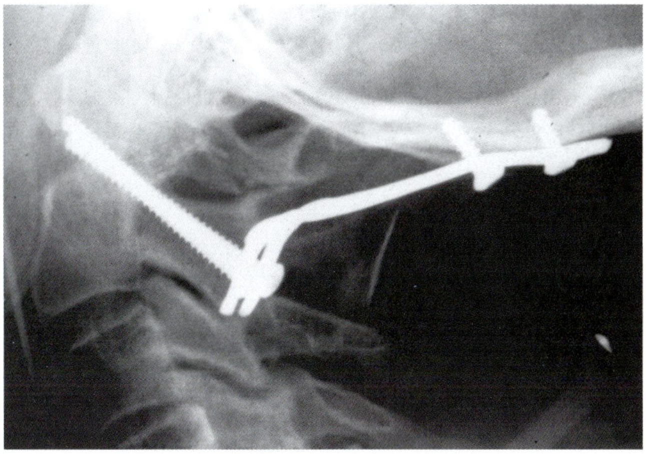

C

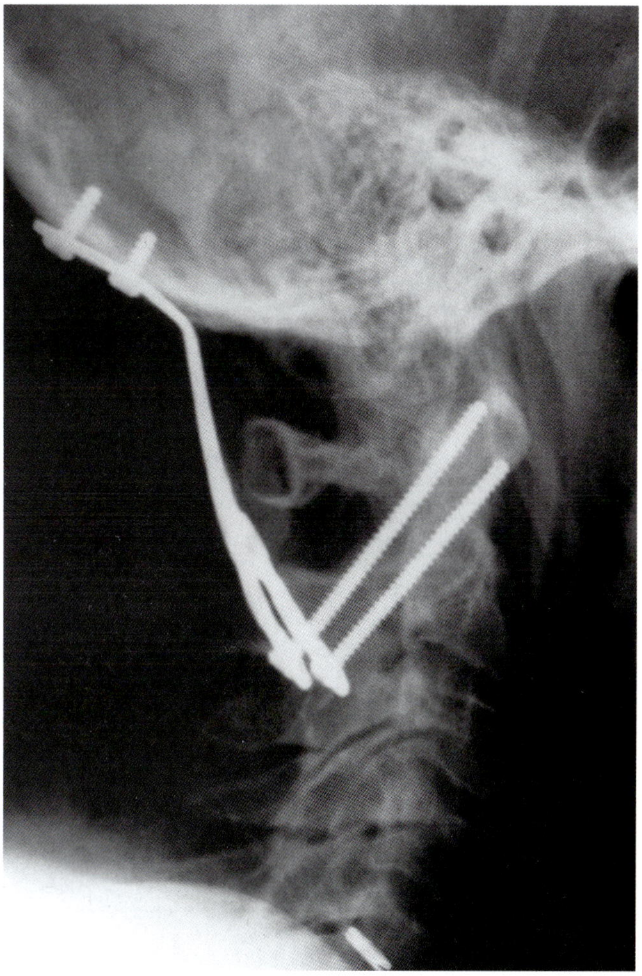

D

Fig. 41.1 *(continued)* **(C,D)** Postoperative lateral cervical radiographs in two different patients stabilized with occipitocervical Y-plates. (Reprinted with permission from Barrow Neurological Institute.)

systems evolved, newer occipital keel plates of different sizes and angles were developed. These plates are fixed to the occiput with screws and have built-in connectors that attach to cervical rods (**Fig. 41.2**). The use of occipital keel plates and polyaxial screws in the cervical spine has greatly reduced the time spent on intraoperative contouring and bending of hardware before implantation and requires less exact mating of hardware to bone surfaces compared with wiring or other plating techniques. Multiple construct variations may be utilized with a wide selection of connectors and rod diameters, providing extension of constructs down the cervical spine or to the thoracic spine, if needed. Recent instrumentation has involved the use of hinged rods that allow the rod to be mated first to the occipital plate and then to the cervical instrumentation. After final adjustments for any distraction or compression are made, the hinge is "locked" at the ideal angle between the occiput and cervical spine, again eliminating an often tedious rod-contouring process (**Fig. 41.3**).

The occipital anatomy must be analyzed before screw insertion. Penetrating the dura can cause cerebrospinal fluid leakage, cerebellar injury, or venous sinus injury. Precise screw insertion techniques are mandatory to avoid complications. The occipital bone is thickest in the midline at the level of the nuchal line, with an average thickness of 14 mm (range 10 to 18 mm).[22,25] The thickness of the bone rapidly decreases lateral to the midline. Therefore, occipital screws are best placed in the midline crest rather than in a paramedian position. The occipital squamosa is very thin laterally and does not hold screws well. To assess an individual's occipital bone, the thickness is measured preoperatively with CT. The screw depths are measured precisely to avoid intradural penetration, and self-drilling or self-tapping screws are typically avoided in this location.

Several alternatives can be used to anchor the screw plates or rods to the cervical spine. Posterior atlantoaxial facet screws and subaxial lateral mass screws can be inserted. Screws incorporating C2 can be placed in the pars, pedicle, or lamina depending on clinical necessity and anatomical considerations as well as surgeon preference and experience.

C1-C2 Transarticular Screws

Posterior atlantoaxial facet screws provide the most rigid mechanical fixation for the plate. Because the screws cross the C1-C2 joints vertically, they eliminate almost all C1-C2 motion. After pilot holes are drilled for C1-C2 transarticular screws, a plate or rod construct of choice is incorporated and an interposed bone graft is positioned over the surface of

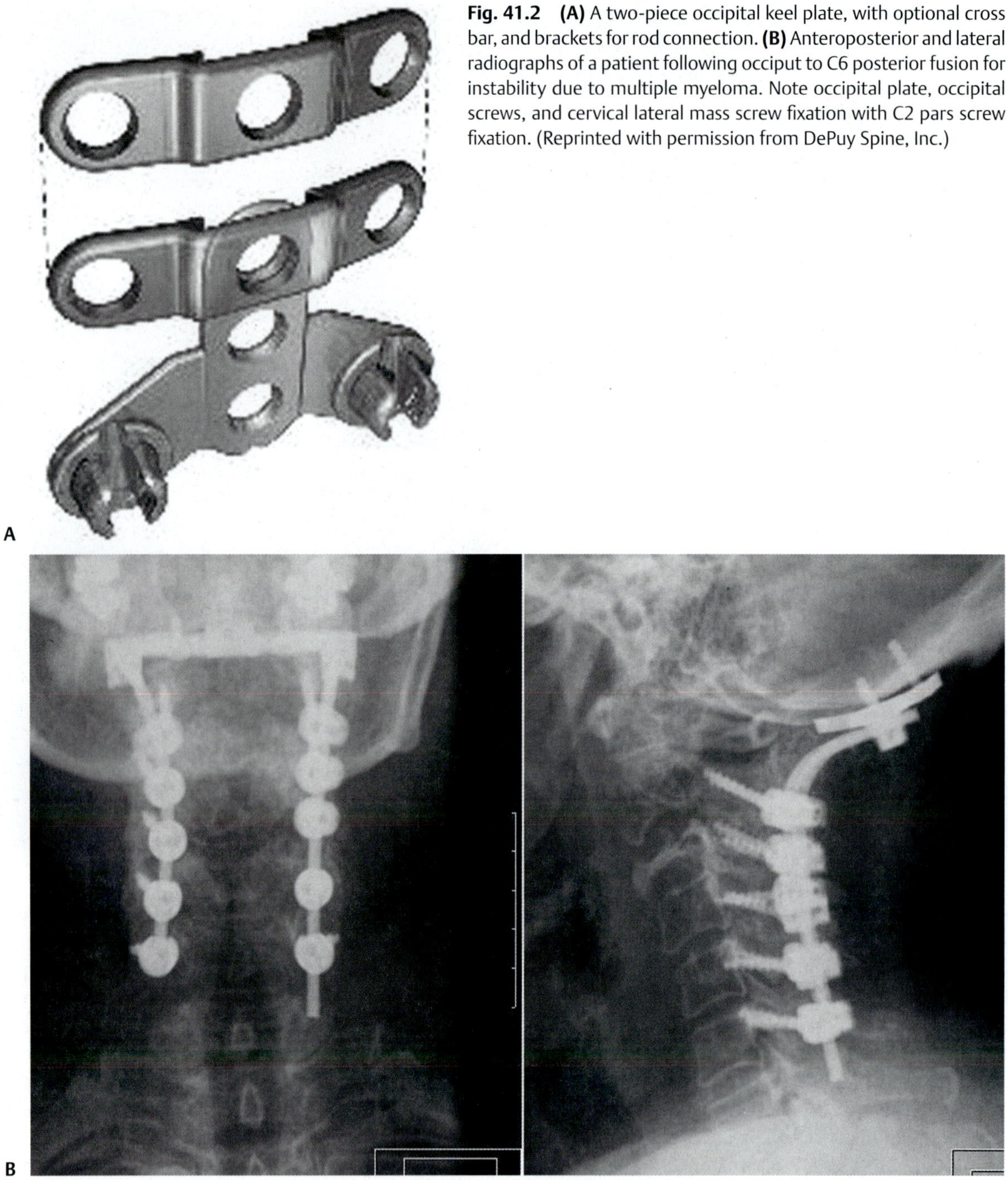

Fig. 41.2 **(A)** A two-piece occipital keel plate, with optional cross bar, and brackets for rod connection. **(B)** Anteroposterior and lateral radiographs of a patient following occiput to C6 posterior fusion for instability due to multiple myeloma. Note occipital plate, occipital screws, and cervical lateral mass screw fixation with C2 pars screw fixation. (Reprinted with permission from DePuy Spine, Inc.)

the occiput, C1, and C2. The plate is cut or the rods are positioned so that they do not extend across unfused segments. The C1-C2 transarticular screws are inserted into the bone. Next, the midline occipital screws are placed. The bone graft is trapped between the plate and bone surfaces. The graft is compressed to facilitate fusion.

Lateral Mass Screws and C2 Pedicle Screws

If C1-C2 transarticular screws cannot be used to anchor a plate, the cervical lateral masses (articular pillars) and C2 pedicle screws are alternatives for screw fixation. Lateral mass and C2 pars screws are short, have a different orientation, and are weaker than C1-C2 transarticular screws. Rather than a single screw site, several lateral mass screws are used on each side to anchor the plate.

Lateral mass screws are placed into the articular pillars of C3 to C6 with similar techniques.[32,34,35] Pilot holes are drilled, beginning 1 mm medial to the center of each lateral mass. The drills and screws are directed 20 to 30 degrees cephalad and 20 to 30 degrees laterally (**Fig. 41.4**). This trajectory avoids the vertebral artery and nerve roots and places the screws bicortically in the lateral masses. Screws should not be inserted in the C7 lateral mass because it is thin and does

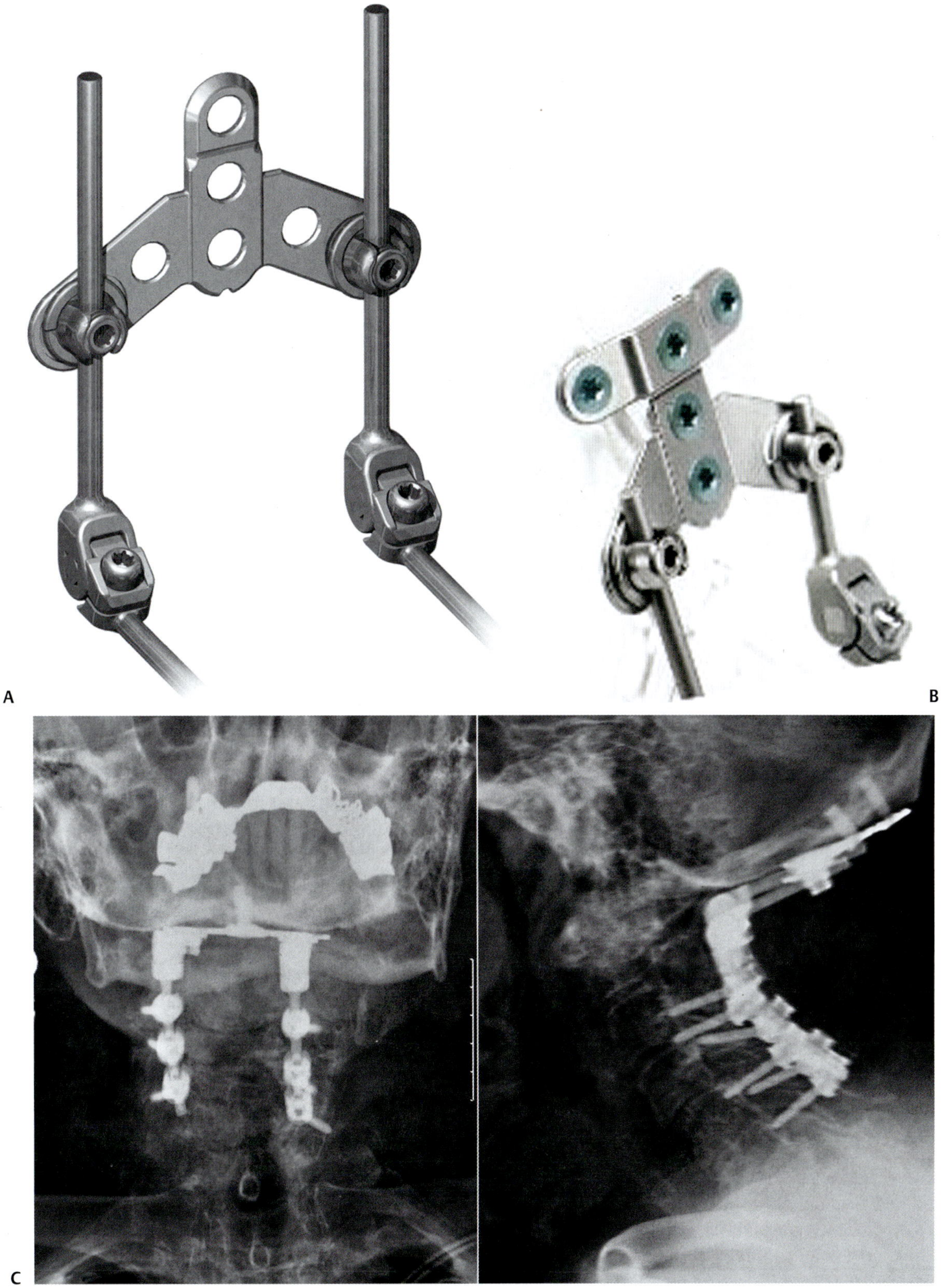

Fig. 41.3 (A,B) An occipital screw-plate device with hinged connector for cervical fixation hardware. **(C)** Anteroposterior and lateral radiographs of a patient following occipital-cervical fixation using a hinged rod connector. (Reprinted with permission from DePuy Spine, Inc.)

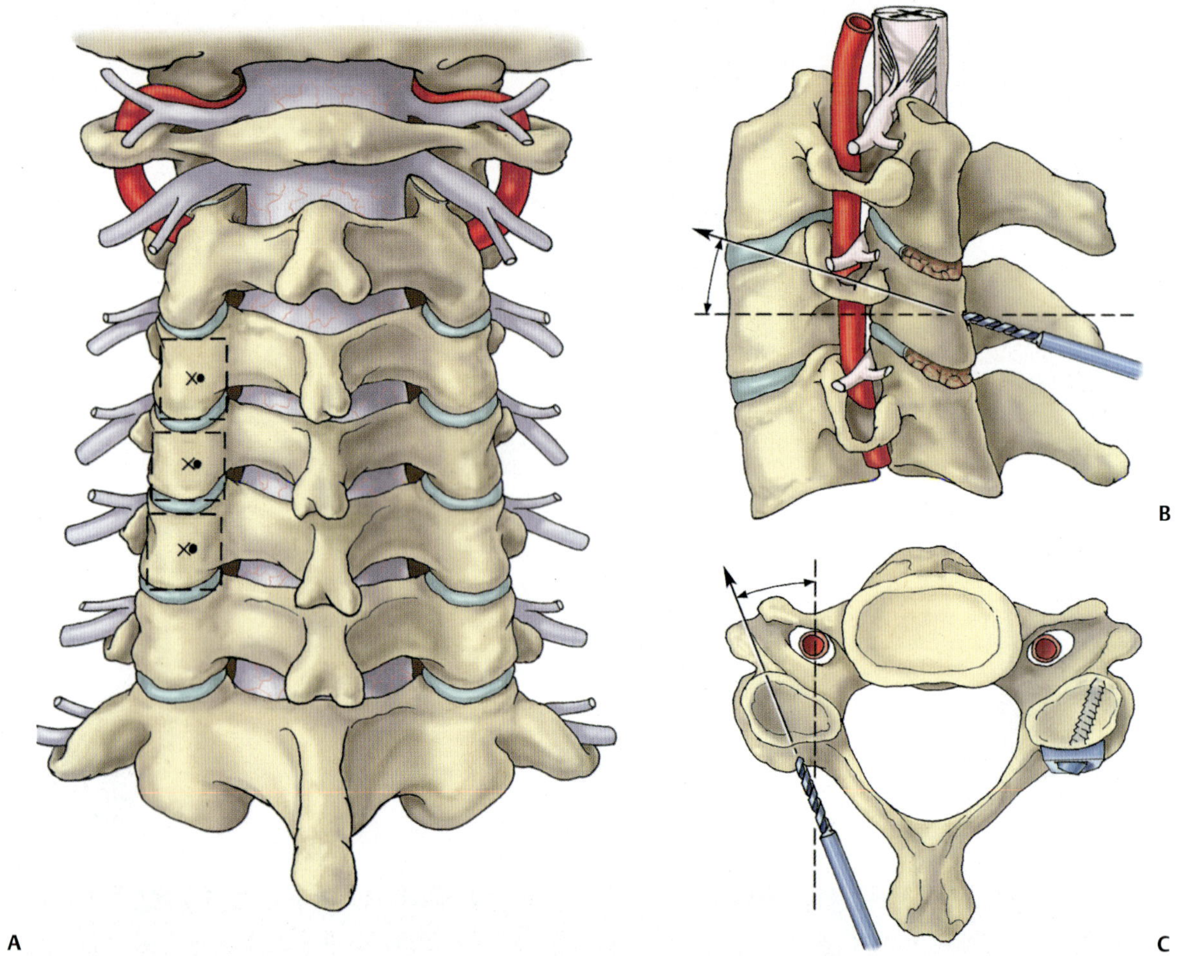

Fig. 41.4 **(A)** Lateral mass screws are inserted into the lower cervical vertebrae (C3 to C7) by entering the bone 1 mm medial to the center of the lateral masses. Bicortical screws are directed **(B)** 20 to 30 degrees cephalad and **(C)** 20 to 30 degrees laterally. This trajectory avoids the nerve roots and vertebral arteries. (Reprinted with permission from Barrow Neurological Institute.)

not hold screws well. The screws also can encroach upon the adjacent nerve roots.

Screws can be placed in the C2 pedicle and have a different trajectory from lateral mass screws (**Fig. 41.5**). C2 pedicle screws are angled 20 to 30 degrees superiorly and 20 to 30 degrees medially into the central axis of the C2 pedicle.

Occipitocervical Wiring Techniques

When screw-rod constructs are impractical or impossible, rod-wire constructs remain an alternative and may be necessary, despite that they are not as strong biomechanically and are more prone to failure than other rigid screw-rod techniques. As with screw placement, the occiput should be wired at locations where the bone is thick (i.e., near the foramen magnum, at the nuchal line, or along the midline crest). To wire the bone adjacent to the foramen magnum, the posterior lip of the foramen magnum is enlarged with a Kerrison rongeur (**Fig. 41.6A**). Two burr holes are placed into the occipital bone 5 mm superior to the rim of the foramen magnum (**Fig. 41.6B**). To prevent intradural wire penetration, the dura is separated from the inner table of the skull between the burr holes and the foramen magnum, and the tip of the wire is bent into a blunt loop. Wire is passed between each burr hole and the foramen magnum. Contoured metallic loops, rectangles, threaded Steinmann pins, or titanium rods can then be used.[17,19,29,36–46]

Threaded Steinmann Pin

A wide (5/32-inch diameter) stainless steel or titanium-threaded Steinmann pin has been used by the authors extensively for occipitocervical fixation (**Figs. 41.7** and **41.8**).[17,39,40,46,47] The Steinmann pin is inexpensive, readily available, and can be custom contoured to fit each patient. The threaded pin prevents settling or "telescoping" of the construct. The Steinmann pin is bent into a U-shape using a rod bender. Secondary bends are placed to match the contour of the occipitocervical region. The curves of the pin need to be smooth because sharp angles create stress risers

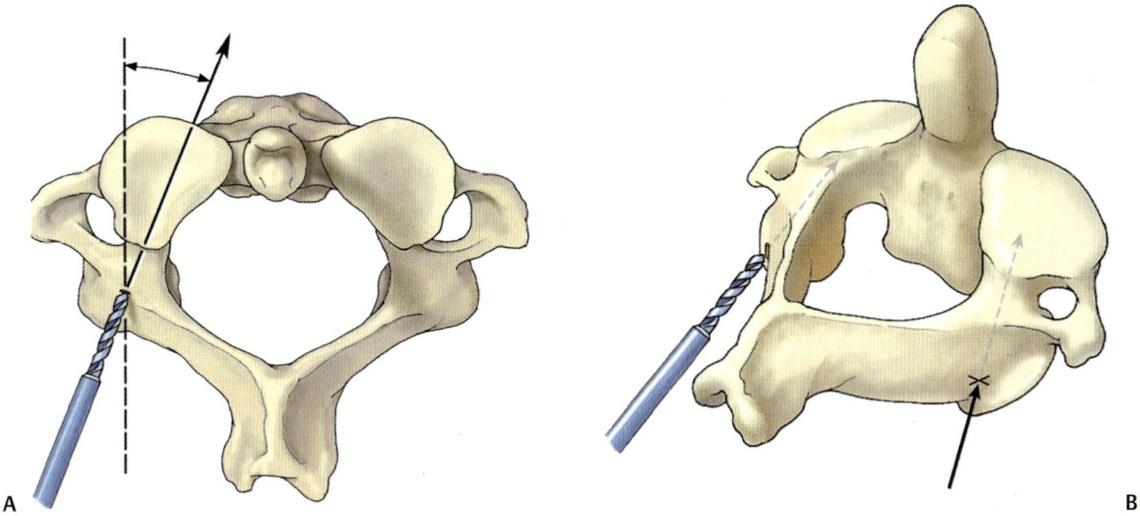

Fig. 41.5 C2 screws can be inserted into the pedicle. The screws are angled **(A)** 20 to 30 degrees medially and **(B)** 20 to 30 degrees rostrally into the center of the C2 pedicle. (Reprinted with permission from Barrow Neurological Institute.)

and encourage pin breakage. The pin length is measured, and the ends are cut so that the pin does not extend beyond the fused segments.

The Steinmann pin is then wired against the occiput and cervical laminae or facets. The laminae are preferred for fixation because they are stronger than the facets in resisting wire pullout and provide more secure stabilization. To achieve optimal fixation, the pin needs to contact the bone surfaces at each level. Gaps between the pin and the bone surfaces fixate the vertebrae loosely, allowing excessive motion.

Following placement of the rod and wires, the occiput and posterior arches of the cervical levels to be fused are segmentally decorticated with a burr, and autologous cancellous bone grafts are compressed against the levels to be fused. If a suboccipital craniotomy or cervical laminectomy has been performed, a plate of cortical iliac crest bone can be sutured or wired to the central portion of the Steinmann pin (**Fig. 41.8**). This bone plate provides a template for the fusion to develop and preserves the dural decompression. A routine multilayered wound closure is performed.

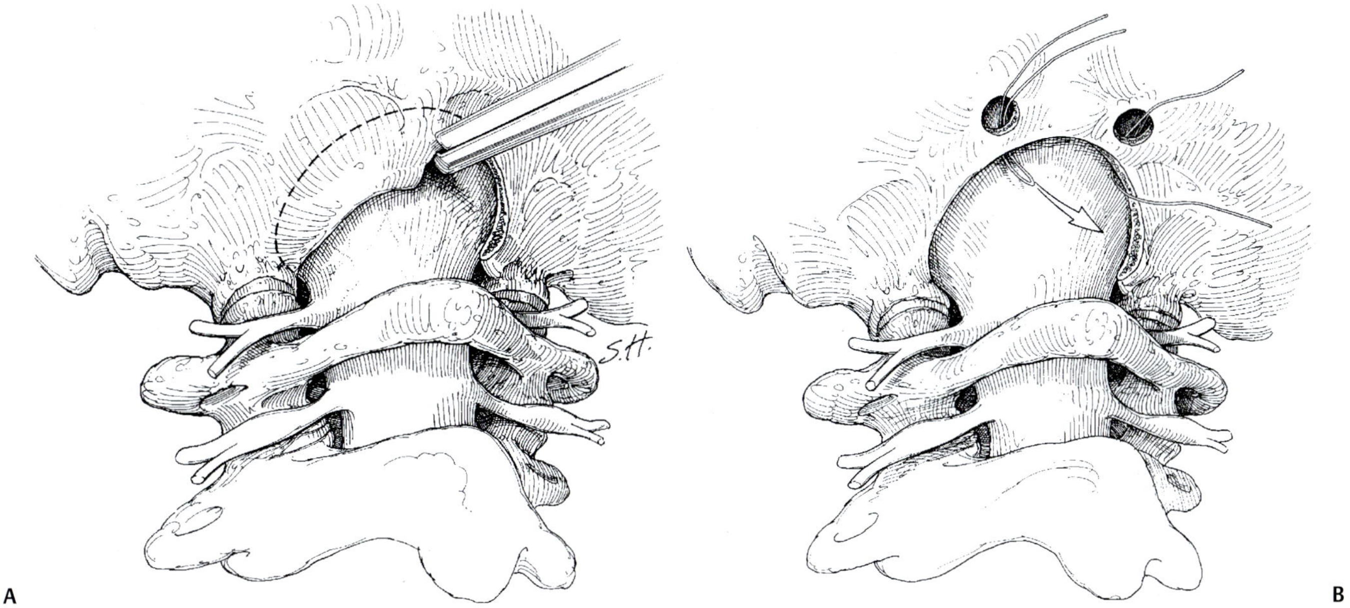

Fig. 41.6 The occiput is wired after **(A)** enlarging the dorsal rim of the foramen magnum. **(B)** Burr holes are placed 5 mm above the edge of the foramen magnum. The dura is separated from the inner table of bone to prevent intradural wire penetration during wire passage. (Reprinted with permission from Barrow Neurological Institute.)

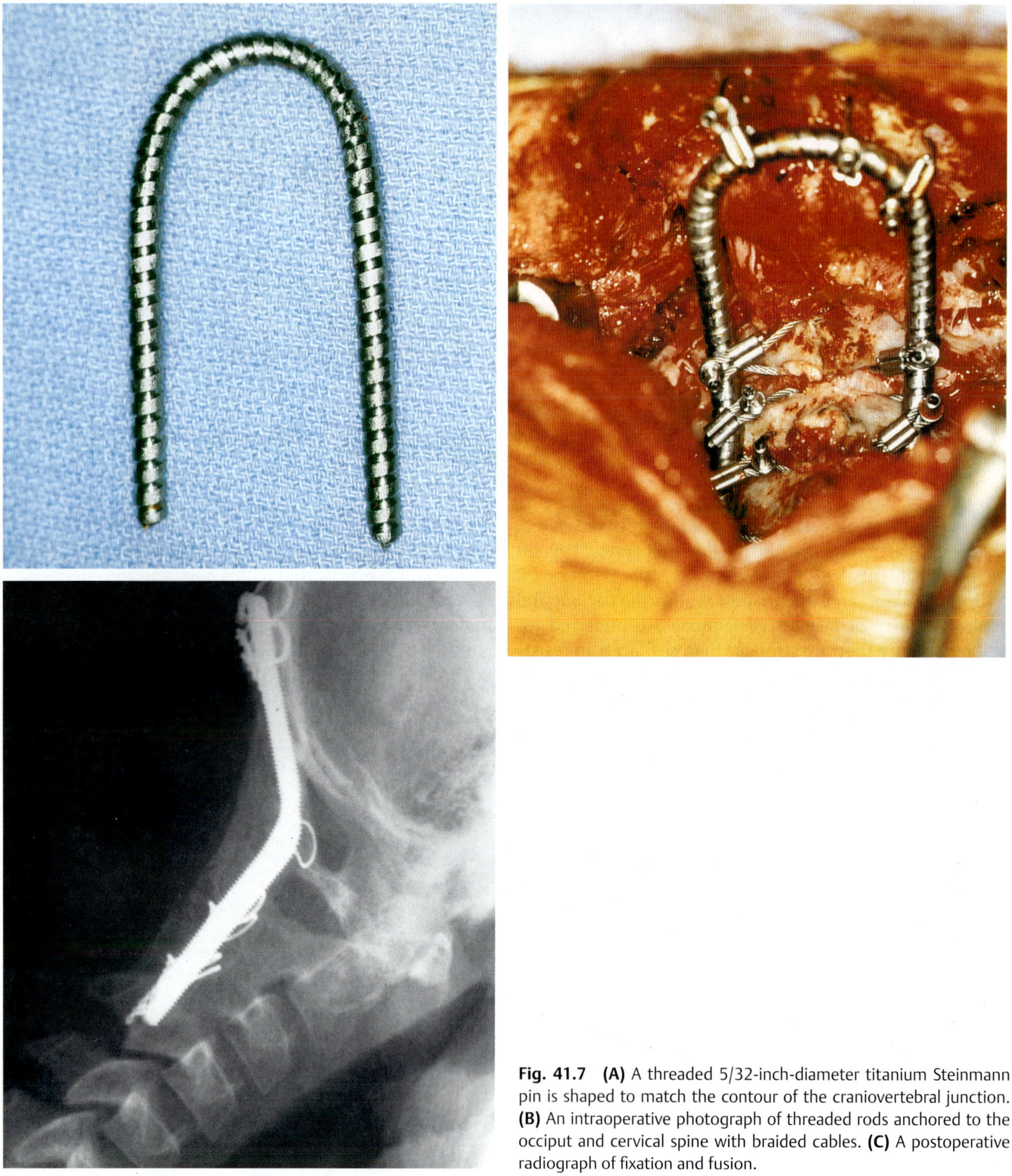

Fig. 41.7 **(A)** A threaded 5/32-inch-diameter titanium Steinmann pin is shaped to match the contour of the craniovertebral junction. **(B)** An intraoperative photograph of threaded rods anchored to the occiput and cervical spine with braided cables. **(C)** A postoperative radiograph of fixation and fusion.

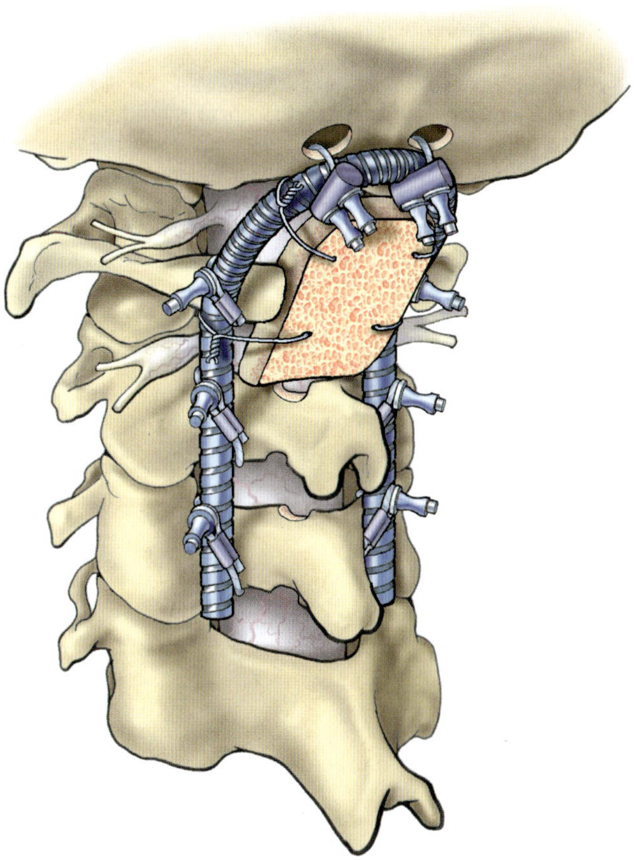

Fig. 41.8 After a suboccipital decompression or cervical laminectomy has been performed, a plate of cortical bone is wired to preserve the decompression and to provide a template for fusion. (Reprinted with permission from Barrow Neurological Institute.)

Other variations of this technique have been described in the literature.[47–52] As a relative advantage, all are technically simpler to perform than screw-rod constructs and may serve as an alternative when extreme osteoporosis or anatomical considerations prevent safe screw placement. Furthermore, due to the higher failure rate associated with wire-rod constructs, an external orthosis is typically utilized in the postoperative period for up to 3 months. A Philadelphia collar or a sterno-occipital-mandibular immobilizer brace may be appropriate when bone quality is good, fixation is strong, and deforming forces are minimal. However, a halo brace or Minerva brace may be needed if there is excessive deformity, soft bone, poor fixation, extensive instability, or excessive loading of the vertebrae. The fixation devices and the postoperative orthoses are specifically tailored to provide appropriate therapy for the individual patient. Nevertheless, the additional morbidity associated with the use of such devices and additional discomfort they may impose are important considerations when choosing a treatment plan for a patient's pathological condition.

Occipitoatlantal Transarticular Screws

In some cases, posterior fixation techniques that rely on midline occipital fixation may be impossible, particularly if the foramen magnum and suboccipital bone have been removed (e.g., in a patient with a previous Chiari decompression). Additionally, in cases of occipitoatlantal (OA) dissociation/dislocation, the primary pathology involves the OA joints and ligaments only. Both of these situations represent ideal cases for OA transarticular screw fixation.

Around 2001 and 2002, a few authors began publishing studies of the anatomy of the occipital condyle, hypoglossal canal, and OA joint.[53–55] In 2003, Gonzalez and colleagues published a detailed biomechanical analysis of the technique and performed it in eight cadaver specimens, with successful placement of 15/16 screws using anteroposterior and lateral fluoroscopy and no violations of the hypoglossal canal.[56] In 2005, the same group provided a case report of a victim of a motor vehicle accident with OA dissociation/dislocation treated successfully with this technique.[20] Patient positioning and intraoperative setup are as described above but with care taken to evaluate the patient's upper thoracic kyphosis and lower cervical lordosis. The very steep superior trajectory exceeds that for C1-C2 transarticular screw fixation and requires percutaneous entry points on the upper thoracic spine to obtain the proper angle, which may be impossible in some patients. A midline skin incision and subperiosteal muscle dissection is performed from the occiput to C3 or lower, if additional fixation is planned. The posterior elements of C1 and C2 are exposed, and the vertebral venous plexus around the C2 nerve root is dissected, exposing the caudal C1 arch laterally where it leads to the posterior aspect of the inferior articular process of C1. The C2 nerve root is retracted caudally. This exposure is identical to the exposure used for placement of C1 lateral mass screws. A drill guide is then advanced percutaneously through the thoracic stab incision and docked at the junction between the base of the C1 posterior arch and the posterior aspect of the inferior articular process of C1. Under fluoroscopic guidance and/or stereotactic navigation, a drill (or K-wire if using a cannulated system) is then advanced at a 45-degree superior angle and at 0 degrees medial-lateral through the C1 lateral mass, across the OA joint, and into the occipital condyle. At a 45-degree angle, the screw tip should stay caudal and anterior to the hypoglossal canal. After appropriate pilot hole preparation, a 28 to 32 mm screw is placed (**Fig. 41.9**). A lag screw can be used to reduce an OA dissociation/dislocation. Based on biomechanical studies done to date, it is recommended that the technique be supplemented with posterior bone strut grafting secured with cables to strengthen the construct in flexion-extension and to provide for long-term bony stability. This technique can also be combined with C1-C2 transarticular screws and other subaxial screw-rod constructs.

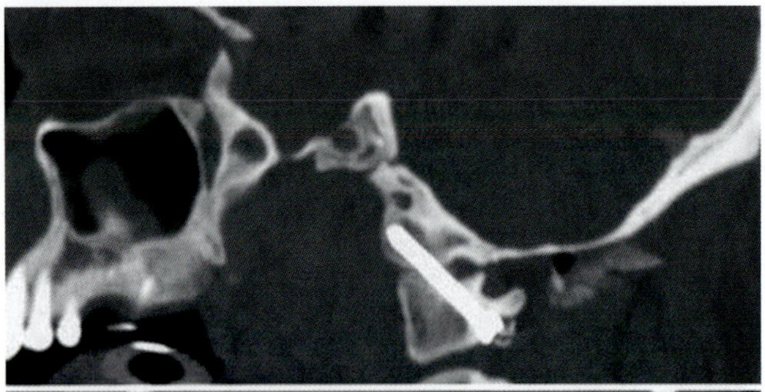

A

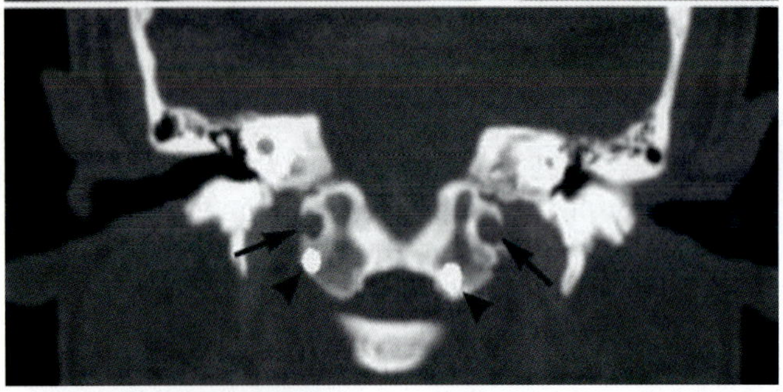

B

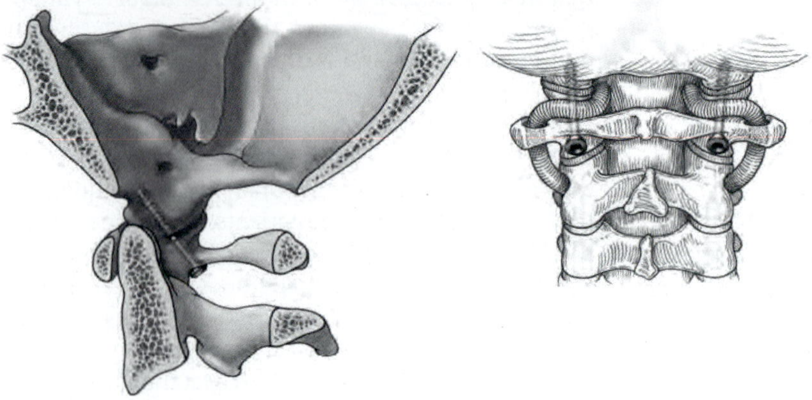

C

Fig. 41.9 **(A)** A sagittal bone-window on a computed tomography (CT) reconstruction of the occipitocervical junction after placement of the posterior transarticular atlanto-occipital screws. **(B)** A coronal bone-window on a CT reconstruction of the craniocervical junction demonstrates the tip of the atlanto-occipital screws in the occipital condyles (*arrowheads*) below the hypoglossal canal (*arrows*). **(C)** Artist's rendition of sagittal and posterior views of successfully placed transarticular occipitoatlantal screws. (Reprinted with permission from Barrow Neurological Institute.)

Conclusion

Modern instrumentation techniques for occipitocervical fusion, including screw-plate, screw-rod, and transarticular screw constructs, provide immediate rigid fixation and avoid sublaminar wire passage and instrumentation in the spinal canal. These techniques are excellent choices for patients who have several absent or fractured laminae that preclude fixation with wires. Softened or diseased bone requires adequate screw purchase sites and may require the use of wire-rod constructs in cases when screw purchase is impossible for anatomic reasons. Fusions can be restructured solely to the involved segments. These methods are technically demanding, require operative precision, and mandate expertise with multiple fixation techniques.

References

1. Fielding JW, Hawkins RJ, Ratzan SA. Spine fusion for atlanto-axial instability. J Bone Joint Surg Am 1976;58(3):400–407
2. Malcolm GP, Ransford AO, Crockard HA. Treatment of non-rheumatoid occipitocervical instability. Internal fixation with the Hartshill-Ransford loop. J Bone Joint Surg Br 1994;76(3):357–366
3. Conaty JP, Mongan ES. Cervical fusion in rheumatoid arthritis. J Bone Joint Surg Am 1981;63(8):1218–1227
4. Elia M, Mazzara JT, Fielding JW. Onlay technique for occipitocervical fusion. Clin Orthop Relat Res 1992;280(280):170–174
5. Newman P, Sweetnam R. Occipito-cervical fusion. An operative technique and its indications. J Bone Joint Surg Br 1969;51(3):423–431
6. Hamblen DL. Occipito-cervical fusion. Indications, technique and results. J Bone Joint Surg Br 1967;49(1):33–45
7. Wertheim SB, Bohlman HH. Occipitocervical fusion. Indications, technique, and long-term results in thirteen patients. J Bone Joint Surg Am 1987;69(6):833–836
8. Menezes AH, VanGilder JC, Graf CJ, McDonnell DE. Craniocervical abnormalities. A comprehensive surgical approach. J Neurosurg 1980;53(4):444–455
9. Lipscomb PR. Cervico-occipital fusion for congenital and post-traumatic anomalies of the atlas and axis. J Bone Joint Surg Am 1957;39-A(6):1289–1301
10. Segal LS, Drummond DS, Zanotti RM, Ecker ML, Mubarak SJ. Complications of posterior arthrodesis of the cervical spine in patients who have Down syndrome. J Bone Joint Surg Am 1991;73(10):1547–1554

11. MacKenzie AI, Uttley D, Marsh HT, Bell BA. Craniocervical stabilization using Luque/Hartshill rectangles. Neurosurgery 1990;26(1):32–36
12. Ransford AO, Crockard HA, Pozo JL, Thomas NP, Nelson IW. Craniocervical instability treated by contoured loop fixation. J Bone Joint Surg Br 1986;68(2):173–177
13. Sakou T, Kawaida H, Morizono Y, Matsunaga S, Fielding JW. Occipitoatlantoaxial fusion utilizing a rectangular rod. Clin Orthop Relat Res 1989;239(239):136–144
14. Heywood AW, Learmonth ID, Thomas M. Internal fixation for occipito-cervical fusion. J Bone Joint Surg Br 1988;70(5):708–711
15. Kaufman HH, Jones E. The principles of bony spinal fusion. Neurosurgery 1989;24(2):264–270
16. Dickman CA, Douglas RA, Sonntag VKH. Occipitocervical fusion: posterior stabilization of the craniovertebral junction and upper cervical spine. BNI Q 1990;6(2):2–14
17. Papadopoulos SM, Dickman CA, Sonntag VK, Rekate HL, Spetzler RF. Traumatic atlantooccipital dislocation with survival. Neurosurgery 1991;28(4):574–579
18. Robinson RA, Southwick WO. Surgical approaches to the cervical spine. In: American Academy of Orthopedic Surgeons, ed. Instructional Course Lectures. St. Louis, MO: CV Mosby; 1960:299–330
19. Fehlings MG, Errico T, Cooper P, Benjamin V, DiBartolo T. Occipitocervical fusion with a five-millimeter malleable rod and segmental fixation. Neurosurgery 1993;32(2):198–207, discussion 207–208
20. Feiz-Erfan I, Gonzalez LF, Dickman CA. Atlantooccipital transarticular screw fixation for the treatment of traumatic occipitoatlantal dislocation. Technical note. J Neurosurg Spine 2005;2(3):381–385
21. Bambakidis NC, Feiz-Erfan I, Horn EM, et al. Biomechanical comparison of occipitoatlantal screw fixation techniques. J Neurosurg Spine 2008;8(2):143–152
22. Grob D, Dvorak J, Panjabi M, Froehlich M, Hayek J. Posterior occipitocervical fusion. A preliminary report of a new technique. Spine 1991;16(3, Suppl):S17–S24
23. Heywood AW, Learmonth ID, Thomas M. Internal fixation for occipito-cervical fusion. J Bone Joint Surg Br 1988;70(5):708–711
24. Sasso RC, Jeanneret B, Fischer K, Magerl F. Occipitocervical fusion with posterior plate and screw instrumentation. A long-term follow-up study. Spine 1994;19(20):2364–2368
25. Grob D, Dvorak J, Panjabi MM, Antinnes JA. The role of plate and screw fixation in occipitocervical fusion in rheumatoid arthritis. Spine 1994;19(22):2545–2551
26. Smith MD, Anderson P, Grady MS. Occipitocervical arthrodesis using contoured plate fixation. An early report on a versatile fixation technique. Spine 1993;18(14):1984–1990
27. Finn MA, Bishop FS, Dailey AT. Surgical treatment of occipitocervical instability. Neurosurgery 2008;63(5):961–968, discussion 968–969
28. Wolfla CE, Salerno SA, Yoganandan N, Pintar FA. Comparison of contemporary occipitocervical instrumentation techniques with and without C1 lateral mass screws. Neurosurgery 2007 61(3, Suppl):87–93, discussion 93
29. Nockels RP, Shaffrey CI, Kanter AS, Azeem S, York JE. Occipitocervical fusion with rigid internal fixation: long-term follow-up data in 69 patients. J Neurosurg Spine 2007;7(2):117–123
30. Anderson RC, Kan P, Gluf WM, Brockmeyer DL. Long-term maintenance of cervical alignment after occipitocervical and atlantoaxial screw fixation in young children. J Neurosurg 2006;105(1, Suppl):55–61
31. Deutsch H, Haid RW Jr, Rodts GE Jr, Mummaneni PV. Occipitocervical fixation: long-term results. Spine 2005;30(5):530–535
32. Roy-Camille R, Saillant G, Mazel C. Internal fixation of the unstable cervical spine by a posterior osteosynthesis with plates and screws. In: Cervical Spine Research Society, ed. The Cervical Spine, 2nd ed. Philadelphia, PA: JB Lippincott; 1989:390–403
33. Dickman CA, Sonntag VKH, Marcotte PJ. Techniques of screw fixation of the cervical spine. BNI Q 1992;8(2):9–26
34. Weidner A. Internal fixation with metal plates and screw. In: Cervical Spine Research Society, ed. The Cervical Spine, 2nd ed. Philadelphia, PA: JB Lippincott; 1989:404–421
35. Heller JG, Carlson GD, Abitbol JJ, Garfin SR. Anatomic comparison of the Roy-Camille and Magerl techniques for screw placement in the lower cervical spine. Spine 1991;16(10, Suppl):S552–S557
36. Geremia GK, Kim KS, Cerullo L, Calenoff L. Complications of sublaminar wiring. Surg Neurol 1985;23(6):629–635
37. Rogers WA. Fractures and dislocations of the cervical spine; an end-result study. J Bone Joint Surg Am 1957;39-A(2):341–376
38. Davey JR, Rorabeck CH, Bailey SI, Bourne RB, Dewar FP. A technique of posterior cervical fusion for instability of the cervical spine. Spine 1985;10(8):722–728
39. Scuderi GJ, Greenberg SS, Cohen DS, Latta LL, Eismont FJ. A biomechanical evaluation of magnetic resonance imaging-compatible wire in cervical spine fixation. Spine 1993;18(14):1991–1994
40. Hanson PB, Montesano PX, Sharkey NA, Rauschning W. Anatomic and biomechanical assessment of transarticular screw fixation for atlantoaxial instability. Spine 1991;16(10):1141–1145
41. Belzberg AJ, Tranmer BI. Stabilization of traumatic atlanto-occipital dislocation. Case report. J Neurosurg 1991;75(3):478–482
42. Dickman CA, Papadopoulos SM, Sonntag VKH, Spetzler RF, Rekate HL, Drabier J. Traumatic occipitoatlantal dislocations. J Spinal Disord 1993;6(4):300–313
43. Itoh T, Tsuji H, Katoh Y, Yonezawa T, Kitagawa H. Occipito-cervical fusion reinforced by Luque's segmental spinal instrumentation for rheumatoid diseases. Spine 1988;13(11):1234–1238
44. Sonntag VKH, Dickman CA. Craniocervical stabilization. Clin Neurosurg 1993;40:243–272
45. Sonntag VKH, Kalfas I. Innovative cervical fusion and instrumentation techniques. Clin Neurosurg 1991;37:636–660
46. Apostolides PJ, Dickman CA, Golfinos JG, Papadopoulos SM, Sonntag VK. Threaded steinmann pin fusion of the craniovertebral junction. Spine 1996;21(14):1630–1637
47. Grantham SA, Dick HM, Thompson RC Jr, Stinchfield FE. Occipitocervical arthrodesis. Indications, technic and results. Clin Orthop Relat Res 1969;65:118–129
48. Lu DC, Roeser AC, Mummaneni VP, Mummaneni PV. Nuances of occipitocervical fixation. Neurosurgery 2010;66(3, Suppl):141–146
49. Couture D, Avery N, Brockmeyer DL. Occipitocervical instrumentation in the pediatric population using a custom loop construct: initial results and long-term follow-up experience. J Neurosurg Pediatr 2010;5(3):285–291
50. Garrido BJ, Puschak TJ, Anderson PA, Sasso RC. Occipitocervical fusion using contoured rods and medial offset connectors: description of a new technique. Orthopedics 2009;32(10)
51. Anderson RC, Ragel BT, Mocco J, Bohman LE, Brockmeyer DL. Selection of a rigid internal fixation construct for stabilization at the craniovertebral junction in pediatric patients. J Neurosurg 2007;107(1, Suppl):36–42
52. Yüksel KZ, Crawford NR, Melton MS, Dickman CA. Augmentation of occipitocervical contoured rod fixation with C1-C2 transarticular screws. Spine J 2007;7(2):180–187
53. Gonzalez LF, Ferreira MA, Deshmukh P, et al. The occipital condyle: A microanatomical study and its surgical relevance. Skull Base 2001;11:19
54. Grob D. Transarticular screw fixation for atlanto-occipital dislocation. Spine 2001;26(6):703–707
55. Gonzalez LF, Sonntag VKH, Dickman CA, Crawford NR. Technique for fixating the atlantooccipital complex with a transarticular screw. Spine 2002;27(2):219–220
56. Gonzalez LF, Crawford NR, Chamberlain RH, et al. Craniovertebral junction fixation with transarticular screws: biomechanical analysis of a novel technique. J Neurosurg 2003;98(2, Suppl): 202–209

42 Craniovertebral Instability: Atlantoaxial Joint Manipulation and Fixation

Atul Goel

Surgical treatment of instability of the craniovertebral junction (CVJ) region requires a three-dimensional (3D) understanding of the anatomy, a high degree of technical competence, and an understanding of biomechanical issues related to the region. Surgical management of CVJ instability is complex due to the relative difficulty in accessing the region, critical relationships of neurovascular structures, and the intricate biomechanical issues involved. While a successful outcome is gratifying, the complications of surgery are potentially lethal. Considering the complexities and intricacies of these issues, the surgeon has to have a complete understanding of the problem and the methodology of treatment prior to treatment. The surgeon should be armed with information related to the subject and to the surgical needs of the patient. Investigations need to be elaborate.

The human spine simulates a pillar that bifurcates in its upper end to support the roof. The bifurcation is at the region of C1-C2 and occipital bone, and C1 and the weight-bearing of the spine in its superior end shifts into the lateral masses. These lateral masses are an intricate formation of ligaments and bone that provides not only stability of the region but its extreme mobility. There is no other joint in the body that has such high mobility and stability. In general, the occipitoaxial joint provides stability, and the atlantoaxial joint provides mobility. Based on our understanding, most craniovertebral instability is related to problems of the atlantoaxial joint.

Atlantoaxial Dislocation

The techniques of craniovertebral fixation evolved during the 20th century as the anatomy and biomechanics of the craniovertebral region became clear. Atlantoaxial dislocation has been treated by various methods of fixation employing autologous bone graft, sublaminar wires, metal loupes, and rectangles. Transarticular and interarticular techniques employing the use of screw implantation in the firm and strong lateral masses of atlas and axis have been successfully employed for more than 20 years.[1–3] In 1988, we suggested an alternative plate and screw technique of fixation of the lateral masses of the atlas and axis and later discussed our 14-year experience with 160 cases of mobile and reducible atlantoaxial dislocation managed by this technique (**Fig. 42.1**).[2,3] Our technique is gaining wide acceptance and is currently used by most large units in which patients with craniovertebral anomalies are treated. The lateral masses of the atlas and axis are considerably larger and stronger than other lateral masses of vertebrae in the spine and can be used effectively for fixation. Firm and multidirectional stabilization is possible with the use of four screws in addition to plates. With our experience now exceeding 600 cases, we are convinced that our technique of atlantoaxial fixation is biomechanically strong, technically easy, and safe for neural structures and that it results in remarkable clinical and radiological improvement (**Fig. 42.2**).

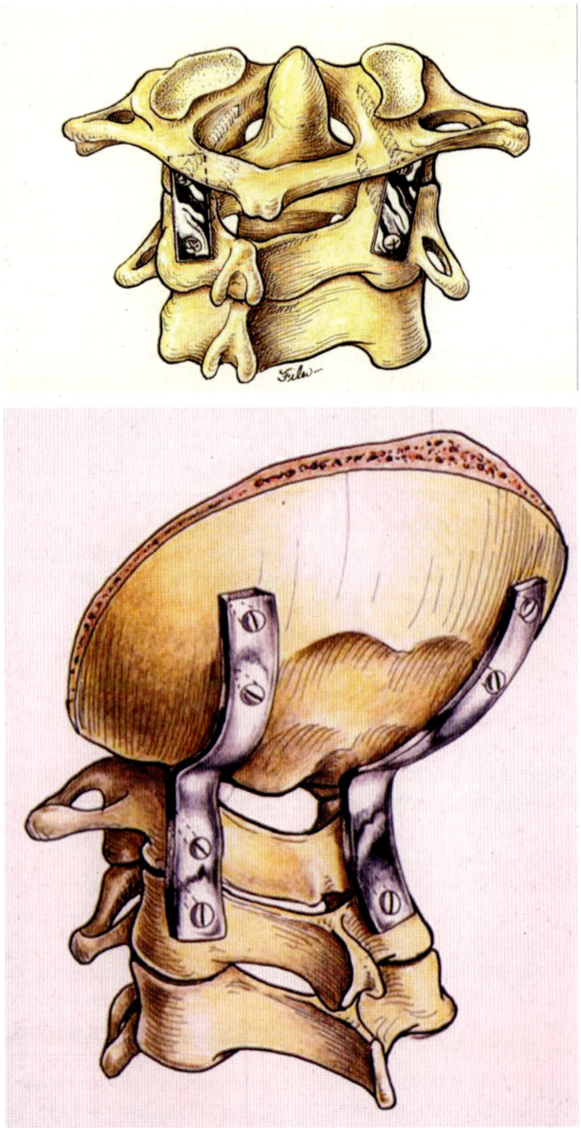

A

B

Fig. 42.1 (A) Lateral mass plate and screw fixation technique. **(B)** Occipitocervical fixation. The occipital end of the plate is fixed with screws. The cervical end of the plate is fixed with a screw in C2 alone or in C1 and C2 lateral mass.

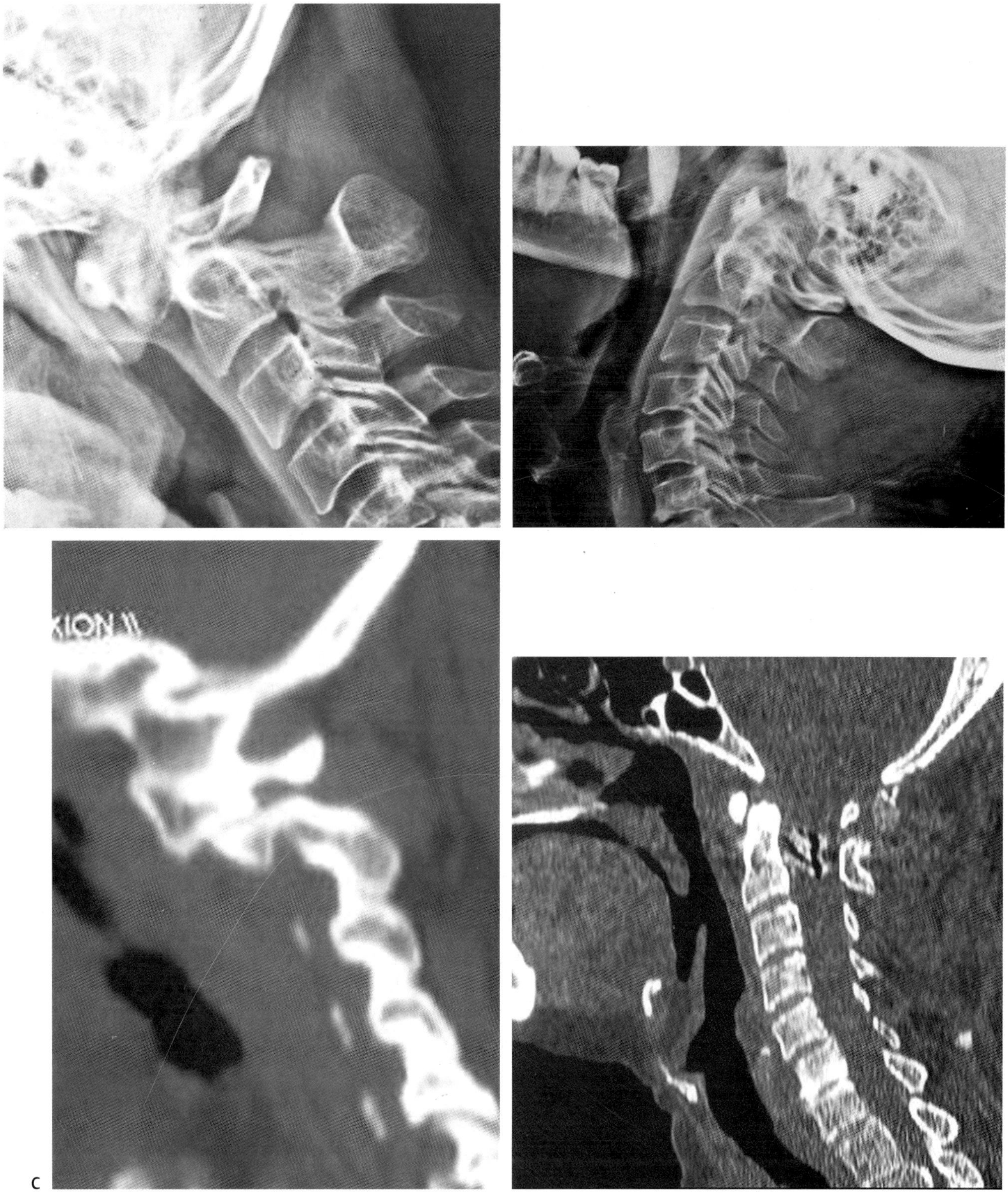

A B C D

Fig. 42.2 **(A)** Lateral plain radiograph with the neck in flexion showing marked atlantoaxial dislocation. **(B)** Lateral radiograph with the head in extension showing complete reduction of the dislocation. **(C)** Sagittal image of computed tomography (CT) scan showing the dislocation of the facet of the atlas over the facet of the axis. **(D)** Postoperative CT scan showing alignment of atlantoaxial region. *(continued)*

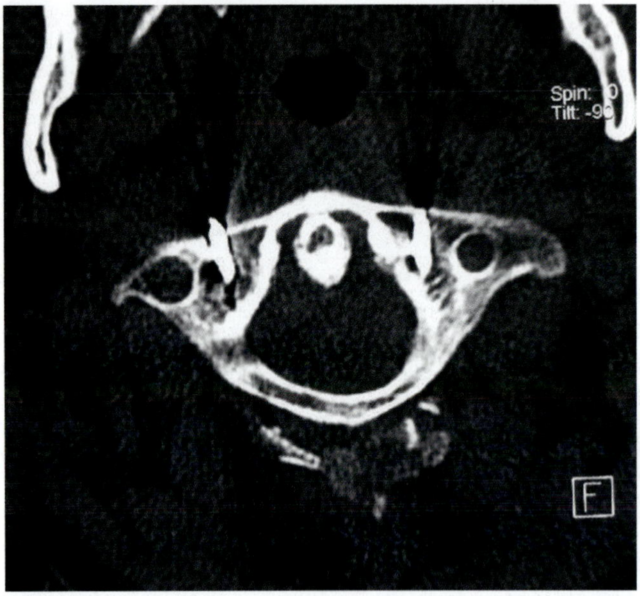

E

Fig. 42.2 *(continued)* **(E)** Axial image showing the screws in the lateral mass of atlas.

Recently, some authors have modified our technique and have recommended polyaxial screws and rods instead of monoaxial screws and plates.

Lateral Mass Plate and Screw Technique

Indications

All cases of atlantoaxial instability are suitable for operation by this technique. Although pathology and deformities of bones in the region may make the operation difficult, an attempt should be made to perform this technique considering the remarkable stability that it provides.[2,3] The procedure can be performed safely even in the presence of torticollis or assimilation of the atlas. Modification of the technique by joint manipulation and facetal distraction can be used in cases with fixed and rotatory dislocation and in group A basilar invagination.

Contraindications

There are no specific contraindications to the performance of lateral mass plate and screw fixation if the lateral masses of the atlas and axis are normal. We have observed that such a fixation is possible even in cases where there is lateral mass destruction, erosion, or significant osteoporosis. The anomalous course of the vertebral artery in the facet of axis and in the vicinity of the posterior arch of the atlas may rarely preclude the use of our technique.

Relevant Surgical Anatomy

Covered with a large plexus of veins, the vertebral artery adopts a serpentine course in relationship to the craniovertebral region. The venous plexuses are the largest in the region lateral to the C1-C2 joint. After a relatively linear ascent of the vertebral artery in the foramen transversarium of C6 to C3, the artery makes a loop medially toward an anteriorly placed superior articular facet of the C2 vertebra, making a deep groove on its inferior surface. The extent of medial extension of the loop varies. The distance of the artery from the midline of the vertebral body of C2 as would be observed during a transoral surgical procedure is 12 mm on average.[4,5] The vertebral artery loops away from the midline underneath the superior articular facet of the C2. The course of the vertebral artery in relationship to the inferior aspect of the superior articular facet of the C2 makes its susceptible to injury during transarticular and interarticular screw implantation techniques.

Operative Technique

Cervical traction is set up prior to induction of anesthesia, and weights are progressively increased to ~5 to 8 kg or a sixth of total body weight. The patient is placed prone with the head end of the table elevated to ~35 degrees. Cervical traction stabilizes the head in an optimally reduced extension position and prevents rotation. The traction also ensures that the weight of the head is directed superiorly toward the direction of the traction and the pressure of the headrest on the face or eyeball is avoided. Although placed on the headrest, the head is essentially floating as the traction pulls it away from the headrest. Elevation of the head end of the table, which acts as countertraction, reduces venous engorgement in the operative field. The suboccipital region and the upper cervical spine are exposed through an ~8-cm, longitudinal, midline skin incision centered on the spinous process of the axis. The process is identified, and the paraspinal muscles attached to it are sharply sectioned. The C2 ganglion is placed transversely over the atlantoaxial joints. The large ganglion is widely exposed and then sectioned and resected. The ganglion is closely related to the vertebral artery on its lateral aspect, and all dissection in the region must be done under direct vision. On some occasions, the ganglion can even be mobilized superiorly or inferiorly, and sectioning can be avoided. However, the author has found that sectioning the ganglion provides a wide and panoramic exposure of the lateral masses of the atlas and axis and the atlantoaxial joint region.[2,3] Such an exposure is essential when manipulation and distraction of the facets are contemplated. Numbness related to the ganglion sectioning is marginal and easily tolerated by the patient (**Fig. 42.3**). Bleeding from the large venous sinuses in the region and in the extradural space can be troublesome. Packing the region with Surgicel (Ethicon, Somerville, NJ) and Gelfoam (DuPuy, Raynham, MA) can assist in the control of venous bleeding. The joint capsule is cut sharply, and the articular surfaces of the joint are exposed. The adjacent synovial articular surfaces of the atlantoaxial joint are decorticated widely with a microdrill, and pieces of bone harvested from the iliac crest are stuffed into the joint space. The lateral aspect of the lamina and a part of the

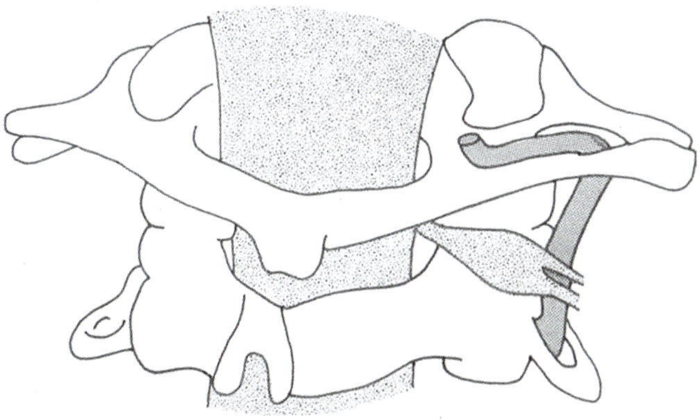

Fig. 42.3 C2 ganglion and its relationship with the joint, vertebral artery, and spinal canal.

pars of the axis are drilled to make the posterior surface of the lateral mass of the axis relatively flat so that the metal plate can be placed snugly and parallel to the bone. Drilling helps reduce the length of the plate and places the screw superiorly and almost directly into the lateral mass of the axis. Actual vertebral artery exposure is unnecessary lateral to the pars of the axis or superior to the arch of the atlas.

Screws are implanted in the previously created guide holes in the lateral mass of the atlas and axis through a two-holed (~2 cm in length) stainless steel or titanium plate (**Fig. 42.1A**). First, a screw is placed into the atlas and directed at an angle of ~15 degrees medial to the sagittal plane and 15 degrees superior to the axial plane. The preferred site of screw insertion is at the center of the posterior surface of the facet, 1 to 2 mm above the articular surface. Whenever necessary, careful drilling of the inferior surface of the lateral aspect of the posterior arch of the atlas in relation to its lateral mass can provide additional space for the placement of the plate and screw implantation. The screw may be implanted by choosing an insertion point on the posterior surface of the posterior arch of the atlas, just superior to the facet or even through the articular surface of the lateral mass of the atlas. Such sites are useful more frequently in children than in adults.

Screw implantation in the axis is relatively unsafe because of the intimacy of vertebral artery relationships. The preferred site of screw implantation in the lateral mass of the axis is in the medial and superior third of the pars. The direction of screw implantation must be sharply medial and superior and should be toward the superior aspect of the body of the axis vertebra toward the midline. The medial surface of the pars/pedicle of the axis is identified before the implantation of the screw. The screw is directed at an angle ~25 degrees medial to the sagittal plane and 15 degrees superior to the axial plane. The angle of screw insertion varies, depending on the local anatomy and size of the bones. The quality of cancellous bone in the lateral masses of the atlas and axis in the proposed trajectory of screw implantation is generally good, providing an excellent purchase of the screw and avoiding the vertebral artery.

The screws are 2.9 mm in diameter in adult patients and 2.7 mm in diameter in pediatric patients. The length of the required screw is calculated on the basis of the size of the lateral masses observed on the preoperative radiological studies. The approximate lengths of the atlas screws are 26 mm in adults and 22 mm in children. The screws in the atlas and axis are similar in length. One of the criteria of good screw placement includes engagement of anterior and posterior cortices of the lateral masses. Some authors have recently reported dangers to the carotid artery in the prevertebral region. However, we have never encountered this complication. It appears that, even if the screw is extra long, it will displace the soft tissues and carotid artery rather than cause injury. Intraoperative fluoroscopic control and neuronavigation was found to be helpful but not essential in determining the state of the screws. Large pieces of corticocancellous bone graft from the iliac crest bone are then placed over the adequately prepared posterior elements of the atlas and axis. After the wound is closed, cervical traction is discontinued. Patients are mobilized as soon as possible and advised to wear a hard cervical collar for 3 months.

Vertebral Artery Management

The most dreaded complication of the procedure is injury to the vertebral artery. Appropriate anatomical information of the region in general and of the case in question is required to avoid this injury. The vertebral artery can be injured during the process of lateral dissection of the C2 ganglion. A second potential site of injury is during insertion of the screw in the axis. To control the bleeding in the second situation, one has to pack the bleeding bone hole with bone wax. One can then insert the screw through the same hole, prepare for an alternative site of screw insertion, or use an alternative method of atlantoaxial fixation. Suturing the artery should be attempted whenever the injury is during its course outside the confines of the bones. Respect and care of all neural and vascular tissues and employment of precise technique are critical to success.[6]

This technique of lateral mass fixation and opening the joint provides an opportunity for manipulating the atlas and axis independently by obtaining fixation points in their strongest elements and, hence, has very versatile applications (**Table 42.1**).

Occipitocervical Fixation

In 1988, we described the use of lateral mass of the axis and atlas for screw implantation for stabilization of the cervical end of the occipitocervical plate.[2] The occipital end of the plate could be fixed with the help of occipital screws or wires (**Fig. 42.1B**). We were among the initial authors to describe screw fixation of the occipital end of the occipitocervical implant. Most of craniovertebral instability is related to the atlantoaxial joint that needs stabilization. In cases having atlantoaxial dislocation, inclusion of the occipital bone and subaxial cervical spine for fixation is suboptimal fixation.

Table 42.1 Advantages of the Authors' Technique

The principle advantages of our technique include the following:
Direct treatment to the fulcrum of the movements located at the atlantoaxial joint is provided.
Removal of the articular cartilage and stuffing of bone graft in the joint obstructs all movements, provides stabilization to the region by itself, and provides additional space for bone fusion.
Fusion is segmental. *The problem is atlantoaxial dislocation, and the treatment is atlantoaxial fixation.*
Fixation is firm and rigid because it involves screw implantation in the tough and strong bones of the facets of the atlas and axis. Such fixation provides an appropriate environment for bone fusion.
Method can be used in children even when other methods are not possible.[36,37]
All midline procedures can be additionally performed.
Manipulating and distracting the facets may affect reduction of mobile and fixed atlantoaxial dislocation and of basilar invagination.[9,11,13,28]
Atlantoaxial fixation can be done even in cases where there is assimilation or occipitalization of the atlas.[38]
Technique is safer for the vertebral artery than other procedures because screw implantation is performed separately in the facet of the atlas and pars of the axis.
Entire procedure is away from neural structures. The avoidance of the introduction of any wire underneath the arch of the atlas and axis adds remarkable safety. As tightening of wires is not involved, the dangers of incomplete tightening and overtightening are avoided.

Double Insurance Fixation

This method of atlantoaxial fixation combines a transarticular method of fixation and the interarticular fixation technique.[7] The technique combines the biomechanical strengths of the more commonly used techniques of fixation and provides maximal stability to the implants (**Fig. 42.4**).

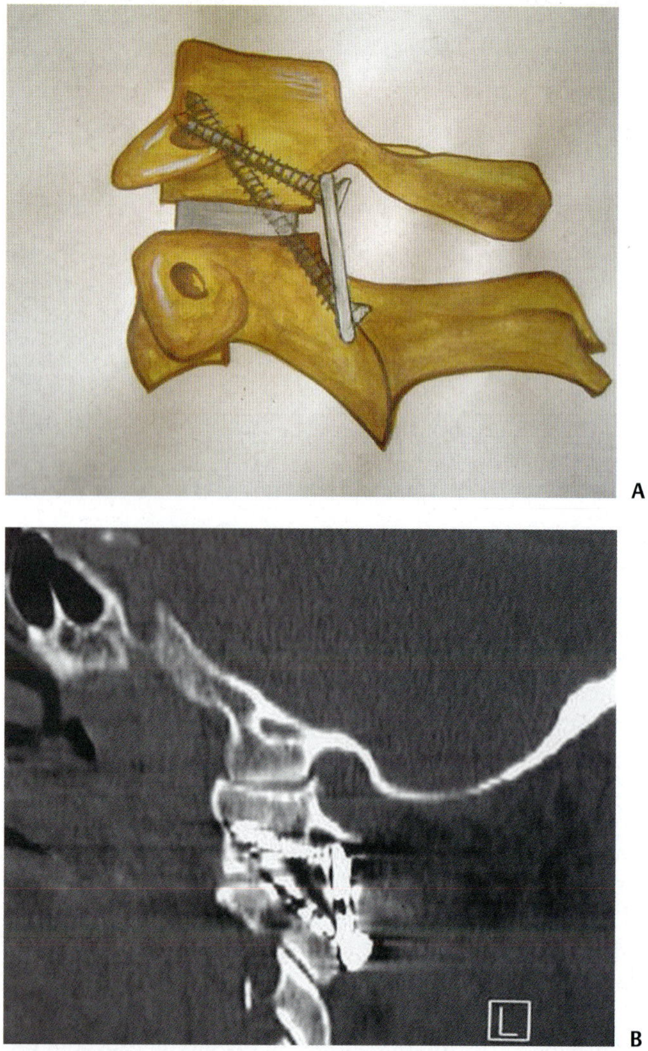

Fig. 42.4 **(A)** Line drawing showing "double insurance" plate and screw fixation. The atlas screw is implanted into the lateral mass of the atlas while the C2 screw is transarticular. **(B)** Sagittal scan through the lateral masses showing double insurance fixation.

Trans-Spinous Process, Trans-Spinolaminar, and Trans-Laminar C2 Screws

The feasibility of direct screw implantation in the spinous process or in the spinolaminar region was first described by Goel in 2004.[8] Screws that are implanted into the base of the spinous process and spinolaminar junction as well as those screws that extend into the substance of the lamina are the strongest in their purchase. Preoperative computed tomography and intraoperative navigation assist in the identification of the thickness of the spinous process and in determining the best site and direction of screw implantation. The relatively strong and stubby spinous process of the axis, particularly in cases with occipitalization of the atlas, facilitates screw implantation. The screw implantation in the spinous process, spinolaminar junction, and lamina provides a firm and stable option for stabilization of the cervical end of the occipitocervical fixation.

Joint-Jamming Technique

The technique of atlantoaxial joint jamming can be a useful method of fixation (**Figs. 42.5** and **42.6**).[9] In this technique, the joint is opened and distracted, and spiked titanium Goel spacers are impacted into it. Bone graft is placed in the joint cavity. No plate, screws, or wires are used in the fixation process. The indication for surgery is subtle atlantoaxial instability following trauma. The joint-jamming technique is also suitable for treatment of instability related to degenerative arthritis. Marked or long-standing instability that is seen in cases with congenital atlantoaxial dislocation may not be suitable for joint jamming. The use of joint spacers can be recommended only as an additional stabilizing method to be used in combination with other fixation techniques. However, direct stabilization of the site of movement of the atlantoaxial joint

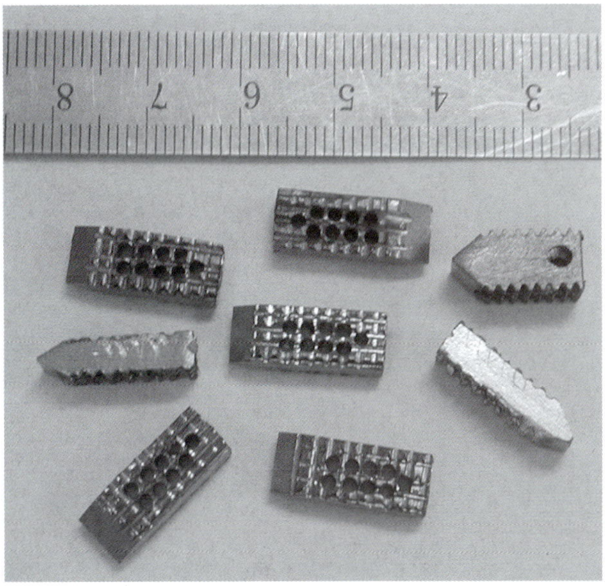

Fig. 42.5 Interarticular spacers.

provides an opportunity for firm and lasting control of abnormal movements in the region.

Fixed or Irreducible Atlantoaxial Dislocation

Atlantoaxial dislocation is described as fixed or irreducible when there is no radiographic reduction of the dislocation on full neck extension or after institution of cervical traction (**Fig. 42.7**). Fixed atlantoaxial dislocation can be congenital in nature or can be secondary to trauma to the region. We recently identified degenerative arthritis and formation of paradens ossification as one of the frequent causes of fixed atlantoaxial dislocation.[10] Congenital os odontoideum and fracture at the base of the odontoid process are frequent accompaniments of fixed atlantoaxial dislocation. According to our current hypothesis based on observations in surgically treated cases, we believe that most patients with fixed dislocations have pathologically abnormal movements that cause micromotion and cord compression.

Various authors have suggested a transoral decompression followed by a posterior fixation as the safest method of treatment of this complex anomaly. Treatment by posterior decompressive procedures has been reported to be associated with a high complication rate.

Direct atlantoaxial facet distraction can result in reduction of the fixed dislocation in a significant number of cases. An attempt can be made toward manipulation of the atlantoaxial joint, craniovertebral realignment, and reduction and fixation of the dislocation. It has been observed that anatomical reduction can be better achieved in cases that have fixed atlantoaxial subluxation in the presence of os odontoideum or odontoid fracture. In cases not associated with the above features, it is generally observed that the reduction is partial probably due to the presence of the relatively unyielding nature of the organized fibrous tissue in the predental region. In our experience, there may be a place for reduction of the fixed atlantoaxial dislocation and subsequent fixation, without the removal of any bony spinal element.[11] Such a treatment can be adopted even in cases with spondyloptosis of the atlas over the axis.[12] As there is no vertebral body of the atlas, spondyloptosis can be labeled as a clinical condition when the facet of the atlas is dislocated anterior to the facet of the axis.

A

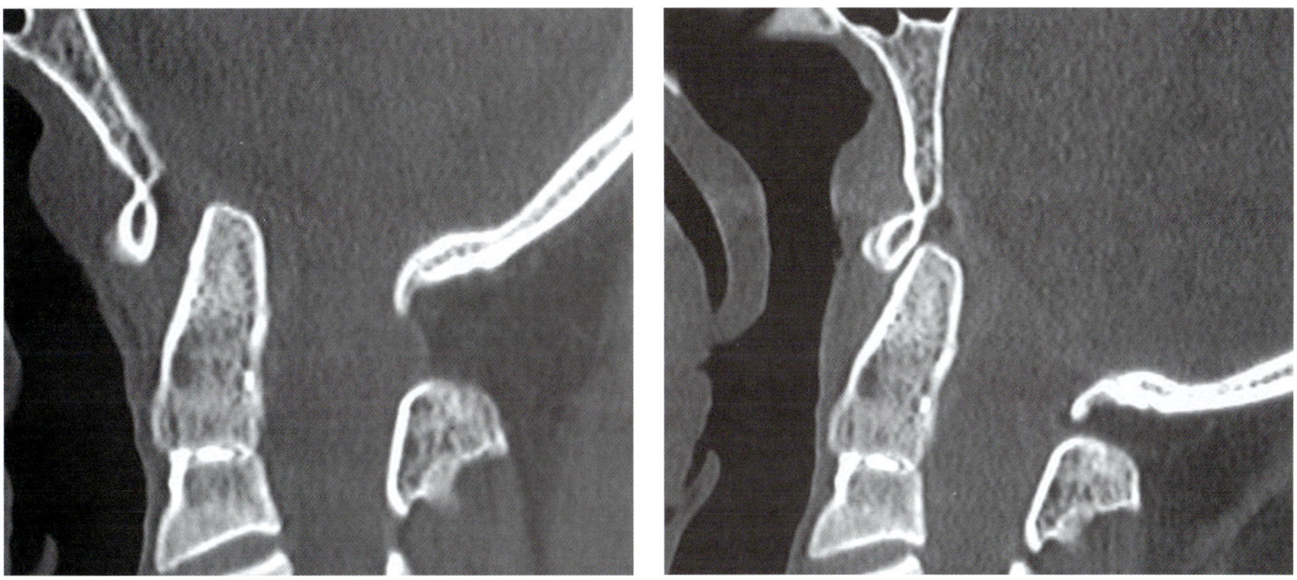

B

Fig. 42.6 **(A)** Computed tomography (CT) scan with the head in flexion showing atlantoaxial dislocation. **(B)** CT scan with the head in extension showing reduction of the dislocation. *(continued)*

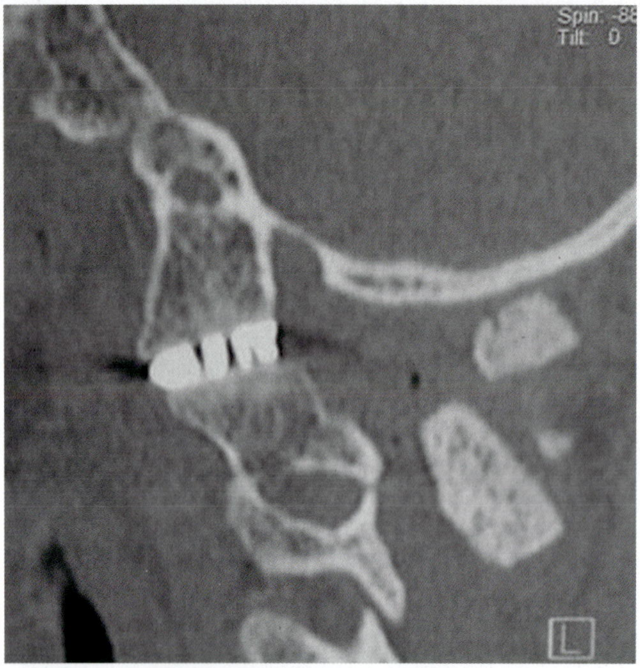

C

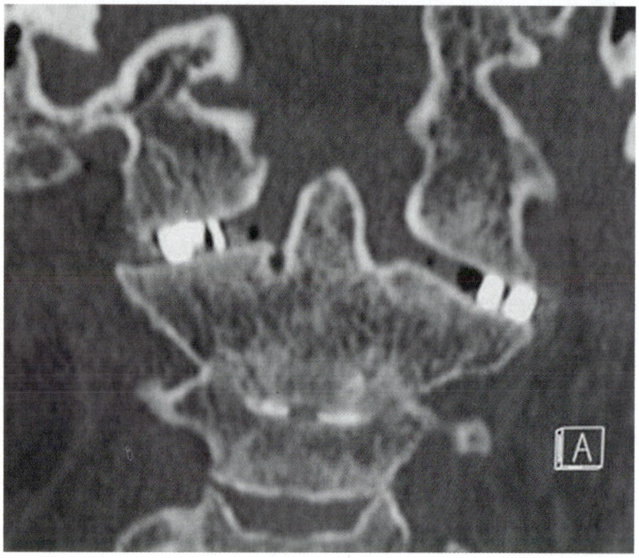

D

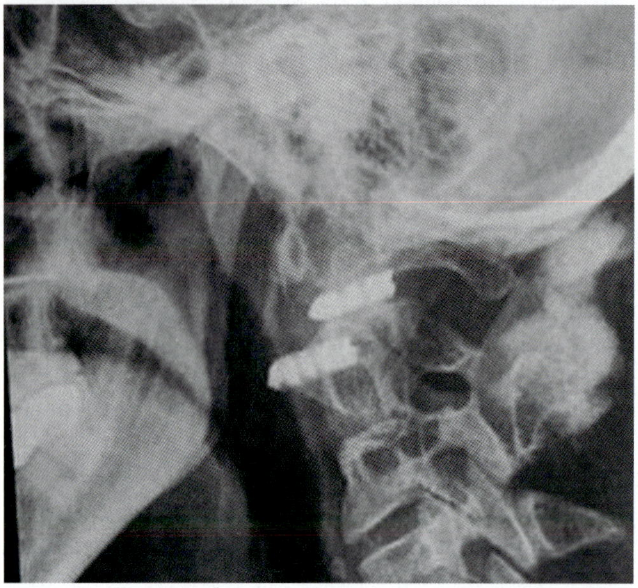

E

Fig. 42.6 *(continued)* **(C)** Sagittal CT scan showing the spacer in the atlantoaxial joint. **(D)** Coronal scan showing the spacers in the joint. **(E)** Postoperative radiograph showing reduction of the dislocation. Spacers in the joint can be seen.

■ Basilar Invagination: Classification into Group A and B

Basilar invagination can be divided into two groups.[13] In group A basilar invagination, there is clinical and radiological evidence of instability of the CVJ. The instability of the region is manifested by distancing the odontoid process away from the anterior arch of the atlas. The tip of the odontoid process "invaginates" into the foramen magnum and is above Chamberlain's line,[14] McRae's line of the foramen magnum,[15] and Wackenheim's clival line.[16,17] The definition of basilar invagination of prolapse of the cervical spine into the base of the skull, as suggested by von Torklus,[18] is suitable for this group of patients (**Fig. 42.8**). In group B basilar invagination, the odontoid process and clivus remain anatomically aligned despite the presence of basilar invagination and other associated anomalies. In this group, the tip of the odontoid process is above Chamberlain's line but below McRae's and Wackenheim's lines.

Radiological findings suggest that the odontoid process in group A patients results in direct compression of the brainstem. In this group, the atlantoaxial joints are active and their orientation is oblique rather than in the normal horizontal orientation. We have found similarities of such a position of the C1-C2 facets with spondylolisthesis seen in the subaxial spine.[19] It appears that the atlantoaxial joint in such cases is in an abnormal position as a result of mechanical instability,

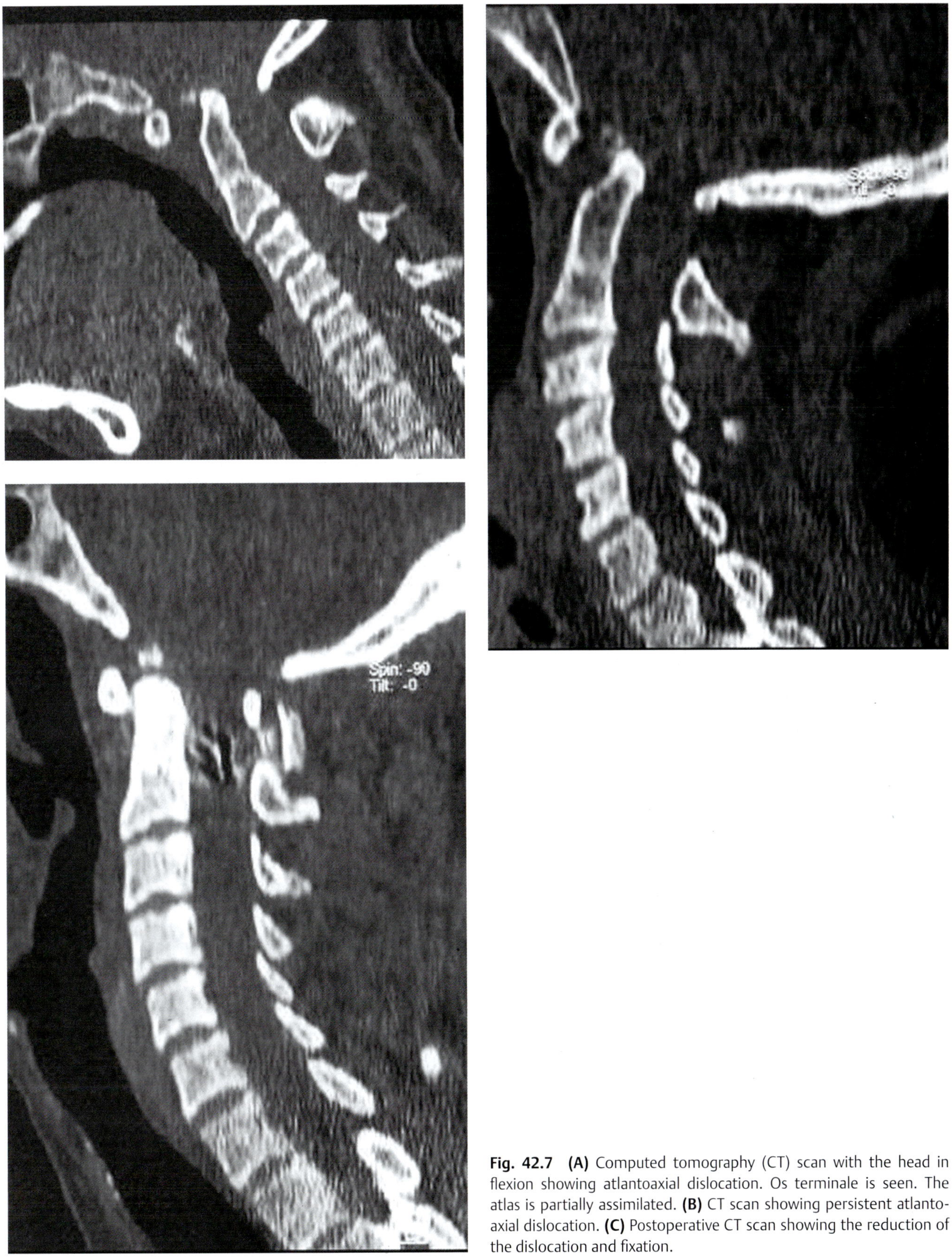

A

B

C

Fig. 42.7 **(A)** Computed tomography (CT) scan with the head in flexion showing atlantoaxial dislocation. Os terminale is seen. The atlas is partially assimilated. **(B)** CT scan showing persistent atlantoaxial dislocation. **(C)** Postoperative CT scan showing the reduction of the dislocation and fixation.

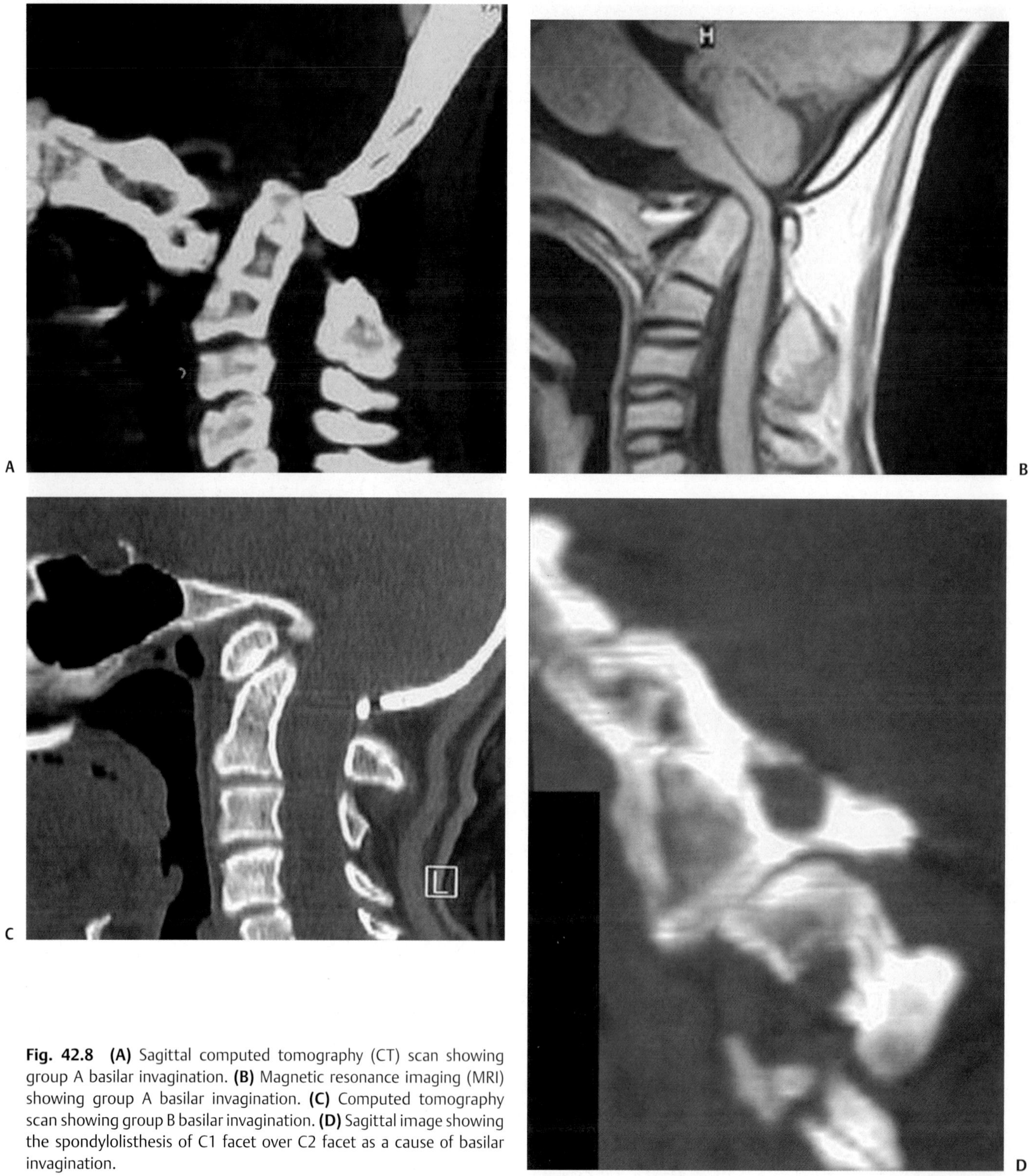

Fig. 42.8 **(A)** Sagittal computed tomography (CT) scan showing group A basilar invagination. **(B)** Magnetic resonance imaging (MRI) showing group A basilar invagination. **(C)** Computed tomography scan showing group B basilar invagination. **(D)** Sagittal image showing the spondylolisthesis of C1 facet over C2 facet as a cause of basilar invagination.

and progressive worsening of the dislocation is probably secondary to increasing slippage of the facets of the atlas over the facets of the axis.[19,20] In our experience handling atlantoaxial joints, the joint in these cases is not fixed or fused but is mobile and, in some cases, hypermobile and probably the prime cause for the basilar invagination. The history of trauma preceding the clinical events, predominant complaint of pain in the neck, and improvement in neurological symptoms following institution of cervical traction suggest vertical instability of the craniovertebral region. In group B, the atlantoaxial joints are normally aligned. In some cases, the joints are entirely fused. The pathogenesis of basilar invagination appears to be different in the two groups. Although it appears that group A basilar invagination may be related to mechanical instability, group B basilar invagination appears to be secondary to a congenital abnormality.

Vertical Atlantoaxial Dislocation/Mobile Basilar Invagination

A select group of patients with group A basilar invagination exhibits complete reduction of basilar invagination on extension of the head without the need of cervical traction. We label this group of patients as having vertical mobile and reducible atlantoaxial dislocation.[21] Incompetence of the lateral masses is the prime cause for such a pathological event. Considering that the imaging characteristics with the head in flexed position are of group A basilar invagination, the term *mobile and reducible basilar invagination* can be used to classify the clinical condition. It is critical to differentiate this group of patients from the other group A basilar invagination cases that have fixed atlantoaxial dislocation because the treatment of the two clinical entities is discrete.

Several bone and soft tissue anomalies are associated with basilar invagination, such as short neck, torticollis, platybasia, spondylotic spinal changes, restriction of neck movements, and cervical vertebral body fusion (Klippel-Feil abnormality),[22,23] including assimilation of the atlas. Several of these abnormalities are reversible following decompression and stabilization of the region.[23] Considering that several physical features associated with this group of basilar invagination are reversible, the pathogenesis in such cases may be due to mechanical factors more than congenital causes or embryological dysgenesis. The common teaching on the subject is that the short neck and torticollis are a result of embryological dysgenesis, effectively resulting in indentation of the odontoid process into the cervicomedullary cord. Our analysis reveals that odontoid compression of the cord is the primary event, and all musculoskeletal alterations are secondary protective mechanisms of the body aimed at reducing the effect of neural compression. These secondary physical abnormalities are reversible following surgery for decompression of the cord and stabilization of the region. Essentially, these abnormalities are not a result of embryonic dysgenesis and only secondary natural adaptive changes. Pain, restriction of neck movements, and hyperlordosis of the neck indicate the presence of instability of the CVJ.

Craniovertebral Realignment for Group A Basilar Invagination

The standard and most accepted form of treatment of group A basilar invagination is transoral decompression.[24–26] The majority of authors recommends a posterior occipitocervical fixation following the anterior decompression (**Fig. 42.9**).

Transoral odontoidectomy and resection of the superior half or third of the C2 body is a gratifying surgical procedure in group A patients.[25,26] However, the long-term clinical outcome following the twin operation of transoral decompression followed by posterior stabilization is inferior to the clinical outcome following our current operation involving craniovertebral realignment without bone, dural, or neural decompression.

When we attempt to reduce basilar invagination by performing occipitocervical fixation following cervical traction,[24,25] the cases treated in this manner subsequently need transoral decompression because the reduction of the basilar invagination and atlantoaxial dislocation cannot be sustained by the implant. The technique of craniovertebral realignment by wide removal of the atlantoaxial joint capsule and articular cartilage by drilling and subsequent distraction of the joint by manual manipulation provides a unique opportunity to obtain reduction of the basilar invagination and fixation of the atlantoaxial joint.[2,3,13] Our current experience with the technique in more than 250 cases convinces us that distraction and direct lateral mass fixation of the atlantoaxial joint is the ideal form of treatment in cases of group A basilar invagination; transoral surgery can be avoided entirely. The technique results in realignment of the facets into horizontal position and in realignment of the entire CVJ.

Craniovertebral Realignment for Group A Basilar Invagination Associated with Syringomyelia

We classify syringomyelia and suggest a specific treatment protocol on the basis of possible pathogenetic factors.[27] We suggest that syringomyelia is a tertiary response to primary craniovertebral anomaly in the form of basilar invagination that leads to secondary Chiari I malformation as a result of reduction in the posterior cranial fossa volume. Accordingly, a posterior fossa bony decompression is considered optimum in the treatment of this subgroup of patients.

In some cases of syringomyelia, associated bony abnormalities of the craniovertebral region include fixed atlantoaxial dislocation or those having Group A basilar invagination. This select group of patients is treated by attempts to reduce the atlantoaxial dislocation and basilar invagination and by direct lateral mass plate and screw atlantoaxial fixation.[28] No bony or dural decompression or neural manipulation is done in these cases.

Foramen Magnum Decompression for Group B Patients

In group B, the assembly of the odontoid process, the anterior arch of the atlas, and the clivus migrates superiorly in unison, resulting in reduction of the posterior cranial fossa volume, which is the primary pathology in these cases.[13] Chiari malformation or herniation of the cerebellar tonsil is considered to be a result of reduction in the posterior cranial fossa volume. In 1997, we defined the clinical implication of association of small posterior cranial fossa volume and Chiari malformation.[25]

Patients in group B benefit by decompression of the bony foramen magnum. The procedure results in amelioration of

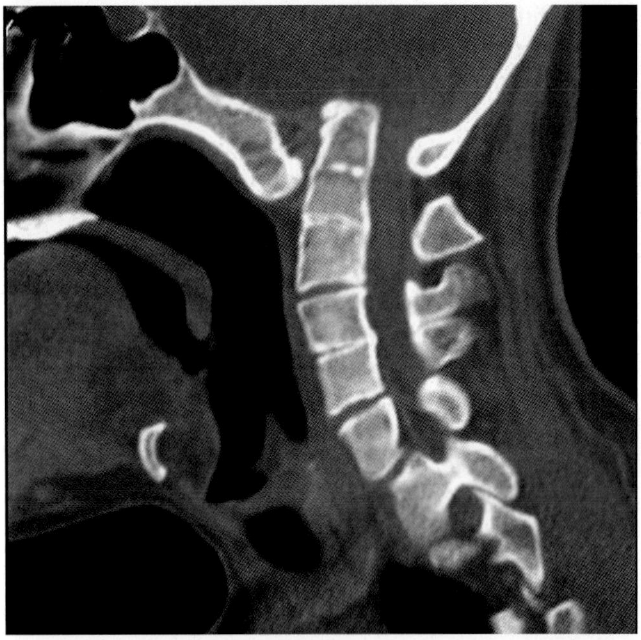
A

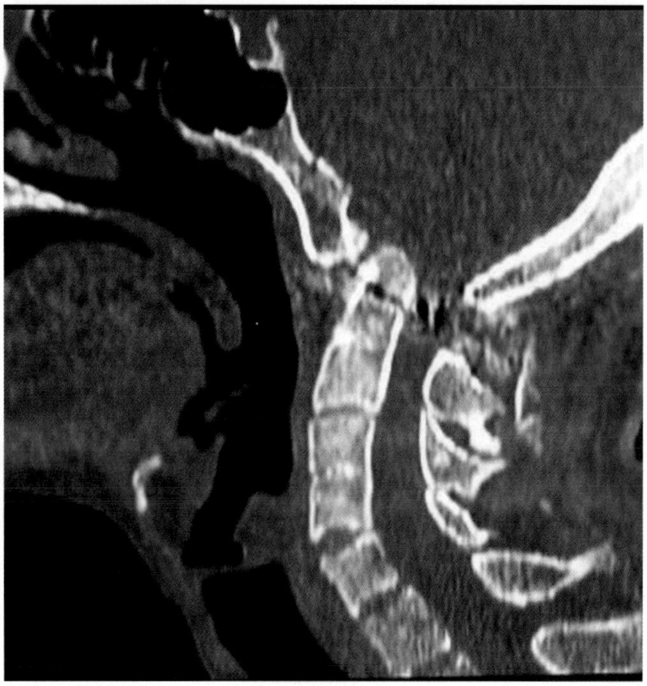
B

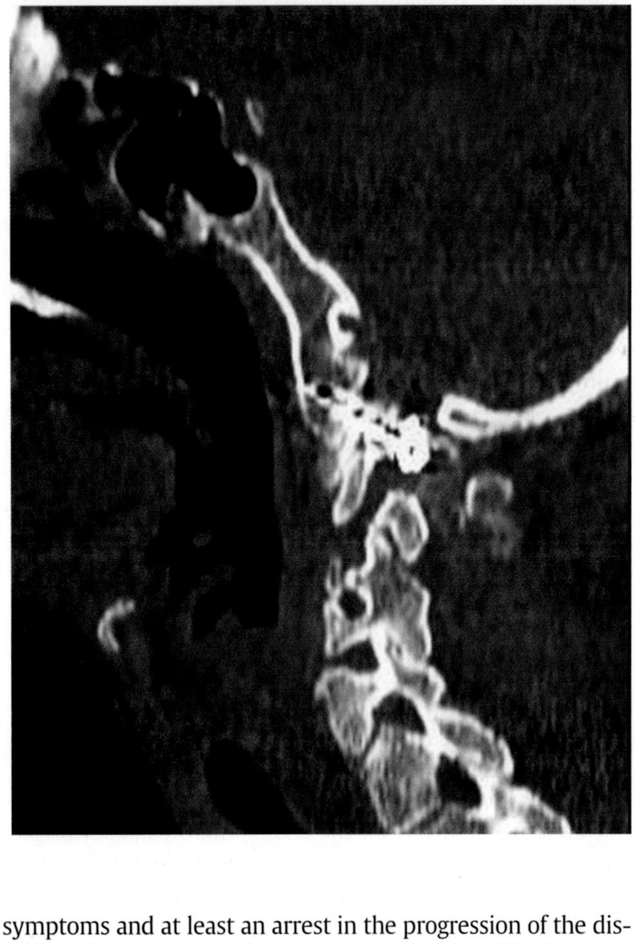
C

Fig. 42.9 **(A)** Preoperative computed tomography (CT) scan of a 10-year-old boy showing marked group A basilar invagination. **(B)** Postoperative CT scan showing reduction of the basilar invagination and realignment of the craniovertebral junction. **(C)** Sagittal image of postoperative CT scan showing the plate and screw fixation and realignment of the facets.

symptoms and at least an arrest in the progression of the disability. The suboccipital bone and posterior rim of the foramen magnum and the dura overlying the herniated cerebellar tissue are thin in a significant number of cases,[29] which is probably related to chronic pressure changes secondary to reduced posterior cranial fossa volume. Various authors recommend that, to achieve maximal decompression, it is necessary to open the dura mater and cut all constrictive dural and arachnoidal bands. Some authors recommend leaving the dura open, whereas others recommend the placement of a graft. Current papers do not recommend resection of herniating tonsils or sectioning of adhesions around them.[30] That dural opening is not necessary while performing posterior fossa or foramen magnum decompression was first described by us in 1997.[25]

This finding is based on the understanding that the dura is an expansile structure and can never be a compressive factor.[31] Opening the dura is not only unnecessary but subjects the patient to an increased risk of cerebrospinal fluid fistula. It makes an otherwise simple surgery a relatively complex and dangerous surgical maneuver. Our experience suggests that bony decompression of the foramen magnum is sufficient even in cases with Chiari malformation associated with syringomyelia. Foramen magnotomy, a procedure that involves reversal of the suboccipital bone flap and placement in the region in a manner that the convex posterior surface of the occipital bone faces outwards, can be effectively used in such a situation. The flap provides an area for bone fusion and curves away from the neural structures to provide neural decompression.[24]

Treatment of Basilar Invagination and Atlantoaxial Dislocation in Cases with Rheumatoid Arthritis

Basilar invagination is commonly associated with atlantoaxial dislocation and results in a significant degree of neck pain and myelopathy, adding considerably to the secondary disability of other joints. Several treatment options are available, including drug therapy and nonoperative treatment. Craniovertebral region bone alignment, distraction of the facets of the atlas and axis, and direct lateral mass plate and screw atlantoaxial fixation are feasible for managing basilar invagination and atlantoaxial dislocation secondary to rheumatoid arthritis.[32,33] Our operation of craniovertebral realignment and stabilization without bone decompression can be successfully employed in cases with atlantoaxial dislocation in the presence or absence of retro-odontoid pannus and in cases with basilar invagination. Patients show a remarkable and sustained neurological and radiological improvement.

Following atlantoaxial joint distraction, there is immediate postoperative reversal of retro-odontoid pannus in addition to reduction of atlantoaxial dislocation and basilar invagination.[34] This finding suggests that retro-odontoid pannus, basilar invagination, and atlantoaxial dislocation are related to atlantoaxial joint arthritis, lateral mass collapse, and reduction of joint space. The laxity of the posterior longitudinal ligament results in its posterior bulging. The exact role of inflammation in the formation of the pannus needs to be reevaluated. Distraction of the facets results in stretching the posterior longitudinal ligament and reducing the pannus, basilar invagination, and atlantoaxial dislocation.

Treatment of Craniovertebral Junction Tuberculosis

Our analysis and review of the literature suggest that tuberculosis frequently starts unilaterally by involving the cancellous part of the facet of the atlas.[35] Less frequently, the cancellous portion of the facet of the axis and odontoid process is where the disease begins. Joint involvement is a result of the extension of the inflammatory reaction. The incompetence of the joint and osseous and the adjoining ligamentous destruction in such a situation has been known to result in subluxation of the atlantoaxial facets. However, due to the presence of a normal atlantoaxial joint on the contralateral side, the region is not alarmingly unstable, and the patient generally presents with symptoms of pain and torticollis. Neurological deficits are notably delayed and less pronounced despite aggressive destruction by the disease. Due to the presence of the relatively stable craniovertebral region, surgery for fixation is not universally recommended in such cases despite the unilateral facetal destruction and effectiveness of modern antituberculous drugs. Management of tuberculosis involving the CVJ and the need for surgery in such cases, particularly when there is atlantoaxial dislocation, is a debated subject.

When the facets of the atlas and axis are destroyed on one side, it appears that the alar and transverse ligament becomes unilaterally incompetent. The contralateral facets are normal for a significant period of time and can be used for stabilization of the region. The shift of balance on the contralateral side and the obliquity of the inclination of the facet of the atlas in the atlantoaxial joint can result in its lateral dislocation over the facet of the axis. Under the circumstances, unilateral fixation of the atlantoaxial joint with or without the addition of distraction of the facets can result in stabilization of the region and realignment of the distorted anatomy. Such a unilateral treatment of the joint in cases with tuberculosis of the CVJ can be a reasonable surgical option in several patients having tuberculosis of the CVJ. Lateral dislocation of the atlas over the axis secondary to osteoligamentous incompetence can be a defined and treatable pathological entity.[35]

Facetal Distraction Treatment for Degenerative Arthritis of the Craniovertebral Junction

Like all other joints of the body, atlantoaxial joints are subject to arthritis (**Fig. 42.10**). With aging, the issue of arthritis becomes more relevant. Osteoarthritis of the atlantoaxial joint is a well-defined phenomenon that eventually results in atlantoaxial instability. The process of joint degeneration and instability is a progressive phenomenon and extends over several months to years. Degenerative erosion of the facets of the atlas and axis, odontoid process, and body of axis as well as periodontoid ligamentous degenerative changes and abnormal osteophyte-like bone formation are frequent. Degenerative pannus, also termed articular, ganglion, synovial, or juxta-facet cyst, may arise from the degenerating synovial lining of any joint in the body. Pannus related to atlantoaxial joint arthritis probably represents degenerative ligaments and secondary osteophyte-like tissue formation in the periodontoid region. Degenerating tissues are typically isointense on T1-weighted images and iso- to hypointense on T2-weighted images and do not enhance on contrast administration. In some cases, the retro-odontoid mass may give a tumor-like

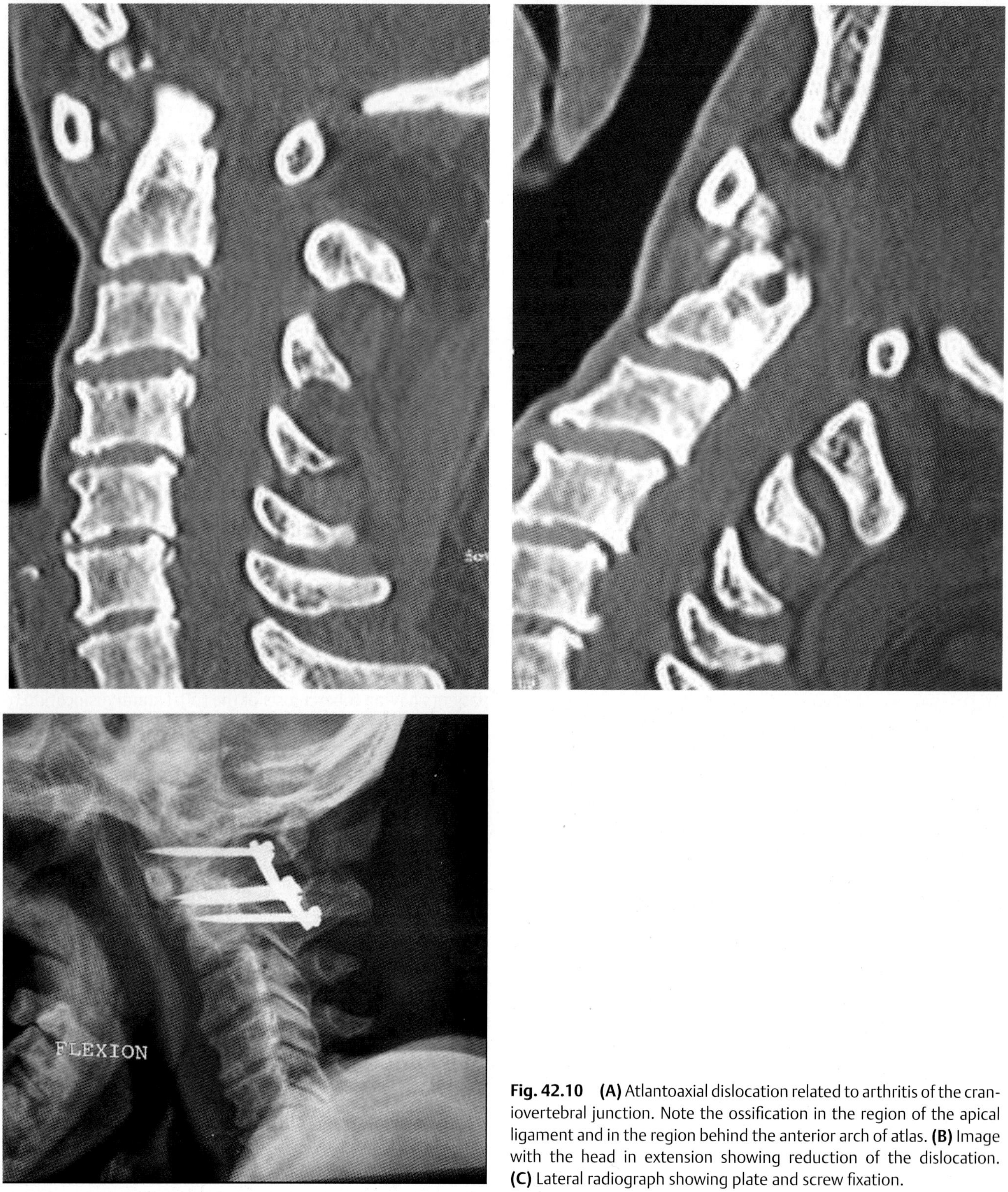

A B C

Fig. 42.10 **(A)** Atlantoaxial dislocation related to arthritis of the craniovertebral junction. Note the ossification in the region of the apical ligament and in the region behind the anterior arch of atlas. **(B)** Image with the head in extension showing reduction of the dislocation. **(C)** Lateral radiograph showing plate and screw fixation.

appearance, resulting in posterior buckling of the posterior longitudinal ligament or the tectorial membrane and indentation of the cord substance. The retro-odontoid ligamentous hypertrophy appears to be related to laxity of ligaments due to reduced atlantoaxial height and secondary to progressive degenerative changes in the region. The pathogenesis of the degenerative changes simulates the formation of posterior osteophytes in cases with spinal degeneration. It appears that the presence of retro-odontoid ligamentous degenerative hypertrophy in an elderly patient can be diagnostic evidence that suggests atlantoaxial instability even when such instability is not clearly visualized on radiological imaging. Atlantoaxial joint arthritis is expected to eventually result in atlantoaxial instability. The dislocation may only be partially reducible due to the presence of nonyielding tissues around the odontoid process. The subtlety of instability may make the diagnosis difficult in some cases. The instability is probably the result of degeneration of the articular cartilage, reduction of the joint space, and secondary incompetence of the ligaments controlling the movements. Surgical treatment in such cases is atlantoaxial fixation. Distraction of the facets not only assists in the reduction and fixation of the atlantoaxial dislocation and basilar invagination but stretches the buckled posterior spinal ligaments that appear to have a significant role in the pathogenesis of retro-odontoid ligamentous degenerative hypertrophic mass.[10]

References

1. Grob D, Magerl F. [Surgical stabilization of C1 and C2 fractures]. Orthopade 1987;16(1):46–54
2. Goel A, Laheri V. Plate and screw fixation for atlanto-axial subluxation. Acta Neurochir (Wien) 1994;129(1–2):47–53
3. Goel A, Desai KI, Muzumdar DP. Atlantoaxial fixation using plate and screw method: a report of 160 treated patients. Neurosurgery 2002;51(6):1351–1356, discussion 1356–1357
4. Cacciola F, Phalke U, Goel A. Vertebral artery in relationship to C1-C2 vertebrae: an anatomical study. Neurol India 2004;52(2):178–184
5. Gupta S, Goel A. Quantitative anatomy of the lateral masses of the atlas and axis vertebrae. Neurol India 2000;48(2):120–125
6. Goel A, Gupta S. Vertebral artery injury with transarticular screws. (Letter) J Neurosurg 1999;90(2):376–377
7. Goel A. Double insurance atlantoaxial fixation. Surg Neurol 2007;67(2):135–139
8. Goel A, Kulkarni AG. Screw implantation in spinous process for occipitoaxial fixation. J Clin Neurosci 2004;11(7):735–737
9. Goel A. Atlantoaxial joint jamming as a treatment for atlantoaxial dislocation: a preliminary report. Technical note. J Neurosurg Spine 2007;7(1):90–94
10. Goel A, Shah A, Gupta SR. Craniovertebral instability due to degenerative osteoarthritis of the atlantoaxial joints: analysis of the management of 108 cases. J Neurosurg Spine 2010;12(6):592–601
11. Goel A, Kulkarni AG, Sharma P. Reduction of fixed atlantoaxial dislocation in 24 cases: technical note. J Neurosurg Spine 2005;2(4):505–509
12. Goel A, Muzumdar D, Dange N. One stage reduction and fixation for atlantoaxial spondyloptosis: report of four cases. Br J Neurosurg 2006;20(4):209–213
13. Goel A. Treatment of basilar invagination by atlantoaxial joint distraction and direct lateral mass fixation. J Neurosurg Spine 2004;1(3):281–286
14. Chamberlain WE. Basilar impression (platybasia). A bizarre developmental anomaly of the occipital bone and upper cervical spine with striking and misleading neurologic manifestations. Yale J Biol Med 1939;11(5):487–496
15. McRAE DL. Bony abnormalities in the region of the foramen magnum: correlation of the anatomic and neurologic findings. Acta Radiol 1953;40(2–3):335–354
16. Klaus E. Rontgendiagnostik der platybasic und basilaren impression. Fortscher Rontgenstr 1957;86:460–469
17. Thiebaut F, Wackenheim A, Vrousos C. [New median sagittal pneumostratigraphical finding concerning the posterior fossa]. J Radiol Electrol Med Nucl 1961;42:1–7
18. Von Torklus D, Gehle W. The Upper Cervical Spine: Regional Anatomy, Pathology, and Traumatology. A Systematic Radiological Atlas and Textbook. New York, NY: Grune & Stratton, 1972:1–98
19. Kothari M, Goel A. Transatlantic odonto-occipital listhesis: the so-called basilar invagination. Neurol India 2007;55(1):6–7
20. Goel A. Progressive basilar invagination after transoral odontoidectomy: treatment by atlantoaxial facet distraction and craniovertebral realignment. Spine 2005;30(18):E551–E555
21. Goel A, Shah A, Rajan S. Vertical mobile and reducible atlantoaxial dislocation. Clinical article. J Neurosurg Spine 2009;11(1):9–14
22. Gunderson CH, Greenspan RH, Glaser GH, Lubs HA. The Klippel-Feil syndrome: genetic and clinical reevaluation of cervical fusion. Medicine (Baltimore) 1967;46(6):491–512
23. Goel A, Shah A. Reversal of longstanding musculoskeletal changes in basilar invagination after surgical decompression and stabilization. J Neurosurg Spine 2009;10(3):220–227
24. Goel A, Achawal S. The surgical treatment of Chiari malformation association with atlantoaxial dislocation. Br J Neurosurg 1995;9(1):67–72
25. Goel A, Bhatjiwale M, Desai K. Basilar invagination: a study based on 190 surgically treated patients. J Neurosurg 1998;88(6):962–968
26. Goel A, Karapurkar AP. Transoral plate and screw fixation of the craniovertebral region—a preliminary report. Br J Neurosurg 1994;8(6):743–745
27. Goel A, Desai KI. Surgery for syringomyelia: an analysis based on 163 surgical cases. Acta Neurochir (Wien) 2000;142(3):293–301, discussion 301–302
28. Goel A, Sharma P. Craniovertebral junction realignment for the treatment of basilar invagination with syringomyelia: preliminary report of 12 cases. Neurol Med Chir (Tokyo) 2005;45(10):512–517, discussion 518
29. Driesen W. [Findings at operation in the central nervous system in basilar impressions and related abnormalities of the atlanto-occipital region]. Acta Neurochir (Wien) 1960;9:9–68 (Ger)
30. Williams B. A critical appraisal of posterior fossa surgery for communicating syringomyelia. Brain 1978;101(2):223–250
31. Kothari M, Goel A. Maternalizing the meninges: a pregnant Arabic legacy. Neurol India 2006;54(4):345–346
32. Goel A, Pareikh S, Sharma P. Atlantoaxial joint distraction for treatment of basilar invagination secondary to rheumatoid arthritis. Neurol India 2005;53(2):238–240
33. Goel A, Sharma P. Craniovertebral realignment for basilar invagination and atlantoaxial dislocation secondary to rheumatoid arthritis. Neurol India 2004;52(3):338–341
34. Goel A, Dange N. Immediate postoperative regression of retro-odontoid pannus after lateral mass reconstruction in a patient with rheumatoid disease of the craniovertebral junction. Case report. J Neurosurg Spine 2008;9(3):273–276
35. Goel A, Shah A. Lateral atlantoaxial facetal dislocation in craniovertebral region tuberculosis: report of a case and analysis of an alternative treatment. Acta Neurochir (Wien) 2010;152(4):709–712
36. Goel A. Craniovertebral junction instability in children. (Letter) J Neurosurg Pediatr 2008;2:173
37. Goel A, Muzumdar D, Dange N. Syringomyelia in infants secondary to mobile ngenital atlantoaxial dislocation. Pediatr Neurosurg 2007;43(1):15–18
38. Goel A, Kulkarni AG. Mobile and reducible atlantoaxial dislocation in presence of occipitalized atlas: report on treatment of eight cases by direct lateral mass plate and screw fixation. Spine 2004;29(22):E520–E523

Index

Note: Page numbers followed by *f* and *t* indicate material in figures and tables, respectively.

O

Q

R

T

U

V